Red Book®:

2009 REPORT OF THE COMMITTEE ON INFECTIOUS DISEASES

TWENTY-EIGHTH EDITION

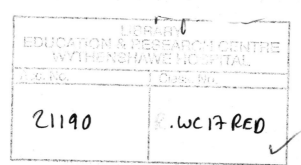

Author: Committee on Infectious Diseases
American Academy of Pediatrics

Larry K. Pickering, MD, FAAP, Editor

Carol J. Baker, MD, FAAP, Associate Editor
David W. Kimberlin, MD, FAAP, Associate Editor
Sarah S. Long, MD, FAAP, Associate Editor

American Academy of Pediatrics
141 Northwest Point Blvd
Elk Grove Village, IL 60007-1098

Suggested Citation: American Academy of Pediatrics. [Chapter title]. In: Pickering LK, Baker CJ, Kimberlin DW, Long SS, eds. *Red Book: 2009 Report of the Committee on Infectious Diseases.* 28th ed. Elk Grove Village, IL: American Academy of Pediatrics; 2009:[page numbers]

28th Edition
1st Edition – 1938
2nd Edition – 1939
3rd Edition – 1940
4th Edition – 1942
5th Edition – 1943
6th Edition – 1944
7th Edition – 1945
8th Edition – 1947
9th Edition – 1951
10th Edition – 1952
11th Edition – 1955
12th Edition – 1957
13th Edition – 1961
14th Edition – 1964
15th Edition – 1966
16th Edition – 1970
16th Edition Revised – 1971
17th Edition – 1974
18th Edition – 1977
19th Edition – 1982
20th Edition – 1986
21st Edition – 1988
22nd Edition – 1991
23rd Edition – 1994
24th Edition – 1997
25th Edition – 2000
26th Edition – 2003
27th Edition – 2006

ISSN No. 1080-0131
ISBN No. 978-1-58110-306-9
MA0450

Quantity prices on request. Address all inquiries to:
American Academy of Pediatrics
PO Box 927, 141 Northwest Point Blvd
Elk Grove Village, IL 60007-1098

or Phone:
1-888-227-1770 Publications

3-208/0509
1 2 3 4 5 6 7 8 9 10

Committee on Infectious Diseases 2007–2009

Robert S. Baltimore, MD
Henry H. Bernstein, DO
Joseph A. Bocchini, Jr, MD
John S. Bradley, MD
Michael T. Brady, MD
Carrie L. Byington, MD
Penelope H. Dennehy, MD
Robert W. Frenck, Jr, MD

Mary P. Glode, MD
Harry L. Keyserling, M D
David W. Kimberlin, MD,
   Red Book Associate Editor
Julia A. McMillan, MD
Walter A. Orenstein, MD
Lorry G. Rubin, MD

Ex-officio

Larry K. Pickering, MD, *Red Book* Editor
Carol J. Baker, MD, *Red Book* Associate Editor
Sarah S. Long, MD, *Red Book* Associate Editor

Liaisons

Beth P. Bell, MD, MPH	Centers for Disease Control and Prevention
Robert Bortolussi, MD	Canadian Paediatric Society
Richard D. Clover, MD	American Academy of Family Physicians
Joanne Embree, MD	Canadian Paediatric Society
Marc A. Fischer, MD	Centers for Disease Control and Prevention
Richard L. Gorman, MD	National Institutes of Health
Lucia Lee, MD	Food and Drug Administration
R. Douglas Pratt, MD	Food and Drug Administration
Jennifer S. Read, MD, MS, MPH, DTM&H	National Institute of Child Health and Human Development
Anne Schuchat, MD	Centers for Disease Control and Prevention
Benjamin Schwartz, MD	National Vaccine Program Office
Jeffrey R. Starke, MD	American Thoracic Society

Consultants

Edgar O. Ledbetter, MD
H. Cody Meissner, MD

AAP Liaisons

Margaret C. Fisher, MD	Section on Infectious Diseases
Jack Swanson, MD	Practice Action Group

Collaborators

Mark Abdy, DVM, PhD, US Department of Health and Human Services, Washington, DC

Emily S. Abernathy, MS, Centers for Disease Control and Prevention, Atlanta, GA

Mark Abzug, MD, University of Colorado School of Medicine, Children's Hospital, Denver, CO

Jennifer Adjemian, PhD, Centers for Disease Control and Prevention, Atlanta, GA

James P. Alexander, Jr, MD, MA, MEd, Centers for Disease Control and Prevention, Atlanta, GA

John J. Alexander, MD, MPH, Food and Drug Administration, Washington, DC

Manual R. Amieva, MD, Stanford University School of Medicine, Stanford, CA

Krow Ampofo, MD, University of Utah, Salt Lake City, UT

Alicia D. Anderson, Centers for Disease Control and Prevention, Atlanta, GA

Larry J. Anderson, MD, Centers for Disease Control and Prevention, Atlanta, GA

Warren A. Andiman, MD, Yale School of Medicine, New Haven, CT

Nelson Arboleda, MD, MPH, Centers for Disease Control and Prevention, Atlanta, GA

John C. Arnold, MD, Rady Children's Hospital, San Diego, CA

Stephen S. Arnon, MD, California Department of Public Health, Richmond, CA

David M. Asher, MD, Food and Drug Administration, Kensington, MD

Shai Ashkenazi, MD, Schneider Children's Medical Center of Israel, Petah-Tikva, Israel

Chintamani D. Atreva, PhD, Food and Drug Administration, Rockville, MD

Kassa Avalew, MD, Food and Drug Administration, Silver Spring, MD

James Baggs, Centers for Disease Control and Prevention, Atlanta, GA

Robert Ball, MD, MPH, ScM, Food and Drug Administration, Rockville, MD

Robert Baltimore, MD, Yale University School of Medicine, New Haven, CT

Albert E. Barskev, IV, MPH, Centers for Disease Control and Prevention, Atlanta, GA

Ezra J. Barzilay, MD, Centers for Disease Control and Prevention, Atlanta, GA

Margaret C. Bash, MD, MPH, Food and Drug Administration, Rockville, MD

Brigid Batten, MPH, Centers for Disease Control and Prevention, Atlanta, GA

Melisse S. Baylor, MD, Food and Drug Administration, Rockville, MD

Michael Beach, Centers for Disease Control and Prevention, Atlanta, GA

Judy Beeler, MD, Food and Drug Administration, Rockville, MD

Ermias D. Belay, MD, Centers for Disease Control and Prevention, Atlanta, GA

Ozlem Belen, MD, MPH, Food and Drug Administration, Silver Spring, MD

Yodit Belew, MD, Food and Drug Administration, Silver Spring, MD

Beth P. Bell, MD, MPH, Centers for Disease Control and Prevention, Atlanta, GA

Elise M. Beltramini, MD, MPH, Centers for Disease Control and Prevention, Atlanta, GA

Jeffrey Bender, MD, University of Utah, Salt Lake City, UT

Latanya T. Benjamin, MD, University of Miami Miller School of Medicine, Cooper City, FL

Stuart M. Berman, MD, ScM, Centers for Disease Control and Prevention, Atlanta, GA

Caryn Bern, MD, MPH, Centers for Disease Control and Prevention, Atlanta, GA

Henry H. Bernstein, MD, Dartmouth Hitchcock Medical Center, Lebanon, NH

Stephanie R. Bialek, MD, MPH, Centers for Disease Control and Prevention, Atlanta, GA

Robin M. Biswas, MD, Food and Drug Administration, Rockville, MD

Margaret Blythe, MD, Indiana University School of Medicine, Indianapolis, IN

Elizabeth A. Bolvard, RN, MPH, Centers for Disease Control and Prevention, Atlanta, GA

Suresh B. Boppana, MD, University of Alabama at Birmingham, Birmingham, AL

Robert Bortolussi, MD, Dalhousie University, Halifax, Nova Scotia

Anna B. Bowen, MD, MPH, Centers for Disease Control and Prevention, Atlanta, GA

Kenneth M. Boyer, MD, University Medical Center, Chicago, IL

John S. Bradley, MD, Children's Hospital of San Diego, San Diego, CA

Michael T. Brady, MD, Children's Hospital Columbus, Ohio State University, Columbus, OH

Mary E. Brandt, PhD, Centers for Disease Control and Prevention, Atlanta, GA

M. Miles Braun, MD, MPH, Food and Drug Administration, Rockville, MD

Joseph S. Bresee, Centers for Disease Control and Prevention, Atlanta, GA

Karen R. Broder, Centers for Disease Control and Prevention, Decatur, GA

Gary W. Brunette, MD, MS, Centers for Disease Control and Prevention, Duluth, GA

Jane L. Burns, MD, University of Washington, Seattle, WA

Jay Butler, Centers for Disease Control and Prevention, Atlanta, GA

Carrie L. Byington, MD, University of Utah, Salt Lake City, UT

Angela Calugar, MD, MPH, Centers for Disease Control and Prevention, Atlanta, GA

D. William Cameron, MD, The Ottawa Hospital, Ottawa, Ontario, Canada

Michael J. Cannon, PhD, Centers for Disease Control and Prevention, Atlanta, GA

Michael Cappello, MD, Yale Child Health Research Center, New Haven, CT

Corey Casper, MD, MPH, University of Washington, Seattle, WA

Tom M. Chiller, MD, MPH, Centers for Disease Control and Prevention, Atlanta, GA

Lance Chilton, MD, University of New Mexico School of Medicine, Albuquerque, NM

Thomas Clark, MD, MPH, Centers for Disease Control and Prevention, Atlanta, GA

Thomas G. Cleary, MD, University of Texas Medical School, Houston, TX

Adam L. Cohen, MD, MPH, Centers for Disease Control and Prevention, Atlanta, GA

Amanda C. Cohn, MD, Centers for Disease Control and Prevention, Atlanta, GA

Felicia L. Collins, MD, MPH, Food and Drug Administration, Silver Spring, MD

Charles K. Cooper, MD, Food and Drug Administration, Silver Spring, MD

Julie Ann Crewalk, MD, Food and Drug Administration, Silver Spring, MD

James E. Crowe, Jr, MD, Vanderbilt University School of Medicine, Nashville, TN

Kimberly M. Cushing, MPH, Centers for Disease Control and Prevention, Greenland, NH

Therese A. Cvetkovich, MD, Food and Drug Administration, Rockville, MD

Ron Dagan, MD, Soroka University Medical Center, Beer-Sheva, Israel

Inger Damon, MD, PhD, Centers for Disease Control and Prevention, Atlanta, GA

Gregory A. Dasch, PhD, Centers for Disease Control and Prevention, Atlanta, GA

S. Deblina Datta, Centers for Disease Control and Prevention, Atlanta, GA

Jon R. Daugherty, PhD, Food and Drug Administration, Rockville, MD

Alma C. Davidson, MD, Food and Drug Administration, Silver Spring, MD

Rajeshwar Dayal, MD, DNB, DCH, S N Medical College, Rajamandi, Agra, India

Michael S. Deming, MD, MPH, Centers for Disease Control and Prevention, Atlanta, GA

Gail J. Demmler, MD, Baylor College of Medicine, Texas Children's Hospital, Houston, TX

Penelope Dennehy, MD, Rhode Island Hospital, Providence, RI

Meredith Deutschler, MD, Centers for Disease Control and Prevention, Atlanta, GA

Pamela S. Diaz, MD, Centers for Disease Control and Prevention, Atlanta, GA

Kenneth L. Dominguez, MD, MPH, Centers for Disease Control and Prevention, Atlanta, GA

Eileen F. Dunne, MD, MPH, Centers for Disease Control and Prevention, Atlanta, GA

Mark L. Eberhard, PhD, Centers for Disease Control and Prevention, Atlanta, GA

Morven S. Edwards, MD, Baylor College of Medicine, Houston, TX

Lawrence F. Eichenfield, MD, University of California San Diego School of Medicine, San Diego, CA

Joanne Embree, MD, University of Manitoba, Winnipeg, Manitoba, Canada

Dean Erdman, DrPH, Centers for Disease Control and Prevention, Atlanta, GA

Marina Eremeeva, PhD, Centers for Disease Control and Prevention, Atlanta, GA

Geoffrey Evans, MD, National Vaccine Injury Compensation Program, Department of Health and Human Services, Rockville, MD

Karen M. Farizo, MD, Food and Drug Administration, Rockville, MD

Mahmood Farshid, PhD, Food and Drug Administration, Rockville, MD

Stephen M. Feinstone, MD, Food and Drug Administration, Bethesda, MD

Theresa M. Finn, PhD, Food and Drug Administration, Rockville, MD

Anthony E. Fiore, MD, MPH, Centers for Disease Control and Prevention, Atlanta, GA

Gayle E. Fischer, MD, MPH, Centers for Disease Control and Prevention, Atlanta, GA

Marc Fischer, MD, MPH, Centers for Disease Control and Prevention, Fort Collins, CO

Margaret Fisher, MD, Monmouth Medical Center, Long Branch, NJ

Collette Fitzgerald, PhD, Centers for Disease Control and Prevention, Atlanta, GA

Patricia M. Flynn, MD, MS, St. Jude's Children's Research Hospital, Memphis, TN

Leanne M. Fox, MD, MPH, DTM, Centers for Disease Control and Prevention, Atlanta, GA

Robert W. Frenck, Jr, MD, Cincinnati Children's Hospital Medical Center, Cincinnati, OH

Cindy R. Friedman, MD, Centers for Disease Control and Prevention, Atlanta, GA

Julianne Gee, Centers for Disease Control and Prevention, Atlanta, GA

Michael A. Gerber, MD, Cincinnati Children's Hospital Medical Center, Cincinnati, OH

Anne A. Gershon, MD, Columbia University Medical Center, New York, NY

Jane Gidudu, Centers for Disease Control and Prevention, Atlanta, GA

Francis Gigliotti, MD, University of Rochester School of Medicine, Rochester, NY

Janet Gilsdorf, MD, Women's Hospital, University of Michigan Medical Center, Ann Arbor, MI

Steve Gitterman, Food and Drug Administration, Silver Spring, MD

Laurence B. Givner, MD, Wake Forest University School of Medicine, Winston-Salem, NC

M. Kathleen Glynn, DVM, MPVM, Centers for Disease Control and Prevention, Atlanta, GA

Bess G. Gold, MD, Children's Hospitals and Clinics of Minnesota, St. Louis Park, MN

Rachel Gorwitz, Centers for Disease Control and Prevention, Atlanta, GA

Patricia M. Griffin, MD, Centers for Disease Control and Prevention, Atlanta, GA

Kevin S. Griffith, MD, MPH, Centers for Disease Control and Prevention, Fort Collins, CO

Charles Grose, MD, Children's Hospital, University of Iowa, Iowa City, IA

Marion F. Gruber, PhD, Food and Drug Administration, Rockville, MD

Marta A. Guerra, DVM, MPH, PhD, Centers for Disease Control and Prevention, Atlanta, GA

Penina Haber, MPH, Centers for Disease Control and Prevention, Atlanta, GA

Jeffrey C. Hageman, MHS, Centers for Disease Control and Prevention, Atlanta, GA

Scott A. Halperin, MD, Dalhousie University, Halifax, Nova Scotia

Neal A. Halsey, MD, Johns Hopkins University Bloomberg School of Public Health, Baltimore, MD

Theresa Anne Harrington, MD, MPH, Centers for Disease Control and Prevention, Atlanta, GA

Julie R. Harris, PhD, MPH, Centers for Disease Control and Prevention, Atlanta, GA

Edward B. Hayes, MD, Centers for Disease Control and Prevention, Fort Collins, CO

Thomas W. Hennessey, MD, MPH, Centers for Disease Control and Prevention, Anchorage, AK

Barbara L. Herwaldt, MD, MPH, Centers for Disease Control and Prevention, Atlanta, GA

Beth F. Hibbs, RN, MPH, Centers for Disease Control and Prevention, Atlanta, GA

Sheila Hickey, MD, University of New Mexico School of Medicine, Albuquerque, NM

Lauri Hicks, Centers for Disease Control and Prevention, Atlanta, GA

Michelle Hlavsa, Centers for Disease Control and Prevention, Atlanta, GA

Scott D. Holmberg, MD, MPH, Centers for Disease Control and Prevention, Atlanta, GA

Karen Hoover, MD, MPH, Centers for Disease Control and Prevention, Atlanta, GA

Peter J. Hotez, MD, PhD, George Washington University and Sabin Vaccine Institute, Washington, DC

Wan-Ting Huang, Centers for Disease Control and Prevention, Atlanta, GA

Joseph P. Icenogle, PhD, Centers for Disease Control and Prevention, Atlanta, GA

Menfo A. Imoisili, MD, MPH, Food and Drug Administration, Ellicott City, MD

John K. Iskander, MD, MPH, Centers for Disease Control and Prevention, Atlanta, GA

Martha Iwamoto, Centers for Disease Control and Prevention, Atlanta, GA

Hector Izurieta, MD, MPH, Food and Drug Administration, Rockville, MD

Richard F. Jacobs, MD, Arkansas Children's Hospital, Little Rock, AR

John A. Jereb, MD, Centers for Disease Control and Prevention, Atlanta, GA

John A. Jernigan, MD, MS, Centers for Disease Control and Prevention, Atlanta, GA

Robert E. Johnson, MD, MPH, Centers for Disease Control and Prevention, Atlanta, GA

Jeffrey L. Jones, MD, MPH, Centers for Disease Control and Prevention, Atlanta, GA

M. Patricia Joyce, MD, Centers for Disease Control and Prevention, Atlanta, GA

Aisha Jumaan, Centers for Disease Control and Prevention, Atlanta, GA

Alexander J. Kallen, MD, MPH, Centers for Disease Control and Prevention, Atlanta, GA

Nino Khetsuriani, MD, PhD, Centers for Disease Control and Prevention, Decatur, GA

Tina Khoie, MD, Food and Drug Administration, Rockville, MD

Peter W. Kim, MD, MS, Food and Drug Administration, Silver Spring, MD

Paul Kitsutani, MD, MPH, Food and Drug Administration, Rockville, MD

Martin B. Kleiman, MD, Indiana University, Indianapolis, IN

Emilia Helen A. Koumans, MD, MPH, Centers for Disease Control and Prevention, Atlanta, GA

Phyllis E. Kozarsky, MD, Centers for Disease Control and Prevention, Atlanta, GA

Philip R. Krause, MD, Food and Drug Administration, Bethesda, MD

John W. Krebs, MS, Centers for Disease Control and Prevention, Atlanta, GA

Andrew T. Kroger, MD, MPH, Centers for Disease Control and Prevention, Atlanta, GA

Matt Kuehnert, Centers for Disease Control and Prevention, Atlanta, GA

John A. Leake, MD, MPH, Children's Hospital–San Diego, San Diego, CA

Lucia H. Lee, MD, Food and Drug Administration, Rockville, MD

Nicole M. A. Le Saux, MD, Children's Hospital of Eastern Ontario, Ottawa, Ontario, Canada

Rebecca E. Levorson, MD, Food and Drug Administration, Silver Spring, MD

Linda L. Lewis, MD, Food and Drug Administration, Silver Spring, MD

Jay M. Lieberman, MD, University of California Irvine, Irvine, CA

Sue Lim, MD, Food and Drug Administration, Silver Spring, MD

Brandi Limbago, PhD, Centers for Disease Control and Prevention, Atlanta, GA

Mark N. Lobato, MD, Centers for Disease Control and Prevention, Hartford, CT

Cherie M. Long, MPH, Centers for Disease Control and Prevention, Atlanta, GA

Shari L. Lydy, BS, MS, PhD, Centers for Disease Control and Prevention, Atlanta, GA

Michael F. Lynch, MD, MPH, Centers for Disease Control and Prevention, Atlanta, GA

Noni E. MacDonald, MD, MSc, Dalhousie University, Halifax, Nova Scotia

Shelley Sylvester Magill, MD, PhD, Centers for Disease Control and Prevention, Atlanta, GA

Yvonne Aida Maldonado, MD, Stanford University School of Medicine, Stanford, CA

Susan E. Manning, MD, MPH, Massachusetts Department of Public Health, Boston, MA

Nina Marano, Centers for Disease Control and Prevention, Atlanta, GA

Mona Marin, MD, Centers for Disease Control and Prevention, Atlanta, GA

Stacene R. Maroushek, MD, PhD, Hennepin County Medical Center, Minneapolis, MN

Robert Massung, PhD, Centers for Disease Control and Prevention, Atlanta, GA

Els Mathieu, MD, MPH, Centers for Disease Control and Prevention, Atlanta, GA

Lisa Mathis, MD, Food and Drug Administration, Silver Spring, MD

Anne E. McCarthy, MD, MSc, FRCPC, DTM&H, Ottawa Hospital General Campus, Ottawa, Ontario, Canada

George H. McCracken, Jr, MD, University of Texas Southwestern Medical Center at Dallas, Dallas, TX

L. Clifford McDonald, MD, Centers for Disease Control and Prevention, Atlanta, GA

Julia A. McMillan, MD, Johns Hopkins Hospital, Baltimore, MD

Meredith L. McMorrow, MD, MPH, Centers for Disease Control and Prevention, Atlanta, GA

Jennifer H. McQuiston, DVM, MS, Centers for Disease Control and Prevention, Atlanta, GA

Paul S. Mead, MD, MPH, Centers for Disease Control and Prevention, Fort Collins, CO

Felicita M. Medalla, MD, MS, Centers for Disease Control and Prevention, Atlanta, GA

H. Cody Meissner, MD, New England Medical Center, Boston, MA

David Menschik, MD, Food and Drug Administration, Rockville, MD
Joette M. Meyer, PharmD, Food and Drug Administration, Silver Spring, MD
Nancy B. Miller, MD, Food and Drug Administration, Rockville, MD
Elaine R. Miller, RN, MPH, Centers for Disease Control and Prevention, Atlanta, GA
Eric D. Mintz, MD, MPH, Centers for Disease Control and Prevention, Atlanta, GA
Roque Miramontes, PA-C, MPH, Centers for Disease Control and Prevention,
    Atlanta, GA
John F. Modlin, MD, Dartmouth Hitchcock Medical Center, Lebanon, NH
Lynne M. Mofenson, MD, Eunice Kennedy Shriver National Institute of Child Health
    and Human Development, National Institutes of Health, Rockville, MD
Nasim Moledina, MD, Food and Drug Administration, Silver Spring, MD
Susan P. Montgomery, DVM, MPH, Centers for Disease Control and Prevention,
    Atlanta, GA
Anne C. Moore, MD, PhD, Centers for Disease Control and Prevention, Atlanta, GA
Gina T. Mootrey, DO, MPH, Centers for Disease Control and Prevention, Atlanta, GA
Riyadh D. Muhammad, MD, MPH, Centers for Disease Control and Prevention,
    Stockbridge, GA
Kenneth L. Muldrew, MD, MPH, Yale University School of Medicine, New Haven, CT
Jean Mulinde, MD, Food and Drug Administration, Silver Spring, MD
Dennis L. Murray, MD, Medical College of Georgia Children's Medical Center,
    Augusta, GA
Sumathi Nambiar, MD, Food and Drug Administration, Silver Spring, MD
Santosh Nanda, DVM, PhD, Food and Drug Administration, Bethesda, MD
Roger S. Nasci, PhD, Centers for Disease Control and Prevention, Fort Collins, CO
James P. Nataro, MD, PhD, MBA, University of Maryland School of Medicine,
    Baltimore, MD
Steven R. Nesheim, MD, Centers for Disease Control and Prevention, Atlanta, GA
Kathleen Neuzil, MD, MPH, University of Washington School of Medicine, Seattle, WA
Jane W. Newburger, MD, MPH, Children's Hospital Boston, Harvard Medical School,
    Boston, MA
Lori M. Newman, MD, Centers for Disease Control and Prevention, Atlanta, GA
William L. Nicholson, BS, MS, PhD, Centers for Disease Control and Prevention,
    Atlanta, GA
Ryan T. Novak, PhD, Centers for Disease Control and Prevention, Atlanta, GA
J. Pekka Nuorti, MD, DSc, Centers for Disease Control and Prevention, Atlanta, GA
M. Steven Oberste, PhD, Centers for Disease Control and Prevention, Atlanta, GA
Masahiro Ohashi, MD, Food and Drug Administration, Bethesda, MD
Rosalyn E. O'Loughlin, MSc, PhD, Centers for Disease Control and Prevention,
    Atlanta, GA
Ciarra E. O'Reilly, PhD, Centers for Disease Control and Prevention, Atlanta, GA
Walter A. Orenstein, MD, Emory University School of Medicine, Emory Vaccine Center,
    Atlanta, GA
Miguel O'Ryan, MD, University of Chile, Santiago, Chile
Elizabeth M. O'Shaughnessy, MD, Food and Drug Administration, Silver Spring, MD
Gary D. Overturf, MD, TriCore Reference Laboratories, Albuquerque, NM
Christopher D. Paddock, MD, Centers for Disease Control and Prevention, Atlanta, GA
Elijah Paintsil, MD, Yale University School of Medicine, New Haven, CT

Debra L. Palazzi, MD, Baylor College of Medicine, Houston, TX

Mark A. Pallansch, PhD, Centers for Disease Control and Prevention, Atlanta, GA

Adelisa L. Panlilio, MD, MPH, Centers for Disease Control and Prevention, Atlanta, GA

Umesh D. Parashar, MBBS, MPH, Centers for Disease Control and Prevention, Atlanta, GA

Monica E. Parise, MD, Centers for Disease Control and Prevention, Atlanta, GA

Ben J. Park, MD, Centers for Disease Control and Prevention, Atlanta, GA

Amy A. Parker, MSN, MPH, Centers for Disease Control and Prevention, Atlanta, GA

Robert Pass, MD, University of Alabama at Birmingham, Department of Pediatrics, Birmingham, AL

Mary E. Patrick, MPH, Centers for Disease Control and Prevention, Atlanta, GA

Andrew T. Pavia, MD, University of Utah, Salt Lake City, UT

Joseph F. Perz, MA, DrPH, Centers for Disease Control and Prevention, Atlanta, GA

Nicki T. Pesik, MD, Centers for Disease Control and Prevention, Decatur, GA

Georges Peter, MD, Brown University, Brookline, MA

Thomas A. Peterman, MD, MSc, Centers for Disease Control and Prevention, Atlanta, GA

John R. Peters, MD, Food and Drug Administration, Silver Spring, MD

Larry K. Pickering, MD, Centers for Disease Control and Prevention, Atlanta, GA

Andreas Pikis, MD, Food and Drug Administration, Silver Spring, MD

Andrew J. Pollard, MD, PhD, University of Oxford, Children's Hospital, Oxford, United Kingdom

R. Douglas Pratt, MD, Food and Drug Administration, Rockville, MD

Charles G. Prober, MD, Stanford University, Stanford, CA

Octavio Ramilo, MD, University of Texas Southwestern Medical Center, Dallas, TX

Gopa Raychaudhuri, PhD, Food and Drug Administration, National Institutes of Allergy and Infectious Diseases, Bethesda, MD

Jennifer S. Read, MD, MS, MPH, DTM&H, National Institute of Child Health and Human Development, National Institutes of Health, Bethesda, MD

Stephen Redd, Centers for Disease Control and Prevention, Atlanta, GA

Susan E. Reef, MD, Centers for Disease Control and Prevention, Atlanta, GA

Frank O. Richards, Jr, MD, Centers for Disease Control and Prevention, Atlanta, GA

Tony Richardson, MS, MPH, CPHA, Centers for Disease Control and Prevention, Atlanta, GA

Pierre E. Rollin, MD, Centers for Disease Control and Prevention, Atlanta, GA

Jennifer B. Rosen, MD, Centers for Disease Control and Prevention, Atlanta, GA

Steven Rosenthal, MD, MPH, Food and Drug Administration, Rockville, MD

Jennifer Ross, PhD, Food and Drug Administration, Rockville, MD

Lawrence A. Ross, MD, Keck School of Medicine at the University of Southern California, Los Angeles, CA

Sandra W. Roush, MT, MPH, Centers for Disease Control and Prevention, Atlanta, GA

Sharon L. Roy, MD, MPH, Centers for Disease Control and Prevention, Atlanta, GA

Lorry G. Rubin, MD, Schneider Children's Hospital, New Hyde Park, NY

Charles E. Rupprecht, VMD, MS, PhD, Centers for Disease Control and Prevention, Atlanta, GA

Hari C. Sachs, MD, Food and Drug Administration, Silver Spring, MD

Leonard Sacks, MD, Food and Drug Administration, Silver Spring, MD

Pablo J. Sanchez, MD, Utah Southwestern Medical Center, Dallas, TX

Jason B. Sauberan, University of California San Diego, San Diego, CA

Mark H. Sawyer, MD, University of California San Diego School of Medicine, San Diego, CA

Elaine J. Scallan, MA, PhD, Centers for Disease Control and Prevention, Atlanta, GA

Urs B. Schaad, MD, University Children's Hospital, Basel, Switzerland

Peter M. Schantz, Centers for Disease Control and Prevention, Atlanta, GA

Lawrence B. Schonberger, MD, MPH, Centers for Disease Control and Prevention, Atlanta, GA

Stephanie Schrag, PhD, Centers for Disease Control and Prevention, Atlanta, GA

Lewis Schrager, MD, Food and Drug Administration, Rockville, MD

Gordon E. Schutze, MD, Texas Children's Hospital, Houston, TX

Ann T. Schwartz, MD, Food and Drug Administration, Rockville, MD

Dorothy Scott, MD, Food and Drug Administration, Bethesda, MD

James J. Seivar, MD, Centers for Disease Control and Prevention, Atlanta, GA

Jane F. Seward, MBBS, MPH, Centers for Disease Control and Prevention, Atlanta, GA

Sean V. Shadomv, DVM, MPH, Centers for Disease Control and Prevention, Atlanta, GA

Andi L. Shane, MD, MPH, Emory University School of Medicine, Atlanta, GA

Alan Shapiro, MD, PhD, Food and Drug Administration, Silver Spring, MD

Eugene D. Shapiro, MD, Yale Department of Pediatrics, New Haven, CT

Stanford T. Shulman, MD, Children's Memorial Hospital, Chicago, IL

Toby A. Silverman, MD, Food and Drug Administration, Rockville, MD

Mary E. Singer, MD, PhD, Food and Drug Administration, Silver Spring, MD

Barbara A. Slade, MD, Centers for Disease Control and Prevention, Atlanta, GA

Laurence Slutsker, MD, MPH, Centers for Disease Control and Prevention, Atlanta, GA

Theresa L. Smith, MD, MPH, Centers for Disease Control and Prevention, Atlanta, GA

Thomas D. Smith, MD, Food and Drug Administration, Silver Spring, MD

Alfred F. Sorbello, DO, MPH, Food and Drug Administration, Silver Spring, MD

Mark J. Sotir, PhD, MPH, Centers for Disease Control and Prevention, Atlanta, GA

Ariun Srinivasan, MD, Centers for Disease Control and Prevention, Atlanta, GA

Mary Allen Staat, MD, MPH, Children's Hospital Medical Center, Cincinnati, OH

J. Erin Staples, MD, PhD, Centers for Disease Control and Prevention, Fort Collins, CO

Jeffrey R. Starke, MD, Baylor College of Medicine, Texas Children's Hospital, Houston, TX

William J. Steinbach, MD, Duke University, Durham, NC

E. Richard Stiehm, MD, University of California Los Angeles Medical Center, Los Angeles, CA

Shannon K. Stokley, MPH, Centers for Disease Control and Prevention, Atlanta, GA

Nancy Strockbine, Centers for Disease Control and Prevention, Atlanta, GA

David L. Swerdlow, MD, Centers for Disease Control and Prevention, Atlanta, GA

Shuang Tang, PhD, Food and Drug Administration, Bethesda, MD

Amy M. Taylor, MD, MHS, Food and Drug Administration, Silver Spring, MD

Tracy N. Thomas, MPH, MSc, Centers for Disease Control and Prevention, Atlanta, GA

Susan D. Thompson, MD, Food and Drug Administration, Silver Spring, MD

Evasu Habtu Teshale, MD, Centers for Disease Control and Prevention, Atlanta, GA

Rosemary Tiernan, MD, MPH, Food and Drug Administration, Rockville, MD

Maureen R. Tierney, MD, MSc, Food and Drug Administration, Potomac, MD

Tejpratap S. P. Tiwari, MD, Centers for Disease Control and Prevention, Atlanta, GA

James K. Todd, MD, The Children's Hospital, Denver, CO

Joseph G. Toerner, MD, MPH, Food and Drug Administration, Rockville, MD

Christine Uhlenhaut, PhD, Food and Drug Administration, Bethesda, MD

Elizabeth R. Unger, PhD, MD, Centers for Disease Control and Prevention, Atlanta, GA

Gary A. Urquhart, MPH, Centers for Disease Control and Prevention, Atlanta, GA

Julienne Vaillancourt, BS, Pharm, MPH, Food and Drug Administration, Rockville, MD

Chris A. Van Beneden, MD, MPH, Centers for Disease Control and Prevention, Atlanta, GA

Jennifer R. Verani, MD, MPH, Centers for Disease Control and Prevention, Atlanta, GA

Govinda S. Visvesvara, PhD, Centers for Disease Control and Prevention, Atlanta, GA

Ellen R. Wald, MD, University of Wisconsin School of Medicine and Public Health, Madison, WI

Gregory S. Wallace, MD, MS, MPH, Centers for Disease Control and Prevention, Atlanta, GA

Richard J. Wallace, MD, University of Texas Health Center, Tyler, TX

Nicholas D. Walter, MD, MSc, Centers for Disease Control and Prevention, Atlanta, GA

Elaine Wang, MD, Replidyne Inc, Milford, CT

Diane W. Wara, MD, University of California San Francisco, San Francisco, CA

Annemarie Wasley, Centers for Disease Control and Prevention, Atlanta, GA

John C. Watson, MD, MPH, Centers for Disease Control and Prevention, Atlanta, GA

Donna L. Weaver, RN, MN, Centers for Disease Control and Prevention, Atlanta, GA

Stanley Wei, Centers for Disease Control and Prevention, Atlanta, GA

Cindy M. Weinbaum, MD, MPH, Centers for Disease Control and Prevention, Atlanta, GA

Michele S. Weinberg, MD, MPH, Centers for Disease Control and Prevention, Atlanta, GA

Leonard B. Weiner, MD, SUNY Upstate Medical University, Syracuse, NY

Eric S. Weintraub, MPH, Centers for Disease Control and Prevention, Atlanta, GA

Richard J. Whitley, MD, The University of Alabama at Birmingham, Children's Hospital, Birmingham, AL

Cynthia G. Whitney, MD, MPH, Centers for Disease Control and Prevention, Atlanta, GA

Marc-Alain Widdowson, MD, Centers for Disease Control and Prevention, Atlanta, GA

Ian Williams, Centers for Disease Control and Prevention, Atlanta, GA

John V. Williams, MD, Vanderbilt University Medical Center, Nashville, TN

Emily Woo, MD, MPH, Food and Drug Administration, Rockville, MD

Kimberly Workowski, MD, Centers for Disease Control and Prevention, Atlanta, GA

Alexandra Worobec, MD, US Food and Drug Administration, Rockville, MD

Jennifer Wright, Centers for Disease Control and Prevention, Atlanta, GA

Henry M. Wu, MD, Centers for Disease Control and Prevention, Atlanta, GA

Yuliya I. Yasinskava, MD, Food and Drug Administration, Silver Spring, MD

Zhiping Ye, MD, Food and Drug Administration, Bethesda, MD

Eileen L. Yee, MD, Centers for Disease Control and Prevention, Atlanta, GA

Emily C. Zielinski-Gutierrez, MPH, DrPH, Centers for Disease Control and Prevention, Fort Collins, CO

Committee on Infectious Diseases, 2007–2009

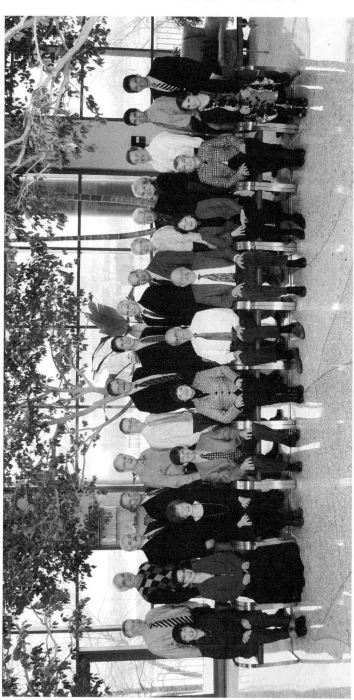

SEATED, LEFT TO RIGHT: Lucia Lee, Carrie L. Byington, Mary P. Glode, David W. Kimberlin, Carol J. Baker, Larry K. Pickering, Joseph A. Bocchini, Jr, Sarah S. Long, Penelope H. Dennehy, Alison Siwek

STANDING, LEFT TO RIGHT: Jack Swanson, Robert Bortolussi, Richard L. Gorman, John S. Bradley, Jeffrey R. Starke, H. Cody Meissner, Robert W. Frenck, Jr, Benjamin Schwartz, Michael T. Brady, Harry Keyserling, Margaret C. Fisher, Edgar O. Ledbetter, Beth P. Bell, Henry H. Bernstein, Marc A. Fischer, Lorry G. Rubin

NOT PICTURED: Robert S. Baltimore, Julia A. McMillan, Walter A. Orenstein, Richard D. Clover, R. Douglas Pratt, Jennifer S. Read, Anne Schuchat

2009 *Red Book* Dedication For Ralph D. Feigin, MD, FAAP (1938–2008)

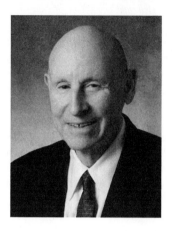

This edition of the *Red Book* is dedicated to Ralph D. Feigin, MD, FAAP. Although Ralph never served on the AAP Committee on Infectious Diseases, there are very few chapters in this book that were not influenced by his considerable body of work or that of his trainees. In fact, a true listing of his accomplishments in pediatrics and pediatric infectious diseases would likely require a book this size. Ralph planned on being a general pediatrician, but entered the field of infectious diseases almost by accident. As a medical student, he learned how to measure amino acids in human blood, a relatively new science at the time. When he entered the military in 1965, he was assigned to the US Army Research Institute of Infectious Diseases at Fort Detrick, Maryland, where he performed ground-breaking work on the circadian periodicity of amino acid metabolism during infection. Thus, a great career was launched. A few of his subsequent contributions to the understanding of infectious diseases and their management in children include:

- Defining many of the metabolic changes that occur during the incubation period and early phases of clinical infectious diseases
- Using animal models to document that the time of day when a viral or bacterial infection occurs may have a marked effect on morbidity and mortality
- Providing one of the first descriptions of the effectiveness of clindamycin for methicillin-susceptible *Staphylococcus aureus* infections
- Defining the stability of antimicrobial agents in parenteral solutions, which still serves as the basis for most manufacturers' recommendations for intravenous use
- Contributing to epidemiologic studies showing that a single dose of measles vaccine would not be an effective strategy to eradicate measles and documenting the development of atypical measles syndrome in previously immunized children
- Defining the pharmacokinetics of cefazolin in children
- Reporting detailed epidemiologic studies of the occurrence of leptospirosis in urban populations and documenting transmission from healthy immunized dogs to humans

- Performing detailed sequential long-term (5–20 years) prospective evaluations of children with bacterial meningitis to determine how epidemiology and pathogenesis related to clinical manifestations and sequelae
- Delineating the role of the syndrome of inappropriate antidiuretic hormone secretion in children with bacterial meningitis
- Contributing to defining adherence of *Haemophilus influenzae* to epithelial cells as a necessary requirement for colonization and/or invasion

Impressive as these accomplishments are, they only scratch the surface of Ralph's contribution to pediatrics. He served as President of the Society for Pediatric Research, the American Pediatric Society, and the Association of Medical School Pediatric Department Chairs. He authored or coauthored 15 books, including 6 editions of the *Textbook of Pediatric Infectious Diseases*, and was coeditor of *Oski's Pediatrics: Principles and Practice*. He served as the Associate Editor of *Pediatrics* and Editor for the Pediatric Division of *Up-To-Date, Inc.* Beginning in 1974, he served as a consultant to the Surgeon General of the US Army on defense of the United States against biologic warfare. He was a vocal advocate for the need to consider the special needs of children in disaster planning, including events of biological terrorism. He also served as a member of the Board of Governors and the Finance Committee for the Clinical Center of the National Institutes of Health, again advocating for promotion and funding of pediatric research. Ralph's many accomplishments were recognized in 2007 with his receipt of the John Howland Award, the penultimate award in pediatrics.

Anyone who knew Ralph understands that his greatest professional passion was teaching. The fabled "Feigin rounds" were a truly unique experience in the art of differential diagnosis. He won the "Outstanding Teacher Award" from the medical students so often that he had to be retired from competition. When Ralph was asked how he built the pediatrics program at Baylor College of Medicine into the largest one in the United States, he emphatically stated that it started with the residency program. In his 31 years as a department chairman, Ralph helped train more than 1000 residents, and his department trained more than 900 fellows. His graduates are members of the faculty at 109 US medical schools and include 55 division heads and 5 department chairs or deans of medical schools. As recognition of his prowess, he received the Lifetime Educational Achievement Award from the American Academy of Pediatrics.

Although his professional accomplishments speak volumes, they reflect only one part of the man himself. Ralph was noted for his boundless energy and limitless optimism. He was one of the rare leaders who turned his personal vision of excellence into reality, but maintained his sense of proportion and humanity. He was kind, gentle, and compassionate in the best tradition of pediatricians. He was generous with his wisdom and his time, with his door always open to friends and colleagues, residents, and students. He also was devoted to his family. With his wife Judy (the "other Dr. Feigin"), he raised 2 daughters and a son and has 6 grandchildren, all of whom live in Houston.

It is difficult to think of anyone who has contributed more to pediatrics and the study of infectious diseases in the last 4 decades than Ralph Feigin. He was a brilliant clinician, accomplished researcher, creative administrator, unparalleled teacher, devoted family man, and revered mentor. He has forever changed the study of pediatric infectious diseases. This edition of the *Red Book* is dedicated to Ralph to thank him on behalf of all the children and pediatricians whose lives he has touched.

Preface

The *Red Book* is a unique source of information on immunizations and infectious diseases for practitioners. The practice of pediatric infectious diseases is changing rapidly. With the limited time available to the practitioner, the ability to quickly obtain up-to-date information about new vaccines and vaccine recommendations, emerging infectious diseases, new diagnostic modalities, and treatment recommendations is essential. The Committee on Infectious Diseases of the American Academy of Pediatrics (AAP) and the editors of the *Red Book* are dedicated to providing the most current and accurate information available in the concise, practical format for which the *Red Book* is known.

The value of the *Red Book* is further enhanced by the *Red Book* Online (**www. aapredbook.org),** where statements and recommendations from the AAP and other important information that becomes available during the 3 years between editions of *Red Book* are provided. Another important resource is the visual library of *Red Book* Online, which has been updated and expanded to include more images of infectious diseases, examples of classic radiologic and other findings, and recent epidemiology of infectious diseases.

The Committee on Infectious Diseases relies on information and advice from many experts, as evidenced by the lengthy list of contributors to *Red Book*. We especially are indebted to the many contributors from other AAP committees, the Centers for Disease Control and Prevention, the Food and Drug Administration, the National Institutes of Health, the Canadian Paediatric Society, the World Health Organization, and many other organizations and individuals who have made this edition possible. In addition, suggestions made by individual AAP members to improve the presentation of information on specific issues and on topic selection have been incorporated into this edition.

Most important to the success of this edition is the dedication and work of the editors, whose commitment to excellence is unparalleled. Under the able leadership of Larry K. Pickering, MD, editor, with associate editors Carol J. Baker, MD, David W. Kimberlin, MD, and Sarah S. Long, MD, this new edition was made possible. We also are indebted to Edgar O. Ledbetter, MD, for his invaluable and untiring efforts to gather and organize the slide materials that make up the visual library of *Red Book* Online and are part of the electronic versions of the *Red Book*.

As noted in previous editions of the *Red Book*, some omissions and errors are inevitable in a book of this type. We ask that AAP members continue to assist the committee actively by suggesting specific ways to improve the quality of future editions.

Joseph A. Bocchini, Jr, MD, FAAP
Chairperson, Committee on Infectious Diseases

Introduction

The Committee on Infectious Diseases (COID) of the American Academy of Pediatrics (AAP) is responsible for developing and revising guidelines for the AAP for control of infectious diseases in children. At intervals of approximately 3 years, the committee issues the *Red Book: Report of the Committee on Infectious Diseases*, which contains a composite summary of current AAP recommendations concerning infectious diseases in and immunizations for infants, children, and adolescents. These recommendations represent a consensus of opinions developed by members of the committee in conjunction with liaison representatives from the Centers for Disease Control and Prevention (CDC), the Food and Drug Administration (FDA), the National Institutes of Health, the National Vaccine Program Office, the Canadian Paediatric Society, the American Thoracic Society, *Red Book* consultants, and numerous collaborators. This edition is based on information available as of January 2009.

Unanswered scientific questions, the complexity of medical practice and technology, continuous new information, and inevitable differences of opinion among experts result in inherent limitations of the *Red Book*. In the context of these limitations, the committee endeavors to provide current, relevant, science-based recommendations for prevention and management of infectious diseases in infants, children, and adolescents. In some cases, other committees and experts may differ in their interpretation of data and resulting recommendations. In some instances, no single recommendation can be made because several options for management are equally acceptable.

In making recommendations in the *Red Book*, the committee acknowledges these differences in viewpoints by use of the phrases "most experts recommend..." and "some experts recommend..." Both phrases indicate valid recommendations, but the first signifies more support among experts, and the second, less support. Hence "some experts recommend..." indicates a minority view that is based on data and/or experience and is sufficiently valid to warrant consideration.

Inevitably in clinical practice, questions arise that cannot be answered on the basis of currently available data. In such cases, the committee attempts to provide guidelines and information that, in conjunction with clinical judgment, will facilitate well-reasoned decisions. We appreciate questions, different perspectives, and alternative recommendations that we have received, and encourage any suggestions or correspondence that will improve future editions of the *Red Book*. Through this process, the committee seeks to provide a practical and authoritative guide for physicians and other health care professionals in their care of infants, children, and adolescents.

To aid physicians and other health care professionals in assimilating current changes in recommendations in the *Red Book*, a list of major changes has been compiled (see Summary of Major Changes, p xxix). However, this listing only begins to cover changes that have occurred in each chapter and section. Health care professionals should consult individual chapters and sections of the book for current guidelines. In addition, new information inevitably begins to outdate some recommendations in the *Red Book*, and necessitates that health care professionals remain informed of new developments and resulting changes in recommendations. Between editions, the AAP publishes new recommendations from the committee in *Pediatrics*, in *AAP News*, and on the *Red Book* Online

Web site (**www.aapredbook.org**). In this edition, we continue to provide Web site addresses throughout the text to enable rapid access to new information. The *Red Book* Online Web site provides access to important *Red Book* errata that may have occurred. On *Red Book* Online, you can enroll for e-mail alerts to be notified automatically when new errata have been announced.

When using antimicrobial agents, physicians should review the package inserts (product labels) prepared by manufacturers, particularly for information concerning contraindications and adverse events. No attempt has been made in the *Red Book* to provide this information, because it is available readily in the *Physicians' Desk Reference,* online (**www.pdr.net**), and in package inserts (product labels). As in previous editions, recommended dosage schedules for antimicrobial agents are given (see Section 4, Antimicrobial Agents and Related Therapy). Recommendations in the *Red Book* for drug dosages may differ from those of the manufacturer in the package insert. Physicians also should be familiar with information in the package insert for vaccines and immune globulins as well as recommendations of other committees (see Sources of Vaccine Information, p 2).

This book could not have been prepared without the dedicated professional competence of many people. Edgar O. Ledbetter, MD, H. Cody Meissner, MD, and Jon R. Almquist, MD, served as *Red Book* reviewers appointed by the AAP Board of Directors. Dr Ledbetter also led the charge in gathering and organizing the new slide materials for the electronic part of the *Red Book.* The AAP staff has been outstanding in its committed work and contributions, particularly Alison Siwek and Hope Hurley, managers, who served as the administrative directors for the committee and coordinated preparation of the *Red Book;* Jennifer Pane, senior medical copy editor, who improved every aspect of the *Red Book;* Darlene Mattefs, department assistant; Barbara Drelicharz, division assistant; Peg Mulcahy, graphic designer; and Jeff Mahony, Mark Ruthman, and Mark Grimes, Department of Marketing, who make the *Red Book* Online and other *Red Book* products possible. Special appreciation is given to Stephanie Renna, assistant to the editor, for her work, patience, and support. Marc Fischer, MD, of the CDC, and R. Douglas Pratt, MD, and Lisa Lee, MD, of the FDA, devoted time and effort in providing input from their organizations. I am especially indebted to the associate editors Carol J. Baker, MD, Sarah S. Long, MD, and David W. Kimberlin, MD, for their expertise, tireless work, good humor, and immense contributions in their editorial and committee work. Georges Peter, MD, continues to provide constant support and advice and has left his imprint on all future editions of the *Red Book.* Members of the committee contributed countless hours and deserve appropriate recognition for their patience, dedication, revisions, and reviews. As a committee, we particularly appreciate the guidance and dedication of the current committee chairperson, Joseph A. Bocchini, MD, whose knowledge, dedication, insight, and leadership are reflected in the quality and productivity of the committee's work. I thank Mimi for always being there and for her patience, understanding, and never-ending support.

There are many other contributors whose professional work and commitment have been essential in the committee's preparation of the *Red Book.* Of special note is the person to whom this edition of the *Red Book* is dedicated, Ralph D. Feigin, MD, who was an exceptional leader, a constant inspiration, and a good friend. His death leaves a void in all of our lives.

Larry K. Pickering, MD, FAAP
Editor

Table of Contents

SECTION 2
RECOMMENDATIONS FOR CARE OF CHILDREN IN SPECIAL CIRCUMSTANCES

SECTION 3
SUMMARIES OF INFECTIOUS DISEASES

SECTION 4
ANTIMICROBIAL AGENTS AND RELATED THERAPY

SECTION 5
ANTIMICROBIAL PROPHYLAXIS

APPENDICES

Summary of Major Changes in the 2009 *Red Book*

MAJOR CHANGES: GENERAL

1. **The use of the dash** (-) has been eliminated and replaced by the word "through" when referring to inclusive ages (eg, 6 through 12 months of age).
2. **All Web sites and telephone numbers** have been updated and verified to be accurate at the time of publication.
3. **References to policy recommendations of the American Academy of Pediatrics, Advisory Committee on Immunization Practices, and other select societies** have been updated throughout.
4. **Standardized vaccine abbreviations (www.cdc.gov/vaccines/recs/acip/vac-abbrev.htm)** are used throughout.

SECTION 1. ACTIVE AND PASSIVE IMMUNIZATION

1. **Table 1.1, showing morbidity from 10 vaccine preventable diseases,** has been updated to include data from 2007.
2. The Web site for the interactive **catch-up immunization scheduler** for children 0 through 6 years of age has been added (**www.cdc.gov/vaccines/programs/default.htm#catchup**).
3. **Table 1.3** has been updated to include vaccines licensed since publication of the 2006 *Red Book*, including DTaP-IPV, DTaP-IPV/Hib, HPV, meningococcal conjugate, rotavirus and zoster vaccines. In addition, references to single-antigen measles, mumps, and rubella vaccines have been removed, because these vaccines currently are not produced in the United States.
4. The table showing **recommended storage temperatures of commonly used vaccines** has been eliminated and replaced with a Web site where this information can be obtained (**www.cdc.gov/vaccines/pubs/downloads/bk-vac-mgt.pdf**).
5. The **2009 childhood and adolescent immunization schedule** has been added (Fig 1.1–1.3), as has the Web site for access to future, updated childhood and adult immunization schedules.
6. The **Combination Vaccines** section has been updated, including addition of a table that shows combination vaccines available in the United States, the age group for which they are licensed, and recommendations for use.
7. The description of **the Vaccine Adverse Event Reporting System (VAERS)** has been revised.
8. **The vaccine contraindications and precautions** section has been revised.
9. The **Common Misconceptions About Immunizations** section has been revised to include addition of Table 1.8, which shows common misconceptions about immunizations.

10. **Hepatitis A prophylaxis.** The use of hepatitis A vaccine and Immune Globulin for postexposure prophylaxis and for international travel has been updated to reflect current recommendations.

11. A new section describing **Immune Globulin Subcutaneous** for children with primary immunodeficiencies has been added.

12. **Pregnancy.** Recommendations for dealing with a woman if a dose of human papillomavirus (HPV) vaccine is administered inadvertently during pregnancy have been added.

13. **The definition and management of anaphylaxis** has been updated to concur with recommendations of the second National Institutes of Health (NIH)-National Institute of Allergy and Infectious Diseases symposium.

14. **Immunization recommendations for human immunodeficiency virus (HIV)-infected or -exposed children** were updated to be consistent with the guidelines of the Centers for Disease Control and Prevention, NIH, and Infectious Diseases Society of America (IDSA) for diagnosis and treatment of opportunistic infections in HIV infected children (*MMWR Early Release* 2009;58(March 24, 2009):1–207).

15. The section on **American Indian/Alaska Native Children** has been updated to reflect changes in vaccine recommendations for these high-risk groups.

16. The **Adolescent and College Populations** section has been updated to include all vaccines recommended for adolescents.

17. The section titled **Misconceptions About Vaccine Contraindications** has been deleted. Information has been incorporated into the **Vaccine Contraindications and Precautions** section.

SECTION 2. RECOMMENDATIONS FOR CARE OF CHILDREN IN SPECIAL CLINICAL CIRCUMSTANCES

1. **Biological Terrorism.** The table detailing biological weapons has been removed, and Table 2.1, providing emergency contacts and educational resources, has been updated.

2. **Transmitted infections.** The Red Cross Web site where blood donor information is available has been added (**www.redcross.org,** then click Blood services, then Blood Donor eligibility guidelines). In addition, blood screening information has been provided for West Nile virus, bacterial contamination, *Trypanosoma cruzi* (Chagas disease), and the variant form of Creutzfeldt-Jakob disease (vCJD).

3. **Human Milk, Human Immunodeficiency Virus (HIV).** The recommendation for routine screening of pregnant women for HIV as well as an update on prevention of HIV during breastfeeding in resource-limited countries have been added. Guidelines for what to do when a child mistakenly has been fed expressed milk from another mother are provided.

4. **Antimicrobial agents in human milk.** The table showing antimicrobial agents taken by mothers that may be cause for concern has been replaced by a Web site that provides current information (**www.toxnet.nlm.nih.gov/help/ LactMedRecordFormat.htm**).

5. **Children in Out-of-Home Child Care.** General recommendations for exclusion of children in out-of-home care have been placed into tables 2.5 and 2.6. Hepatitis A vaccine is recommended for all susceptible close personal contacts of children internationally adopted from a country with high or intermediate hepatitis A endemicity in the first 60 days after arrival in the United States.

6. **School Health.** Immunization recommendations for school-aged children and adolescents have been updated. Recommendations for management of infections spread by direct contact, including methicillin-resistant *Staphylococcus aureus* (MRSA), herpes simplex, *Tinea capitis,* and scabies, have been updated. Guidelines on control and prevention of MRSA in athletic and other school settings have been added.

7. **Infection Control for Hospitalized Children.** The text and Table 2.7 have been updated to include new elements of Standard Precautions.

8. **Sexually Transmitted Infections (STIs) in Adolescents and Children.** Recommendations for use of HPV vaccine beginning at the health care visit at 11- through 12-years of age has been added.

9. **Hepatitis and Youth Correctional Settings.** Rates of hepatitis A, hepatitis B, and hepatitis C in adolescents in youth correctional settings have been updated.

10. **Medical Evaluation of Internationally Adopted Children.** The epidemiology, diagnosis, and prevention aspects of the viral hepatitis section have been revised. Consideration and diagnosis of Chagas disease and *Schistosoma* infections in children from countries with endemic infection and strongyloidiasis in any child with eosinophilia has been added. A description of the Immigration and Nationality Act and how it relates to adopted children has been added.

11. **Table 2.17,** showing approaches to evaluation and immunization of internationally adopted children, has been revised.

12. **Prevention of Mosquitoborne Infections.** An update on the use of picaridin and oil of lemon eucalyptus as insect repellents has been added.

13. **Prevention of Illnesses Associated With Recreational Water Use.** This section was revised to include updated surveillance data from the CDC report on waterborne diseases associated with recreational water use.

14. **Diseases Transmitted From Animals (Zoonoses)** has been added as a new section, which includes tables showing nontraditional pets and animals in public settings and guidelines for prevention of human diseases from exposure to pets, nontraditional pets, and animals in public settings.

SECTION 3. SUMMARIES OF INFECTIOUS DISEASES

1. **Adenovirus.** New methods to detect adenovirus have been added to the "Diagnostic Tests" section. Information about adenovirus serotype 14, an emerging cause of severe pneumonia, has been added.

2. **Amebiasis.** The enzyme immunoassay (EIA) test has replaced the indirect hemagglutination test for routine serodiagnosis of amebiasis.

3. **Anthrax.** Treatment and prevention sections have been updated to include changes in vaccine administration.

4. **Arboviruses.** This chapter has been rewritten. West Nile virus has been moved to form an independent chapter; 2 new tables, one showing clinical manifestations and the other showing genus, geographic location, vectors, and average number of cases for domestic and international arboviral disease, have been created; proposed recommendations for the Japanese encephalitis vaccine being considered by the Food and Drug Administration have been added, as have recommendations from the ACIP statement on Japanese encephalitis.

5. **Candidiasis.** This chapter has been updated to include use of newer antifungal agents in children, including newborn infants and to reflect clinical practice guidelines from the Infectious Diseases Society of America.

6. ***Clostridium difficile.*** A previously uncommon, fluoroquinolone-resistant strain of *C difficile* with variation in toxin genes has emerged. Initial therapy of children with severe disease attributable to *C difficile* has been updated.

7. **Cytomegalovirus.** This chapter has been updated extensively to include outcomes following congenital infection, the role of maternal reinfection as the cause of some cases of congenital infection, diagnostic approaches in congenital infection, treatment options for congenitally infected infants with symptomatic cytomegalovirus (CMV) disease, treatment options for perinatally acquired CMV infection in very preterm infants, new recommendations for treatment and prophylaxis of CMV in HIV-infected patients, and specific details for preparing human milk to prevent perinatal transmission in at-risk preterm infants.

8. ***Ehrlichia* and *Anaplasma* Infections.** Previously referred to collectively as ehrlichiosis, ehrlichiosis and anaplasmosis now are used to describe infections caused by *Ehrlichia* and *Anaplasma* species, respectively.

9. **Enteroviruses.** The classification system for human enteroviruses (HEVs) into HEV A, HEV B, HEV C, and HEV D has been included. Diagnostic tests available have been updated.

10. **Epstein-Barr Virus Infections.** A figure showing the evolution of development of antibodies to Epstein Barr virus antigens has been added.

11. ***Fusobacterium* infections, including Lemierre Disease** has been added as a new chapter.

12. **Gonococcal Infections.** Because of an increase in resistance of *Neisseria gonorrhoeae* to fluoroquinolones, these drugs no longer are recommended to treat gonorrhea. An extended-spectrum cephalosporin is recommended as initial therapy for children, adolescents, and adults for treatment of gonorrhea. Tables 3.7 and 3.8 clarify treatment recommendations.

13. ***Haemophilus influenzae* Infections.** The text and Table 3.10, describing *Haemophilus influenzae* type b (Hib)-containing vaccines licensed for use in the United States, have been updated to include DTaP-IPV/Hib. Information has been added about interim recommendations for use of Hib conjugate vaccines during a Hib vaccine shortage and the importance of completing the primary Hib immunization series.

14. **Hepatitis A.** The text and Table 3.13 have been updated to include changes in recommendations for use of hepatitis A vaccine for both postexposure prophylaxis and for international travelers journeying to countries with endemic hepatitis A infection. In addition, the alternative dose of the combined hepatitis A-hepatitis B vaccine has been added.

15. **Hepatitis B.** The text and Table 3.17 have been updated to include recommended uses of hepatitis B-containing vaccines. Two new tables have been added. One shows the estimated HBsAg prevalence by regions of the world, and the second provides categories of adults at high risk recommended to receive hepatitis B vaccine.

16. **Herpes Simplex.** The chapter has been revised significantly to include risks of neonatal herpes following exposure during delivery; the diagnostic workup of an infant suspected of having neonatal herpes; the care of newborn infants whose mothers have active genital lesions; and the care of newborn infants whose mothers have a history of genital herpes but no active genital lesions at delivery.

17. **Histoplasmosis** has been updated to include recommendations from the Infectious Diseases Society of America.

18. **Human Bocavirus,** a cause of respiratory tract diseases in children, has been added as a new chapter.

19. **Human Immunodeficiency Virus Infection.** This chapter has been updated extensively to include information on new guidelines from CDC/NIH/IDSA on prevention and treatment of opportunistic infections (OIs), changes in occurrence of OIs, expanded description of HIV-1 and HIV-2 epidemiology, including transmission, and new information on diagnosis, treatment, and control measures.

20. **Human Papillomaviruses.** Diagnostic methods and prevention, including use of the US Food and Drug Administration (FDA)-licensed and -submitted vaccines to prevent HPV infections, have been added.

21. **The Influenza** chapter has been updated to include information about the etiology and epidemiology of avian influenza and pediatric influenza; antiviral drug resistance, including oseltamivir resistance; and current immunization recommendations, including immunization of children from 6 months through 18 years of age.

22. **Kawasaki Disease.** This chapter has been updated to include an algorithm from the American Heart Association for evaluation of patients with suspected incomplete disease.

23. **Malaria.** Patterns of resistance of drugs used to treat malaria have been updated with concomitant updates to the treatment and chemoprophylaxis sections.

24. **Measles.** The epidemiology section has been updated, recommendations of the World Health Organization for use of vitamin A for all children with acute measles have been added, information about measles-mumps-rubella-varicella (MMRV) vaccine has been included, and an update on the lack of production of single-antigen measles vaccine in the United States has been added.

25. **Meningococcal Infections.** Use of meningococcal conjugate vaccine (MCV4) has been updated to reflect recommendations for use in people 11 through 18 years of age, and a recommendation not to use MCV4 routinely in children 2 through 10 years of age (only for high risk) has been added. The report of resistance to ciprofloxacin used for chemoprophylaxis has been added.

26. **Mumps.** The epidemiology section, including the increase in cases in 2006, and the diagnostic section have been updated, and recommendations for 2 doses of mumps-containing vaccine (measles-mumps-rubella [MMR]) have been emphasized. Lack of monovalent mumps vaccine, which currently is not produced in the United States, has been added.

27. The **Pediculosis Capitis** chapter has been updated to be consistent with the forthcoming AAP statement on head lice.

28. **Pelvic Inflammatory Disease.** Because of resistance, fluoroquinolones no longer are recommended to treat *N gonorrhoeae*. Reference to recommendations for partner-services for programs for HIV infection, syphilis, gonorrhea, and chlamydia have been added.

29. The **Pertussis** chapter has been updated to clarify recommendations for Tdap use in the text, and Table 3.47 shows special situation recommendations for use of Tdap in adolescents. Information about additional pertussis-containing vaccines (Tdap, DTaP-IPV/Hib, and DTaP-IPV), addition of all pertussis-containing vaccines to Table 3.45, and tables showing contraindications and precautions of DTaP (Table 3.46) and Tdap (Table 3.48) have been added.

30. **Pneumococcal Infections.** The epidemiology of pneumococcal disease since licensure of the heptavalent pneumococcal conjugate (PCV7) vaccine has been updated, including addition of children with cochlear implants in the high-risk category. Additional updates include immunization recommendations for children 24 through 59 months of age who are not completely immunized, high-risk children 10 years of age and younger, and American Indian/Alaska native children 24 through 59 months of age. Case reporting criteria have been updated, as have high-risk criteria for invasive pneumococcal infection. The new Clinical Laboratory Standards Institute (CLSI) definitions of in vitro susceptibility have been added to Table 3.50.

31. *Pneumocystis jirovecii* **Infections.** This chapter has been updated to conform with "Guidelines for Prevention and Treatment of Opportunistic Infections in HIV-Exposed and HIV-Infected Children" published by the CDC/NIH/IDSA.

32. The **Polyomaviruses** (BK virus and JC virus) chapter is new to this edition.

33. **Rabies.** This chapter has been updated to include current information on epidemiology, recommendations for rabies preexposure and postexposure prophylaxis, and information regarding treatment considerations for human rabies patients.

34. **Respiratory Syncytial Virus.** This chapter has been updated to include new information on epidemiology, diagnostic testing, management of infected children, and infection-control measures. New recommendations are provided for the number of doses of palivizumab as well as new eligibility criteria for prophylaxis of high-risk groups.

35. **Rickettsial Diseases.** The section dealing with other spotted fever infections has been updated to include epidemiologically distinct but clinically similar tickborne infections.

36. **Rotavirus.** This chapter has been updated to include recommendations for use of the 2 FDA-licensed rotavirus vaccines in infants in the United States.

37. **Rubella.** Monovalent rubella vaccine currently is not produced in the United States. Rubella immunization recommendations have been adjusted to reflect this.

38. The **Sporotrichosis** chapter has been updated to include recommendations in the Infectious Diseases Society of America guidelines.

39. **Staphylococcal Infections.** The toxic shock chapter has been deleted, and updated information on staphylococcal toxic shock syndrome has been added to this chapter. In addition, current information on the epidemiology, diagnosis, treatment, and prevention of MRSA has been added. An algorithm for initial management of skin and soft tissue infections caused by *S aureus* has been added.

40. **Group A Streptococcal Infections.** This chapter has been updated to include information about toxic shock syndrome attributable to group A streptococcal infections, current American Heart Association guidelines for prevention of bacterial endocarditis, and a table showing the Jones criteria for rheumatic fever.

41. **Syphilis.** An algorithm for evaluation and treatment of infants born to mothers with reactive serologic tests for syphilis has been added, and the text has been updated.

42. **Tuberculosis.** The approach to patients with multiple drug-resistant and extensively drug-resistant tuberculosis, use of interferon-gamma release assays for diagnosis, and infection attributable to *Mycobacterium bovis* have been added.

43. **Diseases Caused by Nontuberculous Mycobacteria.** Diagnosis, treatment, and prevention of nontuberculous mycobacterial diseases have been updated to follow guidelines of the American Thoracic Society/IDSA. A table providing criteria for discontinuing and restarting prophylaxis for *Mycobacterium avium* complex in HIV-infected children has been added.

44. **Varicella-Zoster Infections.** This chapter has been updated to include recommendations for a routine 2-dose varicella immunization program; a second-dose catch-up varicella immunization program; routine immunization for all healthy people 13 years of age or older without evidence of varicella immunity; prenatal assessment and postpartum immunization; expanding the use of varicella vaccines in HIV-infected children; establishing middle school, high school, and college entry immunization requirements; and criteria for and evidence of immunity to varicella.

45. **Toxic Shock Syndrome.** This chapter has been eliminated, and the information has been placed in the Staphylococcal Infections and Group A Streptococcal Infections chapters.

SECTION 4. ANTIMICROBIAL AGENTS AND RELATED THERAPY

1. A section on antimicrobial agents used in adults for serious infections and their potential use in children has been added.

2. **Drug Interactions.** The section on drug interactions has been reduced, including elimination of the accompanying table, which has been replaced with a Web site where information can be obtained (**www.fda.gov/cder/drug/drugInteractions/default.htm**).

3. **Tables** of antibacterial (Tables 4.1 and 4.2), antifungal (Tables 4.5–4.7), antiviral (Table 4.8), and other agents recommended to treat sexually transmitted infections (Table 4.3) have been updated.

4. The **Drugs for Parasitic Infections** tables, reproduced with permission from *The Medical Letter,* have been updated to the most recent versions.

SECTION 5. ANTIMICROBIAL PROPHYLAXIS

1. **Antimicrobial Prophylaxis.** Table 5.1, showing site, exposed host, and vulnerable host categories where antimicrobial chemoprophylaxis is most likely to be successful, has been added.

2. **Prevention of Bacterial Endocarditis.** The American Heart Association guidelines for prevention of infective endocarditis have been included. Antimicrobial prophylaxis for dental procedures now is recommended only for patients at highest risk of severe consequences from endocarditis who are undergoing the highest-risk procedures. Drug regimens are provided in Table 5.3.

3. **Prevention of Neonatal Ophthalmia.** Silver nitrate no longer is recommended for prophylaxis of ocular gonorrheal infection.

APPENDICES

1. **Appendix I** has been updated to include recent contact information of organizations that are listed.

2. **Appendix IV:** The National Childhood Vaccine Injury Act reporting and compensation table has been updated to include vaccines licensed and added to the table since the last edition.

3. **Appendix VI:** Contraindications and precautions of vaccines licensed since the last edition have been added.

4. **Appendix IX:** Newly recognized vehicles of foodborne disease associated with causative agents and additional classical syndromes of foodborne diseases have been added.

5. **New Appendices.** Two new appendices have been added. One (Appendix II) shows dates of vaccines licensed by the FDA, and the other (Appendix III) shows *Current Procedural Terminology* (CPT) and *International Classification of Diseases* (ICD-9) codes for administering licensed vaccines in the United States.

Active and Passive Immunization

·················
PROLOGUE

The ultimate goal of immunization is eradication or elimination of disease; the immediate goal is prevention of disease in people or groups. To accomplish these goals, physicians must make timely immunization, including active and passive immunoprophylaxis, a high priority in the care of infants, children, adolescents, and adults. The global eradication of smallpox in 1977, elimination of poliomyelitis disease from the Americas in 1991, elimination of ongoing measles transmission in 2000, and elimination of rubella and congenital rubella syndrome in 2004 from the United States serve as models for fulfilling the promise of disease control through immunization. These accomplishments were achieved by combining a comprehensive immunization program providing consistent, high levels of vaccine coverage with intensive surveillance and effective public health disease control measures. Future success in the worldwide elimination of polio, measles, rubella, and hepatitis B is possible through implementation of similar prevention strategies.

High immunization rates have reduced dramatically the incidence of diphtheria, measles, mumps, polio, rubella (congenital and acquired), tetanus, and *Haemophilus influenzae* type b disease (see Table 1.1, p 2) in the United States. Declines in the incidence of varicella, invasive pneumococcal disease, and hepatitis A also have occurred. Yet, because organisms that cause these diseases persist in the United States and elsewhere around the world, continued immunization efforts must be maintained and strengthened. Discoveries in immunology, molecular biology, and medical genetics have resulted in burgeoning vaccine research. Licensing of new, improved, and safer vaccines; anticipated arrival of additional combination vaccines; establishment of an adolescent immunization platform; and application of novel vaccine delivery systems promise a new era of preventive medicine. The advent of population-based postlicensure studies of new vaccines facilitates detection of rare adverse events temporally associated with immunization that were undetected during prelicensure clinical trials. Studies of the rare occurrence of intussusception after administration of the first licensed oral rhesus rotavirus vaccine confirmed the value of such surveillance systems. Physicians must regularly update their knowledge about specific vaccines, including information about their recommended use, safety, and effectiveness.

Each edition of the *Red Book* provides recommendations for immunization of infants, children, and adolescents. These recommendations, which are harmonized among the American Academy of Pediatrics (AAP), the Advisory Committee on Immunization Practices of the Centers for Disease Control and Prevention, and the American Academy of Family Physicians, are based on careful analysis of disease epidemiology, the benefits and risks of immunization, and the feasibility of implementation. Whereas immunization recommendations represent the best approach to disease prevention on a population basis, in rare circumstances, individual considerations may warrant a different approach.

Table 1.1. Baseline 20th Century Annual Morbidity and 2007 Morbidity From 10 Infectious Diseases With Vaccines Recommended Before 1990 for Universal Use in Children: United States[a]

Disease	Baseline 20th Century Annual Morbidity	2007 Morbidity	% Decrease
Smallpox	48 164[b]	0	100
Diphtheria	175 885[c]	0	100
Pertussis	147 271[d]	10 454	93
Tetanus	1314[e]	28	98
Poliomyelitis (paralytic)	16 316[f]	0	100
Measles	503 282[g]	43	>99
Mumps	152 209[h]	800	>99
Rubella	47 745[i]	12	>99
Congenital rubella syndrome	823[j]	0	100
Haemophilus influenzae type b	20 000[k]	22[l]	>99

[a] Adapted from Centers for Disease Control and Prevention. Impact of vaccines universally recommended for children—United States, 1990–1998. *MMWR Morb Mortal Wkly Rep.* 1999;48(12):243–248; and Centers for Disease Control and Prevention. Notice to readers: final 2007 reports of nationally notifiable infectious diseases. *MMWR Morb Mortal Wkly Rep.* 2008;57(33):901, 903–913.

[b] Average annual number of cases during 1900–1904.

[c] Average annual number of reported cases during 1920–1922, 3 years before vaccine development.

[d] Average annual number of reported cases during 1922–1925, 4 years before vaccine development.

[e] Estimated number of cases based on reported number of deaths during 1922–1926, assuming a case-fatality rate of 90%.

[f] Average annual number of reported cases during 1951–1954, 4 years before vaccine licensure.

[g] Average annual number of reported cases during 1958–1962, 5 years before vaccine licensure.

[h] Number of reported cases in 1968, the first year reporting began and the first year after vaccine licensure.

[i] Average annual number of reported cases during 1966–1968, 3 years before vaccine licensure.

[j] Estimated number of cases based on seroprevalence data in the population and on the risk that women infected during a childbearing year would have a fetus with congenital rubella syndrome.

[k] Estimated number of cases from population-based surveillance studies before vaccine licensure in 1985.

[l] Represents invasive disease in children younger than 5 years of age; does not include 180 *H influenzae* strains of unknown serotype.

Use of trade names and commercial sources in the *Red Book* is for identification purposes only and does not imply endorsement by the AAP. Internet sites referenced in the *Red Book* are provided as a service to readers and may change without notice; citation of Web sites does not constitute AAP endorsement.

SOURCES OF VACCINE INFORMATION

In addition to the *Red Book*, which is published at intervals of approximately 3 years, physicians should use evidence-based literature and other sources for data to answer specific vaccine questions encountered in practice. Such sources include the following:

- *Pediatrics.* Policy statements developed by the Committee on Infectious Diseases providing updated recommendations are published in *Pediatrics* between editions of the *Red Book.* Policy statements also may be accessed via the American Academy of Pediatrics (AAP) Web site (**http://aappolicy.aappublications.org/**). Recommendations of the Committee on Infectious Diseases are not official until approved by the Board of Directors of the AAP.

  The updated recommended childhood and adolescent immunization schedules for the United States are published annually in the January issue of *Pediatrics* and elsewhere (see Scheduling Immunizations, p 21).
- *AAP News.* Policy statements (or statement summaries) from the COID often are published initially in *AAP News,* the monthly newsmagazine of the AAP (**www. aapnews.org**), to inform the membership promptly of new recommendations.
- *Morbidity and Mortality Weekly Report (MMWR).* Published weekly by the Centers for Disease Control and Prevention (CDC), the *MMWR* contains current vaccine recommendations; reports of specific disease activity; alerts concerning vaccine availability; changes in vaccine formulations, vaccine safety issues, and policy statements; and other infectious disease and vaccine information. Recommendations of the Advisory Committee on Immunization Practices (ACIP) of the CDC are published periodically, often as supplements to the *MMWR,* and are posted on the CDC Web site (**www.cdc.gov/mmwr**). Recommendations of the ACIP are not official until approved by the CDC director and the Department of Health and Human Services and published in the *MMWR.*
- **Manufacturers' package inserts (product labels).** Manufacturers provide product-specific information with each vaccine product. This information also is available in the *Physicians' Desk Reference,* which is published annually. The product label must be in full compliance with US Food and Drug Administration (FDA) regulations pertaining to labeling for prescription drugs, including indications and usage, dosages, routes of administration, clinical pharmacology, contraindications, and adverse events. Each package insert lists contents of the vaccine, including preservatives, stabilizers, antimicrobial agents, adjuvants, and suspending fluids. Health care professionals should be familiar with the label for each product they administer. All vaccine product labels are accessible through the FDA Web site (**www.fda.gov/cber/vaccines.htm**). Most manufacturers maintain Web sites with current information concerning new vaccine releases and changes in labeling. Additionally, 24-hour contact telephone numbers for medical questions are available in the *Physicians' Desk Reference* (**www.pdr.net**).
- *Health Information for International Travel.* This useful monograph is published approximately every 2 years by the CDC as a guide to requirements of various countries for specific immunizations. The monograph also provides information about other vaccines recommended for travel in specific areas and other information for travelers. This document can be purchased from the Superintendent of Documents, US Government Printing Office, Washington, DC 20402–9235. This information also is available on the CDC Web site (**wwwn.cdc.gov/travel/default.aspx**). For additional sources of information on international travel, see International Travel (p 98).
- *CDC materials.* The National Center for Immunization and Respiratory Diseases (NCIRD) of the CDC maintains a comprehensive Web site (**www.cdc.gov/vaccines**) that includes a section for health care professionals that facilitates immunization delivery. Among the resources available are ACIP provisional recommendations that can

assist health care professionals in making decisions on use of new vaccines before publication of final recommendations. A CDC textbook, *Epidemiology and Prevention of Vaccine-Preventable Diseases*, also referred to as the Pink Book, provides comprehensive information on use and administration of childhood vaccines as well as selected ACIP statements and other vaccine-related information (for purchase of the Pink Book, contact the Public Health Foundation at 877-252-1200 or visit **www.cdc.gov/vaccines/ pubs/#text**). A CDC publication titled *Manual for Surveillance of Vaccine-Preventable Diseases* provides insight into principles used to investigate and control outbreaks of disease when immunization levels decrease. The NCIRD publishes a series of brochures on immunization topics and produces a CD-ROM that contains a wide range of resources, including vaccine information statements (VISs) and the complete text of the Pink Book. To obtain CDC materials, contact the CDC information center at 1-800-CDC-INFO (1-800-232-4636), or visit the NCIRD Web site (**www.cdc.gov/ ncird**).

- **Satellite broadcasts and Web-based training courses.** The NCIRD, in conjunction with the Public Health Training Network, conducts several immunization-related "train the trainer" courses live via satellite and over the Internet each year. Annual course offerings include the Immunization Update, Vaccines for International Travel, Influenza, and a 4-part introductory course on the Epidemiology and Prevention of Vaccine-Preventable Diseases. The course schedule, slide sets, and written materials can be accessed on the Internet (**http://www.cdc.gov/vaccines/ ed/default.htm**).
- **Immunization information e-mail–based inquiry system.** This system responds to immunization-related questions submitted from health care professionals and members of the public. Individualized responses to inquiries typically are sent within 24 hours. Inquiries should be sent by completing a form available at **www.cdc. gov/vaccines/about/contact/NIPINFO_contact_form.htm**.
- **CDC Telephone Hot Line.** The hot line is a telephone-based resource available to answer immunization-related questions from health care professionals and members of the public. The hot line can be reached at 1-800-CDC-INFO (1-800-232-4636) and is available in English and Spanish.

    Printed information on immunizations also can be obtained from the NCIRD through the CDC Web site (**www.cdc.gov/vaccines**).
- **Independent sources of reliable immunization information.** Appendix I (p 831) provides a list of reliable immunization information resources, including facts concerning vaccine efficacy, clinical applications, schedules, and unbiased information about safety. Two organizations particularly are comprehensive in addressing concerns of practicing physicians: the National Network for Immunization Information (**www.immunizationinfo.org**) and the Immunization Action Coalition (**www.immunize.org**).
- **Vaccine price list.** Information about pediatric and adolescent vaccines, types of packaging, and CDC and private-sector costs are available at **www.cdc.gov/ vaccines/programs/vfc/cdc-vac-price-list.htm**.

Other resources[1] include the FDA and Institute of Medicine; infectious disease and vaccine experts at university-affiliated hospitals, at medical schools, and in private practice; and state immunization programs and local public health departments. Information can be obtained from state and local health departments about current epidemiology of diseases; immunization recommendations; legal requirements; public health policies; and nursery school, child care, and school health concerns or requirements. Information regarding global health matters can be obtained from the World Health Organization (**www.who.int/**).

- **Immunization schedules.** An online catch-up immunization scheduler is available (**www.cdc.gov/vaccines/recs/scheduler/catchup.htm**) for use by parents and health care professionals. The scheduler is based on the recommended immunization schedule for children 0 through 6 years of age. The scheduler, which can be downloaded, allows the user to determine the vaccines a child needs and especially is useful for quickly viewing missed or skipped vaccines according to the recommended childhood immunization schedule.

INFORMING PATIENTS AND PARENTS

Parents and patients should be informed about the benefits and risks of disease-preventive and therapeutic procedures, including immunization. The patient, parents, and/or legal guardian should be informed about benefits to be derived from vaccines in preventing diseases in immunized people and in the community where they live and about risks of those vaccines. Questions should be encouraged, and adequate time should be allowed so that information is understood.

The National Childhood Vaccine Injury Act (NCVIA) of 1986 included requirements for notifying *all* patients and parents about vaccine benefits and risks. Whether vaccines are purchased with private or public funds, this legislation mandates that a vaccine information statement (VIS) be provided *each* time a vaccine covered under the National Vaccine Injury Compensation Program (VICP) is administered (see Table 1.2, p 6). This applies in all settings, including clinics, offices, and hospitals (eg, for the birth dose of hepatitis B vaccine). Providing this information before the day of immunization is desirable. For vaccines not yet included in the VICP, VISs are available but are not mandated unless the vaccine is purchased through a contract with the Centers for Disease Control and Prevention (CDC [ie, the Vaccines for Children Program, state immunization grants, or state purchases through the CDC]). Copies of current VISs are available online from the CDC (**www.cdc.gov/vaccines/pubs/VIS/default.htm**) and the Immunization Action Coalition Web site (**www.immunize.org**) in English and many other languages. Copies also can be obtained from the American Academy of Pediatrics (AAP), state and local health departments, and vaccine manufacturers or by calling the CDC telephone hotline (1-800-232-4636). Information is available in English and in Spanish. Physicians need to ensure that the VIS provided is the current version by noting the date of publication. The latest version can be determined by calling the CDC telephone hotline or viewing the CDC VIS Web site.

---

[1] Appendix I, Directory of Resources, p 831.

Table 1.2. Guidance in Using Vaccine Information Statements (VISs)[a]

Distribution	Documentation in the Patient's Medical Record
Must be provided each time a VICP-covered vaccine is administered[b]	Vaccine manufacturer, lot number, and date of administration[b]
Given to patient (nonminor), parent, and/or legal guardian[b,c]	Name and business address of the health care professional administering the vaccine[b]
Must be the current version[d]	Date that VIS is provided (and VIS publication date[d])
Can provide (not substitute) other written materials or audiovisual aids in addition to VISs	Site (eg, deltoid area) and route (eg, intramuscular) of administration and expiration date of the vaccine[e]

VICP indicates Vaccine Injury Compensation Program.
[a] VISs are available at **www.cdc.gov/vaccines/pubs/vis/default.htm**.
[b] Required under the National Childhood Vaccine Injury Act.
[c] Consenting adolescent may vary by state.
[d] Required by Centers for Disease Control and Prevention (CDC) regulations for vaccines purchased through CDC contract. See the VIS Web site for current versions.
[e] Recommended by the American Academy of Pediatrics.

The NCVIA requires physicians administering vaccines covered by the VICP, whether purchased with private or public funds, to record in the patient's medical record information shown in Table 1.2 as well as confirmation that the relevant VIS was provided at the time of each immunization (see Record Keeping and Immunization Information Systems, p 38). For vaccines purchased through CDC contract, physicians are required to record the VIS date of publication as well as the date on which the VIS was provided to the patient, parent, and/or legal guardian. Although VIS distribution and vaccine record-keeping requirements do not apply to privately purchased vaccines not covered by the VICP, the AAP recommends following the same record-keeping practices for all vaccines. The AAP also recommends recording the site and route of administration and vaccine expiration date when administering any vaccine. Health care professionals also should be aware of local confidentiality laws involving adolescents.

New VISs do not require parents' or patients' signatures to indicate that they have read and understood the material. However, the health care professional has the option to obtain a signature. Health care professionals should be familiar with requirements of the state in which they practice. Whether or not a signature is obtained, health care professionals should document in the chart that the VIS has been provided and discussed with the patient, parent, and/or legal guardian.

Parental Concerns About Immunization

Health care professionals should anticipate that some parents will question the need for or the safety of immunizations, refuse certain vaccines, or even decide to reject all immunizations for their child. Some parents may have religious or philosophic objections to immunization, which are permitted by some states. Other parents want only to enter into a dialogue with their child's physician about the risks and benefits of one or more of the vaccines. Several factors contribute to parental vaccine concerns or lack of understanding of the benefits of vaccines, including: (1) lack of information about the vaccine being given and about immunizations in general; (2) opposing information from other sources (eg, alternative medicine practitioners, antivaccination organizations, and some religious groups); (3) mistrust of the source of information (eg, vaccine manufacturer); (4) perceived risk of serious vaccine adverse events; (5) concern regarding number of injections or the vaccine schedule; (6) information being delivered in a way that does not recognize cultural differences or that is not tailored to individual concern; (7) information being delivered at an inconvenient time; (8) not perceiving risk of vaccines accurately; and (9) lack of appreciation of the severity of vaccine-preventable diseases. One important aspect physicians can control is their relationship with patients and their parents. Physicians are the most trusted source of health information for parents. If parents trust their child's physician, information presented to them by the physician in support of vaccines is accepted more readily. A nonjudgmental approach is best for parents who question the need for immunizations. Ideally, health care professionals should determine in general terms what parents understand about vaccines their children will be receiving, the nature of their concerns, their health beliefs, and what information they find credible.

People understand and react to vaccine information on the basis of a variety of factors, including previous experiences, attitudes, health beliefs, personal values, and education. The method in which data are presented about immunizations as well as a person's perceptions of the risks of disease, perceived ability to control those risks, and risk preference also contribute to understanding of immunizations. For some people, the risk of immunization can be viewed as disproportionately greater so that immunization is not perceived as beneficial, in part because of the relative infrequency of vaccine-preventable diseases in the United States. Others can dwell on sociopolitical issues, such as mandatory immunization, informed consent, and the primacy of individual rights over that of societal benefit.

Parents may be aware through the media or information from alternative Web sites about controversial issues concerning vaccines their child is scheduled to receive. Many issues about childhood vaccines communicated by these means are presented incompletely or inaccurately. When a parent initiates discussion about a vaccine controversy, the health care professional should listen carefully and then calmly and nonjudgmentally discuss specific concerns. Health care professionals always should provide factual information and use language appropriate for parents and other caregivers. Through direct dialogue with parents and use of available resources, health care professionals can help reduce and possibly prevent acceptance of inaccurate media reports and information from nonauthoritative sources. Encouraging a dialogue may be the most important step to eventual vaccine acceptance.

Helpful information sources that can be provided to parents or to which parents can be directed include the National Center for Immunization and Respiratory Diseases' "Parent's Guide to Childhood Immunization" (**www.cdc.gov/vaccines** or contact the CDC telephone hot line at 1-800-232-4636), the Vaccine Education Center at Children's Hospital of Philadelphia (**www.vaccine.chop.edu**), and the AAP Immunization Initiatives Web site (**www.cispimmunize.org/fam/fam_main.html**).

Parents who refuse vaccines should be advised of state laws pertaining to school or child care entry, which can require that unimmunized children stay home from school during disease outbreaks. Documentation of such discussions in the patient's record may help to decrease any potential liability should a vaccine-preventable disease occur in an unimmunized patient. This *informed refusal* documentation should note that the parent was informed why the immunization was recommended, the risks and benefits of immunization, and the possible consequences of not allowing the vaccine to be administered. A sample Refusal to Vaccinate form can be found on the AAP Web site at **www.cispimmunize.org/pro/ParentalRefusaltoVaccinate.html.**

PARENTAL REFUSAL OF IMMUNIZATION

The approach of a health care professional to a parent who refuses immunization of his or her child is complex and should be based on the reason for the refusal and the knowledge of the parent. Suggested responses to parental refusals of immunization of children are outlined as follows[1]:

- The pediatrician should listen carefully and respectfully to the parent's concerns, recognizing that some parents may not use the same decision criteria as the physician and may weigh evidence differently than does the physician.
- The pediatrician should share honestly what is and is not known about the risks and benefits of the vaccine in question and attempt to correct any misperceptions and misinformation.
- The pediatrician should assist parents in understanding that the risks of any vaccine should not be considered in isolation but in comparison with the risks to the child and community should the child remain unimmunized.
- Parents can be referred to one of several reputable and data-based Web sites for additional information on specific immunizations and the diseases they prevent (see Internet Resources for Immunization Information, p 53). Physicians can access information on this topic at **www.cispimmunize.org.**
- Many parents have concerns related to 1 or 2 specific vaccines. The pediatrician should discuss the benefits and risks of each vaccine, because a parent who is reluctant to accept administration of 1 vaccine may be willing to accept others.
- Parents who have concerns about administering multiple vaccines to a child in a single visit may have their concerns addressed by using methods to reduce the pain of injection (see Managing Injection Pain, p 20) or by developing a schedule of immunizations that does not require multiple injections at a single visit. Any alternative schedule should adhere to age ranges of vaccine administration provided for many vaccines in the Recommended Childhood and Adolescent Immunization schedules (p 24–28).
- Physicians also should explore the possibility that cost is a reason for refusing immunization and assist parents by helping them obtain recommended immunizations for their children.
- For all cases in which parents refuse vaccine administration, pediatricians should take advantage of their ongoing relationship with the family and revisit the immunization discussion on subsequent visits.
- Continued refusal after adequate discussion should be respected unless the child is put at significant risk of serious harm (eg, during an epidemic). Only then should state agencies be involved to override parental discretion on the basis of medical neglect.

[1]Diekema DS; American Academy of Pediatrics, Committee on Bioethics. Responding to parental refusals of immunization of children. *Pediatrics.* 2005;115(5):1428–1431

- Physician concerns about liability should be addressed by appropriate documentation of the discussion of benefits of immunization and risks to the child and risks to other children (eg, children too young to be immunized or certain children who are immunocompromised) associated with remaining unimmunized.
- Physicians also may wish to consider having the parents sign a refusal waiver (a sample refusal-to-vaccinate waiver can be found at **www.cispimmunize.org/pro/ParentalRefusaltoVaccinate.html**).
- When significant differences in philosophy of care emerge, a substantial level of distrust develops, or poor quality of communication persists, the pediatrician can choose to encourage the family to find another physician or practice after providing sufficient advance notice in writing to the patient or custodial parent or legal guardian to permit another health care professional to be secured.

ACTIVE IMMUNIZATION

Active immunization involves administration of all or part of a microorganism or a modified product of that microorganism (eg, a toxoid, a purified antigen, or an antigen produced by genetic engineering) to evoke an immunologic response that mimics that of natural infection but that usually presents little or no risk to the recipient. Immunization can result in antitoxin, antiadherence, anti-invasive, or neutralizing activity or other types of protective humoral or cellular responses in the recipient. Some immunizing agents provide nearly complete and lifelong protection against disease, some provide partial protection, and some must be readministered at regular intervals to maintain protection. The effectiveness of a vaccine is assessed by evidence of protection against the natural disease. Induction of antibodies commonly is an indirect measure of protection (eg, antitoxin against *Clostridium tetani* or neutralizing antibody against measles virus), but for some conditions (eg, pertussis), the immunologic response that correlates with protection is poorly understood, and serum antibody concentration does not always predict protection.

Vaccines incorporating an intact infectious agent may contain live-attenuated (weakened), killed (inactivated), or genetically engineered subunits. Vaccines licensed for use in the United States are listed in Table 1.3 (p 10). The US Food and Drug Administration (FDA) maintains and updates a Web site listing vaccines licensed for immunization in the United States (**www.fda.gov/cber/vaccine/licvacc.htm**). Appendix II shows the years of licensure of vaccines available in the United States, and Appendix III provides the *Current Procedural Terminology* (CPT) and *International Classification of Diseases* (ICD-9) codes used for vaccine administration. Many viral vaccines contain live-attenuated virus. Although active infection (with viral replication) ensues after administration of these vaccines, usually little or no adverse host reaction occurs. The vaccines for some viruses (eg, hepatitis A and hepatitis B, human papillomavirus) and most bacteria are inactivated (killed) components, subunit (purified components) preparations, or inactivated toxins or are conjugated chemically to immunobiologically active proteins (eg, tetanus toxoid, nontoxic variant of mutant diphtheria toxin, meningococcal outer membrane protein complex). Viruses and bacteria in inactivated, subunit, and conjugate vaccine preparations are not capable of replicating in the host; therefore, these vaccines must contain a sufficient antigenic mass to stimulate a desired response. Maintenance of long-lasting immunity with inactivated viral or bacterial vaccines may require periodic administration of booster

Table 1.3. Vaccines Licensed for Immunization and Distributed in the United States and Their Routes of Administration[a]

Vaccine	Type	Route
BCG	Live bacteria	ID (preferred) or SC
Diphtheria-tetanus (DT, Td)	Toxoids	IM
DTaP	Toxoids and inactivated bacterial components	IM
DTaP, hepatitis B, and IPV	Toxoids and inactivated bacterial components, recombinant viral antigen, inactivated virus	IM
DTaP/Hib conjugate (PRP-T[b] reconstituted with DTaP)	Toxoids and inactivated bacterial components with polysaccharide-protein conjugate	IM
DTaP-IPV	Toxoids and inactivated bacterial components, inactivated virus	IM
DTaP-IPV/Hib (PRP-T reconstituted with DTaP-IPV)	Toxoids and inactivated bacterial components, polysaccharide-protein conjugate, inactivated virus	IM
Hepatitis A	Inactivated viral antigen	IM
Hepatitis B	Recombinant viral antigen	IM
Hepatitis A-hepatitis B	Inactivated and recombinant viral antigens	IM
Hib conjugates[b]	Polysaccharide-protein conjugate	IM
Hib conjugate (PRP-OMP[b]) -hepatitis B	Polysaccharide-protein conjugate with recombinant viral antigen	IM
Human papillomavirus (HPV)	Recombinant viral antigens	IM
Influenza	Inactivated viral components	IM
Influenza	Live-attenuated viruses	Intranasal
Japanese encephalitis	Inactivated virus	SC
Meningococcal	Polysaccharide	SC
Meningococcal conjugate	Polysaccharide-protein conjugate	IM
MMR	Live-attenuated viruses	SC

Table 1.3. Vaccines Licensed for Immunization and Distributed in the United States and Their Routes of Administration,[a] continued

Vaccine	Type	Route
MMRV	Live-attenuated viruses	SC
Pneumococcal	Polysaccharide	IM or SC
Pneumococcal conjugate	Polysaccharide-protein conjugate	IM
Poliovirus (IPV)	Inactivated viruses	SC or IM
Rabies	Inactivated virus	IM
Rotavirus	Live-attenuated virus	Oral
Tdap	Toxoids and inactivated bacterial component	IM
Tetanus	Toxoid	IM
Typhoid	Capsular polysaccharide	IM
Typhoid	Live-attenuated bacteria	Oral
Varicella	Live-attenuated virus	SC
Zoster	Live-attenuated virus	SC
Yellow fever	Live-attenuated virus	SC

BCG indicates bacille Calmette-Guérin; ID, intradermal; SC, subcutaneous; DT, diphtheria and tetanus toxoids (for children 7 years of age or older and adults); IM, intramuscular; DTaP, diphtheria and tetanus toxoids and acellular pertussis; Td, diphtheria and tetanus toxoids (for children younger than 7 years of age); T, tetanus toxoid; PRP-T, polyribosylribitol phosphate-tetanus toxoid; IPV, inactivated poliovirus; Hib, *Haemophilus influenzae* type b; PRP-OMP, polyribosylribitol phosphate-meningococcal outer membrane protein; MMR, live measles-mumps-rubella; MMRV, live measles-mumps-rubella-varicella (monovalent measles, mumps, and rubella components are not being produced in the United States); Tdap, tetanus toxoid, reduced diphtheria toxoid, and acellular pertussis.

[a] Other vaccines licensed in the United States but not distributed include anthrax, smallpox, oral poliovirus (OPV), and H5N1 influenza vaccines. The FDA maintains a Web site listing currently licensed vaccines in the United States (**www.fda.gov/cber/vaccine/licvacc.htm**). The AAP maintains a Web site (**www.aapredbook.org/news/vaccstatus.shtml**) showing status of licensure and recommendations for new vaccines.

[b] See Table 3.11, p 319.

doses. Although inactivated vaccines may not elicit the range of immunologic response provided by live-attenuated agents, efficacy of licensed vaccines is high. For example, an injected inactivated viral vaccine may evoke sufficient serum antibody or cell-mediated immunity but evoke only minimal local antibody in the form of secretory immunoglobulin (Ig) A. Mucosal protection after administration of inactivated vaccines generally is inferior to mucosal immunity induced by live vaccines. Inactivated bacterial polysaccharide conjugate vaccines (eg, *Haemophilus* and pneumococcal conjugate vaccines) reduce nasopharyngeal colonization through exudated IgG. However, viruses and bacteria in inactivated vaccines cannot replicate in or be excreted by the vaccine recipient as infectious agents and, thereby, cannot adversely affect immunosuppressed vaccinees or contacts of vaccinees.

Recommendations for dose, vaccine storage and handling (see Vaccine Handling and Storage, p 13), route and technique of administration (see Vaccine Administration, p 17), and immunization schedules should be followed for predictable, effective immunization (see also disease-specific chapters in Section 3). Adherence to recommended guidelines is critical to the success of immunization practices.

Immunizing Antigens

Physicians should be familiar with the major constituents of the products they use. The major constituents, including cell line derivation or animal derivatives, as relevant, are listed in the package inserts. If a vaccine is produced by different manufacturers, differences may exist in the active and/or inert ingredients and the relative amounts contained in the various products. The major constituents of vaccines include the following:

- *Active immunizing antigens.* Some vaccines consist of a single antigen that is a highly defined constituent (eg, tetanus or diphtheria toxoid). In other vaccines, antigens that provoke protective immune responses vary substantially in chemical composition and number (eg, acellular pertussis components, *Haemophilus influenzae* type b, and pneumococcal and meningococcal products). Vaccines containing live-attenuated viruses (eg, measles-mumps-rubella [MMR], measles-mumps-rubella-varicella [MMRV], varicella, oral poliovirus [OPV], live-attenuated influenza vaccine, oral rotavirus vaccine), killed viruses or portions of virus (eg, enhanced inactivated poliovirus [IPV], hepatitis A, and inactivated influenza vaccines), and viral proteins incorporated into a vaccine through recombinant technology (eg, hepatitis B vaccine, human papillomavirus [HPV] vaccine) produce both humoral and cellular-mediated responses to ensure long-term protection.

- *Conjugating agents.* Carrier proteins of proven immunologic potential (eg, tetanus toxoid, nontoxic variant of diphtheria toxin, meningococcal outer membrane protein complex), when chemically combined to less immunogenic polysaccharide antigens (eg, *H influenzae* type b, meningococcal and pneumococcal polysaccharides), enhance the type and magnitude of immune responses, particularly in people with immature immune systems, such as children younger than 2 years of age.

- *Suspending fluid.* The suspending fluid commonly is as simple as sterile water for injection or saline solution, but it may be a complex tissue-culture fluid. This fluid may contain proteins or other constituents derived from the medium and biological system in which the vaccine is produced (eg, egg antigens, gelatin, or cell culture-derived antigens).

- ***Preservatives, stabilizers, and antimicrobial agents.*** Some vaccines and immune globulin preparations contain added substances (eg, preservatives or stabilizers) or residual materials from the manufacturing process (eg, antibiotics or other chemicals, including trace amounts of thimerosal). Allergic reactions may occur if the recipient is sensitive to one or more of these additives. Whenever feasible, these reactions should be anticipated by screening the potential vaccinee for known severe allergy to specific vaccine components. Standardized forms are available to assist clinicians in screening for allergies and other potential contraindications to immunization (**www.immunize. org/catg.d/p4060.pdf**).

- ***Thimerosal.*** All routinely recommended vaccines for infants and children in the United States are available only as thimerosal-free formulations or contain only trace amounts of thimerosal, with the exception of some inactivated influenza vaccines. Inactivated influenza vaccine for pediatric use is available as a thimerosal preservative-containing formulation, a trace thimerosal-containing formulation, and a thimerosal-free formulation. Information about the thimerosal content of vaccines is available from the FDA (**www.fda.gov/cber/vaccine/thimerosal.htm**).

   The only nonvaccine biological agents that contain thimerosal in active production and distribution in the United States are certain antivenins. Immune Globulin Intravenous does not contain thimerosal or other preservatives, and none of the Rho (D) Immune Globulin (Human) products contain thimerosal (**www.fda.gov/cber/ blood/mercplasma.htm**).

- ***Adjuvants.*** An aluminum salt commonly is used in varying amounts to increase immunogenicity and to prolong the stimulatory effect, particularly for vaccines containing inactivated microorganisms or their products (eg, hepatitis B and diphtheria and tetanus toxoids). New adjuvant technology permits use of molecules that stimulate innate immune responses to enhance immunogenicity of vaccine antigens and, thus, broaden the possibilities of vaccines to prevent diseases (eg, deacylated monophosphoryl lipid A plus aluminum hydroxide [ASO[4]], as used in one HPV vaccine) or spare the amount of antigen required when vast numbers of doses are needed (eg, pandemic influenza).

Vaccine Handling and Storage

Vaccines should be transported and stored at recommended temperatures. Inattention to vaccine handling and storage conditions can contribute to vaccine failure. Live-virus vaccines, including MMR, MMRV, varicella, yellow fever, live-attenuated influenza, rotavirus, and OPV vaccines, are sensitive to increased temperature (heat sensitive). Exposure of inactivated vaccines to freezing temperature (0.0°C [32.0°F] or colder) is the most common storage error. Inactivated vaccines may tolerate limited exposure to elevated temperatures but are damaged rapidly by freezing (cold sensitive). Examples of cold-sensitive vaccines include diphtheria and tetanus toxoids and acellular pertussis (DTaP) and tetanus toxoid, reduced diphtheria toxoid, and acellular pertussis (Tdap) vaccines; IPV vaccine; *H influenzae* type b (Hib) vaccine; pneumococcal polysaccharide and conjugate vaccines; hepatitis A and hepatitis B vaccines; inactivated influenza vaccine; and meningococcal polysaccharide and conjugate vaccines. Some vaccines must be protected from light. This can be done by keeping each vial or syringe in its original carton while in recommended storage and until immediate use. Some products may show physical evidence of altered integrity, and others may retain their normal appearance despite a loss of potency. Physical appearance is not an appropriate basis for determining vaccine acceptability. Therefore, all personnel responsible for handling vaccines in an office or clinic setting should be familiar with standard procedures designed to minimize risk of vaccine failure.

Recommendations for handling and storage of selected biologicals are summarized in several areas, including the package insert for each product; in a publication titled *Vaccine Management*, available from the Centers for Disease Control and Prevention (CDC)[1] at **www.cdc.gov/vaccines/pubs/downloads/bk-vac-mgt.pdf;** and in a Web-based toolkit available at **www2a.cdc.gov/nip/isd/shtoolkit/splash.html.** The most current information about recommended vaccine storage conditions and handling instructions can be obtained directly from manufacturers; their telephone numbers are listed in product labels (package inserts) and in the *Physicians' Desk Reference*, which is published yearly. The following guidelines are suggested as part of a quality-control system for safe handling and storage of vaccines in an office or clinic setting.

PERSONNEL

- Designate one person as the vaccine coordinator, and assign responsibility for ensuring that vaccines and other biological agents and products are handled and stored in a careful, safe, recommended, and documentable manner. Assign a backup person to assume these responsibilities during times of illness or vacation.
- Inform all people who will be handling vaccines about specific storage requirements and stability limitations of the products they will encounter. The details of proper storage conditions should be posted on or near each refrigerator or freezer used for vaccine storage or should be readily available to staff.

Receptionists, mail clerks, and other staff members who may receive shipments also should be educated.

EQUIPMENT

- Ensure that refrigerators and freezers in which vaccines are to be stored are working properly and are capable of meeting storage requirements.
- Do not connect refrigerators or freezers to an outlet with a ground-flow circuit interrupter or one activated by a wall switch. Use plug guards and warning signs to prevent accidental dislodging of the wall plug. Post **"Do Not Unplug"** warning signs on circuit breakers.
- Avoid using compact refrigerators intended for dormitory use to store vaccines. Instead, refrigerator-freezers with separate doors and well-sealed compartments for refrigeration and freezing should be used. Alternatively, separate refrigerator and freezer units can be used.
- Equip each refrigerator and freezer compartment with a certified thermometer located at the center of the storage compartment. A certified thermometer has been individually tested against a reference standard, such as the National Institute of Standards and Technology or American Society for Testing and Materials International. These thermometers are sold with an individually numbered certificate documenting this testing. A calibrated, constant-recording thermometer with graphical readings or a thermometer that indicates upper and lower extremes of temperature during an

---

[1]Centers for Disease Control and Prevention. *Vaccine Management: Recommendations for Handling and Storage of Selected Biologicals.* Atlanta, GA: US Department of Health and Human Services, Public Health Service; 2007

observation period ("minimum-maximum" thermometer) will provide more information as to whether vaccines have been exposed to potentially harmful temperatures
than will single-reading thermometers. Placement of vaccine cold-chain monitor cards[1]
in refrigerators and freezers can serve to detect potentially harmful increases in temperature but should not be a substitute for use of certified thermometers.
- Maintain a logbook in which temperature readings are recorded at the beginning and
  end of the clinic day and in which the date, time, and duration of any mechanical mal-
  functions or power outages are noted. The current temperature log should be posted on
  the door to remind staff to monitor and record temperatures. Previous logs should be
  stored for a minimum of 3 years.
- Place all opened vials of vaccine in a refrigerator tray. To avoid mishaps, do not store
  other pharmaceutical products in the same tray. Store unopened vials in the original
  packaging. This facilitates inventory management and rotation of vaccine by expiration
  date. Store opened vials of light-sensitive vaccines, such as MMR and MMRV, in original
  packaging, and mark the outside with a large "X" to indicate that it has been opened.
- Equip refrigerators with several bottles of chilled water and freezers with several ice
  trays or ice packs to fill empty space, which will help to minimize temperature fluctuations during brief electrical or mechanical failures.

PROCEDURES
- Acceptance of vaccine on receipt of shipment:
  - Ensure that the expiration date of the delivered product has not passed.
  - Examine the merchandise and its shipping container for any evidence of damage
    during transport.
  - Consider whether the interval between shipment from the supplier and arrival of
    the product at its destination is excessive (more than 48 hours) and whether the
    product has been exposed to excessive heat or cold that might alter its integrity.
    Review vaccine time and temperature indicators, both chemical and electronic, if
    included in the vaccine shipment.
  - Do not accept the shipment if reasonable suspicion exists that the delivered product
    may have been damaged by environmental insult or improper handling during transport.
  - Contact the vaccine supplier or manufacturer when unusual circumstances raise
    questions about the stability of a delivered vaccine. Store suspect vaccine under proper
    conditions and label it **"Do Not Use"** until the viability has been determined.
- Refrigerator and freezer inspection:
  - Measure the temperature of the central part of the storage compartment twice
    a day, and record this temperature on a temperature log. A minimum-maximum
    thermometer is preferred to record extremes in temperature fluctuation and reset
    to baseline. Consider use of an alarm system to monitor temperature fluctuations.
    The refrigerator temperature should be maintained between 2°C and 8°C (35°F
    and 46°F) with a target temperature of 40°F, and the freezer temperature should
    be −15°C (5°F) or colder.
  - Train staff to respond immediately to temperature recordings outside the recom-
    mended range and to document response and outcome.

---

[1]Available from 3M Pharmaceuticals.

- Inspect the unit weekly for outdated vaccine and either dispose of or return expired products appropriately.
- Routine procedures:
  - Store vaccines according to temperatures recommended in the package insert.
  - Rotate vaccine supplies so that the shortest-dated vaccines are in front to reduce wastage because of expiration.
  - Promptly remove expired (outdated) vaccines from the refrigerator or freezer and dispose of them appropriately or return to manufacturer to avoid accidental use.
  - Keep opened vials of vaccine in a tray so that they are readily identifiable.
  - Store unopened vials in the original packaging.
  - Store light-sensitive vaccines in their original packaging. Mark the original packaging of an opened vial with a large "X" and store it with other open vials in a tray.
  - Indicate on the label of each vaccine vial the date and time the vaccine was reconstituted or first opened.
  - Unless immediate use is planned, avoid reconstituting multiple doses of vaccine or drawing up multiple doses of vaccine in multiple syringes. Predrawing vaccine increases the possibility of medication errors and causes uncertainty of vaccine stability.
  - Because there may be more than one vaccine product for vaccine antigens (eg, DTaP and Tdap or meningococcal polysaccharide vaccine [MPSV4] or meningococcal conjugate vaccine [MCV4]), care should be taken during storage to ensure that the different products are stored separately in a manner to avoid confusion.
  - When feasible, use prefilled unit-dose syringes to prevent contamination of multidose vials and errors in labeling syringes.
  - Discard reconstituted live-virus and other vaccines if not used within the interval specified in the package insert. Examples of discard times include varicella vaccine after 30 minutes and MMR vaccine after 8 hours. All reconstituted vaccines should be refrigerated during the interval in which they may be used.
  - Always store vaccines in the refrigerator or freezer as indicated, including throughout the office day.
  - Do not open more than 1 vial of a specific vaccine at a time.
  - Store vaccine only in the central storage area of the refrigerator, not on the door shelf or in peripheral areas, where temperature fluctuations are greater.
  - Do not keep food or drink in refrigerators in which vaccine is stored; this will limit frequent opening of the unit that leads to thermal instability.
  - Do not store radioactive materials in the same refrigerator in which vaccines are stored.
  - Discuss with all clinic or office personnel any violation of protocol for handling vaccines or any accidental storage problem (eg, electrical failure), and contact vaccine suppliers for information about disposition of the affected vaccine.
  - Develop a written plan for emergency storage of vaccine in the event of a catastrophic occurrence. Office personnel should have a written and easily accessible procedure that outlines vaccine packing and transport. Vaccines that have been exposed to temperatures outside the recommended storage range may be ineffective. Vaccines should be packed in an appropriate insulated storage box and moved to a location where the appropriate storage temperatures can be maintained. Office personnel need to be aware of alternate storage sites and trained in the correct techniques to store and transport vaccines to avoid warming vaccines that need to

be refrigerated or frozen and to avoid freezing vaccines that should be refrigerated. Recommended storage conditions for commonly used vaccines can be found at **www.cdc.gov/vaccines/pubs/downloads/bk-vac-mgt.pdf.** After a power outage or mechanical failure, do not assume that vaccine exposed to temperature outside the recommended range is unusable. Contact the vaccine manufacturer for guidance before discarding vaccine.

Other resources on vaccine storage and handling are available, including a video from the CDC National Immunization Program, "How to Protect Your Vaccine Supply" (available at **www.cdc.gov/vaccines/pubs/videos-webcasts.htm#satbrd**). Additional materials are available at **www.cdc.gov/vaccines/recs/default.htm.**

Vaccine Administration

GENERAL INSTRUCTIONS FOR VACCINE ADMINISTRATION

Personnel administering vaccines should take appropriate precautions to minimize risk of spread of disease to or from patients. Hand hygiene should be used before and after each new patient contact. Gloves are not required when administering vaccines unless the health care professional has open hand lesions or will come into contact with potentially infectious body fluids. Syringes and needles must be sterile and disposable. To prevent inadvertent needlesticks or reuse, a needle should **not** be recapped after use, and disposable needles and syringes should be discarded promptly in puncture-proof, labeled containers placed in the room where the vaccine is administered. Changing needles between drawing a vaccine into a syringe and injecting it into the child is not necessary. A patient should be restrained adequately if indicated before any injection. Different vaccines should not be mixed in the same syringe unless specifically licensed and labeled for such use.

Because of the rare possibility of a severe allergic reaction to a vaccine component, people administering vaccines or other biological products should be prepared to recognize and treat allergic reactions, including anaphylaxis (see Hypersensitivity Reactions After Immunization, p 47). Facilities and personnel should be available for treating immediate allergic reactions. This recommendation does not preclude administration of vaccines in school-based or other nonclinic settings.

Syncope may occur following immunization, particularly in adolescents and young adults. Personnel should be aware of presyncopal manifestations and take appropriate measures to prevent injuries if weakness, dizziness, or loss of consciousness occurs. The relatively rapid onset of syncope in most cases suggests that health care professionals should consider observing adolescents for 15 minutes after they are immunized. Having vaccine recipients *sit or lie down for 15 minutes* after immunization could avert many syncopal episodes and secondary injuries. If syncope develops, patients should be observed until symptoms resolve.[1] Syncope following receipt of a vaccine is not a contraindication to subsequent doses.

---

[1]Centers for Disease Control and Prevention. Syncope after immunization—United States, January 2005–July 2007. *MMWR Morb Mortal Wkly Rep.* 2008;57(17):457–460

SITE AND ROUTE OF IMMUNIZATION (ACTIVE AND PASSIVE)

ORAL VACCINES. Breastfeeding does not interfere with successful immunization with OPV or rotavirus vaccines. Vomiting within 10 minutes of receiving an oral dose is an indication for repeating the dose of OPV but not rotavirus vaccine. If the second dose of OPV vaccine is not retained, neither dose should be counted, and the vaccine should be readministered. OPV is not available for use in the United States.

INTRANASAL VACCINE. Live-attenuated influenza vaccine is the only vaccine licensed for intranasal administration. This vaccine is licensed for healthy, nonpregnant people 2 through 49 years of age. With the recipient in the upright position, approximately 0.1 mL (ie, half of the total sprayer contents) is sprayed into one nostril. An attached dose-divider clip is removed from the sprayer to administer the second half of the dose into the other nostril. If the recipient sneezes after administration, the dose should not be repeated. The vaccine can be administered during minor illnesses. However, if clinical judgment indicates that nasal congestion might impede delivery of the vaccine to the nasopharyngeal mucosa, vaccine deferral should be considered until resolution of the illness.

PARENTERAL VACCINES.[1] Injectable vaccines should be administered using aseptic technique in a site as free as possible from risk of local neural, vascular, or tissue injury. Data do not warrant recommendation of a single preferred site for all injections, and product recommendations of many manufacturers allow flexibility in the site of injection. Preferred sites for vaccines administered subcutaneously (SC) or intramuscularly (IM) include the anterolateral aspect of the upper thigh (SC or IM); upper, outer triceps area of the upper arm (SC); and the deltoid area of the upper arm (IM).

Recommended routes of administration are included in package inserts of vaccines and are listed in Table 1.3 (p 10). The recommended route is based on studies designed to demonstrate maximum safety and efficacy. To minimize untoward local or systemic effects and ensure optimal efficacy of the immunizing procedure, vaccines should be given by the recommended route.

For IM injections, the choice of site is based on the volume of the injected material and the size of the muscle, and the needle should be directed at a 90° angle. In children younger than 1 year of age (ie, infants), the anterolateral aspect of the thigh provides the largest muscle and is the preferred site. In older children, the deltoid muscle usually is large enough for IM injection.

Ordinarily, the upper, outer aspect of the buttocks should not be used for active immunization, because the gluteal region is covered by a significant layer of subcutaneous fat and because of the possibility of damaging the sciatic nerve. However, clinical information on the use of this area is limited. Because of diminished immunogenicity, hepatitis B and rabies vaccines should not be given in the buttocks at any age. People, especially adults, who were given hepatitis B vaccine in the buttocks should be tested for immunity and reimmunized if antibody concentrations are inadequate (see Hepatitis B, p 337).

When the upper, outer quadrant of the buttocks is used for large-volume passive immunization, such as IM administration of large volumes of Immune Globulin (IG), care must be taken to avoid injury to the sciatic nerve. The site selected should be well

---

[1]For a review on intramuscular injections, see Centers for Disease Control and Prevention. *Epidemiology and Prevention of Vaccine-Preventable Diseases (Pink Book)*. Atlanta, GA: Centers for Disease Control and Prevention; 2008. For copies, contact the Public Health Foundation at 877-252-1200 or visit **www.cdc.gov/vaccines/ pubs/pinkbook/default.htm.**

into the upper, outer quadrant of the gluteus maximus, away from the central region of the buttocks, and the needle should be directed anteriorly—that is, if the patient is lying prone, the needle is directed perpendicular to the table's surface, not perpendicular to the skin plane. The ventrogluteal site may be less hazardous for IM injection, because it is free of major nerves and vessels. This site is the center of a triangle for which the boundaries are the anterior superior iliac spine, the tubercle of the iliac crest, and the upper border of the greater trochanter.

Vaccines containing adjuvants (eg, aluminum present in vaccines recommended for IM injection) must be injected deep into the muscle mass. These vaccines should not be administered subcutaneously or intracutaneously, because they can cause local irritation, inflammation, granuloma formation, and tissue necrosis. IG, Rabies Immune Globulin (RIG), Hepatitis B Immune Globulin (HBIG), palivizumab, and other similar products for passive immunoprophylaxis also are injected intramuscularly, except when RIG is infiltrated around the site of a bite wound.

Needles used for IM injections should be long enough to reach the muscle mass to prevent vaccine from seeping into subcutaneous tissue and, therefore, minimize local reactions and not so long as to involve underlying nerves, blood vessels, or bone. Suggested needle lengths are shown in Table 1.4 (below).

Serious complications resulting from IM injections are rare. Reported adverse events include broken needles, muscle contracture, nerve injury, bacterial (staphylococcal, streptococcal, and clostridial) abscesses, sterile abscesses, skin pigmentation, hemorrhage, cellulitis, tissue necrosis, gangrene, local atrophy, periostitis, cyst or scar formation, and inadvertent injection into a joint space.

SC injections can be administered at a 45° angle into the anterolateral aspect of the thigh or the upper, outer triceps area by inserting the needle in a pinched-up fold of skin and SC tissue. A 23- or 25-gauge needle, ⅝ to ¾ inch long, is recommended. Immune responses after SC administration of hepatitis B or recombinant rabies vaccine

Table 1.4. Site and Needle Length by Age for Intramuscular Immunization

Age Group	Needle Length, inches (mm)[a]	Suggested Injection Site
Newborns (preterm and term) and infants <2 mo of age	⅝ (16)	Anterolateral thigh muscle
Term infants, 2–12 mo of age	1 (25)	Anterolateral thigh muscle
Toddlers and children	⅝ (16)	Deltoid muscle of the arm
	1–1¼ (25–32)	Anterolateral thigh muscle
Adolescents and young adults		
Female and male, weight <60 kg	⅝ (16)	Deltoid muscle of the arm
Female, weight 60–90 kg	1 (25)	Deltoid muscle of the arm
Female, weight >90 kg	1½ (38)	Deltoid muscle of the arm
Male, weight 60–118 kg	1 (25)	Deltoid muscle of the arm
Male, weight >118 kg	1½ (38)	Deltoid muscle of the arm

[a]Assumes that needle is inserted fully.

are decreased compared with those after IM administration of either of these vaccines; therefore, these vaccines should not be given subcutaneously. MPSV4 vaccine is administered subcutaneously, whereas MCV4 vaccine is administered intramuscularly. In patients with a bleeding diathesis, the risk of bleeding after IM injection can be minimized by vaccine administration immediately after the patient's receipt of replacement factor, use of a 23-gauge (or smaller) needle, and immediate application of direct pressure to the immunization site for at least 2 minutes. Certain vaccines (eg, Hib vaccines except polyribosylribitol phosphate-meningococcal outer membrane protein [PRP-OMP; PedvaxHIB]) recommended for IM injection may be given subcutaneously to people at risk of hemorrhage after IM injection, such as people with hemophilia. For these vaccines, immune responses and clinical reactions after IM or SC injection generally have been reported to be similar.

Intradermal injections usually are given on the volar surface of the forearm. Because of the decreased antigenic mass administered with intradermal injections, attention to technique is essential to ensure that material is not injected subcutaneously. A 25- or 27-gauge needle is recommended.

When multiple vaccines are administered, separate sites ordinarily should be used if possible, especially if one of the vaccines contains DTaP. When necessary, 2 or more vaccines can be given in the same limb at a single visit. The anterolateral aspect of the thigh is the preferred site for multiple simultaneous IM injections because of its greater muscle mass. The distance separating the injections is arbitrary but should be at least 1 inch, if possible, so that local reactions are unlikely to overlap. Multiple vaccines should not be mixed in a single syringe unless specifically licensed and labeled for administration in 1 syringe. A different needle and syringe should be used for each injection.

Aspiration before injection of vaccines or toxoids (ie, pulling back on the syringe plunger after needle insertion, before injection) is not recommended, because no large blood vessels are located at the preferred injection sites, and rapid plunge may reduce pain.

A brief period of bleeding at the injection site is common and usually can be controlled by applying gentle pressure.

Managing Injection Pain

Concerns and resulting anxiety about injections are common at any age. Recommended childhood immunization schedules sometimes require children to receive multiple injections during a single visit. Although most children older than 5 years of age usually accept immunization with minimal opposition, some children react vigorously or refuse to receive injections. Effective practical techniques can be used to ameliorate some discomfort of injections.

A planned approach to managing the child before, during, and after immunization is helpful for children of any age.[1] Truthful and empathetic preparation for injections is beneficial. Parents should be advised not to threaten children with injections or use them as a punishment for inappropriate behavior. If possible, parents should have a role in comforting rather than restraining their child. For younger children, parents may soothe, stroke, and calm the child. For older children, parents should be coached to distract the child (see Nonpharmacologic Techniques, p 21).

---

[1]Schechter NL, Zempsky WT, Cohen LL, McGrath PJ, McMurtry CM, Bright NS. Pain reduction during pediatric immunizations: evidence-based review and recommendations. *Pediatrics*. 2007;119(5):e1184–e1198

INJECTION TECHNIQUE AND POSITION

A rapid plunge of the needle through the skin without aspirating may decrease discomfort associated with skin penetration. The limb should be positioned to allow relaxation of the muscle to be injected. For the deltoid, some flexion of the arm may be required. For the anterolateral thigh, some degree of internal rotation may be helpful. Infants may exhibit less pain behavior when held on the lap of a parent or other caregiver. Older children may be more comfortable sitting on a parent's lap or examination table edge, hugging their parent chest to chest, while an immunization is administered.

If multiple injections are to be given, having different health care professionals administer them simultaneously at multiple sites (eg, right and left anterolateral thighs) may lessen anticipation of the next injection. Allowing older children some choice in selecting the injection site may be helpful by allowing a degree of control.

TOPICAL ANESTHETIC TECHNIQUES

Some physical techniques and topically applied agents reduce the pain of injection. Applying pressure at the site for 10 seconds or a vapocoolant before injection may reduce the pain of injection. Topical anesthetics have been evaluated in placebo-controlled, randomized clinical trials and have been demonstrated to provide pain relief. Because currently available topical anesthetics require 30 to 60 minutes to provide adequate anesthesia, planning is necessary, such as applying the cream before an office visit or immediately on arrival. Additional studies need to be performed on the use of local anesthetic agents to better establish their safety and effectiveness when used to manage injection pain and to ensure that their use does not interfere with the immune response, particularly to SC injections.

NONPHARMACOLOGIC TECHNIQUES

The parent can play an important role in mitigating injection-related pain. Skin-to-skin contact between mothers and their infants has been shown to reduce crying and lower heart rate significantly during heel stick. In addition, breastfeeding is a potent analgesic intervention in newborn infants during blood collection. Administration of sucrose solution just before the injection reduces crying time in infants younger than 6 months of age. Nonnutritive sucking on a pacifier also may have analgesic properties. Stroking or rocking a child after an injection decreases crying and other pain behaviors. For older children, parent demeanor affects the child's pain behavior. Humor and distraction techniques tend to decrease distress, whereas excessive parental reassurance or apology tends to increase distress. Breathing and distraction techniques, such as "blowing the pain away," use of pinwheels or soap bubbles, telling children stories, reading books, or use of music, all are effective. Techniques that involve the child in a fantasy or reframe the experience with the use of suggestion ("magic love" or "pain switch") also are effective but may require training.

Scheduling Immunizations

A vaccine is intended to be administered to a person who is capable of an appropriate immunologic response and who likely will benefit from the protection given. However, optimal immunologic response for the person must be balanced against the need to achieve effective protection against disease. For example, pertussis-containing vaccines may be less immunogenic in early infancy than in later infancy, but the benefit of conferring protection in young infants mandates that immunization should be given early despite a lessened serum antibody response. For this reason, in some developing countries, OPV vaccine is given at birth, in accordance with recommendations of the World Health Organization.

With parenterally administered live-virus vaccines, the inhibitory effect of residual specific maternal antibody determines the optimal age of administration. For example, live-virus measles-containing vaccine in use in the United States provides suboptimal rates of seroconversion during the first year of life mainly because of interference by transplacentally acquired maternal antibody. If a measles-containing vaccine is administered before 12 months of age, the child should be reimmunized at 12 through 15 months of age with a measles-containing vaccine; a third dose of a measles-containing vaccine is indicated at 4 through 6 years of age but may be administered as early as 4 weeks after the second dose.

An additional factor in selecting an immunization schedule is the need to achieve a uniform and regular response. With some products, a response is achieved after 1 dose. For example, live-virus rubella vaccine evokes a predictable response at high rates after a single dose. A single dose of some vaccines confers less-than-optimal response in the recipient. As a result, several doses are needed to complete primary immunization. For example, some people respond only to 1 or 2 types of poliovirus after a single dose of poliovirus vaccine, so multiple doses are given to produce antibody against all 3 types, thereby ensuring complete protection for the person and maximum response rates for the population. For some vaccines, periodic booster doses (eg, with tetanus and diphtheria toxoids and acellular pertussis antigen) are administered to maintain protection.

Most vaccines are safe and effective when administered simultaneously. This information is particularly important for scheduling immunizations for children with lapsed or missed immunizations and for people preparing for international travel (see Simultaneous Administration of Multiple Vaccines, p 33). Data indicate possible impaired immune responses when 2 or more live-virus vaccines are not given simultaneously but within 28 days of each other; therefore, live-virus vaccines not administered on the same day should be given at least 28 days (4 weeks) apart whenever possible (Table 1.5).

Table 1.5. Guidelines for Spacing of Live and Inactivated Antigens

Antigen Combination	Recommended Minimum Interval Between Doses
2 or more inactivated[a]	None; can be administered simultaneously or at any interval between doses
Inactivated and live	None; can be administered simultaneously or at any interval between doses
2 or more live[b]	28-day minimum interval if not administered at the same visit

[a]If simultaneous administration of tetanus toxoid, reduced diphtheria toxoid, and acellular pertussis (Tdap) vaccine and meningococcal conjugate vaccine (MCV4) is not feasible (ie, one of the vaccines is not available), the American Academy of Pediatrics recommends that administration be separated by at least 28 days.
[b]Some live oral vaccines (eg, Ty21a typhoid vaccine, oral poliovirus vaccine, rotavirus vaccine) can be administered simultaneously or at any interval before or after inactivated or live parenteral vaccines.

The recommended childhood (0 through 6 years of age), adolescent (7 through 18 years of age), and catch-up immunization schedules in Fig 1.1–1.3 (p 24–28) represent a consensus of the American Academy of Pediatrics (AAP), the Advisory Committee on Immunization Practices (ACIP) of the CDC, and the American Academy of Family Physicians. These schedules are reviewed regularly, and updated national schedules are issued annually in January. In 2007, the format of the immunization schedule was changed to provide a table for children from birth through 6 years of age and a second table for children and adolescents from 7 through 18 years of age. Interim recommendations occasionally may be made when issues such as a shortage of a product or a safety concern arises or to incorporate a new vaccine. Special attention should be given to footnotes on the schedule, which summarize major recommendations for routine childhood immunizations. Combination vaccine products may be given whenever any component of the combination is indicated and its other components are not contraindicated, provided they are licensed by the FDA for that dose in the schedule for each component vaccine and for the child's age. A Web-based childhood immunization scheduler using the current vaccine recommendations is available for parents, caregivers, and health care professionals to make instant immunization schedules for any child 6 years of age or younger (**www.cdc.gov/vaccines/recs/scheduler/catchup.htm**). An adult immunization schedule, which is updated annually, also is available (**www.cdc.gov/vaccines/**).

Fig 1.3 (p 28) gives the recommended catch-up schedule for children who were not immunized appropriately during the first year of life.

For children in whom early or rapid immunization is urgent or for children not immunized on schedule, simultaneous immunization with multiple products allows for more rapid protection. In addition, in some circumstances, immunization can be initiated earlier than at the usually recommended time or schedule and doses can be given at shorter intervals than are recommended routinely (for guidelines, see Table 1.6, p 29, and the immunization recommendations in the disease-specific chapters in Section 3). Some states or localities have chosen to implement a compressed schedule to improve immunization rates, noting that immunization completion tends to decline after 12 months of age (eg, New Mexico's "Done By One" schedule, available at **www.health. state.nm.us/immunize/Pages/Public/sched/2008DBO.pdf**). Physicians or localities using such a compressed schedule should be certain to observe the 6-month minimum interval between doses 3 and 4 of DTaP vaccine as well as other minimal interval recommendations.

Influenza vaccine should be administered before the start of influenza season but also provides benefit if administered at any time influenza disease is present in a local area (ie, usually through March) (see Influenza, Timing of Vaccine Administration, p 409).

The immunization schedule issued by the AAP, ACIP, and American Academy of Family Physicians primarily is intended for children in the United States. In many instances, the guidelines will be applicable to children in other countries, but individual pediatricians and recommending committees in each country are responsible for determining the appropriateness of the recommendations for their setting. The schedule recommended by the Expanded Programme on Immunization of the World Health Organization should be consulted (**www.who.int**). Modifications may be made by the ministries of health in individual countries on the basis of local considerations.

FIGURE 1.1 RECOMMENDED IMMUNIZATION SCHEDULE FOR PERSONS AGED 0 THROUGH 6 YEARS

Recommended Immunization Schedule for Persons Aged 0 Through 6 Years—United States • 2009

For those who fall behind or start late, see the catch-up schedule

Vaccine ▼ Age ▶	Birth	1 month	2 months	4 months	6 months	12 months	15 months	18 months	19–23 months	2–3 years	4–6 years
Hepatitis B[1]	HepB	HepB		see footnote1		HepB					
Rotavirus[2]			RV	RV	RV[2]						
Diphtheria, Tetanus, Pertussis[3]			DTaP	DTaP	DTaP		DTaP				DTaP
Haemophilus influenzae type b[4]			Hib	Hib	Hib[4]	see footnote3 / Hib					
Pneumococcal[5]			PCV	PCV	PCV	PCV				PPSV	
Inactivated Poliovirus			IPV	IPV		IPV					IPV
Influenza[6]						Influenza (Yearly)					
Measles, Mumps, Rubella[7]						MMR		see footnote7			MMR
Varicella[8]						Varicella		see footnote8			Varicella
Hepatitis A[9]						HepA (2 doses)				HepA Series	
Meningococcal[10]										MCV	

Range of recommended ages

Certain high-risk groups

This schedule indicates the recommended ages for routine administration of currently licensed vaccines, as of December 1, 2008, for children aged 0 through 6 years. Any dose not administered at the recommended age should be administered at a subsequent visit, when indicated and feasible. Licensed combination vaccines may be used whenever any component of the combination is indicated and other components are not contraindicated and if approved by the Food and Drug Administration for that dose of the series. Providers should consult the relevant Advisory Committee on Immunization Practices statement for detailed recommendations, including high-risk conditions: http://www.cdc.gov/vaccines/pubs/acip-list.htm. Clinically significant adverse events that follow immunization should be reported to the Vaccine Adverse Event Reporting System (VAERS). Guidance about how to obtain and complete a VAERS form is available at http://www.vaers.hhs.gov or by telephone, 800-822-7967.

FIGURE 1.1 RECOMMENDED IMMUNIZATION SCHEDULE FOR PERSONS AGED 0 THROUGH 6 YEARS, CONTINUED

1. Hepatitis B vaccine (HepB). *(Minimum age: birth)*

At birth:
- Administer monovalent HepB to all newborns before hospital discharge.
- If mother is hepatitis B surface antigen (HBsAg)-positive, administer HepB and 0.5 mL of hepatitis B immune globulin (HBIG) within 12 hours of birth.
- If mother's HBsAg status is unknown, administer HepB within 12 hours of birth. Determine mother's HBsAg status as soon as possible and, if HBsAg-positive, administer HBIG (no later than age 1 week).

After the birth dose:
- The HepB series should be completed with either monovalent HepB or a combination vaccine containing HepB. The second dose should be administered at age 1 or 2 months. The final dose should be administered no earlier than age 24 weeks.
- Infants born to HBsAg-positive mothers should be tested for HBsAg and antibody to HBsAg (anti-HBs) after completion of at least 3 doses of the HepB series, at age 9 through 18 months (generally at the next well-child visit).

4-month dose:
- Administration of 4 doses of HepB to infants is permissible when combination vaccines containing HepB are administered after the birth dose.

2. Rotavirus vaccine (RV). *(Minimum age: 6 weeks)*
- Administer the first dose at age 6 through 14 weeks (maximum age: 14 weeks 6 days). Vaccination should not be initiated for infants aged 15 weeks or older (i.e., 15 weeks, 0 days or older).
- Administer the final dose in the series by age 8 months 0 days.
- If Rotarix® is administered at ages 2 and 4 months, a dose at 6 months is not indicated.

3. Diphtheria and tetanus toxoids and acellular pertussis vaccine (DTaP). *(Minimum age: 6 weeks)*
- The fourth dose may be administered as early as age 12 months, provided at least 6 months have elapsed since the third dose.
- Administer the final dose in the series at age 4 through 6 years.

4. Haemophilus influenzae type b conjugate vaccine (Hib). *(Minimum age: 6 weeks)*
- If PRP-OMP (PedvaxHIB® or Comvax® [HepB-Hib]) is administered at ages 2 and 4 months, a dose at age 6 months is not indicated.
- TriHiBit® (DTaP/Hib) should not be used for doses at ages 2, 4, or 6 months but can be used as the final dose in children aged 12 months or older.

5. Pneumococcal vaccine. *(Minimum age: 6 weeks for pneumococcal conjugate vaccine [PCV]; 2 years for pneumococcal polysaccharide vaccine [PPSV])*
- PCV is recommended for all children aged younger than 5 years. Administer 1 dose of PCV to all healthy children aged 24 through 59 months who are not completely vaccinated for their age.

- Administer PPSV to children aged 2 years or older with certain underlying medical conditions (see *MMWR* 2000;49[No. RR-9]), including a cochlear implant.

6. Influenza vaccine. *(Minimum age: 6 months for trivalent inactivated influenza vaccine [TIV]; 2 years for live, attenuated influenza vaccine [LAIV])*
- Administer annually to children aged 6 months through 18 years.
- For healthy nonpregnant persons (i.e., those who do not have underlying medical conditions that predispose them to influenza complications) aged 2 through 49 years, either LAIV or TIV may be used.
- Children receiving TIV should receive 0.25 mL if aged 6 through 35 months or 0.5 mL if aged 3 years or older.
- Administer 2 doses (separated by at least 4 weeks) to children aged younger than 9 years who are receiving influenza vaccine for the first time or who were vaccinated for the first time during the previous influenza season but only received 1 dose.

7. Measles, mumps, and rubella vaccine (MMR). *(Minimum age: 12 months)*
- Administer the second dose at age 4 through 6 years. However, the second dose may be administered before age 4, provided at least 28 days have elapsed since the first dose.

8. Varicella vaccine. *(Minimum age: 12 months)*
- Administer the second dose at age 4 through 6 years. However, the second dose may be administered before age 4, provided at least 3 months have elapsed since the first dose.
- For children aged 12 months through 12 years the minimum interval between doses is 3 months. However, if the second dose was administered at least 28 days after the first dose, it can be accepted as valid.

9. Hepatitis A vaccine (HepA). *(Minimum age: 12 months)*
- Administer to all children aged 1 year (i.e., aged 12 through 23 months). Administer 2 doses at least 6 months apart.
- Children not fully vaccinated by age 2 years can be vaccinated at subsequent visits.
- HepA also is recommended for children older than 1 year who live in areas where vaccination programs target older children or who are at increased risk of infection. See *MMWR* 2006;55(No. RR-7).

10. Meningococcal vaccine. *(Minimum age: 2 years for meningococcal conjugate vaccine [MCV] and for meningococcal polysaccharide vaccine [MPSV])*
- Administer MCV to children aged 2 through 10 years with terminal complement component deficiency, anatomic or functional asplenia, and certain other high-risk groups. See *MMWR* 2005;54(No. RR-7).
- Persons who received MPSV 3 or more years previously and who remain at increased risk for meningococcal disease should be revaccinated with MCV.

The Recommended Immunization Schedules for Persons Aged 0 Through 18 Years are approved by the Advisory Committee on Immunization Practices (www.cdc.gov/vaccines/recs/acip), the American Academy of Pediatrics (http://www.aap.org), and the American Academy of Family Physicians (http://www.aafp.org).

Department of Health and Human Services • Centers for Disease Control and Prevention

CS103164

FIGURE 1.2 RECOMMENDED IMMUNIZATION SCHEDULE FOR PERSONS AGED 7 THROUGH 18 YEARS

Recommended Immunization Schedule for Persons Aged 7 Through 18 Years—United States • 2009

For those who fall behind or start late, see the schedule below and the catch-up schedule

Vaccine ▼ Age ▶	7–10 years	11–12 years	13–18 years
Tetanus, Diphtheria, Pertussis[1]	*see footnote 1*	Tdap	Tdap
Human Papillomavirus[2]	*see footnote 2*	HPV (3 doses)	HPV Series
Meningococcal[3]	MCV	MCV	MCV
Influenza[4]	Influenza (Yearly)	Influenza (Yearly)	Influenza (Yearly)
Pneumococcal[5]	PPSV	PPSV	PPSV
Hepatitis A[6]	HepA Series	HepA Series	HepA Series
Hepatitis B[7]	HepB Series	HepB Series	HepB Series
Inactivated Poliovirus[8]	IPV Series	IPV Series	IPV Series
Measles, Mumps, Rubella[9]	MMR Series	MMR Series	MMR Series
Varicella[10]	Varicella Series	Varicella Series	Varicella Series

Range of recommended ages

Catch-up immunization

Certain high-risk groups

This schedule indicates the recommended ages for routine administration of currently licensed vaccines, as of December 1, 2008, for children aged 7 through 18 years. Any dose not administered at the recommended age should be administered at a subsequent visit, when indicated and feasible. Licensed combination vaccines may be used whenever any component of the combination is indicated and other components are not contraindicated and if approved by the Food and Drug Administration for that dose of the series. Providers should consult the relevant Advisory Committee on Immunization Practices statement for detailed recommendations, including high-risk conditions: http://www.cdc.gov/vaccines/pubs/acip-list.htm. Clinically significant adverse events that follow immunization should be reported to the Vaccine Adverse Event Reporting System (VAERS). Guidance about how to obtain and complete a VAERS form is available at http://www.vaers.hhs.gov or by telephone, 800-822-7967.

FIGURE 1.2 RECOMMENDED IMMUNIZATION SCHEDULE FOR PERSONS AGED 7 THROUGH 18 YEARS, CONTINUED

1. **Tetanus and diphtheria toxoids and acellular pertussis vaccine(Tdap).** *(Minimum age: 10 years for BOOSTRIX® and 11 years for ADACEL®)*
   - Administer at age 11 or 12 years for those who have completed the recommended childhood DTP/DTaP vaccination series and have not received a tetanus and diphtheria toxoid (Td) booster dose.
   - Persons aged 13 through 18 years who have not received Tdap should receive a dose.
   - A 5-year interval from the last Td dose is encouraged when Tdap is used as a booster dose; however, a shorter interval may be used if pertussis immunity is needed.

2. **Human papillomavirus vaccine (HPV).** *(Minimum age: 9 years)*
   - Administer the first dose to females at age 11 or 12 years.
   - Administer the second dose 2 months after the first dose and the third dose 6 months after the first dose (at least 24 weeks after the first dose).
   - Administer the series to females at age 13 through 18 years if not previously vaccinated.

3. **Meningococcal conjugate vaccine (MCV).**
   - Administer at age 11 or 12 years, or at age 13 through 18 years if not previously vaccinated.
   - Administer to previously unvaccinated college freshmen living in a dormitory.
   - MCV is recommended for children aged 2 through 10 years with terminal complement component deficiency, anatomic or functionalasplenia, and certain other groups at high risk. See *MMWR* 2005;54(No. RR-7).
   - Persons who received MPSV 5 or more years previously and remain at increased risk for meningococcal disease should be revaccinated with MCV.

4. **Influenza vaccine.**
   - Administer annually to children aged 6 months through 18 years.
   - For healthy nonpregnant persons (i.e., those who do not have underlying medical conditions that predispose them to influenza complications) aged 2 through 49 years, either LAIV or TIV may be used.
   - Administer 2 doses (separated by at least 4 weeks) to children aged younger than 9 years who are receiving influenza vaccine for the first time or who were vaccinated for the first time during the previous influenza season but only received 1 dose.

5. **Pneumococcal polysaccharide vaccine (PPSV).**
   - Administer to children with certain underlying medical conditions (see *MMWR* 1997;46[No. RR-8]), including a cochlear implant. A single revaccination should be administered to children with functional or anatomic asplenia or other immunocompromising condition after 5 years.

6. **Hepatitis A vaccine (HepA).**
   - Administer 2 doses at least 6 months apart.
   - HepA is recommended for children older than 1 year who live in areas where vaccination programs target older children or who are at increased risk of infection. See *MMWR* 2006;55(No. RR-7).

7. **Hepatitis B vaccine (HepB).**
   - Administer the 3-dose series to those not previously vaccinated.
   - A 2-dose series (separated by at least 4 months) of adult formulationRecombivax HB® is licensed for children aged 11 through 15 years.

8. **Inactivated poliovirus vaccine (IPV).**
   - For children who received an all-IPV or all-oral poliovirus (OPV) series, a fourth dose is not necessary if the third dose was administered at age 4 years or older.
   - If both OPV and IPV were administered as part of a series, a total of 4 doses should be administered, regardless of the child's current age.

9. **Measles, mumps, and rubella vaccine (MMR).**
   - If not previously vaccinated, administer 2 doses or the second dose for those who have received only 1 dose, with at least 28 days between doses.

10. **Varicella vaccine.**
    - For persons aged 7 through 18 years without evidence of immunity (see *MMWR* 2007;56[No. RR-4]), administer 2 doses if not previouslyvaccinated or the second dose if they have received only 1 dose.
    - For persons aged 7 through 12 years, the minimum interval between doses is 3 months. However, if the second dose was administered at least 28 days after the first dose, it can be accepted as valid.
    - For persons aged 13 years and older, the minimum interval between doses is 28 days.

The **Recommended Immunization Schedules for Persons Aged 0 Through 18 Years** are approved by the Advisory Committee on Immunization Practices (www.cdc.gov/vaccines/recs/acip), the American Academy of Pediatrics (http://www.aap.org), and the American Academy of Family Physicians (http://www.aafp.org).

Department of Health and Human Services • Centers for Disease Control and Prevention

CS103164

FIGURE 1.3 CATCH-UP IMMUNIZATION SCHEDULE FOR PERSONS AGED 4 MONTHS THROUGH 18 YEARS WHO START LATE OR WHO ARE MORE THAN 1 MONTH BEHIND

Catch-up Immunization Schedule for Persons Aged 4 Months Through 18 Years Who Start Late or Who Are More Than 1 Month Behind—United States • 2009

The table below provides catch-up schedules and minimum intervals between doses for children whose vaccinations have been delayed. A vaccine series does not need to be restarted, regardless of the time that has elapsed between doses. Use the section appropriate for the child's age.

Vaccine	Minimum Age for Dose 1	Minimum Interval Between Doses			
		Dose 1 to Dose 2	Dose 2 to Dose 3	Dose 3 to Dose 4	Dose 4 to Dose 5
CATCH-UP SCHEDULE FOR PERSONS AGED 4 MONTHS THROUGH 6 YEARS					
Hepatitis B[1]	Birth	4 weeks	**8 weeks** (and at least 16 weeks after first dose)		
Rotavirus[2]	6 wks	4 weeks	**4 weeks[2]**		
Diphtheria, Tetanus, Pertussis[3]	6 wks	4 weeks	4 weeks	6 months	6 months[3]
Haemophilus influenzae type b[4]	6 wks	**4 weeks** if first dose administered at younger than 12 months of age **8 weeks (as final dose)** if first dose administered at age 12-14 months **No further doses needed** if first dose administered at age 15 months or older	**4 weeks[4]** if current age is younger than 12 months **8 weeks (as final dose)[4]** if current age is 12 months or older and second dose administered at younger than 15 months of age **No further doses needed** if previous dose administered at age 15 months or older	**8 weeks (as final dose)** This dose only necessary for children aged 12 months through 59 months who received 3 doses before age 12 months	
Pneumococcal[5]	6 wks	**4 weeks** if first dose administered at younger than 12 months of age **8 weeks (as final dose for healthy children)** if first dose administered at age 12 months or older or current age 24 through 59 months **No further doses needed** for healthy children if first dose administered at age 24 months or older	**4 weeks** if current age is younger than 12 months **8 weeks (as final dose for healthy children)** if current age is 12 months or older **No further doses needed** for healthy children if previous dose administered at age 24 months or older	**8 weeks (as final dose)** This dose only necessary for children aged 12 months through 59 months who received 3 doses before 12 months of age or for high-risk children who received 3 doses at any age	
Inactivated Poliovirus[6]	6 wks	4 weeks	4 weeks	4 weeks[6]	
Measles, Mumps, Rubella[7]	12 mos	4 weeks			
Varicella[8]	12 mos	3 months			
Hepatitis A[9]	12 mos	6 months			
CATCH-UP SCHEDULE FOR PERSONS AGED 7 THROUGH 18 YEARS					
Tetanus, Diphtheria/ Tetanus, Diphtheria, Pertussis[10]	7 yrs[10]	4 weeks	**4 weeks** if first dose administered at younger than 12 months of age **6 months** if first dose administered at age 12 months or older	**6 months** if first dose administered at younger than 12 months of age	
Human Papillomavirus[11]	9 yrs	Routine dosing intervals are recommended[11]			
Hepatitis A[9]	12 mos	6 months			
Hepatitis B[1]	Birth	4 weeks	**8 weeks** (and at least 16 weeks after first dose)		
Inactivated Poliovirus[6]	6 wks	4 weeks	4 weeks	4 weeks[6]	
Measles, Mumps, Rubella[7]	12 mos	4 weeks			
Varicella[8]	12 mos	**3 months** if the person is younger than 13 years of age **4 weeks** if the person is aged 13 years or older			

1. Hepatitis B vaccine (HepB).
- Administer the 3-dose series to those not previously vaccinated.
- A 2-dose series (separated by at least 4 months) of adult formulation Recombivax HB® is licensed for children aged 11 through 15 years.

2. Rotavirus vaccine (RV).
- The maximum age for the first dose is 14 weeks 6 days. Vaccination should not be initiated for infants aged 15 weeks or older (i.e., 15 weeks 0 days or older).
- Administer the final dose in the series by age 8 months 0 days.
- If Rotarix® was administered for the first and second doses, a third dose is not indicated.

3. Diphtheria and tetanus toxoids and acellular pertussis vaccine (DTaP).
- The fifth dose is not necessary if the fourth dose was administered at age 4 years or older.

4. Haemophilus influenzae type b conjugate vaccine (Hib).
- Hib vaccine is not generally recommended for persons aged 5 years or older. No efficacy data are available on which to base a recommendation concerning use of Hib vaccine for older children and adults. However, studies suggest good immunogenicity in persons who have sickle cell disease, leukemia, or HIV infection, or who have had a splenectomy; administering 1 dose of Hib vaccine to these persons is not contraindicated.
- If the first 2 doses were PRP-OMP (PedvaxHIB® or Comvax®), and administered at age 11 months or younger, the third (and final) dose should be administered at age 12 through 15 months and at least 8 weeks after the second dose.
- If the first dose was administered at age 7 through 11 months, administer 2 doses separated by 4 weeks and a final dose at age 12 through 15 months.

5. Pneumococcal vaccine.
- Administer 1 dose of pneumococcal conjugate vaccine (PCV) to all healthy children aged 24 through 59 months who have not received at least 1 dose of PCV on or after age 12 months.
- For children aged 24 through 59 months with underlying medical conditions, administer 1 dose of PCV if 3 doses were received previously or administer 2 doses of PCV at least 8 weeks apart if fewer than 3 doses were received previously.
- Administer pneumococcal polysaccharide vaccine (PPSV) to children aged 2 years or older with certain underlying medical conditions (see MMWR 2000;49[No. RR-9]), including a cochlear implant, at least 8 weeks after the last dose of PCV.

6. Inactivated poliovirus vaccine (IPV).
- For children who received an all-IPV or all-oral poliovirus (OPV) series, a fourth dose is not necessary if the third dose was administered at age 4 years or older.
- If both OPV and IPV were administered as part of a series, a total of 4 doses should be administered, regardless of the child's current age.

7. Measles, mumps, and rubella vaccine (MMR).
- Administer the second dose at age 4 through 6 years. However, the second dose may be administered before age 4, provided at least 28 days have elapsed since the first dose.
- If not previously vaccinated, administer 2 doses with at least 28 days between doses.

8. Varicella vaccine.
- Administer the second dose at age 4 through 6 years. However, the second dose may be administered before age 4, provided at least 3 months have elapsed since the first dose.
- For persons aged 12 months through 12 years, the minimum interval between doses is 3 months. However, if the second dose was administered at least 28 days after the first dose, it can be accepted as valid.
- For persons aged 13 years and older, the minimum interval between doses is 28 days.

9. Hepatitis A vaccine (HepA).
- HepA is recommended for children older than 1 year who live in areas where vaccination programs target older children or who are at increased risk of infection. See MMWR 2006;55(No. RR-7).

10. Tetanus and diphtheria toxoids vaccine (Td) and tetanus and diphtheria toxoids and acellular pertussis vaccine (Tdap).
- Doses of DTaP are counted as part of the Td/Tdap series
- Tdap should be substituted for a single dose of Td in the catch-up series or as a booster for children aged 10 through 18 years; use Td for other doses.

11. Human papillomavirus vaccine (HPV).
- Administer the series to females at age 13 through 18 years if not previously vaccinated.
- Use recommended routine dosing intervals for series catch-up (i.e., the second and third doses should be administered at 2 and 6 months after the first dose). However, the minimum interval between the first and second doses is 4 weeks. The minimum interval between the second and third doses is 12 weeks, and the third dose should be given at least 24 weeks after the first dose.

Information about reporting reactions after immunization is available online at http://www.vaers.hhs.gov or by telephone, 800-822-7967. Suspected cases of vaccine-preventable diseases should be reported to the state or local health department. Additional information, including precautions and contraindications for immunization, is available from the National Center for Immunization and Respiratory Diseases at http://www.cdc.gov/vaccines or telephone, 800-CDC-INFO (800-232-4636).

DEPARTMENT OF HEALTH AND HUMAN SERVICES • CENTERS FOR DISEASE CONTROL AND PREVENTION

Table 1.6.   Recommended and Minimum Ages and Intervals Between Vaccine Doses[a,b]

Vaccine and Dose No.	Recommended Age for This Dose	Minimum Age for This Dose	Recommended Interval to Next Dose	Minimum Interval to Next Dose
Hepatitis B (HepB)-1[c]	Birth	Birth	1–4 mo	4 wk
HepB-2	1–2 mo	4 wk	2–17 mo	8 wk
HepB-3[d]	6–18 mo	24 wk	…	…
Diphtheria-tetanus-acellular pertussis (DTaP)-1[c]	2 mo	6 wk	2 mo	4 wk
DTaP-2	4 mo	10 wk	2 mo	4 wk
DTaP-3	6 mo	14 wk	6–12 mo	6 mo[e,f]
DTaP-4	15–18 mo	12 mo	3 y	6 mo[e]
DTaP-5	4–6 y	4 y	…	…
Haemophilus influenzae type b (Hib)-1[c,g]	2 mo	6 wk	2 mo	4 wk
Hib-2	4 mo	10 wk	2 mo	4 wk
Hib-3[h]	6 mo	14 wk	6–9 mo	8 wk
Hib-4	12–15 mo	12 mo	…	…
Inactivated poliovirus (IPV)-1[c]	2 mo	6 wk	2 mo	4 wk
IPV-2	4 mo	10 wk	2–14 mo	4 wk
IPV-3	6–18 mo	14 wk	3–5 y	4 wk
IPV-4	4–6 y	18 wk	…	…
Pneumococcal conjugate (PCV)-1[g]	2 mo	6 wk	2 mo	4 wk
PCV-2	4 mo	10 wk	2 mo	4 wk
PCV-3	6 mo	14 wk	6 mo	8 wk
PCV-4	12–15 mo	12 mo	…	…
Measles-mumps-rubella (MMR)-1[i]	12–15 mo	12 mo	3–5 y	4 wk

Table 1.6. Recommended and Minimum Ages and Intervals Between Vaccine Doses,[a,b] continued

Vaccine and Dose No.	Recommended Age for This Dose	Minimum Age for This Dose	Recommended Interval to Next Dose	Minimum Interval to Next Dose
MMR-2[i]	4–6 y	13 mo	...	...
Varicella (Var)-1[i]	12–15 mo	12 mo	3–5 y	12 wk[j]
Var-2[i]	4–6 y	15 mo	...	...
Hepatitis A (HepA)-1	12–23 mo	12 mo	6–18 mo[e]	6 mo[e]
HepA-2	18–41 mo	18 mo	...	...
Influenza inactivated (TIV)[k]	6 mo–18 y	6 mo[l]	1 mo	4 wk
Influenza live-attenuated (LAIV)[k]	24 mo–18 y	24 mo	1 mo	4 wk
Meningococcal conjugate (MCV)	11–12 y	2 y	...	...
Meningococcal polysaccharide (MPSV)-1	...	2 y	5 y[m]	5 y[m]
MPSV-2[n]	...	7 y	...	...
Td	11–12 y	7 y	10 y	5 y
Tdap[o]	≥11 y	10 y	...	...
Pneumococcal polysaccharide (PPV)-1	...	2 y	5 y	5 y
PPV-2[p]	...	7 y	...	...
Human papillomavirus (HPV)-1[q]	11–12 y	9 y	2 mo	4 wk
HPV-2	11–12 y (+2 mo)	109 mo	4 mo	12 wk[r]
HPV-3[r]	11–12 y (+6 mo)	114 mo	...	...
Rotavirus (RV)-1[s]	2 mo	6 wk	2 mo	4 wk
RV-2	4 mo	10 wk	2 mo	4 wk

Table 1.6. Recommended and Minimum Ages and Intervals Between Vaccine Doses,[a,b] continued

Vaccine and Dose No.	Recommended Age for This Dose	Minimum Age for This Dose	Recommended Interval to Next Dose	Minimum Interval to Next Dose
RV-3[t]	6 mo	14 wk	…	…
Herpes zoster[u]	60 y	60 y	…	…

DTaP indicates diphtheria and tetanus toxoids and acellular pertussis vaccine; MMR, measles-mumps-rubella; TIV, trivalent (inactivated) influenza vaccine; Td, tetanus and reduced diphtheria toxoids; Tdap, tetanus toxoid, reduced diphtheria toxoid, and reduced acellular pertussis vaccine.

[a] Combination vaccines are available and may be used to reduce the number of injections. When administering combination vaccines, the minimum age for administration is the oldest age for any of the individual components; the minimum interval between doses is equal to the greatest interval of any of the individual components.

[b] For travel vaccines, including typhoid, Japanese encephalitis, and yellow fever, see www.cdc.gov/travel.

[c] Combination vaccines containing the hepatitis B component are available (HepB-Hib, DTaP-HepB-IPV, and HepA-HepB). These vaccines should not be administered to infants younger than 6 weeks of age because of the other components (ie, Hib, DTaP, HepA, and IPV).

[d] HepB-3 should be administered at least 8 weeks after HepB-2 and at least 16 weeks after HepB-1 and should not be administered before 24 weeks of age.

[e] Calendar months.

[f] The minimum recommended interval between DTaP-3 and DTaP-4 is 6 months. However, DTaP-4 need not be repeated if administered at least 4 months after DTaP-3.

[g] For Hib and PCV, children receiving the first dose of vaccine at 7 months of age or older require fewer doses to complete the series (see Fig 1.1–1.3, p 24–28).

[h] If PRP-OMP (Pedvax-Hib) was administered at 2 and 4 months of age, a dose at 6 months of age is not required.

[i] Combination measles-mumps-rubella-varicella (MMRV) vaccine can be used for children 12 months through 12 years of age.

[j] The minimum interval from VAR-1 to VAR-2 for people beginning the series at 13 years of age or older is 4 weeks.

[k] One dose of influenza vaccine per season is recommended for most people. Children younger than 9 years of age who are receiving influenza for the first time or received only 1 dose the previous season (if it was their first immunization season) should receive 2 doses this season.

[l] The minimum age for inactivated influenza vaccine varies by vaccine manufacturer (see Influenza, p 400).

[m] Some experts recommend a second dose of MPSV 3 years after the first dose for people at increased risk of meningococcal disease (see Meningococcal Infections, p 455).

[n] A second dose of meningococcal vaccine is recommended for people previously immunized with MPSV who remain at high risk of meningococcal disease. MCV is preferred when reimmunizing people 2 through 55 years of age, but a second dose of MPSV is acceptable.

[o] Only one dose of Tdap is recommended. Subsequent doses should be given as Td. If immunization to prevent tetanus and/or diphtheria disease is required for children 7 through 9 years of age, Td should be administered (minimum age for Td is 7 years). For one brand of Tdap, minimum age is 11 years. The preferred interval between Tdap and a previous dose of Td is 5 years. In people who have received a primary series of tetanus-toxoid containing vaccine, for management of a tetanus-prone wound, the minimum interval after a previous dose of any tetanus-containing vaccine is 5 years.

[p] A second dose of PPV is recommended for people at highest risk of serious pneumococcal infection and those who are likely to have a rapid decline in pneumococcal antibody concentration (see Pneumococcal Infections, p 524).

[q] HPV is approved only for females 9 through 26 years of age.

[r] HPV-3 should be administered at least 12 weeks after HPV-2 and at least 24 weeks after HPV-1.

[s] The first dose of RV should be administered at 6 through 14 weeks of age. The vaccine series should not be started at 15 weeks of age or older. RV should not be administered to children older than 8 calendar months of age regardless of the number of doses received between 6 weeks and 8 calendar months of age.

[t] If Rotarix is administered as age appropriate, a third dose is not necessary.

[u] Herpes zoster vaccine is approved as a single dose for people 60 years of age and older.

Minimum Ages and Minimum Intervals Between Vaccine Doses

Immunizations are recommended for members of the youngest age group at risk of experiencing the disease for whom efficacy, immunogenicity, and safety have been demonstrated. Most vaccines in the childhood and adolescent immunization schedule require 2 or more doses for stimulation of an adequate and persisting antibody response. Studies have demonstrated that the recommended age and interval between doses of the same antigen(s) provide optimal protection and efficacy. Table 1.6 (p 29) lists recommended minimum ages and intervals between immunizations for vaccines in the recommended childhood and adolescent immunization schedules. Administering doses of a multidose vaccine at intervals shorter than those in the recommended childhood and adolescent immunization schedules might be necessary in circumstances in which an infant or child is behind schedule and needs to be brought up to date quickly or when international travel is pending. In these cases, an accelerated schedule using minimum age or interval criteria can be used. These accelerated schedules should not be used routinely.

Vaccines should not be administered at intervals less than the recommended minimum or at an earlier age than the recommended minimum (eg, accelerated schedules). Two exceptions to this may occur. The first is for measles vaccine during a measles outbreak, in which case the vaccine may be administered before 12 months of age. However, if a measles-containing vaccine is administered before 12 months of age, the dose is not counted toward the 2-dose measles vaccine series, and the child should be reimmunized at 12 through 15 months of age with a measles-containing vaccine. A third dose of a measles-containing vaccine is indicated at 4 through 6 years of age but can be administered as early as 4 weeks after the second dose (see Measles, p 444). The second consideration involves administering a dose a few days earlier than the minimum interval or age, which is unlikely to have a substantially negative effect on the immune response to that dose. Although immunizations should not be scheduled at an interval or age less than the minimums listed in Table 1.6 (p 29), a child may be in the office early or for an appointment not specifically for immunization (eg, recheck of otitis media). In this situation, the clinician can consider administering the vaccine before the minimum interval or age. If the child is known to the clinician, rescheduling the child for immunization closer to the recommended interval is preferred. If the parent or child is not known to the clinician or follow-up cannot be ensured (eg, habitually misses appointments), administration of the vaccine at that visit rather than rescheduling the child for a later visit is preferable. Vaccine doses administered 4 days or fewer before the minimum interval or age can be counted as valid. This 4-day recommendation does not apply to rabies vaccine because of the unique schedule for this vaccine. Doses administered 5 days or more before the minimum interval or age should not be counted as valid doses and should be repeated as age appropriate. The repeat dose should be spaced after the invalid dose by at least 4 weeks (Table 1.6, p 29). In certain situations, local or state requirements might mandate that doses of selected vaccines (in particular, MMR) be administered on or after specific ages, precluding these 4-day recommendations.

Interchangeability of Vaccine Products

Similar vaccines made by different manufacturers can differ in the number and amount of their specific antigenic components and formulation of adjuvants and conjugating agents, thereby eliciting different degrees of immune response. However, such vaccines have been considered interchangeable by most experts when administered according to their licensed indications, although data documenting the effects of interchangeability are limited. Licensed vaccines that may be used interchangeably during a vaccine series from different manufacturers, according to recommendations from the ACIP or AAP, include diphtheria and tetanus toxoids vaccines, hepatitis A vaccines, hepatitis B (HepB) vaccines for infants, and rabies vaccines (see Rabies, p 552). An example of similar vaccines used in different schedules that are not recommended as interchangeable is the 2-dose HepB vaccine option currently available for adolescents 11 through 15 years of age. Adolescent patients begun on a 3-dose HepB regimen are not candidates to complete their series with HepB vaccine used in the 2-dose protocol, and vice versa, and the 2-dose schedule is applicable only to Recombivax HB (see Hepatitis B, p 337).

Licensed Hib conjugate vaccines are considered interchangeable for primary as well as for booster immunization as long as recommendations concerning conversion from a 3-dose regimen (PRP-OMP) to a 4-dose regimen (all other conjugated PRP preparations) are followed (see *Haemophilus influenzae* Infections, p 314). Licensed rotavirus (RV) vaccines are considered interchangeable as long as recommendations concerning conversion from a 2-dose regimen (RV1) to a 3-dose regimen (RV5) are followed (see Rotavirus, p 576).

Minimal data on safety and immunogenicity and no data on efficacy are available for different DTaP vaccines when administered interchangeably (see Pertussis, p 504). However, in circumstances in which the type of DTaP product(s) received previously is not known or the previously administered product(s) is not readily available, any of the DTaP vaccines may be used according to licensure for dose and age. Matching of adolescent Tdap manufacturer with pediatric DTaP manufacturer is not necessary. For interchangeability of combination vaccines, including DTaP-HepB-IPV and DTaP-IPV/Hib combination vaccines, see Combination Vaccines (p 34). These recommendations may change as additional data become available.

Simultaneous Administration of Multiple Vaccines

Simultaneous administration of most vaccines is safe and effective. Infants and children have sufficient immunologic capacity to respond to multiple vaccines. No contraindications to the simultaneous administration of multiple vaccines routinely recommended for infants and children are known. Immune response to one vaccine generally does not interfere with responses to other vaccines. Simultaneous administration of IPV, MMR, varicella, or DTaP vaccines results in rates of seroconversion and of adverse effects similar to those observed when the vaccines are administered at separate visits. For some other routinely administered vaccines, data on simultaneous administration are limited or not available. Because simultaneous administration of common vaccines is not known to affect the effectiveness or safety of any of the recommended childhood vaccines, simultaneous administration of all vaccines that are appropriate for the age and immunization status of the recipient is recommended.[1] When vaccines are administered simultaneously, separate syringes and separate sites should be used, and injections into the same extremity should be separated by at least 1 inch so that any local reactions can be differentiated. Simultaneous administration of multiple vaccines can increase immunization rates significantly. Individual vaccines should never be mixed in the same syringe unless they are

---

[1] Centers for Disease Control and Prevention. General recommendations on immunization. Recommendations of the Advisory Committee Immunization Practices. *MMWR Recomm Rep.* 2009; in press

specifically licensed and labeled for administration in one syringe. For people preparing for international travel, multiple vaccines can be given concurrently. If live-virus vaccines are not administered concurrently, 4 weeks should elapse between sequential immunizations. There is no required interval between administration of a live-virus vaccine and an inactivated vaccine or between inactivated vaccines. If an inactivated vaccine and an Immune Globulin product are indicated concurrently (eg, hepatitis B vaccine and HBIG, rabies vaccine and RIG), they should be administered at separate anatomic sites.

Combination Vaccines

An increasing number of new vaccines to prevent childhood diseases have been or will be licensed and recommended for use. Combination vaccines represent one solution to the issue of increased numbers of injections during single clinic visits. Parenteral combination vaccines may be administered instead of their equivalent component vaccines if licensed and indicated for the patient's age. Table 1.7 lists combination vaccines licensed for use in the United States for which individual components also are available. Health care professionals who provide immunizations should stock sufficient types of combination and monovalent vaccines needed to immunize children against all diseases for which vaccines are recommended, but they need not stock all available types or brand-name products. It is recognized that health care professionals' decisions to implement use of new combination vaccines involve complex economic and logistical considerations. When patients have received the recommended immunizations for some of the components in a combination vaccine, administering the extra antigen(s) in the combination vaccine is permissible if they are not contraindicated and doing so will reduce the number of injections required. Excessive doses of toxoid vaccines (diphtheria and tetanus) may result in extensive local reactions. To overcome recording errors and ambiguities in the names of vaccine combinations, improved systems are needed to enhance the convenience and accuracy of transferring vaccine-identifying information into medical records and immunization information systems.

Lapsed Immunizations

A lapse in the immunization schedule does not require reinitiation of the entire series or addition of doses to the series for any vaccine in the recommended schedule. If a dose of DTaP, IPV, Hib, pneumococcal conjugate, hepatitis A, hepatitis B, HPV, MMR, varicella, or rotavirus (RV) vaccine is missed, subsequent immunizations should be given at the next visit as if the usual interval had elapsed. For RV vaccine, the doses to be administered are age limited (see Rotavirus, p 576). See specific influenza vaccine recommendations for children younger than 9 years of age whose first 2 doses were not administered in the same season. The medical charts of children in whom immunizations have been missed or postponed should be flagged to remind health care professionals to resume the child's immunization regimen at the next available opportunity. Minimum age and interval recommendations should be followed for administration of all doses (see Table 1.6, p 29). A Web site is available that can be used to determine vaccines that a child 6 years of age and younger needs, including timing of missed or skipped vaccines, according to the childhood immunization schedule (**www.cdc.gov/vaccines/recs/scheduler/catchup.htm**).

Table 1.7. Combination Vaccines Licensed by the US Food and Drug Administration (FDA)[a]

Vaccine[b]	Trade Name (Year Licensed)	FDA Licensure	
		Age Group	Recommendations
Hib-HepB	Comvax (1996)	6 wk through 71 mo	Three-dose schedule given at 2, 4, and 12 through 15 mo of age.
DTaP/Hib	TriHIBit (1996)	Fourth dose of Hib and DTaP series	15 through 18 mo of age.
Hep A-HepB	Twinrix (2001)	≥18 y	Three doses on a 0-, 1-, and 6-mo schedule.
DTaP-HepB-IPV	Pediarix (2002)	6 wk through 6 y	Three-dose series at 2, 4, and 6 mo of age.
MMRV	ProQuad (2005)	12 mo through 12 y	Two doses 28 days apart on or after first birthday.
DTaP-IPV	Kinrix (2008)	4 through 6 y	Booster for fifth dose of DTaP and fourth dose of IPV.
DTaP-IPV/Hib	Pentacel (2008)	6 wk through 4 y	Four-dose series at 2, 4, 6, and 15 through 18 mo of age.

Hib indicates *Haemophilus influenzae* type b vaccine; HepB, hepatitis B vaccine; DTaP indicates diphtheria and tetanus toxoids and acellular pertussis vaccine; HepA, hepatitis A vaccine; IPV/Hib trivalent inactivated polio vaccine and *Haemophilus influenzae* type b vaccine; MMRV, measles-mumps-rubella-varicella vaccine.

[a] Excludes measles-mumps-rubella (MMR), DTaP, Tdap, and IPV vaccines, for which individual components are not available.

[b] Dash (-) indicates products are supplied in their final form by the manufacturer and do not require mixing or reconstitution by user; slash (/) indicates products are mixed or reconstituted by user.

Unknown or Uncertain Immunization Status

A physician may encounter children with an uncertain immunization status. Many children, adolescents, and young adults do not have adequate documentation of their immunizations. Parent or guardian recollection of a child's immunization history and the specific vaccines used may not be accurate. Only written, dated records should be accepted as evidence of immunization. In general, when in doubt, a person with unknown or uncertain immunization status should be considered disease susceptible, and recommended immunizations should be initiated without delay on a schedule commensurate with the person's current age. No evidence suggests that administration of most vaccines to already immune recipients is harmful. In general, initiation of revaccination with an age-appropriate schedule of diphtheria and tetanus toxoid-containing vaccine is appropriate, with performance of serologic testing for specific IgG antibody only if a severe local reaction occurs.[1] Adult-type tetanus and diphtheria toxoids (Td), rather than DTaP, should be given to people 7 years of age or older, and Tdap should be used for a single dose of Td-containing vaccine for people 10 through 64 years of age (see Pertussis, p 504, for specific recommendations for different Tdap vaccines).

Immunizations Received Outside the United States

People immunized in other countries, including internationally adopted children, refugees, and exchange students, should be immunized according to recommended schedules (including minimal ages and intervals) in the United States for healthy infants, children, and adolescents (see Fig 1.1–1.3, p 24–28). In general, only written documentation should be accepted as evidence of previous immunization. Written records may be considered valid if the vaccines, dates of administration, numbers of doses, intervals between doses, and age of the patient at the time of immunization are comparable with those of the current US or World Health Organization schedules. Although some vaccines with inadequate potency have been produced in other countries, most vaccines used worldwide are produced with adequate quality-control standards and are reliable. However, immunization records for certain children, especially children from orphanages, may not accurately reflect protection because of inaccuracies, lack of vaccine potency, or other problems, such as recording MMR vaccine but giving a product that did not contain one or more of the components (eg, mumps and/or rubella). Therefore, serologic testing or reimmunization may be reasonable for these children (see Unknown or Uncertain Immunization Status, p 35). If serologic testing is not available and receipt of immunogenic vaccines cannot be ensured, the prudent course is to repeat administration of the immunizations in question (see Medical Evaluation of Internationally Adopted Children, p 177).

Vaccine Dose

Reduced or divided doses of DTaP or any other vaccine, including vaccines given to preterm or low birth weight infants, should not be administered. The efficacy of this practice in decreasing the frequency of adverse events has not been demonstrated. Also, such a practice may confer less protection against disease than that achieved with recommended doses. A diminished antibody response in both term and preterm infants to reduced doses of diphtheria and tetanus and whole-cell pertussis (DTP) has been reported. A previous immunization with a dose that was less than the standard dose or one administered by a nonstandard route should not be counted, and the person should be reimmunized as recommended for age; a general exception is that repeating doses of vaccine administered by the IM route rather than by the SC route is unnecessary. Exceeding a recommended dose volume also may be hazardous. Excessive local concentrations of injectable inactivated vaccines might result in enhanced tissue or systemic reactions, whereas administering an increased dose of a live vaccine constitutes a theoretical but unproven risk.

[1]Centers for Disease Control and Prevention. General recommendations on immunization: recommendations of the Advisory Committee on Immunization Practices (ACIP). *MMWR Recomm Rep.* 2009; in press

Active Immunization of People Who Recently Received Immune Globulin

Live-virus vaccines may have diminished immunogenicity when given shortly before or during the several months after receipt of IG (both specific and nonspecific intramuscular as well as intravenous preparations). In particular, IG administration has been demonstrated to inhibit the response to measles vaccine for a prolonged period. Inhibition of immune response to rubella vaccine also has been demonstrated. The appropriate interval between IG administration and measles immunization varies with the dose of IG and the specific product; suggested intervals are given in Table 3.34 (p 448). The effect of administration of IG on antibody response to varicella vaccine is not known. Because of potential inhibition, varicella vaccine administration should be delayed after receipt of an IG preparation or a blood product (except washed Red Blood Cells), as recommended for measles vaccine (see Table 3.34, p 448). If IG must be given within 14 days after administration of measles- or varicella-containing vaccines, these live-virus vaccines should be administered again after the period specified in Table 3.34 (p 448) unless serologic testing at an appropriate interval after IG administration indicates that adequate serum antibodies were produced.

Administration of IG preparations does not interfere with antibody responses to yellow fever, OPV, or oral rotavirus vaccines and is not expected to affect response to live-attenuated influenza vaccine. Hence, these vaccines can be administered simultaneously with or at any time before or after IG.

In contrast to some live-virus vaccines, administration of IG preparations has not been demonstrated to cause significant inhibition of the immune responses to inactivated vaccines and toxoids. Concurrent administration of recommended doses of HBIG, Tetanus Immune Globulin, or RIG and the corresponding inactivated vaccine or toxoid for postexposure prophylaxis does not impair the efficacy of vaccine and provides immediate and long-term immunity. Standard doses of the corresponding vaccines are recommended. Increases in vaccine dose volume or number of immunizations are not indicated. Vaccines should be administered at a separate body site from that of intramuscularly administered IG. For further information, see chapters on specific diseases in Section 3.

Administration of hepatitis A vaccine generally is preferred to IG (with or without vaccine) for postexposure prophylaxis of hepatitis A contacts (see Hepatitis A, p 329). Specific monoclonal antibody products (eg, the respiratory syncytial virus monoclonal antibody [palivizumab]) does not interfere with response to inactivated or live vaccines.

Tuberculin Testing

Recommendations for use of the tuberculin skin test (see Tuberculosis, p 680) are independent of those for immunization. Tuberculin testing at any age is not required before administration of live-virus vaccines. A tuberculin skin test (TST) can be applied at the same visit during which these vaccines are administered. If not administered concurrently, measles vaccine temporarily can suppress tuberculin reactivity for at least 4 to 6 weeks. The effect of live-virus varicella, yellow fever, and live-attenuated influenza vaccines on TST reactivity is not known. In the absence of data, the same TST spacing recommendation should be applied to these vaccines as described for MMR. The effect of live-virus vaccines on interferon-release assays for tuberculosis is unknown. Until data are available, it may be prudent to space testing as for measles vaccine. There is no evidence that inactivated vaccines, polysaccharide vaccines, or recombinant or subunit vaccines or toxoids interfere with immune response to TST.

Record Keeping and Immunization Information Systems

The National Vaccine Advisory Committee in 1993 recommended a set of standards to improve immunization practices for health care professionals serving children and revised the standards in 2002 (see p 854). The standards include the recommendation that immunizations of patients be documented through use of immunization records that are accurate, complete, and easily accessible. In addition, the standards also recommend use of tracking systems to provide reminder/recall notices to parents/guardians and physicians when immunizations are due or overdue. Immunization information systems address record-keeping needs and tracking functions and have additional capacities, such as adverse event reporting, interoperability with electronic medical records, emergency preparedness functions, and linkage with other public health programs. Additional information about immunization information systems can be found at **www.cdc.gov/ vaccines/programs/iis/default.htm.**

PERSONAL IMMUNIZATION RECORDS OF PATIENTS

The AAP and state health departments have developed an official immunization record. This record should be given to parents of every newborn infant and should be accorded the status of a birth certificate or passport and retained with vital documents for subsequent referral. Physicians should cooperate with this endeavor by recording immunization data in this record and by encouraging patients not only to preserve the record but also to present it at each visit to a health care professional.

The immunization record especially is important for people who frequently move or change health care professionals. The record facilitates maintaining an accurate patient medical history, enables the physician to evaluate a child's immunization status, and fulfills the need for documentation of immunizations for child care and school attendance and for admission to other institutions and organizations.

Although still used, paper-based immunization records are not always kept up-to-date and may be misplaced or destroyed. The absence of an immunization card can result in missed opportunities, extra immunizations, or inability to meet legal requirements.

All states and some large metropolitan areas are developing population-based computerized immunization information systems to record and track immunizations regardless of where in the state or metropolitan area the immunization services are provided. Most immunization information systems can consolidate records from physician offices, help remind parents and health care professionals when immunizations are due or overdue, help health care professionals determine the immunization needs of their patients at each visit, and generate official immunization records to meet child care or school requirements. Immunization information systems also can provide measurements of immunization coverage and rates by age, immunization series, and physician or clinic practice. The AAP urges physicians to cooperate with state and local health officials in providing immunization data for state or local immunization information systems.

IMMUNIZATION RECORDS OF PHYSICIANS

Every physician should ensure that the immunization history of each patient is maintained in a permanent, confidential record that can be reviewed easily and updated when subsequent immunizations are administered. The medical record maintained by the primary health care professional and in some states by their Immunization Information Systems (see Record Keeping and Immunization Information Systems, p 38) should document all vaccines received, including vaccines received in another health care setting. The format of the record should facilitate identification and recall of patients in need of immunization.

Records of children whose immunizations have been delayed or missed should be flagged to indicate the need to complete immunizations. For data that are required by the National Childhood Vaccine Injury Act of 1986 as well as data recommended by the AAP to be recorded in each patient's medical record for each immunization, see Informing Patients and Parents (p 5).

Interest in the use of electronic health record (EHR) systems prompted the AAP to issue a revised statement in 2007 outlining functions that would need to be performed in a pediatric practice for EHR systems to be useful.[1] An executive federal order calls for the widespread adoption of interoperable EHRs. EHR systems that can send and receive data from population-based immunization information systems enhance complete immunization record keeping and facilitate reminder/recall functions to ensure complete immunization coverage and prevent administration of excessive doses.

Vaccine Shortages

When vaccine shortages occur, temporary changes in childhood or adolescent immunization recommendations by the AAP and CDC may be necessary, including temporary deferral of certain immunizations, establishment of vaccine priorities for high-risk children, and suspension in some states of school and child care entry immunization requirements. Several national committees and organizations, including the National Center for Immunization and Respiratory Diseases, National Vaccine Advisory Committee, and the US Government Accountability Office, have proposed comprehensive strategies to prevent future shortages and encourage key stakeholders to work together to develop corrective action.

When vaccines are in short supply, physicians and other health care professionals should maintain lists of children and adolescents who do not receive vaccines at the recommended time or age so they can be recalled when the vaccine supply becomes adequate. For current information about vaccine shortages and resulting recommendations, see the Web sites of the CDC (**www.cdc.gov/vaccines/vac-gen/shortages/default.htm**), FDA (**www.fda.gov/cber/vaccines.htm**), or *Red Book* online (**http://aapredbook.aappublications.org**). For analyses of vaccine shortages and recommended solutions, see the published recommendations from the National Vaccine Advisory Committee.[2]

---

[1] American Academy of Pediatrics, Council on Clinical Information Technology. Special requirements of electronic health record systems in pediatrics. *Pediatrics.* 2007;119(3):631–637

[2] Santoli JM, Peter G, Arvin AM, et al. Strengthening the supply of routinely recommended vaccines in the United States: recommendations from the National Vaccine Advisory Committee. *JAMA.* 2003;290(23):3122–3128

Vaccine Safety and Contraindications

RISKS AND ADVERSE EVENTS

All licensed vaccines in the United States are safe and effective, but no vaccine is completely safe and effective in every person. Some vaccine recipients will have an adverse event, and some will not be protected fully. The goal of vaccine development is to achieve the highest degree of protection with the lowest rate of adverse events. Adverse events following immunization include both true vaccine events and coincidental events that would have occurred without vaccination. As immunizations successfully eliminate their target vaccine-preventable diseases, vaccine safety issues have received more attention, increasing the need for immunization providers to communicate risks and benefits of immunizations to a population whose first-hand experience with vaccine-preventable diseases increasingly is rare. Many families lack awareness of the continued threat of vaccine-preventable diseases (eg, pertussis, measles, mumps, invasive *H influenzae*) among unimmunized people.

Risks of immunization may vary from minor and inconvenient to severe and life threatening. Rarely, serious adverse events following immunization occur, resulting in permanent sequelae or life-threatening illness. When developing immunization recommendations, vaccine benefits and risks are weighed against the risks of natural disease to the person and the community. Recommendations are made to maximize protection and minimize risk by providing specific advice on dose, route, and timing of the vaccine and by identifying people who should be immunized and circumstances that warrant revaccination, deferral, precaution, or contraindication to immunization.

Common vaccine adverse events usually are mild to moderate in severity (eg, fever or injection site reactions, such as swelling, redness, and pain) and have no permanent sequelae. Examples include local inflammation after administration of DTaP, Td, or Tdap vaccines and fever and rash 1 to 2 weeks after administration of MMR or MMRV vaccines.

The occurrence of an adverse event following immunization does not prove that the vaccine caused the symptoms or signs. Vaccines are administered to infants and children during a period in their lives when certain conditions most commonly become clinically apparent (eg, seizure disorders). Because chance temporal association of an adverse event to the timing of administration of a specific vaccine commonly occurs, a true causal association requires that the event occur at a significantly higher rate in vaccine recipients than in unimmunized groups of similar age and residence. This excess risk can be demonstrated in prelicensure clinical trials or in postlicensure epidemiologic studies. More rarely, recovery of a vaccine virus from the ill child with compatible symptoms may provide support for a causal link with a live-virus vaccine (eg, vaccine-associated polio with OPV). Clustering in time of unusual adverse events following immunizations or recurrence of the adverse event with another dose of the same vaccine (eg, rarely but well-documented instances of Guillain-Barré syndrome after administration of tetanus toxoid-containing vaccines) also suggest a causal relationship.

Reporting of any clinically significant adverse event following immunization to the Vaccine Adverse Event Reporting System (VAERS, see p 42) is important, because when analyzed in conjunction with other reports, this information may provide clues to an unanticipated adverse event. Health care professionals are mandated to report serious adverse events to VAERS, as specified in the Reportable Events Table (Appendix IV, p 842) (**http://vaers.hhs.gov/pdf/ReportableEventsTable.pdf**). A reportable vaccine-preventable disease that occurs in a child or adolescent at any time, including after immunization (vaccine failure), should be reported to the local or state health department (see Appendix V, p 845).

INSTITUTE OF MEDICINE IMMUNIZATION SAFETY REVIEW COMMITTEE

The CDC and the National Institutes of Health commissioned the National Academy of Sciences' Institute of Medicine (IOM) to convene an Immunization Safety Review Committee in 2000. This committee, comprising 15 members with diverse expertise, was charged with providing independent advice to vaccine policy makers as well as health care professionals, the public, and the media. Specifically, the committee reviewed the scientific plausibility of possible causal associations between vaccines and various adverse events. The committee reviewed the following 8 specific topics about existing and emerging vaccine safety concerns.

* Measles-Mumps-Rubella Vaccine and Autism (April 2001)
* Thimerosal-Containing Vaccines and Neurodevelopmental Disorders (October 2001)
* Multiple Immunizations and Immune Dysfunction (February 2002)
* Hepatitis B Vaccine and Demyelinating Neurologic Disorders (May 2002)
* SV40 Contamination of Polio Vaccine and Cancer (October 2002)
* Vaccinations and Sudden Unexpected Death in Infancy (March 2003)
* Influenza Vaccines and Neurologic Complications (October 2003)
* Vaccines and Autism (May 2004)

For each topic, the committee found the evidence to be inconclusive or favored rejection of causal associations between vaccines and the adverse events reviewed. On the basis of the conclusions, the committee made recommendations for future activities in the areas of surveillance, research, policy, and communication regarding safety concerns. The committee did not recommend a policy review of the childhood and adolescent immunization schedule or of recommendations for administration of routine childhood vaccines. Executive summaries of each of the committee's 8 reports are available online (**www.iom.edu/imsafety**).

THE BRIGHTON COLLABORATION

The Brighton Collaboration is an international voluntary collaboration formed to develop globally accepted and standardized case definitions for adverse events following immunization, known as the Brighton Standardized Case Definitions for use in surveillance and research. The project began in 2000 with formation of a steering committee and creation of work groups, composed of international volunteers with expertise in vaccine safety, patient care, pharmaceuticals, regulatory affairs, public health, and vaccine delivery. The guidelines for collecting, analyzing, and presenting safety data developed by the collaboration will facilitate sharing and comparison of vaccine data among vaccine safety professionals worldwide. Additional information, including current definitions and updates of progress, can be found online (**www.brightoncollaboration.org/**) after completion of a quick registration process. As of January 2009, a total of 27 case definitions have been completed, and all definitions can be accessed online.

Reporting of Adverse Events

Before administering a dose of any vaccine, health care professionals should ask parents and patients if they have experienced adverse events following immunization with previous doses. Although extensive safety testing is required before vaccine licensure, these prelicensure studies may not be large enough to detect rare adverse events or determine the rate of adverse events previously linked with the vaccine. Unexpected events after administration of any vaccine, particularly events judged to be clinically significant, should be described in detail in the patient's medical record and subsequently submitted to the VAERS (**http://vaers.hhs.gov**). There is no time limit for reporting an adverse event. The FDA and CDC encourage reporting of any significant adverse event following an immunization, even if it is uncertain that the event was caused by the vaccine.

The National Childhood Vaccine Injury Act of 1986 requires physicians and other health care professionals who administer vaccines covered under the National Vaccine Injury Compensation Program to maintain permanent immunization records and to report to the VAERS any condition listed on the reportable events table (see Appendix IV, p 842) or listed in the manufacturer's package insert as a contraindication to additional doses of vaccine. The antigens to which these requirements apply, as of January 2009, are measles, mumps, rubella, varicella, poliovirus, hepatitis A, hepatitis B, pertussis, diphtheria, tetanus, rotavirus, Hib, pneumococcal conjugate, meningococcal (conjugate and polysaccharide), human papillomavirus, and influenza (inactivated and live intranasal) vaccines (see Record Keeping and Immunization Information Systems, p 38).

VACCINE ADVERSE EVENT REPORTING SYSTEM (VAERS)

VAERS is a national passive surveillance system that monitors vaccines licensed for use in the United States. Jointly administered by the CDC and the FDA, VAERS accepts reports of suspected adverse events after administration of any vaccine. The strength of VAERS is its ability to detect previously unrecognized adverse events, monitor known reactions, identify possible risk factors, and evaluate lot-specific frequencies of adverse events. Like all passive surveillance systems, VAERS is subject to limitations, including underreporting, reporting of temporal (but not causal) associations or unconfirmed diagnoses, lack of denominator data, and absence of an unimmunized control group. Because of these limitations, determining causal associations between vaccines and adverse events from VAERS reports usually is not possible.

Vaccine providers are required to report certain adverse events that occur after immunization with vaccines covered under the National Vaccine Injury Compensation Program to VAERS (Appendix IV, p 842). VAERS also encourages reporting of any clinically significant adverse event that occurs after administration of any vaccine licensed for use in the United States. In addition, vaccine failures (disease in an immunized person who received 1 or more dose of vaccine) and vaccine administration errors may be reported. VAERS forms (see Fig 1.4, p 43) are available by calling 1-800-822-7967 or downloading from the Web site (**http://vaers.hhs.gov**). Reports can be submitted by mail, facsimile, or telephone or through a secure online system at **https://secure. vaers.org.** VAERS data, excluding personal identifiers, are made available to the public and are made accessible through the VAERS Web site.

FIGURE 1.4 VAERS FORM

FOR DIRECTIONS FOR COMPLETING FORM AND FOR A NEW
ELECTRONIC REPORTING FORM, SEE HTTP://VAERS.HHS.GOV.

WEBSITE: www.vaers.hhs.gov   E-MAIL: info@vaers.org   FAX: 1-877-721-0366

VACCINE ADVERSE EVENT REPORTING SYSTEM
24 Hour Toll-Free Information 1-800-822-7967
P.O. Box 1100, Rockville, MD 20849-1100
PATIENT IDENTITY KEPT CONFIDENTIAL

For CDC/FDA Use Only
VAERS Number _____
Date Received _____

Patient Name:

Last   First   M.I.

Address

City   State   Zip

Telephone no. (____) _____

Vaccine administered by (Name):

Responsible
Physician _____
Facility Name/Address

City   State   Zip

Telephone no. (____) _____

Form completed by (Name):

Relation   ☐ Vaccine Provider   ☐ Patient/Parent
to Patient   ☐ Manufacturer   ☐ Other
Address *(if different from patient or provider)*

City   State   Zip

Telephone no. (____) _____

1. State	2. County where administered	3. Date of birth mm / dd / yy	4. Patient age	5. Sex ☐M ☐F	6. Date form completed mm / dd / yy

7. Describe adverse events(s) (symptoms, signs, time course) and treatment, if any

8. Check all appropriate:
☐ Patient died   (date ___/___/___)   mm / dd / yy
☐ Life threatening illness
☐ Required emergency room/doctor visit
☐ Required hospitalization (_____days)
☐ Resulted in prolongation of hospitalization
☐ Resulted in permanent disability
☐ None of the above

9. Patient recovered   ☐ YES ☐ NO ☐ UNKNOWN

10. Date of vaccination mm / dd / yy Time _____ AM PM	11. Adverse event onset mm / dd / yy Time _____ AM PM

12. Relevant diagnostic tests/laboratory data

13. Enter all vaccines given on date listed in no. 10

	Vaccine (type)	Manufacturer	Lot number	Route/Site	No. Previous Doses
a.					
b.					
c.					
d.					

14. Any other vaccinations within 4 weeks prior to the date listed in no. 10

	Vaccine (type)	Manufacturer	Lot number	Route/Site	No. Previous doses	Date given
a.						
b.						

15. Vaccinated at:
☐ Private doctor's office/hospital   ☐ Military clinic/hospital
☐ Public health clinic/hospital   ☐ Other/unknown

16. Vaccine purchased with:
☐ Private funds   ☐ Military funds
☐ Public funds   ☐ Other/unknown

17. Other medications

18. Illness at time of vaccination (specify)

19. Pre-existing physician-diagnosed allergies, birth defects, medical conditions (specify)

20. Have you reported this adverse event previously?   ☐ No   ☐ To health department   ☐ To doctor   ☐ To manufacturer

Only for children 5 and under

22. Birth weight _____ lb. _____ oz.

23. No. of brothers and sisters

21. Adverse event following prior vaccination (check all applicable, specify)

	Adverse Event	Onset Age	Type Vaccine	Dose no. in series
☐ In patient				
☐ In brother or sister				

Only for reports submitted by manufacturer/immunization project

24. Mfr./imm. proj. report no.

25. Date received by mfr./imm.proj.

26. 15 day report?   ☐ Yes   ☐ No

27. Report type   ☐ Initial   ☐ Follow-Up

Health care providers and manufacturers are required by law (42 USC 300aa-25) to report reactions to vaccines listed in the Table of Reportable Events Following Immunization. Reports for reactions to other vaccines are voluntary except when required as a condition of immunization grant awards.

Form VAERS-1(FDA)

Reports may be submitted by anyone suspecting that an adverse event might have been caused by immunization. Submission of a report does not necessarily indicate that the vaccine caused the adverse event. All patient-identifying information is kept confidential. Written notification that the report has been received is provided to the person submitting the form or the electronic report.

All reports of serious adverse events and death following immunization are reviewed by FDA medical officers when received and are evaluated to detect adverse event reporting by vaccine lot. Reports of serious adverse events, including reports of death, may be followed up by VAERS staff to obtain additional information about the event. The report is classified as serious if at least one of the following is indicated to occur after vaccination: death, life-threatening illness, hospitalization, prolongation of hospitalization, or permanent disability. The FDA and CDC periodically prepare vaccine and adverse event-specific surveillance summaries, which describe reported adverse events and look for unexpected patterns ("signals") that might suggest a possible causal link between a vaccine and an adverse event. Vaccine safety concerns identified through adverse event monitoring nearly always require confirmation using an epidemiologic or other type of study by the Vaccine Safety Datalink, by the Clinical Immunization Safety Assessment (CISA) Network, or by other means.

VACCINE SAFETY DATALINK PROJECT

To supplement the Vaccine Adverse Event Reporting System (VAERS) program, which is a passive surveillance system, the CDC in 1990 formed partnerships with several large managed-care organizations to establish the Vaccine Safety Datalink (VSD) project, an active surveillance system designed to evaluate vaccine safety continuously. The VSD project includes comprehensive medical and immunization histories on more than 5.5 million people. These histories are derived from participating managed-care organizations that contain more than 9 million members. Data from the study population can be monitored for potential adverse events resulting from immunization. The VSD project allows for both retrospective and prospective observational vaccine safety studies as well as for timely investigations of newly licensed vaccines or emerging vaccine safety concerns. The VSD allows calculation of rates of adverse events following immunization that can be compared with rates in other intervals or unvaccinated populations when available. The VSD concept to evaluate vaccine safety has been proven to be valuable for many vaccines. Information about the VSD can be found at **www.cdc.gov/od/science/iso/vsd.**

CLINICAL IMMUNIZATION SAFETY ASSESSMENT (CISA) NETWORK

Serious and other uncommon clinically significant adverse events following immunization rarely occur in prelicensure clinical trials, and health care professionals see them too infrequently to be able to provide standardized evaluation, diagnosis, and management. The CISA Network was established by the CDC in 2001 with primary goals including: (1) developing research protocols for clinical evaluation, diagnosis, and management of adverse events following immunization; (2) improving understanding of adverse events following immunization at the individual level, including determining possible genetic and other risk factors for predisposed people and high-risk subpopulations; (3) developing evidence-based guidelines for immunization of people at risk of serious adverse events following immunization; and (4) serving as public health regional referral centers for clinical vaccine safety inquiries. The CISA Network comprises 6 academic centers with expertise in neurology, infectious diseases, virology, allergy and immunology, biostatistics, epidemiology, computer programming, pediatrics, internal medicine, health economics, preventative medicine, genetics, dermatology, and gastroenterology. Patients with rare and serious adverse events following immunization can be referred to the CISA Network for inclusion in the CISA Vaccine Consult Registry and Repository so that they may be enrolled in future vaccine safety studies.

The CISA Network advises clinicians on the evaluation, diagnosis, and management of adverse events after immunization. The network conducts research through establishment of a registry for clinical consultations, creation of standardized protocols for evaluation of specific events, and direct patient evaluation to generate increased case series of clinically significant adverse events following immunization. CISA Network data will be used to improve the scientific understanding of these adverse events and to develop protocols or guidelines for health care professionals that will assist in evaluation, diagnosis, and management of similarly affected people. In addition, the CISA Network provides regional clinical vaccine safety resources for clinicians. Current information about the CISA Network can be found online (**http://www.cdc.gov/vaccinesafety/cisa/**).

VACCINE INJURY COMPENSATION

The National Vaccine Injury Compensation Program is a no-fault system in which people may seek compensation if they are thought to have suffered an injury or if a vaccine recipient is thought to have died as a result of administration of a covered vaccine. Claims must be filed within 36 months after the first symptom appeared after immunization, and death claims must be filed within 24 months of the death and within 48 months after onset of the vaccine-related injury from which death occurred. Claims arising from covered vaccines must be adjudicated through the program before civil litigation can be pursued. Developed as an alternative to civil litigation and operational since 1988, the program has decreased the number of lawsuits against health care professionals and vaccine manufacturers and has assisted establishment of a stable vaccine supply and marketplace while ensuring access to compensation for vaccine-associated injury and death.

The program is based on the Vaccine Injury Table (VIT [see Appendix IV, p 842] or **www.hrsa.gov/vaccinecompensation/table.htm**), which lists the vaccines covered by the program, as well as injuries, disabilities, illnesses, and conditions (including death) for which compensation may be awarded. The VIT defines the time during which the first symptoms or significant aggravation of an injury must appear after immunization. If an injury listed in the VIT is proven, claimants receive a "legal presumption of causation," thus avoiding the need to prove causation in an individual case. If the claim pertains to conditions not listed in the VIT, claimants may prevail if they prove causation. Any vaccine that is recommended by the CDC for routine use in children and has an excise tax placed on it by Congress is eligible for coverage by the program.

Program and contact information about the National Vaccine Injury Compensation Program and the VIT are in Appendix I (p 831):

Parklawn Building
5600 Fishers Lane
Room 11C-26
Rockville, MD 20857
Telephone: 800-338-2382
Web site: **www.hrsa.gov/vaccinecompensation**

People wishing to file a claim for a vaccine injury should telephone or write to the following:

United States Court of Federal Claims
717 Madison Place, NW
Washington, DC 20005-1011
Telephone: 202-219-9657

VACCINE CONTRAINDICATIONS AND PRECAUTIONS

A contraindication to immunization is a condition in a recipient that increases the risk of a serious adverse reaction. For example, a history of anaphylactic allergy to egg protein is a contraindication for influenza vaccine, because it could cause serious illness or death in the vaccinee. A vaccine should not be administered when a contraindication is present. In contrast, a precaution is a condition in a recipient that might increase the risk of a serious adverse reaction or that might compromise the ability of the vaccine to produce immunity. However, immunization might be indicated in the presence of a precaution, because the benefit of protection from the vaccine outweighs the risk of an adverse reaction or incomplete response. Usually, precautions are temporary conditions (eg, moderate or severe illness), and a vaccine can be administered at a later time. Failure to understand true contraindications and precautions can result in administration of a vaccine when it should be withheld (see Immunocompromised Children, p 72). Misconceptions about vaccine contraindications can result in missed opportunities to provide vaccines and protect people from serious diseases. Contraindications, precautions, and reasons for deferral of immunizations are addressed in pathogen-specific chapters.

Common conditions or circumstances that are NOT contraindications, precautions, or reasons for deferral include:

- Recent exposure to an infectious disease.
- Mild acute illness with low-grade fever (eg, upper respiratory tract illness, otitis media) or mild diarrheal illness in an otherwise well child. Most evidence does not indicate an increased risk of adverse events or decrease in effectiveness associated with use of inactivated, subunit, or live-attenuated vaccines administered during a minor illness with or without fever. For optimal safety, vaccines should not be administered if an adverse reaction to the vaccine could affect seriously or be confused with an intercurrent illness. A child with frequent febrile illnesses that are moderate or severe, leading to deferrals of immunization, should be asked to return as soon as the illness subsides so that missed vaccines can be administered and the child can remain on the usual schedule.
- The convalescent phase of an illness.

- Currently receiving antimicrobial therapy. Administration of certain antimalaria drugs can reduce efficacy of oral typhoid vaccine, and certain antiviral drugs reduce the efficacy of live varicella virus or live-attenuated influenza virus vaccines (see specific pathogen chapters).
- Preterm birth. The appropriate age for initiating most immunizations in the preterm infant is the recommended chronologic age; vaccine doses should not be reduced for preterm infants (see Preterm and Low Birth Weight Infants, p 68, and Hepatitis B, p 337).
- Pregnancy in a household contact. Pregnancy in a household contact is not a contraindication to administration of any routinely recommended live-virus vaccines, including MMR, MMRV, varicella, rotavirus, or live-attenuated influenza vaccine, to a child or other nonpregnant household contact. Vaccine viruses in MMR vaccine are not transmitted by vaccine recipients, and although varicella vaccine virus and influenza vaccine virus (in live-virus vaccines only) can be transmitted by healthy vaccine recipients to contacts, the frequency is low, and only mild or asymptomatic infection has been reported (see Varicella-Zoster Infections, p 714 and Influenza, p 400).
- Breastfeeding. The only vaccine virus that has been isolated from human milk is rubella; no evidence indicates that human milk from women immunized against rubella is harmful to infants. If rubella infection does occur in an infant as a result of exposure to the vaccine virus in human milk, infection likely would be well tolerated, because the vaccine virus is attenuated.
- Immunosuppression of a household contact. Immunosuppression of a household contact is not a contraindication to administration of any routinely recommended live-virus vaccine, including MMR, MMRV, varicella, and rotavirus. Inactivated influenza vaccines, when available, are preferred to live-attenuated influenza vaccine for household contacts of people who are severely immunosuppressed.
- History of nonspecific allergies or relatives with allergies, including history of a nonanaphylactic allergy to a vaccine component (such as egg). Only anaphylactic allergy to a vaccine component is a true contraindication to immunization.
- History of allergies to penicillin or any other antimicrobial agent, except anaphylactic reactions to neomycin, gentamicin, or streptomycin (see Hypersensitivity Reactions After Immunization, p 47). These reactions occur rarely, if ever. No vaccine licensed for use in the United States contains penicillin.
- Allergies to duck meat or duck feathers. No vaccine licensed for use in the United States is produced in substrates containing duck antigens.
- Family history of seizures (see Children With a Personal or Family History of Seizures, p 86).
- Family history of sudden infant death syndrome.
- Family history of an adverse event following immunization.
- Malnutrition.

HYPERSENSITIVITY REACTIONS AFTER IMMUNIZATION

Hypersensitivity reactions to constituents of vaccines are rare. Facilities and health care professionals should be available for treating immediate hypersensitivity reactions in all settings in which vaccines are administered. This recommendation includes administration of vaccines in school-based or other complementary or nontraditional settings.

The 4 types of hypersensitivity reactions considered related to vaccine constituents are (1) allergic reactions to egg-related antigens; (2) mercury sensitivity to thimerosal-containing vaccines (see the paragraph in which thimerosal is discussed on p 49); (3) antimicrobial-induced allergic reactions; and (4) hypersensitivity to other vaccine components, including gelatin, yeast protein, and the infectious agent itself.

ALLERGIC REACTIONS TO EGG-RELATED ANTIGENS. Current measles and mumps vaccines are derived from chicken embryo fibroblast tissue cultures but do not contain significant amounts of egg cross-reacting proteins. Studies indicate that children with egg allergy, even children with severe hypersensitivity, are at low risk of anaphylactic reactions to these vaccines, singly or in combination (eg, MMR or MMRV), and that skin testing with dilute vaccine is not predictive of an allergic reaction to immunization. Most immediate hypersensitivity reactions after measles or mumps immunization appear to be reactions to other vaccine components, such as gelatin or neomycin. Therefore, children with egg allergy may be given MMR or MMRV vaccines without previous skin testing.

Yellow fever and inactivated and live-attenuated influenza vaccines prepared in eggs contain egg proteins and, on rare occasions, may induce immediate allergic reactions, including anaphylaxis. Skin testing with yellow fever vaccines is recommended before administration to people with a history of systemic anaphylactic symptoms (generalized urticaria, hypotension, or manifestations of upper or lower airway obstruction) after egg ingestion. Skin testing also has been used for children with severe anaphylactic reactions to eggs who are to receive inactivated influenza vaccine. However, these children generally should not receive inactivated or live-attenuated influenza vaccines because of a risk of adverse reaction, the likely need for yearly immunization, and availability of chemoprophylaxis against influenza infection (see Influenza, p 400). History of severe egg allergy in a family member is not a contraindication to influenza vaccines. Less severe or local manifestations of allergy to egg or feathers are not contraindications to administration of yellow fever or influenza vaccines and do not warrant vaccine skin testing.

An egg-sensitive person can be tested with vaccine (eg, inactivated influenza or yellow fever vaccines) before use of the vaccine as follows.

- ***Scratch, prick, or puncture test.*** A drop of a 1:10 dilution of vaccine in physiologic saline solution is applied at the site of a superficial scratch, prick, or puncture on the volar surface of the forearm. Positive (histamine) and negative (physiologic saline solution) control tests also should be used. The test is read after 15 to 20 minutes. A positive test result is a wheal 3 mm larger than that of the saline control area, usually with surrounding erythema. The histamine control test result must be positive for valid interpretation. If the result of this test is negative, an intradermal test is performed.

- ***Intradermal test.*** A dose of 0.02 mL of a 1:100 dilution of the vaccine in physiologic saline solution is injected intradermally on the volar surface of the forearm; positive- and negative-control skin tests are performed concurrently as described previously. A wheal 5 mm or larger than the negative control area with surrounding erythema is considered a positive reaction.

If these test results are negative, the vaccine may be given. If the child's test result is positive, the vaccine still may be given using a desensitization procedure if immunization is considered warranted because of a person's risk of complications resulting from the disease. A suggested protocol is subcutaneous administration of the following successive doses of vaccine at 15- to 20-minute intervals:

1. 0.05 mL of a 1:10 dilution
2. 0.05 mL of full-strength vaccine
3. 0.10 mL of full-strength vaccine
4. 0.15 mL of full-strength vaccine
5. 0.20 mL of full-strength vaccine

Scratch, prick, or puncture tests with other allergens have resulted in fatalities in highly allergic people. Although such untoward effects have not been reported for vaccine testing, all skin tests and desensitization procedures should be performed by trained personnel experienced in management of anaphylaxis. Necessary medications and equipment for treatment of anaphylaxis should be readily available (see Treatment of Anaphylactic Reactions, p 65).

Allergy to thimerosal, which is unusual, consists of delayed type (cell-mediated) hypersensitivity reactions. A localized or delayed type hypersensitivity reaction to thimerosal is not a contraindication to receive a vaccine that contains thimerosal.

ANTIMICROBIAL-INDUCED ALLERGIC REACTIONS. Antimicrobial-induced reactions have been suspected in people with known allergies who received vaccines containing trace amounts of antimicrobial agents (see package insert for each product for specific listing). Proof of a causal relationship often is impossible to confirm.

The IPV vaccine contains trace amounts of streptomycin, neomycin, and polymyxin B. Live-attenuated measles, mumps, rubella, and varicella-containing vaccines contain a trace quantity of neomycin. People who are allergic to neomycin usually develop a delayed-type local reaction 48 to 96 hours after administration of IPV, MMR, MMRV, or varicella vaccines rather than anaphylaxis. The reaction consists of an erythematous, pruritic papule. This minor reaction is of little importance compared with the benefit of immunization and should not be considered a contraindication. However, if a person has a history of anaphylactic reaction to neomycin, neomycin-containing vaccines should not be used. No vaccine currently licensed for use in the United States contains penicillin or its derivatives.

HYPERSENSITIVITY TO OTHER VACCINE COMPONENTS

Antigen(s)/infectious agents themselves. Some live-virus vaccines, such as MMR, MMRV, varicella, and yellow fever vaccines, contain gelatin as a stabilizer. People with a history of food allergy to gelatin rarely develop anaphylaxis after receipt of gelatin-containing vaccines. Skin testing is a consideration for these people before administration of a gelatin-containing vaccine, but no protocol or reported experience is available. Because gelatin used in the United States as a vaccine stabilizer usually is porcine and food gelatins may be derived solely from bovine sources, a negative food history does not exclude the possibility of an immunization reaction.

Hepatitis B vaccines are manufactured using recombinant technology by harvesting purified hepatitis B surface antigen from genetically engineered yeast cells containing the hepatitis B surface antigen. HPV4 is a noninfectious recombinant vaccine prepared from highly purified virus-like particles of the major capsid, L1, protein of the 4 HPV types in the vaccine. The L1 proteins are produced by separate fermentations in recombinant yeast cells and self-assembled into viral-like proteins, which are adsorbed on preformed aluminum-containing adjuvant. Purification results in a substantial reduction of yeast protein contained in the vaccines, but in rare instances, vaccine recipients with a significant hypersensitivity to yeast products may experience an allergic reaction to hepatitis B or HPV4 vaccine that would contraindicate receiving additional doses.

Reactions occur with DTaP vaccines but are much less common than with DTP vaccines. On occasion, urticarial or anaphylactic reactions have occurred in recipients of DTP, DTaP, DT (diphtheria and tetanus toxoids for children younger than 7 years of age), Td, or tetanus toxoid-containing vaccines. Tetanus and diphtheria antigen-specific antibodies of the IgE type have been identified in some of these patients. Although attributing a specific sensitivity to vaccine components is difficult, an immediate, severe, or anaphylactic allergic reaction to any vaccine or vaccine component is a contraindication to subsequent immunization of the patient with the specific component(s). A transient urticarial rash, however, is not a contraindication to further doses (see Appendix VI, p 847).

People who have high serum concentrations of tetanus IgG antibody, usually as the result of frequent booster immunizations, have an increased incidence and severity of adverse reactions to subsequent vaccine administration (see Tetanus, p 655). These Arthus-like (immune complex-mediated) reactions present as extensive painful swelling, often from shoulder to elbow.

Measles vaccines, including MMR and MMRV, and rabies vaccines contain albumin, a derivative of human blood. Reactions resembling serum sickness have been reported in approximately 6% of patients after a booster dose of human diploid rabies vaccine, probably resulting from sensitization to human albumin that had been altered chemically by the virus-inactivating agent.

The inactivated mouse brain-derived Japanese encephalitis virus vaccine, which was licensed for use in the United States in 1992, has been associated with generalized urticaria and angioedema and sometimes with respiratory distress and hypotension, occurring within minutes of immunization to as long as 2 weeks after immunization. This vaccine will be replaced by new-generation Japanese encephalitis virus vaccines to be used for certain people traveling to areas with endemic infection (see Control Measures in Arboviruses, p 214).

ADJUVANTS

Sterile abscesses have occurred at the site of injection of certain inactivated vaccines. Generally, these abscesses result from a hypersensitivity response to the vaccine or its adjuvant (especially alum); in some instances, these reactions may be caused by inadvertent SC inoculation of a vaccine intended for IM use. Alum-related abscesses frequently recur with subsequent dose(s) of vaccines containing alum. Administration of bacille Calmette-Guérin vaccine often is followed by occurrence of local cysts, abscesses, and/or regional lymphadenopathy that will resolve spontaneously (see Tuberculosis, p 680).

LATEX ALLERGY

Latex frequently is used to produce vaccine vial stoppers and syringe plungers. It contains naturally occurring impurities (eg, plant proteins and peptides) that may be responsible for allergies. Information about latex used in vaccine packaging is available in the manufacturer's package insert.

Hypersensitivity reactions to latex after immunization procedures are rare. Vaccines supplied in vials or syringes that contain latex should not be administered to a person reporting a severe allergy to latex unless the benefit of immunization outweighs the risk of anaphylaxis. However, vaccines can be administered to people with reactions other than anaphylaxis to latex.

Reporting of Vaccine-Preventable Diseases

Most vaccine-preventable diseases are reportable throughout the United States (see Appendix V, p 845). Public health officials depend on health care professionals to report promptly to state or local health departments suspected cases of vaccine-preventable disease. These reports are transmitted weekly to the CDC and are used to detect outbreaks, monitor disease-control strategies, and evaluate national immunization practices and policies. Reports provide useful information about vaccine efficacy, changing or current epidemiology of vaccine-preventable diseases, and possible epidemics that could threaten public health. Reporting confirmed and suspected vaccine-preventable diseases is a legal obligation of the physician.

Standards for Child and Adolescent Immunization Practices (see Appendix VII, p 854)

The national *Standards for Pediatric Immunization Practices* were revised by the National Vaccine Advisory Committee, endorsed by the AAP and numerous other medical and public health organizations, and published in *Pediatrics*.[1] As part of this revision, the standards were renamed *Standards for Child and Adolescent Immunization Practices*. These standards include the most essential and desirable immunization practices and are recommended for use by all health care professionals providing care in public or private health care settings who are involved in administration of vaccines or management of immunization services for children. Their use is intended to help identify needed changes in office practices, to improve preschool immunization rates, to prevent vaccine-preventable disease outbreaks, and to achieve national objectives for immunization. The revised standards reflect the increasing role of private practitioners, the importance of adolescent immunization, and recent increases in vaccine safety concerns among the general public.

Common Misconceptions About Immunizations

Misconceptions about the need for and safety of recommended childhood and adolescent immunizations are potential causes of delayed immunization, underimmunization, or both. The National Network for Immunization Information has published a resource kit (**www.immunizationinfo.org**) that includes common misinformed claims, facts, and links to scientific information. Table 1.8 (p 52) outlines several of these misconceptions.

The concerns about potential associations of MMR vaccine and autism, as well as thimerosal-containing vaccines and autism, have been evaluated in many studies. Evidence from several studies examining trends in vaccine use and changes in the frequency of autism does not support such an association. In addition, the Immunization Safety Review Committee of the IOM examined the hypothesis that MMR vaccine and thimerosal-containing vaccines are associated with autism (see IOM Immunization Safety Review Committee, p 41). The IOM Immunization Safety Review Committee developed and published several conclusions and recommendations, including the following:

---

[1] The National Vaccine Advisory Committee. Standards for child and adolescent immunization practices. *Pediatrics*. 2003;112(4):958–963

Table 1.8 Common Misconceptions About Immunizations[a]

Claims	Facts
Natural methods of enhancing immunity are better than vaccinations.	The only "natural way" to be immune is to have the disease. Immunity from a preventive vaccine provides protection against disease when a person is exposed to it in the future. That immunity is usually similar to what is acquired from natural infection, although several doses of a vaccine may have to be given for a child to develop a full immune response.
Epidemiology—often used to establish vaccine safety—is not science but number crunching.	Epidemiology is a well-established scientific discipline that, among other things, identifies the cause of diseases and factors that increase a person's risk for a disease.
Giving multiple vaccines at the same time causes an "overload" of the immune system.	Vaccination does not overburden a child's immune system; the recommended vaccines use only a small portion of the immune system's "memory."
Vaccines are ineffective.	Vaccines have spared millions of people the effects of devastating diseases.
Prior to the use of vaccinations, these diseases had begun to decline because of improved nutrition and hygiene.	In the 19th and 20th centuries, some infectious diseases began to be better controlled because of improvements in sanitation, clean water, pasteurized milk, and pest control. However, vaccine-preventable diseases decreased dramatically after the vaccines for those diseases were licensed and were given to large numbers of children.
Vaccines cause poorly understood illnesses or disorders, such as autism, sudden infant death syndrome (SIDS), immune dysfunction, diabetes, neurologic disorders, allergic rhinitis, eczema, and asthma.	Scientific evidence does not support these claims.[1] See IOM reports.
Vaccines weaken the immune system.	If vaccines weakened the immune system, vaccinated children would be at greater risk from diseases not prevented by vaccines. Several studies have shown that this is not the case. Importantly, natural infections like influenza, measles, and chickenpox do weaken the immune system, increasing the risk of other infections.
Giving many vaccines at the same time is untested.	Concomitant use studies require all new vaccines to be tested with existing vaccines. These studies are performed to ensure that new vaccines do not affect the safety or effectiveness of existing vaccines given at the same time and that existing vaccines administered at the same time do not affect the safety or effectiveness of new vaccines.

Adapted from: Myers MG, Pineda D. *Do Vaccines Cause That? A Guide for Evaluating Vaccine Safety Concerns.* Galveston, TX: Immunizations for Public Health; 2008:79

[a]See IOM Immunization Safety Review Committee (p 41).

- Scientific evidence favors rejection of a causal relationship between thimerosal-containing vaccines and autism.
- Scientific evidence favors rejection of a causal relationship between MMR vaccine and autism.
- Available funding for autism research should be channeled to more promising areas of inquiry.
- Risk-benefit communication requires attention to the needs of both the scientific community and the public.

Each person understands and reacts to information regarding vaccines on the basis of many factors, including past experience, education, perception of risk of disease and vaccine offered, perception of his or her ability to control risk, and personal values. Although parents receive information from multiple sources, they consider health care professionals their most trusted source of health information. Health care professionals should obtain and distribute copies of available AAP and CDC immunization documents, as well as the required VISs, to parents to address their questions and concerns. These materials are written in understandable language and can help parents make informed decisions about immunizing their children. Other sources of objective vaccine information are available (see the list of selected authoritative Web sites, below) that can help health care professionals respond to questions and misconceptions about immunizations and vaccine-preventable diseases. Various approaches to informing patients and parents about the benefits and risks of disease prevention, including immunizations (see Informing Patients and Parents, p 5), and approaches to parents who refuse immunizations for their child (see Parental Refusal of Immunization, p 8) are available.

The National Network for Immunization Information (NNii) provides up-to-date, science-based information to health care professionals, the media, policy makers, and the public. The NNii also provides additional reliable resources for current immunization information and has published a resource kit, "Communicating With Patients About Immunization." Immunization information can be found on the NNii Web site (**www.immunizationinfo.org**).

INTERNET RESOURCES FOR IMMUNIZATION INFORMATION

Several health professional associations, nonprofit groups, universities, and government organizations provide Internet resources containing immunization information.

HEALTH PROFESSIONAL ASSOCIATIONS

American Academy of Family Physicians (AAFP)
www.familydoctor.org
American Academy of Pediatrics (AAP)
www.aap.org
www.cispimmunize.org (AAP Childhood Immunization Support Program)
American Medical Association (AMA)
www.ama-assn.org
American Nurses Association (ANA)
www.nursingworld.org
Association of State and Territorial Health Officials (ASTHO)
www.astho.org

Association of Teachers of Preventive Medicine (ATPM)
www.atpm.org/prof_dev/ed.html
National Medical Association (NMA)
www.nmanet.org

NONPROFIT GROUPS AND UNIVERSITIES

Albert B. Sabin Vaccine Institute
www.sabin.org
Allied Vaccine Group (AVG)
www.vaccine.org
Every Child By Two (ECBT)
www.ecbt.org
www.vaccinateyourbaby.org
GAVI Alliance
www.vaccinealliance.org
Health on the Net Foundation (HON)
www.hon.ch
National Healthy Mothers, Healthy Babies Coalition (HMHB)
www.hmhb.org
Immunization Action Coalition (IAC)
www.immunize.org
Institute for Vaccine Safety (IVS), Johns Hopkins University
www.vaccinesafety.edu
Institute of Medicine (IOM)
www.iom.edu/?ID=4705
National Alliance for Hispanic Health
www.hispanichealth.org
National Network for Immunization Information (NNii)
www.immunizationinfo.org
Parents of Kids with Infectious Diseases (PKIDS)
www.pkids.org
Texas Children's Hospital Vaccine Center
www.vaccine.texaschildrenshospital.org
The Vaccine Education Center at the Children's Hospital of Philadelphia
www.vaccine.chop.edu
The Vaccine Page
www.vaccines.com
University of Pennsylvania
www.vaccineethics.org
World Health Organization
www.who.int/topics/immunization/en/

GOVERNMENT ORGANIZATIONS

Centers for Disease Control and Prevention (CDC)
www.cdc.gov/vaccines
www.cdc.gov/vaccinesafety

Food and Drug Administration (FDA)
www.fda.gov/cber/vaccines.htm
National Vaccine Program Office (NVPO)
www.hhs.gov/nvpo/
National Institute of Allergy and Infectious Diseases (NIAID)
www3.niaid.nih.gov/topics/vaccines/default.htm

PASSIVE IMMUNIZATION

Passive immunization entails administration of preformed antibody to a recipient. Passive immunization is indicated in the following general circumstances for prevention or amelioration of infectious diseases:

- When people are deficient in synthesis of antibody as a result of congenital or acquired B-lymphocyte defects, alone or in combination with other immunodeficiencies.
- Prophylactically, when a person susceptible to a disease is exposed to or has a high likelihood of exposure to that infection, especially when that person has a high risk of complications from the disease or when time does not permit adequate protection by active immunization alone.
- Therapeutically, when a disease is already present, antibody may ameliorate or aid in suppressing the effects of a toxin (eg, foodborne or wound botulism, diphtheria, or tetanus) or suppress the inflammatory response (eg, Kawasaki disease).

Passive immunization has been accomplished with several types of products. The choice is dictated by the types of products available, the type of antibody desired, the route of administration, timing, and other considerations. These products include Immune Globulin (IG) and specific ("hyperimmune") IG preparations given intramuscularly, Immune Globulin Intravenous (IGIV), specific (hyperimmune) IG given by the intravenous (IV) route (eg, Botulism Immune Globulin, Cytomegalovirus Immune Globulin [CMV-IGIV]), and antibodies of animal origin and monoclonal antibodies. Immune Globulin Subcutaneous (Human) has been approved for treatment of patients with primary immune deficiency states.

Indications for administration of IG preparations other than those relevant to infectious diseases are not reviewed in the *Red Book*.

Whole blood and blood components for transfusion (including plasma) from US registered blood banks are released only after appropriate donor screening and testing for the presence of bloodborne pathogens, including syphilis, hepatitis B virus, hepatitis C virus (HCV), human immunodeficiency virus (HIV)-1, HIV-2, human T-lymphotropic virus (HTLV)-1, and HTLV-2; most donations for *Trypanosoma cruzi* (Chagas disease); and selected donations for CMV. Whole blood and blood components also are batch tested for West Nile virus; during an outbreak in a particular geographic area, units may be tested by individual unit nucleic acid amplification testing (see Blood Safety, p 106; and West Nile Virus, p 730). A similar array of tests is performed by US-licensed establishments that collect plasma used only to manufacture plasma derivatives, such as IGIV, IG, and specific immune globulins. IG and specific immune globulin preparations licensed in the United States have not been associated with transmission of any of these diseases. HCV transmission in 1994 was associated with administration of IGIV produced by a single manufacturer. The US Food and Drug Administration (FDA) now requires that IGIV and other immune globulin preparations for IV or intramuscular (IM) administration undergo additional manufacturing procedures that inactivate or remove viruses.

Immune Globulin (Intramuscular)

IG (IM) is derived from pooled plasma of adults by an alcohol-fractionation procedure. IG consists primarily of the immunoglobulin (Ig) fraction (at least 96% IgG and trace amounts of IgA and IgM), is sterile, and is not known to transmit hepatotropic viruses, HIV, or any other infectious disease agents. IG is a concentrated protein solution (approximately 16.5% or 165 mg/mL) containing specific antibodies that reflect the infectious and immunization experience of the population from whose plasma the IG was prepared. Many donors (at least 1000 donors per lot of final product) are used to include a broad spectrum of antibodies.

IG is licensed and recommended for IM administration. Therefore, IG should be administered deep into a large muscle mass, usually in the gluteal region or anterior thigh of a child (see Site and Route of Immunization, p 18). Ordinarily, no more than 5 mL should be administered at one site in an adult, adolescent, or large child; a lesser volume per site (1–3 mL) should be given to small children and infants. Health care professionals should refer to the package insert for total maximal dose at one time. Serum concentrations of antibodies usually are achieved 3 to 5 days after IM administration.

Intravenous use of human IG is contraindicated. Intradermal use of IG is not recommended. Subcutaneous administration has been shown to be safe and effective in children and adults with primary immunodeficiency (see Immune Globulin Subcutaneous, p 61).

INDICATIONS FOR THE USE OF IG

REPLACEMENT THERAPY IN ANTIBODY DEFICIENCY DISORDERS. The usual dose (limited by muscle mass and the volume that should be administered) is 100 mg/kg (equivalent to 0.66 mL/kg) per month intramuscularly. Customary practice is to administer twice this dose initially and to adjust the interval between administration of the doses (2–4 weeks) on the basis of trough IgG concentrations and clinical response (absence of or decrease in infections). For most cases, IG administered intramuscularly has been replaced by IGIV or subcutaneously administered IG, because higher plasma Ig concentrations and greater efficacy can be achieved.

HEPATITIS A PROPHYLAXIS. In people 12 months through 40 years of age, hepatitis A immunization is preferred over IG for postexposure prophylaxis against hepatitis A virus infection and for protection of travelers going to areas with endemic hepatitis A infection. For people younger than 12 months or older than 40 years of age, immunocompromised people of all ages, and people who have chronic liver disease, IG is preferred (see Hepatitis A, p 329).

MEASLES PROPHYLAXIS. IG administered to exposed, measles-susceptible people will prevent or attenuate infection if given within 6 days of exposure (see Measles, p 444).

RUBELLA PROPHYLAXIS. IG administered to rubella-susceptible pregnant women after rubella exposure may decrease the risk of fetal infection (see Rubella, p 579).

ADVERSE REACTIONS TO IG

- Most recipients experience local discomfort, and some experience pain at the site of IG administration (which are lessened if the preparation is at room temperature at the time of injection). Less common reactions include flushing, headache, chills, and nausea.
- Serious reactions are uncommon; these reactions may involve chest pain or constriction, dyspnea, anaphylaxis, or hypotension and shock. An increased risk of systemic reaction results from inadvertent IV administration. People requiring repeated doses of IG have been reported to experience systemic reactions, such as fever, chills, sweating, and shock.
- Because IG contains trace amounts of IgA, people who have IgA deficiency can develop anti-IgA antibodies on rare occasions and react to a subsequent dose of IG. These reactions include systemic symptoms such as chills, fever, and shock-like symptoms. In rare cases in which reactions related to anti-IgA antibodies have occurred, use of IgA-depleted IGIV preparations may decrease the likelihood of further reactions. Because these reactions are rare, routine screening for IgA deficiency is not recommended.

PRECAUTIONS FOR THE USE OF IG

- Caution should be used when giving IG to a patient with a history of adverse reactions to IG.
- Although systemic reactions to IG are rare (see Adverse Reactions to IG, above), epinephrine and other means of treating serious acute reactions should be available immediately. Health care professionals administering IG should have training to manage emergencies appropriately.
- IG should not be used in patients with severe thrombocytopenia or any coagulation disorder that would preclude IM injection. In such cases, use of IGIV is recommended.

Specific Immune Globulins

Specific immune globulins, termed "hyperimmune globulins," differ from other preparations in selection of donors and may differ in number of donors whose plasma is included in the pool from which the product is prepared. Donors known to have high titers of the desired antibody, naturally acquired or stimulated by immunization, are selected. Specific immune globulins are prepared by the same procedure as other immune globulin preparations. Specific immune globulin preparations for use in infectious diseases include Hepatitis B Immune Globulin, Rabies Immune Globulin, Tetanus Immune Globulin, investigational Varicella-Zoster Immune Globulin, CMV-IGIV, and Botulism Immune Globulin Intravenous (for infant botulism). Recommendations for use of these immune globulins are provided in the discussions of specific diseases in Section 3. The precautions and adverse reactions for IG and IGIV are applicable to specific immune globulins. An intramuscularly administered humanized mouse monoclonal antibody preparation for prevention of respiratory syncytial virus is available.

Immune Globulin Intravenous

IGIV is made by individual manufacturers from pooled plasma of adults using methods designed to prepare a product suitable for IV use. The FDA recommends that the number of donors contributing to a pool used for IGIV be greater than 15 000 but no more than 60 000 donors. IGIV consists of more than 95% IgG and trace amounts of IgA and IgM. IGIV is available in lyophilized powder or as a premixed liquid solution, with final concentrations of IgG of 3% to 12% depending on the products. IGIV does not contain thimerosal. IGIV products vary in their sodium content, type and concentration of sugar, osmolarity and osmolality, pH, IgA content, volume load, and infusion rate. Each of these factors may contribute to tolerability. The FDA specifies that all IGIV preparations must have a minimum concentration of antibodies to measles virus, *Corynebacterium diphtheriae*, poliovirus, and hepatitis B virus. Antibody concentrations against other pathogens, such as *Streptococcus pneumoniae*, vary widely among products and even among lots from the same manufacturer.

INDICATIONS FOR THE USE OF IGIV

Initially, IGIV was developed as an infusion product that allowed patients with primary immunodeficiencies to receive enough IG at monthly intervals to protect them from infection until their next infusion. IGIV currently is approved by the FDA in the United States for 6 conditions (Table 1.9, p 59). IGIV products also may be useful for other conditions, although demonstrated efficacy from controlled trials is not available in all cases.

Licensure by the FDA of specific indications for a manufacturer's IGIV product is based on availability of data from one or more clinical trials that demonstrate that the product has the effect it is represented to have under the conditions of use specified in the labeling. All IGIV products are licensed for primary immunodeficiencies and most are licensed for immune-mediated thrombocytopenia, but not all licensed products are approved for the other indications listed in Table 1.9. In some cases, only a single product has the indication in its product label. Therapeutic differences among IGIV products from different manufacturers are likely to exist but may not have been demonstrated in any clinical trials designed to determine whether such differences exist. Among the licensed IGIV products, but not necessarily for each product individually, indications for prevention or treatment of infectious diseases in children and adolescents include the following:

- **Replacement therapy in antibody-deficiency disorders.** The usual dosage of IGIV in immune-deficiency syndromes is 400 to 600 mg/kg, administered approximately every 21 to 28 days by infusion. Effective dosages have ranged from 200 to 800 mg/kg monthly. Maintenance of a trough IgG concentration of at least 500 mg/dL (5 g/L) has been demonstrated to correlate with clinical response. Studies in children with agammaglobulinemia suggest that IgG trough concentrations maintained at greater than 800 mg/dL prevented serious bacterial illnesses and enteroviral meningoencephalitis. Dosage and frequency of infusions should be based on clinical effectiveness in the individual patient and in conjunction with an expert on immunodeficiency disorders.
- **Kawasaki disease.** Administration of IGIV at a dose of 2 g/kg as a single dose within the first 10 days of onset of fever decreases the frequency of coronary artery abnormalities and shortens the duration of symptoms (see Kawasaki Disease, p 413).

Table 1.9. Uses of Immune Globulin Intravenous (IGIV) for Which There is Approval by the US Food and Drug Administration[a]

Primary immunodeficiency states

Kawasaki disease

Immune-mediated thrombocytopenia

Pediatric human immunodeficiency virus infection

Secondary immunodeficiency in chronic lymphocytic leukemia

Prevention of graft-versus-host disease and infection in hematopoietic cell transplantation in adults

[a]Therapeutic differences among IGIV products from different manufacturers are likely to exist.

- *Pediatric HIV infection.* In children with HIV infection and hypogammaglobulinemia, IGIV may be used to prevent serious bacterial infection. IGIV also might be considered for HIV-infected children who have recurrent serious bacterial infection[1] (see Human Immunodeficiency Virus Infection, p 380).
- *Hypogammaglobulinemia in chronic B-cell lymphocytic leukemia.* Administration of IGIV to adults with this disease has been demonstrated to decrease the incidence of serious bacterial infections, although its cost-effectiveness has been questioned.
- *Stem cell transplantation.* IGIV may decrease the incidence of infection and death but does not decrease the incidence of acute graft-versus-host disease (GVHD) in pediatric stem cell transplant recipients. In adult transplant recipients, IGIV decreases the incidence of interstitial pneumonia (presumably caused by cytomegalovirus [CMV]), decreases the risk of sepsis and other bacterial infections, decreases the incidence of acute GVHD (but not overall mortality), and in conjunction with ganciclovir, is effective in treatment of some patients with CMV pneumonia.
- *Varicella postexposure prophylaxis.* If Varicella-Zoster Immune Globulin (VariZIG) is not available, IGIV should be considered as an alternative for certain people up to 96 hours after exposure to varicella (see Varicella-Zoster Infections, p 714). For maximum benefit, it should be administered as soon as possible after exposure.

  IGIV also has been used for many other conditions, some of which are listed below.
- *Low birth weight infants.* Results of most clinical trials have indicated that IGIV does not decrease the incidence or mortality rate of late-onset infections in infants who weigh less than 1500 g at birth. Trials have varied in IGIV dosage, time of administration, and other aspects of study design. IGIV is not recommended for routine use in preterm infants to prevent late-onset infection.

---

[1]Centers for Disease Control and Prevention. Guidelines for prevention and treatment of opportunistic infections among HIV-exposed and HIV-infected children. Recommendations from CDC, the National Institutes of Health, the HIV Medical Association of the Infectious Diseases Society of America, the Pediatric Infectious Diseases Society, and the American Academy of Pediatrics. *MMWR*. 2009; in press

- *Guillain-Barré syndrome and chronic inflammatory demyelinating poly-neuropathy.* In Guillain-Barré syndrome and chronic inflammatory demyelinating polyneuropathy, IGIV treatment has been demonstrated to have efficacy equivalent to that of plasmapheresis.
- *Toxic shock syndrome.* IGIV has been administered to patients with severe staphylococcal or streptococcal toxic shock syndrome and necrotizing fasciitis. Therapy appears most likely to be beneficial when used early in the course of illness.
- *Other potential uses.* IGIV may be useful for severe anemia caused by parvovirus B19 infection and for neonatal alloimmune thrombocytopenia that is unresponsive to other treatments, immune-mediated neutropenia, decompensation in myasthenia gravis, dermatomyositis, polymyositis, and severe thrombocytopenia that is unresponsive to other treatments.

For several years after November 1997, periodic shortages of IGIV existed in the United States because of production impediments related to compliance and product recall based on the theoretical risk of contamination with the Creutzfeldt-Jakob disease (CJD) agent. Other problems that may cause short supply of IGIV include increased administration for approved and unapproved uses, wastage, and exportation of IGIV to other countries. The FDA is using several methods to improve IGIV distribution to patients. Clinicians should review their IGIV use to ensure consistency with current recommendations. Off-label use of IGIV should be limited until there is adequate scientific evidence of effectiveness.

An outbreak of HCV infection occurred in the United States in 1994 among recipients of IGIV lots from a single domestic manufacturer. Changes in the preparation of IGIV, including additional viral inactivation steps (ie, solvent/detergent exposure, pH 4 incubation, nanofiltration, and partitioning), subsequent to this episode have been instituted to prevent transmission of HCV by IGIV infusion. All products currently available in the United States are believed to be free of known pathogens. HIV infection never has been transmitted by IGIV.

ADVERSE REACTIONS TO IGIV

Reactions such as fever, headache, myalgia, chills, nausea, and vomiting often are related to the rate of IGIV infusion and usually are mild to moderate and self-limited. These reactions may result from formation of IgG aggregates during manufacture or storage. There may be product-to-product variations in adverse effects among individual patients. Isoimmune hemolytic reaction is described rarely, especially if large doses of IGIV are infused. Less common but severe reactions include hypersensitivity and anaphylactoid reactions marked by flushing, changes in blood pressure, and tachycardia; thromboembolic events; aseptic meningitis; and renal insufficiency and failure. The causes of these reactions are unknown. Adverse events often can be decreased by following the package insert for the individual product carefully with regard to rate of administration. Aseptic meningitis associated with pleocytosis may occur, especially among patients receiving high doses of IGIV (2 g/kg). Acute renal failure has been reported rarely following IGIV infusions, particularly among patients with preexisting renal disease who receive IGIV products containing sucrose.

Anaphylactic reactions induced by anti-IgA can occur in patients with primary antibody deficiency who have a total absence of circulating IgA and develop IgG antibodies to IgA. These reactions are rare in patients with panhypogammaglobulinemia and potentially are more common in patients with selective IgA deficiency and subclass IgG deficiencies. In rare instances in which reactions related to anti-IgA antibodies have occurred, use of IgA-depleted IGIV preparations may decrease the likelihood of further reactions. Because of the extreme rarity of these reactions, however, screening for IgA deficiency and anti-IgA antibodies is not recommended routinely.

PRECAUTIONS FOR THE USE OF IGIV

- Caution should be used when giving IGIV to a patient with a history of adverse reactions to IG.
- Because systemic reactions to IGIV may occur (see Adverse Reactions to IGIV), epinephrine and other means of treating acute reactions should be available immediately.
- Adverse reactions often can be alleviated by reducing either the rate or the volume of infusion. For patients with repeated severe reactions unresponsive to these measures, hydrocortisone (Solu-Cortef: 5–6 mg/kg in children or 100–150 mg in adults, or Solu-Medrol: 2 mg/kg) can be given intravenously 30 minutes before infusion. Using a different IGIV preparation or pretreatment with prednisone, diphenhydramine, acetaminophen, a nonsteroidal anti-inflammatory agent, or aspirin may modify or relieve symptoms.
- Seriously ill patients with compromised cardiac function who are receiving large volumes of IGIV may be at increased risk of vasomotor or cardiac complications manifested by elevated blood pressure, cardiac failure, or both.
- Screening for IgA deficiency is not recommended routinely for potential recipients of IGIV (see Adverse Reactions to IGIV).

Immune Globulin Subcutaneous

Subcutaneous (SC) administration of Immune Globulin using battery-driven pumps has been shown to be safe and effective in adults and children with primary immunodeficiencies. Smaller doses, administered more frequently (ie, weekly), result in more even serum IgG concentrations over time. Systemic reactions are less frequent than with IV therapy, and some parents or patients can be taught to infuse at home. The most common adverse effects of SC administration of IG are injection-site reactions, including local swelling, redness, itching, soreness, induration, and local heat. There is only one product licensed in the United States for SC use. There are no data on administration of IgG by the SC route for conditions requiring high-dose Immune Globulin, such as Kawasaki disease and idiopathic thrombocytopenic purpura.

Antibodies of Animal Origin (Animal Antisera)

Products of animal origin used for neutralization of toxins or prophylaxis of infectious diseases are derived from serum of horses immunized with the agent/toxoid of interest. Experimental products prepared in other species also may be available. These products are derived by concentrating the serum globulin fraction with ammonium sulfate. Some, but not all, products are subjected to an enzyme digestion process to decrease clinical reactions to administered foreign proteins. These animal-derived immunoglobulin products are referred to here as serum, for convenience.

Use of the following products is discussed in the disease-specific chapters in Section 3:

- Botulism Antitoxin (Equine), available from the Centers for Disease Control and Prevention (CDC).
- Diphtheria Antitoxin (Equine), available from the CDC. The currently available product is manufactured in Brazil and is available only under an investigational new drug protocol.

INDICATIONS FOR USE OF ANIMAL ANTISERA

Antibody-containing products prepared from animal sera pose a special risk to the recipient, and the use of such products should be limited strictly to certain indications for which specific IG preparations of human origin are not available (eg, diphtheria and botulism other than infant botulism).

REACTIONS TO ANIMAL SERA

Before any animal serum is injected, the patient must be questioned about his or her history of asthma, allergic rhinitis, and urticaria after previous exposure to animals or injections of animal sera. Patients with a history of asthma or allergic symptoms, especially from exposure to horses, can be dangerously sensitive to equine sera and should be given these products with the utmost caution. People who previously have received animal sera are at increased risk of developing allergic reactions and serum sickness after administration of sera from the same animal species.

SENSITIVITY TESTS FOR REACTIONS TO ANIMAL SERA

Each patient who is to be given animal serum should be skin tested before administration of that animal serum. Intradermal (ID) skin tests have resulted in fatalities, but the scratch test usually is safe. Therefore, scratch tests always should precede ID tests. Nevertheless, any sensitivity test must be performed by trained personnel familiar with treatment of acute anaphylaxis; necessary medications and equipment should be available readily (see Treatment of Anaphylactic Reactions, p 65).

SCRATCH, PRICK, OR PUNCTURE TEST.[1] Apply 1 drop of a 1:100 dilution of serum in preservative-free isotonic sodium chloride solution to the site of a superficial scratch, prick, or puncture on the volar aspect of the forearm. Positive (histamine) and negative (physiologic saline solution) control tests for the scratch test also should be applied. A positive test result is a wheal with surrounding erythema at least 3 mm larger than the negative control test area, read at 15 to 20 minutes. The histamine control must be positive for valid interpretation. If the scratch test result is negative, an ID test is performed.

INTRADERMAL TEST.[1] A dose of 0.02 mL of a 1:1000 dilution of serum in preservative-free isotonic saline-diluted serum (enough to raise a small wheal) is administered. Positive and negative control tests, as described for the scratch test, also should be applied. If the test result is negative, it should be repeated using a 1:100 dilution. For people with negative history for both animal allergy and previous exposure to animal serum, the 1:100 dilution may be used initially if a scratch, prick, or puncture test result with the serum is negative. Interpretation is the same as for the scratch test.

---

[1]Antihistamines may inhibit reactions in the scratch, prick, or puncture test and in the ID test; hence, testing should not be performed for at least 24 hours or, preferably, 48 hours after receipt of these drugs.

Positive test results not attributable to an irritant reaction indicate sensitivity, but a negative skin test result is not an absolute guarantee of lack of sensitivity. Therefore, animal sera should be administered with caution even to people whose test results are negative. Immediate hypersensitivity testing is performed to identify IgE-mediated disease and does not predict other immune reactions, such as serum sickness.

If the ID test result is positive or if the history of systemic anaphylaxis after previous administration of serum is highly suggestive in a person for whom the need for serum is unquestioned, desensitization can be undertaken (see Desensitization to Animal Sera).

If history and sensitivity test results are negative, the indicated dose of serum can be given intramuscularly. The patient should be observed afterward for at least 30 minutes. IV administration may be indicated if a high concentration of serum antibody is imperative, such as for treatment of diphtheria or botulism. In these instances, serum should be diluted and slowly administered intravenously according to the manufacturer's instructions. The patient should be monitored carefully for signs or symptoms of anaphylaxis.

DESENSITIZATION TO ANIMAL SERA

Tables 1.10 (p 64) and 1.11 (p 64) serve as guides for desensitization procedures for administration of animal sera. IV (Table 1.10) or ID, subcutaneous, or IM (Table 1.11) regimens may be chosen. The IV route is considered safest, because it offers better control. The desensitization procedure must be performed by trained personnel familiar with treatment of anaphylaxis and with appropriate drugs and available equipment (see Treatment of Anaphylactic Reactions, p 65). Some physicians advocate concurrent use of an oral or parenteral antihistamine (such as diphenhydramine) during the procedure, with or without IV hydrocortisone or methylprednisolone. If signs of anaphylaxis occur, aqueous epinephrine should be administered immediately (see Treatment of Anaphylactic Reactions, p 65). Administration of sera during a desensitization procedure must be continuous, because if administration is interrupted, protection achieved by desensitization will be lost.

TYPES OF REACTIONS TO ANIMAL SERA

The following reactions can occur as the result of administration of animal sera. Of these, only anaphylaxis is mediated by IgE antibodies, and thus, occurrence can be predicted by previous skin testing results.

ACUTE FEBRILE REACTIONS. These reactions usually are mild and can be treated with antipyretic agents. Severe febrile reactions should be treated with antipyretic agents or other safe available methods to decrease temperature physically.

SERUM SICKNESS. Manifestations, which usually begin 7 to 10 days (occasionally as late as 3 weeks) after primary exposure to the foreign protein, consist of fever, urticaria, or a maculopapular rash (90% of cases); arthritis or arthralgia; and lymphadenopathy. Local edema can occur at the serum injection site a few days before systemic signs and symptoms appear. Angioedema, glomerulonephritis, Guillain-Barré syndrome, peripheral neuritis, and myocarditis also can occur. However, serum sickness may be mild and resolve spontaneously within a few days to 2 weeks. People who previously have received serum injections are at increased risk after readministration; manifestations in these patients usually occur shortly (from hours to 3 days) after administration of serum. Antihistamines can be helpful for management of serum sickness for alleviation of pruritus, edema, and

Table 1.10. Desensitization to Serum—Intravenous (IV) Route

Dose Number[a]	Dilution of Serum in Isotonic Sodium Chloride	Amount of IV Injection, mL
1	1:1000	0.1
2	1:1000	0.3
3	1:1000	0.6
4	1:100	0.1
5	1:100	0.3
6	1:100	0.6
7	1:10	0.1
8	1:10	0.3
9	1:10	0.6
10	Undiluted	0.1
11	Undiluted	0.3
12	Undiluted	0.6
13	Undiluted	1.0

[a]Administer consistently at 15-minute intervals.

Table 1.11. Desensitization to Serum—Intradermal (ID), Subcutaneous (SC), and Intramuscular (IM) Routes

Dose Number[a]	Route of Administration	Dilution of Serum in Isotonic Sodium Chloride	Amount of ID, SC, or IM Injection, mL
1	ID	1:1000	0.1
2	ID	1:1000	0.3
3	SC	1:1000	0.6
4	SC	1:100	0.1
5	SC	1:100	0.3
6	SC	1:100	0.6
7	SC	1:10	0.1
8	SC	1:10	0.3
9	SC	1:10	0.6
10	SC	Undiluted	0.1
11	SC	Undiluted	0.3
12	IM	Undiluted	0.6
13	IM	Undiluted	1.0

[a]Administer consistently at 15-minute intervals.

urticaria. Fever, malaise, arthralgia, and arthritis can be controlled in most patients by administration of aspirin or other nonsteroidal anti-inflammatory agents. Corticosteroids may be helpful for controlling serious manifestations that are controlled poorly by other agents; prednisone or prednisolone in therapeutic dosages (1.5–2 mg/kg per day; maximum 60 mg/day) for 5 to 7 days is an appropriate regimen.

ANAPHYLAXIS. The rapidity of onset and overall severity of anaphylaxis may vary considerably. Anaphylaxis usually begins within minutes of exposure to the causative agent, and in general, the more rapid the onset, the more severe the overall course. Major symptomatic manifestations include (1) cutaneous: pruritus, flushing, urticaria, and angioedema; (2) respiratory: hoarse voice and stridor, cough, wheeze, dyspnea, and cyanosis; (3) cardiovascular: rapid weak pulse, hypotension, and arrhythmias; and (4) gastrointestinal: cramps, vomiting, diarrhea, and dry mouth. Anaphylaxis is a medical emergency.

Treatment of Anaphylactic Reactions

Personnel administering biological products or serum must be able to recognize and be prepared to treat systemic anaphylaxis. Medications, equipment, and competent staff necessary to maintain the patency of the airway and to manage cardiovascular collapse must be available.[1]

The emergency treatment of systemic anaphylactic reactions is based on the type of reaction. In all instances, epinephrine is the primary drug. Mild symptoms of skin reaction alone (eg, pruritus, erythema, urticaria, or angioedema) intrinsically are not dangerous and can be treated with antihistamines (Table 1.12, p 66), but using clinical judgment, injection of epinephrine may be given (Table 1.13, p 67). Epinephrine should be injected promptly for anaphylaxis (eg, onset of symptoms minutes to several hours with involvement of skin, mucosal tissue, or both after administration of biological product or serum), which is likely (though not exclusively) occurring if the patient has: (1) skin symptoms (generalized hives, itch-flush, swollen lips/tongue/uvula) and respiratory compromise (dyspnea, wheeze, bronchospasm, stridor, or hypoxemia); or (2) 2 or more organ systems involved, including skin symptoms or respiratory compromise as described above, plus gastrointestinal tract symptoms (eg, persistent gastrointestinal tract symptoms, such as crampy abdominal pain or vomiting) or cardiovascular symptoms (eg, reduced blood pressure, syncope, collapse, hypotonia, incontinence). If a patient is known to have had a previous allergic reaction to the biological product/serum, onset of cardiovascular symptoms alone may warrant treatment with epinephrine.[2] Aqueous epinephrine, 0.01 mg/kg (maximum dose, 0.5 mg), usually is administered intramuscularly every 5 to 15 minutes as necessary to control symptoms and maintain blood pressure. Injections can be given at shorter than 5-minute intervals if deemed necessary. Because concentrations of epinephrine are higher and achieved more rapidly after IM administration, SC administration no longer is recommended. When the patient's condition improves and remains stable, oral

[1]Hegenbarth MA; American Academy of Pediatrics, Committee on Drugs. Preparing for pediatric emergencies: drugs to consider. *Pediatrics.* 2008;121(2):433–443

[2]Sampson HA, Munoz-Furlong A, Campbell RL, Adkinson NF, Jr, Bock SA, Branum A, et al. Second Symposium on the Definition and Management of Anaphylaxis: Summary Report-Second National Institute of Allergy and Infectious Disease/Food Allergy and Anaphylaxis Network Symposium. *J Allergy Clin Immunol.* 2006;117(2):391–397

Table 1.12. Epinephrine in the Treatment of Anaphylaxis[a]

Intramuscular (IM) administration
Epinephrine 1:1000 (aqueous): 0.01 mL/kg per dose, up to 0.5 mL, repeated every 10–20 min, up to 3 doses.[b]

Intravenous (IV) administration
An initial bolus of IV epinephrine is given to patients not responding to IM epinephrine using a dilution of 1:10 000 rather than a dilution of 1:1000. This dilution can be made using 1 mL of the 1:1000 dilution in 9 mL of physiologic saline solution. The dose is 0.01 mg/kg or 0.1 mL/kg of the 1:10 000 dilution. A continuous infusion should be started if repeated doses are required. One milligram (1 mL) of 1:1000 dilution of epinephrine added to 250 mL of 5% dextrose in water, resulting in a concentration of 4 μg/mL, is infused initially at a rate of 0.1 μg/kg per minute and increased gradually to 1.5 μg/kg per minute to maintain blood pressure.

[a]In addition to epinephrine, maintenance of the airway and administration of oxygen are critical.
[b]If agent causing anaphylactic reaction was given by injection, epinephrine can be injected into the same site to slow absorption.

antihistamines and possibly oral corticosteroids (1.5–2.0 mg/kg per day of prednisone; maximum 60 mg/day) can be given for an additional 24 to 48 hours.

Severe or potentially life-threatening systemic anaphylaxis involving severe bronchospasm, laryngeal edema, other airway compromise, shock, and cardiovascular collapse necessitates additional therapy. Maintenance of the airway and administration of oxygen should be instituted promptly. Epinephrine is administered intramuscularly immediately while IV access is being established. IV epinephrine may be indicated; for this use, the epinephrine must be diluted from 1:1000 aqueous base to a dilution of 1:10 000 using physiologic saline solution (see Table 1.12, above). Administration of epinephrine intravenously can lead to lethal arrhythmia; cardiac monitoring is recommended. A slow, continuous, low-dose infusion is preferable to repeated bolus administration, because the dose can be titrated to the desired effect, and accidental administration of large boluses of epinephrine can be avoided. Nebulized albuterol is indicated for bronchospasm (see Table 1.13, p 67). Rapid IV infusion of physiologic saline solution, lactated Ringer solution, or other isotonic solution adequate to maintain blood pressure must be instituted to compensate for the loss of circulating intravascular volume.

In some cases, the use of inotropic agents, such as dopamine (see Table 1.13, p 67), may be necessary for blood pressure support. The combination of histamine H_1 and H_2 receptor-blocking agents (see Table 1.12, above) can be synergistic in effect and should be used. Corticosteroids should be used in all cases of anaphylaxis except cases that are mild and have responded promptly to initial therapy (see Table 1.12, above). However, no data support the usefulness of corticosteroids in treating anaphylaxis, and therefore, they should not be considered primary drugs.

All patients showing signs and symptoms of systemic anaphylaxis, regardless of severity, should be observed for several hours in an appropriate facility. Biphasic and protracted anaphylaxis may be mitigated with early administration of oral corticosteroids; however, usefulness of corticosteroids for these 2 conditions has not been established fully. Therefore, patients should be observed even after remission of immediate symptoms. Although a specific period of observation has not been established, a period of observa-

Table 1.13. Dosages of Commonly Used Secondary Drugs in the Treatment of Anaphylaxis

Drug	Dose
H$_1$ receptor-blocking agents (antihistamines)	
Diphenhydramine	Oral, IM, IV: 1–2 mg/kg, every 4–6 h (100 mg, maximum single dose)
Hydroxyzine	Oral, IM: 0.5–1 mg/kg, every 4–6 h (100 mg, maximum single dose)
H$_2$ receptor-blocking agents (also antihistamines)	
Cimetidine	IV: 5 mg/kg, slowly over a 15-min period, every 6–8 h (300 mg, maximum single dose)
Ranitidine	IV: 1 mg/kg, slowly over a 15-min period, every 6–8 h (50 mg, maximum single dose)
Corticosteroids	
Hydrocortisone	IV: 100–200 mg, every 4–6 h
Methylprednisolone	IV: 1.5–2 mg/kg, every 4–6 h (60 mg, maximum single dose)
Prednisone	Oral: 1.5–2 mg/kg, single morning dose (60 mg, maximum single dose); use corticosteroids as long as needed
B$_2$-agonist	
Albuterol	Nebulizer solution: 0.5% (5 mg/mL), 0.05–0.15 mg/kg per dose in 2–3 mL isotonic sodium chloride solution, maximum 5 mg/dose every 20 min over a 1-h to 2-h period or 0.5 mg/kg/h by continuous nebulization (15 mg/h, maximum dose)
Other	
Dopamine	IV: 5–20 µg/kg per minute. Mixing 150 mg of dopamine with 250 mL of saline solution or 5% dextrose in water will produce a solution that, if infused at the rate of 1 mL/kg/h, will deliver 10 µg/kg/min. The solution must be free of bicarbonate, which may inactivate dopamine.

IM indicates intramuscular; IV, intravenous.

tion of 4 hours would be reasonable for mild episodes and as long as 24 hours would be reasonable for severe episodes.

Anaphylaxis occurring in people who are already taking beta-adrenergic–blocking agents presents a unique situation. In such people, the manifestations are likely to be more profound and significantly less responsive to epinephrine and other beta-adrenergic agonist drugs. More aggressive therapy with epinephrine may override receptor blockade in some patients. Some experts recommend use of IV glucagon for cardiovascular manifestations and inhaled atropine for management of bradycardia or bronchospasm.

....
IMMUNIZATION IN SPECIAL CLINICAL CIRCUMSTANCES

Preterm and Low Birth Weight Infants[1]

Preterm infants born at less than 37 weeks' gestation and infants of low birth weight (less than 2500 g) should, with few exceptions, receive all routinely recommended childhood vaccines at the same chronologic age as term infants. Gestational age and birth weight are not limiting factors when deciding whether a clinically stable preterm infant is to be immunized on schedule. Although studies have shown decreased immune responses to several vaccines given to very low birth weight (less than 1500 g) and very early gestational age (less than 29 weeks) neonates, most preterm infants, including infants who receive dexamethasone for chronic lung disease, produce sufficient vaccine-induced immunity to prevent disease. Vaccine dosages given to term infants should not be reduced or divided when given to preterm or low birth weight infants.

Preterm and low birth weight infants tolerate most childhood vaccines as well as term infants do. Apnea, reported to have occurred in some extremely low birth weight (less than 1000 g) infants after use of diphtheria and tetanus toxoids and whole-cell per-tussis vaccine (DTP), has not been reported after use of acellular pertussis-containing vaccines in small numbers of extremely low birth weight infants. However, preterm infants given heptavalent pneumococcal conjugate vaccine (PCV7) concomitantly with DTP and *Haemophilus influenzae* type b (Hib) vaccine were reported to experience benign febrile seizures more frequently than were term infants given the same vaccines. Cardiorespiratory events, including apnea and bradycardia with oxygen desaturation, frequently increase in very low birth weight infants given combination diphtheria and tetanus toxoids and acellular pertussis (DTaP), inactivated poliovirus, hepatitis B, and Hib conjugate vaccine. However, these episodes do not have a detrimental effect on the clinical course of immunized infants.

Medically stable preterm infants who remain in the hospital at 2 months of chronologic age should be given all inactivated vaccines recommended at that age (see Recommended Childhood and Adolescent Immunization Schedule, Fig 1.1–1.3, p 24–28). A medically stable infant is defined as one who does not require ongoing management for serious infection; metabolic disease; or acute renal, cardiovascular, neurologic, or respiratory tract illness and who demonstrates a clinical course of sustained recovery and pattern of steady growth. All immunizations required at 2 months of age can be admin-istered simultaneously to preterm or low birth weight infants. The number of injections at 2 months of age can be minimized by using combination vaccines. When it is difficult to administer 3 or 4 injections simultaneously to hospitalized preterm infants because of limited injection sites, the vaccines recommended at 2 months of age can be administered at different times. However, the same volume of vaccine used for term infants is appropri-ate for medically stable preterm infants. Because recommended vaccines are inactivated, any interval between doses is acceptable. However, to avoid superimposing local reactions, 2-week intervals may be reasonable. The choice of needle lengths used for intramuscular

---

[1]American Academy of Pediatrics, Committee on Infectious Diseases. Immunization of preterm and low birth weight infants. *Pediatrics.* 2003;112(1 Pt 1):193–198 (Reaffirmed May 2006)

vaccine administration is determined by available muscle mass of the preterm or low birth weight infant (see Table 1.4, p 19).

Hepatitis B vaccine given to preterm or low birth weight infants weighing more than 2000 g at birth produces an immune response comparable to that in term infants. Therefore, medically stable preterm or low birth weight infants weighing more than 2000 g born to hepatitis B surface antigen (HBsAg)-negative mothers can receive the first dose of hepatitis B vaccine at birth or shortly thereafter. For medically unstable preterm infants weighing more than 2000 g born to HBsAg-negative mothers, hepatitis B immunization can be deferred until their clinical condition has stabilized. Seroconversion rates and antibody concentrations in infants weighing 2000 g or less at birth immunized with hepatitis B vaccine shortly after birth are often lower than those seen in full-term infants immunized at birth and in preterm infants immunized at a later age. Nonetheless, hepatitis B vaccine appears to protect infants born to HBsAg-positive mothers from complications related to perinatal exposure to hepatitis B infection, and studies confirm that chronologic age at the time of the first dose of hepatitis B vaccine is the best predictor of successful seroconversion, regardless of birth weight or gestational age at birth. Consistent weight gain by preterm infants before receipt of the first dose of hepatitis B vaccine also is predictive of immune responsiveness.

Medically stable, thriving infants weighing less than 2000 g demonstrate predictable, consistent, and sufficient hepatitis B antibody responses and should receive the first dose of hepatitis B vaccine as early as 30 days of chronologic age, regardless of gestational age or birth weight. Preterm infants weighing less than 2000 g who are healthy enough to be released from the hospital before a chronologic age of 30 days can receive hepatitis B vaccine at discharge (see Hepatitis B, p 337). Starting the hepatitis B series at 1 month of age or earlier, regardless of the weight of the preterm infant, offers more options for implementing the immunization schedule in the special care nursery setting, lessens the number of simultaneous injections at 2 months of age (when other recommended childhood immunizations are due), provides earlier protection to vulnerable preterm infants more likely to receive multiple blood products and undergo surgical interventions, and decreases the risk of horizontal transmission from occult hepatitis B chronic carriers among family members, hospital visitors, and other caregivers. Studies have shown that the closer hepatitis B vaccine is given to the infant's birth, the greater the likelihood the complement of childhood vaccines will be completed on time.

All preterm or low birth weight infants born to HBsAg-positive mothers should receive Hepatitis B Immune Globulin (HBIG) within 12 hours of birth and hepatitis B vaccine (see Hepatitis B, p 337). If maternal HBsAg status is unknown at birth, preterm or low birth weight infants should receive hepatitis B vaccine in accordance with recommendations for infants born to HBsAg-positive mothers. Preterm or low birth weight infants given a birth dose of hepatitis B vaccine should receive 3 additional doses. For hepatitis B immunoprophylaxis schemes for preterm or low birth weight infants born to mothers who are HBsAg negative, HBsAg positive, and HBsAg unknown, see Table 3.19 (p 349) and Hepatitis B, Special Considerations (p 347).

Only monovalent hepatitis B vaccine should be used for infants from birth to 6 weeks of age. Giving a birth dose of monovalent hepatitis B vaccine when a combination vaccine containing hepatitis B vaccine subsequently is used means that 4 total doses will be administered. Combination vaccines containing a hepatitis B component have not been assessed for efficacy when given to infants born to HBsAg-positive mothers.

Because all preterm infants are considered at increased risk of complications of influenza, 2 doses of inactivated influenza vaccine given 1 month apart should be offered for preterm infants beginning at 6 months of chronologic age as soon as vaccine is available (see Influenza, p 400). Because preterm infants younger than 6 months of age and infants of any age with chronic complications of preterm birth are extremely vulnerable when exposed to influenza virus, household contacts, child care providers, and hospital nursery personnel caring for preterm infants should receive influenza vaccine annually (see Influenza, p 400). Appropriately selected preterm infants born at less than 32 weeks of gestational age, infants with chronic lung disease and prematurity, and infants with specified cardiovascular conditions up to 2 years of age may benefit from monthly immunoprophylaxis with palivizumab (respiratory syncytial virus monoclonal antibody) during respiratory syncytial virus season (see Respiratory Syncytial Virus, p 560). Palivizumab use does not interfere with immune response to routine childhood immunizations in preterm or low birth weight infants.

Preterm infants can receive rotavirus vaccine under the following circumstances: the infant is at least 6 weeks and less than 15 weeks, 0 days of chronologic age, the infant is medically stable, and the first dose is given at the time of hospital discharge or after hospital discharge.

Pregnancy[1]

Immunization during pregnancy poses theoretical risks to the developing fetus. Although no evidence indicates that vaccines currently in use have detrimental effects on the fetus, pregnant women should receive a vaccine only when the vaccine is unlikely to cause harm, the risk of disease exposure is high, and the infection would pose a significant risk to the mother or fetus. When a vaccine is to be given during pregnancy, delaying administration until the second or third trimester, when possible, is a reasonable precaution to minimize theoretical concern about possible teratogenicity.

The only vaccines recommended for routine administration during pregnancy in the United States, provided they are indicated (either for primary or booster immunization), are adult-type tetanus and diphtheria toxoids (Td) and inactivated influenza vaccines. The American Academy of Pediatrics (AAP) recommends that pregnant women who have not received a Td-containing booster during the previous 2 years should be given tetanus toxoid, reduced diphtheria toxoid, and acellular pertussis (Tdap) vaccine, and women who are unimmunized or only partially immunized should complete the primary series. For complete recommendations regarding use of Td and Tdap vaccines in pregnancy, see Pertussis, p 504. In developing countries with a high incidence of neonatal tetanus, Td vaccine routinely is administered during pregnancy without evidence of adverse effects and with striking decreases in the occurrence of neonatal tetanus.

Studies indicate that women who are pregnant with absence of other underlying medical conditions are at increased risk of complications and hospitalization from influenza. Therefore, inactivated influenza vaccine should be administered to all women who will be pregnant during the influenza season, regardless of trimester (see Influenza, p 400). Influenza immunization of pregnant women also protects infants younger than 6 months of age who cannot be actively immunized or receive antiviral prophylaxis, because neither vaccine nor antiviral agents are approved for use in infants younger

---

[1]See adult immunization schedule available at **www.cdc.gov/vaccines.**

than 6 months of age. Live-attenuated influenza vaccine should not be given to pregnant women.

Pneumococcal and meningococcal vaccines can be given to a pregnant woman at high risk of serious or complicated illness from infection with *Streptococcus pneumoniae* or *Neisseria meningitidis.* Meningococcal conjugate (preferred) or meningococcal polysaccharide vaccines can be given to a pregnant woman when there is increased risk of disease, such as during epidemics or travel to an area with hyperendemic infection. Infection with hepatitis A or hepatitis B in a pregnant woman can result in severe disease in the mother and, in the case of hepatitis B, chronic infection in the newborn infant. Hepatitis A or hepatitis B immunizations, if indicated, can be given to pregnant women. Although data on safety of these vaccines for a pregnant woman or developing fetus are not available, no risk would be expected. Inactivated poliovirus (IPV) vaccine can be given to pregnant women who never have received poliovirus vaccine, are partially immunized, or are immunized completely but require a booster dose (see Poliovirus Infections, p 541).

Pregnancy is a contraindication to administration of all live-virus vaccines, except when susceptibility and exposure are highly probable and the disease to be prevented poses a greater threat to the woman or fetus than does the vaccine. Although only a theoretical risk to the fetus exists with a live-virus vaccine, the background rate of anomalies in uncomplicated pregnancies may result in a defect that could be attributed inappropriately to a vaccine. Therefore, live-virus vaccines should be avoided during pregnancy.

Because measles, mumps, rubella, and varicella vaccines are contraindicated for pregnant women, efforts should be made to immunize susceptible women against these illnesses before they become pregnant or after pregnancy. Although of theoretical concern, no case of embryopathy caused by the attenuated rubella vaccine strain has been reported. Although no infants have been reported with congenital defects attributable to inadvertent administration of rubella vaccine to pregnant women, a rare theoretical risk of embryopathy cannot be excluded. The effect of varicella vaccine on the fetus, if any, is unknown. The manufacturer, in collaboration with the Centers for Disease Control and Prevention (CDC), established the VARIVAX Pregnancy Registry to monitor the maternal and fetal outcomes of women who inadvertently are given varicella vaccine during the 3 months before or at any time during pregnancy. From March 1995 to March 2008, there were 684 women in the registry (161 were seronegative and 523 were unknown or seropositive) who inadvertently received varicella vaccine within 3 months before or during pregnancy and whose pregnancy outcomes are known, available for analysis, and considered complete. No offspring had clinical features consistent with congenital varicella, and there were no birth defects consistent with congenital varicella syndrome in reports of pregnancies that ended in spontaneous abortion or elective termination. The prevalence estimates of birth defects was compatible with the background number of congenital anomalies expected in the general population. Reporting of instances of inadvertent immunization during pregnancy by telephone is encouraged (1-800-986-8999). A pregnant mother or other household member is not a contraindication for varicella immunization of a child in that household. Transmission of vaccine virus from an immunocompetent vaccine recipient to a susceptible person has been reported only rarely and only in the presence of a vaccine-associated rash in the vaccinee (see Varicella-Zoster Infections, p 714). Breastfeeding is not a contraindication for immunization of varicella-susceptible women after pregnancy. Varicella has not been detected by polymerase chain reaction assay in human milk specimens after immunization, and infants breastfed by mothers immunized with varicella vaccine do not seroconvert to varicella.

Pregnant women at risk of exposure to unusual pathogens should be considered for immunization when the potential benefits outweigh the potential risks to the mother and fetus.

- Vaccinia virus vaccine should be given only when there is a definite and significant exposure to smallpox. Because smallpox causes more severe disease in pregnant than nonpregnant women, the potential risks of immunization may be outweighed by the risk of disease. Immunized household contacts should avoid contact with pregnant women until the vaccine site is healed.

- Rabies vaccine should be given to pregnant women after exposure to rabies under the same circumstances as nonpregnant women. There has been no reported association between rabies immunization and adverse fetal outcomes.

- Yellow fever vaccine is a live-attenuated virus vaccine, but if travel of a pregnant woman cannot be postponed and mosquito exposure cannot be avoided, immunization should be considered.[1]

- Japanese encephalitis virus vaccine previously available in the United States no longer is being produced. A vero cell-derived Japanese encephalitis vaccine may be available within 1 to 2 years for use in adult travelers, but no safety data exist for pregnant women. Women should be immunized before conception, if possible, but Japanese encephalitis virus vaccine should be considered if travel to regions with endemic infection and mosquito exposure are unavoidable (see Arboviruses, p 214).

- The parenteral typhoid vaccine should be considered on a case-by-case basis; oral typhoid vaccine is a live-attenuated vaccine and should not be administered to pregnant women.[1]

- Anthrax vaccine contains no live bacteria and no theoretical risk to the fetus, but the vaccine has not been evaluated for safety in pregnant women (see Anthrax, p 211).

- Human papillomavirus (HPV) vaccine contains no live virus, but data on immunization during pregnancy are limited. Initiation of the vaccine series should be delayed until after completion of the pregnancy. If a woman is found to be pregnant after initiating the immunization series, the remainder of the 3-dose regimen should be delayed until after completion of the pregnancy. If a vaccine dose has been administered during pregnancy, no intervention is needed. A vaccine registry has been established for reporting exposure to HPV vaccine during pregnancy (telephone: 800-986-8999).

Immunocompromised Children

PRIMARY AND SECONDARY IMMUNE DEFICIENCIES

The safety and effectiveness of vaccines in people with immune deficiency are determined by the nature and degree of immunosuppression. Immunocompromised people vary in their degree of immunosuppression and susceptibility to infection. Immunocompromised children represent a heterogeneous population with regard to immunization. Immuno-deficiency conditions can be grouped into primary and secondary (acquired) disorders. Primary disorders of the immune system generally are inherited, usually as single-gene disorders; may involve any part of the immune defenses, including B-lymphocyte

---

[1]wwwn.cdc.gov/travel/contentDiseases.aspx

(humoral) immunity, T-lymphocyte (cell)-mediated immunity, complement, and phago-cytic function as well as other, unique abnormalities of innate immunity; and share the common feature of susceptibility to infection.[1] Secondary disorders of the immune system are acquired and occur in people with human immunodeficiency virus (HIV) infection/acquired immunodeficiency syndrome (AIDS) or malignant neoplasms; people who have undergone transplantation or splenectomy; people receiving immunosuppressive, antimetabolic, or radiation therapy; and people with a variety of other illnesses, such as severe malnutrition, protein loss, and uremia (see Table 1.14, p 74). Published studies of experience with vaccine administration in immunocompromised children are limited. In most situations, theoretical considerations are the primary guide to vaccine administra-tion, because experience with specific vaccines in people with a specific disorder is lacking. However, considerable experience in HIV-infected children provides reassurance about the low risk of adverse events in these children after immunization.

LIVE VACCINES. In general, people who are severely immunocompromised or in whom immune status is uncertain should not receive live vaccines, either viral or bacterial, because of the risk of disease caused by the vaccine strains. Although precautions, con-traindications, and suboptimal efficacy of immunizations in less severely immunocom-promised children and adolescents are of concern, benefits may outweigh risks for use of routinely recommended live vaccines.

INACTIVATED VACCINES AND PASSIVE IMMUNIZATION. Inactivated vaccines and Immune Globulin (IG) preparations should be used when appropriate, because the risk of complications from these preparations is not increased in immunocompromised people. However, immune responses of immunocompromised children to inactivated vaccines (eg, DTaP, Tdap, hepatitis B, hepatitis A, IPV, Hib, pneumococcal, meningo-coccal, and influenza) may be inadequate. In children with secondary immunodeficiency, the ability to develop an adequate immunologic response depends on the presence of immunosuppression during or within 2 weeks of immunization. In children in whom immunosuppressive therapy is discontinued, an adequate response usually occurs between 3 months and 1 year after discontinuation. Inactivated influenza vaccine should be given yearly to immunosuppressed children 6 months of age and older before each influenza season. In children with malignant neoplasms, if possible, inactivated influenza immunization should be given no sooner than 3 to 4 weeks after a course of chemotherapy is discontinued and when peripheral granulocyte and lymphocyte counts >1000 cells/μL (1.0×10^9/L) are achieved.

All children and adolescents with primary and secondary immunodeficiencies should receive an annual age-appropriate influenza vaccine to prevent influenza and secondary bacterial infections associated with influenza disease.

PRIMARY IMMUNODEFICIENCIES. Measles and varicella vaccines should be considered for children with B-lymphocyte disorders. However, optimal antibody response may not occur because of the underlying disease and because the patient may be receiving Immune Globulin Intravenous (IGIV) periodically. Oral poliovirus (OPV) vaccine, which no longer is available in the United States, is contraindicated, because it has been associ-ated with an increased incidence of paralytic disease in people with B-lymphocyte or

---

[1]Centers for Disease Control and Prevention. Applying public health strategies to primary immunodeficiency diseases: a potential approach to genetic disorders. *MMWR Recomm Rep.* 2004;53(RR-1):1–29

Table 1.14. Immunization of Children and Adolescents With Primary and Secondary Immune Deficiencies

Category	Example of Specific Immunodeficiency	Vaccine Contraindications	Effectiveness and Comments
Primary[a]			
B lymphocyte (humoral)	Severe antibody deficiencies (eg, X-linked agammaglobulinemia and common variable immunodeficiency)	OPV,[b] smallpox, LAIV, yellow fever, and live-bacteria vaccines[c]; consider measles vaccine; no data for varicella or rotavirus vaccines	Effectiveness of any vaccine dependent only on humoral response is doubtful; IGIV therapy interferes with measles and possibly varicella immune response.
	Less severe antibody deficiencies (eg, selective IgA deficiency and IgG subclass deficiencies)	OPV,[b] other live vaccines[d] appear to be safe, but caution is urged	All vaccines probably effective. Immune response may be attenuated.
T lymphocyte (cell-mediated and humoral)	Complete defects (eg, severe combined immunodeficiency, complete DiGeorge syndrome)	All live vaccines[c,d]	All vaccines ineffective.
	Partial defects (eg, most patients with DiGeorge syndrome, Wiskott-Aldrich syndrome, ataxia telangiectasia)	All live vaccines[c,d]	Effectiveness of any vaccine depends on degree of immune suppression. Recommend inactivated vaccines.
Complement	Deficiency of early components (C1, C4, C2, C3)	None	All routine vaccines probably effective. Pneumococcal and meningococcal vaccines are recommended.
	Deficiency of late components (C5–C9), properdin, factor B	None	All routine vaccines probably effective. Meningococcal and pneumococcal vaccines are recommended.
Phagocytic function	Chronic granulomatous disease, leukocyte adhesion defects, myeloperoxidase deficiency	Live-bacteria vaccinesc	All inactivated vaccines safe and probably effective. Live-virus vaccines probably safe and effective.

Table 1.14. Immunization of Children and Adolescents With Primary and Secondary Immune Deficiencies, continued

Category	Example of Specific Immunodeficiency	Vaccine Contraindications	Effectiveness and Comments
Secondary[a]			
	HIV/AIDS	OPV,[b] smallpox, BCG, LAIV[d]; withhold MMR and varicella in severely immunocompromised children	MMR, varicella, rotavirus, and all inactivated vaccines, including inactivated influenza, may be effective.[e]
	Malignant neoplasm, transplantation, autoimmune disease, immunosuppressive or radiation therapy	Live-virus and -bacteria, depending on immune status[c,d]	Effectiveness of any vaccine depends on degree of immune suppression.

OPV indicates oral poliovirus; LAIV, live-attenuated influenza vaccine; IGIV, Immune Globulin Intravenous; Ig, immunoglobulin; HIV, human immunodeficiency virus; AIDS, acquired immunodeficiency syndrome; BCG, bacille Calmette-Guérin; MMR, measles-mumps-rubella.

[a] All children and adolescents should receive an annual age-appropriate inactivated influenza vaccine. LAIV is indicated only for healthy people 5 to 49 years of age.

[b] OPV vaccine no longer is recommended for routine use in the United States.

[c] Live-bacteria vaccines: BCG and Ty21a *Salmonella typhi* vaccine.

[d] Live-virus vaccines: LAIV, MMR, measles-mumps-rubella-varicella (MMRV), herpes zoster (ZOS), OPV, varicella, yellow fever, vaccinia (smallpox), and rotavirus.

[e] HIV-infected children should receive Immune Globulin after exposure to measles (see Measles, p 444) and may receive varicella vaccine if CD4+ lymphocyte count ≥15% of expected for age (see Varicella-Zoster Infections, p 714).

combined immunodeficiency disorders. Other live vaccines also are contraindicated for most patients with B-lymphocyte defects except immunoglobulin A deficiency. Live vaccines are contraindicated for all patients with T-lymphocyte–mediated disorders of immune function (see Table 1.14, p 74). Fatal or chronic poliomyelitis, measles, and vaccinia after smallpox immunization have occurred in children with disorders of T-lymphocyte function after administration of the respective live-virus vaccines. Inactivated poliovirus vaccine should be administered. Live-attenuated influenza vaccine (LAIV) should not be given to children or adolescents with immunodeficiencies. These patients should be given trivalent inactivated influenza vaccine. Children with deficiency in antibody-synthesizing capacity may be incapable of developing an antibody response to vaccines and may benefit from regular doses of IG (usually IGIV) to provide passive protection against many infectious diseases. Specific immune globulins are available for postexposure prophylaxis for some infections (see Specific Immune Globulins, p 57). Children with milder B-lymphocyte and antibody deficiencies have an intermediate degree of vaccine responsiveness and may require monitoring of postimmunization antibody concentrations to confirm vaccine immunogenicity.

The live-attenuated vaccines for rotavirus are of unproven safety in infants with immunodeficiencies, including primary and acquired immunodeficiency conditions, infants with blood dyscrasias, infants on immunosuppressive therapy, or infants who are HIV exposed or infected. Because these vaccines are recommended for infants beginning at 6 weeks of age, some recipients will have these as-yet undiagnosed diseases and have the potential for prolonged shedding and systemic illness. Health care professionals should consider the potential risks and benefits of administering rotavirus vaccine to infants with known or suspected altered immunocompetence (see Rotavirus, p 576).[1]

Most experts believe that live-virus vaccines are safe to administer to children with complement deficiencies and disorders of phagocyte function. Children with early or late complement deficiencies can receive all immunizations, including live vaccines. Children with phagocytic function disorders, including chronic granulomatous disease and leukocyte adhesion defects, can receive all immunizations except live-bacteria vaccines (bacille Calmette-Guérin [BCG] and Ty21a *Salmonella typhi*).

SECONDARY (ACQUIRED) IMMUNODEFICIENCIES. Several factors should be considered in immunization of children with secondary immunodeficiencies, including the underlying disease, the specific immunosuppressive regimen (dose and schedule), and the infectious disease and immunization history of the person. Live vaccines generally are contraindicated because of an increased risk of serious adverse effects. Exceptions are children 1 through 8 years of age with HIV infection who are in CDC clinical categories N, A, and B, in whom measles-mumps-rubella (MMR) vaccine is recommended (see Human Immunodeficiency Virus Infection, p 380) and in whom varicella vaccine should be considered if CD4+ T-lymphocyte counts are 15% or greater than expected for age (see Varicella-Zoster Infections, p 714). Immunization with MMR and varicella vaccines of people 9 years of age and older who have CD4+ T-lymphocyte counts 200 cells/mm^3

[1]Centers for Disease Control and Prevention. Prevention of rotavirus gastroenteritis among infants and children: recommendations of the Advisory Committee on Immunization Practices (ACIP). *MMWR Recomm Rep.* 2009; 58(RR-2):1–25

or greater can be considered.[1] The use of varicella vaccine in children with acute lymphocytic leukemia in remission should be considered, because the risk of natural varicella disease outweighs the risk associated with the live-attenuated vaccine virus (see Varicella-Zoster Infections, p 714).

Live-virus vaccines usually are withheld for an interval of at least 3 months after immunosuppressive cancer chemotherapy has been discontinued. For corticosteroid therapy (see Corticosteroids, p 78), the interval is based on the assumption that immune response will have been restored in 3 months and that the underlying disease for which immunosuppressive therapy was given is in remission or under control. Immunodeficiency that follows use of recombinant human proteins with antiinflammatory properties, including tumor necrosis factor alpha antagonists (eg, adalimumab, infliximab, and etanercept) or anti–B-lymphocyte monoclonal antibodies (eg, rituximab), appears to be prolonged. The interval until immune reconstitution varies with the intensity and type of immunosuppressive therapy, radiation therapy, underlying disease, and other factors. Therefore, often it is not possible to make a definitive recommendation for an interval after cessation of immunosuppressive therapy when live-virus vaccines can be administered safely and effectively.

OTHER CONSIDERATIONS. Because patients with congenital or acquired immunodeficiencies may not have an adequate response to an immunizing agent, they may remain susceptible despite having received an appropriate vaccine. If there is an available test for a known antibody correlate of protection, specific serum antibody titers should be determined 4 to 6 weeks after immunization to assess immune response and guide further immunization and management of future exposures.

People with certain immune deficiencies may benefit from specific immunizations directed at preventing infections by organisms to which they are particularly susceptible. Examples include administration of pneumococcal and meningococcal vaccines to people with splenic dysfunction, asplenia (see Children With Asplenia, p 84), and complement deficiencies, because they are at increased risk of infection with encapsulated bacteria. Also, annual inactivated influenza immunization is indicated for children 6 months of age and older with immune deficiencies, including splenic dysfunction, asplenia, and phagocyte function deficiencies, to prevent influenza and decrease the risk of secondary bacterial infections (see Influenza, p 400).

HOUSEHOLD CONTACTS. Immunocompetent siblings and other household contacts of people with an immunologic deficiency should not receive smallpox vaccine or OPV vaccines, because vaccine virus may be transmitted to immunocompromised people. However, siblings and household contacts should receive MMR, varicella, and rotavirus vaccines if indicated, because transmission of the vaccine viruses rarely occurs. Household contacts 6 months of age and older should receive yearly inactivated influenza vaccine to prevent infection and subsequent transmission to the immunocompromised person. Limited data are available assessing the risk of transmission of LAIV virus from vaccine recipients to immunosuppressed contacts, although this appears to be a rare event. Inactivated influenza vaccine is recommended for immunizing household

---

[1]Centers for Disease Control and Prevention. Guidelines for prevention and treatment of opportunistic infections among HIV-exposed and HIV-infected children. Recommendations from CDC, the National Institutes of Health, the HIV Medical Association of the Infectious Diseases Society of America, the Pediatric Infectious Diseases Society, and the American Academy of Pediatrics. *MMWR.* 2009; in press.

members of immunosuppressed people. Varicella vaccine is recommended for susceptible contacts of immunocompromised children, because transmission of varicella vaccine virus from healthy people is rare, and vaccine-associated illness, if it develops, is mild. No precautions need to be taken after immunization unless the vaccine recipient develops a rash, particularly a vesicular rash. In such instances, the vaccine recipient should avoid direct contact with immunocompromised, susceptible hosts for the duration of the rash. If contact occurs inadvertently, risk of transmission is low. Therefore, administration of Varicella-Zoster Immune Globulin (VariZIG) or IGIV is not indicated. Also, when transmission has occurred, the virus has maintained its attenuated characteristics. In most instances, antiviral therapy is not necessary but can be initiated if illness occurs (see Varicella-Zoster Infections, p 714).

CORTICOSTEROIDS

Children who receive systemic corticosteroid therapy can become immunocompromised. The minimal amount of systemic corticosteroids and duration of administration sufficient to cause immunosuppression in an otherwise healthy child are not well defined. The frequency and route of administration of corticosteroids, the underlying disease, and concurrent therapies are additional factors affecting immunosuppression. Despite these uncertainties, sufficient experience exists to recommend empiric guidelines for administration of attenuated live-virus vaccines to previously healthy children receiving corticosteroid therapy. A dosage equivalent to ≥2 mg/kg per day of prednisone or equivalent to a total of ≥20 mg/day for children who weigh more than 10 kg, particularly when given for more than 14 days, is considered sufficient to raise concern about the safety of immunization with attenuated live-virus vaccines. Accordingly, guidelines for administration of attenuated live-virus vaccines to recipients of corticosteroids are as follows:

- *Topical therapy, local injections, or aerosol use of corticosteroids.* Application of low-potency topical corticosteroids to focal areas on the skin; administration by aerosolization in the respiratory tract; application on conjunctiva; or intraarticular, bursal, or tendon injections of corticosteroids usually do not result in immunosuppression that would contraindicate administration of attenuated live-virus vaccines. However, attenuated live-virus vaccines should not be administered if clinical or laboratory evidence of systemic immunosuppression results from prolonged application until corticosteroid therapy has been discontinued for at least 1 month.
- *Physiologic maintenance doses of corticosteroids.* Children who are receiving only maintenance physiologic doses of corticosteroids can receive attenuated live-virus vaccines during corticosteroid treatment.
- *Low or moderate doses of systemic corticosteroids given daily or on alternate days.* Children receiving <2 mg/kg per day of prednisone or its equivalent, or <20 mg/day if they weigh more than 10 kg, can receive attenuated live-virus vaccines during corticosteroid treatment.
- *High doses of systemic corticosteroids given daily or on alternate days for fewer than 14 days.* Children receiving ≥2 mg/kg per day of prednisone or its equivalent, or ≥20 mg/day if they weigh more than 10 kg, can receive attenuated live-virus vaccines immediately after discontinuation of treatment. Some experts, however, would delay immunization until 2 weeks after corticosteroid therapy has been discontinued, if possible (ie, if the patient's condition allows temporary cessation).

- *High doses of systemic corticosteroids given daily or on alternate days for 14 days or more.* Children receiving ≥ 2 mg/kg per day of prednisone or its equivalent, or ≥ 20 mg/day if they weigh more than 10 kg, should not receive attenuated live-virus vaccines until corticosteroid therapy has been discontinued for at least 1 month.
- *Children who have a disease that, in itself, is considered to suppress the immune response and who are receiving systemic or locally administered corticosteroids.* These children should not be given attenuated live-virus vaccines, except in special circumstances.

These guidelines are based on concerns about vaccine safety in recipients of high doses of corticosteroids. When deciding whether to administer attenuated live-virus vaccines, the potential benefits and risks of immunization for an individual patient and the specific circumstances should be considered.

The guidelines also are based on considerations of safety concerning attenuated live-virus vaccines and do not necessarily correlate with those for optimal vaccine immunogenicity. For example, some children receiving moderate doses of prednisone, such as 1.5 mg/kg per day for several weeks or longer, may have a less-than-optimal immune response to some vaccine antigens. In contrast, some children receiving relatively high doses of corticosteroids (eg, 30 mg/day of prednisone) may respond adequately to immunization. Immunization can be deferred temporarily until corticosteroids are discontinued if timely return for immunization is ensured. Otherwise, children should be immunized despite corticosteroid use to enhance the likelihood of protection in the case of exposure to disease.

HEMATOPOIETIC STEM CELL AND OTHER TRANSPLANT RECIPIENTS

Many factors can affect immunity to vaccine-preventable diseases for a child recovering from successful hematopoietic stem cell transplantation (HSCT), including bone marrow transplantation. These include the donor's immunity, type of transplantation (ie, autologous or allogeneic, blood or hematopoietic stem cell[1]), interval since the transplantation, receipt of immunosuppressive medications, and presence of graft-versus-host disease (GVHD). Although many children who are transplant recipients acquire the immunity of the donor, some will lose serologic evidence of immunity. Retention of donor immune memory can be facilitated if recalled by antigenic stimulation soon after transplantation. Clinical studies of stem cell transplant recipients indicate that administration of diphtheria and tetanus toxoids to the donor before harvest and immediate administration to the recipient after transplantation can facilitate response to these antigens; serum antibody titers did not increase when immunization of the recipient was delayed until 5 weeks after transplantation. In theory, these results could be expected with other inactivated vaccine antigens, including pertussis, Hib, influenza, hepatitis B, hepatitis A, IPV, and pneumococcal and meningococcal conjugate and polysaccharide vaccines.

The risk of acquiring diphtheria or tetanus during the year after HSCT is low. Some experts elect to reimmunize all children without serologic evaluation, and others base the decision to reimmunize against diphtheria and tetanus on adequacy of serologic titers

---

[1]Centers for Disease Control and Prevention, Infectious Disease Society of America, and the American Society of Blood and Marrow Transplantation. Guidelines for preventing opportunistic infections among hematopoietic stem cell transplant recipients. *MMWR Recomm Rep.* 2000;49(RR-10):1–125, CE1–CE7

obtained 1 year after transplantation. Adequate immune responses can be obtained with 3 doses of Td at 12, 14, and 24 months after transplantation in people 7 years of age or older. In people younger than 7 years of age, DTaP or DT (diphtheria and tetanus toxoids for children younger than 7 years of age) should be used. No data are available on safety and immunogenicity of pertussis immunization for stem cell transplant recipients. People with tetanus-prone wounds sustained during the first year after transplantation should be given Tetanus Immune Globulin, regardless of their tetanus immunization status.

Data on which to base recommendations for reimmunization against Hib or *S pneumoniae* are limited. Doses of Hib conjugate vaccine appear to provide some protection if given at 12, 14, and 24 months after HSCT for recipients of any age. In one study, time after transplantation was the most important factor in determining the immune response to pneumococcal polysaccharide vaccine, with the greatest response observed when the vaccine was administered 2 or more years after transplantation. In another study, Hib conjugate and tetanus toxoid vaccines given 12 and 24 months after HSCT induced adequate immune responses. Some experts recommend a multiple-dose schedule of pneumococcal conjugate and/or polysaccharide vaccine at 12 and 24 months after transplantation, depending on the age of the person (see Pneumococcal Infections, p 524). The second dose of pneumococcal vaccine provides a second opportunity for pneumococcal immunization for people who fail to respond to the first dose. In patients undergoing autologous HSCT, preharvest immunization with Hib conjugate vaccine resulted in higher anti-Hib antibody concentrations for 2 years after transplantation, compared with patients who were not immunized before harvest. Similar benefit in transplant recipients was noted when allogenic stem cell donors were immunized before harvest.

Recovery of immune function after HSCT is variable depending on interaction of several factors. Relying on a generalized schedule for immunization is problematic. Some experts suggest a trial of assessing antibody response to tetanus or diphtheria and tetanus toxoids; a positive result would indicate probable safety of administration of live-virus vaccines. Receipt of IGIV may compromise interpretation of this test. Data indicate that healthy survivors can be immunized with inactivated bacterial and viral vaccines 1 year after HSCT and can receive MMR vaccine 2 years after HSCT. Insufficient data are available for recommendations regarding varicella-zoster virus vaccine. Inactivated influenza vaccine can be given 6 months or longer after HSCT. A second dose of MMR vaccine should be given 28 days or more after the first dose unless serologic response to measles is demonstrated after the first dose. The benefit of a second dose in this population has not been evaluated. Patients with chronic GVHD should not receive MMR vaccine because of concern about resulting latent virus infection and its sequelae. Susceptible people who are exposed to measles should receive passive immunoprophylaxis (see Measles, p 444). Varicella vaccine is contraindicated for stem cell transplant recipients less than 24 months after transplantation. Use of varicella vaccine for stem cell transplant recipients is restricted to research protocols in which the vaccine may be considered 24 months or more after HSCT for recipients who are presumed immunocompetent. Passive immunization is recommended for susceptible people with known exposure to varicella (see Varicella-Zoster Infections, p 714).

IPV vaccine can be given to transplant recipients and their household contacts. Stem cell transplant recipients should be immunized with IPV vaccine at 12, 14, and 24 months after transplantation. The effectiveness of giving additional doses is not known; more data are needed on optimal methods and timing of IPV immunization. Recipients can be tested for type-specific antibodies, but serologic tests for antibody titers against polioviruses are not readily available.

Inactivated influenza vaccine is not effective when given within the initial 6 months after HSCT, but immunization may provide protection when given 1 year after HSCT. Because the risk of disease is substantial, inactivated influenza vaccine should be administered annually during early autumn (see Influenza, p 400) to people who underwent HSCT more than 6 months previously, even if the interval is fewer than 12 months. For children and adolescents for whom fewer than 6 months have elapsed after HSCT, influenza chemoprophylaxis should be considered (see Influenza, p 400). Live-attenuated influenza vaccine should not be administered to children and adolescents who have undergone HSCT.

The immunogenicity of hepatitis B vaccine in stem cell transplant recipients has not been assessed adequately. On the basis of the response of these patients to other protein antigens, initiation of a 3-dose series at 12, 14, and 24 months after HSCT followed by postimmunization serologic testing for antibody to HBsAg is reasonable. Additional doses (maximum of 3) should be given to vaccine nonresponders. Administration of hepatitis A vaccine may be considered 12 months or longer after HSCT for people who have chronic liver disease or chronic GVHD or people from areas with endemic infection or outbreaks of hepatitis A. Hepatitis A immunization requires 2 doses (see Hepatitis A, p 329). Household and health care professional contacts of stem cell and solid organ transplant recipients should have immunity to or be immunized against poliovirus, measles, mumps, rubella, varicella, influenza, and hepatitis A.

SOLID ORGAN TRANSPLANT RECIPIENTS

Children and adolescents being considered for solid organ transplantation should receive immunizations recommended for their age before the transplantation is performed. In general, vaccines will be more immunogenic before transplantation, because the medications given after transplantation to prevent and treat organ rejection adversely affect numbers and/or function of T and B lymphocytes. Live-virus vaccines should be given at least 1 month before transplantation and, in general, should not be given to patients receiving immunosuppressive medications after transplantation. MMR vaccine may be given before transplantation to patients as young as 6 months of age if transplantation is anticipated before 12 through 15 months of age. For transplantation candidates who are older than 12 months of age, if previously immunized, serum concentrations of antibody to measles, mumps, rubella, and varicella should be measured. Children who are susceptible should be immunized before transplantation.

Information about use of live-virus vaccines in patients after solid organ transplantation is limited. Some transplant centers have reported administration of live-virus vaccines (eg, MMR and varicella vaccines) in patients who are stable at least 6 months after transplantation, who are receiving minimal immunosuppressive agents, and who have not had recent episodes of organ rejection. No serious adverse reactions have been reported among these children, but too few children have been studied to recommend general use of live-virus vaccines in this population. MMR vaccine may be considered for susceptible solid organ transplant recipients in the event of an outbreak of measles, mumps, or rubella in the local community. Serum antibody concentrations for measles, mumps, rubella, and varicella should be measured in all patients 1 year or more after transplantation. Household and close contacts of a solid organ recipient should receive MMR and varicella vaccines, if susceptible, to reduce the risk of transmission of wild-type virus to the immunosuppressed child. Oral poliovirus vaccine, which is not available in the United States, is contraindicated for transplant recipients and their household contacts. Inactivated poliovirus should be used for protection against poliovirus. Live-bacteria vaccines (eg, BCG and Ty21a *S typhi*) are contraindicated in patients receiving immunosuppressive medications after transplantation.

Killed and subunit vaccines should not pose a risk to solid organ transplant recipients. After transplantation, DTaP, Hib, hepatitis B, hepatitis A, inactivated influenza, and pneumococcal and meningococcal conjugate and polysaccharide vaccines can be administered, if indicated. Safety and immunogenicity data for these vaccines in children after transplantation are limited. Most experts wait at least 6 months after transplantation, when immune suppression is less intense, for resumption of immunization schedules. However, immunization schedules vary in different transplant centers, and immune responses to some inactivated vaccines are diminished compared with healthy controls. Hepatitis A vaccine should be administered to patients undergoing liver transplantation because of increased disease severity associated with hepatitis A infection in patients with chronic liver disease. Annual influenza immunization with inactivated vaccine is indicated before and after solid organ transplantation. Live-attenuated influenza vaccine is contraindicated for solid organ transplant recipients. Solid organ transplant recipients at highest risk of infection with *S pneumoniae* appear to be those who have undergone cardiac transplantation or splenectomy. Pneumococcal conjugate or polysaccharide vaccine should be considered in all transplant recipients (see Pneumococcal Infections, p 524).

The decision to use passive immunization with an IG preparation (see Passive Immunization, p 55) should be made on the basis of serologic evidence of susceptibility and exposure to disease. Household and health care contacts of stem cell and solid organ transplant recipients should have immunity to or be immunized against poliovirus, measles, mumps, rubella, varicella, influenza, and hepatitis A.

HIV INFECTION (SEE ALSO HUMAN IMMUNODEFICIENCY VIRUS INFECTION, P 380)

Although data on use of currently available live-virus vaccines in HIV-infected children are limited, studies are available on safety and immunogenicity for many childhood vaccines. An ACIP-approved vaccine schedule for HIV-exposed and infected children and adolescents is available.[1] Complications have been reported after BCG, measles, and varicella immunizations in severely immunocompromised children, including vaccine-related measles pneumonitis in a severely immunocompromised child 1 year after measles immunization. Because there have been reports of severe wild-type measles in symptomatic HIV-infected children, with fatalities in as many as 40% of cases, measles immunization (given as MMR vaccine) is recommended for HIV-infected children with CD4+ T-lymphocyte counts 15% or greater. MMR vaccine should be given at 12 months of age to enhance the likelihood of an appropriate immune response. The second dose after the 12-month immunization can be administered as soon as 28 days later to induce seroconversion as early as possible. In a measles epidemic, MMR may be given to infants

---

[1] Centers for Disease Control and Prevention. Guidelines for prevention and treatment of opportunistic infections among HIV-exposed and HIV-infected children. Recommendations from CDC, the National Institutes of Health, the HIV Medical Association of the Infectious Diseases Society of America, the Pediatric Infectious Diseases Society, and the American Academy of Pediatrics. *MMWR*. 2009; in press

as young as 6 months of age. Children immunized before their first birthday should be immunized with 2 additional doses of MMR vaccine (see Measles, Immunization During an Outbreak, p 451). Severely immunocompromised patients with HIV infection, as defined by age-specific low CD4+ T-lymphocyte counts or low percentage of total circulating lymphocytes, should not receive measles vaccine (see Human Immunodeficiency Virus Infection, p 380, and Table 3.27, p 386).

No safety or efficacy data are available for administration of rotavirus vaccine to infants who potentially are immunocompromised, including infants who are HIV positive. However, the following considerations support immunization of HIV-exposed or HIV-infected infants: (1) the HIV diagnosis may not be established in infants born to HIV-positive mothers before the age when the first rotavirus vaccine dose is due, and only 1.5% to 3% of HIV-exposed infants in the United States eventually will have positive HIV test results; and (2) rotavirus vaccines are considerably attenuated.

Because children infected with HIV are at increased risk of morbidity from varicella and zoster compared with children not infected with HIV, after the potential risks and benefits are weighed, monovalent varicella vaccine (2 doses, 3 months apart) should be considered for HIV-infected children and adolescents with CD4+ T-lymphocyte counts of 15% or more of the expected for age or 200 cells/mm^3 (see Varicella-Zoster Infections, p 714). Data are not available regarding safety, immunogenicity, or efficacy of measles-mumps-rubella-varicella (MMRV) vaccine in HIV-infected children; MMRV vaccine should not be administered as a substitute for monovalent varicella vaccine when vaccinating these children.

Children and adolescents with asymptomatic or symptomatic HIV infection should receive all routinely recommended inactivated vaccines, including DTaP, Tdap, IPV, hepatitis B, hepatitis A, Hib, and pneumococcal and meningococcal conjugate and/or polysaccharide vaccines, according to the recommended childhood and adolescent immunization schedule (see Fig 1.1–1.3, p 24–28). Annual inactivated influenza immunization of HIV-infected children 6 months of age or older and adolescents is recommended; LAIV is not licensed for use in this population (see Influenza, p 400). Household contacts of any child infected with HIV should receive influenza vaccine annually. Immunization with pneumococcal conjugate and/or polysaccharide vaccine is indicated on the basis of age and- vaccine-specific recommendations (see Pneumococcal Infections, p 524).

In the United States, BCG vaccine is contraindicated for HIV-infected patients. In areas of the world with a high incidence of tuberculosis, the World Health Organization (WHO) recommends giving BCG vaccine to HIV-infected children who are asymptomatic.

Routine or widespread screening to detect HIV infection in asymptomatic children before routine immunizations is not recommended. Children without clinical manifestations of or known risk factors for HIV infection should be immunized in accordance with the recommended childhood and adolescent immunization schedule. For screening of newborn infants for HIV infection, see Human Immunodeficiency Virus Infection (p 380).

Because the ability of HIV-infected children to respond to vaccine antigens likely is related to the degree of immunosuppression at the time of immunization and may be inadequate, these children should be considered potentially susceptible to vaccine-preventable diseases, even after appropriate immunization, unless a recent serologic test demonstrates adequate antibody concentrations. Hence, passive immunoprophylaxis or chemoprophylaxis after exposure to these diseases should be considered, even if the child previously has received the recommended vaccines. Children with HIV infection given recommended vaccines when they had high HIV RNA concentrations and/or low CD4+ T lymphocyte percentages (eg, before the diagnosis of HIV infection was made or before institution of therapy) may benefit from reimmunization after improvement of their immune status (eg, after institution of highly active antiretroviral therapy).

Vaccine-strain varicella-zoster virus rarely has been transmitted from healthy people. Therefore, household contacts of HIV-infected people can be immunized with live-virus varicella vaccine (see Varicella-Zoster Infections, p 714). No precautions are needed after immunization of healthy children who do not develop a rash. Vaccine recipients who develop a rash should avoid direct contact with susceptible immunocompromised hosts for the duration of the rash. If the immunocompromised contact develops varicella caused by the vaccine strain, disease likely will be mild, and use of VariZIG, if available, or IGIV to prevent transmission is not indicated.

CHILDREN WITH ASPLENIA OR FUNCTIONAL ASPLENIA

The asplenic state results from the following: (1) surgical removal of the spleen (eg, after trauma, for staging of Hodgkin disease, for treatment of hemolytic conditions); (2) certain diseases, such as sickle cell disease (functional asplenia); or (3) congenital asplenia. All infants, children, adolescents, and adults with asplenia, regardless of the reason for the asplenic state, have an increased risk of fulminant bacteremia, especially associated with encapsulated bacteria, which is associated with a high mortality rate. In comparison with immunocompetent children who have not undergone splenectomy, the incidence of and mortality rate from septicemia are increased in children who have had splenectomy after trauma and in children with sickle cell disease by as much as 350-fold, and the rate may be even higher in children who have had splenectomy for thalassemia. The risk of bacteremia is higher in younger children than in older children, and risk may be greater during the years immediately after splenectomy. Fulminant septicemia, however, has been reported in adults as long as 25 years after splenectomy.

Streptococcus pneumoniae is the most common pathogen that causes bacteremia in children with asplenia. Less common causes of bacteremia include Hib, *N meningitidis,* other streptococci, *Escherichia coli, Staphylococcus aureus,* and gram-negative bacilli, such as *Salmonella* species, *Klebsiella* species, and *Pseudomonas aeruginosa.* People with functional or anatomic asplenia also are at increased risk of fatal malaria and severe babesiosis.

Pneumococcal conjugate and/or polysaccharide vaccine is indicated for all children with asplenia at the recommended age (see Pneumococcal Infections, p 524). For children with asplenia who received conjugate and/or polysaccharide vaccine before 24 months of age, additional immunization should be considered in reference to age and products received (see Pneumococcal Infections, p 524). Immunization against Hib infections should be initiated at 2 months of age, as recommended for otherwise healthy young children (see Fig 1.1–1.3, p 24–28) and for all previously unimmunized children with asplenia. Tetravalent meningococcal conjugate vaccine also should be administered to children with asplenia from 2 years of age through adolescence (see Meningococcal Infections, p 455), although the efficacy of meningococcal vaccines in children with asplenia has not been established. No known contraindication exists to giving these vaccines at the same time in separate syringes at different sites.

Daily antimicrobial prophylaxis against pneumococcal infections is recommended for many children with asplenia, regardless of immunization status. For infants with sickle cell anemia, oral penicillin prophylaxis against invasive pneumococcal disease should be initiated as soon as the diagnosis is established and preferably by 2 months of age. Although the efficacy of antimicrobial prophylaxis has been proven only in patients with sickle cell anemia, other children with asplenia at particularly high risk, such as children with malignant neoplasms or thalassemia, also should receive daily chemoprophylaxis. Less agreement exists about the need for prophylaxis for children who have had splenectomy after trauma. In general, antimicrobial prophylaxis (in addition to immunization) should be considered for all children with asplenia younger than 5 years of age and for at least 1 year after splenectomy.

The age at which chemoprophylaxis is discontinued often is an empiric decision. On the basis of a multicenter study, prophylactic penicillin can be discontinued at 5 years of age in children with sickle cell anemia who are receiving regular medical attention and who have not had a severe pneumococcal infection or surgical splenectomy. The appropriate duration of prophylaxis for children with asplenia attributable to other causes is unknown. Some experts continue prophylaxis throughout childhood and into adulthood for particularly high-risk patients with asplenia.

For antimicrobial prophylaxis, oral penicillin V (125 mg, twice a day, for children younger than 5 years of age; and 250 mg, twice a day, for children 5 years of age and older) is recommended. Some experts recommend amoxicillin (20 mg/kg per day). In recent years, the proportion of pneumococcal isolates that have intermediate or high-level resistance to penicillin has increased in most areas of the United States. Administration of pneumococcal conjugate vaccine reduces carriage of penicillin-nonsusceptible vaccine strains of pneumococci. Ongoing surveillance for resistant pneumococci is needed to determine whether changes to the recommended chemoprophylaxis will be required.

When antimicrobial prophylaxis is used, the limitations must be stressed to parents and patients, who should recognize that some bacteria capable of causing fulminant septicemia are not susceptible to the antimicrobial agents given for prophylaxis. Parents should be aware that all febrile illnesses potentially are serious in children with asplenia and that immediate medical attention should be sought, because the initial signs and symptoms of fulminant septicemia can be subtle. When bacteremia or septicemia is a possibility, the health care professional should consider hospitalizing the child, obtain specimens for blood and other cultures as indicated, and immediately begin treatment with an antimicrobial regimen effective against *S pneumoniae*, Hib, and *N meningitidis*. In some clinical situations, other antimicrobial agents, such as aminoglycosides, may be indicated. If a child with asplenia travels to or resides in an area where medical care is not accessible, an appropriate antimicrobial agent should be readily available, and the child's caregiver should be instructed in appropriate use.

Whenever possible, alternatives to splenectomy should be considered. Management options include postponement of splenectomy for as long as possible in congenital hemolytic anemias, preservation of accessory spleens, performance of partial splenectomy for benign tumors of the spleen, conservative (nonoperative) management of splenic trauma, or when feasible, repair rather than removal and, if possible, avoidance of splenectomy when immunodeficiency is present (eg, Wiskott-Aldrich syndrome). When surgical splenectomy is planned, immunization status for Hib, pneumococcus, and meningococcus should be ascertained, and needed vaccines should be administered at least 2 weeks before surgery if possible. If splenectomy is emergent, immediate administration of needed vaccines is recommended.

Children With a Personal or Family History of Seizures

Infants and children with a personal or family history of seizures are at increased risk of having a seizure after receipt of DTP or measles- or varicella-containing vaccines. In most cases, these seizures are brief, self-limited, and generalized and occur in conjunction with fever, indicating that such vaccine-associated seizures usually are febrile seizures. No evidence indicates that febrile seizures cause permanent brain damage or epilepsy, aggravate neurologic disorders, or affect the prognosis for children with underlying disorders. Universal use of DTaP has reduced greatly the incidence of febrile seizures associated with DTP immunization.

In the case of pertussis immunization during infancy, administration of DTaP could coincide with or hasten the recognition of a disorder associated with seizures, such as infantile spasms, and cause confusion about the role of pertussis immunization. Hence, pertussis immunization in infants with a history of recent seizures should be deferred until a progressive neurologic disorder is excluded or the cause of the earlier seizure has been determined. In contrast, measles or varicella immunization is given at an age when the cause and nature of any seizures and related neurologic status are more likely to have been established. This difference provides the basis for the recommendation that measles immunization should not be deferred for children with a history of recent seizures.

A family history of a seizure disorder is not a contraindication to pertussis, measles, or varicella immunization or a reason to defer immunization. Postimmunization seizures in these children are uncommon, and if they occur, usually are febrile in origin, have a benign outcome, and are not likely to be confused with manifestations of a previously unrecognized neurologic disorder. In addition, many children have a family history of seizures and would remain susceptible to pertussis, measles, or varicella if family history were a contraindication to immunization.

Specific recommendations for pertussis and measles immunization of children with a personal or family history of seizures are given in the respective disease-specific chapters (see Pertussis, p 504, and Measles, p 444); a detailed discussion and recommendations about pertussis immunization of children with neurologic disorders also are given in the chapter on Pertussis (p 504).

Children With Chronic Diseases

Chronic diseases may make children more susceptible to the severe manifestations and complications of common infections. Unless specifically contraindicated, immunizations recommended for healthy children should be given to children with chronic diseases. An exception is children with immunologic disorders in whom live-virus vaccines usually are contraindicated; the major exceptions are MMR and varicella vaccines for HIV-infected children who are not severely immunocompromised (see Immunocompromised Children, p 72). For children with conditions that may require organ transplantation or immunosuppression, administering recommended immunizations before the start of immunosuppressive therapy is important. Children with certain chronic diseases (eg, cardiorespiratory, allergic, hematologic, metabolic, and renal disorders; cystic fibrosis; and diabetes mellitus) are at increased risk of complications of influenza, varicella, and pneumococcal infection and should receive inactivated influenza vaccine and live varicella vaccine and/or pneumococcal conjugate or polysaccharide vaccine as recommended for age and immunization status (see Influenza, p 400, Varicella-Zoster Infections, p 714, and Pneumococcal Infections, p 524). People with chronic liver disease are at risk of severe clinical manifestations of acute infection with hepatitis viruses and should receive hepatitis A and hepatitis B vaccines on a catch-up schedule if they have not received vaccines routinely (see Hepatitis A, p 329, and Hepatitis B, p 337). Siblings of children with chronic diseases and children in households of adults with chronic diseases should receive recommended vaccines (see Fig 1.1–1.3, p 24–28, and Immunocompromised Children, p 72).

Active Immunization After Exposure to Disease

Because not all susceptible people receive vaccines before exposure, active immunization may be considered for a person who has been exposed to a specific disease. The following situations are the most commonly encountered (see the disease-specific chapters in Section 3 for detailed recommendations).

- *Measles.* Live-virus measles vaccine given to susceptible (ie, lack of antibody or receipt of fewer than 2 doses of measles virus-containing vaccine after 12 months of age) immunocompetent children 12 months of age and older, adolescents, and adults within 72 hours of exposure will provide protection against measles in some cases (see Measles, p 444). Determining the time of exposure may be difficult, because measles can be spread from 4 days before to 4 days after onset of the rash.

  Immune Globulin (IG), administered intramuscularly within 6 days of exposure, also can prevent or attenuate measles in an immunocompetent or immunocompromised susceptible person (see Measles, p 444). Because measles morbidity rate is high in children younger than 1 year of age, administration of IG is recommended for infants, immunocompromised people at any age, and pregnant women exposed to measles. Immunocompromised children who receive IGIV regularly are considered to be protected against measles.

- *Varicella.* Susceptible (ie, lack of antibody, lack of a reliable history of varicella, or receipt of fewer than 2 doses of varicella-virus containing vaccine after 12 months of age) immunocompetent children 12 months of age or older and household contacts exposed to a person with varicella disease should be given varicella vaccine within 72 hours of the appearance of the rash in the index case (see Varicella-Zoster Infections, p 714). Immunization is safe even in the event that the exposure results in clinical varicella disease. Susceptible immunocompromised children should receive passive immunoprophylaxis as soon as possible but within 96 hours after contact with an infected person or acyclovir preemptively starting 7 days after exposure (see Varicella-Zoster Infections, p 714). Immunocompromised children who receive IGIV regularly are considered to be protected against varicella.

- *Hepatitis B.* Postexposure immunization is highly effective if combined with administration of HBIG. Administration of HBIG does not inhibit active immunization from hepatitis B vaccine. For postexposure prophylaxis in a newborn infant whose mother is an HBsAg carrier, administration of HBIG and hepatitis B immunization is essential. For percutaneous or mucosal exposure to hepatitis B virus (HBV), combined active and passive immunization is recommended for susceptible people (see Hepatitis B, p 337). People with continuing household or sexual contact with an HBsAg carrier also should be immunized.

- **Hepatitis A.** Availability of highly effective inactivated hepatitis A vaccines and results from a randomized, double-blind noninferiority clinical trial comparing the efficacy of hepatitis A vaccine and IG after exposure to hepatitis A virus (HAV) led to a change in recommendations of postexposure prophylaxis (see Hepatitis A, p 329).[1]

  People who recently have been exposed to HAV and who previously have not received hepatitis A vaccine should receive a single dose of single-antigen hepatitis A vaccine (or IG, 0.02 mL/kg, if not a vaccine candidate and exposure was within 2 weeks [see Hepatitis A, p 329]).

  - For healthy people 12 months through 40 years of age, single-antigen hepatitis A vaccine at the age-appropriate dose is preferred.
  - For people older than 40 years of age, IG is preferred; vaccine can be used if IG cannot be obtained.
  - For infants younger than 12 months of age, immunocompromised people, people who have chronic liver disease, and people for whom vaccine is contraindicated, IG should be used.

- **Tetanus.** In wound management, cleaning and débriding all dirty wounds as soon as possible is essential. Unimmunized and incompletely immunized people or people who have not received a booster dose in the past 5 years should be given a tetanus toxoid-containing vaccine immediately. Some people may require Tetanus Immune Globulin in addition to immunization (see Table 3.77, p 657).

- **Rabies.** Thorough local cleansing and débridement of the wound and postexposure active and passive immunization are essential aspects of immunoprophylaxis for rabies after proven or suspected exposure to rabid animals (see Rabies, p 552).

- **Mumps and Rubella.** Exposed susceptible people are not necessarily protected by postexposure administration of live-virus vaccine. However, a common practice for people exposed to mumps or rubella is to administer vaccine to presumed susceptible people so that permanent immunity will be afforded by immunization if mumps or rubella does not result from the current exposure. Administration of live-virus vaccine is recommended for exposed adults born in the United States in 1957 or after who previously have not been immunized against or had mumps or rubella.

American Indian/Alaska Native Children

Compared with children from other ethnic groups, American Indian/Alaska Native (AI/AN) children historically have been at greater risk of acquiring certain vaccine-preventable diseases, such as hepatitis A, hepatitis B, Hib, and *S pneumoniae* infections, and being hospitalized for respiratory syncytial virus infection and other lower respiratory tract infections. The rate of diarrhea-associated hospitalizations is significantly higher in AI/AN infants than in other US infants. AN women have a rate of cervical cancer 3.4 times that of white women in the United States, indicating a high rate of infection with HPV and lack of preventive care.

Geographic differences exist in disease risk. Increased risk of acquiring vaccine-preventable diseases has been demonstrated among AI/AN infants and children who live on reservations or in traditional rural villages, and the increased risk may be related

---

[1]Centers for Disease Control and Prevention. Update: prevention of hepatitis A after exposure to hepatitis A virus and in international travelers: updated recommendations of the Advisory Committee on Immunization Practices (ACIP). *MMWR Morb Mortal Wkly Rep.* 2007;56(41):1080–1084

to crowded living conditions and lack of indoor plumbing. However, high incidences of hepatitis A and hepatitis B infections also have been demonstrated among urban AI/AN children, which may result from high-risk behaviors or frequent visits to extended family members.

During the past decade, universal childhood immunization for hepatitis B and targeted immunization for hepatitis A in the United States have eliminated disease disparities for these pathogens in most AI/AN child populations, and significant decreases in disease have been demonstrated for Hib and *S pneumoniae*. Continued immunization is critical to maintaining this success and eliminating other disparities. It particularly is important that recommendations for universal immunization for hepatitis A and hepatitis B, *S pneumoniae*, HPV, rotavirus, influenza, and Hib are implemented optimally in AI/AN children because of high rates of infection and severe disease. Children in AI/AN communities should be specifically targeted to receive immunizations on time and to receive the full schedule of immunizations even in times of vaccine shortages. Specific vulnerabilities are noted here.

- **Respiratory Syncytial Virus.** The rates of hospitalization for respiratory syncytial virus (RSV) are higher for AI/AN children in the Alaska and southwestern Indian Health Service regions (71 and 48 RSV hospitalizations per 1000 births, respectively) compared with other US children (27 per 1000 births). Use of RSV-specific monoclonal antibody prophylaxis, as recommended by the AAP, should be optimized among high-risk AI/AN infants (see Respiratory Syncytial Virus, p 560). AI/AN infants born at 32 and 35 weeks' gestation often have several risk factors for severe RSV disease. Additionally, one third of rural Alaska Native communities lack in-home running water and flush toilets, and this lack of availability of water service is associated with increased risk of hospitalization for lower respiratory tract infections. RSV season length is prolonged in northern latitudes, including Alaska, and RSV prophylaxis should reflect local seasonality.

- ***Haemophilus influenzae* type B.** Hib immunization requires consideration regarding preferred vaccine product for AI/AN children. Before availability and public use of conjugated Hib vaccines, the incidence of invasive Hib disease was approximately 10 times higher among young AI/AN children compared with the general US population. Because of the high risk of invasive Hib disease within the first 6 months of life in many AI/AN infant populations, the Indian Health Service and AAP recommend that the first dose of Hib conjugate vaccine contain polyribosylribitol phosphate-meningococcal outer membrane protein (PRP-OMP) as a single-antigen vaccine or in a combination vaccine with other antigens. The administration of a PRP-OMP–containing vaccine leads to more rapid seroconversion to protective concentrations of antibody within the first 6 months of life, and failure to use vaccine containing PRP-OMP has been associated with excess cases of Hib disease in young infants in this population. For subsequent doses, PRP-OMP or any of the other Hib conjugate vaccines can be used with apparently equal efficacy (see *Haemophilus influenzae* Infections, p 314). Because availability of more than one Hib vaccine in a clinic can be confusing, strict attention must be paid to vaccine type. To avoid confusion for health care professionals who serve AI/AN children predominantly, it may be prudent to use only a PRP-OMP–containing Hib vaccine.

- **Streptococcus pneumoniae.** Recommendations for PCV7 for AI/AN children are the same as for other US children. However, in special situations, public health authorities may recommend use of PPSV23 after PCV7 for AI/AN children 24 through 59 months of age who are living in areas in which risk of invasive pneumococcal disease is increased. The incidence of invasive pneumococcal disease (IPD) in certain AI/AN children was 5 to 24 times higher than the incidence among other US children before use of PCV7. Use of PCV7 in AI/AN infants has resulted in decreased incidence of IPD in AI/AN children. However, AI/AN children continue to have an increased risk of acquiring IPD—more than twice the national average. Therefore, AN and AI children in Alaska and the southwest should receive the standard 4-dose PCV7 series, even in times of vaccine shortages, as recommended by the AAP and the Advisory Committee on Immunization Practices (ACIP) of the CDC.
- **Hepatitis viruses.** Before the advent of immunization initiatives, rates of hepatitis A and hepatitis B in the AI/AN population exceeded those of the general US population. Universal immunization reduced incidence of hepatitis A and hepatitis B to that of the general US population. Sustained routine immunization of all young AI/AN children will be necessary to maintain high levels of population immunity and low disease rates currently observed in AI/AN communities. In addition, special efforts should be made to ensure catch-up hepatitis B immunization of previously unimmunized adolescents. In 2006, the ACIP approved the recommendation that unimmunized adults at high risk of hepatitis B infection and all adults seeking protection from hepatitis B should be immunized.

Children in Residential Institutions

Children housed in institutions pose special problems for control of certain infectious diseases. Ensuring appropriate immunization is important because of the risk of transmission within the facility and because conditions that led to institutionalization can increase the risk of complications from the disease. All children entering a residential institution should have received recommended immunizations for their age (see Fig 1.1–1.3, p 24–28). If they have not been immunized appropriately, arrangements should be made to administer these immunizations as soon as possible. Staff members should be familiar with standard precautions and procedures for handling blood and body fluids that might be contaminated by blood. For residents who acquire potentially transmissible infectious agents while living in an institution, isolation precautions similar to those recommended for hospitalized patients should be followed (see Infection Control for Hospitalized Children, p 148). Specific diseases of concern include the following (see the disease-specific chapters in Section 3 for detailed recommendations).

- **Measles.** Epidemics can occur among susceptible children in institutional settings. Recommendations for managing children in an institutional setting when a case of measles is recognized are as follows: (1) within 72 hours of exposure, administer live measles virus vaccine (as MMR) to all susceptible children 12 months of age or older for whom immunization is not contraindicated; and (2) administer IG to immunocompromised children (see Measles, p 444) as soon as possible and within 6 days of exposure to all exposed susceptible children younger than 1 year of age. These IG recipients also will require live-virus vaccine (as MMR vaccine) at 12 months of age or thereafter, depending on the age and dose of IG administration (see Table 3.34, p 448, for the appropriate interval between IG administration and MMR immunization).

- **Mumps.** Epidemics can occur among susceptible children in institutions. Major hazards are disruption of activities, the need for acute nursing care in difficult settings, and occasional serious complications (eg, in susceptible adult staff).

  If mumps is introduced, prophylaxis is not available to limit the spread or to attenuate the disease in a susceptible person. IG is not effective, and Mumps Immune Globulin is not available. Although mumps virus vaccine may not be effective after exposure, the vaccine should be administered to people who lack documentation of immunity to protect against infection from future exposures.

- **Influenza.** Influenza can be unusually severe in a residential or custodial institutional setting. Rapid spread, intensive exposure, and underlying disease can result in a high risk of severe illness that may affect many residents simultaneously or in close sequence. Current measures for control of influenza in institutions include: (1) a program of annual influenza immunization of residents and staff; and (2) appropriate use of chemoprophylaxis during influenza epidemics; and (3) initiation of an appropriate infection-control policy (see Influenza, p 400).

- **Pertussis.** Because progressive neurologic disorders may have resulted in a deferral of pertussis immunization, many children in an institutional setting may not be appropriately immunized against pertussis. Because pertussis vaccine does not cause progressive neurologic disease and because pertussis disease poses a greater risk than does pertussis immunization, children who are not immunized fully and who are younger than 7 years of age or 10 years of age and older should be immunized against pertussis. If pertussis is recognized, infected people and their close contacts should receive chemoprophylaxis (see Pertussis, p 504).

- **Hepatitis A.** Outbreaks of hepatitis A affecting residents and staff can occur in institutions for custodial care by fecal-oral transmission. Infection usually is mild or asymptomatic in young children but can be severe in adults. Hepatitis A vaccine may be indicated for postexposure prophylaxis (PEP) for staff and people 12 months through 40 years of age in institutions in which a hepatitis A outbreak is occurring. Hepatitis A vaccine is preferable to IG for PEP of contacts in this age range. Contacts under 12 months of age and people older than 40 years of age should receive IG if PEP is indicated (see Hepatitis A, p 329).

- **Hepatitis B.** Children with developmental disabilities living in residential institutions and their caregivers are assumed to be at increased risk of acquiring HBV infection. The high prevalence of markers of HBV infection among children living in these facilities indicates that HBV infections have the propensity for spread in an institutional setting, presumably by exposure to blood and body fluids containing HBV. Factors associated with high prevalence of HBV markers include crowding, high resident-to-staff ratios, and lack of in-service educational programs for staff. In the presence of such factors, the prevalence of HBV infection increases with the duration of time spent at the institution. Thus, susceptible residents entering or already residing and staff in institutions for children with developmental disabilities should be immunized against HBV; preimmunization serologic screening for HBV probably is not cost-effective.

  After parenteral or sexual exposure to an institutionalized patient recognized to be an HBsAg carrier, contacts who are unimmunized and susceptible should receive active and passive immunoprophylaxis (see also Hepatitis B, p 337, for recommendations for previously immunized people).

- **Pneumococcal Infections.** Children 6 years of age or older with severe physical or mental disabilities, particularly children who are bedridden, who suffer from a compromised respiratory status, or who are capable of only limited physical activity, may benefit from pneumococcal conjugate or polysaccharide vaccine (see Pneumococcal Infections, p 524).
- **Varicella.** Because varicella is highly contagious, disease can occur in a large proportion of susceptible people in an institutional setting. All healthy people 12 months of age or older who lack a reliable history of varicella disease or immunization should be immunized (see Varicella-Zoster Infections, p 714). In addition, during a varicella outbreak, a dose of varicella vaccine is recommended for people who have not received 2 doses of varicella vaccine, provided that the appropriate interval has elapsed since the first dose (3 months for people 12 months through 12 years of age and at least 4 weeks for people 13 years of age and older). If varicella vaccine is administered to a child from 12 months through 12 years of age 28 days or more after the first dose, the second dose does not need to be repeated. Passive immunization during outbreaks currently is recommended only for immunocompromised, susceptible children at risk of serious complications or death from varicella (see Varicella-Zoster Infections, p 714).
- **Other Infections.** Other organisms causing diseases that spread in institutions and for which no immunizations are available include *Shigella* species, *E coli* O157:H7, *C difficile*, other enteric pathogens, *Streptococcus pyogenes, S aureus,* respiratory tract viruses other than influenza, cytomegalovirus, scabies, and lice.

Children Living Outside the United States

In general, children living outside the United States require the same immunizations as children living in the United States and may require additional vaccines related to regional pathogens. If delay in any immunization occurs for any reason, parents should be warned that the risk of contracting diseases in countries where immunization is not administered routinely is substantial. For children and adolescents living or traveling internationally, the risk of exposure to HAV, HBV, measles, pertussis, diphtheria, *N meningitidis*, poliovirus, yellow fever, Japanese encephalitis, and other organisms or infections may be increased and may necessitate additional immunizations (see International Travel, p 98). In these instances, the choice of immunizations will be dictated by the country of proposed residence, duration of residence abroad, expected itinerary, and age and health of the child. For information on the risk of specific diseases in different countries and preventive measures, see International Travel (p 98) or consult the CDC Web site (**wwwn.cdc.gov/travel/default.aspx**) or the WHO Web site (**www.who.int/ith**). For children (especially children younger than 5 years of age) who will reside for a year or longer in countries with high rates of endemic tuberculosis, some experts recommend BCG immunization. Other methods of preventing tuberculosis exposure and disease often are not practical or available. In many cases, it may be desirable for the child to receive the BCG vaccine as soon as possible after entering the foreign country.

Adolescent and College Populations

Adolescents and young adults may not be protected against all vaccine-preventable diseases. Lack of protection may occur in people who have escaped natural infection and who (1) were not immunized with all recommended vaccines and doses; (2) received appropriate vaccines but at too young an age (eg, measles vaccine before 12 months of age); (3) failed to respond to vaccines administered at appropriate ages; or (4) have waned immunity despite appropriate immunization.

The adolescent population presents many challenges with regard to immunization, including the infrequent visits that adolescents have with health care professionals. As a result, many adolescents do not receive the routine preventive care that provides an opportunity for immunization.

For many years, the adolescent immunization schedule was relatively simple, consisting of only routine administration of the tetanus-diphtheria booster. However, new vaccines have been added to the adolescent immunization schedule, and recommendations for other vaccines have been expanded. In January 2007, the childhood and adolescent immunization schedule was divided into 2 separate tables; one of the tables provides recommendations for people from 7 through 18 years of age (see Childhood and Adolescent Immunization Schedules, Fig 1.2, p 26–27). The adult immunization schedule includes people 19 years of age and older (**www.cdc.gov/vaccines/recs/ schedules/adult-schedule.htm**).

Recommended vaccines for adolescents can be grouped into 3 categories:
- Vaccines for routine administration:
  - Human papillomavirus (3 dose primary series for females)
  - Meningococcal conjugate vaccine (1 primary dose)
  - Tetanus, diphtheria, and acellular pertussis (1 booster dose)
  - Influenza (annual dose)
- Catch-up vaccines:
  - Hepatitis B
  - Inactivated poliovirus
  - MMR
  - Varicella
- Vaccines for certain high-risk adolescents:
  - Hepatitis A
  - Pneumococcal polysaccharide

To ensure age-appropriate immunization, all children should have a routine appointment at 11 through 12 years of age for administration of appropriate vaccines and to provide other preventive health care services that are indicated.[1] During all adolescent visits, immunization status should be reviewed and deficiencies should be corrected. Specific indications for each of these vaccines are given in the respective disease-specific chapters in Section 3.

School immunization laws encourage "catch-up" programs for older adolescents. Accordingly, school and college health services should establish a system to ensure that all students are protected against vaccine-preventable diseases. Because outbreaks of vaccine-preventable diseases, including measles, mumps, and meningococcal disease,

---

[1] American Academy of Pediatrics, Committee on Practice and Ambulatory Medicine and Bright Futures Steering Committee. Recommendations for preventive pediatric health care. *Pediatrics.* 2007;120(6):1376

have occurred at colleges and universities, many colleges and universities are implementing the American College Health Association recommendations for prematriculation
immunization requirements, mandating protection against measles, mumps, rubella,
tetanus, diphtheria, poliovirus, varicella, and HBV (**www.acha.org**). In addition,
N meningitidis vaccine is required by some colleges and universities for people who have
not been immunized previously. Information regarding state laws requiring prematriculation immunization is available at **www.immunize.org/laws.**

Because adolescents and young adults commonly travel internationally, their immunization status and travel plans should be reviewed 2 or more months before departure to allow time to administer any needed vaccines (see International Travel, p 98).
Pediatricians should assist in providing information on benefits and risks of immunization
to ensure that adolescents are appropriately immunized. Vaccine refusal should be documented after emphasis of the importance of immunization.

The possible occurrence of illness attributable to a vaccine-preventable disease in a
school or college should be reported promptly to local health officials according to individual state guidelines (see Appendix V, p 845).

Health Care Personnel[1]

Adults whose occupations place them in contact with patients with contagious diseases are
at increased risk of contracting vaccine-preventable diseases and, if infected, transmitting
them to their patients. All health care personnel should protect themselves and susceptible
patients by receiving appropriate immunizations. Physicians, health care facilities, and
schools for health care professionals should play an active role in implementing policies to
maximize immunization of health care personnel. Vaccine-preventable diseases of special
concern to people involved in the health care of children are as follows (see the disease-
specific chapters in Section 3 for further recommendations).

- *Rubella.* Outbreaks of rubella among health care personnel have been reported.
  Although the disease is mild in adults, the risk to a fetus necessitates documentation
  of rubella immunity in health care personnel of both sexes. People should be considered immune on the basis of a positive serologic test result for rubella antibody or
  documented proof of rubella immunization on or after the first birthday. A history
  of rubella disease is unreliable and should not be used in determining immune status.
  All susceptible people should be immunized with MMR and varicella vaccines before
  initial or continuing contact with pregnant patients.

- *Measles.* Because measles in health care personnel has contributed to spread of this
  disease during outbreaks, evidence of immunity to measles should be required for
  health care personnel. Proof of immunity is established by physician-documented
  measles, a positive serologic test result for measles antibody, or documented receipt of
  2 doses of live virus-containing measles vaccine, the first of which is given on or after
  the first birthday. Health care personnel born before 1957 generally have been considered immune to measles. However, because measles cases have occurred in health care
  personnel in this age group, health care facilities should consider offering at least 1 dose

[1]Centers for Disease Control and Prevention. Immunization of health-care workers: recommendations of the
Advisory Committee on Immunization Practices (ACIP) and the Hospital Infection Control Practices Advisory
Committee (HICPAC). *MMWR Recomm Rep.* 1997;46(RR-18):1–42

of measles-containing vaccine to health care personnel who lack proof of immunity to measles, particularly in communities with documented measles outbreaks.

- **Mumps.** Transmission of mumps in health care facilities can be disruptive and costly. All people who work in health care facilities should be immune to mumps. Adequate mumps immunization for health care personnel born during or after 1957 consists of 2 doses of MMR vaccine. Health care personnel with no history of mumps immunization and no other evidence of immunity should receive 2 doses (at a minimum interval of 28 days between doses) of MMR. Health care personnel who have received only 1 dose previously should receive a second dose. Because birth before 1957 is only presumptive evidence of immunity, health care facilities should consider recommending 1 dose of MMR vaccine for unimmunized health care personnel born before 1957 who do not have a history of physician-diagnosed mumps or laboratory evidence of mumps immunity.[1]

- **Hepatitis B.** Vaccine is recommended for all health care personnel who are likely to be exposed to blood or blood-containing body fluids. The Occupational Safety and Health Administration of the US Department of Labor issued a regulation requiring employers of personnel at risk of occupational exposure to HBV to offer hepatitis B immunization to personnel at the employer's expense. Personnel who refuse recommended immunizations should sign a refusal document.

  In some cases, susceptible health care personnel immunized appropriately with hepatitis B vaccines fail to develop serologic evidence of immunity (antibody to HBsAg [anti-HBs]). Serologic evidence of immunity is defined as serum anti-HBs concentration ≥ 10 mIU/mL. People who do not respond to the primary immunization series should complete a second 3-dose vaccine series with reevaluation of anti-HBs titers 1 to 2 months after the series is completed. People who do not respond to the second series and are HBsAg negative should be considered susceptible to HBV infection and will need to receive HBIG prophylaxis after any known or probable exposure to blood or body fluids infected with HBV.[2]

- **Influenza.** Because health care personnel can transmit influenza to their patients and because health care-associated outbreaks do occur, influenza immunization should be recommended and encouraged for all hospital personnel and other health care personnel with direct patient contact. Health care personnel should be educated about the benefits of influenza immunization and the potential health consequences of influenza illness for themselves and patients at their facilities. Influenza vaccine should be offered at no cost annually to all eligible people and should be available to personnel on all shifts in a convenient manner and location, such as through use of mobile immunization carts. A signed refusal document should be obtained from personnel who decline for reasons other than medical contraindications.[3] Inactivated vaccine or live-attenuated

[1]Centers for Disease Control and Prevention. Notice to readers: updated recommendations of the Advisory Committee on Immunization Practices (ACIP) for the control and elimination of mumps. *MMWR Morb Mortal Wkly Rep.* 2006;55(22):629–630

[2]Centers for Disease Control and Prevention. A comprehensive immunization strategy to eliminate transmission of hepatitis B virus infection in the US. Recommendations of the Advisory Committee on Immunization Practices (ACIP). Part II: immunization of adults. *MMWR Recomm Rep.* 2006;55(RR-16):1–25

[3]Centers for Disease Control and Prevention. Influenza vaccination of health-care personnel: recommendation of the Healthcare Infection Control Practices Advisory Committee (HICPAC) and the Advisory Committee on Immunization Practices (ACIP). *MMWR Recomm Rep.* 2006;55(RR-2):1–16

vaccine (according to age and health status limitations) is appropriate. Live-attenuated vaccine should not be used for personnel who have direct contact with severely immunocompromised people, such as hematopoietic stem cell recipients.

- **Varicella.** Proof of varicella immunity is recommended for all health care personnel. In health care institutions, serologic screening of personnel who have an uncorroborated negative or uncertain history of varicella before immunization is likely to be cost-effective but need not be performed. All health care personnel without evidence of immunity to varicella should receive 2 doses of varicella vaccine. Evidence of immunity to varicella in adults includes any of the following: (1) documentation of 2 doses of varicella vaccine at least 4 weeks apart; (2) having been born in the United States before 1980 (although for health care personnel and pregnant women, having been born in the United States before 1980 should not be considered definitive evidence of immunity); (3) history of varicella diagnosed or verified by a health care professional (for a patient reporting a history of or presenting with an atypical case, a mild case, or both, health care professionals should seek either an epidemiologic link with a typical varicella case or evidence of laboratory confirmation, if it was performed at the time of acute disease); (4) history of herpes zoster diagnosed by a health care professional; or (5) laboratory evidence of immunity or laboratory confirmation of disease.

- **Pertussis.** Pertussis outbreaks involving adults occur in the community and the workplace. Health care personnel frequently are exposed to *Bordetella pertussis* and have substantial risk of illness and can be sources for spread of infection to patients, colleagues, their families, and the community. Health care personnel in hospitals or ambulatory-care settings who have direct patient contact should receive a single dose of Tdap as soon as is feasible if they have not previously received Tdap. An interval as short as 2 years from the last dose of Td is recommended. Other health care personnel should receive a single dose of Tdap to replace the next scheduled Td dose. Hospitals and ambulatory-care facilities should provide Tdap for health care personnel using approaches that maximize immunization rates.[1]

- **Tuberculosis.** Early detection and treatment of patients (or visitors) with communicable tuberculosis is recommended to prevent tuberculosis infection in health care personnel. The risk of transmission of tuberculosis in hospitals varies greatly and is determined by multiple factors (eg, the community profile of tuberculosis disease and the types of environmental controls in place). Policies for tuberculin skin testing for health care personnel should conform to CDC guidelines.[2] Each health care setting should have a tuberculosis infection-control plan based on initial and ongoing evaluations of the risk for transmission of *Mycobacterium tuberculosis* in the specific setting. The need for screening and frequency of screening should be based on the risk classification (ie, low, moderate, or high). Most pediatric settings will be low risk; more details are available in the CDC guidelines. Even in a low-risk setting, all health care personnel

---

[1] Centers for Disease Control and Prevention. Preventing tetanus, diphtheria, and pertussis among adults: use of tetanus toxoid, reduced diphtheria toxoid and acellular pertussis vaccine recommendations of the Advisory Committee on Immunization Practices (ACIP) and recommendation of ACIP, supported by the Healthcare Infection Control Practices Advisory Committee (HICPAC), for use of Tdap among health-care personnel. *MMWR Recomm Rep.* 2006;55(RR-17):1–37

[2] Centers for Disease Control and Prevention. Guidelines for preventing the transmission of *Mycobacterium tuberculosis* in health-care settings, 2005. *MMWR Recomm Rep.* 2005;54(17):1–141

should receive baseline tuberculosis screening using a 2-step tuberculin skin test or a single blood assay for *M tuberculosis.*[1]

Refugees and Immigrants

Prevention of infectious diseases in refugee and immigrant children presents special challenges because of the diseases to which these children may have been exposed and the different immunization practices in their native countries. In addition, other aspects of providing care (including testing for exposure to environmental toxins, such as lead) to immigrant, refugee, homeless, and immigrant children should be considered.[2] In 1996, Congress amended the Immigration and Nationality Act (INA), requiring immigrant visa applicants to provide "proof of vaccination" with at least the first dose of ACIP-recommended vaccines before entry into the United States. Although these regulations apply to most immigrant children entering the United States, internationally adopted children who are 10 years of age or younger may obtain an exemption from these requirements. Adoptive parents are required to sign a waiver indicating their intention to comply with the ACIP immunization requirements within 30 days after the child's arrival in the United States. Refugees are not required to meet immunization requirements of the INA at the time of initial entry into the United States but must show proof of immunization when they apply for permanent residency, typically 1 year after arrival. However, in outbreak settings, selected refugees bound for the United States are immunized in their country of origin before arrival in the United States. Clinicians should review the CDC Refugee Health Web site (**www.cdc.gov/ncidod/dq/refugee/index.htm**) for information about which refugee populations currently are receiving immunization outside the United States. Information about immunization requirements for immigrants is available at **www.cdc.gov/ncidod/dq/panel_vaccine_2007.htm.**

Children who have resided in refugee processing camps for a few months often have had access to medical and treatment services, which may have included some immunizations. However, these children almost universally are incompletely immunized and often have no immunization records. For refugee children whose immunizations are not up-to-date, as documented by a written immunization record (see Immunizations Received Outside the United States, p 36), vaccines as recommended for their age should be administered (see Fig 1.1–1.3, p 24–28). For children without documentation of immunizations, a new vaccine schedule may be initiated. Alternatively, measurement of antibody concentrations to diphtheria, tetanus, measles, mumps, rubella, varicella, and poliovirus (each serotype) as well as anti-HBs, HBsAg, and antibody to hepatitis B core antigen (anti-HBc), if from an area with endemic hepatitis B infection, may be considered to determine whether the child needs additional immunizations or initiation of the immunization schedule appropriate for that child's age (see Table 2.17, Approaches to the Evaluation and Immunization of Internationally Adopted Children, p 185). Although many children will have received DTP, poliovirus, measles, and hepatitis B vaccines, most will not have received Hib, pneumococcal, hepatitis A, rubella, mumps, and varicella vaccines. Measles antibody may be measured to determine whether the child is immune; however, many

---

[1]Centers for Disease Control and Prevention. Guidelines for preventing the transmission of *Mycobacterium tuberculosis* in health-care settings, 2005. *MMWR Recomm Rep.* 2005;54(17):1–141

[2]American Academy of Pediatrics, Committee on Community Health Services. Providing care for immigrant, homeless, and migrant children. *Pediatrics.* 2005;115(4):1095–1100

children may need a dose of mumps and rubella vaccines, because these vaccines are not given routinely in developing countries. A clinical diagnosis of rubella without serologic testing should not be accepted as evidence of rubella immunity. Varicella vaccine is not administered in most countries, and history of varicella infection may be unavailable or unreliable in these populations; therefore, children should be immunized for varicella or have antibody testing performed.

All refugees and immigrants from areas with endemic hepatitis B infection, particularly Asia and Africa, should be screened for hepatitis B with serologic tests for HBsAg, anti-HBs, and anti-HBc. A child who has positive test results for HBsAg has active infection and may be defined as a chronic carrier if the HBsAg persists for longer than 6 months. Most children who are HBsAg carriers are asymptomatic. Therefore, screening is important to identify children who need follow-up and management and to limit transmission of disease. Transmission risks should be minimal among children in the United States because of universal infant HBV immunization programs. However, unimmunized adult caregivers should be given hepatitis B vaccine if they are susceptible and HBIG if they have had a significant exposure to blood of a carrier (see Hepatitis B, p 337). Serologic screening of all pregnant refugees and immigrants for HBsAg is imperative to identify women whose infants need passive as well as active immunoprophylaxis.

Tuberculosis and HIV infection are important public health concerns, because many refugees and immigrants come from countries with high prevalences of tuberculosis and HIV infection. Tuberculosis cases in foreign-born people now account for more than 50% of all tuberculosis cases in the United States. Although tuberculosis rates have decreased among children born in the United States in the last decade, rates remain high among children from developing countries. The overseas screening requirements for tuberculosis for immigrants and refugees bound for the United States underwent a major revision in 2007, including tuberculosis screening for all people, and are in the process of being implemented. Information about the screening and implementation is available at **www.cdc.gov/ncidod/dq/panel_2007.htm.** The risk of HIV infection among refugees and immigrants depends on the country of origin and on individual risk factors, especially among vulnerable refugee populations. As part of the required overseas medical assessment, HIV testing is performed on all immigrants and refugees 15 years of age and older. Children younger than 15 years of age are tested for HIV if history or examination raises concern about possible HIV infection (eg, maternal history of HIV infection, history of rape or sexual assault). The decision to screen children for HIV after arrival in the United States should depend on history and risk factors (eg, receipt of blood products, maternal drug use), physical examination findings, and prevalence of HIV infection in the child's country of origin (**www.who.int/hiv/countries**). If there is a suspicion of HIV infection, testing should be performed before administration of live vaccines.

International Travel

Children and adolescents should be up-to-date on routinely recommended immunizations before international travel. In addition, travel requires consideration of additional vaccines to prevent hepatitis A, yellow fever, meningococcal disease, typhoid fever, rabies, and Japanese encephalitis. Vaccines may be required or recommended depending on the destination and type of international travel (see Table 1.15, p 101). Travelers to tropical and subtropical areas often risk exposure to malaria, dengue fever, other vectorborne pathogens, leptospirosis, diarrhea, and other diseases for which vaccines are not available. For travelers to areas with endemic malaria, antimalarial chemoprophylaxis and insect precautions are vitally important (see Malaria, p 438). Attention to hand hygiene and choosing safer foods and beverages for consumption also can reduce travelers' risk of acquiring other communicable diseases.

Up-to-date information, including alerts about current disease outbreaks that may affect international travelers, is available on the CDC Travelers' Health Web site at **wwwn.cdc.gov/travel/default.aspx** or the WHO Web site at **www.who.int/ith/**. *Health Information for International Travel* (the "Yellow Book") is revised every 2 years by the CDC and is an excellent reference for travelers and for practitioners who advise international travelers of health risks. To enhance the usefulness of travel notices, the CDC Travelers' Health Web site issues and removes travel notices under 1 of 4 levels: in the news, outbreak notice, travel health precaution, and travel health warning. Travel information and recommendations can be obtained from the CDC (877-FYI-TRIP). Local and state health departments and travel clinics also can provide updated information. Information about cruise ship sanitation inspection scores and reports can be found at **www.cdc.gov/nceh/vsp/default.htm.** In June 2007, federal agencies developed a public health Do Not Board (DNB) list, enabling domestic and international public health officials to request that people with communicable diseases who meet specific criteria and pose a serious threat to the public be restricted from boarding commercial aircraft from or arriving in the United States.[1]

RECOMMENDED IMMUNIZATIONS

Infants and children embarking on international travel should be up-to-date on receipt of immunizations recommended for their age. For travel to any developing country, immunization against HAV also is recommended for any child or adolescent not immunized previously (see Hepatitis A, p 329). To optimize immunity before departure, vaccines may need to be given on an accelerated schedule (see Table 1.15, p 101).

POLIOVIRUS. Although poliovirus eradication previously had been targeted for 2005, polio remains endemic in a few countries in Africa and Asia (an up-to-date listing of polio cases can be found at **www.polioeradication.org**). The Western Hemisphere was declared free of wild-type poliovirus in 1994, and the Western Pacific Region was declared free in 2000. The finding of vaccine-derived poliovirus in stool samples from several asymptomatic unimmunized people in a community is the first occurrence of vaccine-derived poliovirus transmission in a community in the United States since OPV immunizations were discontinued in 2000.[2] This finding raises concerns about the risk of transmission to other communities with a low level of transmission and the risk of a polio outbreak occurring in the United States. To ensure protection, all children, including pediatric travelers, should be immunized fully against poliovirus. Three doses of IPV vaccine should be administered before departure as shown in the recommended childhood and adolescent immunization schedules (Fig 1.1–1.3, p 24–28). If necessary, the doses may be given at 4-week intervals, although 6- to 8-week intervals are preferred. Children

---

[1]Centers for Disease Control and Prevention. Federal air travel restrictions for public health purposes—United States, June 2007–May 2008. *MMWR Morb Mortal Wkly Rep.* 2008;57(37):10009–1012

[2]Centers for Disease Control and Prevention. Poliovirus infections in four unvaccinated children—Minnesota, August–October 2005. *MMWR Morb Mortal Wkly Rep.* 2005;54(41):1053–1055

should receive a supplemental fourth dose at 4 to 6 years of age (see Poliovirus Infections, p 541).

MEASLES. People traveling abroad should be immune to measles to provide personal protection and minimize importation of the infection. Importation of measles remains an important source for measles cases in the United States.[1] People should be considered susceptible to measles unless they have documentation of appropriate immunization, physician-diagnosed measles, or laboratory evidence of immunity to measles or were born in the United States before 1957. For people born in the United States in 1957 or after, 2 doses of measles vaccine, the first administered at or after 12 months of age, are required to ensure immunity (see Measles, p 444). The age of initiation of measles immunization can be lowered for children traveling to areas with a high rate of measles transmission. Infants 6 through 11 months of age should receive 1 dose of a measles-containing vaccine. Children receiving measles vaccine before 12 months of age require 2 additional doses of a measles-containing vaccine separated by at least 1 month starting at 12 through 15 months of age.

HEPATITIS B. Hepatitis B vaccine is recommended routinely for all children in the United States and should be considered for susceptible travelers of all ages visiting areas where hepatitis B infection is endemic, such as countries in Asia, Africa, and some parts of South America (see Hepatitis B, p 337). An accelerated dosing schedule is licensed for one hepatitis B vaccine (Engerix-B), during which the first 3 doses are given at 0, 1, and 2 months. This schedule may benefit travelers who have insufficient time (ie, less than 6 months) to complete a standard 3-dose schedule before departure. If the accelerated schedule is used, a fourth dose should be given 12 months after the third dose (see Hepatitis B, p 337). A combination hepatitis A-hepatitis B vaccine is available for people 18 years of age and older.

REQUIRED OR RECOMMENDED TRAVEL-RELATED IMMUNIZATIONS

Depending on the destination, planned activity, and length of stay, other immunizations may be required or recommended (see Table 1.15, p 101, and disease-specific chapters in Section 3).

HEPATITIS A. Immunoprophylaxis against HAV infection is indicated for susceptible people traveling internationally to areas with intermediate or high rates of HAV infection. These include all areas of the world except Australia, Canada, Japan, New Zealand, and Western Europe. Inactivated vaccine is used for immunoprophylaxis for people 1 year of age and older. For children younger than 1 year of age, IG is indicated, because hepatitis A vaccine is not licensed in the United States for use in this age group. Administration of IG may interfere with the immune response to varicella and MMR vaccines for up to 6 months.

YELLOW FEVER. Yellow fever vaccine, a live-attenuated virus vaccine, is required by some countries as a condition of entry, including travelers arriving from regions with endemic infection.[2] The vaccine is available in the United States only in centers designated by

---

[1]Centers for Disease Control and Prevention. Update: measles—United States, January–July 2008. *MMWR Morb Mortal Wkly Rep.* 2008;57(33):893–896

[2]Centers for Disease Control and Prevention. Yellow fever vaccine. Recommendations of the Advisory Committee on Immunization Practices, 2002. *MMWR Recomm Rep.* 2002;51(RR-17):1–10

Table 1.15. Recommended Immunizations for Travelers to Developing Countries[a]

Immunizations	Length of Travel		
	Brief, <2 wk	Intermediate, 2 wk through 3 mo	Long-term Residential, >3 mo
Review and complete age-appropriate childhood schedule (see text for details) • DTaP, poliovirus, pneumococcal, and *Haemophilus influenzae* type b vaccines may be given at 4-wk intervals if necessary to complete the recommended schedule before departure • Measles: 2 additional doses given if younger than 12 mo of age at first dose • Varicella • Hepatitis B[b]	+	+	+
Yellow fever[c]	+	+	+
Hepatitis A[d]	+	+	+
Typhoid fever[e]	±	+	+
Meningococcal disease[f]	±	±	±
Rabies[g]	±	+	+
Japanese encephalitis[h]	±	±	+

DTaP indicates diphtheria and tetanus toxoids and acellular pertussis; +, recommended; ±, consider.

[a]See disease-specific chapters in Section 3 for details. For further sources of information, see text.

[b]If insufficient time to complete 6-month primary series, accelerated series can be given (see text for details).

[c]For regions with endemic infection (see *Health Information for International Travel*, p 3).

[d]Indicated for travelers to areas with intermediate or high endemic rates of HAV infection.

[e]Indicated for travelers who will consume food and liquids in areas of poor sanitation.

[f]Recommended for regions of Africa with endemic infection and during local epidemics and required for travel to Saudi Arabia for the Hajj.

[g]Indicated for people with high risk of animal exposure (especially to dogs) and for travelers to countries with endemic infection.

[h]For regions with endemic infection (see *Health Information for International Travel*, p 3). For high-risk activities in areas experiencing outbreaks, vaccine is recommended, even for brief travel.

state health departments. Current requirements and recommendations for yellow fever immunization on the basis of travel destination can be obtained from the CDC Travelers' Health Web site (**wwwn.cdc.gov/travel/default.aspx**) or from the CDC Yellow Book, *Health Information for International Travel*. Yellow fever occurs year-round in predominantly rural areas of sub-Saharan Africa and South America; in recent years, outbreaks have been reported, including in some urban areas. Although rare, yellow fever continues to be reported among unimmunized travelers and may be fatal. Prevention measures against yellow fever should include immunization and protection against mosquito bites (see Prevention of Mosquitoborne Infections, p 193). Yellow fever vaccine generally is considered to be a safe and effective vaccine. However, the vaccine rarely has been found to be associated with a risk of viscerotropic disease (multiple organ system failure) and neurotropic disease (postvaccinal encephalitis). There is increased risk of adverse events in people of any age with thymic dysfunction and people older than 60 years of age. The vaccine should not be used in infants younger than 6 months of age and should be used with caution in infants younger than 9 months of age and only after consultation with a travel medicine expert or the CDC Division of Vector-Borne Infectious Diseases (970-221-6400) or the Division of Global Migration and Quarantine (404-498-1600) to weigh risks and benefits. Whenever possible, immunization should be delayed until 9 months of age to minimize the risk of vaccine-associated encephalitis. People who cannot receive yellow fever vaccine because of contraindications should consider alternative itineraries or destinations or should wait until infants reach an appropriate age to be immunized before traveling to an area with endemic infection. The CDC has stated that, given the risk of serious illness and death attributable to yellow fever, potential for transmission of the disease, and the known effectiveness of the vaccine, clinicians should continue to use yellow fever vaccine to protect travelers. However, the CDC recommends that health care professionals carefully review travel itineraries so that only people traveling to areas with endemic yellow fever infection or areas where there is reported yellow fever activity receive yellow fever vaccine.

CHOLERA. The whole-cell inactivated cholera vaccine no longer is produced in the United States. According to WHO regulations, no country may require cholera immunization as a condition for entry. However, despite WHO recommendations, some local authorities may require documentation of immunization. In such cases, a notation of vaccine contraindication should be sufficient to satisfy local requirements.

TYPHOID. Typhoid vaccine is recommended for travelers who may be exposed to contaminated food or water. In particular, people with anticipated long-term travel or residence in areas with poor sanitation and people who visit remote areas are at greatest risk. Two typhoid vaccines are available for civilian use in the United States: an oral vaccine containing live-attenuated *Salmonella typhi* (Ty21a strain) and a parenteral Vi capsular polysaccharide (ViCPS) vaccine. For specific recommendations, see *Salmonella* Infections (p 584). Mefloquine or chloroquine may be administered simultaneously with oral Ty21a vaccine. The oral vaccine capsules should be refrigerated. Because the vaccine is not completely efficacious, typhoid immunization is not a substitute for careful selection of food and drink.

MENINGOCOCCUS. Meningococcal tetravalent (groups A, C, Y, and W-135) vaccine (polysaccharide or conjugate) should be offered for travelers to areas where epidemics of meningococcal infection occur frequently, such as sub-Saharan Africa, and countries with current meningococcal epidemics. Saudi Arabia requires a certificate of immunization for pilgrims to Mecca or Medina, where outbreaks with meningococcal serogroups A and W-135 have been reported in travelers participating in the Hajj.

RABIES.[1] Rabies immunization should be considered for children who will be traveling to areas where they may encounter wild or domestic animals (particularly dogs in developing countries) or where they may engage in activities involving increased risk of rabies transmission (eg, spelunking and camping), especially because children are less likely to report having been scratched or bitten. The 3-dose preexposure series is given by IM injection (see Rabies, p 552). In the event of a bite by a potentially rabid animal, all travelers (whether they have received preexposure rabies vaccine or not) should be counseled

[1]Centers for Disease Control and Prevention. Human rabies prevention—United States, 2008: recommendations of the Advisory Committee on Immunization Practices. *MMWR Recomm Rep.* 2008;57(RR-3):1–28

to clean the wound thoroughly with soap and water and then promptly receive post-exposure management, including Rabies Immune Globulin and the immunization series if not immunized previously or booster doses of rabies vaccine if immunized previously.

JAPANESE ENCEPHALITIS. Japanese encephalitis (JE) virus, a mosquitoborne flavivirus, is the most common cause of encephalitis in Asia. Among an estimated 35 000 to 50 000 annual cases of JE, approximately 20% to 30% of patients die and 30% to 50% of survivors have neurologic sequelae. JE virus transmission occurs principally in rural agricultural areas, often associated with rice production. In temperate areas of Asia, JE cases usually peak in summer and fall. In the tropics, transmission varies with monsoon rains and irrigation practices, and cases may occur year-round. In countries with endemic infection, JE primarily is a disease of children However, travel-associated JE can occur among people of any age. The risk of JE for most travelers to Asia is low but varies on the basis of season, destination, duration, and activities. The overall incidence of JE reported among people from countries without endemic infection traveling to Asia is less than 1 case per million travelers. However, expatriates and travelers staying for prolonged periods in rural areas with active JE virus transmission likely are at similar risk as the susceptible resident population (0.1 to 2 cases per 100 000 people per week). Short-term travelers whose visits are restricted to major urban areas are at minimal risk of JE. For additional information on JE vaccine and preventing arboviral diseases, see Arboviruses (p 214).

INFLUENZA. In addition to routine annual influenza immunization, vaccine may be warranted for international travelers, depending on the destination, duration of travel, risk of acquisition of disease (in part on the basis of the season of the year), and the traveler's underlying health status. Because the influenza season is different in the northern and southern hemispheres and epidemic strains may differ, the antigenic composition of influenza vaccines used in North America may be different from those used in the southern hemisphere, and timing of administration may vary (see Influenza, p 400).

TUBERCULOSIS. The risk of acquiring latent tuberculosis infection (LTBI) during international travel depends on the activities of the traveler and the epidemiology of tuberculosis in the areas in which travel occurs. In general, the risk of acquiring LTBI during usual tourism activities appears to be low, and no pre- or post-travel testing is recommended routinely. When travelers live or work among the general population of a high-prevalence country, the risk may be appreciably higher. In most high-prevalence countries, contact investigation of tuberculosis cases is not performed, and treatment of LTBI is not available. Children returning to the United States who have signs or symptoms compatible with tuberculosis should be evaluated appropriately for tuberculosis disease. It may be prudent to perform a tuberculin skin test 8 to 12 weeks after return for children who spent 3 months or longer in a high-prevalence country. Pretravel administration of BCG vaccine generally is not recommended. However, some countries may require BCG vaccine for issuance of work and residency permits for expatriate workers and their families.

OTHER CONSIDERATIONS. In addition to vaccine-preventable diseases, travelers to the tropics will be exposed to other diseases, such as malaria, which can be life threatening. Prevention strategies for malaria are twofold: prevention of mosquito bites and use of antimalarial chemoprophylaxis. For recommendations on appropriate use of chemoprophylaxis, including recommendations for pregnant women, infants, and breastfeeding mothers, see Malaria (p 438). Prevention of mosquito bites will decrease the risk of malaria, dengue fever, and other mosquito-transmitted diseases (see Prevention of Mosquitoborne Infections, p 193). Appropriate personal protective measures, particularly during the malaria mosquito-biting period from dusk to dawn, can be highly effective. These preventive measures include wearing long-sleeved shirts and long trousers; application of insect repellent, such as diethyltoluamide (DEET), to exposed skin; and use of window screens and bed nets. Insect sprays and soaks containing the residual insecticide permethrin may be applied to clothing and bed nets.

Traveler's diarrhea is a significant problem that may be mitigated by attention to foods and beverages ingested and by appropriately treating suspected water sources. Chemoprophylaxis generally is not recommended. Educating families about self-treatment, particularly oral rehydration, is critical. Packets of oral rehydration salts can be obtained before travel or are readily available in most pharmacies throughout the world, especially in developing countries where diarrheal diseases are most common. During international travel, families may want to carry an antimicrobial agent (eg, fluoroquinolone for people 16 years of age and older and azithromycin for younger children) for treatment of significant diarrheal symptoms. Antimotility agents may be considered for older children and adolescents (see *Escherichia coli* Diarrhea, p 294) but should not be used if diarrhea is bloody.

Travelers should be aware of potential acquisition of respiratory tract viruses, including avian influenza. They should be counseled on hand hygiene and avoidance of close contact with animals (dead or live). Swimming, other recreational water sports, and ecotourism carry risks of acquisition of infections from environmental contamination.

Recommendations for Care of Children in Special Circumstances

BIOLOGICAL TERRORISM

Some infectious agents have the potential to be used in acts of bioterrorism. The Centers for Disease Control and Prevention (CDC) has designated 3 categories of biological agents to stratify the risk to civilians and guide national public health bioterrorism preparedness and response.[1] The highest-priority agents are designated category A, because they can be disseminated or transmitted person-to-person easily, cause high rates of mortality with potential for major public health effects, could cause public panic and social disruption, and require special action for public health preparedness. Category A agents are transmitted easily and cause high morbidity and mortality rates. Organisms in category A cause anthrax, smallpox, plague, tularemia, botulism, and viral hemorrhagic fevers, including Ebola, Marburg, Lassa, Junin, and other related viruses. Category B agents are moderately easy to disseminate, cause moderate morbidity and low mortality rates, and require enhanced diagnostic capacity and disease surveillance. These agents include *Coxiella burnetii* (Q fever), *Brucella* species (brucellosis), *Burkholderia mallei* (glanders), *Burkholderia pseudomallei* (melioidosis), alphaviruses (Venezuelan equine, eastern equine, and western equine encephalomyelitis), *Rickettsia prowazekii* (typhus), *Chlamydophila psittaci* (psittacosis), and toxins (toxic syndromes including those caused by ricin toxin from *Ricinus communis* [castor beans], epsilon toxin of *Clostridium perfringens*, and *Staphylococcus* enterotoxin B). Additional category B agents that are foodborne or waterborne safety threats include, but are not limited to, *Salmonella* species, *Shigella dysenteriae*, *Escherichia coli* O157:H7, *Vibrio cholerae*, and *Cryptosporidium parvum*. Category C agents include emerging pathogens that could be engineered for mass dissemination in the future because of availability, ease of production and dissemination, and potential for high morbidity and mortality rates and major health effects. Examples include Nipah virus, hantavirus, tickborne hemorrhagic fever viruses, tickborne encephalitis viruses, yellow fever virus, and multidrug-resistant *Mycobacterium tuberculosis*.

Children may be particularly vulnerable to a bioterrorist attack, because children have a more rapid respiratory rate, increased skin permeability, higher ratio of skin surface area to mass, and less fluid reserve compared with adults. Accurate and rapid diagnosis may be more difficult in children because of their inability to describe symptoms. In addition, the adults on whom children depend for their health and safety may become ill or require quarantine during a bioterrorist event. Many preventive and therapeutic agents recommended for adults exposed or potentially exposed to agents of bioterrorism have not been studied in infants and children, and pediatric doses have not been

---

[1]Centers for Disease Control and Prevention. Biological and chemical terrorism: strategic plan for preparedness and response. Recommendations of the CDC Strategic Planning Workgroup. *MMWR Recomm Rep.* 2000;49(RR-4):1–14

established or approved by the US Food and Drug Administration for use in children.[1] Children also may be at risk of unique adverse effects from preventive and therapeutic agents that are recommended for treating exposure to agents of bioterrorism. Further, availability of appropriate pediatric formulations of medical countermeasures may be limited. Parents, pediatricians, and other adults should be cognizant of the psychological responses of children to a disaster or terrorist incident to reduce the possibility of long-term psychological morbidity.[2]

Fever, malaise, headache, vomiting, and diarrhea are common early manifestations of illness caused by many bioterrorist agents and other infectious diseases. Some bioterrorist agents can cause typical distinctive signs and symptoms and incubation periods and require unique diagnostic tests, isolation, and recommended treatment and prophylaxis. Agents are discussed in Section 3 under specific pathogens, and extensive information and advice are available elsewhere. Table 2.1 (p 107) lists resources, including telephone numbers and Internet sites, that provide updated information concerning clinical recognition, prevention, diagnosis, and treatment of illness caused by potential agents of bioterrorism.

Clinicians should be familiar with the reporting requirements within their public health jurisdiction for these conditions. When clinicians suspect that illness is caused by an act of biological terrorism, they should contact their local public health authority immediately so that appropriate infection-control measures and outbreak investigations can begin. In the event of a biological terrorist attack, clinicians should review the CDC Emergency Preparedness and Response Web site (**http://emergency.cdc. gov/bioterrorism**) for current information and specific prophylaxis and treatment guidelines. Public health authorities should be contacted before obtaining and submitting patient specimens for identification of suspected agents of bioterrorism.

The American Academy of Pediatrics and Agency for Healthcare Research and Quality have prepared a resource document outlining recommendations to pediatricians and the government to ensure that the needs of children and families are met in the event of chemical or biological terrorism.[3]

....

BLOOD SAFETY: REDUCING THE RISK OF TRANSFUSION-TRANSMITTED INFECTIONS

In the United States, the risk of transmission of infectious agents through transfusion of blood components (Red Blood Cells, Platelets, and Plasma) and plasma derivatives (clotting factor concentrates, immune globulins, and protein-containing plasma volume expanders) is extremely low. Nevertheless, continued vigilance, including improved surveillance and reporting, is crucial, because no uniform system for transfusion reaction surveillance exists in the United States, and the blood supply remains vulnerable to

---

[1]American Academy of Pediatrics, Committee on Environmental Health and Committee on Infectious Diseases. Chemical-biological terrorism and its impact on children. *Pediatrics.* 2006;118(3):1267–1278

[2]Hagan JF Jr, and American Academy of Pediatrics, Committee on Psychosocial Aspects of Child and Family Health. Psychosocial implications of disaster or terrorism on children: a guide for the pediatrician. *Pediatrics.* 2005;116(3):787–795

[3]American Academy of Pediatrics. *Pediatric Terrorism and Disaster Preparedness: A Resource for Pediatricians.* AHRQ Publication No. 06(07)-0056 and 06(07)-0056-1. Rockville, MD: Agency for Healthcare Research and Quality; October 2006. Available at: **www.ahrq.gov/research/pedprep/resource.htm**

Table 2.1. Emergency Contacts and Educational Resources

Health Department Information

- State Health Department Web sites: **www.cdc.gov/mmwr/international/relres.html**

Emergency Contacts

- Centers for Disease Control and Prevention (CDC) 24-Hour Emergency Operations Center: **770-488-7100**
- US Army Medical Research Institute of Infectious Disease (USAMRIID) Emergency Response Line: **888-872-7443**
- National Response Center: **800-424-8802** or **202-267-2675**
- National Disaster Medical System: **800-USA-NDMS** or **www.ndms.dhhs.gov**

Selected Web Information Resources

- American Academy of Pediatrics bioterrorism information: **www.aap.org/terrorism**
- CDC Emergency Preparedness and Response: **http://emergency.cdc.gov**
- Infectious Diseases Society of America Web site: **www.idsociety.org/BT/ToC.htm**
- American Society for Microbiology Web site: **www.asm.org/Policy/index.asp?bid 20**
- University of Pittsburgh Medical Center, Center for Biosecurity: **www.upmc-biosecurity.org**
- USAMRIID: **www.usamriid.army.mil/**
- US Food and Drug Administration (FDA) Drug Preparedness: **www.fda.gov/cder/drugprepare/default.htm#Pediatrics**

organisms associated with newly identified or emerging infections. This chapter reviews blood and plasma collection procedures in the United States, factors that have contributed to enhancing the safety of the blood supply, some of the known and emerging infectious agents and related blood safety concerns, and approaches to decreasing the risk of transfusion-transmitted infections.

Blood Components and Plasma Derivatives

Blood collection, preparation, and testing are regulated by the US Food and Drug Administration (FDA). In the United States, whole blood is collected from volunteer donors and separated into **components,** including Red Blood Cells, Platelets, Plasma, and White Blood Cells. Platelets and, less commonly, Red Blood Cells and Plasma can be collected through apheresis, in which blood passes through a machine that separates blood components and returns uncollected components to the donor. Plasma for transfusion or further manufacturing into plasma derivatives can be prepared from Whole Blood or collected by apheresis. Most Plasma in the United States is obtained from paid donors at specialized collection centers. **Plasma derivatives** are prepared by pooling plasma from many donors and subjecting the plasma to a fractionation process that separates the desired proteins, including Gamma Globulin and clotting factors.

From an infectious disease standpoint, plasma derivatives differ from blood components in several ways. For economic and therapeutic reasons, plasma from thousands of donors is pooled, and therefore, recipients of plasma derivatives have vastly greater donor exposure than do blood component recipients. However, plasma derivatives are able to withstand vigorous viral inactivation processes that would destroy Red Blood Cells and Platelets. Most recognized infectious organisms, with the notable exception of non–lipid-enveloped viruses and prions, have been shown to be inactivated easily by plasma processing methods. Development and evaluation of various strategies for inactivation of infectious agents are ongoing.

Current Blood Safety Measures

The safety of the blood supply relies on multiple steps, including donor interview and selection, donor screening by serologic tests, screening of collected blood components for markers of infection, inactivation procedures for plasma-derived products, and leukodepletion of certain blood components (see Tables 2.2, p 109, and 2.3, p 110).[1] Blood donors are interviewed to exclude people with a history of exposures or behaviors that increase the risk that their blood will contain an infectious agent. All blood donations are tested routinely for syphilis, hepatitis B virus (HBV), hepatitis C virus (HCV), human T-lymphotropic virus (HTLV) types 1 and 2, and human immunodeficiency virus (HIV) types 1 and 2; selected donations are tested for cytomegalovirus (CMV). Since July 2003, most donations are tested for West Nile virus. Since January 2007, most donations were tested on an investigational basis for *Trypanosoma cruzi*, the etiologic agent of Chagas disease.

Transfusion-Transmitted Agents: Known Threats and Potential Pathogens

Any infectious agent that has an infectious blood phase potentially can be transmitted by blood transfusion. Factors that influence the risk of transmission by transfusion of an infectious agent and development of clinical disease in the recipient include prevalence and incidence of the agent in donors, duration of hematogenous phase, tolerance of the agent to processing and storage, infectivity and pathogenicity of the agent, and recipient's health status. Table 2.3 (p 110) lists major known transfusion-transmitted infections and some of the emerging agents under investigation.

VIRUSES

HIV (P 380), HCV (P 357), HBV (P 337). The probability of infection in recipients who are exposed to HIV, HCV, or HBV in transfused blood products is approximately 90%. Although blood donations are screened for these viruses, there is a small residual risk of infection resulting almost exclusively from donations collected during the "window period" of infection—the period soon after infection during which a blood donor is infectious but screening results are negative.

To decrease the time period when donor HIV and HCV infection may be undetected, routine nucleic acid amplification (NAA) testing of blood and plasma donations was implemented beginning in 1999 in the United States and is performed on blood and plasma donations. At present, NAA testing for HBV is an optional donor screening test. Various estimates suggest that NAA testing on pooled units can decrease the preantibody seroconversion "window period" from 22 days to 13 to 15 days for HIV and from 70 days to 10 to 29 days for HCV. Mathematical models have been developed to estimate the cur-

---

[1] www.redcross.org/services/biomed/0,1082,0_557_,00.html

Table 2.2. Blood Donor Screening Measures[a]

Measure	Targeted Infectious Agents
General interview and screening	Bloodborne phase of multiple agents
• Previous donor history (ie, no deferral in effect)	
• General health, current illness, temperature at time of donation	
• Donor confidential unit exclusion option[b]	
• Remember to notify blood collector of illness (eg, fever, diarrhea after donation, or any other pertinent information recalled)	
Specific risk factor history	
• High-risk sexual behaviors or injection drug use in donor or donor's partner(s)	HIV, HCV, HBV, HTLV
• Geographic risks (travel and residence)	Malaria, vCJD, leishmaniasis
• History of specific infections	HIV, HBV, HCV, other hepatitis agents, parasites (those causing malaria, Chagas disease, babesiosis, and leishmaniasis)
• Previous parenteral exposure to blood via transfusion or occupational exposure; not lifetime deferral	HIV, HCV, HBV
Laboratory screening	HIV-1 and HIV-2 (HIV antibody and HIV-1 NAA), HCV (antibody), HIV and HCV NAA; HBV (HBsAg and anti-HBc, ALT sometimes is performed but not recommended by the FDA), HTLV-1 and HTLV-2 (antibodies), syphilis (antibodies), WNV (NAA), screens for bacteria

HIV indicates human immunodeficiency virus; HCV, hepatitis C virus; HBV, hepatitis B virus; HTLV, human T-lymphotropic virus; vCJD, variant Creutzfeldt-Jakob disease; NAA, nucleic acid amplification (test); HBsAg, hepatitis B surface antigen; anti-HBc, antibody to hepatitis B core antigen; ALT alanine transaminase; FDA, US Food and Drug Administration; WNV, West Nile Virus.

[a]Screening of Source Plasma (paid) donors is similar but not identical. For example, because HTLV-1 and HTLV-2 are cell-associated agents, Plasma donations are not tested for anti-HTLV-1 and anti-HTLV-2. Donors are tested for syphilis at least every 4 months.

[b]Donor is given the opportunity during the screening process to exclude himself or herself without disclosing the reason.

rent very low risks of transfusion transmission of HIV, HCV, and HBV using currently accepted screening policies (Table 2.3, p 110).

HTLV-1 AND HTLV-2. Infections with HTLV are relatively common in certain geographic areas of the world and in specific populations. For example, HTLV-1 is more common in Japan, the Caribbean, and the southern United States, and HTLV-2 is more common in indigenous people of North America, Central America, and South America and among injection drug users in the United States and Europe. HTLV-1 and HTLV-2 are transmitted by transfusion of cellular components of blood but not by plasma or plasma derivatives. The risk of HTLV transmission from screened blood donated during the "window period" has been estimated at 1 per 641 000 units screened. However, transmission of

Table 2.3. Selected Known and Potential Transfusion-Transmitted Agents[a]

Agents and Products	Transfusion-Transmitted	Pathogenic	Estimated per-Unit Risk of Contamination (US Studies, Except as Noted)
Viruses for which all blood donors tested			
HIV	Yes	Yes	1 in 675 000
HCV	Yes	Yes	1 in 100 000
HBV	Yes	Yes	1 in 63 000–500 000
HTLV-1 and HTLV-2	Yes	Yes	1 in 641 000
Other viruses			
CMV	Yes	Yes	Most donors harbor virus
Parvovirus B19	Yes	Yes	1 in 10 000
HAV	Yes	Yes	Less than 1 in 1 million contaminated per units transfused
TT virus	Yes	Unknown	1 in 10 (Japan), 1 in 50 (Scotland)
SEN virus	Yes	Unknown	Unknown
HHV-8	Probable	Yes	Unknown
Bacteria			
Red Blood Cells: *Yersinia enterocolitica* and other gram-negative bacteria	Yes	Yes	1 in 5 million units
Platelets: *Staphylococcus epidermidis, Bacillus* species, *Staphylococcus aureus, Salmonella* species, *Serratia* species	Yes	Yes	1 in 100 000 units
Parasites[b]			
Malaria *(Plasmodium falciparum)*	Yes	Yes	Varies widely depending on location
Chagas disease *(Trypanosoma cruzi)*	Yes	Yes	Unknown
Prion diseases			
CJD/vCJD	Yes	Yes	Unknown
Tickborne (in nature)			
Babesia species	Yes	Yes	Unknown
Rickettsia rickettsii	Yes	Yes	Unknown
Colorado tick fever virus	Yes	Yes	Unknown
Borrelia burgdorferi	Unknown	Yes	Unknown
Ehrlichia species	Unknown	Yes	Unknown
Mosquitoborne			
West Nile virus	Yes	Yes	Variable (depends on epidemic year)

HIV indicates human immunodeficiency virus; HCV, hepatitis C virus; HBV, hepatitis B virus; HTLV, human T-lymphotropic virus; CMV, cytomegalovirus; HAV, hepatitis A virus; HHV, human herpesvirus; CJD, Creutzfeldt-Jakob disease; and vCJD, variant CJD. (TT and SEN viruses were named for the initials of patients from whom the viruses first were isolated.)

[a]For additional information, see Goodnough LT, Brecher ME, Kanter MH, AuBuchon JP. Transfusion medicine. First of two parts: blood transfusion. *N Engl J Med.* 1999;340(7):438–447; and Goodnough LT, Brecher ME, Kanter MH, AuBuchon JP. Transfusion medicine. Second of two parts: blood conservation. *N Engl J Med.* 1999;340(7):525–533.

[b]Other transfusion-transmitted agents include *Toxoplasma gondii* and leishmanial species.

HTLV is less likely to lead to infection than is transmission of HIV, HBV, or HCV, with an approximate 27% seroconversion rate in people in the United States who receive non-leukocyte reduced cellular blood components from infected donors.

CYTOMEGALOVIRUS (P 275). Immunocompromised people, including preterm infants, stem cell and solid organ transplant recipients, and others, are at risk of severe, life-threatening illness from transfusion-transmitted CMV. Consequently, in many centers, only blood from donors who lack CMV antibodies is given to people in these categories. Leukoreduction decreases the risk of CMV transmission, because CMV resides in a latent phase within white blood cells.

PARVOVIRUS B19 (P 491). Blood donations are not screened universally for parvovirus B19, because infection with this virus is common in humans. Seroprevalence rates in adult blood donors range from 29% to 79%. Estimates of parvovirus B19 viremia in blood donors have ranged from 0 to 2.6 per 10 000. Parvovirus, like CMV, usually does not cause severe disease in immunocompetent hosts but may be a threat to certain groups (eg, fetuses of nonimmune pregnant women; people with hemoglobinopathies, such as sickle cell disease and thalassemia; and immunocompromised patients). The risk of transmission of parvovirus B19 from whole blood donations is unknown but thought to be rare. However, pooled plasma derivatives commonly test positive for parvovirus B19 DNA, because parvovirus B19 lacks a lipid envelope, making it resistant to solvent/detergent treatment. To increase safety, manufacturers of plasma derivatives test plasma minipools for parvovirus DNA and exclude those containing parvovirus above a threshold concentration.

HEPATITIS A VIRUS (P 329). As with parvovirus, hepatitis A virus (HAV) lacks a lipid envelope and may survive solvent/detergent treatment. Infection with HAV leads to a relatively short period of viremia, and a chronic carrier state does not occur. Cases of transfusion-transmitted HAV infection have been reported but are rare. Clusters of HAV infections transmitted from clotting factor concentrates occurred among people with hemophilia in Europe during the early 1990s, in South Africa, and more recently, in the United States.

NON-A THROUGH -E HEPATITIS VIRUSES. A small proportion of people with post-transfusion hepatitis as well as community-acquired hepatitis will have negative test results for all known hepatitis agents. Several other viruses have been evaluated as possible etiologic agents. Although 3 of these viruses—hepatitis G virus/GB virus type C (strain variants of a member of the *Flaviviridae* family), TT virus (named for the patient from whom the virus was first isolated in Japan), and SEN virus—can be found in blood donors and can be transmitted by transfusion, none of these viruses have been found to be associated with development of post-transfusion hepatitis; hence, technically they are not "hepatitis" viruses. No test has been approved for screening donors for any of these viruses, and no data suggest that such tests would be beneficial.

HUMAN HERPESVIRUS 8. Human herpesvirus 8 (HHV-8) is associated with Kaposi sarcoma in people with HIV infection, non-HIV Kaposi sarcoma, and certain rare malignant neoplasms. The predominant modes of transmission are male-to-male sexual contact in the United States and close, nonsexual contact in Africa. Because HHV-8 DNA has been detected in peripheral blood mononuclear cells and serum specimens, there is concern that HHV-8 could be transmitted through blood and blood products. Serologic evidence of HHV-8 infection has been associated with receipt of transfused and nonleukoreduced blood components as well as with injection drug use. However, HHV-8 transmission has not been detected in some studies of small numbers of recipients of blood from known HHV-8–seropositive donors. Among people with exposure to blood and blood products (eg, people with hemophilia), HHV-8 seroprevalence generally is comparable with that among healthy, HIV-seronegative people. Research on larger populations of recipients of blood or blood products from HHV-8–positive people will be needed to evaluate more completely this risk. An epidemiology study in Uganda, where HHV-8 is endemic, has provided evidence that HHV-8 can be transmitted by blood transfusion.

WEST NILE VIRUS. West Nile virus (WNV) has been shown to be transmitted through blood transfusions. To reduce transfusion-associated transmission, blood collection agencies have implemented NAA testing for WNV. Blood collection agencies primarily use an algorithm starting with minipools of donation samples. Donations making up a reactive minipool are retested individually and removed from the blood supply if results still are positive. If there is evidence of local epidemic WNV transmission, local blood collection agencies switch to individual donation testing to improve the sensitivity of finding blood donations containing WNV. These steps have reduced but not eliminated the risk of WNV transmission via blood products. Cases of WNV disease in patients who have received blood transfusions within 28 days before illness onset should be reported promptly to the Centers for Disease Control and Prevention (CDC) through state and local public health authorities. Serum and tissue samples should be retained for later studies. In addition, cases of WNV disease diagnosed in people who have donated blood within 2 weeks before the onset of illness should be reported promptly.

BACTERIA

Although major advances in blood safety have been made, bacterial contamination of blood products remains an important cause of transfusion reaction. Bacterial contamination can occur during collection, processing, and transfusion of blood components.

Platelets are stored at room temperature, which can facilitate growth of contaminating bacteria. Bacterial contamination of blood products previously was underestimated. The predominant bacterium that contaminates Platelets is *Staphylococcus epidermidis. Bacillus* species; more virulent organisms, such as *Staphylococcus aureus;* and various gram-negative bacteria, including *Salmonella* and *Serratia* species, also have been reported. Transfusion reactions attributable to contaminated Platelets potentially are underrecognized, because episodes of bacteremia with skin organisms are common in patients requiring Platelets, and the link to the transfusion may not be suspected.

On March 1, 2004, the AABB (formerly known as the American Association of Blood Banks) adopted a new standard that requires member blood banks and transfusion services to implement measures to detect and limit bacterial contamination of all Platelet components. As a result, most apheresis platelets are screened using liquid culture methods, while pooled platelets generally are screened using less-sensitive methods. All widely used detection methods have been reported to fail, so no method is failsafe. The American Red Cross has estimated that current culture methods may detect only 50% of bacterial contamination. Hospitals should ensure that protocols are in place to communicate results of bacterial contamination, both for quarantine of components from individual donors and prompt treatment of any transfused recipients. Post-transfusion notification of appropriate personnel is required if cultures identify slow-growing bacteria after product release or transfusion. If bacterial contamination of a component is suspected, the transfusion should be stopped immediately, the unit should be saved for further testing, and blood cultures should be obtained from the recipient. Bacterial isolates from cultures of the recipient and unit should be saved for further investigation. The AABB should be consulted for management guidance (**www.aabb.org/**). In 2007, the FDA cleared for marketing a rapid test to screen for bacterial contamination of Platelets before transfusion (**www.fda.gov/bbs/topics/NEWS/2007/NEW01702.html**).

Red Blood Cell units are much less likely than are Platelets to contain bacteria at the time of transfusion, because refrigeration kills or inhibits growth of many bacteria. However, certain bacteria, most notably gram-negative organisms, such as *Yersinia enterocolitica*, may contaminate Red Blood Cells, because they survive cold storage. Cases of septic shock and death attributable to transfusion-transmitted *Y enterocolitica* and other gram-negative organisms have been documented.

Reported rates of transfusion-associated bacterial sepsis have varied widely depending on study methodology and microbial detection methods used. A prospective, multisite study (the Assessment of the Frequency of Blood Component Bacterial Contamination Associated with Transfusion Reaction [BaCon] Study) estimated the rate of transfusion-transmitted sepsis to be 1 in 100 000 units for single-donor and pooled Platelets and 1 in 5 million units for Red Blood Cells. Other studies that did not require matching bacterial cultures and/or molecular typing of both the component and the recipient's blood, as in the BaCon Study, or which included less severe recipient reactions in addition to sepsis have found higher rates of infection.

PARASITES

Several parasitic agents have been reported to cause transfusion-transmitted infections, including malaria, Chagas disease, babesiosis, toxoplasmosis, and leishmaniasis. Increasing travel to and immigration from areas with endemic infection have led to a need for increased vigilance in the United States. Babesiosis and toxoplasmosis are endemic in the United States.

MALARIA (SEE P 438). The incidence of transfusion-associated malaria has decreased over the last 30 years in the United States. During the last decade, the rate has ranged from 0 to 0.18 cases per million units transfused—that is, no more than 1 to 2 cases per year. Most cases are attributed to infectious donors who have immigrated to the United States rather than people born in the United States who traveled to areas with endemic infection. *Plasmodium falciparum* is the species most commonly transmitted. Prevention of transfusion-transmitted malaria relies on interviewing donors for risk factors related to residence in or travel to areas with endemic infection or previous treatment for malaria. Donation should be delayed until 3 years after either completing treatment of malaria or living in a country where malaria is found and 12 months after returning from a trip to an area where malaria is found. There is no approved laboratory test to screen donated blood for malaria.

CHAGAS DISEASE (SEE AMERICAN TRYPANOSOMIASIS, P 678). The immigration of millions of people from areas with endemic *T cruzi* infection (parts of Central America, South America, and Mexico) and increased international travel have raised concern about the potential for transfusion-transmitted Chagas disease. To date, fewer than 10 cases of transfusion-transmitted Chagas disease have been reported in North America. However, studies of blood donors likely to have been born in or to have traveled to areas with endemic infection have found antibodies to *T cruzi* in as many as 0.5% of people tested. Although recognized transfusion transmissions of *T cruzi* in the United States have been rare, in some areas of the United States, the prevalence of Chagas disease estimated by detection of antibodies, appears to have increased in recent years. Screening for Chagas disease by donor history has not been adequately sensitive or specific. In December 2006, the FDA licensed a test for *T cruzi* (**www.fda.gov/bbs/topics/NEWS/2006/ NEW01524.html**). The American Red Cross tested approximately 150 000 samples from areas of the United States where some blood donors were expected to have undiagnosed Chagas disease and found that 61 donors were repeatedly reactive for antibodies to *T cruzi* (**www.cdc.gov/mmwr/preview/mmwrhtml/mm5607a2.htm**). The AABB offered recommendations to member facilities regarding appropriate use of the test. The American Red Cross and Blood Systems, Inc began screening all blood donations in January 2008. As of November 2007, the FDA concluded that the test offers an important new safety measure and is expected to issue specific guidance for appropriate use of the test for all blood donations.

BABESIOSIS (P 226). The most commonly reported transfusion-associated tickborne infection in the United States is babesiosis. More than 30 cases of transfusion-induced babesiosis have been documented; most were attributed to *Babesia microti*, but the WA1-type *Babesia* parasite also has been implicated. *Babesia* organisms are intracellular parasites that infect red blood cells. However, at least 4 cases have been associated with receipt of Platelets, which often contain a small number of red blood cells. Although most infections are asymptomatic, *Babesia* infection can cause severe, life-threatening disease, particularly in elderly or splenectomized patients. Severe infection can result in hemolytic anemia, thrombocytopenia, and renal failure. Surveys using indirect immunofluorescent antibody assays in areas of Connecticut and New York with highly endemic infection have revealed seropositivity rates for *B microti* in approximately 1% and 4%, respectively. In a study of blood donors in Connecticut, 19 (56%) of 34 seropositive donors had positive results for nucleic acid, as determined by polymerase chain reaction (PCR) assay. Blood from 3 (20%) of 15 donors with positive PCR assay results was infectious when inoculated into hamsters, and infection was transmitted to recipients of blood from approximately 1 in 4 donors with positive PCR assay results.

No licensed test is available to screen donors for *Babesia* organisms. Donors with a history of babesiosis are deferred indefinitely from future donation. Although people with acute illness or fever are not eligible to donate, infected people commonly are asymptomatic or experience only mild and nonspecific clinical symptoms. In addition, *Babesia* species can cause asymptomatic infection for months and even years in untreated, otherwise healthy people. Questioning donors about recent tick bites has been shown to be ineffective, because donors who are seropositive for antibody to tickborne agents are no more likely than seronegative donors to recall tick bites.

TRANSMISSIBLE SPONGIFORM ENCEPHALOPATHIES: PRION DISEASE

CREUTZFELDT-JAKOB DISEASE AND VARIANT CREUTZFELDT-JAKOB DISEASE

(P 547). Creutzfeldt-Jakob disease (CJD) and variant CJD (vCJD) are fatal neurologic illnesses caused by unique infectious agents known as prions (see Transmissible Spongiform Encephalopathies, p 547).

SPORADIC CJD. The risk of transmitting most forms of CJD through blood has been considered theoretical. No cases of CJD resulting from receipt of blood transfusion from donors who later developed sporadic, familial, or iatrogenic forms of CJD have been documented, and case-control studies have not found an association between receipt of blood and development of CJD.

Nevertheless, because blood of animals with a number of naturally acquired and experimental transmissible spongiform encephalopathies (TSEs) may be infective, concerns have remained about the theoretical risk of transmitting CJD by blood transfusion. Since 1987, the FDA has recommended that certain people at increased risk of having CJD be deferred as blood donors. Concern increased after 4 reports of transfusion-transmitted vCJD (see next paragraph). People with signs of CJD or who are at increased risk of other forms of CJD (eg, receipt of pituitary-derived growth hormone or dura mater transplant or family history of CJD) should be deferred from donation. In addition, if postdonation information reveals that a donor should have been deferred because of increased CJD risk, in-date Whole Blood and components, including unpooled Plasma remaining from previous donations, should be retrieved and discarded; if those units already have been distributed, a biological product deviation report should be submitted to the FDA by the blood establishment. However, since 1998, withdrawal of plasma derivatives no longer has been recommended in that situation, because epidemiologic and laboratory data suggest that most plasma derivatives are much less likely to transmit TSE agents than are blood components, because Plasma undergoes extensive processing during fractionation.

VARIANT CJD. In 1996, cases of a new clinically and histopathologically distinct variant form of CJD (vCJD) first were reported in the United Kingdom. The agent causing this new TSE is believed to be the same as that of bovine spongiform encephalopathy (BSE). BSE in cattle first was recognized in the United Kingdom in 1986 and later in more than 20 other countries.

Transmission of vCJD to 4 elderly people in the United Kingdom presumptively has been attributed to transfusions years earlier with nonleukoreduced Red Blood Cells from healthy donors who became ill with vCJD 16 months to 3.5 years after the donations. Three of the recipients had typical vCJD, and a fourth had evidence of preclinical or subclinical infection. The asymptomatic incubation periods in the clinically ill recipients lasted from 6.3 to 8.5 years; the patient with evidence of preclinical infection died of an unrelated illness approximately 5 years after receiving the implicated transfusion. Recipients of blood components from other donors later diagnosed with vCJD remain under surveillance in the United Kingdom and France. As a precaution, authorities in the United Kingdom have notified recipients of plasma derivatives that they also may be at increased risk of vCJD; the magnitude of that risk is uncertain, and at the time of this writing, no case of vCJD has been attributed to treatment with a plasma derivative.

In the United States, the following categories of potential blood and plasma donors are deferred indefinitely: people who received a blood or blood component transfusion in the United Kingdom after January 1, 1980, when the BSE epidemic is believed to have begun; people who have lived in the United Kingdom for any combined period of 3 months or more from the beginning of 1980 until the end of 1996 (after which rigorous food protection measures were implemented fully throughout the United Kingdom); people who spent a total of 5 years or more in most other European countries (excluding countries of the former Soviet Union) from 1980 to the present; people injected with bovine insulin, unless it is confirmed that the insulin was not manufactured from cattle in the United Kingdom; and military personnel, civilian employees, and dependents who resided or worked on US military bases from 1980 through the end of 1990 in northern Europe or the end of 1996 in southern Europe (as defined by the US Department of Defense). Policies regarding CJD donor deferral may change, and blood and Plasma programs are expected to remain informed about such changes, which are announced promptly by trade organizations and the FDA.

Improving Blood Safety

A number of strategies have been proposed or implemented to further decrease the risk of transmission of infectious agents through blood and blood products. Various safety strategies are as follows.

ELIMINATION OF INFECTIOUS AGENTS

AGENT INACTIVATION. Virtually all Plasma derivatives, including Immune Globulin Intravenous (IGIV) and clotting factors, are treated to eliminate infectious agents that may be present despite screening measures. Methods used for this include wet and dry heat and treatment with a solvent/detergent. Solvent/detergent-treated pooled Plasma for transfusion no longer is marketed in the United States, but methods of treating single-donor Plasma are under study. Solvent/detergent treatment dissolves the lipid envelope of HIV, HBV, and HCV but is not effective against non–lipid-enveloped viruses, such as HAV and parvovirus B19. Transmission of HIV through administration of IGIV never has been documented.

Because of the fragility of Red Blood Cells and Platelets, pathogen inactivation is more difficult. However, several methods have been developed, such as addition of psoralens followed by exposure to ultraviolet A, which binds nucleic acids and blocks replication of bacteria and viruses. Clinical trials of these treated components are underway.

AGENT REMOVAL. Leukoreduction, whereby filters are used to remove donor white blood cells, is performed increasingly in the United States. Benefits of this process include decreasing febrile transfusion reactions related to white blood cells and their products and decreasing the immune modulation associated with transfusion. Leukoreduction also decreases cell-associated agents (eg, intracellular viruses, such as CMV, Epstein-Barr virus, HHV-8, and HTLV). Several countries have adopted this practice.

DECREASING EXPOSURE TO BLOOD PRODUCTS

Current screening policies have decreased the risk of transfusion associated infections dramatically, but blood products remain a source of known and potentially unknown infection agents.

ALTERNATIVES TO HUMAN BLOOD PRODUCTS. Many alternatives to human blood products have been developed. Established alternatives include recombinant clotting factors for patients with hemophilia and factors such as erythropoietin used to stimulate red blood cell production. Physicians should use the lowest erythropoiesis-stimulating agent (ESA) dose that will increase the hemoglobin level gradually to a concentration not exceeding 12 g/dL. Increased risks of death and serious cardiovascular and thrombotic events have been described when ESAs were administered to achieve a target hemoglobin concentration greater than 12 g/dL in people with chronic kidney failure and surgical candidates. These adverse safety outcomes and shortened time to tumor progression have been observed in certain patients with cancer with chemotherapy-related anemia, such as people with advanced head and neck cancer receiving radiation therapy and metastatic breast cancer.

Other agents currently in clinical trials include hemoglobin-based oxygen carriers, Red Blood Cell substitutes, such as human hemoglobin extracted from Red Blood Cells, recombinant human hemoglobin, animal hemoglobin, and various oxygen-carrying chemicals.

AUTOLOGOUS TRANSFUSION. Another means of decreasing recipient exposure is autologous transfusion. Blood may be donated by the patient several weeks before a surgical procedure (preoperative autologous donation) or, alternatively, donated immediately before surgery and replaced with a volume expander (acute normovolemic hemodilution). In either case, the patient's blood can be reinfused if needed. Autologous blood is not completely risk free, because bacterial contamination may occur.

Blood recycling techniques (autotransfusion) also are in this category. During surgery, blood lost by the patient may be collected, processed, and reinfused to the patient.

SURVEILLANCE FOR TRANSFUSION-TRANSMITTED INFECTION

Transfusion-transmitted infection surveillance is crucial and must be coupled with the capacity to investigate reported cases rapidly and to implement measures needed to prevent additional infections. The AABB and CDC have begun a collaboration to develop a blood transfusion adverse event module in the National Healthcare Safety Network, a voluntary prospective surveillance system. Serious adverse reactions and product problems should be reported to the manufacturer (or, alternatively, to the supplier for transmission to the manufacturer). Health care professionals also may report such information directly to the FDA through MedWatch. This can be done by telephone (1-800-FDA-1088), fax (1-800-FDA-0178), Internet (**www.fda.gov/medwatch/ report/hcp.htm**), or mail (see MedWatch, p 817). Voluntary reporting is considered vital for monitoring product safety.

ORGAN AND TISSUE TRANSPLANTATION

More than 25 000 organ and 2 000 000 tissue transplantations (eg, musculoskeletal allografts, cornea, and skin) and numerous cell therapy infusions (eg, bone marrow and peripheral stem cell transplants) occur each year in the United States. The proliferation of these products also has increased the opportunities for transmission of infectious pathogens, including bacteria, viruses, and parasites. Transmission of Chagas disease, *Mycobacterium tuberculosis*, lymphocytic choriomeningitis virus, rabies, WNV, HIV, and HCV have been reported through organ transplantation.

In 2005, the FDA final rule, Current Good Tissue Practice for Human Cells, Tissues, and Cellular and Tissue-Based Products (HCT/Ps), became effective. The purpose of this rule is to improve the safety of HCT/Ps by preventing introduction, transmission, and spread of communicable disease through transplantation of HCT/Ps.[1] The Joint Commission adopted some of these standards, which will apply to accredited organizations that store or use tissue. In addition, The Transplantation Transmission Sentinel Network is a system under development to facilitate recognition of adverse events associated with transplanted allografts (organs, tissues, and eyes). Along with receiving mandatory reports of adverse events from HCT/P establishments that manufacture tissue, the FDA encourages direct voluntary reporting through its MedWatch program by using MedWatch Form FDA-3500 (available at **www.fda.gov/medwatch**). Additional information about the FDA and HCT/Ps is available at **www.fda.gov/cber/tiss.htm**.

HUMAN MILK

Breastfeeding provides numerous health benefits to infants, including protection against morbidity and mortality from infectious diseases of bacterial, viral, and parasitic origin. In addition to providing an ideal source of infant nutrition, human milk contains immune-modulating factors, including secretory antibodies, glycoconjugates, anti-inflammatory components, and other factors. Breastfed infants have high concentrations of protective bifidobacteria and lactobacilli in their gastrointestinal tracts, which prevent colonization and infection with pathogenic organisms. Protection by human milk is established most clearly for pathogens causing gastrointestinal tract infection. In addition, human milk seems to provide protection against otitis media, invasive *Haemophilus influenzae* type b infection, and other causes of upper and lower respiratory tract infections. Evidence also indicates that human milk may modulate development of the immune system of infants.

The American Academy of Pediatrics (AAP) publishes policy statements and a manual on infant feeding[2] that provide further information about the benefits of breastfeeding, recommended feeding practices, and potential contaminants of human milk. In the *Pediatric Nutrition Handbook*[3] and in the AAP policy statement on human milk,[4] issues regarding immunization of lactating mothers and breastfeeding infants, transmission of infectious agents via human milk, and potential effects on breastfed infants of antimicrobial agents administered to lactating mothers are addressed.

[1]Centers for Disease Control and Prevention. Notice to Readers: FDA Rule for Current Good Tissue Practice for Human Cells, Tissues, and Cellular and Tissue-Based Products. *MMWR Morb Mortal Wkly Rep.* 2005;54(19):490

[2]American Academy of Pediatrics. *Breastfeeding Handbook for Physicians.* Schanler RJ, Gartner LM, Krebs NF, Dooley S, Mass SB, eds. Elk Grove Village, IL: American Academy of Pediatrics; 2006

[3]American Academy of Pediatrics, Committee on Nutrition. *Pediatric Nutrition Handbook.* 6th ed. Elk Grove Village, IL: American Academy of Pediatrics; 2009

[4]American Academy of Pediatrics, Section on Breastfeeding. Breastfeeding and the use of human milk. *Pediatrics.* 2005;115(2):496–506

Immunization of Mothers and Infants

EFFECT OF MATERNAL IMMUNIZATION

Women who have not received recommended immunizations before or during pregnancy may be immunized during the postpartum period regardless of lactation status. No evidence exists to validate concern about the potential presence of live viruses from vaccines in maternal milk if the mother is immunized during lactation. Lactating women may be immunized as recommended for adults and adolescents to protect against many infectious diseases (**www.cdc.gov/vaccines** [see adult immunization schedule]). If previously unimmunized or if traveling to an area with endemic infection, a lactating mother may be given inactivated poliovirus vaccine. Rubella-seronegative mothers who could not be immunized during pregnancy should be immunized during the early postpartum period. Women should receive a dose of tetanus toxoid, reduced diphtheria toxoid, and acellular pertussis (Tdap) vaccine in the immediate postpartum period if they previously have not received Tdap.[1,2]

EFFICACY OF IMMUNIZATION IN BREASTFED INFANTS

Infants should be immunized according to the recommended childhood and adolescent immunization schedule regardless of the mode of infant feeding. The immunogenicity of some recommended vaccines is enhanced by breastfeeding, but data are lacking as to whether the efficacy of these vaccines is enhanced. Although high concentrations of anti-poliovirus antibody in milk of some mothers theoretically could interfere with the immunogenicity of oral poliovirus vaccine, no such association has been demonstrated, and this is not a concern with inactivated poliovirus vaccine. The effectiveness of rotavirus vaccine in breastfed infants is comparable to that in nonbreastfed infants.

Transmission of Infectious Agents via Human Milk

BACTERIA

Postpartum mastitis occurs in one third of breastfeeding women in the United States and leads to breast abscesses in 10% of cases. Mastitis and breast abscesses have been associated with the presence of bacterial pathogens in human milk. Breast abscesses have the potential to rupture into the ductal system, releasing large numbers of organisms, such as *Staphylococcus aureus*, into milk. Although an increase in community-acquired methicillin-resistant *S aureus* (MRSA)-associated mastitis corresponding to an increase in community-acquired MRSA prevalence in a community has been noted, cases of infant infection were not increased in a single-center cohort study from 1998–2005. Temporary discontinuation of breastfeeding on the affected breast for 24 to 48 hours after surgical drainage and appropriate antimicrobial therapy may be necessary. In general, infectious mastitis resolves with continued lactation during appropriate antimicrobial therapy and does not

---

[1]American Academy of Pediatrics, Committee on Infectious Diseases. Prevention of pertussis among adolescents: recommendations for use of tetanus toxoid, reduced diphtheria toxoid, and acellular pertussis (Tdap) vaccine. *Pediatrics*. 2006;117(3):965–978

[2]Centers for Disease Control and Prevention. Prevention of pertussis, tetanus, and diphtheria among pregnant women and their infants. Recommendations of the Advisory Committee on Immunization Practices (ACIP). *MMWR Recomm Rep.* 2008;57(RR-4):1–47, 51

pose a significant risk for the healthy term infant. Even when breastfeeding is interrupted on the affected breast, breastfeeding may continue on the unaffected breast.

Women with tuberculosis who have been treated appropriately for 2 or more weeks and who are not considered contagious may breastfeed. Women with tuberculosis disease suspected of being contagious should refrain from breastfeeding and other close contact with the infant because of potential transmission through respiratory tract droplets (see Tuberculosis, p 680). *Mycobacterium tuberculosis* rarely causes mastitis or a breast abscess, but if a breast abscess caused by *M tuberculosis* is present, breastfeeding should be discontinued until the mother has received treatment and no longer is considered to be contagious.

Expressed human milk can become contaminated with a variety of bacterial pathogens, including *Staphylococcus* species and gram-negative bacilli. Outbreaks of gram-negative bacterial infections in neonatal intensive care units occasionally have been attributed to contaminated human milk specimens that have been collected or stored improperly. Expressed human milk may be a reservoir for multiresistant *S aureus* and other pathogens. Human milk fed to infants from women other than the biologic mother should be treated according to the guidelines of the Human Milk Banking Association of North America (**www.hmbana.org**). Routine culturing or heat treatment of a mother's milk fed to her infant has not been demonstrated to be necessary or cost-effective (see Human Milk Banks, p 123).

VIRUSES

CYTOMEGALOVIRUS. Cytomegalovirus (CMV) may be shed intermittently in human milk. Although transmission of CMV through human milk has occurred, disease in neonates who acquire CMV by this route is uncommon, presumably because of passively transferred maternal antibody. Very low birth weight preterm infants, however, are at greater potential risk of symptomatic disease. Decisions about breastfeeding of preterm infants by mothers known to be CMV seropositive should include consideration of the potential benefits of human milk and the risk of CMV transmission. Holder pasteurization (62.5°C [144.5°F] for 30 minutes) and short-term pasteurization (72°C [161.6°F] for 5 seconds) of milk seems to inactivate CMV; short-term pasteurization may be less harmful to the beneficial constituents of human milk. Freezing milk at −20°C (−4°F) will decrease viral titers but does not eliminate CMV reliably.

HEPATITIS B VIRUS. Hepatitis B surface antigen (HBsAg) has been detected in milk from HBsAg-positive women. However, studies from Taiwan and England have indicated that breastfeeding by HBsAg-positive women does not increase significantly the risk of infection among their infants. In the United States, infants born to known HBsAg-positive women should receive Hepatitis B Immune Globulin and the recommended series of 3 doses of hepatitis B vaccine, effectively eliminating any theoretical risk of transmission through breastfeeding. Immunoprophylaxis of infants with hepatitis B vaccine alone also provides protection, but optimal therapy of infants born to HBsAg-positive mothers includes Hepatitis B Immune Globulin within 12 hours of birth and initiation of the 3-dose series of hepatitis B vaccine before hospital discharge (see Hepatitis B, p 337). There is no need to delay initiation of breastfeeding until after the infant is immunized.

HEPATITIS C VIRUS. Hepatitis C virus (HCV) RNA and antibody to HCV have been detected in milk from mothers infected with HCV. Transmission of HCV via breastfeeding has not been documented in mothers who have positive test results for anti-HCV but negative test results for human immunodeficiency virus (HIV) antibody. Mothers infected with HCV should be counseled that transmission of HCV by breastfeeding theoretically is possible but has not been documented. Mothers infected with HCV should consider abstaining from breastfeeding from a breast with cracked or bleeding nipples. According to current guidelines of the US Public Health Service, maternal HCV infection is not a contraindication to breastfeeding. The decision to breastfeed should be based on informed discussion between a mother and her health care professional.

HUMAN IMMUNODEFICIENCY VIRUS. HIV has been isolated from human milk and can be transmitted through breastfeeding. The risk of transmission is higher for women who acquire HIV infection during lactation (ie, postpartum) than for women with preexisting infection. In populations such as the United States, in which the risk of infant mortality from infectious diseases and malnutrition is low and in which safe and effective alternative sources of feeding are available readily, HIV-infected women, including women receiving antiretroviral therapy, should be counseled not to breastfeed their infants or donate their milk. It is not yet known whether maternal highly active antiretroviral therapy (HAART) will reduce human milk transmission to the infant, although ongoing studies are evaluating this. Available data indicate that various antiretroviral drugs have differential penetration into human milk; some antiretroviral drugs have concentrations in human milk that are much higher than those in maternal plasma, and other drugs have concentrations in human milk that are much lower than those in plasma or are not detectable. This raises potential concerns regarding infant toxicity as well as the potential for selection of drug-resistant virus within human milk.

All pregnant women in the United States should be screened for HIV infection to allow implementation of effective interventions to prevent mother-to-child HIV transmission (eg, antiretroviral prophylaxis and elective cesarean delivery) should the woman be found to have HIV infection and to permit appropriate counseling of the woman regarding breastfeeding.[1] Screening should occur after a woman is notified that HIV screening is recommended for all pregnant patients and that she will receive an HIV test as part of the routine panel of prenatal tests unless she declines (see Human Immunodeficiency Virus Infection, p 380).

In areas where infectious diseases and malnutrition are important causes of mortality early in life and where safe, affordable, and sustainable infant replacement feeding may not be available, infant feeding decisions are more complex. In such countries, women whose HIV status is unknown are encouraged to continue breastfeeding, because the morbidity associated with artificial feeding is unacceptably high in resource-poor locations. For HIV-infected mothers, studies in Africa found that exclusive breastfeeding for the first 3 to 6 months after birth appeared to lower the risk of human milk transmission compared with infants who received mixed feedings (breastfeeding and other foods or milks), although postnatal transmission is not eliminated and transmission is higher than in infants who receive only replacement feeding from birth. Current World Health Organization, UNICEF, and UNAIDS infant feeding guidelines state that if replacement feeding is affordable, feasible, acceptable, sustainable, and safe, replacement of human milk from HIV-infected women with nutritional substitutes is recommended to decrease the risk of HIV transmission. If these criteria are not met, HIV-infected women are

---

[1]Centers for Disease Control and Prevention. Revised recommendations for HIV testing of adults, adolescents, and pregnant women in health-care settings. *MMWR Recomm Rep.* 2006;55(RR-14):1–17

recommended to breastfeed exclusively for the first 6 months of life, with weaning after that time when replacement feeding meets the affordable, feasible, acceptable, sustainable, and safe criteria. Thus, in resource-poor countries, the most appropriate feeding option for an HIV-infected mother needs to be based on her individual circumstances and should weigh the multifactional benefits of breastfeeding against the risk of transmission of HIV through breastfeeding (see Human Immunodeficiency Virus Infection, p 380).

HUMAN T-LYMPHOTROPIC VIRUS TYPE 1. Human T-lymphotropic virus (HTLV) type 1, which is endemic in Japan, the Caribbean, and parts of South America, is associated with development of malignant neoplasms and neurologic disorders among adults. Epidemiologic and laboratory studies suggest that mother-to-infant transmission of human HTLV-1 occurs primarily through breastfeeding, although freezing/thawing of expressed human milk may decrease infectivity of human milk. Women in the United States who are HTLV-1 seropositive should be advised not to breastfeed. Routine screening for HTLV-1 or HTLV-2 during pregnancy is not recommended.

HUMAN T-LYMPHOTROPIC VIRUS TYPE 2. HTLV type 2, also a retrovirus, has been detected among American and European injection drug users and some American Indian/Alaska Native groups. Although apparent maternal-infant transmission has been reported, the rate and timing of transmission have not been established. Until additional data about possible transmission through breastfeeding become available, women in the United States who are seropositive should be advised not to breastfeed.

HERPES SIMPLEX VIRUS TYPE 1. Women with herpetic lesions may transmit herpes simplex virus (HSV) to their infants by direct contact with the lesions. Whenever a woman has herpes lesions, she must use careful hand hygiene and cover any lesions with which the infant might come into contact. Women with herpetic lesions on a breast or nipple should refrain from breastfeeding an infant from the affected breast until lesions have resolved.

RUBELLA. Wild and vaccine strains of rubella virus have been isolated from human milk. However, the presence of rubella virus in human milk has not been associated with significant disease in infants, and transmission is more likely to occur via other routes. Women with rubella or women who have been immunized recently with live-attenuated rubella virus vaccine need not refrain from breastfeeding.

VARICELLA. Whether varicella vaccine virus is secreted in human milk or whether the virus would infect a breastfeeding infant is unknown. Varicella vaccine may be considered for a susceptible breastfeeding mother if the risk of exposure to natural varicella-zoster virus is high. Recommendations for use of passive immunization and varicella vaccine for breastfeeding mothers who have had contact with people in whom varicella has developed or for contacts of a breastfeeding mother in whom varicella has developed are available (see Varicella-Zoster Infections, p 714).

WEST NILE VIRUS. West Nile virus RNA has been detected in human milk collected from a woman with disease attributable to West Nile virus; her breastfed infant developed West Nile virus immunoglobulin M antibodies but remained asymptomatic. Animal experiments have shown that West Nile virus can be transmitted in animal milk, and other related flaviviruses can be transmitted to humans via unpasteurized milk from ruminants. The degree to which West Nile virus is transmitted in human milk and the extent to which breastfeeding infants become infected are unknown. Because the health benefits of breastfeeding have been established and the risk of West Nile virus transmission through breastfeeding is unknown, women who reside in an area with endemic West Nile virus infection may continue to breastfeed.

HUMAN MILK BANKS

Some circumstances, such as preterm delivery, may preclude breastfeeding, but infants in these circumstances still may be fed milk collected from their own mothers or from individual donors. The potential for transmission of infectious agents through donor human milk requires appropriate selection and screening of donors and careful collection, processing, and storage of milk. Currently, US donor milk banks that belong to the Human Milk Banking Association of North America voluntarily follow guidelines drafted in consultation with the US Food and Drug Administration and the Centers for Disease Control and Prevention. These guidelines include screening of all donors for HBsAg and antibodies to HIV-1, HIV-2, HTLV-1, HTLV-2, hepatitis C, and syphilis. Donor milk is dispensed only by prescription after it is heat treated at 62.5°C (144.5°F) for 30 minutes and bacterial cultures reveal no growth of pathogenic organisms. Milk from the birth mother of a preterm infant does not require processing if fed to her infant, but proper collection and storage procedures should be followed. Some neonatal intensive care units have adopted policies to deal with occasions when an infant inadvertently is fed expressed human milk not obtained from his or her mother. These policies require documentation, counseling, and observation of the affected infant for signs of infection and potential testing of the source mother for infections that could be transmitted via human milk. In addition, information can be found at **www.cdc.gov/breastfeeding/ recommendations/other_mothers_milk.htm.** If an infant mistakenly has been fed another infant's bottle of expressed human milk, the situation should be treated just as if an accidental exposure to other body fluids has occurred. The health care professional should do the following:

1. Inform the mother who expressed the human milk about the bottle switch, and ask:
   + Whether she has had an HIV test and, if so, would she be willing to share the results with the parents of the infant given the incorrect milk?
   + If she does not know results of an HIV test for herself, would she be willing to be tested and share those results with parents of the other infant?
2. Discuss administration of the mistaken milk with the parents of the infant who was fed the wrong bottle.
   + Inform the parents that their infant received another infant's bottle of expressed human milk and that the risk of transmission of infection is low.
   + Inform the parents that their infant soon should undergo a baseline test for HIV.

Heat treatment at 56°C or greater (133°F or greater) for 30 minutes reliably eliminates bacteria, inactivates HIV, and decreases titers of other viruses but may not eliminate CMV completely. Holder pasteurization (62.5°C [144.5°F] for 30 minutes) reliably inactivates HIV and CMV and eliminates or decreases significantly titers of most other viruses. Short-term pasteurization (72°C [161.6°F] for 5 seconds) also appears to inactivate CMV.

Freezing at −20°C (−4°F) eliminates HTLV-1 and decreases the concentration of CMV but does not destroy most other viruses or bacteria. Microbiologic quality standards for fresh, unpasteurized, expressed milk are not available. The presence of gram-negative bacteria, S aureus, or alpha- or beta-hemolytic streptococci may preclude use of expressed milk. Routine culture of milk that a birth mother provides to her own infant is not warranted.

Antimicrobial Agents in Human Milk

Antimicrobial agents often are prescribed for lactating women. Although these drugs may appear in milk, the potential risk to an infant must be weighed against the known benefits of continued breastfeeding. As a general guideline, an antimicrobial agent is safe to administer to a lactating woman if it is safe to administer to an infant. Only in rare cases will interruption of breastfeeding be necessary because of maternal medications.

The amount of drug an infant receives from a lactating mother depends on a number of factors, including maternal dose, frequency and duration of administration, absorption, and distribution characteristics of the drug. When a lactating woman receives appropriate doses of an antimicrobial agent, the concentration of the compound in her milk usually is less than the equivalent of a therapeutic dose for the infant. A breastfed infant who requires antimicrobial therapy should receive the recommended doses, independent of administration of the agent to the mother.

Current information about drugs and lactation can be found at the Toxicology Data Network Web site **www.toxnet.nlm.nih.gov/help/LactMedRecordFormat. htm**). Data for drugs, including antimicrobial agents, administered to lactating women are provided in several categories, including maternal and infant drug levels, effects in breastfed infants, possible effects on lactation, the category into which the drug has been placed, alternative drugs to consider, and references.

CHILDREN IN OUT-OF-HOME CHILD CARE[1]

Infants and young children who are cared for in group settings have an increased rate of communicable infectious diseases and an increased risk of acquiring antimicrobial-resistant organisms. Prevention and control of infection in out-of-home child care settings is influenced by several factors, including the following: (1) caregivers' practice of personal hygiene and immunization status; (2) environmental sanitation; (3) food-handling procedures; (4) ages and immunization status of children; (5) ratio of children to caregivers; (6) physical space and quality of facilities; (7) frequency of use of antimicrobial agents in children in child care; and (8) adherence to standard precautions for infection control. Adequately addressing problems of infection control in child care settings requires collaborative efforts of public health officials, licensing agencies, child care providers, physicians, nurses, parents, employers, and other members of the community.

Child care programs should require that all enrollees and staff members receive age-appropriate immunizations and routine health care. In addition, these programs have the opportunity to provide parents with ongoing instruction in child development, hygiene, appropriate nutrition, and management of minor illnesses. Many early education and child care programs have access to health consultants who can assist providers and parents with these issues.

[1]American Academy of Pediatrics. *Managing Infectious Diseases in Child Care and Schools: A Quick Reference Guide.* Aronson SS, Shope TR, eds. 2nd ed. Elk Grove Village, IL: American Academy of Pediatrics; 2009

Classification of Care Service

Child care services commonly are classified by the type of setting, number of children in care, and ages and health status of the children. **Small family child care homes** provide care and education for up to 6 children simultaneously, including any preschool-aged relatives of the care provider, in a residence that usually is the home of the care provider. **Large family child care homes** provide care and education for between 7 and 12 children at a time, including any preschool-aged relatives of the care provider, in a residence that usually is the home of one of the care providers. A **child care center** is a facility that provides care and education to any number of children in a nonresidential setting or to 13 or more children in any setting if the facility is open on a regular basis. A **facility for ill children** provides care for 1 or more children who temporarily are excluded from their regular child care setting for health reasons. A facility for children with special needs provides specialized care and education for 1 child or more who cannot be accommodated in a setting with typically developing children. All 50 states license out-of-home child care; however, licensing is directed toward center-based child care; few states or municipalities license small or large family child care homes. Licensing requirements for every state can be accessed through the Web sites of the National Resource Center for Health and Safety in Child Care and Early Education (**www.nrckids.org**) and AAP (**www.healthychildcare.org/**).

Grouping of children by age varies, but in child care centers, common groups consist of **infants** (birth through 12 months of age), **toddlers** (13 through 35 months of age), **preschoolers** (36 through 59 months of age), and **school-aged children** (5 through 12 years of age).

Age grouping reflects developmental status. Infants and toddlers who require diapering or assistance in using a toilet have significant hands-on contact with care providers. Furthermore, they have oral contact with the environment, have poor control over their secretions and excretions, and have immunity to fewer common pathogens. Toddlers also have frequent direct contact with each other and with secretions of other toddlers. Therefore, child care programs that provide infant and toddler care should emphasize infection-control measures.

Management and Prevention of Illness

Modes of transmission of bacteria, viruses, parasites, and fungi within child care settings are listed in Table 2.4 (p 126). In most instances, the risk of introducing an infectious agent into a child care group is related directly to prevalence of the agent in the population and to the number of susceptible children in that group. Transmission of an agent within the group depends on the following: (1) characteristics of the organism, such as mode of spread, infective dose, and survival in the environment; (2) frequency of asymptomatic infection or carrier state; and (3) immunity to the respective pathogen. Transmission also can be affected by behaviors of the child care providers, particularly hygienic aspects of child handling; by environmental sanitation practices; and by age and immunization status of children enrolled. Children infected in a child care group can transmit organisms not only within the group but also within their households and the community. Appropriate hand hygiene is the most important factor for decreasing transmission of disease in child care settings.

Table 2.4. Modes of Transmission of Organisms in Child Care Settings

Usual Route of Transmission[a]	Bacteria	Viruses	Other[b]
Fecal-oral	*Campylobacter* organisms, *Clostridium difficile*, *Escherichia coli* O157:H7, *Salmonella* organisms, *Shigella* organisms	Astrovirus, norovirus, enteric adenovirus, enteroviruses, hepatitis A virus, rotaviruses	*Cryptosporidium* species, *Enterobius vermicularis*, *Giardia intestinalis*
Respiratory	*Bordetella pertussis, Haemophilus influenzae* type b, *Mycobacterium tuberculosis, Neisseria meningitidis,* *Streptococcus* pneumoniae, group A streptococcus, *Kingella kingae*	Adenovirus, influenza virus, human meta-pneumovirus, measles virus, mumps virus, parainfluenza virus, parvovirus B19, respiratory syncytial virus, rhinovirus, rubella virus, varicella-zoster virus	...
Person-to-person contact	Group A streptococcus, *Staphylococcus aureus*	Herpes simplex virus, varicella-zoster virus	Agents causing pediculosis, scabies, and ringworm[c]
Contact with blood, urine, and/or saliva	...	Cytomegalovirus, herpes simplex virus	...
Bloodborne	...	Hepatitis B virus	...

[a]The potential for transmission of microorganisms in the child care setting by food and animals also exists (see Appendix IX, Clinical Syndromes Associated With Foodborne Diseases, p 860, and Appendix X, Diseases Transmitted by Animals, p 864, and Diseases Transmitted by Animals [Zoonoses]: Household Pets, Including Nontraditional Pets, and Exposure to Animals in Public Settings, p 198).

[b]Parasites, fungi, mites, and lice.

[c]Transmission also may occur from contact with objects in the environment.

Options for management of ill or infected children in child care and for reducing transmission of pathogens include the following: (1) antimicrobial treatment or prophylaxis when appropriate; (2) immunization when appropriate; (3) exclusion of ill or infected children from the facility; (4) provision of alternative care at a separate site; (5) cohorting to provide care (eg, segregation of infected children in a group with separate staff and facilities); (6) limiting new admissions; and (7) closing the facility (a rarely exercised option). Recommendations for controlling spread of specific infectious agents differ according to the epidemiology of the pathogen (see disease-specific chapters in Section 3) and characteristics of the setting.

Infection-control procedures in child care programs that decrease acquisition and transmission of communicable diseases include: (1) periodic review of center-maintained child and employee illness records, including current immunization status; (2) hygienic and sanitary procedures for toilet use, toilet training, and diaper changing; (3) review and enforcement of hand-hygiene procedures; (4) environmental sanitation; (5) personal hygiene for children and staff; (6) sanitary preparation and handling of food; (7) communicable disease surveillance and reporting; and (8) appropriate handling of pets. Policies that include training procedures for full- and part-time employees and staff illness exclusion policies also aid in control of infectious diseases. Health departments should have plans for responding to reportable and nonreportable communicable diseases in child care programs and should provide training, written information, and technical consultation to child care programs when requested. Evaluation of the health status of each child should be performed by a trained staff member each day as the child enters the site and throughout the day. Parents should be required to report their child's immunization status on an ongoing basis and should be encouraged to share information with child care staff about their child's acute and chronic illnesses and medication use.

Recommendations for Inclusion or Exclusion

Mild illness is common among children. Most children will not need to be excluded from their usual source of care for mild respiratory tract illnesses, because transmission is likely to have occurred before symptoms developed in the child. Disease may occur as a result of contact with children with asymptomatic infection. The risk of illness can be decreased by following common-sense hygienic practices.

Exclusion of sick children and adults from out-of-home child care settings has been recommended when such exclusion could decrease the likelihood of secondary cases. In many situations, the expertise of the program's medical consultant and that of the responsible local and state public health authorities are helpful for determining the benefits and risks of excluding children from their usual care program. Most states have laws about isolation of people with specific communicable diseases. Local or state health departments should be contacted about these laws, and public health authorities in these areas should be notified about cases of nationally notifiable infectious diseases and unusual outbreaks of other illnesses involving children or adults in the child care environment (see Appendix V, Nationally Notifiable Infectious Diseases in the United States, p 845).

General recommendations for exclusion of children in out-of-home care are shown in Table 2.5 (p 128). Disease- or condition-specific recommendations for exclusion from out-of-home care and management of contacts are shown in Table 2.6 (p 129).

Table 2.5. General Recommendations for Exclusion of Children in Out-Of-Home Child Care

Symptom(s)	Management
Illness preventing participation in activities, as determined by child care staff	Exclusion until illness resolves and able to participate in activities
Illness that requires a need for care that is greater than staff can provide without compromising health and safety of others	Exclusion or placement in care environment where appropriate care can be provided, without compromising care of others
Severe illness suggested by fever with behavior changes, lethargy, irritability, persistent crying, difficulty breathing, progressive rash	Medical evaluation and exclusion until symptoms have resolved
Rash with fever or behavioral change	Medical evaluation and exclusion until illness is determined not to be communicable
Persistent abdominal pain (2 hours or more) or intermittent abdominal pain associated with fever, dehydration, or other systemic signs and symptoms	Medical evaluation and exclusion until symptoms have resolved
Vomiting 2 or more times in preceding 24 hours	Exclusion until symptoms have resolved, unless vomiting is determined to be caused by a noncommunicable condition and child is able to remain hydrated and participate in activities
Diarrhea or stools containing blood or mucus	Medical evaluation and exclusion until symptoms have resolved
Oral lesions	Exclusion until child or staff member is considered to be noninfectious (lesions crusted and dry)

Most minor illnesses do not constitute a reason for excluding a child from child care. Examples of illnesses and conditions that do not necessitate exclusion include the following:
- Nonpustular rash without fever and without behavioral change.
- Parvovirus B19 infection in an immunoc)ompetent host.
- Cytomegalovirus (CMV) infection.
- Chronic hepatitis B virus (HBV) infection (see p 135 for possible exceptions).
- Conjunctivitis without fever and without behavioral change; if 2 or more children in a group care setting develop conjunctivitis in the same period, seek advice from the program's health consultant or public health authority.
- Human immunodeficiency virus (HIV) infection (see p 136 for possible exceptions).
- Known methicillin-resistant *Staphylococcus aureus* (MRSA) carriers or children with colonization of MRSA but without an illness that would otherwise require exclusion.

Asymptomatic children who excrete an enteropathogen usually do not need to be excluded, except when an infection with Shiga toxin-producing *Escherichia coli*, *Shigella* species, or *Salmonella* serotype Typhi has occurred in the child care program. Because these infections are transmitted easily and can be severe, exclusion is warranted until

Table 2.6. Disease- or Condition-Specific Recommendations for Exclusion of Children in Out-Of-Home Child Care

Condition	Management of Case	Management of Contacts
Hepatitis A virus (HAV) infection	Serologic testing to confirm HAV infection in suspected cases. Exclusion until 1 week after onset of jaundice.	If ≥1 case confirmed in child or staff attendees or ≥2 cases in households of staff or attendees, HAV vaccine or Immune Globulin (IG) should be administered within 14 days of exposure to unimmunized staff and attendees. In centers without diapered children, HAV vaccine or IG should be given to unimmunized classroom contacts of index case. Asymptomatic IG recipients may return after receipt of IG (see Hepatitis A, p 329).
Impetigo	Exclusion until 24 hours after treatment has been initiated. Lesions on exposed skin covered with watertight dressing.	No intervention unless additional lesions develop.
Measles	Exclusion until 4 days after beginning of rash and when the child is able to participate.	Immunize exposed children without evidence of immunity within 72 hours of exposure. Children who do not receive vaccine within 72 hours or who remain unimmunized after exposure should be excluded until at least 2 weeks after onset of rash in the last case of measles. For use of IG, see Measles (p 444).
Mumps	Exclusion until 5 days after onset of parotid gland swelling.	In outbreak setting, people without documentation of immunity should be immunized or excluded. Immediate readmission may occur following immunization. Unimmunized people should be excluded for ≥26 days following onset of parotitis in last case.
Pediculosis capitis (head lice)	Treatment at end of program day and readmission on completion of first treatment.	Household and close contacts should be examined and treated if infested. No exclusion necessary.
Pertussis	Exclusion until 5 days of appropriate antimicrobial therapy course have been completed (see Pertussis, p 504).	Immunization and chemoprophylaxis should be administered as recommended for household contacts. Symptomatic children and staff should be excluded until completion of 5 days of antimicrobial therapy course. Untreated adults should be excluded until 21 days after onset of cough (see Pertussis Infections, p 504).
Rubella	Exclusion until 6 days after onset of rash for postnatal infection.	Pregnant contacts should be evaluated (see Rubella, p 579).

Table 2.6. Disease- or Condition-Specific Recommendations for Exclusion of Children in Out-Of-Home Child Care, continued

Condition	Management of Case	Management of Contacts
Salmonella serotype Typhi infection	Exclusion until diarrhea resolves. Three negative stool culture results required before readmission.	Stool cultures should be performed for attendees and staff; infected people should be excluded on the basis of age (see *Salmonella* Infections, p 584).
Non-serotype Typhi *Salmonella* infection	Exclusion until diarrhea resolves. Negative stool culture results not required for non-serotype Typhi *Salmonella* species.	Symptomatic contacts should be excluded until symptoms resolve. Stool cultures are not required for asymptomatic contacts. Antimicrobial therapy is not recommended for asymptomatic infection or uncomplicated diarrhea or for contacts.
Scabies	Exclusion until after treatment given.	Close contacts with prolonged skin-to-skin contact should have prophylactic therapy. Bedding and clothing in contact with skin of infected people should be laundered (see Scabies, p 589).
Shiga toxin-producing *Escherichia coli* (STEC), including *E coli* O157:H7, or *Shigella* infection	Exclusion until diarrhea resolves and results of 2 stool cultures are negative for these organisms, depending on state regulations.	Meticulous hand hygiene; stool cultures should be performed for contacts. Center(s) with cases should be closed to new admissions during *E coli* O157:H7 outbreak (see *Escherichia coli* diarrhea, p 294, and *Shigella* infections, p 593).
Staphylococcus aureus skin infections	Exclusion only if skin lesions are draining and cannot be covered with a watertight dressing.	Meticulous hand hygiene; cultures of contacts are not recommended.
Streptococcal pharyngitis	Exclusion until 24 hours after treatment has been initiated and the child is able to participate in activities.	Symptomatic contacts of documented cases of group A streptococcal infection should be tested and treated if test results are positive.
Tuberculosis	For active disease, exclusion until determined to be noninfectious by physician or health department authority. May return to activities after therapy is instituted, symptoms have diminished, and adherence to therapy is documented. No exclusion for latent tuberculosis infection (LTBI).	Local health department personnel should be informed for contact investigation (see Tuberculosis, p 680).
Varicella (see Varicella-Zoster Infections, p 714)	Exclusion until all lesions have dried and crusted (usually 6 days after onset of rash in immunocompetent people; may be longer in immunocompromised people).	Varicella vaccine should be administered by 3 to 5 days after exposure, and Varicella-Zoster Immune Globulin should be administered up to 96 hours after exposure when indicated.

results of 2 stool cultures are negative for Shiga toxin-producing *E coli* or *Shigella* species (see *Escherichia coli* Diarrhea, p 294, *Shigella* Infections, p 593) and results of 3 stool cultures are negative for *Salmonella* serotype Typhi (see *Salmonella* Infections, p 584). Other *Salmonella* types do not require negative test results from stool cultures. Local health ordinances may differ with respect to number and timing of specimens.

During the course of an identified outbreak of any communicable illness in a child care setting, a child determined to be contributing to transmission of organisms causing the illness at the program may be excluded. The child may be readmitted when the risk of transmission no longer is present.

Infectious Diseases—Epidemiology and Control[1]

(Also see disease-specific chapters in Section 3.)

ENTERIC DISEASES

The close personal contact and suboptimal hygiene of young children provide ready opportunities for spread of enteric bacteria, viruses, and parasites in child care settings. Enteric pathogens transmitted by the person-to-person route, such as rotaviruses, enteric adenoviruses, astroviruses, noroviruses, *Shigella* species, *E coli* O157:H7, *Giardia intestinalis*, *Cryptosporidium* species, and hepatitis A virus (HAV), have been the principal organisms implicated in outbreaks. *Salmonella* species, *Clostridium difficile*, and *Campylobacter* species infrequently have been associated with outbreaks of disease in children in child care.

Human-animal contact involving family and classroom pets, animal displays, and petting zoos expose children to pathogens harbored by these animals. Most reptiles and many rodents (eg, hamsters, mice, rats) are colonized with *Salmonella* organisms, lymphocytic choriomeningitis virus, and other viruses that may be transmitted to children via contact (see Diseases Transmitted by Animals [Zoonoses]: Household Pets, Including Nontraditional Pets, and Exposure to Animals in Public Settings, p 198). Optimal hand hygiene is essential to prevent transmission of zoonoses in the child care setting.

Young children who are not toilet trained have an increased frequency of diarrhea and of HAV infection. Fecal contamination of the environment is common in child care programs and is highest in infant and toddler areas, especially among partially toilet trained attendees. Enteropathogens are spread by the fecal-oral route, either directly by person-to-person transmission or indirectly via fomites, environmental surfaces, and food. The risk of food contamination can be increased when staff members who assist with toilet use and diaper-changing activities also prepare or serve food. Several enteric pathogens, including rotaviruses, HAV, *G intestinalis* cysts, and *Cryptosporidium* oocysts, survive on environmental surfaces for periods ranging from hours to weeks.

Before universal hepatitis A immunization of children 12 through 23 months of age began in 2006, child care programs were a source of HAV spread within the community. HAV infection differs from most other diseases in child care centers, because symptomatic illness occurs primarily among adult contacts of infected asymptomatic children. To recognize outbreaks and initiate appropriate control measures, health care professionals and child care providers need to be aware of this epidemiologic characteristic (see Hepatitis A, p 329). Hepatitis A vaccine should be considered for the staff of child care centers with

[1]Also see American Academy of Pediatrics. *Managing Infectious Diseases in Child Care and Schools: A Quick Reference Guide*. Aronson SS, Shope TR, eds. 2nd ed. Elk Grove Village, IL: American Academy of Pediatrics; 2009

ongoing or recurrent outbreaks, in communities where cases in a child care center are a major source of HAV infection, and routinely for all children from 12 through 23 months of age (see Hepatitis A, p 329).

The single most important procedure to minimize fecal-oral transmission is frequent hand hygiene measures combined with staff training and monitoring of staff implementation. A child in whom jaundice develops should not have contact with other children or staff until 7 days after symptom onset. Exclusion criteria are provided in Table 2.5, p 128, and Table 2.6, p 129).

RESPIRATORY TRACT DISEASES

Organisms spread by the respiratory route include organisms causing acute upper respiratory tract infections or bacterial organisms associated with serious infections, such as *Haemophilus influenzae* type b, *Streptococcus pneumoniae*, *Neisseria meningitidis*, *Bordetella pertussis*, *Mycobacterium tuberculosis*, and *Kingella kingae*. Possible modes of spread of respiratory tract viruses include aerosols, respiratory droplets, and direct hand contact with contaminated secretions and fomites. The viral pathogens responsible for respiratory tract disease in child care settings are those that cause disease in the community, including respiratory syncytial virus, parainfluenza virus, influenza virus, human metapneumovirus, adenovirus, and rhinovirus. The incidence of viral infections of the respiratory tract is increased in child care settings. Hand hygiene measures can decrease the incidence of acute respiratory tract disease among children in child care (see Recommendations for Inclusion and Exclusion, p 127).

Transmission of *H influenzae* type b may occur among unimmunized young children in group child care settings, especially children younger than 24 months of age. In an outbreak of invasive *H influenzae* type b disease in child care, rifampin prophylaxis may be indicated for all nonpregnant contacts (see *Haemophilus influenzae* Infections, p 314), especially when unimmunized or incompletely immunized children attend the child care facility.

Infections caused by *N meningitidis* occur in all age groups. The age group experiencing the highest incidence is children younger than 1 year of age. Extended close contact between children and staff exposed to an index case of meningococcal disease predisposes to secondary transmission. Because outbreaks may occur in child care settings, chemoprophylaxis is indicated for exposed child care contacts (see Meningococcal Infections, p 455).

The risk of primary invasive disease attributable to *S pneumoniae* among children in child care settings is increased compared with children not in child care settings. Secondary spread of *S pneumoniae* in child care centers has been reported, but the degree of risk of secondary spread in child care facilities is unknown. Prophylaxis for contacts after the occurrence of one or more cases of invasive *S pneumoniae* disease is not recommended. Use of *S pneumoniae* conjugate vaccine has decreased the incidence of both invasive disease and pneumonia and has decreased carriage of the 7 serotypes of *S pneumoniae* contained in the pneumococcal conjugate vaccine.

Group A streptococcal infection among children in child care has been reported. A child with proven group A streptococcal infection should be excluded from classroom contact until 24 hours after initiation of antimicrobial therapy. Although outbreaks of streptococcal pharyngitis in these settings have occurred, the risk of secondary transmission after a single case of mild or even severe invasive group A streptococcal infection remains low. Chemoprophylaxis for contacts after group A streptococcal infection in child care facilities generally is not recommended (see Group A Streptococcal Infections, p 616).

Infants and young children with tuberculosis disease are not as contagious as are adults, because children are less likely to have cavitary pulmonary lesions and are unable to expel large numbers of organisms into the air forcefully. If approved by health officials, children with tuberculosis disease may attend group child care if the following criteria are met: (1) chemotherapy has begun; (2) ongoing adherence to therapy is documented; (3) clinical symptoms have resolved; (4) they are considered noninfectious to others; and (5) they are able to participate in activities. Because an adult with tuberculosis disease poses a hazard to children in group child care, tuberculin screening with a tuberculin skin test (TST) or an interferon-gamma release blood assay of all adults who have contact with children in a child care setting is recommended before caregiving activities are initiated. This includes noncare providers present in family child care homes. However, adults with tuberculosis, especially adults with diminished or altered immunologic function, may not have a reaction to a TST, and further evaluation may be required (see Tuberculosis, p 680). The need for periodic subsequent TSTs for people without clinically important reactions should be determined on the basis of their risk of acquiring a new infection and local or state health department recommendations. Adults with symptoms compatible with tuberculosis should be evaluated for the disease as soon as possible. Child care providers found to have tuberculosis disease should be excluded from the center and should not be allowed to care for children until chemotherapy has rendered them noninfectious (see Tuberculosis, p 680). The need for subsequent periodic TSTs for adults with an initial negative test result and no clinical symptoms of disease should be determined on the basis of their risk of acquiring a new infection and local or state health department recommendations.

OTHER CONDITIONS

PARVOVIRUS B19. Isolation or exclusion of immunocompetent people with parvovirus B19 infection in child care settings is unwarranted, because little or no virus is present in respiratory tract secretions at the time of occurrence of the rash of erythema infectiosum. In addition, because fewer than 1% of pregnant teachers during erythema infectiosum outbreaks would be expected to experience an adverse fetal outcome, exclusion of pregnant women from employment in child care or teaching is not recommended (see Parvovirus B19, p 491). Also, during outbreaks in the community, there is risk of acquisition of parvovirus B19 from a source not affiliated with the child care center.

VARICELLA-ZOSTER VIRUS. Children with varicella who have been excluded from child care may return after all lesions have dried and crusted, which usually occurs on the sixth day after onset of rash. All staff members and parents should be notified when a case of varicella occurs; they should be informed about the greater likelihood of serious infection in susceptible adults and adolescents and in susceptible immunocompromised people in addition to the potential for fetal sequelae if infection occurs during the pregnancy of a susceptible woman. Less than 5% of adults may be susceptible to varicella-zoster virus. Susceptible adults should be offered 2 doses of varicella vaccine unless contraindicated. Susceptible child care staff members who are pregnant and exposed to children with varicella should be referred promptly to a qualified physician or other health care professional for counseling and management. The American Academy of Pediatrics and Centers for Disease Control and Prevention (CDC) recommend use of varicella vaccine in nonpregnant immunocompetent susceptible people 12 months of age or older within 72 and possibly up to 96 hours after exposure to varicella (see Varicella-Zoster Infections, p 714). During a varicella outbreak, people who have received 1 dose of varicella vaccine should, resources permitting, receive a second dose of vaccine, provided the appropriate interval has elapsed since the first dose (3 months for children 12 months through 12 years of age and at least 4 weeks for people 13 years of age and older).

The decision to exclude staff members or children with herpes zoster infection (shingles) whose lesions cannot be covered should be made on the basis of criteria similar to criteria for varicella. Herpes zoster lesions that can be covered pose a minimal risk, because transmission usually occurs as a result of direct contact with fluid from lesions (see Varicella-Zoster Infections, p 714).

HERPES SIMPLEX VIRUS. Children with herpes simplex virus (HSV) gingivostomatitis who do not have control of oral secretions (drooling) should be excluded from child care when active lesions are present. Although HSV can be transmitted from a mother to her fetus or newborn infant, maternal HSV infections that are a threat to offspring usually are acquired by the infant during birth from genital tract infection of the mother. Exposure of a pregnant woman to HSV in a child care setting carries little risk for her fetus. Child care providers should be educated on the importance of hand hygiene and other measures for limiting transfer of infected material from children with varicella-zoster virus or HSV infection (eg, saliva, tissue fluid, or fluid from a skin lesion).

CMV INFECTION. Spread of CMV from asymptomatic infected children in child care to their mothers or to child care providers is the most important consequence of child care-related CMV infection (see Cytomegalovirus Infection, p 275). Children enrolled in child care programs are more likely to acquire CMV than are children primarily cared for at home. The highest rates (eg, 70%) of viral shedding in oral secretions and urine occur in children between 1 and 3 years of age, and excretion commonly continues (sometimes intermittently) for years. Studies of CMV seroconversion among child care providers have found annualized seroconversion rates of 8% to 20%. Women who are or who may become pregnant and who are CMV naive are at risk of being infected during pregnancy and delivering an infant with CMV disease.

In view of the risk of CMV infection in child care staff and the potential consequences of gestational CMV infection, child care staff members should be counseled about risks. This counseling may include testing for serum antibody to CMV to determine the child care provider's protection against primary CMV infection, but routine serologic testing is not recommended. CMV excretion is so prevalent that attempts at isolation or segregation of children who excrete CMV are impractical and inappropriate. Similarly, testing of children to detect CMV excretion is inappropriate, because excretion often is intermittent, and results of testing can be misleading.

BLOODBORNE VIRUS INFECTIONS

HBV, HIV, and hepatitis C virus (HCV) are bloodborne pathogens. Although the risk of contact with blood containing one of these viruses is low in the child care setting, appropriate infection-control practices will prevent transmission of bloodborne pathogens if exposure occurs. All child care providers should receive regular training on how to prevent transmission of bloodborne diseases and how to respond should an exposure occur.

HEPATITIS B VIRUS. Transmission of HBV in the child care setting has been described but occurs rarely. Because of the low risk of transmission, high immunization rates against HBV in children, and implementation of infection-control measures, children known to have chronic HBV infection (hepatitis B surface antigen [HBsAg] positive) may attend child care in most circumstances.

Transmission of HBV in a child care setting is most likely to occur through direct exposure to blood after an injury or from bites or scratches that break the skin and introduce blood or body secretions from an HBV carrier into another person. Indirect transmission through environmental contamination with blood or saliva is possible. This occurrence has not been documented in a child care setting in the United States. Because saliva contains much less virus than does blood, the potential infectivity of saliva is low. Infectivity of saliva has been demonstrated only when inoculated through the skin of gibbons and chimpanzees.

On the basis of limited data, the risk of disease transmission from a child or staff member who has chronic HBV infection but who behaves normally and is without injury, generalized dermatitis, or bleeding problems is minimal. This slight risk usually does not justify exclusion of a child who has chronic HBV infection from child care or the necessity of HBV immunization of the child's contacts at the care program, most of whom already should be protected by previous HBV immunization as part of their recommended immunization schedule.

Routine screening of children for HBsAg before admission to child care is not justified. Admission of a child previously identified to have chronic HBV infection with one or more risk factors for transmission of bloodborne pathogens (eg, biting, frequent scratching, generalized dermatitis, or bleeding problems) should be determined by the child's physician, child care provider, or program director. The responsible public health authority or child care health consultant should be consulted when appropriate. Regular assessment of behavioral risk factors and medical conditions of enrolled children with chronic HBV infection is necessary.

Children who bite pose an additional concern. Existing data in humans suggest a small risk of HBV transmission from the bite of a child with chronic HBV infection. For a susceptible child (not fully immunized with HBV vaccine) who is bitten by a child with chronic HBV infection, prophylaxis with Hepatitis B Immune Globulin (HBIG) and hepatitis B immunization is recommended (see Hepatitis B, p 337).

The risk of HBV acquisition when a susceptible child bites a child who has chronic HBV infection is unknown. A theoretical risk exists if HBsAg-positive blood enters the oral cavity of the biter, but transmission by this route has not been reported. Most experts would initiate the hepatitis B vaccine series but not give HBIG to a susceptible biting child (not fully immunized with HBV vaccine) who does not have oral mucosal disease when the amount of blood transferred from a child with chronic HBV infection is small.

In the common circumstance in which the HBsAg status of both the biting child and the victim is unknown, the risk of HBV transmission is extremely low because of the expected low seroprevalence of HBsAg in most groups of preschool-aged children, the low efficiency of disease transmission from bites, and routine HepB immunization of preschool children. Serologic testing generally is not warranted for the biting child or the recipient of the bite, but each situation should be evaluated individually.

Efforts to decrease the risk of HBV transmission in child care through hygienic and environmental standards generally should focus on precautions for blood exposures and limiting potential saliva contamination of the environment. Toothbrushes and pacifiers should be labeled individually and should not be shared among children. Accidents that lead to bleeding or contamination with blood-containing body fluids by any child should be handled as follows: (1) disposable gloves should be used when cleaning or removing any blood or blood-containing body fluid spills; (2) the material should be absorbed using disposable towels or tissues; (3) the area should be disinfected with a freshly prepared solution of a 1:10 dilution of household bleach, applied for at least 30 seconds and wiped after the minimum contact time; (4) people involved in cleaning contaminated surfaces should avoid exposure of open skin lesions or mucous membranes to blood or blood-containing body fluids and to wound or tissue exudates; (5) hands should be washed thoroughly after exposure to blood or blood-containing body fluids after gloves are removed and discarded properly; (6) disposable towels or tissues should be used and discarded properly, and mops should be rinsed in disinfectant; (7) blood-contaminated paper towels, diapers, gloves, and other materials should be placed in a leak-proof plastic bag with a secure tie for disposal; and (8) staff members should be educated about standard precautions for handling blood or blood-containing material.

HIV INFECTION (SEE ALSO HUMAN IMMUNODEFICIENCY VIRUS INFECTION, P 380). Children who enter child care should not be required to be tested for HIV or to disclose their HIV status. There is no need to restrict placement of HIV-infected children without risk factors for transmission of bloodborne pathogens in child care facilities to protect other children or staff members in these settings. Because HIV-infected children whose status is unknown may attend child care, standard precautions should be adopted for handling all spills of blood and blood-containing body fluids and wound exudates of all children, as described in the preceding HBV section.

The decision to admit known HIV-infected children to child care is best made on an individual basis by qualified people, including the child's physician, who are able to evaluate whether the child will receive optimal care in the program and whether an HIV-infected child poses a significant risk to others. Specifically, admission of each HIV-infected child with one or more potential risk factors for transmission of blood-borne pathogens (eg, biting, frequent scratching, generalized dermatitis, or bleeding problems) should be assessed by the child's physician and the program director. A responsible public health authority should be consulted as appropriate. If a bite results in blood exposure to either person involved, the US Public Health Service recommends postexposure follow-up, including consideration of postexposure prophylaxis (see Human Immunodeficiency Virus Infection, p 380). Information about a child who has immunodeficiency, regardless of cause, should be available to care providers who need to know how to help protect the child against other infections. For example, immunodeficient children exposed to measles or varicella should receive postexposure immunoprophylaxis as soon as possible (see Measles, p 444, and Varicella-Zoster Infections, p 714).

HIV-infected adults who do not have open and uncoverable skin lesions, other conditions that would allow contact with their body fluids, or a transmissible infectious disease may care for children in child care programs. However, immunosuppressed adults with HIV infection may be at increased risk of acquiring infectious agents from children and should consult their physician about the safety of continuing to work in child care. All child care providers, especially providers known to be HIV-infected, should be notified immediately if they have been exposed to varicella, parvovirus B19, tuberculosis, diarrheal disease, or measles through children or other adults in the facility.

HEPATITIS C VIRUS. Transmission risks of HCV infection in child care settings are unknown. The general risk of HCV infection from percutaneous exposure to infected blood is estimated to be 10 times greater than that of HIV but lower than that of HBV. The risk of transmission of HCV via contamination of mucous membranes or broken skin probably is between the risk of transmission of HIV and the risk of transmission of HBV via contaminated blood. Standard precautions (see Hepatitis C, p 357) should be followed to prevent infection with HCV.

IMMUNIZATIONS

Routine immunization at appropriate ages is important for children in child care, because preschool-aged children can have high age-specific incidence rates of measles, rubella, *H influenzae* type b disease, hepatitis A, varicella, pertussis, rotavirus, influenza, and invasive *S pneumoniae* disease attributable to serotypes contained in respective vaccines.

Written documentation of immunizations appropriate for age should be provided by parents or guardians of all children enrolling in child care. Unless contraindications exist or children have received medical, religious, or philosophic exemptions, immunization records should demonstrate immunizations as shown in the recommended childhood and adolescent immunization schedules (see Fig 1.1–1.3, p 24–28). Immunization mandates by state for children in child care can be found online (**www.immunize.org/laws**).

Children who have not received recommended age-appropriate immunizations before enrollment should be immunized as soon as possible, and the series should be completed according to Fig 1.1–1.3 (p 24–28). In the interim, unimmunized or inadequately immunized children should be allowed to attend child care unless a vaccine-preventable disease to which they may be susceptible occurs in the child care program. In such a situation, all underimmunized children should be excluded for the duration of possible exposure or until they have completed their immunizations.

Child care providers and staff members should have received all immunizations routinely recommended for adults (**www.cdc.gov/vaccines** [see adult immunization schedule]) according to guidelines for adult immunization of the Advisory Committee on Immunization Practices of the CDC, the American College of Physicians, the American College of Obstetricians and Gynecologists, and the American Academy of Family Physicians. Child care providers should be immunized against influenza annually and should be immunized appropriately against measles as shown in the adult immunization schedule. Hepatitis B immunization also should be considered, especially for providers who may manage blood-containing fluids. All child care providers should receive written information about hepatitis B disease and its complications as well as means of prevention.

Child care providers should be asked to document history of varicella disease or immunization. Child care providers with a negative or uncertain history of varicella and no history of immunization should be immunized with 2 doses of varicella vaccine or undergo serologic testing for susceptibility; providers who are not immune should be offered 2 doses of varicella vaccine unless it is contraindicated medically. All child care providers should receive written information about varicella, particularly disease manifestations in adults, complications, and means of prevention.

Because HAV can cause symptomatic illness in adult contacts and because child care programs have been a source of infection in the community, hepatitis A vaccine in some circumstances may be justified (see Hepatitis A, p 329). However, because the prevalence of HAV infection does not seem significantly increased in staff members of child care centers in comparison with the prevalence in the general population and because routine HAV immunization of children 12 through 23 months of age is indicated, routine immunization of staff members is not recommended. During HAV outbreaks, immunization should be considered (see Hepatitis A, p 329).

Adult child care providers younger than 65 years of age who received their last dose of Td (diphtheria and tetanus toxoids for children 7 years of age or older and adults) vaccine 10 years or more earlier should receive a single dose of Tdap (tetanus toxoid, reduced diphtheria toxoid, and acellular pertussis) vaccine to replace a single dose of Td for booster immunization against tetanus, diphtheria, and pertussis. For other recommendations for Tdap vaccine use in adults, see Pertussis (p 504).

General Practices

The following practices are recommended to decrease transmission of infectious agents in a child care setting:

- Each child care facility should have **written policies** for managing child and provider illness in child care.
- **Toilet areas and toilet-training equipment** should be maintained in sanitary condition.
- **Diaper-changing surfaces** should be nonporous and sanitized between uses. The diaper-changing surface should be covered with nonabsorbent paper liners large enough to cover the changing surface from the child's shoulders to beyond the child's feet. The liner is discarded after each use. If the surface becomes wet or soiled, it should be cleaned and sanitized.
- **Diaper-changing procedures** should be posted at the changing area. Soiled disposable diapers and soiled disposable wiping cloths should be discarded in a secure, foot-activated, plastic-lined container. Diapers should contain all urine and stool and minimize fecal contamination of children, child care providers, environmental surfaces, and objects in the child care environment. Diapers that should be used are modern disposable paper diapers with absorbent gelling material or carboxymethylcellulose or single-unit reusable systems with an inner cotton lining attached to an outer waterproof covering that are changed as a unit. Clothes should be worn over diapers while the child is in the child care facility. Soiled clothing should be bagged and sent home for laundering. Both the child's and caregiver's hands should be sanitized after a diaper change.
- **Diaper-changing areas** never should be located in food preparation areas and never should be used for temporary placement of food, drinks, or eating utensils.
- The use of **child-sized toilets** or access to steps and modified toilet seats that provide for easier maintenance should be encouraged. The use of potty chairs should be discouraged, but if used, potty chairs should be emptied into a toilet, cleaned in a utility sink, and disinfected after each use. Staff members should sanitize potty chairs, toilets, and diaper-changing areas with a freshly prepared solution of a 1:64 dilution of household bleach (one quarter cup of bleach diluted in 1 gallon of water) applied for at least 2 minutes, rinsed, and dried.

- **Written procedures for hand hygiene** should be established and enforced.[1] Hand-washing sinks should be adjacent to all diaper-changing and toilet areas. These sinks should be washed and disinfected at least daily and should not be used for food preparation. Food and drinking utensils should not be washed in sinks in diaper-changing areas. Hand-washing sinks should not be used for rinsing soiled clothing or for cleaning potty chairs. Children should have access to height-appropriate sinks, soap dispensers, and disposable paper towels and should be supervised when using alcohol-based hand sanitizing gels.

Written **personal hygiene policies** for staff and children are necessary.

Written **environmental sanitation policies and procedures** should include cleaning and disinfecting floors, covering sandboxes, cleaning and sanitizing play tables, and cleaning and disinfecting spills of blood or body fluids and wound or tissue exudates. In general, routine housekeeping procedures using a freshly prepared solution of commercially available cleaner (eg, detergents, disinfectant detergents, or chemical germicides) compatible with most surfaces are satisfactory for cleaning spills of vomitus, urine, and feces. For spills of blood or blood-containing body fluids and of wound and tissue exudates, the material should be removed using gloves to avoid contamination of hands, and the area then should be disinfected using a freshly prepared solution of a 1:10 dilution of household bleach applied for at least 30 seconds and wiped with a disposable cloth after the minimum contact time.

Each item of **sleep equipment** should be used only by a single child and should be cleaned and sanitized before being assigned to another child. Crib mattresses should have a nonporous easy-to-wipe surface and should be cleaned and sanitized when soiled or wet. Sleeping cots should be stored so that contact with the sleeping surface of another mat does not occur. Bedding (sheets and blankets) should be assigned to each child and cleaned and sanitized when soiled or wet.

Optimally, **toys** that are placed in children's mouths or otherwise contaminated by body secretions should be cleaned with water and detergent, disinfected, rinsed and air-dried before handling by another child. All frequently touched toys in rooms that house infants and toddlers should be cleaned and disinfected daily. Toys in rooms for older continent children should be cleaned at least weekly and when soiled. Soft, nonwashable toys should not be used in infant and toddler areas of child care programs.

Food should be handled safely and appropriately to prevent growth of bacteria and to prevent contamination by enteropathogens, insects, or rodents.[2] Tables and countertops used for food preparation and food service should be cleaned and sanitized between uses, between preparation of raw and cooked food, and before and after eating. People with signs or symptoms of illness, including vomiting, diarrhea, jaundice, or infectious skin lesions that cannot be covered, or with potential foodborne pathogen infections should not be responsible for food handling. Hands should be washed using soap and water before handling food. Because of their frequent exposure to feces and children with enteric diseases, staff members who work with diapered children or assist with toilet use should not prepare food. Caregivers who prepare food for infants should be aware of

---

[1]Centers for Disease Control and Prevention. Guideline for hand hygiene in health-care settings. Recommendations of the Healthcare Infection Control Practices Advisory Committee and the HICPAC/SHEA/APIC/IDSA Hand Hygiene Task Force. *MMWR Recomm Rep.* 2002;51(RR-16):1–45

[2]Centers for Disease Control and Prevention. Surveillance for foodborne disease outbreaks—United States 1998–2002. *MMWR Recomm Rep.* 2006;55(SS-10):1–42

the importance of careful hand hygiene. When milk, milk products, or juices are served, they must be pasteurized products (see Appendix VIII, Potentially Contaminated Food Products, p 857).

- The living quarters of **pets** should be enclosed and kept clean of waste to decrease the risk of human contact with the waste. Hands should be washed after handling all animals or animal wastes. Dogs and cats should be in good health, immunized appropriately for age, and should be kept away from child play areas and handled only with staff supervision. Such animals should be given flea, tick, and worm control programs. Reptiles and rodents should not be handled by children (see Diseases Transmitted by Animals [Zoonoses]: Household Pets, Including Nontraditional Pets, and Exposure to Animals in Public Settings, p 198).
- Written policies that comply with local and state regulations for filing and regularly updating **immunization records** of each child and child care provider should be maintained.
- Each child care program should use the services of a **health consultant** to assist in development and implementation of written policies for prevention and control of communicable diseases and provision of related health education to children, staff, and parents.
- The child care provider should, when registering each child, **inform parents of the need to share information about illnesses** that could be communicable in the child or in any member of the immediate household to facilitate prompt reporting of disease and institution of any measures necessary to prevent transmission to others. The child care provider or program director, after consulting with the program's health consultant or the responsible public health official, should follow recommendations of the consultant or public health official for **notification of parents** of children who attend the program about exposure of their child to a communicable disease.
- Local and/or state **public health authorities should be notified** about cases of notifiable diseases involving children or care providers in the child care setting.
- In settings where human milk is stored and delivered to infants, there should be a written policy and a quality-improvement program (as is done routinely for blood products) to ensure administration of human milk to the designated infant, monitor the program results, and develop protocols to deal with incidents when human milk inadvertently is fed to an infant other than the designated infant (see Human Milk Banks, p 123). Some neonatal intensive care units have adopted policies to address such incidents. These policies require documentation, counseling, observation of the affected infant for signs of infection, and verification of the donor mother's infectious disease status.

SCHOOL HEALTH

Clustering of children together in a school setting provides opportunities for spread of infectious diseases. Determining the likelihood that infection in one or more children will pose a risk for schoolmates depends on an understanding of several factors: (1) the mechanism by which the organism causing the infection is spread; (2) the ease with which the organism is spread (contagion); and (3) the likelihood that classmates are immune because of immunization or previous infection. Decisions to intervene to prevent spread of infection within a school should be made through collaboration among school officials, local public health officials, and health care professionals, considering the availability and effectiveness of specific methods of prevention and risk of serious complications from infection.

Generic methods for control and prevention of spread of infection in the school setting include the following:

- For vaccine-preventable diseases, documentation of the immunization status of enrolled children should be reviewed. Schools have a legal responsibility to ensure that students have been immunized against vaccine-preventable diseases at the time of enrollment, in accordance with state requirements (see Appendix XI, State Immunization Requirements for School Attendance, p 871). Although specific laws vary by state, most states require proof of protection against poliomyelitis, tetanus, pertussis, diphtheria, measles, mumps, and rubella. Hepatitis B immunization and immunization against varicella and meningococcal disease are mandatory in many states (**www.immunize. org/laws** or **www.cdc.gov/other.htm#states**). Hepatitis A virus (HAV) immunization is required for school entry in some states. In 2007, the Centers for Disease Control and Prevention recommended that all states require that children entering elementary school have received 2 doses of varicella vaccine or have other evidence of immunity to varicella. Policies established by state health departments concerning exclusion of unimmunized children and exemptions for children with certain underlying medical conditions and families with religious or philosophic objection to immunization should be followed. Exemption rates by state can be found at **www2. cdc.gov/nip/schoolsurv/rptgmenu.asp.**
- Infected children should be excluded from school until they no longer are considered contagious (for recommendations on specific diseases, see relevant disease-specific chapters in Section 3).
- In some instances, administration of appropriate antimicrobial therapy will limit further spread of infection (eg, streptococcal pharyngitis and pertussis).
- Antimicrobial prophylaxis given to close contacts of children with infections caused by specific pathogens may be warranted in some circumstances (eg, meningococcal infection).
- Temporary school closing can be used in limited circumstances: (1) to prevent spread of infection; (2) when an infection is expected to affect a large number of susceptible students and available control measures are considered inadequate (eg, outbreak of influenza); or (3) when an infection is expected to have a high rate of morbidity or mortality.

Physicians involved with school health should be aware of current public health guidelines to prevent and control infectious diseases. In all circumstances requiring intervention to prevent spread of infection within the school setting, the privacy of children who are infected should be protected.

Diseases Preventable by Routine Childhood Immunization

Children and adolescents immunized according to the recommended childhood and adolescent immunization schedule (see Fig 1.1–1.3, p 24–28) should be considered to be protected against diseases for which they were immunized. Disease-specific chapters should be consulted for details.

Measles and varicella vaccines have been demonstrated to provide protection in some susceptible people if administered within 72 hours after exposure. Measles or varicella immunization should be recommended immediately for all nonimmune people during a measles or varicella outbreak, respectively, except for people with a contraindication to immunization. Students immunized for measles or varicella for the first time under these circumstances should be allowed to return to school after immunization. Susceptible children and adolescents 12 months of age or older exposed to HAV should receive single-antigen hepatitis A vaccine (or Immune Globulin) within 14 days after exposure. People who are immunocompromised, are older than 40 years of age, or have liver disease should receive Immune Globulin (see Hepatitis A, p 329).[1]

Mumps vaccine given after exposure has not been demonstrated to prevent infection among susceptible contacts, but immunization should be administered to unimmunized students to protect them from infection from subsequent exposure.

Infections Spread by the Respiratory Route

Some pathogens that cause severe lower respiratory tract disease in infants and toddlers, such as respiratory syncytial virus, are of less concern in healthy school-aged children. Respiratory tract viruses, however, are associated with exacerbations of reactive airway disease and an increase in the incidence of otitis media and can cause significant complications for children with chronic respiratory tract disease, such as cystic fibrosis, or for children who are immunocompromised.

Influenza virus infection is a common cause of febrile respiratory tract disease and school absenteeism. Annual influenza immunization should be administered to children 6 months through 18 years of age and to all eligible close contacts of children 0 through 59 months of age and contacts of children 5 through 18 years of age who have an underlying medical condition that predisposes them to influenza complications (see Influenza Vaccine, p 405).

Mycoplasma pneumoniae causes upper and lower respiratory tract infection in school-aged children, and outbreaks of *M pneumoniae* infection occur in communities and schools. The nonspecific symptoms and signs of this infection make distinguishing *M pneumoniae* infection from other causes of respiratory tract illness difficult. Antimicrobial therapy does not necessarily eradicate the organism nor prevent spread. Thus, intervention to prevent secondary infection in the school setting is difficult. Mass prophylaxis may be considered in certain limited outbreak situations. Mycoplasma outbreaks in schools should be reported to the local health department.

Symptomatic contacts of students with pharyngitis attributable to group A streptococcal infection should be evaluated and treated if streptococcal infection is demonstrated. Infected students may return to school 24 hours after initiation of antimicrobial therapy. Students awaiting results of culture or antigen-detection tests who are not receiving antimicrobial therapy may attend school during the culture incubation period unless there is an associated fever or the infection involves a child with poor hygiene and poor control of secretions. Asymptomatic contacts usually require neither evaluation nor therapy.

---

[1]Advisory Committee on Immunization Practices (ACIP) Centers for Disease Control and Prevention (CDC). Update: Prevention of hepatitis A after exposure to hepatitis A virus and in international travelers. Updated recommendations of the Advisory Committee on Immunization Practices (ACIP). *MMWR Morb Mortal Wkly Rep.* 2007;56(41):1080–1084

Bacterial meningitis in school-aged children may be caused by *Neisseria meningitidis*. Infected people are not considered contagious after 24 hours of appropriate antimicrobial therapy. After discharge from the hospital, they pose no risk to classmates and may return to school. Prophylactic antimicrobial therapy is not recommended for school contacts in most circumstances. Close observation of contacts is recommended, and they should be evaluated promptly if a febrile illness develops. Students who have been exposed to oral secretions of an infected student, such as through kissing or sharing of food and drink, should receive chemoprophylaxis (see Meningococcal Infections, p 455). Immunization of school contacts with meningococcal conjugate vaccine (MCV4), which in the United States contains antigens for serogroups A, C, Y, and W-135, should be considered, in consultation with local public health authorities, if evidence suggests an outbreak within a school attributable to one of the meningococcal serogroups contained in the vaccine. Immunization recommendations for administration of a single dose of meningococcal conjugate vaccine for all adolescents 11 through 18 years of age and for high-risk groups 2 through 10 years of age and 19 through 55 years of age should be followed (see Meningococcal Infections, p 455).

Students and staff members with documented pertussis should be excluded until they have received at least 5 days of the recommended course of azithromycin, clarithromycin, or erythromycin therapy. In some circumstances, chemoprophylaxis is recommended for their school contacts (see Pertussis, p 504). Tetanus toxoid, reduced diphtheria toxoid, and acellular pertussis (Tdap) should be substituted for a single dose of Td (diphtheria and tetanus toxoids for children 7 years of age or older and adults) in the primary catch-up series or as a booster dose if age appropriate (see Fig 1.1–1.3, p 24–28).

Before adolescence, children with tuberculosis generally are not contagious, but students who are in close contact with a child, teacher, or other adult with tuberculosis should be evaluated for infection, including tuberculin skin testing (see Tuberculosis, p 680). An adolescent or adult with tuberculosis almost always is the source of infection for young children. If an adult source outside the school is identified (eg, parent or grandparent of a student), efforts should be made to determine whether other students have been exposed to the same source and whether they warrant evaluation for infection.

Children with erythema infectiosum should be allowed to attend school, because the period of contagion occurs before a rash is evident. Parvovirus B19 infection poses no risk of significant illness for healthy classmates, although aplastic crisis can develop in infected children with sickle cell disease or other hemoglobinopathies. The relatively low risk of fetal damage should be explained to pregnant students and teachers exposed to children in the early stages of parvovirus B19 infection, 5 to 10 days before appearance of the rash. Exposed pregnant women should be referred to their physician for counseling and possible serologic testing.

Infections Spread by Direct Contact

Infection and infestation of skin, eyes, and hair can spread through direct contact with the infected area or through contact with contaminated hands or fomites, such as hair brushes, hats, and clothing. *Staphylococcus aureus* (including methicillin-resistant *S aureus* [MRSA]) and group A streptococcal organisms may colonize the skin or the oropharynx of asymptomatic people. Lesions may develop when these organisms are passed from a person with infected skin to another person. Organisms also can be transmitted to open skin lesions in the same child or to other children. Although most skin infections attributable to *S aureus* and group A streptococcal organisms are minor and require only topical or oral antimicrobial therapy, person-to-person spread should be interrupted by appropriate treatment whenever lesions are recognized. Local and systemic infections associated with MRSA pose a diagnostic and therapeutic challenge (see Staphylococcal Infections, p 601). Exclusion of any infected child with an open or draining lesion that cannot be covered is recommended.

Herpes simplex virus (HSV) infection of the mouth and skin is common among school-aged children. Infection is spread through direct contact with herpetic lesions or asymptomatic shedding of virus from oral or genital secretions. "Cold sore" lesions of herpes labialis represent active infection, but no evidence suggests that these students pose any greater risk to their classmates than do unidentified asymptomatic shedders. For immunocompromised children and for children with open skin lesions (eg, severe eczema), exposure to another child with HSV infection may pose an increased risk of HSV acquisition and of severe or disseminated infection. Because of the frequency of symptomatic and asymptomatic shedding of HSV among classmates and staff members, careful hygienic practices are the best means of preventing infection (see Herpes Simplex, p 363).

Infectious conjunctivitis can be caused by bacterial (eg, nontypable *Haemophilus influenzae* and *Streptococcus pneumoniae*) or viral (eg, adenoviruses, enteroviruses, and HSV) pathogens. Bacterial conjunctivitis is less common in children older than 5 years of age. Infection occurs through direct contact or through contamination of hands followed by autoinoculation. Respiratory tract spread from large droplets also may occur. Topical antimicrobial therapy is indicated for bacterial conjunctivitis, which usually is distinguished by a purulent exudate. Herpes simplex virus conjunctivitis usually is unilateral and may be accompanied by vesicles on adjacent skin. Evaluation of HSV conjunctivitis by an ophthalmologist and administration of specific antiviral therapy are indicated. Conjunctivitis attributable to adenoviruses or enteroviruses is self-limited and requires no specific antiviral therapy. Spread of infection is minimized by careful hand hygiene, and infected people should be presumed contagious until symptoms have resolved. Except when viral or bacterial conjunctivitis is accompanied by systemic signs of illness, infected children should be allowed to remain in school once any indicated therapy is implemented, unless their behavior is such that close contact with other students cannot be avoided. The local health department should be notified of an outbreak of conjunctivitis.

Fungal infections of the skin and hair are spread by direct person-to-person contact and through contact with contaminated surfaces or objects. *Trichophyton tonsurans,* the predominant cause of tinea capitis, remains viable for long periods on combs, hair brushes, furniture, and fabric. The fungi that cause tinea corporis (ringworm) are transmissible by direct contact. Tinea cruris (jock itch) and tinea pedis (athlete's foot) occur in adolescents and young adults. The fungi that cause these infections have a predilection for moist areas and are spread through direct contact and contact with contaminated surfaces.

Students with fungal infections of the skin or scalp should be encouraged to receive treatment both for their benefit and to prevent spread of infection. However, lack of treatment does not necessitate exclusion from school unless the nature of their contact with other students could potentiate spread. Students with tinea capitis should be instructed not to share combs, hair brushes, hats, or hair ornaments with classmates until they have been treated. Students with tinea pedis should be excluded from swimming pools and from walking barefoot on locker room and shower floors until treatment has been initiated. Spread of infection by students with tinea capitis may be decreased by use of selenium sulfide shampoos, but treatment requires systemic antifungal therapy (see Tinea Capitis, p 661).

Sarcoptes scabiei (scabies) and *Pediculus capitis* (head lice) are transmitted primarily through person-to-person contact. The scabies parasite survives on clothing for only 3 to 4 days without skin contact. Combs, hair brushes, hats, and hair ornaments can transmit head lice, but away from the scalp, lice do not remain viable.

Children identified as having scabies or head lice should be referred for treatment at the end of the school day and subsequently excluded from school only until treatment recommended by the child's health care professional has been started. School contacts generally should not be treated prophylactically. Caregivers who have prolonged skin-to-skin contact with students infested with scabies may benefit from prophylactic treatment (see Scabies, p 589).

Shampooing with an appropriate pediculicide and manually removing nits by combing usually are effective in eradicating viable lice. Manual removal of nits after treatment with a pediculicide is not necessary to prevent reinfestation (see Pediculosis Capitis, p 495).

Infections Spread by the Fecal-Oral Route

For developmentally typical school-aged children, pathogens spread via the fecal-oral route constitute a risk only if the infected person fails to maintain good hygiene, including hand hygiene after toilet use, or if contaminated food is shared between or among schoolmates.

Outbreaks attributable to HAV can occur in schools, but these outbreaks usually are associated with community outbreaks. Schoolroom exposure generally does not pose an appreciable risk of infection, and administration of HAV vaccine or Immune Globulin to susceptible people for postexposure prophylaxis is not indicated. However, if transmission within a school is documented, HAV vaccine should be considered as a means of prophylaxis and prolonged protection for immunocompetent people 12 months through 40 years of age (see Hepatitis A, p 329). If an outbreak occurs, consultation with local public health authorities is indicated before initiating interventions. Ultimately, implementation of the recommended immunization of preschool-aged children with HAV vaccine should help reduce school outbreaks of disease.

Enteroviral infections probably are spread via the oral-oral route as well as by the fecal-oral route. The incidence is so high when outbreaks occur during summer and fall epidemics that control measures specifically aimed at the school classroom likely would be futile. Person-to-person spread of bacterial, viral, and parasitic enteropathogens within school settings occurs infrequently, but foodborne outbreaks attributable to enteric pathogens can occur. Symptomatic people with gastroenteritis attributable to an enteric pathogen should be excluded until symptoms resolve.

Children in diapers at any age and in any setting constitute a far greater risk of spread of gastrointestinal tract infection attributable to enteric pathogens. Guidelines for control of these infections in child care settings should be applied for school-aged students with developmental disabilities who are diapered (see Children in Out-of-Home Child Care, p 124).

Infections Spread by Blood and Body Fluids

Contact with blood and other body fluids of another person requires more intimate exposure than usually occurs in the school setting. The care required for children with developmental disabilities, however, may result in exposure of caregivers to urine, saliva, and in some cases, blood. The application of Standard Precautions for prevention of transmission of bloodborne pathogens, as recommended for children in out-of-home child care, prevents spread of infection from these exposures (see Children in Out-of-Home Child Care, p 124). School staff members who routinely provide acute care for children with epistaxis or bleeding from injury should wear disposable gloves and use appropriate hand hygiene measures immediately after glove removal to protect themselves from bloodborne pathogens. Staff members at the scene of an injury or bleeding incident who do not have access to gloves need to use some type of barrier to avoid exposure to blood or blood-containing materials, use appropriate hand hygiene measures, and adhere to proper protocols for handling contaminated material. Routine use of these precautions helps avoid the necessity of identifying children known to be infected with human immunodeficiency virus (HIV), hepatitis B virus (HBV), or hepatitis C virus (HCV) and acknowledges that an unknown exposure poses at least as much risk as does exposure from an identified infected child.

Students infected with HIV, HBV, or HCV do not need to be identified to school personnel. Because HIV-, HBV-, and HCV-infected children and adolescents will not be identified, policies and procedures to manage all potential exposures to blood or blood-containing materials should be established and implemented. Parents and students should be educated about the types of exposure that present a risk for school contacts. Although a student's right to privacy should be maintained, decisions about activities at school should be made by parents or guardians together with a physician on a case-by-case basis, keeping the health needs of the infected student and the student's classmates in mind.

Prospective studies to aid in determining the risk of transmission of HIV, HBV, or HCV during contact sports among high school students have not been performed, but the available evidence indicates that risk is low. Guidelines for management of bleeding injuries have been developed for college and professional athletes in recognition of the possibility of unidentified HIV, HBV, or HCV infection in any competitor. Recommendations developed by the American Academy of Pediatrics (AAP) for prevention of transmission of HIV and other bloodborne pathogens in the athletic setting were issued in 1999 and reaffirmed in 2005.[1,2]

- Athletes infected with HIV, HBV, or HCV should be allowed to participate in competitive sports.
- The physician should respect the right of infected athletes to confidentiality. The patient's infection status should not be disclosed to other participants or the staff of athletic programs.
- Testing for bloodborne pathogens should not be mandatory for athletes or sports participants.

[1]American Academy of Pediatrics, Committee on Sports Medicine and Fitness. Human immunodeficiency virus and other blood-borne viral pathogens in the athletic setting. *Pediatrics.* 1999;104(6):1400–1403 (Reaffirmed 2005)

[2]Rice SG; American Academy of Pediatrics, Council on Sports Medicine and Fitness. Medical conditions affecting sports participation. *Pediatrics.* 2008;121(4):841–848

- Pediatricians are encouraged to counsel athletes who are infected with HIV, HBV, or HCV and assure them that they have a low risk of infecting other competitors. Infected athletes should consider choosing a sport in which this risk is minimal. This may be protective for other participants and for infected athletes themselves, decreasing their possible exposure to bloodborne pathogens other than the one(s) with which they are infected. Wrestling and boxing probably have the greatest potential for contamination of injured skin by blood. The AAP opposes boxing as a sport for youth for other reasons.
- Athletic programs should inform athletes and their parents that the program is operating under the policies of the aforementioned recommendations and that the athletes have a low risk of becoming infected with a bloodborne pathogen.
- Clinicians and staff of athletic programs should promote HBV immunization among all athletes and among coaches, athletic trainers, equipment handlers, laundry personnel, and any other people at risk of exposure to blood of athletes as an occupational hazard.
- Each coach and athletic trainer must receive training in first aid and emergency care and in prevention of transmission of bloodborne pathogens in the athletic setting. These staff members then can help implement these recommendations.
- Coaches and members of the health care team should educate athletes about precautions described in these recommendations. Such education should include the greater risks of transmission of HIV and other bloodborne pathogens through sexual activity and needle sharing during the use of injection drugs, including anabolic steroids. Athletes should be told not to share personal items, such as razors, toothbrushes, and nail clippers, that might be contaminated with blood.
- Depending on law in some states, schools may need to comply with Occupational Safety and Health Administration (OSHA) regulations[1] for prevention of bloodborne pathogens. The athletic program must determine what rules apply. Compliance with OSHA regulations is a reasonable and recommended precaution even if this is not required specifically by the state.
- The following precautions should be adopted in sports with direct body contact and other sports in which an athlete's blood or other body fluids visibly tinged with blood may contaminate the skin or mucous membranes of other participants or staff members of the athletic program. Even if these precautions are adopted, the risk that a participant or staff member may become infected with a bloodborne pathogen in the athletic setting will not be eliminated entirely.
  - Athletes must cover existing cuts, abrasions, wounds, or other areas of broken skin with an occlusive dressing before and during participation. Caregivers should cover their own damaged skin to prevent transmission of infection to or from an injured athlete.
  - Disposable, water-impervious vinyl or latex gloves should be worn to avoid contact with blood or other body fluids visibly tinged with blood and any objects, such as equipment, bandages, or uniforms, contaminated with these fluids. Hands should be cleaned with soap and water or an alcohol-based antiseptic agent as soon as possible after gloves are removed.

---

[1]Occupational Safety and Health Administration (**www.osha.gov**)

- Athletes with active bleeding should be removed from competition as soon as possible until bleeding is stopped. Wounds should be cleaned with soap and water. Skin antiseptic agents may be used if soap and water are not available. Wounds must be covered with an occlusive dressing that will remain intact and not become soaked through during further play before athletes return to competition.
- Athletes should be advised to report injuries and wounds in a timely fashion before or during competition.
- Minor cuts or abrasions that are not bleeding do not require interruption of play but can be cleaned and covered during scheduled breaks. During these breaks, if an athlete's equipment or uniform fabric is wet with blood, the equipment should be cleaned and disinfected (see next bullet), or the uniform should be replaced.
- Equipment and playing areas contaminated with blood must be cleaned using gloves and disposable absorbent material until all visible blood is gone and then disinfected with an appropriate germicide, such as a freshly made bleach solution containing 1 part bleach in 10 parts of water.[1] The decontaminated equipment or area should be in contact with the bleach solution for at least 30 seconds. The area then may be wiped with a disposable cloth after the minimum contact time or allowed to air dry.
- Emergency care must not be delayed because gloves or other protective equipment are not available. If the caregiver does not have appropriate protective equipment, a towel may be used to cover the wound until an off-the-field location is reached where gloves can be used during more definitive treatment.
- Breathing bags (eg, Ambu manual resuscitators) and oropharyngeal airways should be available for giving resuscitation. Mouth-to-mouth resuscitation is recommended only if this equipment is not available.
- Equipment handlers, laundry personnel, and janitorial staff must be educated in proper procedures for handling washable or disposable materials contaminated with blood.
- For guidelines on control and prevention of MRSA in athletes and other school settings, see Staphylococcal Infections (p 601).

INFECTION CONTROL FOR HOSPITALIZED CHILDREN

Health care-associated infections are a major cause of morbidity and mortality in hospitalized children, particularly children in intensive care units. Hand hygiene before and after each patient contact remains the single most important practice in prevention and control of health care-associated infections. A comprehensive set of guidelines for preventing and controlling health care-associated infections, including isolation precautions, personnel health recommendations, and guidelines for prevention of postoperative and device-related infections, can be found on the Centers for Disease Control and Prevention (CDC) Web site (**www.cdc.gov/ncidod/dhqp/guidelines.html**). Additional guidelines are available from the principal infection control societies in the

---

[1] Centers for Disease Control and Prevention. Guidelines for environmental infection control in health-care facilities. Recommendations of CDC and the Healthcare Infection Control Practices Advisory Committee (HICPAC). *MMWR Recomm Rep.* 2003;52(RR-10):1–42

United States, the Society for Healthcare Epidemiology of America and the Association for Professionals in Infection Control and Epidemiology, as well as specialty societies and regulatory agencies, such as the Occupational Safety and Health Administration (OSHA). The Cystic Fibrosis Foundation published an evidence-based guideline for prevention of transmission of infectious agents among cystic fibrosis patients in 2003. The Joint Commission also has established infection-control standards. Physicians and infection-control professionals should be familiar with this increasingly complex array of guidelines, regulations, and standards. Ongoing educational programs that encompass appropriate aspects of infection control should be implemented, reinforced, documented, and evaluated on a regular basis.

Isolation Precautions

Isolation precautions are designed to protect hospitalized children, health care personnel, and visitors from health care-associated infections. The Healthcare Infection Control Practices Advisory Committee updated evidence-based isolation guidelines in 2007 for preventing transmission of infectious agents in health care settings.[1] Adherence to these isolation policies, supplemented by health care facility policies and procedures for other aspects of infection and environmental control and occupational health, should result in reduced transmission and safe patient care. Adaptations should be made according to the conditions and population served by each facility.

Routine and optimal performance of **Standard Precautions** is appropriate for the care of all patients regardless of their diagnosis or suspected or confirmed infection status. In addition to Standard Precautions, pathogen- and syndrome-based **Transmission-Based Precautions** are used when caring for patients who are infected or colonized with pathogens transmitted by the airborne, droplet, or contact routes.

STANDARD PRECAUTIONS

Standard Precautions are used to prevent transmission of all infectious agents through contact with any body fluid except sweat (regardless of whether these fluids contain visible blood), nonintact skin, or mucous membranes. Barrier techniques are recommended to decrease exposure of health care personnel to body fluids. Precautions are used with all patients when exposure to blood and body fluids is anticipated, because medical history and examination cannot reliably identify all patients infected with human immunodeficiency virus or other infectious agents. Standard Precautions decrease transmission of microorganisms from patients who are not recognized as harboring potential pathogens, such as antimicrobial-resistant bacteria. See Table 2.7, p 150, for new elements added to Standard Precautions (respiratory hygiene/cough etiquette). Standard Precautions include the following practices:

---

[1]Centers for Disease Control and Prevention. Guideline for isolation precautions: preventing transmission of infectious agents in health care settings 2007. Recommendations of the Healthcare Infection Control Practices Advisory Committee. Atlanta, GA: Centers for Disease Control and Prevention; 2007. Available at: **www.cdc. gov/ncidod/dhqp/pdf/guidelines/isolation2007.pdf**

Table 2.7. Recommendations for Application of Standard Precautions for Care of All Patients in All Health Care Settings

Component	Recommendations
Hand hygiene	After touching blood, body fluids, secretions, excretions, or contaminated items; immediately after removing gloves; between patient contacts. Alcohol-containing antiseptic hand rubs preferred except when hands are soiled visibly with blood or other proteinaceous materials or if exposure to spores (eg, *Clostridium difficile, Bacillus anthracis*) is likely to have occurred.
Personal protective equipment (PPE)	
Gloves	For touching blood, body fluids, secretions, excretions, or contaminated items; for touching mucous membranes and nonintact skin.
Gown	During procedures and patient-care activities when contact of clothing/exposed skin with blood/body fluids, secretions, and excretions is anticipated.
Mask, eye protection (goggles), face shield	During procedures and patient-care activities likely to generate splashes or sprays of blood, body fluids, or secretions, especially suctioning and endotracheal intubation, to protect health care personnel. For patient protection, use of a mask by the person inserting an epidural anesthesia needle or performing myelograms when prolonged exposure of the puncture site is likely to occur.
Soiled patient-care equipment	Handle in a manner that prevents transfer of microorganisms to others and to the environment; wear gloves if visibly contaminated; perform hand hygiene.
Environmental control	Develop procedures for routine care, cleaning, and disinfection of environmental surfaces, especially frequently touched surfaces in patient care areas.
Textiles (linens) and laundry	Handle in a manner that prevents transfer of microorganisms to others and the environment.
Injection practices (use of needles and other sharps)	Do not recap, bend, break, or hand manipulate used needles; if recapping is required, use a one-handed scoop technique only; use needle-free safety devices when available; place used sharps in puncture-resistant container. Use a sterile, single-use, disposable needle and syringe for each injection given. Single-dose medication vials are preferred when medications are administered to more than one patient.
Patient resuscitation	Use mouthpiece, resuscitation bag, or other ventilation devices to prevent contact with mouth and oral secretions.

Table 2.7. Recommendations for Application of Standard Precautions for Care of All Patients in All Health Care Settings, continued

Component	Recommendations
Patient placement	Prioritize for single-patient room if patient is at increased risk of transmission, is likely to contaminate the environment, does not maintain appropriate hygiene, or is at increased risk of acquiring infection or developing adverse outcome following infection.
Respiratory hygiene/cough etiquette (source containment of infectious respiratory tract secretions in symptomatic patients) beginning at the initial point of encounter (eg, triage and reception areas in emergency departments and physician offices)	Instruct symptomatic people to cover mouth/nose when sneezing/coughing; use tissues and dispose in no-touch receptacle; observe hand hygiene after soiling of hands with respiratory tract secretions; wear surgical mask if tolerated or maintain spatial separation (more than 3 feet if possible).

- **Hand hygiene**[1] is necessary before and after all patient contacts and after touching blood, body fluids, secretions, excretions, and contaminated items, whether gloves are worn or not. Hand hygiene should be performed either with alcohol-based agents or soap and water immediately after removing gloves, between patient contacts, and when otherwise indicated to avoid transfer of microorganisms to other patients and to items in the environment. When hands are visibly dirty or contaminated with proteinaceous material such as blood or other body fluids, hands should be washed with soap and water. When exposure to spores (eg, *Clostridium difficile*) is likely, handwashing with soap and water is preferred, because alcohol is not sporicidal and the friction of handwashing is more effective in removing spores.
- **Gloves** (clean, nonsterile) should be worn when touching blood, body fluids, secretions, excretions, and items contaminated with these fluids except for wiping a child's tears or nose or for routine diaper changing. Clean gloves should be used before touching mucous membranes and nonintact skin. Gloves should be changed between tasks and procedures on the same patient after contact with material that may contain a high concentration of microorganisms (eg, purulent drainage).
- **Masks, eye protection, and face shields** should be worn to protect mucous membranes of the eyes, nose, and mouth during procedures and patient care activities likely to generate splashes or sprays of blood, body fluids, secretions, or excretions.
- Masks should be worn when placing a catheter or injecting material into the spinal canal or subdural space (eg, during myelograms and spinal or epidural anesthesia).

---

[1]Centers for Disease Control and Prevention. Guideline for hand hygiene in health-care settings. Recommendations of the Healthcare Infection Control Practices Advisory Committee and the HICPAC/SHEA/APIC/IDSA Hand Hygiene Task Force. *MMWR Recomm Rep.* 2002;51(RR-16):1–45

- **Nonsterile gowns** that are fluid-resistant will protect skin and prevent soiling of clothing during procedures and patient care activities likely to generate splashes or sprays of blood, body fluids, secretions, or excretions. Soiled gowns should be removed promptly.
- **Patient care equipment** that has been used should be handled in a manner that prevents skin or mucous membrane exposures and contamination of clothing or the environment.
- **All used textiles (linens)** are considered to be contaminated and should be handled, transported, and processed in a manner that prevents aerosolization of microorganisms, skin and mucous membrane exposure, and contamination of clothing.
- **Safe injection practices:** Bloodborne pathogen exposure of health care personnel should be avoided by taking precautions to prevent injuries caused by needles, scalpels, and other sharp instruments or devices during procedures; when handling sharp instruments after procedures; when cleaning used instruments; and during disposal of used needles. To prevent needlestick injuries, needles should not be recapped, purposely bent or broken by hand, removed from disposable syringes, or otherwise manipulated by hand. After use, disposable syringes and needles, scalpel blades, and other sharp items should be placed in puncture-resistant containers for disposal; the puncture-resistant containers should be located as close as practical to the use area. Large-bore reusable needles should be placed in a puncture-resistant container located close to the site of use for transport to the reprocessing area for maximal patient safety. Sharp devices with safety features are preferred whenever such devices have function equivalent to conventional sharp devices, and should be evaluated and implemented by users. Single-dose vials of medication are preferred.
- **Mouthpieces, resuscitation bags, and other ventilation devices** should be available in all patient care areas and used instead of mouth-to-mouth resuscitation.

TRANSMISSION-BASED PRECAUTIONS[1]

Transmission-Based Precautions are designed for patients documented or suspected to have colonization or infection with pathogens for which additional precautions beyond **Standard Precautions** are recommended to prevent transmission. The 3 types of transmission routes on which these precautions are based are airborne, droplet, and contact.

- **Airborne transmission** occurs by dissemination of airborne droplet nuclei (small-particle residue [≤5 μm in size] of evaporated droplets containing microorganisms that remain suspended in the air for long periods) or small respirable particles containing the infectious agent or spores. Microorganisms transmitted by the airborne route can be dispersed widely by air currents and can be inhaled by a susceptible host within the same room or a long distance from the source patient, depending on environmental factors. Special air handling and ventilation are required to prevent airborne transmission. Examples of microorganisms transmitted by airborne droplet nuclei are *Mycobacterium tuberculosis*, rubeola (measles) virus, and varicella-zoster virus. Specific recommendations for **Airborne Precautions** are as follows:

---

[1]A complete list of recommended precautions for specific pathogens can be found in: Centers for Disease Control and Prevention. Guideline for hand hygiene in health-care settings. Recommendations of the Healthcare Infection Control Practices Advisory Committee and the HICPAC/SHEA/APIC/IDSA Hand Hygiene Task Force. *MMWR Recomm Rep.* 2002;51(RR-16):1–45.

- Provide infected or colonized patients with a single-patient room (if unavailable, consult with an infection-control professional).
- Use special ventilation, including 6 to 12 air changes per hour, air flow direction from surrounding area to the room, and room air exhausted directly to the outside or recirculated through a high-efficiency particulate air (HEPA) filter.
- If infectious pulmonary tuberculosis is suspected or proven, respiratory protective devices (ie, National Institute for Occupational Safety and Health-certified personally "fitted" and "sealing" respirator, such as N95 or N100 respirators, powered air-purifying respirators) should be worn while inside the patient's room.
- Susceptible health care personnel should not enter rooms of patients with measles or varicella-zoster virus infections. If susceptible people must enter the room of a patient with measles or varicella infection or an immunocompromised patient with local or disseminated zoster infection, a mask should be worn. People with proven immunity to these viruses need not wear a mask.

- **Droplet transmission** occurs when droplets containing microorganisms generated from an infected person, primarily during coughing, sneezing, or talking and during the performance of certain procedures, such as suctioning and bronchoscopy, are propelled a short distance (3 feet or less) and deposited on the conjunctivae, nasal mucosa, or mouth. Because these relatively large droplets do not remain suspended in air, special air handling and ventilation are not required to prevent droplet transmission. Droplet transmission should not be confused with airborne transmission via droplet nuclei, which are much smaller. Specific recommendations for **Droplet Precaution**s are as follows:
  - Provide the patient with a single-patient room if possible. If unavailable, consider cohorting patients infected with the same organism. Spatial separation of more than 3 feet should be maintained between the bed of the infected patient and the beds of the other patients in multiple bed rooms. Standard precautions plus a mask should be used.
  - Wear a mask on entry into the room or into the cubical space.

    If a patient with influenza, severe acute respiratory syndrome (SARS), or viral hemorrhagic fever is to undergo an aerosol-generating procedure (eg, bronchoscopy, intubation, nebulizer treatments), N95 or higher respirators should be used by people in the vicinity of the patient, because small droplet nuclei may be generated by such procedures and could be transmitted to others.

    Specific illnesses and infections requiring **Droplet Precautions** include the following:
  - Adenovirus pneumonia
  - Diphtheria (pharyngeal)
  - *Haemophilus influenzae* type b (invasive)
  - Influenza
  - Mumps
  - *Mycoplasma pneumoniae*
  - *Neisseria meningitidis* (invasive)
  - Parvovirus B19 during the phase of illness before onset of rash in immunocompetent patients; see Parvovirus B19 (p 491)
  - Pertussis
  - Plague (pneumonic)

- Rhinovirus
- Rubella
- SARS
- Group A streptococcal pharyngitis, pneumonia, or scarlet fever
- Viral hemorrhagic fevers

- **Contact Transmission** is the most common route of transmission of health care-associated infections. *Direct contact* transmission involves a direct body surface-to-body surface contact and physical transfer of microorganisms between a person with infection or colonization and a susceptible host, such as occurs when a health care professional turns a patient, gives a patient a bath, or performs other patient care activities that require direct personal contact. Direct contact transmission also can occur between 2 patients when one serves as the source of the infectious microorganisms and the other serves as a susceptible host. *Indirect contact* transmission involves contact of a susceptible host with a contaminated intermediate object, usually inanimate, such as contaminated instruments, needles, dressings, toys, or contaminated hands that are not cleansed or gloves that are not changed between patients.

  Specific recommendations for **Contact Precautions** are as follows:
  - Provide the patient with a single-patient room if possible. If unavailable, cohorting patients likely to be infected with the same agent and using standard and contact precautions between contacts with patients is permissible.
  - Gloves (clean, nonsterile) should be used at all times.
  - Hand hygiene should be performed after glove removal.
  - Gowns should be used during direct contact with a patient, environmental surfaces, or items in the patient room. Gowns should be worn on entry into the room and should be removed before leaving the patient's room or area.

  Specific illnesses and infections with organisms requiring **Contact Precautions** include the following:
  - Multidrug-resistant bacteria judged by the infection-control practitioner on the basis of current state, regional, or national recommendations to be of special clinical and epidemiologic significance (eg, vancomycin-resistant enterococci; methicillin-resistant *Staphylococcus aureus;* multidrug-resistant, gram-negative bacilli) or other epidemiologically important susceptible bacteria
  - *C difficile*
  - Conjunctivitis, viral and hemorrhagic
  - Diphtheria (cutaneous)
  - Enteroviruses
  - *Escherichia coli* O157:H7 and other Shiga toxin-producing *E coli*
  - Hepatitis A virus
  - Herpes simplex virus (neonatal, mucocutaneous, or cutaneous)
  - Herpes zoster (localized with no evidence of dissemination)
  - Impetigo
  - Major (noncontained) abscess, cellulitis, or decubitus ulcer
  - Parainfluenza virus
  - Pediculosis (lice)
  - Respiratory syncytial virus
  - Rotavirus
  - Salmonella

- Scabies
- *Shigella*
- *S aureus* (cutaneous or draining wounds)
- Viral hemorrhagic fevers (Ebola, Lassa, or Marburg)

Airborne, Droplet, and **Contact Precautions** should be combined for diseases caused by organisms that have multiple routes of transmission. When used alone or in combination, these transmission-based precautions always are to be used in addition to **Standard Precautions,** which are recommended for all patients. The specifications for these categories of isolation precautions are summarized in Table 2.7 (p 150) and Table 2.8. Table 2.9 (p 156) lists syndromes and conditions that are suggestive of contagious infection and require empiric isolation precautions pending identification of a specific pathogen. When the specific pathogen is known, isolation recommendations and duration of isolation are given in the pathogen- or disease-specific chapters in Section 3.

PEDIATRIC CONSIDERATIONS

Unique differences in pediatric care necessitate modifications of these guidelines, including the following: (1) diaper changing and wiping a child's tears or nose; (2) use of single-patient room isolation; and (3) use of common areas, such as hospital waiting rooms, play rooms, and schoolrooms.

Because diapering or wiping a child's nose or tears does not soil hands routinely, wearing gloves is not mandatory except when gloves are required as part of Transmission-Based Precautions. However, it may be prudent for women who are pregnant or likely to be pregnant to use gloves when changing diapers because of the high prevalence of shedding of cytomegalovirus in the urine of healthy infants and toddlers.

Table 2.8. Transmission-Based Precautions for Hospitalized Patients[a]

Category of Precautions	Single-Patient Room	Respiratory Tract/ Mucous Membrane Protection	Gowns	Gloves
Airborne	Yes, with negative air-pressure ventilation, 6–12 air exchanges per hour, ± HEPA filtration	Respirators: N95 or higher level	No[b]	No[b]
Droplet	Yes[c]	Surgical masks[d]	No[b]	No[b]
Contact	Yes[c]	No	Yes	Yes

HEPA indicates high-efficiency particulate air.

[a]These recommendations are in addition to those for **Standard Precautions** for all patients.

[b]Gowns and gloves may be required as a component of **Standard Precautions** (eg, for blood collection or during procedures likely to cause blood splashes or if there are skin lesions containing transmissible infectious agents).

[c]Preferred. Cohorting of children infected with the same pathogen is acceptable if a single-patient room is not available, a distance of more than 3 feet between patients can be maintained, and precautions are observed between all contacts with different patients in the room.

[d]Masks should be donned on entry into the room.

Table 2.9. Clinical Syndromes or Conditions Warranting Precautions in Addition to *Standard Precautions* to Prevent Transmission of Epidemiologically Important Pathogens Pending Confirmation of Diagnosis[a]

Clinical Syndrome or Condition[b]	Potential Pathogens[c]	Empiric Precautions[d]
Diarrhea		
Acute diarrhea with a likely infectious cause	Enteric pathogens[e]	Contact
Diarrhea in patient with a history of recent antimicrobial use	*Clostridium difficile*	Contact; use soap and water for handwashing
Meningitis	*Neisseria meningitidis*	Droplet
	Enteroviruses	Contact
Rash or exanthems, generalized, cause unknown		
Petechial or ecchymotic with fever	*N meningitidis, Haemophilus influenzae*	Droplet
	Hemorrhagic fever viruses	Add Contact plus face/eye protection
Vesicular	Varicella-zoster virus	Airborne and Contact
Maculopapular with coryza and fever	Measles virus	Airborne
Respiratory tract infections		
Pulmonary cavitary disease	*Mycobacterium tuberculosis*	Airborne
Paroxysmal or severe persistent cough during periods of pertussis activity in the community	*Bordetella pertussis*	Droplet
Viral infections, particularly bronchiolitis and croup, in infants and young children	Respiratory viral pathogens	Contact plus Droplet until adenovirus, pneumonia, rhinovirus, and influenza virus excluded[f]
Risk of multidrug-resistant microorganisms[f]		
History of infection or colonization with multidrug-resistant organisms	Resistant bacteria	Contact
Skin, wound, or urinary tract infection in a patient with a recent stay in a hospital or chronic care facility	Resistant bacteria	Contact until resistant organism is excluded by cultures

Table 2.9. Clinical Syndromes or Conditions Warranting Precautions in Addition to Standard Precautions to Prevent Transmission of Epidemiologically Important Pathogens Pending Confirmation of Diagnosis,[a] continued

Clinical Syndrome or Condition[b]	Potential Pathogens[c]	Empiric Precautions[d]
Skin or wound infection		
Abscess or draining wound that cannot be covered	Staphylococcus aureus, group A Streptococcus	Contact

[a] Infection-control professionals are encouraged to modify or adapt this table according to local conditions. To ensure that appropriate empiric precautions are implemented, hospitals must have systems in place to evaluate patients routinely according to these criteria as part of their preadmission and admission care.

[b] Patients with the syndromes or conditions listed may have atypical signs or symptoms (eg, pertussis in neonates, absence of paroxysmal or severe cough in adults). The clinician's index of suspicion should be guided by the prevalence of specific conditions in the community and clinical judgment.

[c] The organisms listed in this column are not intended to represent the complete or even most likely diagnoses but, rather, possible causative agents that require additional precautions beyond **Standard Precautions** until a causative agent can be excluded.

[d] Duration of isolation varies by agent and the antimicrobial treatment administered.

[e] These pathogens include Shiga toxin–producing Escherichia coli including E coli O157:H7, Shigella organisms, Salmonella organisms, Campylobacter organisms, hepatitis A virus, enteric viruses including rotavirus, Cryptosporidium organisms, and Giardia organisms. Use masks when cleaning vomitus or stool during norovirus outbreak.

[f] Resistant bacteria judged by the infection control program on the basis of current state, regional, or national recommendations to be of special clinical or epidemiologic significance.

Single-patient rooms are recommended for all patients for **Transmission-Based Precautions** (ie, **Airborne, Droplet,** and **Contact**). Patients placed on Transmission-Based Precautions should not leave their rooms to use common areas, such as child life play rooms, schoolrooms, or waiting areas, except under special circumstances as defined by the facility infection-control personnel. The guidelines for **Standard Precautions** state that patients who cannot control body excretions should be in single-patient rooms. Because most young children are incontinent, this recommendation does not apply to routine care of uninfected children.

The CDC isolation guidelines were developed for preventing transmission of infection in hospitals and other settings in which health care is delivered. These recommendations do not apply to schools, out-of-home child care centers, and other settings in which healthy children congregate in shared space.

Occupational Health

Standard Precautions and Transmission-Based Precautions are designed to prevent transmission of infectious agents in health care settings to limit transmission among patients and health care personnel. Transmission of infectious agents within health care settings is facilitated by close contact between patients and health care personnel and lack of hygienic practices by infants and young children.

To limit risks of transmission of organisms between children and health care personnel, health care facilities should have established personnel health policies and services. It is important particularly to ensure that personnel are protected against vaccine-preventable diseases by establishing appropriate screening and immunization policies (see adult immunization schedule at **www.cdc.gov/vaccines/recs/schedules/adult-schedule.htm**).

For infections that are not vaccine preventable, personnel should be counseled about exposures and the possible need for leave if they are exposed to, ill with, or a carrier of a specific pathogen, whether the exposure occurs in the home, community, or health care setting.

The frequency and need for screening of health care personnel for tuberculosis should be determined by local epidemiologic data as described in the CDC guideline for prevention of transmission of tuberculosis in health care settings.[1] People with commonly occurring infections, such as gastroenteritis, dermatitis, herpes simplex lesions on exposed skin, or upper respiratory tract infections, should be evaluated to determine the resulting risk of transmission to patients or to other health care personnel.

Health care personnel, including pregnant women, should be educated about pathogens for which they are at increased risk if they follow Standard Precautions.

Health care personnel education, including understanding of hospital policies, is of paramount importance in infection control. Pediatric health care professionals should be knowledgeable about the modes of transmission of infectious agents, proper hand hygiene techniques, and serious risks to children from certain mild infections in adults. Frequent educational sessions will reinforce safe techniques and the importance of infection-control policies. Written policies and procedures relating to needlestick or sharp injuries are man-

---

[1] Centers for Disease Control and Prevention. Guidelines for preventing the transmission of *Mycobacterium tuberculosis* in health-care settings, 2005. *MMWR Recomm Rep.* 2005;54(RR-17):1–141

dated by OSHA.[1] Recommendations for postinjury prophylaxis are available (see Human Immunodeficiency Virus Infection, p 380, and Table 3.27, p 386).[2,3]

Pregnant health care personnel who follow recommended precautions should not be at increased risk of infections that have possible adverse effects on the fetus (eg, parvovirus B19, cytomegalovirus, rubella, and varicella). Personnel who are immunocompromised and at increased risk of severe infection (eg, *M tuberculosis*, measles virus, herpes simplex virus, and varicella-zoster virus), should seek advice from their primary health care professional.

The consequences to pediatric patients of acquiring infections from adults can be significant. Mild illness in adults, such as viral gastroenteritis, upper respiratory tract viral infection (eg, with respiratory syncytial virus), pertussis, or herpes simplex infection, can cause life-threatening disease in infants and children. People at greatest risk are preterm infants, children who have heart disease or chronic pulmonary disease, and immunocompromised patients.

Sibling Visitation

Sibling visits to birthing centers, postpartum rooms, pediatric wards, and intensive care units are encouraged. Neonatal intensive care, with its increasing sophistication, often results in long hospital stays for the preterm or sick newborn, making family visits important. If guidelines are followed, subsequent infection is not increased in the sick or preterm newborn infant visited by siblings.

Guidelines for sibling visits should be established to maximize opportunities for visiting and to minimize the risks of transmission of pathogens brought into the hospital by young visitors. Guidelines may need to be modified by local nursing, pediatric, obstetric, and infectious diseases staff members to address specific issues in their hospital settings. Basic guidelines for sibling visits to pediatric patients are as follows:
- Sibling visits may benefit hospitalized children.
- Before the visit, a trained health care professional should interview the parents at a site outside the unit to assess the health of each sibling visitor. These interviews should be documented in the patient's record, and approval for each sibling visit should be noted. No child with fever or symptoms of an acute illness, including upper respiratory tract infection, gastroenteritis, or dermatitis, should be allowed to visit. Siblings who recently have been exposed to a person with a known communicable disease and are susceptible should not be allowed to visit.
- Siblings who are visiting should have received all recommended immunizations for age. Before and during influenza season, siblings who visit should have received influenza vaccine.
- Asymptomatic siblings who recently have been exposed to varicella but have been immunized previously can be assumed to be immune.

[1] Occupational Safety and Health Administration (**www.osha.gov**)

[2] American Academy of Pediatrics, Committee on Pediatric AIDS. Postexposure prophylaxis in children and adolescents for nonoccupational exposure to human immunodeficiency virus. *Pediatrics.* 2003;111(5):1475–1489 (Reaffirmed January 2007)

[3] Centers for Disease Control and Prevention. Updated US Public Health Service guidelines for the management of occupational exposures to HIV and recommendations for postexposure prophylaxis. *MMWR Recomm Rep.* 2005;54(RR-9):1–17

- The visiting sibling should visit only his or her sibling and not be allowed in play rooms with groups of patients.
- Children should perform recommended hand hygiene before any patient contact.
- Throughout the visit, sibling activity should be supervised by parents or a responsible adult and limited to the mother's or patient's single-patient room or other designated areas where other patients are not present.

Adult Visitation

Guidelines should be established for visits by other relatives and close friends. Anyone with fever or contagious illnesses ideally should not visit. Medical and nursing staff members should be vigilant about potential communicable diseases in parents and other adult visitors (eg, a relative with a cough who may have pertussis or tuberculosis; a parent with a cold visiting a highly immunosuppressed child). Before and during influenza season, it is prudent to encourage all visitors to receive influenza vaccine. Adherence to these guidelines especially is important for oncology, hematopoietic stem cell transplant units, and neonatal intensive care units.

Pet Visitation

Pet visitation in the health care setting can be separated into 2 categories: visits by a child's personal pet and pet visitation as a part of child life therapeutic programs. Guidelines for pet visitation should be established to minimize risks of transmission of pathogens from pets to humans or injury from animals. The specific health care setting and the level of concern for zoonotic disease will influence establishment of pet visitation policies. The pet visitation policy should be developed in consultation with pediatricians, infection-control professionals, nursing staff, the hospital epidemiologist, and veterinarians. Basic principles for pet visitation policies in health care settings are as follows:

- Personal pets other than cats and dogs should be excluded from the hospital. No reptiles (eg, iguanas, turtles, snakes), amphibians, birds, primates, ferrets, or rodents should be allowed to visit. Exceptions may be made for end-of-life patients who are in single-patient rooms.
- Visiting pets should have a certificate of immunization from a licensed veterinarian and verification that the pet is healthy.
- The pet should be bathed and groomed for the visit.
- Pet visitation is inappropriate in an intensive care unit.
- The visit of a pet should be approved by appropriate personnel (for example, the director of the child life therapy program), who should observe the pet for temperament and general health at the time of visit. The pet should be free of obvious bacterial skin infections, infections caused by superficial dermatophytes, and ectoparasitic infections (fleas and ticks).
- Pet visitation should be confined to designated areas. Contact should be confined to the petting and holding of animals, as appropriate. All contact should be supervised throughout the visit by appropriate personnel and should be followed by hand hygiene performed by all who had contact with the pet. Supervisors should be familiar with institutional policies for managing animal bites and cleaning pet urine, feces, or vomitus.

- Patients having contact with pets must have approval from a physician or physician representative before animal contact. Documented allergy to dogs or cats should be considered before approving contact. For patients who are immunodeficient or for people receiving immunosuppressive therapy, the risks of exposure to the microflora of pets may outweigh the benefits of contact. Contact of children with pets should be approved on a case-by-case basis.
- Care should be taken to protect indwelling catheter sites (eg, central venous catheters, peritoneal dialysis catheters). These sites should have dressings that provide an effective barrier to pet contact, including licking, and be covered with clothing or gown. Concern for contamination of other body sites should be considered on a case-by-case basis.
- Patients should perform appropriate hand hygiene after contact with pets.
- The pet policy should not apply to professionally trained service animals, such as "seeing eye" dogs. These animals are not pets, and separate policies should govern their uses and presence in the hospital.

··

INFECTION CONTROL AND PREVENTION IN AMBULATORY SETTINGS

Infection control is an integral part of pediatric practice in ambulatory care settings as well as in hospitals. All health care professionals should be aware of the routes of transmission and techniques used to prevent transmission of infectious agents. Written policies and procedures for infection control and prevention should be developed, implemented, and reviewed at least every 2 years. Standard Precautions, as outlined for the hospitalized child (see Infection Control for Hospitalized Children, p 148) and by the Centers for Disease Control and Prevention,[1] with a modification by the American Academy of Pediatrics exempting the use of gloves for routine diaper changes and wiping a child's nose or tears,[2] are appropriate for most patient encounters. Key principles of infection control in an outpatient setting are as follows:

- Infection control should begin when the child enters the office or clinic. Standard Precautions should be used when caring for all patients.
- Contact between contagious children and uninfected children should be minimized. Policies for children who are suspected of having contagious infections, such as varicella or measles, should be implemented. Immunocompromised children should be kept away from people with potentially contagious infections.
- In waiting rooms of ambulatory care facilities, use of some or all components of respiratory hygiene/cough etiquette should be considered for patients and accompanying people with suspected respiratory tract infection.[3]

[1]Centers for Disease Control and Prevention. Guideline for isolation precautions: preventing transmission of infectious agents in health care settings 2007. Recommendations of the Healthcare Infection Control Practices Advisory Committee. Atlanta, GA: Centers for Disease Control and Prevention; 2007. Available at: **www.cdc. gov/ncidod/dhqp/pdf/guidelines/isolation2007.pdf**

[2]American Academy of Pediatrics, Committee on Infectious Diseases. Infection prevention and control in pediatric ambulatory settings. *Pediatrics.* 2007;120(3):650–665

[3]Centers for Disease Control and Prevention. Respiratory Hygiene/Cough Etiquette in Healthcare Settings. Available at: **www.cdc.gov/flu/professionals/infectioncontrol/resphygiene.htm**

- All health care professionals should perform hand hygiene before and after each patient contact. In health care settings, alcohol-based hand products are preferred for decontaminating hands routinely. Soap and water are preferred when hands are visibly dirty or contaminated with proteinaceous material, such as blood or other body fluids. Parents and children should be taught the importance of hand hygiene.
- Health care personnel should receive influenza immunization annually as well as immunizations against other vaccine-preventable infections that can be transmitted in an ambulatory setting.
- Health care professionals should be familiar with aseptic technique, particularly regarding insertion or manipulation of intravascular catheters, performance of other invasive procedures, and preparation and administration of parenteral medications.
- Alcohol is preferred for skin preparation before immunization or routine venipuncture. Skin preparation for incision, suture, or collection of blood for culture requires 10% povidone-iodine, 70% alcohol, alcohol tinctures of iodine, or 2% chlorhexidine. After application of iodophor skin preparations, the skin should dry for 2 minutes.
- Needles and sharps should be handled with great care. The use of safer medical devices designed to reduce the risk of needlesticks should be evaluated and implemented. Needle-disposal containers that are impermeable and puncture proof should be available adjacent to the areas where injections or venipunctures are performed. The containers should not be overfilled and should be kept out of reach of young children. Policies should be established for removal and incineration or sterilization of contents consistent with local regulations.
- A written bloodborne pathogens exposure control plan that includes policies for management of exposures to blood and body fluids, such as through needlesticks and exposures of nonintact skin and mucous membranes, should be developed, readily available to all staff, and reviewed regularly (see Hepatitis B, p 337; Hepatitis C, p 357; and Human Immunodeficiency Virus Infection, p 380).
- Standard guidelines for decontamination, disinfection, and sterilization should be followed.
- Appropriate use of antimicrobial agents is essential to limit the emergence and spread of drug-resistant bacteria (see Appropriate Use of Antimicrobial Agents, p 740).
- Policies and procedures should be developed for communication with local and state health authorities about reportable diseases and suspected outbreaks.
- Ongoing educational programs that encompass appropriate aspects of infection control should be implemented, reinforced, documented, and evaluated on a regular basis.
- Physicians should be aware of requirements of government agencies, such as the Occupational Safety and Health Administration, as they relate to the operation of physicians' offices.

SEXUALLY TRANSMITTED INFECTIONS IN ADOLESCENTS AND CHILDREN

Physicians and other health care professionals perform a critical role in preventing and treating sexually transmitted infections (STIs) in the pediatric population. STIs are a major problem for adolescents; an estimated 25% of adolescents will develop an STI before graduating from high school. For infants and children, detection of an STI is an

important warning signal of sexual abuse. Sexual abuse of children has been endemic for generations, but the prevalence and potentially devastating psychologic effects of sexual abuse have been recognized more recently. Whenever sexual abuse is suspected, appropriate social service and law enforcement agencies must be involved to ensure the child's protection and to provide appropriate counseling.

STIs in Adolescents

EPIDEMIOLOGY

Adolescents and young adults continue to have higher rates of STIs when compared with any other age group. Adolescents are at greater risk of STIs, because they frequently have unprotected intercourse, may be more susceptible biologically to infection, often are engaged in multiple sequential monogamous partnerships of limited duration, and face multiple obstacles in accessing confidential health care services.[1] The rate of diagnosed STIs is higher in women than in men by a factor of 3:1, but far fewer sexually active male than female adolescents are screened for STIs. Data underestimate the incidence of STIs among sexually experienced adolescents, because *all* adolescents, including US high school students who never have had sexual intercourse, are included in the denominators used to calculate age-specific STI rates and because many cases are not diagnosed or reported.

MANAGEMENT

Pediatricians should screen for risk of STIs by asking all adolescent patients whether they ever have had sexual intercourse or been sexually active. It is important that adolescents recognize that oral and anal intercourse, as well as vaginal intercourse, put them at risk of STIs. Adolescents at increased risk of STIs are listed in Table 2.10, p 164. Physicians can prepare patients for this sensitive question by educating both parents and adolescents about confidentiality. At each annual checkup and at visits for acute illness, a private interview with an adolescent patient should occur. More detailed recommendations for preventive health care for adolescents are available in the American Academy of Pediatrics' *Bright Futures: Guidelines for Health Supervision of Infants, Children, and Adolescents,* Third Edition.[2] All 50 states allow minors to give their own consent for confidential STI screening, diagnosis, and treatment. Despite the high prevalence of STIs among adolescents, health care professionals frequently fail to inquire about sexual behavior, assess STI risks, counsel about risk reduction, and screen for STIs.

Within 3 years of initiation of consensual or nonconsensual sexual intercourse, all adolescent females should begin having annual Papanicolaou smears to screen for cervical dysplasia associated with human papillomavirus (HPV) infection. For adolescent females who are immunosuppressed or immunocompromised, yearly Papanicolaou smears should begin with the initiation of consensual or nonconsensual sexual intercourse. All young adult females should begin yearly Papanicolaou smear screening by 21 years of

---

[1]Centers for Disease Control and Prevention. Youth risk behavior surveillance—United States, 2007. *MMWR Surveill Summ.* 2008;57(SS-4):1–131

[2]American Academy of Pediatrics, Bright Futures Steering Committee. *Bright Futures: Guidelines for Health Supervision of Infants, Children, and Adolescents.* Hagan JF Jr, Shaw JS, Duncan P, eds. 3rd ed. Elk Grove Village, IL: American Academy of Pediatrics; 2008

Table 2.10. Adolescents Whose History Includes One or More of the Following Features Are Considered at Increased Risk of Contracting a Sexually Transmitted Infection (STI)[a]

- Sexual contact with people with known STI or history of STI
- Symptoms or signs of STI
- Multiple sexual partners
- Street involvement (eg, homelessness)
- Sexual intercourse with new partner during last 2 months
- More than 2 sexual partners during previous 12 months
- No or inconsistent use of barrier contraceptive methods
- Injection drug use
- Males who have sex with males
- "Survival sex" (eg, exchanging sex for money, drugs, shelter, or food)
- Time spent in detention facilities
- Having been a patient of an STI clinic
- Having been pregnant or having requested a pregnancy test

[a]Modified from Health Canada. *Canadian STD Guidelines: 1998 Edition.* Ottawa, Ontario: Population and Public Health Branch, Health Canada; 1998. Available at: **www.phac-aspc.gc.ca/publicat/std-mts98/index.html**

age. Sexually active adolescent females and males should be screened at least annually for chlamydia and gonorrhea. Many experts recommend more frequent screening of females, especially for *Chlamydia* infection in patients with a previous chlamydia diagnosis. The 2006 "Sexually Transmitted Infections Treatment Guidelines" from the Centers for Disease Control and Prevention (**www.cdc.gov/std/treatment**) suggest that screening of asymptomatic sexually active adolescent males should be considered in clinical settings with a high prevalence of chlamydia (eg, adolescent clinics, correctional facilities, and STI clinics). Sexually active adolescents should receive human immunodeficiency virus (HIV) and syphilis prevention counseling at least annually, and screening should be provided for adolescents with a previous STI or with multiple sexual partners and for adolescents requesting screening annually. All adolescents should receive hepatitis B virus immunization if they were not immunized earlier in childhood, and the HPV immunization series should be started for females at the 11- through 12-year visit (or at 13 through 18 years of age if they were not immunized previously). Hepatitis A vaccine should be offered to adolescent males who have sex with males (see Recommended Childhood and Adolescent Immunization Schedules, Fig 1.1–1.3, p 24–28) and others at high risk of hepatitis A virus infection (see Hepatitis A, p 329).

For treatment recommendations for specific STIs, see the disease-specific chapters in Section 3 and Table 4.3, Guidelines for Treatment of Sexually Transmitted Infections in Children and Adolescents According to Syndrome (p 758). Patients and their partners treated for gonorrhea, *Chlamydia trachomatis* infection, and trichomoniasis should be advised to refrain from sexual intercourse for 1 week after completion of appropriate treatment. Retesting to detect therapeutic failure (tests of cure) for patients who receive recommended treatment regimens for *Neisseria gonorrhoeae* or *C trachomatis* infection is not recommended unless therapeutic adherence is in question or symptoms persist. If a

multiple-dose regimen is used, nonadherence is possible. Retesting for chlamydia infection using nonculture techniques fewer than 3 to 4 weeks after treatment may yield false-positive results attributable to residual nonviable organisms. Many experts suggest repeat testing for these infections within 3 months because of the likelihood of reinfection as a result of nontreatment of a current sexual partner and/or from a new sexual partner.

PREVENTION

Pediatricians can contribute to primary prevention of STIs by encouraging adolescent patients to postpone their initiation of sexual intercourse and by preparing adolescents who become sexually active to use barrier methods correctly and consistently for prevention of pregnancy and of STIs beginning with the first intercourse experience. Adolescents should be reminded that barrier methods should be used with all forms of sexual intercourse (vaginal, oral, and anal). Pediatricians should encourage adolescents who already have had sexual intercourse to practice "secondary" abstinence (to be celibate), to minimize their lifetime number of sexual partners, to use barrier methods consistently and correctly to prevent pregnancy and infection, and to be aware of the strong association between alcohol or drug use and failure to appropriately use barrier methods correctly. The correct use of male and female condoms and some strategies for encouraging condom use are reviewed in Table 2.11 (below). A quadrivalent vaccine against HPV types 6, 11, 16, and 18 is available and licensed for females 9 through 26 years of age, and a bivalent HPV vaccine against HPV types 16 and 18 is under consideration by the US Food and Drug Administration. The quadrivalent vaccine also is being evaluated in clinical trials in males and in women 27 through 45 years of age.

Table 2.11. Recommendations for Proper Use of Condoms[a] to Decrease the Risk of Transmission of Sexually Transmitted Infections[b]

Male Condoms
- Use a new condom with each act of sexual intercourse (penile-vaginal, oral, or anal intercourse).
- Carefully handle the condom to avoid damaging it with fingernails, teeth, or other sharp objects.
- Put condom on after the penis is erect and before genital contact with partner.
- Ensure that no air is trapped in the tip of the condom.
- Ensure that adequate lubrication exists during intercourse, possibly requiring the use of external lubricants.
- Use only water-based lubricants with latex condoms. Oil-based lubricants can weaken latex.
- Hold the condom firmly against the base of the penis during withdrawal, and withdraw while penis is still erect to prevent slippage.

Female Condoms
- Lubricated polyurethane sheath with a ring on each end, one of which is inserted into the vagina and rests over the cervix like a diaphragm and the other remains outside the vagina and covers the external genitalia.
- When a male condom cannot be used appropriately, consider use of a female condom. Instructions about insertion may be needed.

[a]Note: Use of both female and male condoms at the same time is not recommended. Friction between the two surfaces may displace the condoms and contribute to loss of protection.
[b]From Centers for Disease Control and Prevention. Sexually transmitted infections treatment guidelines—2006. *MMWR Recomm Rep.* 2006;55(RR-11):1–29 (see **www.cdc.gov/std/treatment**)

Diagnosis and Treatment of STIs in Children[1]

Because of the social and legal implications of the diagnosis, STIs in children must be diagnosed using tests with high specificity, because the low prevalence of STIs in children increases the probability that rapid detection tests for STIs will give false-positive results. Therefore, tests that allow for isolation of the organism and have the highest specificities must be used.

Because of the serious implications of the diagnosis of an STI in a child, antimicrobial therapy for children with suspected STIs may need to be withheld until the final outcome of the diagnostic test is known. Specimens to screen for *N gonorrhoeae* and *C trachomatis* should be obtained for culture from the rectum and vagina of girls and from the rectum and urethra of boys. Specimens to screen for *N gonorrhoeae* also should be obtained for culture from the pharynx, even in the absence of symptoms. Endocervical specimens for culture are not required for prepubertal girls; only vaginal specimens are required. If vaginal discharge is present, specimens for wet mount for *Trichomonas vaginalis* and wet mount or Gram stain for bacterial vaginosis may be obtained as well. Serum specimens for testing for syphilis, HIV, and hepatitis B surface antigen (if receipt of full immunization series cannot be documented) should be obtained. For more detailed diagnosis and treatment recommendations for specific STIs, see Section 3 and Table 4.3, Guidelines for Treatment of Sexually Transmitted Infections in Children and Adolescents According to Syndrome (p 758). If the female being evaluated is pubertal or postmenarcheal, specimens for cultures of *C trachomatis* and *N gonorrhoeae* must be obtained from the endocervix.

Social Implications of STIs in Children

Children can acquire STIs through vertical transmission, by autoinoculation, or by sexual contact. Each of these mechanisms should be given appropriate consideration in the evaluation of a preadolescent child with an STI. Evaluation based solely on suspicion of an STI should not proceed until the STI diagnosis has been confirmed. Factors to be considered in assessing the likelihood of sexual abuse in a child with an STI include whether the child reports a history of sexual victimization, biologic characteristics of the STI in question, and age of the child (see Table 2.12, p 167).

Anogenital gonorrhea in a prepubertal child indicates sexual abuse in virtually every case. All confirmed cases of gonorrhea in prepubertal children beyond the neonatal period should be reported to the local child protective services agency for investigation.

First-episode symptomatic herpes simplex has a short incubation period but can be transmitted by sexual or nonsexual contact with another person or by self-inoculation. In an infant or toddler in diapers, genital herpes may arise from any of these mechanisms. In a prepubertal child whose toilet-use activities are independent, the new occurrence of genital herpes should prompt a careful investigation, including a child protective services investigation, for suspected sexual abuse. Viral typing for herpes simplex virus (HSV)-1 and HSV-2 can yield additional helpful information.

---

[1]Centers for Disease Control and Prevention. Sexually transmitted infections treatment guidelines—2006. *MMWR Recomm Rep.* 2006;55(RR-11):1–29 (see **www.cdc.gov/mmwr**)

Table 2.12. Implications of Commonly Encountered Sexually Transmitted Infections (STIs) for Diagnosis and Reporting of Suspected or Diagnosed Sexual Abuse of Infants and Prepubertal Children[a]

STI Confirmed	Sexual Abuse	Suggested Action
Gonorrhea[b]	Diagnostic[c]	Report[d]
Syphilis[b]	Diagnostic	Report
Human immunodeficiency virus infection[e]	Diagnostic	Report
Chlamydia trachomatis infection[b]	Diagnostic[c]	Report
Trichomonas vaginalis infection	Highly suspicious	Report
Condylomata acuminata infection[b] (anogenital warts)	Suspicious	Report
Herpes (genital location)	Suspicious	Report[f]
Bacterial vaginosis	Inconclusive	Medical follow-up

[a]Adapted from Kellogg N; American Academy of Pediatrics, Committee on Child Abuse and Neglect. The evaluation of sexual abuse in children. *Pediatrics.* 2005;116(2):506–512
[b]If not perinatally acquired and rare nonsexual vertical transmission is excluded.
[c]Athough the culture technique is the "gold standard," studies are investigating the use of nucleic acid amplification testing as an alternative diagnostic method in children.
[d]Report to the agency mandated in the community to receive reports of suspected sexual abuse.
[e]If not acquired perinatally or by transfusion.
[f]Unless there is a clear history of autoinoculation.

Trichomoniasis is transmitted perinatally or by sexual contact. In a perinatally infected infant, vaginal discharge can persist for several weeks; accordingly, intense social investigation may not be warranted. However, a new diagnosis of trichomoniasis in an older infant or child should prompt a careful investigation, including a child protective services investigation, for suspected sexual abuse.

Infections that have long incubation periods (eg, HPV infection) and that can be asymptomatic for a period of time after vertical transmission (eg, syphilis, HIV infection, *C trachomatis* infection, herpes simplex infection) are more problematic. The possibility of vertical transmission should be considered in these cases, but an evaluation of the patient's circumstances by the local child protective services agency usually is warranted.

Although hepatitis B virus, scabies, and pediculosis pubis may be transmitted sexually, other modes of transmission can occur. The discovery of any of these conditions in a prepubertal child does not warrant child protective services involvement unless the clinician finds other information that suggests abuse. The presence of *T vaginalis* does not indicate a diagnosis of bacterial vaginosis (see Bacterial Vaginosis, p 228).

Sexual Victimization and STIs

GENERAL CONSIDERATIONS

Child sexual abuse has been defined as the exploitation of a child, either by physical contact or by other interactions, for the sexual stimulation of an adult or a minor who is in a position of power over the child. Sexual victimization of a child younger than

18 years of age by a caregiver is termed *abuse;* physicians are required by law to report abuse to their state child protective services agency. Sexual victimization of a child or adolescent by a person who is not a caregiver is termed *assault.* In some instances, sexual victimization involves physical contact permitting the transfer of sexually transmitted microorganisms. Approximately 5% of sexually abused children acquire an STI as a result of the victimization.

SCREENING ASYMPTOMATIC SEXUALLY VICTIMIZED CHILDREN FOR STIS

Factors that influence the likelihood that a sexually victimized child will acquire an STI include the regional prevalence of STIs in the adult population, the number of assailants, the type and frequency of physical contact between the perpetrator(s) and the child, the infectivity of various microorganisms, the child's susceptibility to infection, and whether the child has received intercurrent antimicrobial agent treatment. The time interval between a child's physical contact with an assailant and the medical evaluation influences the likelihood that an exposed child will demonstrate signs or symptoms of an STI.

The decision to obtain genital or other specimens from a child who has been victimized sexually to conduct an STI evaluation must be made on an individual basis. The following situations involve a high risk of STIs and constitute a strong indication for testing:

- The child has or has had signs or symptoms of an STI or an infection that can be transmitted sexually, even in the absence of suspicion of sexual abuse.
- A sibling, another child, or an adult in the household or child's immediate environment has an STI.
- A suspected assailant is known to have an STI or to be at high risk of STIs (eg, has had multiple sexual partners or a history of STIs) or has an unknown history.
- The patient or family requests testing.
- Evidence of genital, oral, or anal penetration or ejaculation is present.

See Table 2.13 (p 169) if STI testing of a child is to be performed.

Most experts recommend universal screening of postpubertal patients who have been victims of sexual abuse or assault, because the prevalence of preexisting asymptomatic infection in this group is high. When STI screening is performed, it should focus on likely anatomic sites of infection (as determined by the patient's history or by epidemiologic considerations) and should include assessment for HIV infection if the patient, family, or both consent to serologic screening; assessment for bacterial vaginosis for female patients and trichomoniasis; and testing for *N gonorrhoeae* infection, *C trachomatis* infection, and syphilis. To preserve the "chain of custody" for information that may later constitute legal evidence, specimens for laboratory analysis obtained from sexually victimized patients should be labeled carefully, and standard hospital procedures for transferring specimens from site to site should be followed carefully. Only tests with high specificities (eg, culture), should be used, and specimens should be obtained by health care professionals with experience in the evaluation of children who have been sexually abused or assaulted. Data on the utility of nucleic acid amplification tests are limited, but these tests may be an alternative if confirmation is available and culture systems for *C trachomatis* are unavailable. Confirmation tests should consist of a second US Food and Drug Administration-cleared nucleic acid amplification test that targets a different sequence from the initial test. A follow-up visit approximately 2 to 6 weeks after the most recent sexual exposure may include a repeat physical examination and collection of additional specimens. Another follow-up

Table 2.13. Sexually Transmitted Infection (STI) Testing in a Child[a] When Sexual Abuse Is Suspected

Organism/Syndrome	Specimens
Neisseria gonorrhoeae	Rectal, throat, urethral (male), and/or vaginal cultures[b]
Chlamydia trachomatis	Rectal, urethral (male), and vaginal cultures[b]
Syphilis	Darkfield examination of chancre fluid, if present; blood for serologic tests at time of abuse and 6, 12, and 24 wk later
Human immunodeficiency virus	Serologic testing of abuser (if possible); serologic testing of child at time of abuse and 6, 12, and 24 wk later
Hepatitis B virus	Serum hepatitis B surface antigen testing of abuser or hepatitis B surface antibody testing of child, unless the child has received 3 doses of hepatitis B vaccine
Herpes simplex virus	Culture of lesion specimen; in addition, polymerase chain reaction assay of lesion specimen if lesion crusted
Bacterial vaginosis	Wet mount, pH, and potassium hydroxide testing of vaginal discharge or Gram stain in pubertal and postmenarcheal girls
Human papillomavirus	Biopsy of lesion specimen
Trichomonas vaginalis	Wet mount and culture of vaginal discharge
Pediculus pubis	Identification of eggs, nymphs, and lice with naked eye or using hand lens

[a]See text for indications for testing for STIs (Screening Asymptomatic Sexually Victimized Children for STIs, p 168).
[b]Cervical specimens are not recommended or necessary for prepubertal girls, but cervical specimens must be obtained in pubertal premenarchal and pubertal postmenarcheal girls.

visit at 3 and 6 months after the most recent sexual exposure may be necessary to obtain convalescent sera to test for syphilis, HIV infection, and hepatitis B virus infection.

PROPHYLAXIS AFTER SEXUAL VICTIMIZATION

Most experts do not recommend antimicrobial prophylaxis for asymptomatic prepubertal children who have been sexually abused, because their incidence of STIs is low, the risk of spread to the upper genital tract in prepubertal girls is low, and follow-up usually can be ensured. If a test result for an STI is positive, treatment then can be given. Factors that may increase the likelihood of infection or that constitute an indication for prophylaxis are the same as those listed under Screening Asymptomatic Sexually Victimized Children for STIs (p 168).

Many experts believe that prophylaxis is warranted for postpubertal female patients who seek care within 72 hours after an episode of sexual victimization because of the high prevalence of preexisting asymptomatic infection and the substantial risk of pelvic inflammatory disease in this age group. All patients who receive prophylaxis should be screened for relevant STIs (see Table 2.13, above) before treatment is given. Postmenarcheal patients should be tested for pregnancy before antimicrobial treatment or emergency contraception is given. Regimens for prophylaxis are presented in Tables 2.14 (children [p 170]) and 2.15 (adolescents [p 171]).

Table 2.14. Prophylaxis After Sexual Victimization of Preadolescent Children

Weight <100 lb (<45 kg)		Weight ≥100 lb (≥45 kg)
	For prevention of gonorrhea	
1. Ceftriaxone, 125 mg, intramuscularly, in a single dose		1A. Ceftriaxone, 125 mg, intramuscularly, in a single dose **OR** 1B. Cefixime, 400 mg, orally, in a single dose
PLUS	**For prevention of *Chlamydia trachomatis* infection**	**PLUS**
2A. Azithromycin, 20 mg/kg (maximum 1 g), orally, in a single dose **OR** 2B. Erythromycin base or ethylsuccinate, 50 mg/kg per day, divided into 4 doses for 14 days		2A. Azithromycin, 1 g, orally, in a single dose **OR** 2B. Doxycycline, 100 mg, twice daily, for 7 days (if at least 8 years of age)
PLUS	**For prevention of hepatitis B virus infection**	**PLUS**
3. Begin or complete hepatitis B virus immunization if not fully immunized		3. Begin or complete hepatitis B virus immunization if not fully immunized
PLUS	**For prevention of trichomoniasis and bacterial vaginosis**	**PLUS**
4. Consider adding prophylaxis for trichomoniasis and bacterial vaginosis (metronidazole, 15 mg/kg per day, orally, in 3 divided doses for 7 days; maximum 2 g)		4. Consider adding prophylaxis against trichomoniasis and bacterial vaginosis (metronidazole, 2 g, orally, in a single dose)

See text for human immunodeficiency virus infection prophylaxis in children following sexual abuse or assault.

Because of the demonstrated effectiveness of prophylaxis to prevent HIV infection after perinatal and occupational exposures, the question arises whether HIV prophylaxis is warranted for children and adolescents after sexual assault (see also Human Immunodeficiency Virus Infection, Control Measures, p 396, and Table 3.28, p 397). The risk of HIV transmission from a single sexual assault that involves transfer of secretions and/or blood is low. Prophylaxis may be considered for patients who seek care within 72 hours after an assault if the assault involved the transfer of secretions and particularly if the alleged perpetrator is known or suspected to have HIV infection or to have used injection

Table 2.15. Prophylaxis After Sexual Victimization of Adolescents[a]

Antimicrobial prophylaxis[b] is recommended to include an empiric regimen to prevent *Chlamydia trachomatis* infection, gonorrhea, trichomoniasis, and bacterial vaginosis

For gonorrhea[c]	Ceftriaxone, 125 mg, intramuscularly, in a single dose **OR** Cefixime, 400 mg orally, in a single dose **PLUS**
For *C trachomatis* infection	Azithromycin, 1 g, orally, in a single dose **OR** Doxycycline, 100 mg, orally, twice a day for 7 days (for those ≥8 years of age and not pregnant) **PLUS**
For trichomoniasis and bacterial vaginosis	Metronidazole, 2 g, orally, in a single dose **PLUS**
For hepatitis B virus infection	Hepatitis B virus immunization at time of initial examination, if not fully immunized. Follow-up doses of vaccine should be administered 1–2 and 4–6 mo after the first dose **PLUS**
For human immunodeficiency virus (HIV) infection[b]	Consider offering prophylaxis for HIV, depending on circumstances (see Table 3.28, p 397)

Emergency contraception[d]

Plan B (levonorgestrel 0.75 mg), 2 tablets at the same time
OR
Oral contraceptive pills each containing 20 or 30 µg of ethinyl estradiol plus levonorgestrel 0.1 mg or 0.15 mg or 0.3 mg norgestrel: each of 2 doses must be given 12 h apart. Each dose must contain at least 100–120 µg of ethinyl estradiol and 0.5 to 0.6 mg levonorgestrel or 1 mg norgestrel.
PLUS
An antiemetic (eg, meclizine, 25–50 mg, once before the first dose of oral contraceptive)

[a]Source: Centers for Disease Control and Prevention. Sexually transmitted infections treatment guidelines—2006. *MMWR Recomm Rep.* 2006;55(RR-11):1–29 (see **www.cdc.gov/std/treatment**).
[b]See text for discussion of prophylaxis for human immunodeficiency virus (HIV) infection after sexual abuse or assault.
[c]Fluoroquinolones no longer recommended for treatment of gonococcal infections because of increasing prevalence of resistant organisms (Centers for Disease Control and Prevention. Update to CDC's sexually transmitted diseases treatment guidelines, 2006: fluoroquinolones no longer recommended for treatment of gonococcal infections. *MMWR Recomm Rep.* 2007;56[RR-14]:332–336).
[d]The patient should have a negative pregnancy test result before emergency contraception is given. Although emergency contraception is most effective if taken within 72 hours of event, data suggest it is effective up to 120 hours.

drugs (see Human Immunodeficiency Virus Infection, p 380).[1] Following are recommendations for postexposure assessment of children within 72 hours of sexual assault:

[1]Centers for Disease Control and Prevention. Antiretroviral postexposure prophylaxis after sexual, injection-drug use, or other nonoccupational exposure to HIV in the United States: recommendations from the US Department of Health and Human Services. *MMWR Recomm Rep.* 2005;54(RR-2):1–20

- Review HIV/acquired immunodeficiency syndrome (AIDS) local epidemiology and assess risk of HIV infection in the assailant.
- Evaluate circumstances of assault that may affect risk of HIV transmission.
- Consult with a specialist in treating HIV-infected children if postexposure prophylaxis is considered.
- If the child appears to be at risk of HIV transmission from the assault, discuss postexposure prophylaxis with the caregiver(s), including toxicity and unknown efficacy.
- If caregivers choose for the child to receive antiretroviral postexposure prophylaxis, provide enough medication until the return visit at 3 to 7 days after initial assessment to reevaluate the child and to assess tolerance of medication; dosages should not exceed those for adults.
- Perform HIV antibody test at original assessment and 6, 12, and 24 weeks later.

Hepatitis and Youth in Correctional Settings[1]

Pediatricians should work with state and local public health agencies and administrators of correctional facilities to address the health needs of youth in detention and to protect the community. The number of arrests of juveniles (younger than 18 years of age) in the United States was 2.1 million in 2005, fewer than the number of arrests in 1996 but still a rate of 6350 per 100 000 youths 10 through 17 years of age in the United States. On any given day, approximately 120 000 adolescents are held in juvenile correctional facilities or adult prisons or jails. Incarceration periods of at least 90 days await 60% of juvenile inmates, and 15% can expect to be confined for a year or more behind bars. Males account for approximately 85% of juvenile offenders in residential placement, and 61% of the custodial population are members of ethnic or racial minority groups. Female juveniles in custody represent a much larger proportion of "status" offenders, with offenses including ungovernability, running away, truancy, curfew violation, and underage drinking, than "delinquent" offenders (who have committed offenses against other people or property) in custody (40% vs 14%, respectively).

Juvenile offenders commonly lack regular access to preventive health care in their communities and suffer significantly greater health deficiencies, including psychosocial disorders, chronic illness, exposure to illicit drugs, and physical trauma when compared with adolescents who are not in the juvenile justice system. Detained youth are more likely to have contracted sexually transmitted infections (STIs) early in adolescence, and delayed or incomplete treatment places them at increased risk of chronic complications of chlamydia, gonorrhea, syphilis, and human papillomavirus infections. Tuberculosis (TB) is more common in correctional populations, and although current juvenile detainees continue to have a low prevalence of human immunodeficiency virus (HIV) infection, their lifestyle choices place them at significant risk. Hepatitis A, hepatitis B, and hepatitis C virus infections are of particular concern because of the increased frequency of alcohol and injection drug use and the increased rate of unprotected sex with multiple partners early in life. The rate of juvenile arrests for drug abuse violations increased 47% between

[1]Centers for Disease Control and Prevention. Prevention and control of infections with hepatitis viruses in correctional settings. *MMWR Recomm Rep.* 2003;52(RR-1):1–33

1990 and 2005, and a history of injection drug use has played a major role in explaining the increased incidence of hepatitis C virus infections in adolescent offenders. Infected juveniles place their communities at risk after their release from detention.

Up to 15% of all chronic hepatitis B virus infections and more than 30% of all hepatitis C virus infections known to exist in the United States are found among people with a history of incarceration. High-risk behaviors make adolescents particularly vulnerable to hepatitis A, hepatitis B, and hepatitis C virus infections well before their first incarceration. Fewer than 3% of new hepatitis virus infections of all types are acquired once incarceration has occurred. Most juvenile offenders ultimately are returned to their community and, without intervention, resume a high-risk lifestyle. High recidivism rates lead many juvenile offenders to adult prisons, where the prevalence of hepatitis B and hepatitis C virus infections may be significantly higher than those found in juvenile correctional facilities. Viral hepatitis also can be a comorbid condition with other diseases, including TB and HIV infection. Correctional facilities, in partnership with public health departments and other community resources, have the opportunity to assess, contain, control, and prevent liver infection in a highly vulnerable segment of the population. Hepatitis C virus presents the greatest challenge to correctional facilities overall because of the lack of a vaccine to protect prisoners and the public. The extremely high rate of chronic carriage after infection increases the risk to their communities on their release. The controlled nature of the correctional system facilitates initiation of many hepatitis prevention and treatment strategies for an adolescent population that otherwise is difficult to reach.

Hepatitis A

Correctional facilities in the United States rarely report cases of hepatitis A, and national prevalence data for incarcerated populations are not available. States that have assessed prevalence of past infection in incarcerated populations younger than 20 years of age show a similar ethnic distribution of predominance in American Indian/Alaska Native and Hispanic inmates, as is reflected in the population as a whole. Some estimates suggest an overall seroprevalence of antibody to hepatitis A virus between 22% and 39% in the adult prison population, with up to a 43% prevalence found in older prisoners between 40 and 49 years of age. Risk factors that could contribute to outbreaks of hepatitis A among adolescents include using injection and noninjection street drugs, having multiple sexual partners, and participating in male-with-male sexual activity.

RECOMMENDATIONS FOR CONTROL OF HEPATITIS A VIRUS INFECTIONS IN INCARCERATED YOUTH. Routine screening of incarcerated youth for hepatitis A virus serologic markers is not recommended. However, adolescents who have signs or symptoms of hepatitis should be tested for seromarkers of acute hepatitis A, acute hepatitis B, and hepatitis C. Hepatitis A vaccine (see Hepatitis A Vaccine, p 331) should be given to all adolescents in residential facilities located in states with existing programs for routine hepatitis A immunization of adolescents, generally in states that historically had the highest hepatitis A rates. Correctional facilities in all states should consider routine hepatitis A immunization of all adolescents under their care because of the likelihood that most adolescents in the juvenile correctional system have indications for hepatitis A immunization. If this is not possible, hepatitis A vaccine should be provided to juveniles with high-risk profiles, including illicit drug users and male adolescents who may engage in sex with men. Routine postimmunization serologic testing is not recommended. There is no contraindication to giving hepatitis A vaccine to a person who may be immune as the result of a previous hepatitis A virus infection or immunization. Incarcerated juveniles found to have acute hepatitis A disease should be reported to the local health department, and appropriate postexposure prophylaxis with hepatitis A vaccine should be given to other susceptible residents who may have been exposed (see Hepatitis A, p 329).

Hepatitis B

Hepatitis B virus in the United States is transmitted mainly through exposure to blood, saliva, semen, and vaginal fluid; chronic infection with hepatitis B virus mainly is found among people born in countries with prevalence higher than 2% where most infections are transmitted in the perinatal period or during early childhood (see Hepatitis B, p 337). Adolescents in correctional facilities may include foreign-born (eg, Asia, Africa) residents who can have chronic infection and can transmit infection to susceptible residents. Resident adolescents also can include people with high-risk behaviors, including adolescents engaged in injection drug use with needle sharing; inmates who have had early initiation of sexual intercourse, unprotected sexual activity, multiple sexual partners, or history of STIs; and male adolescents who engage in homosexual activity. Although no published national studies have determined hepatitis B prevalence rates for incarcerated juveniles, rates of hepatitis B seroprevalence in homeless and high-risk street youth are higher when compared with peers lacking risk factors. Studies investigating hepatitis B outbreaks in prison settings also suggest that horizontal transmission may occur when people with chronic hepatitis B virus infection are present. Adolescent female inmates present additional challenges for hepatitis B assessment and management if they are pregnant during incarceration, in which case coordination of care for mother and infant become paramount.

RECOMMENDATIONS FOR CONTROL OF HEPATITIS B VIRUS INFECTIONS IN INCARCERATED YOUTH. Routine screening of juvenile inmates for hepatitis B virus markers generally is not recommended, although testing for chronic infection is recommended in certain populations (see Hepatitis B, p 337). However, in states with school entry laws (**www.immunize.org/laws**) where high levels of adolescent hepatitis B immunization have been achieved, adolescents who entered school when a law was in effect may be considered immunized. In other states, in the absence of proof of immunization, initial testing for hepatitis B immunity may save vaccine costs, provided the timing of testing does not delay hepatitis B immunization should the patient lack immunity. Correctional facilities may wish periodically to survey juvenile inmates for hepatitis B immunity as they enter the institution to approximate hepatitis B prevalence and determine the desirability of preimmunization testing. Adolescent detainees with signs and symptoms of hepatitis disease should be tested for serologic markers for acute hepatitis A, acute hepatitis B, and hepatitis C to determine the presence of acute or chronic infection and coinfection.

All adolescents receiving medical evaluation in a correctional facility should begin the hepatitis B vaccine series or complete a previously begun series unless they have proof of completion of a previous hepatitis B immunization series. Beginning a hepatitis B vaccine series is critical, because a single dose of vaccine may confer protection from infection and subsequent complications of chronic carriage in a high-risk adolescent who may be lost to follow-up. Routine preimmunization and postimmunization serologic screening is not recommended. In states where hepatitis B vaccine school entry requirements are in place, correctional facilities may use a combination of immunization history, immunization registry data, school entry immunization laws, and serologic testing to develop institutional policies regarding the need for hepatitis B immunization in specific age groups of adolescents. Facilities should have mechanisms in place for completion of the hepatitis B series in the community after release of the juvenile. Immunization information should be made available to the inmate, the parents or legal guardian, the state immunization registry, and the patient's future medical home in the community.

Postexposure hepatitis B prophylaxis regimens for unimmunized incarcerated adolescents after potential percutaneous or sexual exposures to hepatitis B virus are available (see Hepatitis B, Care of Exposed People, p 352). Should the source of the exposure be found to be hepatitis B surface antigen (HBsAg) positive, the unimmunized inmate exposed percutaneously should receive Hepatitis B Immune Globulin (HBIG) as soon as possible after exposure (preferably within 24 hours, and not more than 14 days after exposure). Exposed juveniles who have begun but not completed their hepatitis B vaccine series should receive an appropriate dose of HBIG and complete the remainder of the series as scheduled (see Hepatitis B, p 337). If the source of exposure is unknown and not available for HBsAg testing, the exposed person should receive hepatitis B vaccine or complete a vaccine series already initiated.

All pregnant adolescents should be tested for HBsAg at the time a pregnancy is discovered, regardless of hepatitis B immunization history and previous results of tests for HBsAg and antibody to HBsAg. Unimmunized pregnant adolescents who are HBsAg negative should begin the hepatitis B vaccine series as soon as possible during the course of pregnancy. Pregnancy is not a contraindication to receiving hepatitis B vaccine in any trimester. The pregnant adolescent's HBsAg status should be reported to the patient's prenatal care facility, the hospital where she will deliver the infant, and the state health department where case-management assistance will occur. Infants born to HBsAg-positive mothers must receive a dose of hepatitis B vaccine and HBIG within 12 hours of birth (see Hepatitis B, Care of Exposed People, p 352).

Incarcerated adolescents who are found to have evidence of chronic hepatitis B virus infection should be evaluated by a specialist to determine the extent of their liver disease and their eligibility for antiviral therapy. Detainees who are HBsAg positive should be reported to the local health department to facilitate long-term follow-up after release.

All adolescents with chronic liver disease should be immunized with hepatitis A vaccine to prevent fulminant liver disease should infection with hepatitis A virus occur. Adolescents who are chronically infected with hepatitis B virus should be counseled against the use and abuse of alcohol and street drugs, both of which can degrade liver function in patients with hepatitis B-induced cirrhosis. Chronically infected people may remain infectious to sexual and household contacts for life and must be counseled accordingly to protect sexual partners and household contacts.

Hepatitis C

Of the nearly 4 million people chronically infected with hepatitis C virus in the United States, approximately 30% have been incarcerated in one or more of the nation's correctional institutions. The most common mode of acquisition of hepatitis C virus is injection drug use; exposure to multiple sexual partners is a distant second. Up to 80% of inmates who use illicit injection drugs will be infected with hepatitis C virus within 5 years after the onset of their drug use. Tattooing and body piercing in regulated settings are not thought to be significant sources of transmission of hepatitis C virus, but tattoos received in a correctional facility can be associated with hepatitis C. Prevalence studies of hepatitis C virus infection in incarcerated youth are limited but show an approximate two- to fourfold increase over youth who are not in the juvenile justice system. Injection drug use is the predominant hepatitis C virus infection risk factor for detained juveniles.

Testing inmates for hepatitis C virus infection has created conflicts for administrators of correctional facilities. Many do not view the diagnosis and potential treatment of their residents with hepatitis C virus infection as part of the correctional mission. Inmates commonly refuse testing, even when at high risk of hepatitis, to avoid persecution from fellow prisoners. The lack of a vaccine for hepatitis C places a substantial burden on prevention counseling to elicit changes in high-risk behaviors and health maintenance counseling to decrease health risks in people already infected. This includes lifestyle alterations and avoidance of street drug and alcohol abuse, which increase morbidity and mortality from hepatitis C.

RECOMMENDATIONS FOR CONTROL OF HEPATITIS C VIRUS INFECTIONS IN INCARCERATED YOUTH. Routine screening of incarcerated adolescents for hepatitis C virus infection is not recommended. Focused screening of adult inmates on the basis of risk criteria has proven reliable and cost-effective for correctional facilities that use it consistently. Risk factor assessments of newly admitted juvenile inmates being considered for hepatitis C testing might include (1) self-reported history of injection drug use; (2) history of liver disease; (3) presence of antibody to hepatitis B core antigen; (4) increased alanine transaminase concentration; or (5) history of hemodialysis or receipt of clotting factors, blood transfusions, or organ transplants. Testing of detainees with one or more of these factors for antibody to hepatitis C virus can detect more than 90% of hepatitis C virus infections in correctional facilities. Some juvenile offenders may withhold reporting risk behaviors and yet express interest in hepatitis C testing when offered. These requests, in most instances, should be accommodated. Adolescents with signs or symptoms of hepatitis should undergo diagnostic testing for acute hepatitis A, acute hepatitis B, and hepatitis C virus infection.

Adolescents who test positive for antibody to hepatitis C virus should receive ongoing medical attention to determine the likelihood of chronic infection, and cases should be reported to the local health department. The presence of hepatitis C virus antibody and the absence of hepatitis C virus RNA do not preclude the possibility of active liver disease. Hepatitis C virus antigenemia is variable from day to day and occurs in the presence of circulating hepatitis C antibody. Juveniles found to be chronically infected with hepatitis C virus should receive ongoing medical evaluation (in consultation with an expert in caring for chronic live disease) to monitor the course of their liver disease and to determine their suitability for therapeutic interventions (see Hepatitis C, p 357). Incarcerated adolescents with hepatitis C virus infection should be enrolled in a risk-reduction program for drug and alcohol avoidance as indicated and should receive counseling for safe sex practices for the safety of their sexual partners and the protection of the community at large (**www.cdc.gov/ncidod/diseases/hepatitis/resource/index.htm#training**). Incarcerated adolescents with hepatitis C related chronic liver disease or with ongoing risk behaviors should receive hepatitis A and hepatitis B vaccines if not already immunized.

· ·

MEDICAL EVALUATION OF INTERNATIONALLY ADOPTED CHILDREN FOR INFECTIOUS DISEASES[1]

Annually, more than 20 000 children from other countries are adopted by families in the United States. More than 90% of international adoptees are from Asian (China, South Korea, Philippines, Vietnam, and India), Central and South American (Guatemala and Colombia), and Eastern European (Russia, Belarus, Ukraine, Kazakhstan, and Bulgaria) countries. Africa and the Middle East are less common origins for international adoptees, but an increasing minority of children are adopted from Ethiopia, Sierra Leone, Liberia, and other African countries. The diverse birth countries of these children, their unknown medical histories before adoption, their previous living circumstances (eg, orphanages and/or foster care), and the limited availability of reliable health care in some economically developing countries make the medical evaluation of internationally adopted children a challenging but important task.

Internationally adopted children typically differ from refugee children in terms of their access to medical care and treatment before arrival in the United States and in the frequency of certain infectious diseases. Many refugee children may have resided in refugee camps for months before resettlement in the United States and will have had access to limited medical care and treatment services. The history of access to and quality of medical care for international adoptees can be variable. Before admission to the United States, all internationally adopted children are required to have a medical examination performed by a physician designated by the US Department of State in their country of origin. However, this examination is limited to completing legal requirements for screening for certain communicable diseases and examination for serious physical or mental defects that would prevent the issue of a permanent residency visa. Information about this required health assessment is available at **www.cdc.gov/ncidod/ dq/refugee/faq/faq_aliens.htm.** This evaluation is not a comprehensive assessment of the child's health. During preadoption visits, pediatricians can stress to prospective parents the importance of acquiring immunization and other health records. The Immigration and Nationality Act of 1996 requires immigrant visa applicants to provide "proof of vaccination" with vaccines recommended by the Advisory Committee on Immunization Practices (ACIP) before entry into the United States. Internationally adopted children who are 10 years of age and younger may obtain a waiver of exemption from the Immigration and Nationality Act regulations pertaining to immunization of immigrants before arrival in the United States (see Refugees and Immigrants, p 97). When an exemption is granted, adoptive parents are required to sign a waiver indicating their intention to comply with ACIP-recommended immunizations within 30 days after the child arrives in the United States. However, the child should be seen by his or her pediatrician as soon as possible after arrival in the United States to begin all preventive health services, including immunizations.

---

[1]For additional information, see Canadian Paediatric Society. *Children and Youth New to Canada: Health Care Guide.* Ottawa, Ontario: Canadian Paediatric Society; 1999; and the CDC (**www.cdc.gov/travel/default.aspx**) and World Health Organization (**www.who.int**) Web sites.

Infectious diseases are among the most common medical diagnoses identified in international adoptees after arrival in the United States. Children may be asymptomatic, and therefore, the diagnoses must be made by screening tests in addition to history and physical examination. Because of inconsistent use of the birth dose of hepatitis B vaccine; inconsistent perinatal screening for hepatitis B, syphilis, and human immunodeficiency virus (HIV); and the high prevalence of certain intestinal parasites and tuberculosis, all international adoptees should be screened for these infections on arrival in the United States. Suggested screening tests for infectious diseases are listed in Table 2.16 (see also disease-specific chapters in Section 3). In addition to these infections, other medical and developmental issues, including hearing and vision assessment, evaluation of growth and development, nutritional assessment, blood lead concentration, complete blood cell count with red blood cell indices, newborn screening and/or measurement of thyroid-stimulating hormone concentration, and examination for congenital anomalies (including fetal alcohol syndrome), should be part of the initial evaluation of any internationally adopted child.

Parents generally will have limited information about a child before the adoption. Parents should obtain any medical information available and meet with the child's physician before their child arrives home to review available information and to discuss common medical issues regarding internationally adopted children. Parents who have not met with a physician before adoption should notify their physician when their child

Table 2.16. Screening Tests for Infectious Diseases in International Adoptees[a]

Hepatitis B virus serologic testing:
  Hepatitis B surface antigen (HBsAg)

Syphilis serologic testing
  Nontreponemal test (RPR, VDRL, or ART)
  Treponemal test (MHA-TP, FTA-ABS, or TPPA)

Human immunodeficiency virus 1 and 2 serologic testing

Complete blood cell count with red blood cell indices

Stool examination for ova and parasites (3 specimens)[b] with specific request for *Giardia intestinalis* and *Cryptosporidium* species testing

Tuberculin skin test[b]

In children from countries with endemic infection[b]
  Trypanosoma cruzi serologic testing

In children with eosinophilia (absolute eosinophil count exceeding 450 cells/mm^3) and negative stool ova and parasite examinations
  Strongyloides species serologic testing
  Schistosoma species serologic testing (for sub-Saharan African, Southeast Asian, and certain Latin American adoptees)

RPR indicates rapid plasma reagin; VDRL, Venereal Disease Research Laboratories; ART, automated reagin test; MHA-TP, microhemagglutination test for *Treponema pallidum;* FTA-ABS, fluorescent treponemal antibody absorption; TPPA, *T pallidum* particle agglutination.
[a]For evaluation of noninfectious disease conditions, see text.
[b]See text.

arrives so that a timely medical evaluation can be arranged. Internationally adopted children should be examined as soon as possible after arrival in the United States. A list of pediatricians with special interest in adoption and foster care medicine is available on the American Academy of Pediatrics Web site at **www.aap.org/Sections/adoption/ SOAFCAdoptionDirectory2.pdf.**

Viral Hepatitis

In studies conducted primarily during the 1990s, the prevalence of hepatitis B surface antigen (HBsAg) in internationally adopted children ranged from 1% to 5%, depending on the country of origin and the year studied. Hepatitis B virus (HBV) infection was prevalent in adoptees from Asia and Africa, regions of high endemicity, and in some countries of central and Eastern Europe (eg, Romania) and states of the former Soviet Union (eg, Russia and Ukraine). Over the past 5 to 10 years, the number of countries with routine infant hepatitis B immunization programs has increased markedly. By 2006, 163 countries, encompassing 84% of the world's population, had implemented routine infant hepatitis B immunization nationwide. However, administration of a birth dose of hepatitis B vaccine, needed to prevent perinatal transmission from an infected mother, is not routine in many countries, and coverage among infants can be suboptimal. Therefore, all children should be tested for HBsAg to identify cases of chronic infection, regardless of immunization status (see Hepatitis B, p 337). Hepatitis B serologic tests performed in the country of origin may not be useful, because testing may be incomplete and accuracy can vary. Unimmunized children with a negative HBsAg laboratory result should be immunized as soon as possible according to the recommended childhood and adolescent immunization schedules (Fig 1.1–1.3, p 24–28).

Children with a positive HBsAg laboratory result should be reported to the local or state health department. To verify the presence of chronic HBV infection, HBsAg-positive children should be retested. The absence of immunoglobulin M antibody to hepatitis B core antigen (IgM anti-HBc) or the persistence of HBsAg for at least 6 months indicates chronic HBV infection (see Hepatitis B, p 337). Children with chronic HBV infection should be tested for biochemical evidence of liver disease and followed by a specialist who cares for patients with chronic hepatitis B (see Hepatitis B, p 337). All unimmunized household contacts of children with chronic HBV infection should be immunized (see Hepatitis B, p 337).

Hepatitis D virus (HDV), which occurs only in conjunction with the presence of HBsAg, can infect adoptees, particularly from North Africa, parts of South America, and the Mediterranean Basin. Serologic tests for the diagnosis of HDV infection are not available widely (see Hepatitis D, p 361). Routine testing is not recommended but might be included as part of further clinical evaluation of children found to have chronic HBV infection.

Children adopted at 12 through 23 months of age should receive hepatitis A vaccine as recommended according to the routine immunization schedule (Fig 1.1, p 24–25). Many international adoptees may have acquired hepatitis A virus (HAV) infection early in life in their country of origin and be immune. However, because HAV is endemic in many of these countries, internationally adopted children are at ongoing risk of HAV infection while in their countries of origin. These children could be incubating HAV infection at the time of adoption and could transmit the virus to their adoptive families and others on arrival in the United States, as has occurred with adoptees from Ethiopia. Adoptive parents and any accompanying family members should ensure they are immunized or otherwise immune to HAV infection before international travel to pick up their child. In addition, hepatitis A vaccine should be administered to all susceptible nontraveling people who anticipate having close personal contact with a child adopted internationally from a country with high or intermediate hepatitis A endemicity before arrival of the adoptee. Adopted children or their household or other close contacts with symptoms consistent with acute viral hepatitis should be evaluated promptly.

Routine testing for hepatitis C virus (HCV) infection is not recommended. Testing can be considered for children who received blood products or other medical interventions, especially children from countries where HCV infection prevalence is high (eg, Egypt) or where infection-control practices in health care facilities may be suboptimal (eg, Russia, Eastern Europe, China). If testing is performed, an enzyme immunoassay (EIA) should be used. Passively transferred maternal antibody may remain detectable by EIA for up to 18 months (see Hepatitis C, p 357). Also, the predictive value of a positive EIA result is poor in low-prevalence populations, and a positive EIA does not distinguish past from current infection. Therefore, a positive EIA result needs to be confirmed with a more specific assay and scheduled follow-up visits (see Hepatitis C, p 357).

Cytomegalovirus

Routine screening for cytomegalovirus (CMV) is not recommended. Shedding of CMV in young children after postnatal acquisition is common in the United States and worldwide. Parents should use appropriate hand hygiene practices.

Intestinal Pathogens

Fecal examinations for ova and parasites by an experienced laboratory will identify a pathogen in 15% to 35% of internationally adopted children. The prevalence of intestinal parasites varies by age of the child and country of origin. The most common pathogens identified are *Giardia intestinalis, Dientamoeba fragilis, Hymenolepis* species, *Ascaris lumbricoides,* and *Trichuris trichiura. Strongyloides stercoralis, Entamoeba histolytica,* and hookworm are recovered less commonly. One stool specimen may be sufficient to test for intestinal ova and parasites and for *Giardia* antigen in asymptomatic children, although some experts recommend that 3 different daily specimens be tested. If gastrointestinal tract signs or symptoms or malnutrition are present, 3 stool specimens collected daily should be examined for ova and parasites with specific requests for *G intestinalis* and *Cryptosporidium* species testing. Therapy for intestinal parasites generally will be successful, but complete eradication may not occur. Therefore, repeat ova and parasite testing after treatment is important to ensure successful elimination of parasites if symptoms persist. Children with gastrointestinal tract symptoms or signs that occur or recur months or even years after arrival in the United States should be reevaluated for intestinal parasites. In addition, testing stool specimens for *Salmonella* species, *Shigella* species, *Campylobacter* species, and *Escherichia coli* O157:H7 should be considered in children with diarrhea, especially if stools are bloody.

Tuberculosis

Tuberculosis commonly is encountered in international adoptees from all countries. Reported rates of latent *Mycobacterium tuberculosis* infection range from 0.6% to 30%. All immigrants, including international adoptees, are required to have screening for tuberculosis before arriving in the United States. The screening requirements for tuberculosis underwent a major revision in 2007. Information about the screening and implementation requirements is available at **www.cdc.gov/ncidod/dq/panel_2007.htm.**

Because tuberculosis may be more severe in young children and may reactivate in later years, screening with the tuberculin skin test (TST) in all-aged children or an interferon-gamma release assay in children 5 years of age or older is important in this high-risk population (see Tuberculosis, p 680). Routine chest radiography is not indicated in asymptomatic children in whom the TST result is negative. However, some international adoptees may be anergic because of malnutrition, which is common in malnourished children. If malnutrition is suspected, the TST should be repeated once the child is appropriately nourished. Receipt of bacille Calmette-Guérin (BCG) vaccine is not a contraindication to a TST, and a positive TST result should not be attributed to BCG vaccine. In these children, further investigation is necessary to determine whether latent tuberculosis infection or active disease is present and therapy is needed (see Tuberculosis, p 680). Some children will have had recent exposure to a person with tuberculosis disease. Preventive therapy should be considered if such a history is available. Some experts repeat the TST 6 months after a child has left an area with high prevalence of tuberculosis. When tuberculosis is suspected in an international adoptee, efforts to isolate and test the organism for drug susceptibilities are imperative because of the high prevalence of drug resistance in many countries.

Syphilis

Congenital syphilis, especially with involvement of the central nervous system, may not have been diagnosed or may have been treated inadequately in adoptees from some developing countries. Children 15 years of age and older should have had serologic testing for syphilis as part of the required overseas medical assessment. Children who had positive test results are required to complete treatment before arrival in the United States. After arrival in the United States, clinicians should screen each international adoptee for syphilis by reliable nontreponemal and treponemal serologic tests, regardless of history or a report of treatment (see Syphilis, p 638). Children with positive treponemal serologic test results should be evaluated by someone with special expertise to assess the differential diagnosis of pinta, yaws, and syphilis and to determine extent of infection so appropriate treatment can be administered (see Syphilis, p 638).

HIV Infection

The risk of HIV infection in internationally adopted children depends on the country of origin and individual risk factors. Adoptees 15 years of age and older have HIV testing as part of required medical assessment in their country of origin. Because of the rapidly changing epidemiology of HIV infection and because adoptees may come from populations at high risk of infection, screening for HIV should be performed on all internationally adopted children. Although many children will have HIV test results documented in their referral information, test results from the child's country of origin may not be reliable. Transplacentally acquired maternal antibody in the absence of infection can be detected in a child younger than 18 months of age. Hence, positive HIV antibody test results in asymptomatic children of this age require clinical evaluation, further testing, and counseling (see Human Immunodeficiency Virus Infection, p 380).

Chagas Disease (American Trypanosomiasis)

Chagas disease is endemic throughout much of Mexico, Central America, and South America. Risk of Chagas disease varies by region within countries with endemic infection. Although the risk of Chagas disease is low in internationally adopted children from countries with endemic infection, treatment of infected children is highly effective. Countries with endemic Chagas disease include Argentina, Belize, Bolivia, Brazil, Chile, Colombia, Costa Rica, Ecuador, El Salvador, French Guiana, Guatemala, Guyana, Honduras, Mexico, Nicaragua, Panama, Paraguay, Peru, Suriname, Uruguay, and Venezuela. Transmission within countries with endemic infection is focal, but if a child comes from a country with endemic Chagas disease, testing for *Trypanosoma cruzi* should be considered. Serologic testing should be performed only in children 12 months of age or older because of the potential presence of maternal antibody.

Other Infectious Diseases

Skin infections that occur commonly in international adoptees include bacterial (eg, impetigo) and fungal (eg, candidiasis) infections and ectoparasitic infestations (eg, scabies and pediculosis). Adoptive parents should be instructed on how to examine their child for signs of scabies, pediculosis, and tinea so treatment can be initiated and transmission to others can be prevented (see Scabies, p 589, and Pediculosis, p 495–499).

Diseases such as typhoid fever, malaria, leprosy, or melioidosis are encountered infrequently in internationally adopted children. Although routine screening for these diseases is not recommended, findings of fever, splenomegaly, respiratory tract infection, anemia, or eosinophilia should prompt an appropriate evaluation on the basis of the epidemiology of infectious diseases that occur in the child's country of origin. If the child came from a country where malaria is present, malaria should be considered in the differential diagnosis (see Malaria, p 438).

In the United States, multiple outbreaks of measles have been reported in children adopted from China and in their United States contacts. Measles outbreaks among children in orphanages in China also were reported. In 2002 and 2004, adoptions from affected orphanages were suspended temporarily while Chinese authorities implemented measures to control and prevent further transmission of measles among the children. Measles elimination has been achieved only in the Americas; transmission continues in other parts of the world. Prospective parents who are traveling internationally to adopt children, as well as their household contacts, should ensure that they have a history of natural disease or have been immunized adequately for measles according to US guidelines. All people born after 1957 should receive 2 doses of measles-containing vaccine in the absence of documented measles infection or contraindication to the vaccine (see Measles, p 444).

Clinicians should be aware of potential diseases in internationally adopted children and their clinical manifestations. Some diseases, such as central nervous system cysticercosis, may have incubation periods as long as several years and, thus, may not be detected during initial screening. On the basis of findings at the initial evaluation, consideration should be given to a repeat evaluation 6 months after adoption. In most cases, the longer the interval from adoption to development of a clinical syndrome, the less likely the syndrome can be attributed to a pathogen acquired in the country of origin.

In international adoptees who have negative stool ova and parasite examinations and in whom eosinophilia (absolute eosinophil count exceeding 450 cells/mm^3) is found on review of complete blood count, serologic testing for *Strongyloides* and *Schistosoma* organisms should be considered. Serologic testing for *Strongyloides stercoralis* should be performed on all international adoptees with eosinophilia and no identified pathogen commonly associated with an increased eosinophil count, regardless of country of origin. Serologic testing for *Schistosoma* species should be performed on international adoptees with eosinophilia and no identified pathogen commonly associated with eosinophilia who are from Sub-Saharan Africa, South East Asia, or areas of Latin America where schistosomiasis is endemic.

Immunizations

Only written documentation of immunizations received by an adoptee should be accepted. Immunizations such as BCG, diphtheria and tetanus toxoids and pertussis (DTP or DTaP), poliovirus, measles, and hepatitis B vaccines are given routinely in many parts of the world and may be documented in an immunization record. However, because other immunizations such as *Haemophilus influenzae* type b, *Streptococcus pneumoniae*, mumps, rubella, hepatitis A, and varicella vaccines are given less frequently or are not part of the routine immunization schedule in other countries, written documentation may be available less often. Internationally adopted children and adolescents should receive immunizations according to the recommended schedule in the United States for healthy children and adolescents (see Fig 1.1–1.3, p 24–28). Although some vaccines with inadequate potency are used in other countries, most vaccines available worldwide are produced with adequate quality-control standards and are reliable. However, information about storage, handling, site of administration, vaccine potency, and provider generally is not available. In general, written documentation of immunizations can be accepted as evidence of adequacy of previous immunization if the vaccines, dates of administration, number of doses, intervals between doses, and age of the child at the time of immunization are consistent internally and comparable to current US or World Health Organization schedules (see Immunizations Received Outside the United States, p 36). Given the limited data available regarding verification of immunization records from other countries, evaluation of concentrations of antibody to the antigens given repeatedly is an option to ensure that vaccines were given and were immunogenic. Serologic testing may be performed to determine whether protective antibody concentrations are present. An acceptable alternative when doubt exists is to reimmunize the child. Because the rate of more serious local reactions after DTaP vaccine increases with the number of doses administered, serologic testing for antibody to tetanus and diphtheria toxins before reimmunizing (or if a serious reaction occurs) can be considered if appropriate immunization is in question.

Table 2.17 (p 185) lists the vaccines for which antibody testing can be performed, specifies the types of tests to be ordered, and provides recommended and alternative approaches. In children older than 6 months of age with or without written documentation of immunization, serologic testing for antibodies to diphtheria and tetanus toxoids and poliovirus may be considered to determine whether the child has protective antibody concentrations. If the child has protective concentrations, then the immunization series should be completed as appropriate for that child's age. In children older than 12 months of age, hepatitis A, measles, mumps, rubella, and varicella antibody concentrations may be measured to determine whether the child is immune; these antibody tests should not be performed in children younger than 12 months of age because of the potential presence of maternal antibody. Many children will need a dose of mumps and rubella vaccines, because these vaccines are administered infrequently in developing countries. One dose of measles-mumps-rubella (MMR) vaccine could be administered for mumps and rubella coverage, even if measles antibodies are present. At this time, no antibody testing is reliable or available routinely to assess immunity to pertussis. Serologic testing for HBsAg should be performed for all children to identify chronic infection. If serologic testing is not available and receipt of immunogenic vaccines cannot be ensured, the prudent course is to provide the immunization series.

INJURIES FROM DISCARDED NEEDLES IN THE COMMUNITY

Contact with and injuries from hypodermic needles and syringes discarded in public places, presumably by injection drug users, may pose a risk of transmission of bloodborne pathogens, including human immunodeficiency virus (HIV), hepatitis B virus (HBV), and hepatitis C virus (HCV). Although nonoccupational needlestick injuries may pose a lower risk of infection transmission than do occupational needlestick injuries, a person injured by a needle in a nonoccupational setting needs evaluation and counseling. People exposed in this manner may not be aware that they need evaluation. Even if the potential that the discarded syringe contains a bloodborne pathogen can be estimated from the prevalence rates of these infections in the local community, the need to test the injured or exposed person usually is not influenced significantly by this assessment.

Management of people with needlestick injuries includes acute wound care and consideration of the need for antimicrobial prophylaxis. Standard wound cleansing and care is indicated; such wounds rarely require closure. Tetanus toxoid vaccine with or without Tetanus Immune Globulin should be considered as appropriate for the severity of the injury, the immunization status of the exposed person, and the potential for dirt or soil contamination of the needle (see Tetanus, p 655).

Consideration of the need for prophylaxis for HBV and HIV is the next step in exposure management; currently, there is no recommended postexposure prophylaxis for HCV. Risk of acquisition of various pathogens depends on the nature of the wound, the ability of the pathogens to survive on environmental surfaces, the volume of source material, the concentration of virus in the source material, prevalence rates among local injection drug users, the probability that the syringe and needle were used by a local injection drug user, and the immunization status of the exposed person. Unlike an occupational blood or body fluid exposure, in which the status of the exposure source for HBV, HCV,

Table 2.17. Approaches to the Evaluation and Immunization of Children Adopted From Outside the United States[a]

Vaccine	Recommended Approach	Alternative Approach
Hepatitis B	Test for HBsAg. Give age-appropriate immunization if negative.	—
Diphtheria, pertussis and tetanus toxoids (DTaP, Tdap, DT, Td)	Immunize with diphtheria, pertussis, and tetanus-containing vaccine as appropriate for age (see Diphtheria, p 280, Pertussis, p 504, and Tetanus, p 655). Serologic testing for antitoxoid antibodies 4 wk after dose 1 if severe local reaction occurs.	Children whose records indicate receipt of ≥3 doses: serologic testing for antitoxoid antibody to diphtheria and tetanus toxins before administering additional doses or administer a single booster dose of diphtheria and tetanus-containing vaccine, followed by serologic testing after 1 mo for antitoxoid antibody to diphtheria and tetanus toxins with reimmunization as appropriate (see text).
Haemophilus influenzae type b (Hib)	Age-appropriate immunization.	—
Pertussis (DTaP, Tdap)	No serologic test routinely available. May use antibodies to diphtheria or tetanus toxoids as a marker of receipt of diphtheria, tetanus, and pertussis-containing vaccine.	—
Poliovirus	Immunize with inactivated poliovirus (IPV) vaccine.	Serologic testing for neutralizing antibody to poliovirus types 1, 2, and 3 or administration of a single dose of IPV, followed by serologic testing for neutralizing antibody to poliovirus types 1, 2, and 3.
Measles-mumps-rubella (MMR)	Immunize with MMR vaccine or obtain measles antibody and if positive, give MMR vaccine for mumps and rubella protection.	Serologic testing for immunoglobulin G antibody to vaccine viruses indicated by immunization record.
Varicella	Age-appropriate immunization of children who lack reliable history of previous varicella disease or serologic evidence of protection.	—
Pneumococcal	Age-appropriate immunization.	—

[a] Centers for Disease Control and Prevention. General recommendations on immunization. Recommendations of the Advisory Committee on Immunization Practices. *MMWR Recomm Rep.* 2009; in press. Also see Fig 1.1–1.3 (p 24–28).

and HIV often is known, these data usually are not available to help in the decision-making process in a nonoccupational exposure.[1,2]

Hepatitis B virus is the hardiest of the major bloodborne pathogens and can survive on environmental surfaces for at least 7 days. Children who have not completed the 3-dose hepatitis B vaccine series should receive a dose of vaccine and, if indicated, should be scheduled to receive the remaining doses to complete the schedule. Administration of Hepatitis B Immune Globulin usually is not indicated if the child has received the 3-dose regimen of hepatitis B vaccine (see Table 3.22, p 355). However, experts differ in opinion about the need for Hepatitis B Immune Globulin at the time of an injury of an incompletely immunized child. If the child has received 2 doses of hepatitis B vaccine 4 or more months previously, the immediate administration of the third dose of vaccine alone should be sufficient in most cases.

Infection with HIV usually is the greatest concern of the victim and family. The need for initial baseline serologic tests for preexisting HIV infection is controversial. Negative results from these initial tests support the conclusion that any subsequent positive test result likely reflects infection acquired from the needlestick. A positive initial test result in a pediatric patient requires further investigation of the cause, such as perinatal transmission, sexual abuse or activity, or drug use. An alternative option is to obtain and save a baseline serum specimen for later testing for HIV antibody in the unlikely event that a subsequent test result is positive. Counseling is necessary before and after testing (see Human Immunodeficiency Virus Infection, p 380).

The risk of HIV transmission from a needle discarded in public is low. Risk of HIV transmission from a puncture wound caused by a needle found in the community is lower than the 0.3% risk of HIV transmission to a health care professional from a needlestick injury from a person with known HIV infection. As of March 2008, no cases in which HIV was transmitted by needlestick injury outside a health care setting had been reported to the Centers for Disease Control and Prevention. Data are not available on the efficacy of postexposure prophylaxis with antiretroviral drugs in these circumstances for adults or children, and as a result, the US Public Health Service is unable to recommend for or against prophylaxis in this circumstance.[3,4]

Antiretroviral therapy is not without risk and often is associated with significant adverse effects (see Human Immunodeficiency Virus Infection, p 380). Therefore, postexposure prophylaxis is not recommended routinely in this situation. However, some experts recommend that baseline serologic testing for preexisting HIV infection be performed and that antiretroviral chemoprophylaxis be considered if it can be initiated within 72 hours of the puncture wound and if the needle and/or syringe are available and found to

[1]Centers for Disease Control and Prevention. Updated US Public Health Service guidelines for the management of occupational exposures to HBV, HCV, and HIV and recommendations for postexposure prophylaxis. *MMWR Recomm Rep.* 2001;50(RR-11):1–52

[2]US Department of Health and Human Services. Antiretroviral postexposure prophylaxis after sexual, injection-drug use, or other nonoccupational exposure to HIV in the United States: recommendations from the US Department of Health and Human Services. *MMWR Recomm Rep.* 2005;54(RR-2):1–20

[3]Centers for Disease Control and Prevention. Antiretroviral postexposure prophylaxis after sexual injection-drug-use, or other nonoccupational exposure to HIV in the United States: recommendations from the US Department of Health and Human Services. *MMWR Recomm Rep.* 2005;54(RR-2):1–20

[4]American Academy of Pediatrics, Committee on Pediatric AIDS. Postexposure prophylaxis in children and adolescents for nonoccupational exposure to human immunodeficiency virus. *Pediatrics.* 2003;111(6):1475–1489

contain visible blood or the source is known to be an HIV-infected person. Other experts recommend chemoprophylaxis if blood was visible on the syringe or needle, and other experts recommend chemoprophylaxis for any needlestick injury. Testing the syringe for HIV is not practical or reliable and is not recommended. In most reports of occupational HIV transmission by percutaneous injury, needlestick injury occurred shortly after needle withdrawal from the vein or artery of the source patient with HIV infection. Human immunodeficiency virus RNA was detected in only 3 (3.8%) of 80 discarded disposable syringes that had been used by health care professionals for intramuscular or subcutaneous injection of patients with HIV infection, indicating that most syringes will not contain HIV even after being used to draw blood from a person with HIV infection. HIV is susceptible to drying, and when HIV is placed on a surface exposed to air, the 50% tissue culture infective dose decreases by approximately 1 log every 9 hours. A specialist in HIV infection should be consulted before deciding whether to initiate postexposure chemoprophylaxis. If the decision to begin prophylaxis is made, any delay before starting the medications should be minimized (see Human Immunodeficiency Virus Infection, p 380). The suggested medication options are the same as for HIV occupational exposure (see Human Immunodeficiency Virus Infection, p 380).

Follow-up testing of a child to detect HIV seroconversion should include testing for HIV antibody at 6 weeks, 12 weeks, and 6 months after injury. Testing also is indicated if an illness consistent with acute HIV-related syndrome develops before the 6-week testing (see Human Immunodeficiency Virus Infection, p 380).

The third bloodborne pathogen of concern is HCV. Although transmission by sharing syringes among injection drug users is efficient, the risk of transmission from a discarded syringe is likely to be low. The need for testing for HCV is uncertain. If performed, testing for antibody to HCV should be performed at the time of injury and 6 months later. If earlier diagnosis is desired, testing for HCV RNA may be performed at 4 to 6 weeks. Positive test results should be confirmed by supplemental confirmatory laboratory tests (see Hepatitis C, p 357). There is no recommended postexposure prophylaxis for HCV using Immune Globulin preparations (which do not contain antibody to HCV) or antiviral drugs.

Needlestick injuries of both children and adults can be minimized by public health programs on safe needle disposal and by programs for exchange of used syringes and needles from injection drug users for sterile ones. Needle and syringe exchanges decrease improper disposal and the spread of bloodborne pathogens without increasing the rate of injection drug use. The American Academy of Pediatrics supports needle-exchange programs in conjunction with drug treatment and within the context of continuing research to assess their effectiveness.

BITE WOUNDS

As many as 1% of all pediatric visits to emergency departments during summer months are for treatment of human or animal bite wounds. An estimated 4.7 million bites occur annually in the United States; dog bites account for 80% of those wounds. The rate of infection after cat bites is as high as 50%, and rates of infection after dog or human bites are 10% to 15%. The bites of humans, wild animals, or nontraditional pets potentially are sources of serious infection. Parents should be informed to teach children to avoid contact with wild animals and should secure garbage containers so that raccoons and other animals will not be attracted to the home and places where children play. Ferrets and other nontraditional pets are not appropriate pets for children. Concern about potential transmission of rabies should be increased when a bite, particularly unprovoked, is from a wild animal (especially a bat or a carnivore) or from a domestic animal that cannot be observed for 10 days after the bite (see Rabies, p 552). Dead animals should be avoided, because they can harbor rabies virus in their nervous system tissues and saliva and can be infested with arthropods (fleas or ticks) infected with a variety of bacterial, rickettsial, protozoan, or viral agents.

Recommendations for bite wound management are given in Table 2.18 (p 189). Sufficient prospective, controlled studies on which to base recommendations about the closure of bite wounds are lacking. In general, recent, apparently uninfected, low-risk lesions can be sutured after thorough wound cleansing, irrigation, and débridement. Use of local anesthesia can facilitate these procedures. Because suturing can enhance the risk of wound infection, some clinicians prefer that small wounds be managed by approximation of the wound edges with adhesive strips or tissue adhesive. Bite wounds on the face, which have important cosmetic considerations, seldom become infected and should be closed whenever possible. Hand and foot wounds have a higher risk of infection and should be managed in consultation with an appropriate surgical specialist. Specimens for culture should be obtained from wounds that appear infected; anaerobic cultures should be performed for wounds with abscess formation, extensive cellulitis, or devitalized tissue or if the wound exudate has a foul odor. Approximation of margins and closure by delayed primary or secondary intent is prudent for infected nonfacial wounds. Elevation of injured areas to minimize swelling is important.

Limited data exist to guide antimicrobial therapy for patients with wounds that are not overtly infected. The use of an antimicrobial agent within 8 to 12 hours of injury for a 2- to 3-day course of therapy may decrease the rate of infection. Children at high risk of infection (eg, children who are immunocompromised or who have joint penetration) should receive empiric antimicrobial therapy. Patients with mild injuries in which the skin is abraded do not need to be treated with antimicrobial agents. Guidelines for choice of antimicrobial therapy regimen for human and animal bites are given in Table 2.19 (p 190) and reflect the organisms likely to cause infection.[1] Empiric therapy should be modified when culture results become available. The increasing prevalence of community-acquired methicillin-resistant *Staphylococcus aureus* may require a modification of therapy if this organism is isolated from an infected wound (see Staphylococcal Infections, p 601).

Prophylaxis or treatment of the penicillin-allergic child with a human or animal bite wound is problematic. Doxycycline is an alternative agent that has activity against *Pasteurella multocida;* its use in children younger than 8 years of age must be weighed against the risk of dental staining. Azithromycin displays good in vitro activity against organisms that commonly cause bite wound infections, except for some strains of staphylococci, but no clinical trials have documented its efficacy. Oral or parenteral treatment with trimethoprim-sulfamethoxazole, which is effective against *S aureus, P multocida,* and *Eikenella corrodens,* in conjunction with clindamycin, which is active in vitro against anaerobic bacteria, streptococci, and many strains of *S aureus*, may be

---

[1]For a complete listing of antimicrobial agents for infections following animal or human bites, see Stevens DL, Bisno AL, Chambers HF, et al. Practice guidelines for the diagnosis and management of skin and soft-tissue infections. *Clin Infect Dis.* 2005;41(10):1373–1406

Table 2.18. Prophylactic Management of Human or Animal Bite Wounds to Prevent Infection

Category of Management	Management
Cleansing	Sponge away visible dirt. Irrigate with a copious volume of sterile saline solution by high-pressure syringe irrigation.[a] Do not irrigate puncture wounds. Standard Precautions should be used.
Wound culture	No for fresh wounds, unless signs of infection exist. Yes for wounds more than 8–12 h old and wounds that appear infected.[b]
Radiographs	Indicated for penetrating injuries overlying bones or joints, for suspected fracture, or to assess foreign body inoculation.
Débridement	Remove devitalized tissue.
Operative débridement and exploration	Yes if one of the following: • Extensive wounds (devitalized tissue) • Involvement of the metacarpophalangeal joint (closed fist injury) • Cranial bites by large animal
Wound closure	Yes for selected fresh, nonpuncture bite wounds (see text)
Assess tetanus immunization status[c]	Yes
Assess risk of rabies from animal bites[d]	Yes
Assess risk of hepatitis B virus infection from human bites[e]	Yes
Assess risk of human immunodeficiency virus from human bites	Yes
Initiate antimicrobial therapy[g]	Yes for: • Moderate or severe bite wounds, especially if edema or crush injury is present • Puncture wounds, especially if penetration of bone, tendon sheath, or joint has occurred • Facial bites • Hand and foot bites • Genital area bites • Wounds in immunocompromised and asplenic people • Wounds with signs of infection
Follow-up	Inspect wound for signs of infection within 48 h

[a]Use of an 18-gauge needle with a large-volume syringe is effective. Antimicrobial or anti-infective solutions offer no advantage and may increase tissue irritation.
[b]Both aerobic and anaerobic bacterial culture should be performed.
[c]See Tetanus, p 655.
[d]See Rabies, p 552.
[e]See Hepatitis B, p 337.
[f]See Human Immunodeficiency Virus Infection, p 380.
[g]See Table 2.19 (p 190) for suggested drug choices.

Table 2.19. Antimicrobial Agents for Human or Animal Bite Wounds

Source of Bite	Organism(s) Likely to Cause Infection	Antimicrobial Agent			
		Oral Route	Oral Alternatives for Penicillin-Allergic Patients[a]	Intravenous Route	Intravenous Alternatives for Penicillin-Allergic Patients[a]
Dog, cat, or mammal	*Pasteurella* species, *Staphylococcus aureus*, streptococci, anaerobes, *Capnocytophaga* species, *Moraxella* species, *Corynebacterium* species, *Neisseria* species	Amoxicillin-clavulanate	Extended-spectrum cephalosporin or trimethoprim-sulfamethoxazole **PLUS** Clindamycin	Ampicillin-sulbactam[b]	Trimethoprim-sulfamethoxazole **PLUS** Clindamycin **OR** Cefoxitin or meropenem
Reptile	Enteric gram-negative bacteria, anaerobes	Amoxicillin-clavulanate	Extended-spectrum cephalosporin or trimethoprim-sulfamethoxazole **PLUS** Clindamycin	Ampicillin-sulbactam[b] **PLUS** Gentamicin	Clindamycin **PLUS** Gentamicin
Human	Streptococci, *S aureus*, *Eikenella corrodens*, *Haemophilus* species, anaerobes	Amoxicillin-clavulanate	Extended-spectrum cephalosporin or trimethoprim-sulfamethoxazole **PLUS** Clindamycin	Ampicillin-sulbactam[b]	Trimethoprim-sulfamethoxazole **PLUS** Clindamycin **OR** Cefoxitin or meropenem

[a]For patients with history of allergy to penicillin or one of its congeners, alternative drugs are recommended. In some circumstances, a cephalosporin or other beta-lactam–class drug may be acceptable. However, these drugs should not be used for patients with an immediate hypersensitivity (anaphylaxis) to penicillin, because approximately 5% to 15% of penicillin-allergic patients also will be allergic to cephalosporins.

[b]Piperacillin-tazobactam or ticarcillin-clavulanate can be used as alternatives.

effective for preventing bite wound infections. Extended-spectrum cephalosporins, such as cefotaxime or ceftriaxone parenterally or cefpodoxime orally, do not have good anaerobic spectra of activity but can be used in conjunction with clindamycin as alternative therapy for penicillin-allergic patients who can tolerate cephalosporins. A 7- to 10-day course usually is sufficient for soft tissue infections. The duration of treatment for bite wound-associated bone infections is based on location and severity and on the pathogens isolated.

PREVENTION OF TICKBORNE INFECTIONS

Tickborne infectious diseases in the United States include diseases caused by bacteria (eg, tularemia), spirochetes (Lyme disease and relapsing fever), rickettsiae (eg, Rocky Mountain spotted fever, ehrlichiosis, anaplasmosis), viruses (eg, Colorado tick fever, Powassan virus), and protozoa (eg, babesiosis) (see Table 2.20, p 192, and disease-specific chapters in Section 3). Different species of ticks transmit different infectious agents (eg, brown dog ticks transmit the agent of Rocky Mountain spotted fever; black-legged ticks transmit the agent of Lyme disease), and some species of ticks may transmit more than one agent. Physicians should be aware of the epidemiology of tickborne infections in their local areas. Prevention of tickborne diseases is accomplished through avoidance of tick-infested habitats, by decreasing tick populations in the environment, using personal protection against tick bites, and limiting the length of time ticks remain attached to the human host. Control of tick populations in the field often is not practical but can be effective in more defined areas around places where children reside and play. Specific measures for prevention are as follows:
- Physicians, parents, and children should be made aware that ticks can transmit pathogens that cause human and animal diseases.
- Tick-infested areas should be avoided whenever possible. Ticks prefer dense woods with thick growth of shrubs and small trees as well as along the edge of the woods where the woods abut lawns.
- If a tick-infested area is entered, light-colored clothing that covers the arms, legs, and other exposed areas should be worn, pants should be tucked into boots or socks, and long-sleeved shirts should be buttoned at the cuff. In addition, permethrin (a synthetic pyrethroid) can be sprayed onto clothes to decrease tick attachment. Permethrin should not be sprayed onto skin. Some manufacturers now offer permethrin-treated clothing, which will remain effective for up to 20 washings.
- Because of lack of adequate safety and efficacy data regarding clothing that has been treated with permethrin by the manufacturer before sale, its use is not recommended for children.
- Tick and insect repellents that contain diethyltoluamide (DEET) applied to the skin provide additional protection but may require reapplication every 1 to 2 hours for maximum effectiveness. Newer formulations are microencapsulated to increase the time before reapplication to 8 to 12 hours. Although there have been rare reports of serious neurologic complications in children resulting from the frequent and excessive application of DEET-containing insect repellents, the risk is extremely low when these products are used properly. Products containing DEET should be applied as recommended (see Prevention of Mosquitoborne Infections, p 193).

Table 2.20. Some Tick-Transmitted Pathogens (Domestic and Imported)

Human Disease Type	Pathogens in the United States	Pathogens in Other Countries
Bacteria		
Human anaplasmosis	*Anaplasma phagocytophilum*	*A phagocytophilum*
Human ehrlichiosis	*Ehrlichia chaffeensis, Ehrlichia ewingii*	*Ehrlichia muris,* possibly *Ehrlichia canis,* other species
Lyme disease, Lyme borreliosis	*Borrelia burgdorferi*	*B burgdorferi, Borrelia afzelii, Borrelia garinii, Borrelia bissettii*
Q fever (uncommon tick transmission)	*Coxiella burnetii*	*C burnetii*
Spotted fever group of rickettsioses	*Rickettsia rickettsii, Rickettsia parkeri,* perhaps other species	*Rickettsia rickettsii, Rickettsia conorii, Rickettsia africae, Rickettsia honei, Rickettsia japonica, Rickettsia sibirica, Rickettsia slovaca,* other species
Tickborne relapsing fever	*Borrelia hermsii, Borrelia turicatae, Borrelia parkeri*	*Borrelia duttonii,* other species
Tularemia	*Francisella tularensis*	*F tularensis*
Protozoa		
Human babesiosis	*Babesia microti, Babesia* species (MO1) *Babesia duncani* (WA1, CA2)	*B microti, Babesia divergens,* other species
Viruses		
Coltivirus infection	Colorado tick fever virus	European Eyach virus
Flavivirus infection	Powassan virus, Deer tick virus	Powassan virus, tickborne encephalitis virus, Kyasanur Forest disease virus, Russian spring-summer encephalitis virus, Omsk hemorrhagic fever virus

- Picaridin and oil of eucalyptus preparations have been approved for use as repellents by the US Environmental Protection Agency. These may be more acceptable to some families. They do not damage certain synthetic fabrics and plastics as DEET products do occasionally.
- People should inspect themselves and their children's bodies and clothing daily after possible tick exposure. Special attention should be given to the exposed hairy regions of the body where ticks often attach, including the head, neck, and behind the ears in children. Ticks also may attach at areas of tight clothing (eg, belt line, axillae, groin). Ticks should be removed promptly. For removal, a tick should be grasped with a fine tweezers close to the skin and gently pulled straight out without twisting motions. Although not recommended, if fingers are used to remove ticks, they should be protected with a barrier such as tissue and washed after removal of the tick. The bite site should be washed with soap and water to reduce the risk of secondary skin infections.
- Maintaining tick-free pets also will decrease tick exposure. Daily inspection of pets and removal of ticks are indicated, as is the routine use of appropriate veterinary products to prevent ticks on pets. Consult a veterinarian for information.
- Chemoprophylaxis to prevent Lyme disease may be considered only in unusual circumstances (see Lyme Disease, p 430).

PREVENTION OF MOSQUITOBORNE INFECTIONS

Mosquitoborne infectious diseases in the United States are caused by arboviruses (eg, West Nile, La Crosse, St. Louis encephalitis, eastern equine encephalitis, and western equine encephalitis viruses [see Arboviruses, p 214]). International travelers may encounter arboviral or other mosquitoborne infections (eg, malaria, Yellow fever, dengue, Japanese encephalitis) during travel (also see disease-specific chapters in Section 3). Physicians should be aware of the epidemiology of arbovirus infections in their local areas. Prevention involves protection from the bite of an infected mosquito. In areas with arbovirus transmission, protection of children is recommended during outdoor activities, including activities related to school, child care, or camping. Education of families and other caregivers is an important component of prevention. Specific measures include:

- **Eliminate local mosquito sources.** Mosquitoes develop in standing water. Often, large numbers of mosquitoes are produced from sources at or very near the home. Measures to limit mosquito sources around the home include drainage or removal of receptacles for standing water (old tires, toys, flower pots, cans, buckets, barrels, other containers that collect rain water); keeping swimming pools, decorative pools, children's wading pools, and bird-baths clean; and cleaning clogged rain gutters. Under certain circumstances, large-scale mosquito control measures may be conducted by community mosquito-control programs or public health officials. These efforts include drainage of standing water, use of larvicides in waters that are sources of mosquitoes, and use of pesticides to control biting adult mosquitoes.
- **Reduce exposure to mosquitoes.** Avoiding mosquito bites by limiting outdoor activities at times of high mosquito activity, which primarily occur at dusk and dawn, and screening of windows and doors can help reduce exposure to mosquitoes. Many parts of the United States also have mosquitoes that bite during the day, and some of

these have been found to transmit West Nile virus. Mosquito traps, ultrasonic repellers, and other devices marketed to prevent mosquitoes from biting people are not effective and should not be relied on to reduce mosquito biting.

• **Use barriers to protect skin.** Barriers include mosquito nets and screens for baby strollers or other areas where immobile children are placed. Additional protection can be gained, when practical, by using clothing to cover exposed skin (ie, long sleeves, long pants, shoes, and hats).

• **Discourage mosquitoes from biting.** Mosquitoes are attracted to people by odors on the skin and by carbon dioxide from the breath. The active ingredients in repellents make the user unattractive for feeding, but they do not kill the mosquitoes. Repellents should be used during outdoor activities when mosquitoes are present, especially in regions with arbovirus transmission, and should always be used according to the label instructions. Repellents are synthetic compounds or derivatives of plant oils. The most effective repellents for use on skin are products that contain diethyltolu-amide (DEET). Picaridin (KBR 3023), available in 7%, 15%, and 20% formulations in the United States, has been shown to be as effective as lower concentrations of DEET, with higher concentrations offering longer protection. Finally, the plant-based oil of lemon eucalyptus (OLE) and its synthetic equivalent p-menthane-3,8-diol also have been shown to have repellent activity. Products with a higher concentration of active ingredients protect longer and are appropriate for people who will be exposed to mos-quitoes during outdoor activities lasting many hours. Products with lower concentra-tions of active ingredients may be used where more transient protection is required, but they may require repeated applications. Studies in human volunteers document the association of active ingredient concentration with duration of repellent activity. For example, results of one study demonstrated an average duration of protection of 5 hours, 4 hours, 2 hours, and 1.5 hours for products with DEET concentrations of 23.8%, 20%, 6.7%, and 4.5%, respectively. Products containing picaridin may be as effective in repelling mosquitos as products with low concentrations of DEET but also require frequent reapplication for lasting protection. OLE appears to have similar dura-tion of action as products containing lower concentrations of DEET, with a product containing 30% OLE providing protection roughly equivalent to a product containing 15% DEET. All other plant products studied, including those based on citronella, pro-tected for less than 20 minutes. Ingestion of garlic or vitamin B_1 or wearing devices that emit sounds or impregnated wristbands all are ineffective measures.

DEET has been used worldwide since 1957, has been studied more extensively than any other repellent, and has a good safety profile. Concerns about potential toxicity, especially in children, are unfounded. Adverse effects are rare, are most often associated with ingestions; chronic use, or excessive use; and do not appear to be related to DEET concentration used. Urticaria and contact dermatitis have been reported in a small num-ber of people. Reports of encephalopathy have been rare, with 13 cases reported after skin application in children. Encephalopathy also has been reported after unintentional ingestion. DEET is irritating to eyes and mucous membranes. Concentrated formulations can damage plastic and certain fabrics. If used appropriately, DEET does not present a health problem.

Although concentrations of 10% to 15% DEET or lower have been recommended for children, there is no evidence that these concentrations are safer than 30% DEET. Products with DEET concentrations of 10% or less should not be used for exposures lasting more than 1 to 2 hours. There is no evidence that repellents that do not contain DEET are safer, and there are no safety data for other products in children. One approach is to select the lowest concentration that is effective for the amount of time spent outdoors. In 2001, the US Environmental Protection Agency (EPA) concluded that appropriate use of DEET at concentrations of up to 30% posed no significant risk to children or adults but that DEET should not be used in children younger than 2 months of age because of increased skin permeability. The American Academy of Pediatrics has supported this recommendation.[1] The Centers for Disease Control and Prevention currently recommends DEET at concentrations up to 30% for both adults and children older than 2 months of age.

Picaridin-containing compounds have been used as an insect repellent for years in Europe and Australia as a 20% formulation with no serious toxicity reported. Except for eye irritation, products containing oil of eucalyptus appear safe, although the EPA specifies that they should not be used on children younger than 3 years of age.

The EPA recommends the following precautions when using insect repellents. Recommendations for use of any of these insect repellents should be followed for children:

- Do not apply over cuts, wounds, or irritated or sunburned skin. Avoid areas around eyes and mouth.
- Do not spray onto the face; apply with hands.
- Use just enough to cover exposed skin.
- Do not apply to young children's hands, because they may rub it into their eyes or mouth.
- Do not allow young children to apply a product themselves.
- Do not apply under clothing.
- Do not use sprays in enclosed areas or near food.
- Repellents containing DEET, applied according to label instructions, can be used along with a separate sunscreen. No data are available regarding the use of other active repellent ingredients in combination with a sunscreen.
- Reapply if washed off by sweating or by getting wet.
- After returning indoors, wash treated skin with soap and water or bathe. Also, wash treated clothing before wearing again.
- If a child develops a rash or other reaction from any insect repellent, wash the repellent off with soap and water and contact the child's physician or the poison control center (800-222-1222) for guidance.

Permethrin-containing repellents are registered by the EPA for use on clothing, shoes, bed nets, and camping gear. Permethrin is a synthetic pyrethroid that is highly effective both as an insecticide and as a repellent for ticks, mosquitoes, and other arthropods. Permethrin can be sprayed onto clothes but should not be sprayed onto skin. Some manufacturers now offer permethrin-treated clothing, but because of lack of adequate safety and efficacy data, their use is not recommended for children at this time. Repellents should not be used on clothing or mosquito nets that young children may chew or suck.

---

[1] American Academy of Pediatrics Committee on Environmental Health. Pesticides. In: Etzel RA, ed. *Pediatric Environmental Health.* 2nd ed. Elk Grove Village, IL: American Academy of Pediatrics; 2003:323–359

PREVENTION OF ILLNESSES ASSOCIATED WITH RECREATIONAL WATER USE

Disease transmission through consumption or use of recreational water (eg, swimming pools, water slides, splash pools, lakes, oceans) continues to be a source of illness in the United States. Since the mid-1980s, the number of outbreaks related to recreational water activities has increased significantly, particularly in disinfected swimming venues (eg, swimming pools).[1] Therefore, preventing recreational water-related illness increasingly is becoming important for the health of children and adults. Recreational water illnesses (RWIs) are caused by swallowing, breathing, or having contact with contaminated water from swimming pools, spas, lakes, rivers, or oceans. Illnesses caused by recreational water exposure include infections of the gastrointestinal tract, respiratory tract, central nervous system, skin, ears, and eyes. During 2005–2006, 78 waterborne disease outbreaks associated with recreational water were reported in 31 states, causing illness in 4412 people and resulting in 116 hospitalizations and 5 deaths. Of these 78 outbreaks, the majority (74%) were associated with inadequately treated or disinfected recreational water (eg, wading pools intended for children, swimming pools, spas). Of the 78 outbreaks, 48 (62%) were outbreaks of gastroenteritis that resulted from infectious agents or chemicals, 11 (14%) were outbreaks of acute respiratory tract illnesses, and 11 (14%) were outbreaks of dermatitis or other skin conditions. The most common illness associated with treated water venues was gastroenteritis caused by *Cryptosporidium* species.

Swimming is a communal bathing activity by which the same water may be shared by dozens to thousands of people each day, depending on venue size (eg, "kiddy" splash pools, swimming pools, water parks). Fecal contamination of swimming venues is a common occurrence because of the high prevalence of diarrhea and fecal incontinence (particularly in young children) and the presence of residual fecal material on the bodies of swimmers (up to 10 g for young children). The largest outbreaks of waterborne diseases tend to occur during the summer months in treated water venues and result in gastrointestinal tract illness.

Chlorination of water at public swimming venues is one of the most commonly used methods to oxidize fecal matter and pathogens to protect swimmers from transmission of infectious diseases. Although many pathogens are inactivated rapidly by chlorination, several pathogens are moderately to highly resistant to chlorination and can survive for extended periods of time in chlorinated pools. *Cryptosporidium* oocysts can remain infectious for days in chlorine concentrations typically used in swimming pools, thus contributing to the role of *Cryptosporidium* species as the leading cause of pool-associated outbreaks of gastroenteritis. *Giardia* species and norovirus have been shown to survive in water chlorinated at concentrations typically used in swimming pools for up to 30 to 60 minutes and are well documented as causes of pool-associated disease outbreaks.

---

[1]Centers for Disease Control and Prevention. Surveillance for waterborne disease and outbreaks associated with drinking water and water not intended for drinking—United States, 2005–2006. *MMWR Surveill Summ.* 2008;57(SS-9):39–62

Recreational water use is an ideal means of amplifying pathogen transmission within a community because of chlorine-resistant pathogens, coupled with low infectious doses, a high prevalence of diarrhea in the general population, high pathogen excretion concentrations, and heavy use of swimming venues. As a result, one or more swimmers ill with diarrhea can contaminate large volumes of water and expose large numbers of coswimmers to pathogens, particularly if pool disinfection is inadequate or the pathogen is chlorine-resistant. However, RWI outbreaks generally are preventable and can be decreased substantially through a combination of proper pool maintenance, water disinfection, and improved swimmer hygiene and behavior.

CONTROL MEASURES

Swimming continues to be a safe and effective means of exercise. RWI transmission can be prevented by reducing contamination of swimming venues and exposure to contaminated water through adoption of the following practices:

- People with diarrhea should avoid recreational water activities, including swimming.
  - After cessation of symptoms, all people who had diarrhea attributable to *Cryptosporidium* species also should avoid recreational water activities for an additional 2 weeks. This is because of prolonged excretion of *Cryptosporidium* organisms after cessation of symptoms, the potential for intermittent diarrhea that may cause infected people to think symptoms have stopped, and the increased transmission potential in disinfected venues (eg, swimming pools) because of the parasite's high chlorine tolerance.
  - After cessation of symptoms, children who had diarrhea attributable to other potentially waterborne pathogens (eg, *Shigella* species, *Giardia* species, and norovirus) and who have not been toilet trained should avoid recreational water activities for 1 additional week.
- Avoid ingestion of recreational water.
- Practice good swimming hygiene by:
  - Showering, using soap and water, before entering recreational water.
  - Washing children thoroughly, especially the perianal area, with soap and water before allowing them to participate in recreational water activities.
  - Taking young children for regular bathroom breaks or checking diapers often.
  - Washing hands with soap and water after toilet use and diaper-changing activities. These should occur at a distance from the recreational water source.
  - Washing hands with soap and water before and after consumption of food and drink.
  Revised recommendations for responding to fecal accidents in disinfected swimming venues have been published.[1]

---

[1]Centers for Disease Control and Prevention. Notice to readers: revised recommendations for responding to fecal accidents in disinfected swimming venues. *MMWR Morb Mortal Wkly Rep.* 2008;57(6):151–152

Diseases Transmitted by Animals (Zoonoses): Household Pets, Including Nontraditional Pets, and Exposure to Animals in Public Settings[1]

Disease transmission from animals to humans is possible for children who interact with pets or with wild or domestic animals. Important zoonoses that may be encountered in North America, the common animal source or vector, and major modes of transmission are reviewed in disease-specific chapters in Section 3 and are listed in Appendix X (p 864). Most households in the United States contain one pet or more. The number of families with nontraditional pets, defined as (1) imported, nonnative species or species that originally were nonnative but now are bred in the United States; (2) indigenous wildlife; or (3) wildlife hybrids (offspring of wildlife crossbred with domestic animals), has increased in recent years. Infants and children also come in contact with animals at many venues outside the home, including zoos, farms, shopping malls, schools, hospitals, animal swap meets, agricultural fairs, and petting zoos. Examples of nontraditional pets and animals commonly encountered in public settings are listed in Table 2.21, p 199.

Exposure to animals can pose significant infection risks to all people, but children younger than 5 years of age, pregnant women, the elderly, and people of all ages with immunodeficiencies are at higher risk of serious infections. The increased infection risk for children younger than 5 years of age is attributable, in part, to children's less-than-optimal hygiene practices and developing immune systems. Children younger than 5 years of age also are at increased risk of injury from animals because of their size and behavior. Bites, scratches, kicks, falls, and crush injuries to hands or feet or from being pinned between an animal and a fixed object can occur.

Nontraditional pets pose a potential risk of infection and injury. Most imported nonnative animal species are caught in the wild rather than bred in captivity. These animals are held and transported in close contact with multiple other species, thus increasing the transmission risk of potential pathogens for humans and domestic animals. Some nonnative animals are brought into the United States illegally, thus bypassing rules established to reduce introduction of disease and potentially dangerous animals. In addition, as an animal matures, its physical and behavioral characteristics can result in an increased risk of injuries to children. The behavior of captive indigenous wildlife and wildlife hybrids cannot be predicted. These potential risks are enhanced when there is an inadequate understanding of disease transmission and methods to prevent transmission; animal behavior; or how to maintain appropriate facilities, environment, or nutrition for captive animals. Among nontraditional pets, reptiles pose a particular risk because of high carriage rates of *Salmonella* species, the intermittent shedding of *Salmonella* in their feces, and persistence of *Salmonella* organisms in the environment. The US Food and Drug Administration ban on commercial distribution of turtles with shells less than 4 inches long in 1975 resulted in

---

[1]Pickering LK, Marano N, Bocchini JA, Angulo FJ, American Academy of Pediatrics, Committee on Infectious Diseases. Exposure to nontraditional pets at home and to animals in public settings: risks to children. *Pediatrics*. 2008;122(4):876–886

Table 2.21. Nontraditional Pets and/or Animals That May Be Encountered in Public Settings[a]

Category	Examples
Amphibians	Frogs, toads, newts, salamanders
Fish	Many types
Mammals	
Wildlife	Raccoons, skunks, foxes, coyotes, civet cats, tigers, lions, bobcats, bears, nonhuman primates
Domesticated livestock	Cattle, pigs, goats, sheep
Poultry	Baby chicks, ducklings, goslings, and turkeys
Equines	Horses, mules, donkeys, zebras
Weasels	Ferrets, minks, sables, skunks
Lagomorphs	Rabbits, hares, pikas
Rodents	Mice, rats, hamsters, gerbils, guinea pigs, chinchillas, gophers, lemmings, squirrels, chipmunks, prairie dogs, hedgehogs
Feral animals	Cats, dogs, horses, swine
Reptiles	Turtles, lizards, iguanas, snakes, alligators

[a]Pickering LK, Marano N, Bocchini JA, Angulo FJ; American Academy of Pediatrics, Committee on Infectious Diseases. Exposure to nontraditional pets at home and to animals in public settings: risks to children. *Pediatrics.* 2008;122(4):876–886

a sustained reduction of human *Salmonella* infections. *Salmonella* infections also have been described as a result of contact with hedgehogs, hamsters, and rodents and with baby chicks and other baby poultry, including ducklings, goslings, and turkeys.

Infectious diseases, injuries, and other health problems can occur after contact with animals in public settings. Enteric bacteria and parasites pose the highest infection risk. Individual cases and outbreaks associated with *Salmonella* species, *Escherichia coli* O157:H7, *Campylobacter* species, *Giardia* species, and *Cryptosporidium* species have been reported. Ruminant livestock (cattle, sheep, and goats) are the major source of infection, but poultry, rodents, and other domestic and wild animals also are potential sources and often are asymptomatic carriers of potential human pathogens. Direct contact with animals (especially young animals), contamination of the environment or food or water sources, and inadequate hand hygiene facilities at animal exhibits all have been implicated as reasons for infection in these public settings. Unusual infection or exposure has been reported occasionally; rabies has occurred in animals in a petting zoo, pet store, and county fair, necessitating prophylaxis of adults and children.

Contact with animals has numerous positive benefits, including opportunities for education and entertainment. However, many pet owners and people in the process of choosing a pet are unaware of the potential risks posed by pets. Pediatricians, veterinarians, and other health care professionals are in a unique position to offer advice on proper pet selection, provide information about safe pet ownership and responsibility, and minimize risks to infants and children. Pet size and temperament should be matched to the age and behavior of an infant or child. Acquisition and ownership of nontraditional pets should be discouraged in households with young children. Information brochures and posters are available for display in physician and veterinarian offices so parents can be educated about the guidelines available for safe pet selection and appropriate handling (**www.cdc.gov/healthypets/index.htm, www.cdc.healthypets/ health_prof.htm** and **www.avma.org/animal_health/brochures/pet_ selection.asp.**

Young children should be supervised closely when in contact with animals at home or in public settings, and children should be educated about appropriate human-animal interactions. Parents should be made aware of recommendations for prevention of human diseases and injuries from exposure to pets, including nontraditional pets and animals in the home and animals in public settings (Table 2.22).

Questions regarding pet and animal contact should be part of well-child evaluations and the evaluation of a suspected infectious disease.

Table 2.22. Guidelines for Prevention of Human Diseases From Exposure to Pets, Nontraditional Pets, and Animals in Public Settings[a]

General
- Wash hands immediately after contact with animals, animal products, or their environment
- Supervise hand washing for children younger than 5 years of age
- Wash hands after handling animal-derived pet treats
- Never bring wild animals home, and never adopt wild animals as pets
- Teach children never to handle unfamiliar, wild, or domestic animals, even if animals appear friendly
- Avoid rough play with animals to prevent scratches or bites
- Children should not be allowed to kiss pets or put their hands or other objects into their mouths after handling animals
- Do not permit nontraditional pets to roam or fly freely in the house or allow nontraditional or domestic pets to have contact with wild animals
- Do not permit animals in areas where food or drink are prepared or consumed
- Administer rabies vaccine to mammals as appropriate
- Keep animals clean and free of intestinal parasites, fleas, ticks, mites, and lice
- People at increased risk of infection or serious complications of salmonellosis (eg, children younger than 5 years of age, older adults, and immunocompromised hosts) should avoid contact with animal-derived pet treats

Animals Visiting Schools and Child-Care Facilities
- Designate specific areas for animal contact
- Display animals in enclosed cages or under appropriate restraint
- Do not allow food in animal-contact areas
- Always supervise children, especially those younger than 5 y, during interaction with animals
- Obtain a certificate of veterinary inspection for visiting animals and/or proof of rabies immunization according to local or state requirements
- Properly clean and disinfect all areas where animals have been present
- Consult with parents or guardians to determine special considerations needed for children who are immunocompromised or who have allergies or asthma

Table 2.22. Guidelines for Prevention of Human Diseases From Exposure to Pets, Nontraditional Pets, and Animals in Public Settings,[a] continued

- Animals not recommended in schools, child-care settings, and hospitals include nonhuman primates, inherently dangerous animals (lions, tigers, cougars, bears, wolf/dog hybrids), mammals at high risk of transmitting rabies (bats, raccoons, skunks, foxes, and coyotes), aggressive animals or animals with unpredictable behavior, stray animals with unknown health history, reptiles, and amphibians

- Ensure that people who provide animals for educational purposes are knowledgeable regarding animal handling and zoonotic disease issues

Public Settings

- Venue operators must know about risks of disease and injury
- Venue operators and staff must maintain a safe environment
- Venue operators and staff must educate visitors about the risk of disease and injury and provide appropriate preventive measures

Animal Specific

- Children younger than 5 years of age and immunocompromised people should avoid contact in public settings with reptiles, amphibians, rodents, ferrets, baby poultry (chicks, ducklings), and any items that have been in contact with these animals or their environments

- Reptiles, amphibians, rodents, ferrets, and baby poultry (chicks, ducklings) should be kept out of households that contain children younger than 5 years of age, immunocompromised people, or people with sickle cell disease and should not be allowed in child-care centers

- Reptiles, amphibians, rodents, and baby poultry should not be permitted to roam freely throughout a home or living area and should not be permitted in kitchens or other food-preparation areas

- Disposable gloves should be used when cleaning fish aquariums, and aquarium water should not be disposed in sinks used for food preparation or for obtaining drinking water

- Mammals at high risk of transmitting rabies (bats, raccoons, skunks, foxes, and coyotes) should not be touched by children

---

[a]Pickering LK, Marano N, Bocchini JA, Angulo FJ; American Academy of Pediatrics, Committee on Infectious Diseases. Exposure to nontraditional pets at home and to animals in public settings: risks to children. *Pediatrics.* 2008;122(4):876–886

Summaries of Infectious Diseases

Actinomycosis

CLINICAL MANIFESTATIONS: The 3 major anatomic types of disease are cervicofacial, thoracic, and abdominal. **Cervicofacial** lesions are the most common and often occur after tooth extraction, oral surgery, or facial trauma or are associated with carious teeth. Localized pain and induration progress to "woody hard" nodular lesions that can be complicated by draining sinus tracts that usually are located at the angle of the jaw or in the submandibular region. The infection usually spreads by direct invasion of adjacent tissues. Infection also may contribute to chronic obstructive tonsillitis. **Thoracic** disease most commonly is secondary to aspiration of oropharyngeal secretions and occurs rarely after esophageal disruption secondary to surgery or nonpenetrating trauma or may be an extension of cervicofacial infection. Disease manifests as pneumonia, which can be complicated by abscesses, empyema, and rarely, pleurodermal sinuses. Focal or multifocal masses may be mistaken for tumors. **Abdominal** actinomycosis usually is attributable to penetrating trauma or intestinal perforation. The appendix and cecum are the most common sites, and symptoms are similar to those of appendicitis. Slowly developing masses may simulate abdominal or retroperitoneal neoplasms. Intra-abdominal abscesses and peritoneal-dermal draining sinuses occur eventually. Chronic localized disease often forms sinus tracts that drain a purulent discharge. Other sites of actinomycosis infection include the liver, pelvis (which, in some cases, has been linked to use of intrauterine devices), and brain. Primary cutaneous actinomycosis also has been reported.

ETIOLOGY: *Actinomyces israelii* is the usual cause. *A israelii* and at least 5 other *Actinomyces* species are slow-growing, microaerophilic or facultative anaerobic, gram-positive, filamentous branching bacilli that can be part of the normal oral, gastrointestinal, or vaginal flora. *Actinomyces* species frequently are copathogens in tissues harboring multiple species. *Actinobacillus actinomycetemcomitans* is a frequent copathogen, and its isolation may predict the presence of actinomycosis.

EPIDEMIOLOGY: *Actinomyces* species are worldwide in distribution. The organisms are components of the endogenous oral and gastrointestinal tract flora. *Actinomyces* species are opportunistic pathogens, and disease results from penetrating (including human bite wounds) and nonpenetrating trauma. Infection is rare in infants and children. Overt, microbiologically confirmed, monomicrobial disease caused by *Actinomyces* species has become rare in the era of antimicrobial agents.

The **incubation period** varies from several days to several years.

DIAGNOSTIC TESTS: A microscopic demonstration of beaded, branched, gram-positive bacilli in purulent material or tissue specimens suggests the diagnosis. The specimen should be taken only from a normally sterile site. Acid-fast staining can be used to distinguish *Actinomyces* species, which are acid-fast negative, from *Nocardia* species, which are variably acid-fast positive. "Sulfur granules" in drainage or loculations of purulent material usually are yellow and may be visualized microscopically or macroscopically and suggest the diagnosis when present. A Gram stain of sulfur granules discloses a dense reticulum of filaments. Immunofluorescent stains for *Actinomyces* species are available. *Actinomyces* species can be identified in tissue specimens using the 16s rRNA sequencing and polymerase chain reaction assay. Although most *Actinomyces* species are microaerophilic or facultative anaerobic, specimens must be obtained, transported, and cultured anaerobically on semiselective media.

TREATMENT: Initial therapy should include intravenous penicillin G or ampicillin for 4 to 6 weeks followed by high doses of oral penicillin (up to 2 g/day for adults) for a total of 6 to 12 months. Amoxicillin, erythromycin, clindamycin, doxycycline, and tetracycline are alternative antimicrobial choices. Tetracyclines are not recommended for pregnant women or children younger than 8 years of age. Surgical drainage often is a necessary adjunct to medical management and may allow for a shorter duration of antimicrobial treatment.

ISOLATION OF THE HOSPITALIZED PATIENT: Standard precautions are recommended. There is no person-to-person spread.

CONTROL MEASURES: Appropriate oral hygiene, regular dental care, and careful cleansing of wounds, including human bite wounds, can prevent infection.

Adenovirus Infections

CLINICAL MANIFESTATIONS: The most common site of adenovirus infection is the upper respiratory tract. Manifestations include symptoms of the common cold, pharyngitis, tonsillitis, otitis media, and pharyngoconjunctival fever. Life-threatening disseminated infection, severe pneumonia, meningitis, and encephalitis occur occasionally, especially among young infants and immunocompromised hosts. Adenoviruses occasionally cause acute hemorrhagic conjunctivitis, a pertussis-like syndrome, croup, bronchiolitis, exudative tonsillitis, pneumonia, or hemorrhagic cystitis. Enteric adenovirus serotypes cause gastroenteritis.

ETIOLOGY: Adenoviruses are double-stranded, nonenveloped DNA viruses; at least 51 distinct serotypes divided into 6 species (A through F) cause human infections. Some adenovirus serotypes are associated primarily with respiratory tract disease, and others are associated primarily with gastroenteritis (types 40, 41, and to a lesser extent, 31).

Adenovirus serotype 14 is a rarely reported but emerging serotype of adenovirus that can cause severe and sometimes fatal respiratory tract illness in patients of all ages, including healthy young adults. During early 2007, 140 cases of confirmed adenovirus serotype 14 respiratory tract illness were identified in clusters of patients in several states. Of these patients, 38% were hospitalized, including 17% who were admitted to intensive care units; 5% of the patients died. The isolates were distinct from the adenovirus serotype 14 reference strain isolated in 1955, suggesting the emergence and spread of a new adenovirus serotype 14 variant in the United States.[1]

[1] Centers for Disease Control and Prevention. Acute respiratory disease associated with adenovirus serotype 14—four states, 2006–2007 *MMWR Morb Mortal Wkly Rep.* 2007;56(45):1181–1184

EPIDEMIOLOGY: Infection in infants and children can occur at any age. Adenoviruses causing respiratory tract infections usually are transmitted by respiratory tract secretions through person-to-person contact, airborne droplets, and fomites, the latter because adenoviruses are stable in the environment. Other routes of transmission have not been defined clearly. The conjunctiva can provide a portal of entry. Outbreaks of febrile respiratory tract illness can be a common, significant problem in military trainees. Community outbreaks of adenovirus-associated pharyngoconjunctival fever have been attributed to exposure to water from contaminated swimming pools and fomites, such as shared towels. Health care-associated transmission of adenoviral respiratory tract, conjunctival, and gastrointestinal tract infections can occur in hospitals, residential institutions, and nursing homes from exposures between infected health care professionals, patients, or contaminated equipment. Adenovirus infections in transplant recipients can occur from donor tissues. Epidemic keratoconjunctivitis has been associated with equipment used during eye examinations. Enteric strains of adenoviruses are transmitted by the fecal-oral route. Adenoviruses do not demonstrate the marked seasonality of other respiratory tract viruses, although the incidence of adenovirus-induced respiratory tract disease is increased slightly during late winter, spring, and early summer. Enteric disease occurs throughout the year and primarily affects children younger than 4 years of age. Adenovirus infections are most communicable during the first few days of an acute illness, but persistent and intermittent shedding for longer periods, even months, is common. Asymptomatic infections are common. Reinfection can occur.

The **incubation period** for respiratory tract infection varies from 2 to 14 days; for gastroenteritis, the incubation period is 3 to 10 days.

DIAGNOSTIC TESTS: The preferred methods for diagnosis of adenovirus infection include cell culture as well as antigen and DNA detection. Adenoviruses associated with respiratory tract disease can be isolated from pharyngeal and eye secretions and feces by inoculation of specimens into susceptible cell cultures. A pharyngeal or ocular isolate is more suggestive of recent infection than is a fecal isolate, which may indicate prolonged carriage or recent infection. Adenovirus antigens can be detected in less than 30 minutes in a variety of body fluids from infected people by commercial immunoassay techniques. These rapid assays especially are useful for diagnosis of diarrheal disease, because enteric adenovirus types 40 and 41 usually cannot be isolated in standard cell cultures, and for ocular disease. Adenoviruses also can be identified by electron microscopic examination of respiratory or stool specimens. Multiple methods to detect group-reactive hexon antigens of the virus in body secretions and tissue have been developed. Also, viral DNA can be detected and quantitated by polymerase chain reaction assays available from commercial reference laboratories. Adenovirus typing is available from some reference and research laboratories, although its clinical utility is limited. Serotyping can be determined by hemagglutination inhibition or serum neutralization tests with selected antisera or by hexon gene sequence molecular methods. Serodiagnosis is used primarily for epidemiologic studies.

TREATMENT: Treatment of adenovirus infection is supportive. Randomized clinical trials evaluating specific antiviral therapy have not been performed. However, case reports of successful intravenous cidofovir in immunocompromised patients with severe adenovirus disease have been published.

ISOLATION OF THE HOSPITALIZED PATIENT: In addition to standard precautions for young children with respiratory tract infections, contact and droplet precautions are indicated for the duration of hospitalization. For patients with conjunctivitis and for diapered and incontinent children with adenoviral gastroenteritis, contact precautions in addition to standard precautions are indicated for the duration of the illness.

CONTROL MEASURES: Children who participate in group child care, particularly children from 6 months through 2 years of age, are at increased risk of adenoviral respiratory tract infections and gastroenteritis. Effective measures for preventing spread of adenovirus infection in this setting have not been determined, but frequent hand hygiene is recommended. If 2 or more children in a group care setting develop conjunctivitis in the same period, advice should be sought from the program health consultant or state health department.

Adequate chlorination of swimming pools is recommended to prevent pharyngoconjunctival fever. Epidemic keratoconjunctivitis associated with ophthalmologic practice can be difficult to control and requires use of single-dose medication dispensing and strict attention to hand hygiene and instrument sterilization procedures. Effective disinfection can be accomplished by immersing contaminated equipment in a 1% solution of sodium hypochlorite or washing with chlorhexidine gluconate for 10 minutes or by steam autoclaving.

Health care professionals with known or suspected adenoviral conjunctivitis should avoid direct patient contact for 14 days after onset of disease in the most recently involved eye. Because adenoviruses are difficult to inactivate, they can remain viable on skin, fomites, and environmental surfaces. Thus, assiduous adherence to hand hygiene and use of disposable gloves when caring for infected patients are recommended.

Amebiasis

CLINICAL MANIFESTATIONS: Clinical syndromes associated with *Entamoeba histolytica* infection include noninvasive intestinal infection, intestinal amebiasis, ameboma, and liver abscess. Disease is more severe in the very young, the elderly, and pregnant women. Patients with noninvasive intestinal infection may be asymptomatic or may have nonspecific intestinal tract complaints. People with intestinal amebiasis (amebic colitis) generally have 1 to 3 weeks of increasingly severe diarrhea progressing to grossly bloody dysenteric stools with lower abdominal pain and tenesmus. Weight loss is common, but fever occurs only in a minority of patients (8%–38%). Symptoms may be chronic and may mimic inflammatory bowel disease. Progressive involvement of the colon may produce toxic megacolon, fulminant colitis, ulceration of the colon and perianal area, and rarely, perforation. Progression may occur in patients inappropriately treated with corticosteroids or antimotility drugs. An ameboma may occur as an annular lesion of the cecum or ascending colon that may be mistaken for colonic carcinoma or as a tender extrahepatic mass mimicking a pyogenic abscess. Amebomas usually resolve with antiamebic therapy and do not require surgery.

In a small proportion of patients, extraintestinal disease may occur. Although the liver is the most common extraintestinal site, the lungs, pleural space, pericardium, brain, skin, and genitourinary tract also may be involved. Liver abscess may be acute, with fever, abdominal pain, tachypnea, liver tenderness, and hepatomegaly; or chronic, with weight loss, vague abdominal symptoms, and irritability. Rupture of abscesses into the abdomen or chest may lead to death. Evidence of recent intestinal infection usually is absent.

ETIOLOGY: The genus *Entamoeba* includes 6 species that live in human intestine. Three of these species are identical morphologically: *E histolytica, Entamoeba dispar,* and *Entamoeba moshkovskii.* The pathogenic *E histolytica* and the nonpathogenic *E dispar* and *E moshkovskii* are excreted as cysts or trophozoites in stools of infected people.

EPIDEMIOLOGY: *E histolytica* can be found worldwide but is more prevalent in people of lower socioeconomic status who live in economically developing countries, where the prevalence of amebic infection may be as high as 50% in some communities. Groups at increased risk of infection in industrialized countries include immigrants from or long-term visitors to areas with endemic infection, institutionalized people, and men who have sex with men. *E histolytica* is transmitted via amebic cysts by the fecal-oral route. Ingested cysts, which are unaffected by gastric acid, undergo excystation in the alka-line small intestine and produce trophozoites that infect the colon. Cysts that develop subsequently are the source of transmission, especially from asymptomatic cyst excret-ers. Infected patients excrete cysts intermittently, sometimes for years if untreated. Transmission occasionally has been associated with contaminated food, water, and enema equipment. Sexual transmission also may occur.

The **incubation period** is variable, ranging from a few days to months or years but commonly is 2 to 4 weeks.

DIAGNOSTIC TESTS: A presumptive diagnosis of intestinal infection depends on identi-fying trophozoites or cysts in stool specimens. Examination of serial specimens may be necessary. Specimens of stool, endoscopy scrapings (not swabs), and biopsies should be examined by wet mount within 30 minutes of collection and fixed in formalin or polyvi-nyl alcohol (available in kits) for concentration and permanent staining. *E histolytica* is not distinguished easily from the noninvasive and more prevalent *E dispar* and *E moshkovskii,* although trophozoites containing ingested red blood cells are more likely to be *E histolytica.* Polymerase chain reaction, isoenzyme analysis, and monoclonal antibody-based antigen detection assays can differentiate *E histolytica, E dispar,* and *E moshkovskii.*

The indirect hemagglutination (IHA) test has been replaced by commercially avail-able enzyme immunoassay (EIA) test kits for routine serodiagnosis of amebiasis. The EIA test detects antibody specific for *E histolytica* in approximately 95% of patients with extraintestinal amebiasis, 70% of patients with active intestinal infection, and 10% of asymptomatic people who are passing cysts of *E histolytica.* Patients may continue to have positive test results even after adequate therapy.

Ultrasonography and computed tomography can identify effectively liver abscesses and other extraintestinal sites of infection. Aspirates from a liver abscess usually show neither trophozoites nor leukocytes.

TREATMENT[1]: Treatment involves elimination of the tissue-invading trophozoites as well as organisms in the intestinal lumen. *E dispar* and *E moshkovskii* infections do not require treatment. Corticosteroids and antimotility drugs administered to people with amebiasis can worsen symptoms and the disease process. In settings where tests to distinguish species are not available, treatment should be given to symptomatic people on the basis of posi-tive results of microscopic examination. The following regimens are recommended:

---

[1] For further information, see Drugs for Parasitic Infections, p 783.

- **Asymptomatic cyst excreters (intraluminal infections):** treat with a luminal amebicide, such as iodoquinol, paromomycin, or diloxanide.
- **Patients with mild to moderate or severe intestinal symptoms or extraintestinal disease (including liver abscess):** treat with metronidazole or tinidazole, followed by a therapeutic course of a luminal amebicide (iodoquinol or paromomycin). Nitazoxanide also may be effective for mild to moderate intestinal amebiasis, although it is only approved by the US Food and Drug Administration for treatment of diarrhea caused by *Giardia* species or *Cryptosporidium* species.

Dehydroemetine followed by a therapeutic course of a luminal amebicide may be considered for patients for whom treatment of invasive disease has failed or cannot be tolerated. However, dehydroemetine has significant toxicity and should be used with caution. An alternate treatment for liver abscess is chloroquine phosphate concomitantly with metronidazole or tinidazole, followed by a therapeutic course of a luminal amebicide.

Surgical aspiration occasionally may be required when response of the abscess to medical therapy is unsatisfactory. To prevent spontaneous rupture of an abscess, patients with large liver abscesses may benefit from percutaneous or surgical aspiration.

Follow-up stool examination is recommended after completion of therapy, because no pharmacologic regimen is effective in eradicating intestinal infection completely. Household members and other suspected contacts also should have adequate stool examinations performed and be treated if results are positive for *E histolytica*.

ISOLATION OF THE HOSPITALIZED PATIENT: In addition to standard precautions, contact precautions are recommended for the duration of illness.

CONTROL MEASURES: Careful hand hygiene after defecation, sanitary disposal of fecal material, and treatment of drinking water will control the spread of infection. Sexual transmission may be controlled by use of condoms and avoidance of sexual practices that may permit fecal-oral transmission.

Amebic Meningoencephalitis and Keratitis
(*Naegleria fowleri*, *Acanthamoeba* species, and *Balamuthia mandrillaris*)

CLINICAL MANIFESTATIONS: *Naegleria fowleri* can cause a rapidly progressive, almost always fatal, primary amebic meningoencephalitis. Early symptoms include fever, headache, vomiting, and sometimes, disturbances of smell and taste. The illness progresses rapidly to signs of meningoencephalitis, including nuchal rigidity, lethargy, confusion, and altered level of consciousness. Seizures are common. Death occurs within a week of onset of symptoms. No distinct clinical features differentiate this disease from fulminant bacterial meningitis.

Granulomatous amebic encephalitis caused by *Acanthamoeba* species and *Balamuthia mandrillaris* has a more insidious onset and progression of manifestations occurring weeks to months after exposure. Signs and symptoms may include personality changes, seizures, headaches, nuchal rigidity, ataxia, cranial nerve palsies, hemiparesis, and other focal deficits. Fever often is low grade and intermittent. The course may resemble that of a bacterial brain abscess or a brain tumor. Chronic granulomatous skin lesions (pustules, nodules, ulcers) may be present without central nervous system involvement, particularly in patients with acquired immunodeficiency syndrome, and lesions may present on the midface for months before brain involvement in immunocompetent hosts.

Amebic keratitis, usually attributable to *Acanthamoeba* species, occurs primarily in people who wear soft contact lenses. The most common symptoms are pain (often out of proportion to clinical signs), photophobia, tearing, and foreign body sensation. Characteristic clinical findings include radial keratoneuritis and stromal ring infiltrate. Amebic keratitis generally follows an indolent course and initially may resemble herpes simplex or bacterial keratitis; delay in diagnosis is associated with worse outcomes.

ETIOLOGY: *N fowleri*, *Acanthamoeba* species, and *B mandrillaris* are free-living amebae that exist as motile, infectious trophozoites and environmentally hardy cysts.

EPIDEMIOLOGY: *N fowleri* is found in warm fresh water and moist soil. Most infections with *N fowleri* have been associated with swimming in warm, natural bodies of water, such as hot springs, but other sources have included tap water, contaminated and poorly chlorinated swimming pools, and baths. Small outbreaks associated with swimming in a warm lake or swimming pool have been reported. Disease has been reported worldwide but is uncommon. In the United States, infection occurs primarily in the summer and usually affects children and young adults. The trophozoites of the parasite invade the brain directly from the nose along the olfactory nerves via the cribriform plate. In infections with *N fowleri*, trophozoites but not cysts can be visualized in sections of brain.

The **incubation period** for *N fowleri* infection is 1 to 2 weeks.

Acanthamoeba species and *B mandrillaris* cause granulomatous amebic encephalitis. *Acanthamoeba* species are distributed worldwide and are found in soil, fresh and brackish water, dust, hot tubs, and sewage. The environmental niche of *B mandrillaris* is not known clearly, although it has been isolated from soil. Central nervous system infection attributable to *Acanthamoeba* occurs primarily in debilitated and immunocompromised people. However, some patients infected with *B mandrillaris* have had no demonstrable underlying disease or defect. Acquisition probably occurs by inhalation or direct contact with contaminated soil or water. The primary focus of infection most likely is skin or respiratory tract, followed by hematogenous spread to the brain.

Acanthamoeba organisms also cause keratitis, primarily among healthy contact lens users. Poor contact lens hygiene and/or disinfection practices, swimming with contact lenses, and preceding ocular trauma are important risk factors. In 2007, a multipurpose soft contact lens solution was found to be associated strongly with a nationwide increase in cases of *Acanthamoeba* keratitis; the solution, which was found to kill *Acanthamoeba* organisms inadequately, was recalled.[1]

The **incubation period** for these infections is unknown.

DIAGNOSTIC TESTS: *N fowleri* infection can be documented by microscopic demonstration of the motile trophozoites on a wet mount of centrifuged cerebrospinal fluid (CSF). The organism also can be cultured on 1.5% nonnutrient agar layered with gram-negative bacteria held in saline solution. Immunofluorescent and polymerase chain reaction (PCR) assays performed on CSF and biopsy material to determine the species of the organism are available through the Centers for Disease Control and Prevention. CSF shows polymorphonuclear pleocytosis, an increased protein concentration, a normal to very low glucose concentration, and no bacteria.

---

[1]Centers for Disease Control and Prevention. Acanthamoeba keratitis multiple states, 2005–2007. *MMWR Morb Mortal Wkly Rep.* 2007;56(21):532–534

In infection with *Acanthamoeba* species, trophozoites and cysts can be visualized in sections of brain, lungs, skin, or corneal scrapings. Trophozoites and cysts of *B mandrillaris* also are evident in sections of brain, lungs, and skin. CSF typically shows a mononuclear pleocytosis and an increased protein concentration with normal or low glucose but no organisms. *Acanthamoeba* species, but not *Balamuthia* species, can be cultured by the same method used for *N fowleri*. *B mandrillaris* can be cultured on mammalian cell culture. Real-time PCR has been developed by the Centers for Disease Control and Prevention for detection of the nucleic acid of *Acanthamoeba* species, *N fowleri*, and *B mandrillaris* in clinical specimens.

TREATMENT: If meningoencephalitis caused by *N fowleri* is suspected because of the presence of organisms in the CSF, therapy should not be withheld while waiting for results of confirmatory diagnostic tests. Amphotericin B is the drug of choice, although treatment usually is unsuccessful, with only a few cases of complete recovery having been documented. Recovery has occurred after treatment with amphotericin B alone or in combination with other agents, such as miconazole or ornidazole plus rifampin, although rifampin probably has no additional effect. Early diagnosis and institution of high-dose drug therapy is thought to be important for optimizing outcome.

Effective treatment for central nervous system infections caused by *Acanthamoeba* species and *B mandrillaris* has not been established. *Acanthamoeba* species are susceptible in vitro to a variety of antimicrobial agents (eg, pentamidine, flucytosine, ketoconazole, clotrimazole, and to a lesser degree, amphotericin B). The antifungal drug voriconazole and the alkyl phosphocholine agent miltefosine have been shown to be highly active against *Acanthamoeba* species, and several patients treated with these drugs as well as pentamidine have recovered from this infection. Three patients survived *B mandrillaris* infection following treatment with flucytosine, pentamidine, sulfadiazine, fluconazole, and clarithromycin in addition to surgical resection of the central nervous system lesion. Some patients with skin lesions attributable to *Acanthamoeba* species have been treated successfully by first washing lesions with chlorhexidine gluconate and then applying topical ketoconazole cream 3 to 4 times a day. Patients also have been given intravenous pentamidine and oral itraconazole.

Patients with keratitis should be evaluated by an ophthalmologist. Topical chlorhexidine and polyhexamethylene biguanide, either alone or in combination, have been used successfully in a large number of patients. Propamidine isethionate or hexamidine may be combined with either chlorhexidine or polyhexamethylene biguanide. The combination of chlorhexidine, natamycin, and débridement also has been successful. Most cysts are resistant to neomycin, which no longer is recommended. Azole antifungal drugs (ketoconazole, itraconazole) have been used as oral or topical adjuncts. Use of corticosteroids is controversial. Early diagnosis and therapy are important for a good outcome (see Drugs for Parasitic Infections, p 783).

ISOLATION OF THE HOSPITALIZED PATIENT: Standard precautions are recommended.

CONTROL MEASURES: People should avoid swimming in warm, stagnant fresh water. *Acanthamoeba* organisms are resistant to freezing, drying, and the usual concentrations of chlorine found in drinking water and swimming pools.

Soft contact lens users should maintain good contact lens hygiene and disinfection practices, use only sterile solutions to clean lenses, and avoid swimming with lenses.

Anthrax

CLINICAL MANIFESTATIONS: Depending on the route of infection, anthrax can occur in 3 forms: cutaneous, inhalation, and gastrointestinal. **Cutaneous** anthrax begins as a pruritic papule or vesicle that enlarges and ulcerates in 1 to 2 days, with subsequent formation of a central black eschar. The lesion characteristically is painless, with surrounding edema, hyperemia, and regional lymphadenopathy. Patients may have associated fever, malaise, and headache. **Inhalation** anthrax is a frequently lethal form of the disease and is a medical emergency. A nonspecific prodrome of fever, sweats, nonproductive cough, chest pain, headache, myalgia, malaise, and nausea and vomiting may occur initially, but illness progresses to the fulminant phase 2 to 5 days later. In some cases, a period of improvement can intervene between prodromal symptoms and overwhelming illness. Fulminant manifestations include hypotension, dyspnea, hypoxia, cyanosis, and shock occurring as a result of hemorrhagic mediastinal lymphadenitis, hemorrhagic pleural effusions, bacteremia, and toxemia. A widened mediastinum is the classic finding on imaging of the chest. Pleural effusions and hemorrhagic infiltrates can be present, but initially, changes on chest radiography may be subtle. **Gastrointestinal tract** disease can present as 2 clinical syndromes—intestinal or oropharyngeal. Patients with the intestinal form have symptoms of nausea, anorexia, vomiting, and fever progressing to severe abdominal pain, massive ascites, hematemesis, and bloody diarrhea. Oropharyngeal anthrax may include posterior oropharyngeal ulcers that are associated with marked, often unilateral neck swelling, regional adenopathy, fever, and sepsis. Hemorrhagic meningitis can result from hematogenous spread of the organism after acquiring any form of disease and may develop without any other apparent clinical presentation. The case-fatality rate for patients with appropriately treated cutaneous anthrax usually is less than 1%, but for inhalation or gastrointestinal tract disease, mortality often exceeds 50% and approaches 100% for meningitis in the absence of antimicrobial therapy.

ETIOLOGY: *Bacillus anthracis* is an aerobic, gram-positive, encapsulated, spore-forming, nonmotile rod. *B anthracis* has 3 major virulence factors: an antiphagocytic capsule and 2 exotoxins, called lethal and edema toxins. The toxins are responsible for the significant morbidity and clinical manifestations of hemorrhage, edema, and necrosis.

EPIDEMIOLOGY: Anthrax is a zoonotic disease that occurs in many rural regions of the world. *B anthracis* spores can remain viable in the soil for decades, representing a potential source of infection for livestock through ingestion. Natural infection of humans occurs through contact with infected animals or contaminated animal products, including carcasses, hides, hair, wool, meat, and bone meal. Internationally, outbreaks of gastrointestinal tract anthrax have occurred after ingestion of undercooked or raw meat. In the United States, the incidence of naturally occurring human anthrax decreased from an estimated 130 cases annually in the early 1900s to one case in 2006 in a person with inhalation anthrax acquired while processing imported, untreated animal hides and 1 case in 2007 of cutaneous disease from goat hide exposure. The vast majority (more than 95%) of US cases historically have been cutaneous infections among animal handlers or mill workers.

    B anthracis is one of the most likely agents to be used as a biological weapon, because (1) its spores are highly stabile; (2) spores can infect via the respiratory route; and (3) the resulting inhalation anthrax has a high mortality rate. In 1979, an accidental release of *B anthracis* spores from a military microbiology facility in the former Soviet Union resulted in at least 69 deaths. In 2001, 22 cases of anthrax (11 inhalation, 11 cutaneous) were identified in the United States after intentional contamination of the mail; 5 (45%) of the inhalation anthrax cases were fatal. In addition to aerosolization, there is a theoretical health risk associated with *B anthracis* spores being introduced into food products or water supplies. Use of *B anthracis* in a biological attack would require immediate response and mobilization of public health resources. Because naturally occurring anthrax is rare in the United States, every suspected case should be reported immediately to the local or state health department (see Biological Terrorism, p 105).

The **incubation period** typically is 1 week or less for cutaneous or gastrointestinal tract anthrax. However, because of spore dormancy and slow clearance from lungs, the incubation period for inhalation anthrax may be prolonged and has been reported to be up to 42 days in humans and up to 2 months in experimental nonhuman primates. Discharge from cutaneous lesions potentially is infectious, but person-to-person transmission rarely has been reported. Both inhalation and cutaneous anthrax have occurred in laboratory workers.

DIAGNOSTIC TESTS: Depending on the clinical presentation, Gram stain and culture should be performed on specimens of blood, pleural fluid, cerebrospinal fluid, and tissue biopsy specimens or discharge from cutaneous lesions before initiating antimicrobial therapy, because previous treatment with antimicrobial agents makes isolation by culture unlikely. Gram-positive bacilli seen on unspun peripheral blood smears or in cerebrospinal fluid can be an important initial finding. Definitive identification of suspect *B anthracis* isolates can be performed through the Laboratory Response Network (LRN) in each state. Additional diagnostic tests for anthrax, including tissue immunohistochemistry, real-time polymerase chain reaction, time-resolved fluorescent assay, and an enzyme immunoassay that measures immunoglobulin G antibodies against *B anthracis* protective antigen in paired sera, also can be accessed through state health departments. The commercially available QuickELISA Anthrax-PA Kit can be used as a screening test. Clinical evaluation of patients with suspected inhalation anthrax should include a chest radiograph and/or computed tomography scan to evaluate for widened mediastinum and pleural effusion.

TREATMENT: A high index of clinical suspicion and rapid administration of appropriate antimicrobial therapy to people suspected of being infected, along with access to critical care support, are essential for effective treatment of anthrax. No controlled trials in humans have been performed to validate current treatment recommendations for anthrax, and there is limited clinical experience. Case reports suggest that naturally occurring cutaneous disease can be treated effectively with a variety of antimicrobial agents, including penicillins and tetracyclines, for 7 to 10 days. For bioterrorism-associated cutaneous disease in adults or children, ciprofloxacin (30 mg/kg per day, orally, divided 2 times/day for children, not to exceed 1000 mg every 24 hours), levofloxacin (16 mg/kg per day, orally, divided 2 times/day, not to exceed 500 mg every 24 hours), or doxycycline (100 mg, orally, 2 times/day for children 8 years of age or older; or 4.4 mg/kg per day, orally, divided 2 times/day for children younger than 8 years of age) are recommended for initial treatment until antimicrobial susceptibility data are available. Because of the risk of concomitant inhalational exposure, the antimicrobial regimen should be continued for a total of 60 days to provide postexposure prophylaxis, in conjunction with administration of vaccine (see Control Measures).

On the basis of in vitro data and animal studies, ciprofloxacin (400 mg, intravenously, every 8–12 hours) or doxycycline (200 mg, intravenously, every 8–12 hours) is recommended as part of an initial multidrug regimen for treating inhalation anthrax, anthrax meningitis, cutaneous anthrax with systemic signs, and gastrointestinal tract anthrax until results of antimicrobial susceptibility testing are known.[1] Other agents with in vitro activity suggested for use in conjunction with ciprofloxacin or doxycycline include rifampin, penicillin, ampicillin, vancomycin, imipenem, chloramphenicol, clindamycin, and clarithromycin. Other fluoroquinolones, including levofloxacin and ofloxacin, have excellent in vitro activity against *B anthracis*, as do newer agents, such as quinupristin/dalfopristin and the ketolide telithromycin. Ciprofloxacin theoretically may be favorable over doxycycline as the first-line antimicrobial agent because of its bactericidal activity and central nervous system penetration when meningeal inflammation is present. Because of intrinsic resistance, cephalosporins and trimethoprim-sulfamethoxazole should not be used for therapy. Treatment should continue for at least 60 days. Neither ciprofloxacin nor tetracyclines are used routinely in children or pregnant women because of safety concerns. However, ciprofloxacin or doxycycline should be used for treatment of life-threatening anthrax infections in children until antimicrobial susceptibility patterns are known. For severe anthrax, Anthrax-Specific Hyperimmune Globulin 5% should be considered in consultation with the Centers for Disease Control and Prevention under an emergency investigational new drug (IND) use protocol.[2]

ISOLATION OF THE HOSPITALIZED PATIENT: Standard precautions are recommended. In addition, contact precautions should be implemented when draining cutaneous lesions are present. Contaminated dressings and bedclothes should be incinerated or steam sterilized (121°C for 30 minutes) to destroy spores. Autopsies performed on patients with systemic anthrax require special precautions.

CONTROL MEASURES: BioThrax (formerly known as Anthrax Vaccine Adsorbed) is the only human vaccine for prevention of anthrax licensed in the United States and is prepared from a cell-free culture filtrate. Potential new anthrax vaccines are in various stages of development. Biothrax is licensed for use before an event or exposure to provide immunity to those who may be exposed occupationally to aerosolized *B anthracis* spores.[3] The vaccine is not licensed for use in children or pregnant women.

The vaccine efficacy of BioThrax is based on animal studies and a single controlled trial of the alum-precipitated precursor to BioThrax. The alum-precipitated vaccine had a demonstrated 93% efficacy for preventing cutaneous and inhalation anthrax in a controlled study in adult mill workers. Further studies in nonhuman primates have demonstrated the efficacy of the BioThrax vaccine in preventing inhalation anthrax. Adverse

[1]Centers for Disease Control and Prevention. Update: investigation of bioterrorism-related anthrax and interim guidelines for exposure management and antimicrobial therapy, October 2001. *MMWR Morb Mortal Wkly Rep.* 2001;50(42):909–919; and Centers for Disease Control and Prevention. Notice to readers: update: interim recommendations for antimicrobial prophylaxis for children and breastfeeding mothers and treatment of children with anthrax. *MMWR Morb Mortal Wkly Rep.* 2001;50(45):1014–1016

[2]Centers for Disease Control and Prevention. *E-IND Protocol: One Time Emergency Use of Liquid 5% Anthrax Immune Globulin for Treatment of Severe Anthrax.* Atlanta, GA: Centers for Disease Control and Prevention; February 22, 2006

[3]Centers for Disease Control and Prevention. Use of anthrax vaccine in the United States. 2009 recommendations of the Advisory Committee on Immunization Practices (ACIP). *MMWR Morb Mortal Wkly Rep.* 2009; in press

events usually are local injection site reactions with rare systemic symptoms, including fever, chills, muscle aches, and hypersensitivity. Pre-event immunization consists of 5 intramuscular injections at 0 and 4 weeks and 6, 12, and 18 months followed by annual boosters and is recommended for people at risk of repeated exposures to aerosolized *B anthracis* spores, including selected laboratory workers, remediation workers, military personnel, and some responders.[1] In a postexposure setting, a shorter regimen of vaccine administration likely would be employed, with guidance provided at that time by the CDC, because Biothrax is not licensed for postexposure use.

On the basis of limited available data, the best means for prevention of inhalation anthrax after exposure to *B anthracis* spores is prolonged antimicrobial therapy in conjunction with anthrax immunization. BioThrax is not licensed for use in pediatric populations and has not been studied in children. There is, however, no reason to suggest an increased risk of adverse events associated with the use of anthrax vaccine in pediatric populations. The extraordinary morbidity of inhalation anthrax should affect decision making. During an event, appropriate public health authorities will determine whether to offer vaccine to children under the existing IND protocol (No. 10061), which includes children 0 through 18 years of age. Under this IND protocol, in a postexposure setting, 3 doses of vaccine would be administered at 0, 2, and 4 weeks, along with 60 days of appropriate antimicrobial therapy. When no information is available about antimicrobial susceptibility of the implicated strain of *B anthracis*, initial postexposure prophylaxis for adults or children with ciprofloxacin or doxycycline is recommended. Although fluoroquinolones and tetracyclines are not recommended as first-choice drugs in children because of adverse effects, these concerns may be outweighed by the need for prophylaxis to prevent disease in pregnant women and children exposed to *B anthracis* after a biological terrorism event. As soon as susceptibility of the organism to penicillin has been confirmed, prophylactic therapy for children should be changed to oral amoxicillin, 80 mg/kg per day, divided into 3 daily doses administered every 8 hours (each dose not to exceed 500 mg). Because of intrinsic resistance, cephalosporins and trimethoprim-sulfamethoxazole should not be used for prophylaxis.

Arboviruses (also see West Nile Virus, p 730)
(Including Colorado Tick Fever, Dengue, Eastern Equine Encephalitis, California, Powassan, St. Louis Encephalitis, Western Equine Encephalitis, Chikungunya, Japanese Encephalitis, Tickborne Encephalitis, Venezuelan Equine Encephalitis, and Yellow Fever)

CLINICAL MANIFESTATIONS: More than 150 arthropodborne viruses (arboviruses) are known to cause human disease. Although most infections are subclinical, symptomatic illness manifests as 1 of 3 primary clinical syndromes: systemic febrile illness, neuroinvasive disease, or hemorrhagic fever (Table 3.1).

1. **Systemic febrile illness.** Most arboviruses are capable of causing a systemic febrile illness that often includes headache, arthralgia, myalgia, and rash. Some viruses also can cause more severe, prolonged, or characteristic clinical manifestations, including severe joint pain (eg, chikungunya) or jaundice (yellow fever).

---

[1]Centers for Disease Control and Prevention. Use of anthrax vaccine in the United States. 2009 recommendations of the Advisory Committee on Immunization Practice. *MMWR Morb Mortal Wkly Rep.* 2009; in press

Table 3.1. Clinical Manifestations for Select Domestic and International Arboviral Diseases

Virus	Systemic Febrile Illness	Neuroinvasive Disease[a]	Hemorrhagic Fever
Domestic			
Colorado tick fever	Yes	Rare	No
Dengue	Yes	Rare	Yes
Eastern equine encephalitis	Yes	Yes	No
California serogroup[b]	Yes	Yes	No
Powassan	Yes	Yes	No
St. Louis encephalitis	Yes	Yes	No
Western equine encephalitis	Yes	Yes	No
West Nile	Yes	Yes	No
International			
Chikungunya[c]	Yes	Rare	No
Japanese encephalitis	Yes	Yes	No
Tickborne encephalitis	Yes	Yes	No
Venezuelan equine encephalitis	Yes	Yes	No
Yellow fever	Yes	Rare	Yes

[a]Aseptic meningitis, encephalitis, or acute flaccid paralysis.
[b]The most common virus in this group is LaCrosse. Other viruses include California encephalitis, Jamestown Canyon, Keystone, snowshoe hare, and trivittatus.
[c]Most often characterized by sudden onset of high fever and severe joint pain.

2. **Neuroinvasive disease.** Many arboviruses cause neuroinvasive diseases, including aseptic meningitis, encephalitis, or acute flaccid paralysis. Illness usually presents with a prodrome similar to the systemic febrile illness followed by neurologic symptoms. The specific symptoms vary by virus and clinical syndrome but can include vomiting, stiff neck, mental status changes, seizures, or focal neurologic deficits. The severity and long-term outcome of the illness vary by etiologic agent and the underlying characteristics of the host, such as age, immune status, and preexisting medical condition.

3. **Hemorrhagic fever.** Hemorrhagic fevers can be caused by dengue or yellow fever viruses. After several days of nonspecific febrile illness, the patient may develop overt signs of hemorrhage (eg, petechiae, ecchymoses, bleeding from the nose and gums, hematemesis, and melena) and septic shock (eg, decreased peripheral circulation, azotemia, tachycardia, and hypotension). Hemorrhagic fever caused by dengue and yellow fever viruses may be confused with hemorrhagic fevers transmitted by rodents (eg, Argentine hemorrhagic fever, Bolivian hemorrhagic fever, and Lassa fever) or those caused by Ebola or Marburg viruses. For information on other potential infections causing hemorrhagic manifestations, see Hemorrhagic Fevers caused by Arenaviruses

Table 3.2. Genus, Geographic Location, Vectors, and Average Number of Annual Cases for Selected Domestic and International Arboviral Diseases

Virus	Genus	Geographic Location United States	Geographic Location Non-United States	Vectors	Number of Cases/ Year (Range)[a]
Domestic					
Colorado tick fever	*Coltivirus*	Western states	Canada	Ticks	10 (2–23)
Dengue	*Flavivirus*	Puerto Rico, Texas, and Hawaii	Worldwide in tropical areas	Mosquitoes	45 (20–71)[b]
Eastern equine encephalitis	*Alphavirus*	Eastern and gulf states	Canada, Central and South America	Mosquitoes	8 (3–21)
California serogroup	*Bunyavirus*	Widespread, most prevalent in Midwest and southeast states	Canada	Mosquitoes	100 (55–167)
Powassan	*Flavivirus*	Northeast and north central states	Canada, Russia	Ticks	1 (0–7)
St. Louis encephalitis	*Flavivirus*	Widespread	Canada, Caribbean, Mexico, Central and South America	Mosquitoes	22 (2–79)
Western equine encephalitis	*Alphavirus*	Central and western states	Mexico, South America	Mosquitoes	1 or less
West Nile	*Flavivirus*	Widespread	Canada, Europe, Africa, Asia	Mosquitoes	1237 (19–2946)[c]
International					
Chikungunya	*Alphavirus*	Imported only	Europe, Asia, Africa	Mosquitoes	27 (14–39)[d]
Japanese encephalitis	*Flavivirus*	Imported only	Asia	Mosquitoes	Less than 1
Tickborne encephalitis	*Flavivirus*	Imported only	Europe, northern Asia	Ticks	Less than 1
Venezuelan equine encephalitis	*Alphavirus*	Imported only	Mexico, Central and South America	Mosquitoes	Less than 1
Yellow fever	*Flavivirus*	Imported only	South America, Africa	Mosquitoes	Less than 1

[a]Average annual number of domestic and/or imported cases from 1998–2007 unless otherwise noted.
[b]Domestic and imported cases from 1997–2006; excludes indigenous transmission in Puerto Rico.
[c]Neuroinvasive disease only from 1999–2007; for more information, see West Nile Virus (p 730).
[d]Cases imported into the United States in 2006 and 2007 only.

(p 325) and Hemorrhagic Fevers and Related Syndromes Caused by Viruses of the Family Bunyaviridae (p 327).

ETIOLOGY: Arboviruses are RNA viruses that are transmitted to humans primarily through the bites of infected arthropods (mosquitoes, ticks, sand flies, biting midges). The viral families responsible for most arboviral infections in humans are Flaviviridae (genus *Flavivirus*), Togaviridae (genus *Alphavirus*), and Bunyaviridae (genus (*Bunyavirus*). Reoviridae (genus *Coltivirus*) also are responsible for a smaller number of human arboviral infections (eg, Colorado tick fever [Table 3.2]).

EPIDEMIOLOGY: Most arboviruses maintain cycles of transmission between birds or small mammals and arthropod vectors. Humans and domestic animals usually are infected incidentally as "dead-end" hosts (Table 3.2). Important exceptions are dengue, yellow fever, and chikungunya viruses, which can be spread from person-to-arthropod-to-person (anthroponotic transmission). For other arboviruses, humans usually do not develop a sustained or high enough level of viremia to infect arthropod vectors. Direct person-to-person spread of arboviruses can occur through blood transfusion, organ transplantation, intrauterine transmission, and possibly human milk (see Blood Safety, p 106, Human Milk, p 118, and West Nile Virus, p 730). Experimentally, Venezuelan equine encephalitis (VEE) virus also has been spread via the respiratory aerosol route.

In the northern United States, arboviral infections occur during summer and autumn, when mosquitoes and ticks are most active. In the southern United States, cases occur throughout the year because of warmer temperatures, which are conducive to year-round arthropod activity. The number of domestic or imported arboviral disease cases reported in the United States varies greatly by specific etiology and year (Table 3.2).

The **incubation periods** for arboviral diseases typically range between 2 and 15 days. Longer incubation periods can occur in immunocompromised people and for tickborne viruses, such as tickborne encephalitis and Powassan viruses.

DIAGNOSTIC TESTS: Arboviral infections are confirmed most frequently by measurement of virus-specific antibody in serum or cerebrospinal fluid (CSF). Acute-phase serum specimens should be tested for virus-specific immunoglobulin (Ig) M antibody using an enzyme immunoassay (EIA). With clinical and epidemiologic correlation, a positive IgM test has good diagnostic predictive value, but cross-reaction with related arboviruses from the same family can occur. For most arboviral infections, IgM is detectable 3 to 8 days after onset of illness and persists for 30 to 90 days, but longer persistence has been documented. Serum collected within 8 days of illness onset may not have detectable IgM, and the test should be repeated on a convalescent sample to rule out adequately arboviral infection. IgG antibody generally is detectable shortly after IgM and persists for years. Plaque-reduction neutralization tests (PRNT) can be performed to measure virus-specific neutralizing antibodies. A fourfold or greater rise in virus-specific neutralizing antibodies between acute and convalescent serum specimens collected 2 to 3 weeks apart may be used to confirm recent infection or discriminate between cross-reacting antibodies in primary arboviral infections. In patients who have been immunized previously or exposed to another arbovirus from the same virus family (ie, secondary arboviral infections), cross-reactive antibodies in both the EIA and neutralization assays may make it difficult to identify a specific etiologic agent. For some arboviral infections (eg, Colorado tick fever), the immune response may be delayed, with IgM antibodies not appearing until 2 to 3 weeks after onset of illness and neutralizing antibodies taking up to a month to develop. Immunization history, date of onset of symptoms, and information regarding other arboviruses known to circulate in the geographic area that may cross-react in serologic assays need to be considered when interpreting results.

Viral culture and nucleic acid amplification (NAA) tests for RNA can be performed on acute serum, CSF, or tissue specimens. Viruses that are more likely to be detected using culture or NAA tests early in the illness include yellow fever, chikungunya, and dengue viruses. Immunohistochemical staining (IHC) can detect specific antigens in unpreserved or formalin-fixed tissue. Negative results of these tests do not rule out infection.

Antibody testing for common domestic arboviral diseases is performed in most state public health laboratories and in certain commercial or reference laboratories. Confirmatory PRNT, viral culture, NAA testing, IHC, and testing for less common domestic and international arboviruses are performed only in select state public health laboratories and at the Centers for Disease Control and Prevention (CDC) Division of Vector-Borne Infectious Diseases in Colorado (telephone: 970-221-6400).

TREATMENT: The primary treatment for all arboviral disease is supportive. Although various therapies have been evaluated for several arboviral diseases, none have shown specific benefit.

ISOLATION OF THE HOSPITALIZED PATIENT: Standard precautions are recommended.

CONTROL MEASURES: Reduction of vectors in areas with endemic infection is important to reduce risk of infection. Use of certain personal protective strategies can help decrease the risk of human infection. These strategies include using insect repellent, wearing long pants and long-sleeved shirts while outdoors, staying in screened or air-conditioned dwellings, and avoiding outdoor activities during peak vector feeding times. Effective repellents for use on skin include diethyltoluamide (DEET), picaridin, and oil of lemon eucalyptus (see Prevention of Mosquitoborne Infections, p 193). The American Academy of Pediatrics recommends using formulations of no more than 30% DEET on infants and children and not using products containing DEET on infants younger than 2 months of age. Products containing DEET or permethrin also can be applied to clothing.

Select arboviral infections also can be prevented through screening of blood and organ donations and through immunization. The blood supply in the United States has been screened for West Nile virus since 2003. Blood donations from areas with endemic infection also are screened for dengue virus. Vaccines are available in the United States to protect against travel-related yellow fever and Japanese encephalitis.

Yellow Fever Vaccine.[1] Live-attenuated (17D strain) vaccine is available at state-approved immunization centers. A single dose provides protection for 10 years or longer. Unless contraindicated, yellow fever immunization is recommended for all people 9 months of age or older living in or traveling to areas with endemic disease and is required by international regulations for travel to and from certain countries (**wwwn.cdc.gov/travel/default.aspx**). Infants younger than 4 months of age should not be immunized, because they have an increased risk of vaccine-associated encephalitis. The decision to immunize infants between 4 and 9 months of age must balance the infant's risk of exposure with the theoretical risks of vaccine-associated encephalitis.

Yellow fever vaccine is a live-virus vaccine produced in eggs and, thus, is contraindicated in people who have an allergic reaction to eggs, women who are pregnant or breastfeeding, and people who are immunocompromised. These people should be

[1]Centers for Disease Control and Prevention. Yellow fever vaccine: recommendations of the Advisory Committee on Immunization Practices (ACIP), 2002. *MMWR Recomm Rep.* 2002;51(RR-17):1–10

excused from immunization and issued a medical waiver letter to fulfill health regulations unless travel to an area with endemic infection is unavoidable and the risk of exposure outweighs the risks of immunization. Procedures for immunizing people with egg allergy are described in the vaccine package insert. For more detailed information on the yellow fever vaccine, including adverse events, precautions, and contraindications, visit **wwwn. cdc.gov/travel/default.aspx.**

Japanese Encephalitis (JE) Vaccine.[1] Inactivated mouse brain-derived JE vaccine (JE-VAX) is licensed in the United States for use in people 1 year of age and older. The recommended primary immunization series for JE-VAX is 3 doses administered on days 0, 7, and 30. An abbreviated schedule (days 0, 7, and 14) provides similar rates of seroconversion but significantly lower neutralizing antibody titers. The last dose should be administered at least 10 days before beginning travel to ensure an adequate immune response and access to medical care in the event of any delayed adverse reactions. The duration of protection after primary immunization is unknown, but circulating neutralizing antibodies appear to last for approximately 2 to 3 years. JE-VAX no longer is being produced, and available supplies may be exhausted as early as 2009. A new inactivated Vero cell-derived JE vaccine (Ixiaro) has been evaluated in the United States and has been licensed for use in adult travelers (18 years of age or older), but safety and efficacy data are not yet available for children. Therefore, the distributor of JE-VAX is expected to maintain a stockpile for use in children until the new vaccine is licensed for pediatric use.

The risk of JE for most travelers to Asia is low but varies on the basis of season, destination, duration, and activities. Inactivated mouse brain-derived JE vaccine has been associated with allergic hypersensitivity reactions and rare neurologic adverse events. People with a previous history of anaphylaxis, urticaria, or other allergies are significantly more likely to develop a hypersensitivity reaction. Decisions regarding the use of JE vaccine for travelers must balance the low risk of disease and the low probability of serious adverse events. The CDC Advisory Committee on Immunization Practices (ACIP) recommends that JE vaccine should be offered to travelers 1 year of age and older who plan to spend 1 month or longer in areas of Asia with endemic infection during the JE virus transmission season. JE vaccine also should be considered for shorter stays if the travel will include extensive outdoor activities in rural areas with endemic infection. Information on the location of JE virus transmission and detailed information on vaccine recommendations and adverse events can be obtained from the CDC (**wwwn.cdc.gov/travel/ default.aspx**).

Other Arboviral Vaccines. An inactivated vaccine for tickborne encephalitis virus is licensed in Canada and some countries in Europe where the disease is endemic, but this vaccine is not available in the United States. Vaccines also exist against chikungunya virus, Eastern equine encephalitis virus, Venezuelan equine encephalitis virus, and Western equine encephalitis virus but are used primarily to protect laboratory workers and other people with occupational exposure to these viruses and are not available for public use. Dengue and West Nile virus vaccines are under development.

---

[1]Centers for Disease Control and Prevention. Inactivated Japanese encephalitis virus vaccine: recommendations of the Advisory Committee on Immunization Practices (ACIP). *MMWR Recomm Rep.* 2009; in press

REPORTING: Arboviral diseases are nationally notifiable conditions and should be reported to the appropriate local and state health authorities. For select arboviruses (eg, dengue, yellow fever, and chikungunya), patients may remain viremic during their acute illness. Such patients pose a risk for further person-to-arthropod-to-person transmission, increasing the importance of timely reporting.

Arcanobacterium haemolyticum Infections

CLINICAL MANIFESTATIONS: Acute pharyngitis attributable to *Arcanobacterium haemolyticum* often is indistinguishable from that caused by group A streptococci. Fever, pharyngeal exudate, lymphadenopathy, rash, and pruritus are common, but palatal petechiae and strawberry tongue are absent. In almost half of all reported cases, a maculopapular or scarlatiniform exanthem is present, beginning on the extensor surfaces of the distal extremities, spreading centripetally to the chest and back, and sparing the face, palms, and soles. Respiratory tract infections that mimic diphtheria, including membranous pharyngitis, sinusitis, and pneumonia; and skin and soft tissue infections, including chronic ulceration, cellulitis, paronychia, and wound infection have been attributed to *A haemolyticum*. Invasive infections, including septicemia, peritonsillar abscess, Lemierre syndrome, brain abscess, orbital cellulitis, meningitis, endocarditis, pyogenic arthritis, osteomyelitis, urinary tract infection, pneumonia, and pyothorax have been reported. No nonsuppurative sequelae have been reported.

ETIOLOGY: *A haemolyticum* is a catalase-negative, facultative anaerobic gram-positive bacillus formerly classified as *Corynebacterium haemolyticum*.

EPIDEMIOLOGY: Humans are the primary reservoir of *A haemolyticum*, and spread is person to person, presumably via droplet respiratory tract secretions. Severe disease occurs almost exclusively among immunocompromised people. Pharyngitis occurs primarily in adolescents and young adults. Although long-term pharyngeal carriage with *A haemolyticum* has been described after an episode of acute pharyngitis, isolation of the bacterium from the nasopharynx of asymptomatic people is rare. An estimated 0.5% to 3% of acute pharyngitis is attributable to *A haemolyticum*. Case reports also document isolation in combination with other pathogens. Person-to-person spread is inferred from studies of families and epidemiologic reports.

The **incubation period** is unknown.

DIAGNOSTIC TESTS: *A haemolyticum* grows on blood-enriched agar, but colonies are small, have narrow bands of hemolysis, and may not be visible for 48 to 72 hours. The organism will not be detected on routine evaluation of pharyngitis by the antigen test for group A streptococci. Detection is enhanced by culture on rabbit or human blood agar rather than on more commonly used sheep blood agar because of larger colony size and wider zones of hemolysis. Growth also is enhanced by addition of 5% carbon dioxide. Nonstandardized serologic tests for antibodies to *A haemolyticum* have been developed but are not available commercially.

TREATMENT: Erythromycin is the drug of choice for treating tonsillopharyngitis attributable to *A haemolyticum*, but no prospective therapeutic trials have been performed. *A haemolyticum* is susceptible in vitro to erythromycin, clindamycin, and tetracycline; susceptibility to penicillin is variable, and failures in treatment of pharyngitis have been reported, perhaps because of penicillin tolerance. Resistance to trimethoprim-sulfamethoxazole is common. In rare cases of disseminated infection, susceptibility tests should be performed. In disseminated infection, parenteral penicillin plus an aminoglycoside may be used initially as empiric treatment.

ISOLATION OF THE HOSPITALIZED PATIENT: Standard precautions are recommended.

CONTROL MEASURES: None.

Ascaris lumbricoides Infections

CLINICAL MANIFESTATIONS: Most infections with *Ascaris lumbricoides* are asymptomatic, although moderate to heavy infections may lead to malnutrition and nonspecific gastrointestinal tract symptoms. During the larval migratory phase, an acute transient pneumonitis (Löffler syndrome) associated with fever and marked eosinophilia may occur. Acute intestinal obstruction has been associated with heavy infections. Children are prone to this complication because of the small diameter of the intestinal lumen and their propensity to acquire large worm burdens. Worm migration can cause peritonitis, secondary to intestinal wall perforation, and common bile duct obstruction resulting in biliary colic, cholangitis, or pancreatitis. Adult worms can be stimulated to migrate by stressful conditions (eg, fever, illness, or anesthesia) and by some anthelmintic drugs. *A lumbricoides* has been found in the appendiceal lumen in patients with acute appendicitis.

ETIOLOGY: *A lumbricoides* is the most prevalent of all human intestinal nematodes (roundworms), with more than 1 billion people infected worldwide.

EPIDEMIOLOGY: Adult worms live in the lumen of the small intestine. Female worms produce approximately 200 000 eggs per day, which are excreted in stool and must incubate in soil for 2 to 3 weeks for an embryo to become infectious. Following ingestion of embryonated eggs, usually from contaminated soil, larvae hatch in the small intestine, penetrate the mucosa, and are transported passively by portal blood to the liver and lungs. After migrating into the airways, larvae ascend through the tracheobronchial tree to the pharynx, are swallowed, and mature into adults in the small intestine. Infection with *A lumbricoides* is widespread but is most common in the tropics, in areas of poor sanitation, and where human feces are used as fertilizer. If infection is untreated, adult worms can live for 12 to 18 months, resulting in daily fecal excretion of large numbers of ova. Female worms are longer than male worms and can measure 40 cm in length and 6 mm in diameter.

The **incubation period** (interval between ingestion of eggs and development of egg-laying adults) is approximately 8 weeks.

DIAGNOSTIC TESTS: Ova can be detected by microscopic examination of stool. Occasionally, patients pass adult worms from the rectum, from the nose after migration through the nares, and from the mouth, usually in vomitus. Adult worms sometimes are detected by computed tomographic scan of the abdomen or by ultrasonographic examination of the biliary tree.

TREATMENT: Albendazole taken with food in a single dose, mebendazole for 3 days, or ivermectin taken on an empty stomach in a single dose are recommended for treatment of ascariasis (see Drugs for Parasitic Infections, p 783). Although limited data suggest that these drugs are safe in children younger than 2 years of age, the risks and benefits of therapy should be considered before administration. In 1-year-old children, the World Health Organization recommends reducing the albendazole dose to half of that given to older children and adults. Albendazole is not labeled for use for treatment of ascariasis. Nitazoxanide also is effective against *A lumbricoides*, although it also is not approved for this indication. Reexamination of stool specimens 2 weeks after therapy to determine whether the worms have been eliminated is helpful for assessing therapy but is not essential.

Conservative management of small bowel obstruction, including nasogastric suction and intravenous fluids, may result in resolution of major symptoms before administration of anthelminthic therapy. Piperazine, which may relieve intestinal obstruction caused by heavy worm burden, is not available in the United States. Surgical intervention occasionally is necessary to relieve intestinal or biliary tract obstruction or for volvulus or peritonitis secondary to perforation. Endoscopic retrograde cholangiopancreatography has been used successfully for extraction of worms from the biliary tree.

ISOLATION OF THE HOSPITALIZED PATIENT: Standard precautions are recommended, because there is no direct person-to-person transmission.

CONTROL MEASURES: Sanitary disposal of human feces stops transmission. Children's play areas should be given special attention. Vegetables cultivated in areas where uncomposted human feces are used as fertilizer must be thoroughly cooked or soaked in a diluted iodine solution before eating. Despite relatively rapid reinfection, frequent deworming of school-aged children may prevent morbidity (nutritional and cognitive deficits) associated with soil-transmitted nematode infections.

Aspergillosis

CLINICAL MANIFESTATIONS: Aspergillosis manifests as invasive, noninvasive, chronic, or allergic disease depending on the immune status of the host.
- Invasive aspergillosis occurs almost exclusively in immunocompromised patients with prolonged neutropenia (eg, cytotoxic chemotherapy), graft-versus-host disease, or impaired phagocyte function (eg, chronic granulomatous disease, immunosuppressive therapy, corticosteroids). Invasive infection usually involves pulmonary, sinus, cerebral, or cutaneous sites. Rarely, endocarditis, osteomyelitis, meningitis, infection of the eye or orbit, and esophagitis occur. The hallmark of invasive aspergillosis is angioinvasion with resulting thrombosis, dissemination to other organs, and occasionally, erosion of the blood vessel wall with catastrophic hemorrhage. Aspergillosis in patients with chronic granulomatous disease rarely displays angioinvasion.
- Aspergillomas and otomycosis are 2 syndromes of nonallergic colonization by *Aspergillus* species in immunocompetent children. Aspergillomas ("fungal balls") grow in preexisting pulmonary cavities or bronchogenic cysts without invading pulmonary tissue; almost all patients have underlying lung disease, such as cystic fibrosis or tuberculosis. Patients with otomycosis have chronic otitis media with colonization of the external auditory canal by a fungal mat that produces a dark discharge.
- Allergic bronchopulmonary aspergillosis is a hypersensitivity lung disease that manifests as episodic wheezing, expectoration of brown mucus plugs, low-grade fever, eosinophilia, and transient pulmonary infiltrates. This form of aspergillosis occurs most commonly in immunocompetent children with asthma or cystic fibrosis and can be a trigger for asthmatic flares.

- Allergic sinusitis is a far less common allergic response to colonization by *Aspergillus* species than is allergic bronchopulmonary aspergillosis. Allergic sinusitis occurs in children with nasal polyps or previous episodes of sinusitis or children who have undergone sinus surgery. Allergic sinusitis is characterized by symptoms of chronic sinusitis with dark plugs of nasal discharge.

ETIOLOGY: *Aspergillus* species are ubiquitous molds that grow on decaying vegetation and in soil. *Aspergillus fumigatus* is the most common cause of invasive aspergillosis, with *Aspergillus flavus* being the next most common. Several other species, including *Aspergillus terreus, Aspergillus nidulans,* and *Aspergillus niger,* also cause invasive human infections.

EPIDEMIOLOGY: The principal route of transmission is inhalation of conidia (spores), but contaminated aerosolized water supply (eg, shower heads) can cause disease. Incidence of disease in transplant recipients is bimodal, with episodes occurring during periods of neutropenia or, more often, during treatment for graft-versus-host disease. Health care-associated outbreaks of invasive pulmonary aspergillosis in susceptible hosts have occurred in which the probable source of the fungus was a nearby construction site or faulty ventilation system. Transmission by direct inoculation of skin abrasions or wounds is less likely. Person-to-person spread does not occur.

The **incubation period** is unknown.

DIAGNOSTIC TESTS: Dichotomously branched and septate hyphae, identified by microscopic examination of 10% potassium hydroxide wet preparations or of Gomori methenamine-silver nitrate stain of tissue or bronchoalveolar lavage specimens, are suggestive of the diagnosis. Isolation of *Aspergillus* species is required for definitive diagnosis. The organism usually is not recoverable from blood (except *A terreus*) but is isolated readily from lung, sinus, and skin biopsy specimens when cultured on Sabouraud dextrose agar or brain-heart infusion media (without cycloheximide). *Aspergillus* species can be a laboratory contaminant, but when evaluating results from ill, immunocompromised patients, recovery of this organism usually indicates infection. Biopsy of a lesion usually is required to confirm the diagnosis, and care should be taken to distinguish aspergillosis from zygomycosis, which appears similar radiologically. A serologic assay for detection of galactomannan, a molecule found in the cell wall of *Aspergillus* species, is available commercially but has not been evaluated extensively for use in infants and children. A positive test result in adults supports a diagnosis of invasive aspergillosis, and monitoring of serum antigen concentrations twice weekly may be useful to assess response to therapy. False-positive test results have been reported in children and can be related to consumption of food products containing galactomannan (eg, rice and pasta) or from cross-reactivity with antimicrobial agents derived from fungi (eg, penicillins). A negative galactomannan test result does not exclude the diagnosis of invasive aspergillosis. False-negative galactomannan test results consistently occur in patients with chronic granulomatous disease, so the test should not be used in this population. Unlike adults, children frequently do not manifest cavitation or the air crescent or halo signs as pulmonary radiographic findings. In allergic aspergillosis, diagnosis is suggested by a typical clinical syndrome with elevated total concentrations of immunoglobulin (Ig) E (greater than 1000 ng/mL) and *Aspergillus*-specific serum IgE, eosinophilia, and a positive result of a skin test for *Aspergillus* antigens. In people with cystic fibrosis, the diagnosis is more difficult, because wheezing, eosinophilia, and a positive skin test result not associated with allergic bronchopulmonary aspergillosis often are present.

TREATMENT[1]: Voriconazole or amphotericin B in high doses are the drugs of choice for invasive aspergillosis (see Drugs for Invasive and Other Serious Fungal Infections, p 772). Voriconazole has been shown to be superior to amphotericin B in a large, randomized trial in adults. Therapy is continued for at least 12 weeks, but treatment duration should be individualized for each patient. Voriconazole is metabolized in a linear fashion in children (nonlinear in adults), so the recommended adult dosing is thought to be too low for children. The optimal pediatric dose is not yet known. Posaconazole has been used as salvage therapy in adults with invasive aspergillosis.

Caspofungin has been studied as salvage therapy for invasive aspergillosis with good response. The pharmacokinetics of caspofungin differ in children, in whom a body-surface area dosing scheme is preferred to a weight-based dosing regimen. Itraconazole alone is an alternative for mild to moderate cases of aspergillosis, although extensive drug interactions and poor absorption (capsular form) may limit the utility of itraconazole. Lipid formulations of amphotericin B can be considered, but *A terreus* is resistant to all amphotericin B products. Data are limited on the safety and efficacy of voriconazole, itraconazole, posaconazole, and caspofungin in children. Studies are needed to evaluate the benefit and safety of combination antifungal therapy for invasive aspergillosis.

Surgical excision of a localized invasive lesion (eg, cutaneous eschars, a single pulmonary lesion, sinus debris, accessible cerebral lesions) usually is warranted. In pulmonary disease, surgery is indicated only when a mass is impinging on a great vessel. Historically, allergic bronchopulmonary aspergillosis has been treated with corticosteroids. More recently, antifungal therapy has been recommended. Allergic sinus aspergillosis also is treated with corticosteroids, and surgery has been reported to be beneficial in many cases. Antifungal therapy has not been found to be useful.

ISOLATION OF THE HOSPITALIZED PATIENT: Standard precautions are recommended.

CONTROL MEASURES: Outbreaks of invasive aspergillosis have occurred among hospitalized immunosuppressed patients during construction in hospitals or at nearby sites. Environmental measures reported to be effective include erecting suitable barriers between patient care areas and construction sites, routine cleaning of air-handling systems, repair of faulty air flow, and replacement of contaminated air filters. High-efficiency particulate air filters and laminar flow rooms markedly decrease the risk of exposure to conidia in patient care areas. These latter measures may be expensive and difficult for patients to tolerate. Posaconazole has been shown to be effective in prophylaxis against invasive aspergillosis for people 13 years of age and older who have undergone hematopoietic stem cell transplant and have graft-versus-host disease and in patients with hematologic malignancies with prolonged neutropenia in 2 randomized controlled trials. Low-dose amphotericin B, itraconazole, voriconazole, or posaconazole prophylaxis has been reported for other high-risk patients, but controlled trials have not been completed in pediatric patients. Patients at risk of invasive infection should have their home conditions evaluated before discharge and avoid environmental exposure (eg, gardening). People with allergic aspergillosis should take measures to reduce exposure to *Aspergillus* species in the home.

---

[1]Walsh TJ, Anaissie EJ, Denning DW, et al. Treatment of aspergillosis: clinical practice guidelines of the Infectious Diseases Society of America. *Clin Infect Dis.* 2008;46(3):327–360

Astrovirus Infections

CLINICAL MANIFESTATIONS: Illness is characterized by diarrhea of short duration accompanied by vomiting, fever, and occasionally, abdominal pain and mild dehydration. Illness in an immunocompetent host is self-limited, lasting a median of 5 to 6 days. Asymptomatic infections are common.

ETIOLOGY: Astroviruses are nonenveloped, single-stranded RNA viruses with a characteristic starlike appearance when visualized by electron microscopy. Eight human antigenic types are known.

EPIDEMIOLOGY: Human astroviruses have a worldwide distribution. Multiple antigenic types cocirculate in the same region. Astroviruses have been detected in as many as 10% to 34% of sporadic cases of nonbacterial gastroenteritis among young children in the community but appear to cause a lower proportion of cases of more severe childhood gastroenteritis requiring hospitalization. Astrovirus infections occur predominantly in children younger than 4 years of age and have a seasonal peak during the late winter and spring in the United States. Transmission is person to person via the fecal-oral route. Outbreaks tend to occur in closed populations of the young and the elderly, and incidence is high among hospitalized children and children in child care centers. Excretion lasts a median of 5 days after onset of symptoms, but asymptomatic excretion after illness can last for several weeks in healthy children. Persistent excretion may occur in immunocompromised hosts.

The **incubation period** is 1 to 4 days.

DIAGNOSTIC TESTS: Commercial tests for diagnosis are not available in the United States, although enzyme immunoassays are available in many other countries. The following tests are available in some research and reference laboratories: electron microscopy for detection of viral particles in stool, enzyme immunoassay for detection of viral antigen in stool or antibody in serum, latex agglutination in stool, and reverse transcriptase-polymerase chain reaction (RT-PCR) assay for detection of viral RNA in stool. Of these tests, RT-PCR assay is the most sensitive.

TREATMENT: Rehydration with oral or intravenous fluid and electrolyte solutions is recommended.

ISOLATION OF THE HOSPITALIZED PATIENT: In addition to standard precautions, contact precautions are recommended for diapered or incontinent children with possible or proven astrovirus infection for the duration of the illness.

CONTROL MEASURES: No specific control measures are available. The spread of infection in child care settings can be decreased by using general measures for control of diarrhea, such as training caregivers about infection-control procedures, maintaining cleanliness of surfaces and food preparation areas, exercising adequate hand hygiene, cohorting ill children, and excluding ill child care providers, food handlers, and children (see Children in Out-of-Home Child Care, p 124).

Babesiosis

CLINICAL MANIFESTATIONS: *Babesia* infection often is asymptomatic or associated with mild, nonspecific symptoms. The infection also can be severe and life threatening, particularly in people who are asplenic, immunocompromised, or elderly. In general, babesiosis, like malaria, is characterized by the presence of fever and hemolytic anemia. Infected people may have a prodromal illness, with gradual onset of symptoms, such as malaise, anorexia, and fatigue, followed by development of fever and other influenza-like symptoms (eg, chills, sweats, myalgia, arthralgia, headache, anorexia, nausea, vomiting). Less common findings include hyperesthesia, sore throat, abdominal pain, conjunctival injection, photophobia, weight loss, and nonproductive cough. Clinical signs generally are minimal, often consisting only of fever and tachycardia, although mild hepatosplenomegaly may be noted. Thrombocytopenia and a normal or low white blood cell count are common. If untreated, illness can last for several weeks or months; even asymptomatic people can have persistent low-level parasitemia, sometimes for longer than 1 year.

ETIOLOGY: *Babesia* species are intraerythrocytic protozoa. The etiologic agents of babesiosis in the United States include *Babesia microti*, which has caused most of the reported cases, and several other genetically and antigenically distinct organisms.

EPIDEMIOLOGY: Babesiosis predominantly is a tickborne zoonosis. *Babesia* parasites also can be transmitted by blood transfusion and through congenital/perinatal routes. In the United States, the primary reservoir host for *B microti* is the white-footed mouse *(Peromyscus leucopus)*, and the primary vector is the tick *Ixodes scapularis*, which also can transmit *Borrelia burgdorferi*, the causative agent of Lyme disease, and *Anaplasma phagocytophilum*, the causative agent of human granulocytic anaplasmosis. Humans become infected through tick bites, which typically are not noticed. The white-tailed deer *(Odocoileus virginianus)* is an important host for blood meals for the tick but is not a reservoir host of *B microti*. An increase in the deer population in some geographic areas, including some suburban areas, during the past few decades is thought to be a major factor in the spread of *I scapularis* and the increase in numbers of reported cases of babesiosis. The reported vectorborne cases of *B microti* infection have been acquired in the Northeast (particularly, but not exclusively, in Connecticut, Massachusetts, New Jersey, New York, and Rhode Island) and, to a lesser extent, in the upper Midwest (Wisconsin and Minnesota). Occasional human cases of babesiosis caused by other species have been described in various regions of the United States; tick vectors and reservoir hosts for these species have not been identified. Whereas most US vectorborne cases of babesiosis occur during late spring, summer, or autumn, transfusion-associated cases can occur year round.

The **incubation period** ranges from approximately 1 week to several months.

DIAGNOSTIC TESTS: Babesiosis is diagnosed by microscopic identification of the organism on Giemsa- or Wright-stained thick or thin blood smears. If seen, the Maltese cross appearance of the merozoite is pathognomonic. *B microti* and other *Babesia* species can be difficult to distinguish from *Plasmodium falciparum;* examination of blood smears by a reference laboratory should be considered for confirmation of the diagnosis. Serologic and molecular testing are performed at the Centers for Disease Control and Prevention and at some other reference laboratories and are important adjunctive tests. If indicated, the possibility of concurrent *B burgdorferi* or *Anaplasma* infection should be considered.

TREATMENT: Clindamycin plus oral quinine for 7 to 10 days or atovaquone plus azithromycin for 7 to 10 days had comparable efficacy in a controlled clinical trial conducted among adult patients who did not have life-threatening babesiosis (see Drugs for Parasitic Infections, p 783). Therapy with atovaquone plus azithromycin is associated with fewer adverse effects. However, the combination of clindamycin and quinine remains the standard of care for severely ill patients. In addition, exchange blood transfusions should be considered for patients who are critically ill (eg, hemodynamically unstable), especially but not exclusively for patients with parasitemia concentrations 10% or greater.

ISOLATION OF THE HOSPITALIZED PATIENT: Standard precautions are recommended.

CONTROL MEASURES: Specific recommendations concern prevention of tick bites and are similar to those for prevention of Lyme disease and other tickborne infections (see Prevention of Tickborne Infections, p 191).

Bacillus cereus Infections

CLINICAL MANIFESTATIONS: Two clinical syndromes are associated with *Bacillus cereus* foodborne illness. The first is the emetic syndrome, which, like staphylococcal foodborne illness, develops after a short incubation period and is characterized by nausea, vomiting, abdominal cramps, and in approximately 30% of patients, diarrhea. The second is the diarrhea syndrome, which, like *Clostridium perfringens* foodborne illness, has a slightly longer incubation period and is characterized predominantly by moderate to severe abdominal cramps and watery diarrhea, with vomiting in approximately 25% of patients. Both syndromes are mild, usually are not associated with fever, and abate within 24 hours.

B cereus also can cause local skin and wound infections, periodontitis, ocular infections, and invasive disease, including bacteremia, central intravascular catheter-associated infection, endocarditis, osteomyelitis, pneumonia, brain abscess, and meningitis. Ocular involvement includes panophthalmitis, endophthalmitis, and keratitis.

ETIOLOGY: *B cereus* is an aerobic and facultatively anaerobic, spore-forming, gram-positive bacillus. The emetic syndrome is caused by a preformed heat-stable enterotoxin. The emetic toxin is cytotoxic, can cause rhabdomyolysis, and has been associated with fulminant liver failure. The diarrhea syndrome is caused by in vivo production of heat-labile enterotoxins.

EPIDEMIOLOGY: *B cereus* is ubiquitous in the environment. It commonly is present in small numbers in raw, dried, and processed foods but is an uncommon cause of foodborne illness in the United States. Spores of *B cereus* are heat resistant and can survive pasteurization, brief cooking, or boiling. Vegetative forms can grow and produce enterotoxins over a wide range of temperatures, from 25°C to 42°C (77°F–108°F). The emetic syndrome occurs after eating food containing preformed toxin, most commonly fried or recooked rice. Disease can result from eating food contaminated with *B cereus* spores, which produce enterotoxin in the gastrointestinal tract. Spore-associated disease most commonly is caused by contaminated meat or vegetables and manifests as the diarrhea syndrome. Foodborne illness caused by *B cereus* is not transmissible from person-to-person.

Risk factors for invasive disease attributable to *B cereus* include history of injection drug use, presence of indwelling intravascular catheters or implanted devices, neutropenia or immunosuppression, and preterm birth. *B cereus* endophthalmitis has occurred after penetrating ocular trauma and injection drug use.

The **incubation period** for the emetic syndrome is 0.5 to 6 hours; for the diarrhea syndrome, the incubation period is 6 to 24 hours.

DIAGNOSTIC TESTS: For foodborne illness, isolation of *B cereus* in a concentration of 10^5 colony-forming units/g or greater of epidemiologically incriminated food establishes the diagnosis. Because the organism can be recovered from stool specimens from some well people, the presence of *B cereus* in feces or vomitus of ill people is not definitive evidence of infection unless isolates from several ill patients are demonstrated to be the same serotype or unless stool cultures from a matched control group have negative test results. Toxin testing is useful but not widely available. Phage typing, DNA hybridization, plasmid analysis, and enzyme electrophoresis have been used as epidemiologic tools in outbreaks of foodborne illness.

In patients with risk factors for invasive disease, isolation of *B cereus* from wounds, blood, or other usually sterile body fluids is significant.

TREATMENT: People with *B cereus* food poisoning require only supportive treatment. Oral rehydration or, occasionally, intravenous fluid and electrolyte replacement for patients with severe dehydration is indicated. Antimicrobial agents are not indicated.

Patients with invasive disease require antimicrobial therapy. Prompt removal of any potentially infected foreign bodies, such as catheters or implants, is essential. *B cereus* usually is susceptible to vancomycin, which is the drug of choice, and also to alternative drugs, including clindamycin, meropenem, imipenem, and ciprofloxacin. *B cereus* is resistant to beta-lactam antimicrobial agents.

ISOLATION OF THE HOSPITALIZED PATIENT: Standard precautions are recommended.

CONTROL MEASURES: Proper cooking and appropriate storage of foods, particularly rice cooked for later use, will help prevent foodborne outbreaks. Food should be kept at temperatures higher than 60°C (140°F) or rapidly cooled to less than 10°C (50°F) after cooking.

Hand hygiene and strict aseptic technique in caring for immunocompromised patients or patients with indwelling intravascular catheters are important to minimize the risk of invasive disease.

Bacterial Vaginosis

CLINICAL MANIFESTATIONS: Bacterial vaginosis (BV), a syndrome diagnosed primarily in sexually active adolescent and adult females, is characterized by changes in vaginal flora. Signs include a thin white or grey, homogenous, adherent vaginal discharge with a fishy odor. BV can be asymptomatic in up to 84% of cases; the remainder of cases have vaginal discharge that uncommonly is associated with abdominal pain, significant pruritus, or dysuria. However, BV has been associated with chorioamnionitis, preterm delivery, and postpartum endometritis.

Vaginitis and vulvitis in prepubertal girls usually have a nonspecific cause and rarely are manifestations of BV. In prepubertal girls, other predisposing causes of vaginal discharge include foreign bodies or infections attributable to group A streptococci, herpes simplex virus, *Neisseria gonorrhoeae*, *Chlamydia trachomatis*, *Trichomonas vaginalis*, *Candida* species, or enteric bacteria, including *Shigella* species.

ETIOLOGY: The microbiologic cause of BV has not been delineated clearly. Typical microbiologic findings of specimens obtained from the vagina include an increase in concentrations of *Gardnerella vaginalis, Mycoplasma species,* and *Ureaplasma* species, anaerobic bacteria (eg, *Prevotella* species and *Mobiluncus* species), and a marked decrease in the concentration of *Lactobacillus* species.

EPIDEMIOLOGY: BV is the most prevalent vaginal infection in sexually active adolescents and adult females. It can occur with other conditions associated with vaginal discharge, such as trichomoniasis or candidiasis. Although evidence of sexual transmission of BV is inconclusive, the correct and consistent use of condoms reduces the risk of acquisition. An increased prevalence of BV is associated significantly with race or ethnicity (eg, black), increasing number of sexual partners, poverty, and douching. Preexisting symptomatic or asymptomatic BV may be a risk factor for pelvic inflammatory disease. BV increases the risk of acquiring many other sexually transmitted infections.

Sexually active adolescent and adult females with BV should be evaluated for coinfection with other sexually transmitted infections, including syphilis, gonorrhea, *C trachomatis* infection, trichomoniasis, hepatitis B infection, and human immunodeficiency virus (HIV) infection. Presence of *G vaginalis* in vaginal secretions is not, by itself, adequate for diagnosis of BV.

The **incubation period** for BV is unknown.

DIAGNOSTIC TESTS: The clinical diagnosis of BV requires the presence of 3 or more of the following symptoms or signs (Amsel criteria):
- Homogenous, grey or white, noninflammatory vaginal discharge that smoothly coats the vaginal walls
- Vaginal fluid pH greater than 4.5
- A fishy odor (amine test) of vaginal discharge before or after addition of 10% potassium hydroxide (ie, the whiff test)
- Presence of "clue cells" (squamous vaginal epithelial cells covered with bacteria, which cause a stippled or granular appearance and ragged "moth-eaten" borders) on microscopic examination of at least 20% of vaginal epithelial cells.

A Gram stain of vaginal secretions is an alternative means of establishing a diagnosis. A paucity of large gram-positive bacilli consistent with lactobacilli and a predominance of gram-negative and gram-variable rods and cocci (eg, *G vaginalis, Prevotella* species, *Porphyromonas* species, and *Peptostreptococcus* species) and curved gram-negative rods (*Mobiluncus* species) are characteristic. Douching, recent intercourse, menstruation, and coexisting infection can alter findings on Gram stain. Culture for *G vaginalis* is not recommended, because the organism is found in females without BV, including females who are not sexually active.

TREATMENT: The principal goal of treatment is to relieve vaginal symptoms and signs of infection and decrease the risk of infectious complications. All nonpregnant patients who are symptomatic require treatment. Nonpregnant patients with symptoms should be treated with metronidazole, 1.0 g/day, orally, in 2 divided doses for 7 days; tinidazole, 2 g/day orally for 2 days; metronidazole gel, 0.75%, 5 g (1 applicator), intravaginally, once a day for 5 days; or clindamycin cream, 2%, 1 applicator (5 g), intravaginally, at bedtime for 7 days. Clindamycin cream can weaken latex condoms and diaphragms for up to 5 days after completion of therapy. Alternative regimens that have a lower efficacy for BV are single-dose metronidazole, oral clindamycin, or clindamycin intravaginal ovales.

Pregnant women with symptoms of BV should be treated, regardless of other risk factors for adverse pregnancy outcome. Topical intravaginal clindamycin cream is not recommended in the latter part of pregnancy, because it can result in preterm labor. Asymptomatic pregnant women at increased risk of adverse pregnancy outcome in association with BV (eg, previous preterm birth) also should be treated, according to some experts. Metronidazole (1.0 g/day, in 2 divided doses; or 750 mg/day, in 3 divided doses daily for 7 days) is the preferred treatment during pregnancy. An alternative regimen is clindamycin, 600 mg/day, orally, in 2 divided doses for 7 days. Because treatment of BV in high-risk pregnant women who are asymptomatic might prevent adverse pregnancy outcomes, a follow-up evaluation 1 month after completion of treatment should be considered to evaluate whether therapy was successful.

For nonpregnant women, routine follow-up visits on completion of therapy for BV are unnecessary if symptoms resolve. Recurrences are common and can be treated with the same regimen that was given initially. The presence of a foreign body in the vagina should be excluded. Routine treatment of male sexual partners is not indicated, because treatment has no influence on relapse of recurrence rates.

Treatment of BV in females infected with HIV is the same as for HIV-negative patients and especially is important in women who are pregnant, because BV and chorioamnionitis may increase the risk of perinatal transmission of HIV.

ISOLATION OF THE HOSPITALIZED PATIENT: Standard precautions are recommended.

CONTROL MEASURES: None.

Bacteroides and *Prevotella* Infections

CLINICAL MANIFESTATIONS: *Bacteroides* and *Prevotella* organisms from the oral cavity can cause chronic sinusitis, chronic otitis media, dental infection, peritonsillar abscess, cervical adenitis, retropharyngeal space infection, aspiration pneumonia, lung abscess, empyema, or necrotizing pneumonia. Species from the gastrointestinal tract are recovered in patients with peritonitis, intra-abdominal abscess, pelvic inflammatory disease, postoperative wound infection, or vulvovaginal and perianal infections. Soft tissue infections include synergistic bacterial gangrene and necrotizing fasciitis. Invasion of the bloodstream from the oral cavity or intestinal tract can lead to brain abscess, meningitis, endocarditis, arthritis, or osteomyelitis. Skin involvement includes omphalitis in newborn infants, cellulitis at the site of fetal monitors, human bite wounds, infection of burns adjacent to the mouth or rectum, and decubitus ulcers. Neonatal infections, such as conjunctivitis, pneumonia, bacteremia, or meningitis, rarely occur. Most *Bacteroides* infections are polymicrobial.

ETIOLOGY: Most *Bacteroides* and *Prevotella* organisms associated with human disease are pleomorphic, non-spore–forming, facultatively anaerobic, gram-negative bacilli.

EPIDEMIOLOGY: *Bacteroides* species and *Prevotella* species are part of the normal flora of the mouth, gastrointestinal tract, and female genital tract. Members of the *Bacteroides fragilis* group predominate in the gastrointestinal tract flora; members of the *Prevotella melaninogenica* (formerly *Bacteroides melaninogenicus*) and *Prevotella oralis* (formerly *Bacteroides oralis*) groups are more common in the oral cavity. These species cause infection as opportunists, usually after an alteration of the body's physical barrier, and in conjunction with other endogenous species. Endogenous infection results from aspiration, spillage from the bowel, or damage to mucosal surfaces from trauma, surgery, or chemotherapy. Mucosal injury or granulocytopenia predispose to infection. Except in infections resulting from human bites, no evidence of person-to-person transmission exists.

The **incubation period** is variable and depends on the inoculum and the site of involvement but usually is 1 to 5 days.

DIAGNOSTIC TESTS: Anaerobic culture media are necessary for recovery of *Bacteroides* or *Prevotella* species. Because infections usually are polymicrobial, aerobic cultures also should be obtained. A putrid odor suggests anaerobic infection. Use of an anaerobic transport tube or a sealed syringe is recommended for collection of clinical specimens. Rapid diagnostic tests, including polymerase chain reaction and fluorescent in situ hybridization, are available in research laboratories.

TREATMENT: Abscesses should be drained when feasible; abscesses involving the brain, liver, and lungs may resolve with effective antimicrobial therapy. Necrotizing soft tissue lesions should be débrided surgically.

The choice of antimicrobial agent(s) is based on anticipated or known in vitro susceptibility testing. *Bacteroides* infections of the mouth and respiratory tract generally are susceptible to penicillin G, ampicillin, and broad-spectrum penicillins, such as ticarcillin or piperacillin. Clindamycin is active against virtually all mouth and respiratory tract *Bacteroides* and *Prevotella* isolates and is recommended by some experts as the drug of choice for anaerobic infections of the oral cavity and lungs. Some species of *Bacteroides* and almost 50% of *Prevotella* species produce beta-lactamase. A beta-lactam penicillin active against *Bacteroides* species combined with a beta-lactamase inhibitor (ampicillin-sulbactam, amoxicillin-clavulanate, ticarcillin-clavulanate, or piperacillin-tazobactam) can be useful to treat these infections. *Bacteroides* species of the gastrointestinal tract usually are resistant to penicillin G but are susceptible predictably to metronidazole, beta-lactam plus beta-lactamase inhibitors, chloramphenicol, and sometimes, clindamycin. Tigecycline has demonstrated in vitro activity against *Prevotella* species and *Bacteroides* species but is not approved by the US Food and Drug Administration for use in people younger than 18 years of age. More than 80% of isolates are susceptible to cefoxitin, ceftizoxime, linezolid, imipenem, meropenem, and ertapenem. Cefuroxime, cefotaxime, and ceftriaxone are not reliably effective.

ISOLATION OF THE HOSPITALIZED PATIENT: Standard precautions are recommended.

CONTROL MEASURES: None.

Balantidium coli Infections
(Balantidiasis)

CLINICAL MANIFESTATIONS: Most human infections are asymptomatic. Acute symptomatic infection is characterized by rapid onset of nausea, vomiting, abdominal discomfort or pain, and bloody or watery mucoid diarrhea. In many patients, the course is chronic with intermittent episodes of diarrhea, anorexia, and weight loss. Rarely, organisms spread to mesenteric nodes, pleura, or liver. Inflammation of the gastrointestinal tract and local lymphatic vessels can result in bowel dilation, ulceration, and secondary bacterial invasion. Colitis produced by *Balantidium coli* often is indistinguishable from that produced by *Entamoeba histolytica*. Fulminant disease can occur in malnourished or otherwise debilitated or immunocompromised patients.

ETIOLOGY: *B coli*, a ciliated protozoan, is the largest pathogenic protozoan known to infect humans.

EPIDEMIOLOGY: Pigs are the primary host reservoir of *B coli*, but other sources of infection have been reported. Infections have been reported in most areas of the world but are rare in industrialized countries. Cysts excreted in feces can be transmitted directly from hand to mouth or indirectly through fecally contaminated water or food. Excysted trophozoites infect the colon. A person is infectious as long as cysts are excreted in stool. Cysts may remain viable in the environment for months.

The **incubation period** is unknown but may be several days.

DIAGNOSTIC TESTS: Diagnosis of infection is established by scraping lesions via sigmoidoscopy, histologic examination of intestinal biopsy specimens, or ova and parasite examination of stool. The diagnosis usually is established by demonstrating trophozoites in stool or tissue specimens. Stool examination is less sensitive, and repeated stool examination may be necessary to diagnose infection, because shedding of organisms can be intermittent. Microscopic examination of fresh diarrheal stools must be performed promptly, because trophozoites degenerate rapidly.

TREATMENT: The drug of choice is tetracycline, which should not be given to children younger than 8 years of age or during pregnancy unless the benefits of therapy are greater than the risks of dental staining (see Antimicrobial Agents and Related Therapy, p 737). Alternative drugs are metronidazole and iodoquinol (see Drugs for Parasitic Infections, p 783).

ISOLATION OF THE HOSPITALIZED PATIENT: In addition to standard precautions, contact precautions are recommended.

CONTROL MEASURES: Control measures include sanitary disposal of human feces and avoidance of contamination of food and water with porcine feces. Despite chlorination of water, waterborne outbreaks of disease have occurred.

Baylisascaris Infections

CLINICAL MANIFESTATIONS: *Baylisascaris procyonis*, a raccoon roundworm, is a rare cause of acute eosinophilic meningoencephalitis. In a young child, acute central nervous system (CNS) disease (eg, altered mental status and seizures) accompanied by peripheral and/or cerebrospinal fluid (CSF) eosinophilia occurs 2 to 4 weeks after infection. Severe neurologic sequelae or death are typical outcomes. *B procyonis* is a rare cause of predominantly extraneural disease in older children and adults. Ocular larva migrans can result in diffuse unilateral subacute neuroretinitis; direct visualization of worms in the retina sometimes is possible. Visceral larval migrans can present with nonspecific signs, such as macular rash, pneumonitis, and hepatomegaly. Subclinical or asymptomatic infection can occur and is thought to be the most common form of infection.

ETIOLOGY: *B procyonis* is a 10- to 25-cm roundworm (nematode) with a life cycle usually limited to its asymptomatic definitive host, the raccoon, and to soil.

EPIDEMIOLOGY: *B procyonis* is found distributed focally throughout the United States; an estimated 22% to 80% of raccoons harbor the parasite in their intestines. Embryonated eggs containing infective larvae are ingested from the soil by raccoons, rodents, and birds. When the infective eggs or infected host is eaten by a raccoon, the larvae grow to maturity in the small intestine, from which adult female worms shed millions of eggs per day. The eggs are 60 to 80 μm in size and have an outer shell that permits long-term viability in soil. Cases have been reported in the Midwest, northeast, and west coast, where significant raccoon populations live near humans.

Risk factors for *Baylisascaris* infection include contact with raccoon latrines, uncovered sand boxes, geophagia/pica, being younger than 4 years of age, and in older children, developmental delay. Nearly all reported cases have been in males.

DIAGNOSTIC TESTS: *Baylisascaris* infection is confirmed by identification of larvae in biopsy specimens. Serologic assays (serum, CSF) are available only in research laboratories, and their sensitivity and specificity are not known. A presumptive diagnosis can be made only on the basis of clinical (meningoencephalitis, diffuse unilateral subacute neuroretinitis, pseudotumor), epidemiologic (raccoon exposure), and laboratory (blood and CSF eosinophilia) findings. Neuroimaging results can be normal initially, but as larval growth and migration through CNS tissue progress, abnormalities are found in periventricular white matter and elsewhere focally. In people with ocular symptoms, ophthalmologic examination can reveal characteristic, chorioretinal lesions or even larvae. Because eggs are not shed in human feces, the disease is not transmitted from person-to-person, and stool examination is not helpful.

TREATMENT: On the basis of CNS and CSF penetration and in vitro activity, albendazole, in conjunction with high-dose corticosteroids, has been advocated most widely. However, treatment with anthelmintic agents and corticosteroids may not affect clinical outcome once severe CNS disease manifestations are evident. Some experts advocate the use of additional anthelmintic agents. Preventive therapy with albendazole is recommended for children with a history of ingestion of soil potentially contaminated with raccoon feces. Worms localized to the retina can be killed by direct photocoagulation (see Drugs for Parasitic Infections, p 783).

ISOLATION OF THE HOSPITALIZED PATIENT: Standard precautions are recommended.

CONTROL MEASURES: *Baylisascaris* infections are prevented by avoiding ingestion of soil containing stool of infective animal reservoirs, primarily raccoons; avoiding raccoon communal defecation sites, such as flat tree stumps and rocks; handwashing, especially after pet or other animal contact; discouraging raccoon presence by limiting access to human or pet food sources; and decontaminating raccoon latrines, particularly latrines located near homes, with lye.

Blastocystis hominis Infections

CLINICAL MANIFESTATIONS: The importance of *Blastocystis* hominis as a cause of gastrointestinal tract disease is controversial. The asymptomatic carrier state is well documented. *B hominis* has been associated with symptoms of bloating, flatulence, mild to moderate diarrhea without fecal leukocytes or blood, abdominal pain, nausea, and poor growth. When *B hominis* is identified in stool from symptomatic patients, other causes of this symptom complex, particularly *Giardia intestinalis* and *Cryptosporidium parvum*, should be investigated before assuming that *B hominis* is the cause of the signs and symptoms. Polymerase chain reaction fingerprinting suggests that some *B hominis* organisms are disease associated but others are not.

ETIOLOGY: *B hominis* is classified as a protozoan, and multiple forms have been described: vacuolar, which is observed most commonly in clinical specimens; granular; which is seen rarely in fresh stools; ameboid; and cystic.

EPIDEMIOLOGY: *B hominis* is recovered from 1% to 20% of stool specimens examined for ova and parasites. Because transmission is believed to be via the fecal-oral route, presence of the organism may be a marker for presence of other pathogens spread by fecal contamination. Transmission from animals occurs.

The **incubation period** is unknown.

DIAGNOSTIC TESTS: Stool specimens should be preserved in polyvinyl alcohol and stained with trichrome or iron-hematoxylin before microscopic examination. The parasite may be present in varying numbers, and infections may be reported as light to heavy. The presence of 5 or more organisms per high-power ($\times$ 400 magnification) field can indicate heavy infection with many organisms, which, to some experts suggests causation when other enteropathogens are absent. Other experts consider the presence of 10 or more organisms per 10 oil immersion fields ($\times$ 1000 magnification) to represent many organisms.

TREATMENT: Indications for treatment are not established. Some experts recommend that treatment should be reserved for patients who have persistent symptoms and in whom no other pathogen or process is found to explain the gastrointestinal tract symptoms; randomized controlled treatment trials for both nitazoxanide and metronidazole have demonstrated benefit in symptomatic patients. Trimethoprim-sulfamethoxazole and iodoquinol have been used with limited success (see Drugs for Parasitic Infections, p 783). Other experts believe that B hominis does not cause symptomatic disease and recommend only a careful search for other causes of symptoms.

ISOLATION OF THE HOSPITALIZED PATIENT: In addition to standard precautions, contact precautions are recommended for diapered or incontinent children.

CONTROL MEASURES: None.

Blastomycosis

CLINICAL MANIFESTATIONS: Infection can be asymptomatic or associated with acute, chronic, or fulminant disease. The major clinical manifestations of blastomycosis are pulmonary, cutaneous, and disseminated. Children commonly have pulmonary disease that can be associated with a variety of symptoms, and radiographic appearances can be misdiagnosed as bacterial pneumonia, tuberculosis, sarcoidosis, or malignant neoplasm. Skin lesions can be nodular, verrucous, or ulcerative, often with minimal inflammation. Abscesses generally are subcutaneous but can involve any organ. Disseminated blastomycosis usually begins with pulmonary infection and can involve skin, bones, central nervous system (CNS), abdominal viscera, and kidneys. Intrauterine or congenital infections occur rarely.

ETIOLOGY: Blastomycosis is caused by *Blastomyces dermatitidis,* a dimorphic fungus existing in the yeast form at 37°C (98°F), in infected tissues, and in a mycelial form at room temperature and in soil. Conidia, produced from hyphae of the mycelial form, are infectious for humans.

EPIDEMIOLOGY: Infection is acquired through inhalation of conidia from soil. Person-to-person transmission does not occur. Infection may be epidemic or sporadic and has been reported in the United States, Canada, Africa, and India. Areas with endemic infection in the United States are the southeastern and central states and the midwestern states bordering the Great Lakes. Although blastomycosis can occur in immunocompetent and immunocompromised hosts, the disease has been reported rarely in people infected with human immunodeficiency virus.

The **incubation period** is approximately 30 to 45 days.

DIAGNOSTIC TESTS: Thick-walled, figure-of-eight shaped, broad-based, single-budding yeast forms may be seen in sputum, tracheal aspirates, cerebrospinal fluid, urine, or material from lesions processed with 10% potassium hydroxide or a silver stain. Children with pneumonia who are unable to produce sputum may require an invasive procedure (eg, open biopsy or bronchoalveolar lavage) to establish the diagnosis. Organisms can be cultured on brain-heart infusion media and Sabouraud dextrose agar at room temperature. Chemiluminescent DNA probes are available for identification of *B dermatitidis.* Because serologic tests lack adequate sensitivity, every effort should be made to obtain appropriate specimens for culture. An assay to detect *Blastomyces* antigen in urine is available commercially, but cross-reactivity occurs in 70% to 100% of patients with histoplasmosis or paracoccidiodiomycosis and with *Penicillium marneffei* infection.

TREATMENT[1]: Amphotericin B is the treatment of choice for life-threatening or CNS infection (see Drugs for Invasive and Other Serious Fungal Infections, p 772). Oral itraconazole or fluconazole has been used for mild or moderately severe infections alone or after a short course of amphotericin B. Data regarding the efficacy of fluconazole therapy in children are limited. Although itraconazole is indicated for treatment of nonmeningeal, non–life-threatening infections in adults, the safety and efficacy of this agent in children has not been established.

Therapy usually is continued for at least 6 months for pulmonary and extrapulmonary disease. Some experts suggest 1 year of therapy for patients with osteomyelitis.

ISOLATION OF THE HOSPITALIZED PATIENT: Standard precautions are recommended.

CONTROL MEASURES: None.

Borrelia Infections
(Relapsing Fever)

CLINICAL MANIFESTATIONS: Relapsing fever is characterized by the sudden onset of high fever, shaking chills, sweats, headache, muscle and joint pains, and nausea. A fleeting macular rash of the trunk and petechiae of the skin and mucous membranes sometimes occur. Complications include hepatosplenomegaly, jaundice, thrombocytopenia, iridocyclitis, cough with pleuritic pain, pneumonitis, meningitis, and myocarditis. Mortality

---

[1]Chapman SW, Dismukes WE, Proia LA, et al. Clinical guidelines for the management of blastomycosis: 2008 update by the Infectious Diseases Society of America. *Clin Infect Dis.* 2008;46(12):1801–1812

rates are 10% to 70% in untreated louseborne relapsing fever (possibly related to comorbidities in refugee-type settings where this disease typically is found) and 4% to 10% in untreated tickborne relapsing fever, and death occurs predominantly in people with underlying illnesses, infants, and the elderly. Early treatment reduces mortality to less than 5%. Untreated, an initial febrile period of 2 to 7 days terminates spontaneously by crisis. The initial febrile episode is followed by an afebrile period of several days to weeks, then by one relapse or more. Relapses typically become shorter and milder progressively as afebrile periods lengthen. Relapse is associated with expression of new borrelial antigens, and resolution of symptoms is associated with production of antibody specific to those new antigenic determinants. Infection during pregnancy often is severe and can result in preterm birth, abortion, stillbirth, or neonatal infection.

ETIOLOGY: Relapsing fever is caused by certain spirochetes of the genus *Borrelia*. *Borrelia recurrentis* is the only species that causes louseborne (epidemic) relapsing fever, and there is no animal reservoir of *B recurrentis*. Worldwide, at least 14 *Borrelia* species cause tickborne (endemic) relapsing fever, including *Borrelia hermsii*, *Borrelia turicatae*, and *Borrelia parkeri* in North America.

EPIDEMIOLOGY: Louseborne epidemic relapsing fever has been reported in Ethiopia, Eritrea, Somalia, and the Sudan, especially among the homeless and in refugee populations. Epidemic transmission occurs when body lice *(Pediculus humanus)* become infected by feeding on humans with spirochetemia; the infection is transmitted when infected lice are crushed and their body fluids contaminate a bite wound or skin abraded by scratching.

Endemic tickborne relapsing fever is distributed widely throughout the world, is transmitted by soft-bodied ticks (*Ornithodoros* species), and occurs sporadically and in small clusters, often within families. Ticks become infected by feeding on rodents or other small mammals and transmit infection via their saliva and other fluids when they take subsequent blood meals. Ticks may serve as reservoirs of infection as a result of transovarial and trans-stadial transmission. Soft-bodied ticks inflict painless bites and feed briefly (10–30 minutes), usually at night, so people often are unaware of bites.

Most tickborne relapsing fever in the United States is caused by *B hermsii*. Infection typically results from tick exposures in rodent-infested cabins in western mountainous areas, including state and national parks. *B turicatae* infections occur less frequently; most cases have been reported from Texas and often are associated with tick exposures in rodent-infested caves. *B parkeri* causes the lowest number of infections and is associated with burrows, rodent nests, and caves in arid areas or grasslands in the western United States.

Infected body lice and ticks remain alive and infectious for several years without feeding. Relapsing fever is not transmitted between individual humans, but perinatal transmission from an infected mother to her infant does occur and can result in preterm birth, stillbirth, and neonatal death.

The **incubation period** is 2 to 18 days, with a mean of 7 days.

DIAGNOSTIC TESTS: Spirochetes can be observed by dark-field microscopy and in Wright-, Giemsa-, or acridine orange-stained preparations of thin or dehemoglobinized thick smears of peripheral blood or in stained buffy-coat preparations. Organisms often can be detected in blood obtained while the person is febrile. Spirochetes can be cultured from blood in Barbour-Stoenner-Kelly medium or by intraperitoneal inoculation of immature laboratory mice. Serum antibodies to *Borrelia* species can be detected by enzyme immunoassay and Western immunoblot analysis at some reference and commercial specialty laboratories; these tests are not standardized and are affected by antigenic variations among and within *Borrelia* species and strains. Serologic cross-reactions occur with other spirochetes, including *Borrelia burgdorferi*, *Treponema pallidum*, and *Leptospira* species. Biologic specimens for laboratory testing can be sent to the Division of Vector-Borne Infectious Diseases, Centers for Disease Control and Prevention, Fort Collins, CO 80522 (telephone: 970-221-6400).

TREATMENT: Treatment of tickborne relapsing fever with a 5- to 10-day course of one of the tetracyclines, usually doxycycline, produces prompt clearance of spirochetes and remission of symptoms. For children younger than 8 years of age and for pregnant women, penicillin and erythromycin are the preferred drugs. Penicillin G procaine or intravenous penicillin G is recommended as initial therapy for people who are unable to take oral therapy, although penicillin G has been associated with an increased rate of relapse. A Jarisch-Herxheimer reaction (an acute febrile reaction accompanied by headache, myalgia, and an aggravated clinical picture lasting less than 24 hours) commonly is observed during the first few hours after initiating antimicrobial therapy. Because this reaction sometimes is associated with transient hypotension attributable to decreased effective circulating blood volume (especially in louseborne relapsing fever), patients should be monitored closely, particularly during the first 4 hours of treatment. However, the Jarisch-Herxheimer reaction in children typically is mild and usually can be managed with antipyretic agents alone.

Single-dose treatment using a tetracycline, penicillin, or erythromycin is effective for curing louseborne relapsing fever.

ISOLATION OF THE HOSPITALIZED PATIENT: Standard precautions are recommended. If louse infestation is present, contact precautions also are indicated (see Pediculosis, p 495–499).

CONTROL MEASURES: Soft ticks often frequent rodent nests; exposure is best reduced by preventing rodent infestations of homes or cabins by blocking rodent access to foundations and attics, and other forms of rodent control. Dwellings infested with soft ticks should be rodent proofed and treated professionally with chemical agents. When in a louse-infested environment, body lice can be controlled by bathing, washing clothing at frequent intervals, and use of pediculicides (see Pediculosis, p 495–499). Reporting of suspected cases of relapsing fever to health authorities is required in most western states and is important for initiation of prompt investigation and institution of control measures.

Brucellosis

CLINICAL MANIFESTATIONS: Brucellosis in children commonly is a mild self-limited disease compared with the more chronic disease in adults. However, in areas where *Brucella melitensis* is the endemic species, disease can be severe. Onset of illness can be acute or insidious. Manifestations are nonspecific and include fever, night sweats, weakness, malaise, anorexia, weight loss, arthralgia, myalgia, abdominal pain, and headache. Physical findings include lymphadenopathy, hepatosplenomegaly, and occasionally, arthritis. Serious complications include meningitis, endocarditis, and osteomyelitis, especially involving the sacroiliac joint.

ETIOLOGY: *Brucella* species are small, nonmotile, gram-negative coccobacilli. The species that infect humans are *Brucella abortus, B melitensis, Brucella suis,* and rarely, *Brucella canis.*

EPIDEMIOLOGY: Brucellosis is a zoonotic disease of wild and domestic animals. Humans are accidental hosts, contracting the disease by direct contact with infected animals or their carcasses or secretions or by ingesting unpasteurized milk or milk products. People in occupations such as farming, ranching, and veterinary medicine as well as abattoir workers, meat inspectors, and laboratory personnel are at increased risk. Infection is transmitted by inoculation through cuts and abrasions in the skin, inhalation of contaminated aerosols, contact with the conjunctival mucosa, or oral ingestion. One hundred to 150 cases of brucellosis are reported annually in the United States, and 3% to 10% of cases occur in people younger than 19 years of age. Most cases occur in immigrants or travelers returning from areas with endemic infection and result from ingestion of unpasteurized dairy products. Although human-to-human transmission is rare, congenital brucellosis has been reported, and infected mothers can transmit *Brucella* species to their infants through breastfeeding.

The **incubation period** varies from less than 1 week to several months, but most people become ill within 3 to 4 weeks of exposure.

DIAGNOSTIC TESTS: A definitive diagnosis is established by recovery of *Brucella* species from blood, bone marrow, or other tissue. A variety of media will support growth of *Brucella* species, but the physician should contact laboratory personnel and ask them to incubate cultures for a minimum of 4 weeks. In patients with a clinically compatible illness, serologic testing can confirm the diagnosis with a fourfold or greater increase in antibody titers in serum specimens collected at least 2 weeks apart. The serum agglutination test, the most commonly used test, will detect antibodies against *B abortus, B suis,* and *B melitensis,* but not *B canis,* which requires use of *B canis*-specific antigen. Although a single titer is not diagnostic, most patients with active infection in an area without endemic infection have a titer of 1:160 or greater within 2 weeks of clinical disease onset. Lower titers may be found early in the course of infection. Immunoglobulin (Ig) M antibodies are produced within the first week, followed by a gradual increase in IgG synthesis. Low IgM titers may persist for months or years after initial infection. Increased concentrations of IgG agglutinins are found in acute infection, chronic infection, and relapse. When interpreting serum agglutination test results, the possibility of cross-reactions of *Brucella* antibodies with those against other gram-negative bacteria, such as *Yersinia enterocolitica* serotype 09, *Francisella tularensis,* and *Vibrio cholerae,* should be considered. To avoid a prozone phenomenon, serum should be diluted to 1:320 or higher before testing. Enzyme immunoassay is a sensitive method for determining IgG, IgA, and IgM anti-*Brucella* antibodies. Until better standardization is established, enzyme immunoassay should be used only for suspected cases with negative serum agglutination test results or for evaluation of patients with suspected relapse or reinfection. Polymerase chain reaction tests have been developed but are not available in most clinical laboratories.

TREATMENT: Prolonged antimicrobial therapy is imperative for achieving a cure. Relapses generally are not associated with development of *Brucella* resistance but rather with premature discontinuation of therapy. Monotherapy is associated with a high rate of relapse; combination therapy is recommended.

Oral doxycycline (2–4 mg/kg per day, maximum 200 mg/day, in 2 divided doses) or oral tetracycline (30–40 mg/kg per day, maximum 2 g/day, in 4 divided doses) is the drug of choice and should be administered for at least 6 weeks. However, tetracyclines should be avoided, if possible, in children younger than 8 years of age (see Antimicrobial Agents and Related Therapy, p 737). Oral trimethoprim-sulfamethoxazole (trimethoprim, 10 mg/kg per day, maximum 480 mg/day; and sulfamethoxazole, 50 mg/kg per day, maximum 2.4 g/day) divided in 2 doses for 4 to 6 weeks is appropriate therapy for younger children.

To decrease the incidence of relapse, combination therapy with a tetracycline (or trimethoprim-sulfamethoxazole if tetracyclines are contraindicated) and rifampin (15–20 mg/kg per day, maximum 600–900 mg/day, in 1 or 2 divided doses) is recommended. Because of the potential emergence of rifampin resistance, rifampin monotherapy is not recommended.

For treatment of serious infections or complications, including endocarditis, meningitis, and osteomyelitis, streptomycin or gentamicin for the first 14 days of therapy in addition to a tetracycline for 6 weeks (or trimethoprim-sulfamethoxazole if tetracyclines are contraindicated) are recommended. In addition, rifampin can be used with this regimen to decrease the rate of relapse. For life-threatening complications of brucellosis, such as meningitis or endocarditis, the duration of therapy often is extended for 4 to 6 months. Surgical intervention should be considered in patients with complications such as deep tissue abscesses.

The benefit of corticosteroids for people with neurobrucellosis is unproven. Occasionally, a Jarisch-Herxheimer-like reaction (an acute febrile reaction accompanied by headache, myalgia, and an aggravated clinical picture lasting less than 24 hours) occurs shortly after initiation of antimicrobial therapy, but this reaction rarely is severe enough to require corticosteroids.

ISOLATION OF THE HOSPITALIZED PATIENT: In addition to standard precautions, contact precautions are indicated for patients with draining wounds.

CONTROL MEASURES: The control of human brucellosis depends on eradication of *Brucella* species from cattle, goats, swine, and other animals. Pasteurization of milk and milk products for human consumption is important to prevent disease in children. The certification of raw milk does not eliminate the risk of transmission of *Brucella* organisms.

Burkholderia Infections

CLINICAL MANIFESTATIONS: *Burkholderia cepacia* complex has been associated with severe pulmonary infections in patients with cystic fibrosis, with significant bacteremia in preterm infants after prolonged hospitalization, and with infection in children with chronic granulomatous disease, hemoglobinopathies, or malignant neoplasms. Health care-associated infections include wound and urinary tract infections and pneumonia. Pulmonary infections in people with cystic fibrosis occur late in the course of disease, usually after respiratory epithelial damage caused by infection with *Pseudomonas aeruginosa* has been established. Patients with positive culture results can experience no change in the rate of pulmonary decompensation, become chronically infected and exhibit a more rapid decline in pulmonary function, or experience an unexpectedly rapid deterioration in clinical status that results in death. In patients with chronic granulomatous disease, pneumonia is the most common manifestation of *B cepacia* complex infection; lymphadenitis also occurs. Disease onset is insidious, with low-grade fever early in the course and systemic effects occurring 3 to 4 weeks later. Pleural effusion is common, and lung abscess can occur.

Burkholderia pseudomallei is the cause of melioidosis, which is endemic in southeast Asia and northern Australia but also found in other tropical and subtropical areas. Melioidosis can occur in the United States, usually among travelers returning from areas with endemic disease. Melioidosis can manifest as a localized infection or as fulminant septicemia. Localized infection usually is nonfatal and most commonly manifests as pneumonia, but skin, soft tissue, and skeletal infections also occur. In severe cutaneous infection, necrotizing fasciitis has been reported. In disseminated infection, hepatic and splenic abscesses can occur, and relapses are common without prolonged therapy.

ETIOLOGY: *Burkholderia* organisms are nutritionally diverse, oxidase- and catalase-producing, non–lactose-fermenting, gram-negative bacilli. *B cepacia* complex comprises at least 10 species (*B cepacia, Burkholderia multivorans, Burkholderia cenocepacia, Burkholderia stabilis, Burkholderia vietnamiensis, Burkholderia dolosa, Burkholderia ambifaria, Burkholderia anthina, Burkholderia pyrrocinia,* and *Burkholderia ubonensis*). Other species of *Burkholderia* include *Burkholderia gladioli, Burkholderia mallei, Burkholderia thailandensis, Burkholderia oklahomensis,* and *B pseudomallei,* which is the cause of the disease melioidosis.

EPIDEMIOLOGY: *Burkholderia* species are waterborne and soilborne organisms that can survive for prolonged periods in a moist environment. Epidemiologic studies of recreational camps and social events attended by people with cystic fibrosis from different geographic areas have demonstrated person-to-person spread of *B cepacia* complex. The source for acquisition of *B cepacia* complex by patients with chronic granulomatous disease has not been identified. Health care-associated spread of *B cepacia* complex most often is associated with contamination of disinfectant solutions used to clean reusable patient equipment, such as bronchoscopes and pressure transducers, or to disinfect skin. *B gladioli* also has been isolated from sputum from people with cystic fibrosis and may be mistaken for *B cepacia.* The clinical significance of *B gladioli* is not known.

In areas with highly endemic infection, *B pseudomallei* is acquired early in life, with the highest seroconversion rates between 6 and 42 months of age. Disease can be acquired by direct inhalation of aerosolized organisms, from dust particles containing organisms or by percutaneous or wound inoculation with contaminated soil. Symptomatic infection can occur in people as early as 1 year of age. Risk factors for disease include diabetes mellitus and renal insufficiency, but most people with melioidosis in areas with endemic infection have no underlying disease. *B pseudomallei* also has been reported to cause pulmonary infection in people with cystic fibrosis and people traveling to areas with endemic infection as well as septicemia in children with chronic granulomatous disease.

The **incubation period** is 1 to 21 days, with a median of 9 days but can be prolonged (years) for melioidosis.

DIAGNOSTIC TESTS: Culture is the appropriate method to diagnose *B cepacia* complex infection. In cystic fibrosis lung infection, culture of sputum on selective agar is recommended to decrease the potential for overgrowth by mucoid *P aeruginosa. B cepacia* and *B gladioli* can be identified by polymerase chain reaction assay, but this assay is not available routinely. Definitive diagnosis of melioidosis is made by isolation of *B pseudomallei* from blood or other infected sites. The likelihood of successfully isolating the organism is increased by culturing sputum, throat, rectum, and ulcers or skin lesions. A positive result by the indirect hemagglutination assay for a traveler who has returned from an area with endemic infection may support the diagnosis of meliodosis, but definitive diagnosis still requires isolation of *B pseudomallei* from an infected site. Other rapid assays are being developed for diagnosis of melioidosis, but none are available commercially.

TREATMENT: Meropenem is the agent most active against the majority of *B cepacia* complex isolates, although other drugs that may be effective include trimethoprim-sulfamethoxazole, ceftazidime, chloramphenicol, and imipenem. Most experts recommend combinations of antimicrobial agents that provide synergistic activity against *B cepacia* complex. Most *B cepacia* complex isolates are resistant intrinsically to aminoglycosides and polymyxin B.

The drugs of choice for melioidosis include ceftazidime, meropenem, or imipenem. After acute therapy is completed, eradication can be attempted with trimethoprim-sulfamethoxazole and doxycycline for 20 weeks to reduce recurrence, but the optimal duration and regimen remain unclear.

ISOLATION OF THE HOSPITALIZED PATIENT: Contact and droplet precautions are recommended for patients infected with multidrug-resistant strains of *B cepacia* complex. Standard precautions are recommended for people with *B pseudomallei* infection.

CONTROL MEASURES: Because some strains of *B cepacia* complex are highly transmissible and virulence is not well understood, many centers limit contact between *B cepacia* complex-infected and -uninfected patients with cystic fibrosis. This includes inpatient, outpatient, and social settings. For example, patients with cystic fibrosis who are infected with *B cepacia* complex are cared for in single rooms and have unique clinic hours.

Education of patients and families about hand hygiene and appropriate personal hygiene is recommended. Prevention of infection with *B pseudomallei* in areas with endemic infection can be difficult, because contact with contaminated water and soil is common. People with diabetes mellitus and skin lesions should avoid contact with soil and standing water in these areas. Wearing boots and gloves during agricultural work in areas with endemic infection is recommended.

Human Calicivirus Infections (Norovirus and Sapovirus)

CLINICAL MANIFESTATIONS: Abrupt onset of vomiting accompanied by watery diarrhea, abdominal cramps, and nausea are characteristic but not pathognomonic of human calicivirus (HuCV) infections. Mild to moderate diarrhea without vomiting is common in children. Symptoms last from 24 to 60 hours.

ETIOLOGY: Caliciviruses are 20- to 40-nm, noneveloped, single-stranded RNA viruses belonging to the Caliciviridae family. Vesivirus and lagovirus infect animals, in contrast to Norovirus and Sapovirus, which commonly infect humans and are referred to as HuCVs. HuCVs are diverse genetically and antigenically but can be grouped into genogroups and genotypes for epidemiologic purposes.

EPIDEMIOLOGY: HuCVs have a worldwide distribution, with multiple antigenic types circulating simultaneously in the same region. HuCVs, of which most are noroviruses, are a major cause of both sporadic cases and outbreaks of gastroenteritis. Norovirus GII.4 genotype has been predominant during the past decade in the United States, Europe, and Oceania. Sapovirus infections have been less frequently reported, albeit increasingly, mostly from children with sporadic acute diarrhea. Asymptomatic norovirus excretion is common in children. In the United States, noroviruses account for more than 90% of community outbreaks associated with viral gastroenteritis, which occur in all age groups. Outbreaks with high attack rates tend to occur in closed populations, such as child care centers and on cruise ships. Transmission is by person-to-person spread via the fecal-oral route or through contaminated food or water. Common-source outbreaks have been described after ingestion of ice, shellfish, and a variety of ready-to-eat foods, including salads and bakery products, usually contaminated by infected food handlers. Transmission via vomitus has been documented. Exposure to contaminated surfaces and vomitus has been implicated in some outbreaks. Excretion lasts 5 to 7 days after onset of symptoms in approximately 50% of infected people, and in 25%, excretion can be as long as 3 weeks. Prolonged excretion can occur in immunocompromised hosts. Infection occurs year round but is more common during the colder months of the year.

The **incubation period** is 12 to 48 hours.

DIAGNOSTIC TESTS: Commercial assays for diagnosis are not available in the United States. The following tests are available in some research and reference laboratories: electron microscopy for detection of viral particles in stool, enzyme immunoassay for detection of viral antigen in stool or antibody in serum, and reverse transcriptase-polymerase chain reaction (RT-PCR) assay for detection of viral RNA in stool. A complex 3-dimensional tissue-culture model for noroviruses has been developed and is under evaluation. The most sensitive assays utilize real-time RT-PCR; electron microscopy is insensitive compared with RT-PCR assay. Laboratory and epidemiologic support for diagnosis of suspected calicivirus outbreaks is available at the Centers for Disease Control and Prevention, and RT-PCR assays for viral detection in stools increasingly are available at state and local health department laboratories.

TREATMENT: Supportive therapy includes oral or intravenous rehydration solutions to replace fluid and electrolytes.

ISOLATION OF THE HOSPITALIZED PATIENT: In addition to standard precautions, contact precautions are recommended for diapered and incontinent children for the duration of illness.

CONTROL MEASURES: Several factors favor transmission. HuCVs are extremely contagious, large numbers of virus can be excreted, and shedding can last several weeks. The spread of infection can be decreased by standard measures for control of diarrhea, such as educating child care providers and all food handlers about infection control, maintaining cleanliness of surfaces and food preparation areas, using appropriate disinfectants approved by the US Environmental Protection Agency, excluding caregivers or food handlers who are ill, exercising adequate hand hygiene, and excluding or grouping ill children in child care (see Children in Out-of-Home Child Care, p 124). If a mode of transmission can be identified (eg, contaminated food, such as shellfish, or water) during an outbreak, then specific interventions to interrupt transmission can be effective. People with diarrhea caused by this potentially waterborne pathogen should not use recreational water venues (eg, swimming pools, lakes, rivers, the ocean) for 2 weeks after symptoms resolve. The lack of demonstration of protective immunity elicited by natural HuCV infections has curtailed vaccine development to date.

Campylobacter Infections

CLINICAL MANIFESTATIONS: Predominant symptoms of *Campylobacter* infections include diarrhea, abdominal pain, malaise, and fever. Stools can contain visible or occult blood. In neonates and young infants, bloody diarrhea without fever can be the only manifestation of infection. Abdominal pain can mimic that produced by appendicitis or intussusception. Mild infection lasts 1 or 2 days and resembles viral gastroenteritis. Most patients recover in less than 1 week, but 20% have a relapse or a prolonged or severe illness. Severe or persistent infection can mimic acute inflammatory bowel disease. Bacteremia is uncommon but can occur in children, including neonates. Immunocompromised hosts can have prolonged, relapsing, or extraintestinal infections, especially with *Campylobacter fetus* and other species. Immunoreactive complications, such as acute idiopathic polyneuritis (Guillain-Barré syndrome), Miller Fisher syndrome (ophthalmoplegia, areflexia, ataxia), reactive arthritis, Reiter syndrome (arthritis, urethritis, and bilateral conjunctivitis), and erythema nodosum, can occur during convalescence.

ETIOLOGY: *Campylobacter* species are motile, comma-shaped, gram-negative bacilli that cause gastroenteritis. *Campylobacter jejuni* and *Campylobacter coli* are the most common species isolated from patients with diarrhea. *C fetus* predominantly causes systemic illness in neonates and debilitated hosts. Other *Campylobacter* species, including *Campylobacter upsaliensis, Campylobacter lari,* and *Campylobacter hyointestinalis,* can cause similar diarrheal or systemic illnesses in children.

EPIDEMIOLOGY: An estimated 2.4 million cases of *Campylobacter* infection occur in the United States each year, leading to 13 000 hospitalizations and 124 deaths. Data from the Foodborne Diseases Active Surveillance Network (**www.cdc.gov/foodnet**) indicate a 30% decrease in the incidence of infections since 1996. In 2007, the incidence was 12.8 per 100 000 population. The highest rates of infection occur in children younger than 5 years of age, and the incidence is higher in males than in females. In susceptible people, as few as 500 *Campylobacter* organisms can cause infection.

The gastrointestinal tracts of domestic and wild birds and animals are reservoirs of infection. *C jejuni* and *C coli* have been isolated from feces of 30% to 100% of healthy chickens, turkeys, and water fowl. Poultry carcasses usually are contaminated. Many farm animals and meat sources can harbor the organism, and pets (especially young animals), including dogs, cats, hamsters, and birds, are potential sources of infection. Transmission of *C jejuni* and *C coli* occurs by ingestion of contaminated food or by direct contact with fecal material from infected animals or people. Improperly cooked poultry, untreated water, and unpasteurized milk have been the main vehicles of transmission. Outbreaks are rare but have occurred among school children who drank unpasteurized milk, including children who participated in field trips to dairy farms. Person-to-person spread occurs occasionally, particularly among very young children, and outbreaks of diarrhea in child care centers have been reported uncommonly. Person-to-person transmission also has occurred in neonates of infected mothers and has resulted in health care-related outbreaks in nurseries. In perinatal infection, *C jejuni* and *C coli* usually cause neonatal gastroenteritis, whereas *C fetus* often causes neonatal septicemia or meningitis. Enteritis occurs in people of all ages. Communicability is uncommon but is greatest during the acute phase of illness. Excretion of *Campylobacter* organisms typically lasts 2 to 3 weeks without treatment.

The **incubation period** usually is 2 to 5 days but can be longer.

DIAGNOSTIC TESTS: *C jejuni* and *C coli* can be cultured from feces, and *Campylobacter* species, including *C fetus*, can be cultured from blood. Laboratory identification of *C jejuni* and *C coli* in stool specimens requires selective media, microaerophilic conditions, and an incubation temperature of 42°C. Unless the laboratory uses a nonselective isolation technique, such as filtration, many *Campylobacter* species other than *C jejuni* and *C coli* will not be detected. *C upsaliensis, C hyointestinalis,* and *C fetus* may not be isolated because of susceptibility to antimicrobial agents present in routinely used *Campylobacter* selective media. Because many of the species not isolated on routine selective media require increased hydrogen, the filtration method is best used if an atmosphere containing increased hydrogen can be used. The presence of motile, curved, spiral, or S-shaped rods resembling *Vibrio cholerae* by stool phase contrast or darkfield microscopy can provide rapid, presumptive evidence for *Campylobacter* species infection. *Campylobacter* species can be detected directly in stool specimens by commercially available enzyme immunoassay or in research laboratories by polymerase chain reaction assay.

TREATMENT: Rehydration is the mainstay for all children with diarrhea. Erythromycin and azithromycin shorten the duration of illness and excretion of organisms and prevent relapse when given early in gastrointestinal tract infection. Treatment with azithromycin or erythromycin usually eradicates the organism from stool within 2 or 3 days. A fluoroquinolone, such as ciprofloxacin, may be effective, but resistance is common (22% of isolates in the United States in 2005 **[www.cdc.gov/NARMS]**), and fluoroquinolones are not approved for this indication by the US Food and Drug Administration for people younger than 18 years of age (see Antimicrobial Agents and Related Therapy, p 737). If antimicrobial therapy is given for treatment of gastroenteritis, the recommended duration is 5 to 7 days. Antimicrobial agents for bacteremia should be selected on the basis of antimicrobial susceptibility tests. *C fetus* generally is susceptible to aminoglycosides, extended-spectrum cephalosporins, meropenem, imipenem, and ampicillin.

ISOLATION OF THE HOSPITALIZED PATIENT: In addition to standard precautions, contact precautions are recommended for diapered and incontinent children for the duration of illness.

CONTROL MEASURES:
- Exercise hand hygiene after handling raw poultry, wash cutting boards and utensils with soap and water after contact with raw poultry, avoid contact of fruits and vegetables with juices of raw poultry, and cook poultry thoroughly.
- Exercise hand hygiene after contact with feces of dogs and cats, particularly stool of puppies and kittens with diarrhea.
- Pasteurization of milk and chlorination of water supplies are important.
- People with diarrhea should be excluded from food handling, care of patients in hospitals, and care of people in custodial care and child care centers.
- Infected food handlers and hospital employees who are asymptomatic need not be excluded from work if proper personal hygiene measures, including hand hygiene, are maintained.

- Outbreaks are uncommon in child care centers. General measures for interrupting enteric transmission in child care centers are recommended (see Children in Out-of-Home Child Care, p 124). Infants and children in diapers with symptomatic infection should be excluded from child care or cared for in a separate area until diarrhea has subsided. Azithromycin or erythromycin treatment may further limit the potential for transmission.
- Stool cultures of asymptomatic exposed children are not recommended.

Candidiasis
(Moniliasis, Thrush)

CLINICAL MANIFESTATIONS: Mucocutaneous infection results in oral-pharyngeal (thrush) or vaginal candidiasis; intertriginous lesions of the gluteal folds, neck, groin, and axilla; paronychia; and onychia. Dysfunction of T lymphocytes, other immunologic disorders, and endocrinologic diseases are associated with chronic mucocutaneous candidiasis. Chronic or recurrent oral candidiasis may be the presenting sign of human immunodeficiency virus (HIV) infection or primary immunodeficiency. Esophageal and laryngeal candidiasis can occur in immunocompromised patients. Disseminated or invasive candidiasis occurs in very low birth weight newborn infants and in immunocompromised or debilitated hosts, can involve virtually any organ or anatomic site, and can be rapidly fatal. Candidemia can occur with or without systemic disease in patients with indwelling vascular catheters, especially patients receiving prolonged intravenous infusions with parenteral alimentation or lipids. Peritonitis can occur in patients undergoing peritoneal dialysis, especially in patients receiving prolonged broad-spectrum antimicrobial therapy. Candiduria can occur in patients with indwelling urinary catheters, focal renal infection, or disseminated disease.

ETIOLOGY: *Candida* species are yeasts that reproduce by budding. *Candida albicans* and some *Candida tropicalis* are dimorphic and form long chains of elongated yeast forms called pseudohyphae. *C albicans* causes most infections, but in some patient populations, the non-*albicans Candida* species now account for more than half of invasive infections. Other species, including *C tropicalis*, *Candida parapsilosis*, *Candida glabrata*, *Candida krusei*, *Candida guilliermondii*, *Candida lusitaniae*, and *Candida dubliniensis*, also can cause serious infections, especially in immunocompromised and debilitated hosts. *C parapsilosis* is second only to *C albicans* as a cause of systemic candidiasis in very low birth weight neonates.

EPIDEMIOLOGY: *C albicans* is ubiquitous. Like other *Candida* species, *C albicans* is present on skin and in the mouth, intestinal tract, and vagina of immunocompetent people. Vulvovaginal candidiasis is associated with pregnancy, and newborn infants can acquire the organism in utero, during passage through the vagina, or postnatally. Mild mucocutaneous infection is common in healthy infants. Person-to-person transmission occurs rarely. Invasive disease occurs typically in people with impaired immunity, with infection usually arising from colonization sites. Factors such as extreme prematurity, neutropenia, or treatment with corticosteroids or cytotoxic chemotherapy can increase the risk of invasive infection. People with diabetes mellitus generally have localized mucocutaneous lesions. An estimated 5% to 20% of newborn infants weighing less than 1000 g at birth develop invasive candidiasis. Patients with neutrophil defects, such as chronic granulomatous disease or myeloperoxidase deficiency, also are at increased risk. Patients undergoing intravenous alimentation or receiving broad-spectrum antimicrobial agents, especially extended-spectrum cephalosporins, carbapenems, and vancomycin, or requiring long-term indwelling central venous or peritoneal dialysis catheters, have increased susceptibility to infection. Postsurgical patients can be at risk, particularly after cardiothoracic or abdominal procedures.

The **incubation period** is unknown.

DIAGNOSTIC TESTS: The presumptive diagnosis of mucocutaneous candidiasis or thrush usually can be made clinically, but other organisms or trauma also can cause clinically similar lesions. Yeast cells and pseudohyphae can be found in *C albicans*-infected tissue and are identifiable by microscopic examination of scrapings prepared with Gram or calcofluor white stain or suspended in 10% to 20% potassium hydroxide. Endoscopy is useful for diagnosis of esophagitis. Ophthalmologic examination can reveal typical retinal lesions that can result from candidemia. Lesions in the brain, kidney, liver, or spleen may be detected by ultrasonography or computed tomography; however, these lesions may not appear by imaging until late in the course of disease or after neutropenia has resolved.

A definitive diagnosis of invasive candidiasis requires isolation of the organism from a typically sterile body fluid or tissue (eg, blood, cerebrospinal fluid, bone marrow, or biopsy specimen) or demonstration of organisms in a tissue biopsy specimen. Negative results of culture for *Candida* species do not exclude invasive infection in immunocompromised hosts. Recovery of the organism is expedited using blood culture systems that are biphasic or use a lysis-centrifugation method. Special fungal culture media are not needed to grow *Candida* species. A presumptive species identification of *C albicans* can be made by demonstrating germ tube formation. Another method of detection is the assay for (1,3)-beta-D-glucan from fungal cell walls, which does not distinguish *Candida* species from other fungi and currently is not in widespread use but offers promise as a tool for diagnosis of noninvasive disease. Data on use of the assay for children are limited.

TREATMENT[1]:

Mucous Membrane and Skin Infections. Oral candidiasis in immunocompetent hosts is treated with oral nystatin suspension or clotrimazole troches applied to lesions. Troches should not be used in infants.

Fluconazole or itraconazole can be beneficial for immunocompromised patients with oropharyngeal candidiasis. Voriconazole or posaconazole are alternative drugs. Although cure rates with fluconazole are greater than with nystatin, relapse rates are comparable. Safety and efficacy of itraconazole in HIV-infected children with oropharyngeal candidiasis have been demonstrated.

Esophagitis caused by *Candida* species is treated with oral or intravenous fluconazole or oral itraconazole solutions for 14 to 21 days after clinical improvement. Alternatively, voriconazole, intravenous amphotericin B, caspofungin, micafungin, or anidulafungin (18 years of age and older) can be used for refractory, azole-resistant, or severe esophageal candidiasis. Duration of treatment depends on severity of illness and patient factors, such as age and degree of immunocompromise.

---

[1]Infectious Diseases Society of America. Clinical practice guidelines for the management of candidiasis: 2009 update by the Infectious Diseases Society of America. *Clin Infect Dis.* 2009;48(5):503–535

Skin infections are treated with topical nystatin, miconazole, clotrimazole, naftifine, ketoconazole, econazole, or ciclopirox (see Topical Drugs for Superficial Fungal Infections, p 773). Nystatin usually is effective and is the least expensive of these drugs.

Vulvovaginal candidiasis is treated effectively with many topical formulations, including clotrimazole, miconazole, butoconazole, terconazole, and tioconazole. Such topically applied azole drugs are more effective than nystatin. Oral azole agents (fluconazole, itraconazole, and ketoconazole) also are effective and should be considered for recurrent or refractory cases (see Recommended Doses of Parenteral and Oral Antifungal Drugs, p 768).

For chronic mucocutaneous candidiasis, fluconazole, itraconazole and voriconazole are effective drugs. Low-dose amphotericin B given intravenously is effective in severe cases. Relapses are common with any of these agents once therapy is terminated, and treatment should be viewed as a lifelong process, hopefully using only intermittent pulses of antifungal agents. Invasive infections in patients with this condition are rare.

Keratomycosis is treated with corneal baths of amphotericin B (1 mg/mL of sterile water) in conjunction with systemic therapy. Patients with cystitis, especially patients with neutropenia, patients with renal allographs, and patients undergoing urologic manipulation attributable to *Candida* organisms, should be treated with fluconazole because of the concentrating effect of fluconazole in the urinary tract. An alternative is a short course (7 days) of low-dose amphotericin B intravenously (0.3 mg/kg per day). Repeated bladder irrigations with amphotericin B (50 μg/mL of sterile water) have been used to treat patients with candidal cystitis, but this does not treat disease beyond the bladder and is not recommended routinely. A urinary catheter in a patient with candidiasis should be removed or replaced.

Invasive Disease. Treatment of invasive candidiasis should include removal of any infected central vascular or peritoneal catheters and replacement, if necessary, when infection is controlled and, to the extent possible, avoidance or reduction of systemic immunosuppression.

Amphotericin B deoxycholate is the drug of choice for treating neonates with systemic candidiasis; if urinary tract involvement and meningitis are excluded, lipid formulations can be considered. Echinocandins should be used with caution in neonates. Treatment for neonates is 3 weeks. In nonneutropenic children and adults, fluconazole or an echinocandin (caspofungin, micafungin, anidulafungin) is the recommended treatment; amphotericin B deoxycholate or lipid formulations are alternative therapies (see Drugs for Invasive and Other Serious Fungal Infections, p 772). In nonneutropenic patients with candidemia and no metastatic complications, the treatment is 2 weeks after clearance of *Candida* organisms from the bloodstream. In critically ill neutropenic patients, an echinocandin or a lipid formulation of amphotericin B is recommended. In less seriously ill neutropenic patients, fluconazole is the alternative treatment, and voriconazole may be considered. The duration of treament for candidemia without metastatic complications is 2 weeks after documented clearance of *Candida* organisms from the bloodstream and resolution of neutropenia.

Most *Candida* species are susceptible to amphotericin B, although *C lusitaniae* and some strains of *C glabrata* and *C krusei* have decreased susceptibility or resistance. Among patients with persistent candidemia despite appropriate therapy, investigation for a deep focus of infection should be conducted. Short-course therapy (ie, 7–10 days) can be used for intravenous catheter-associated infections, provided the catheter is removed promptly and there is no evidence of invasive disease (ie, negative blood cultures after catheter removal). Lipid-associated preparations of amphotericin B can be used as an alternative to amphotericin B deoxycholate in patients who experience significant toxicity during therapy. Published reports in adults and anecdotal reports in preterm infants indicate that lipid-associated amphotericin B preparations have failed to eradicate renal candidiasis, because these large-molecule drugs may not penetrate well into the renal parenchyma.

Flucytosine can be given with intravenous amphotericin B deoxycholate for *C albicans* infection involving the central nervous system if enteral administration is feasible. The dose of flucytosine should be decreased for patients with renal insufficiency. Serum concentrations of flucytosine should be maintained between 40 and 60 µg/mL; higher concentrations (100 µg/L or greater) predispose to toxic effects, but delays in obtaining assay results often limit their utility. Adverse effects of flucytosine, which are more common in patients with azotemia, include dose-related bone marrow suppression, rash, hepatic and renal dysfunction, diarrhea, gastrointestinal tract bleeding, and ulcerative colitis.

Fluconazole may be appropriate for patients with impaired renal function or for patients with meningitis. However, data on fluconazole use for *Candida* meningitis are limited. Fluconazole is not an appropriate choice for therapy before the infecting *Candida* species is known, because *C krusei* is resistant to fluconazole, and up to 50% of *C glabrata* also can be resistant. Caspofungin, micafungin, and anidulafungin all are active in vitro against most *Candida* species and are appropriate first-line drugs for *Candida* infections in adults (see Echinocandins, p 767). Few data regarding safety and effectiveness of echinocandins in children are available.

Ophthalmologic evaluation is recommended for all patients with candidemia. Evaluation should take place once candidemia is controlled, and in patients with neutropenia, evaluation should be deferred until recovery of the neutrophil count.

Chemoprophylaxis. Chemoprophylaxis of *Candida* infections in immunocompromised patients with oral nystatin and fluconazole has been evaluated. Prospective, randomized, controlled trials in neonates weighing less than 1000 g at birth or less than 1500 g at birth, respectively, demonstrated the safety and efficacy of fluconazole given intravenously for 4 to 6 weeks in preventing *Candida* colonization and systemic infection. Several retrospective cohort studies have reported similar results. None of these studies reported emergence of resistant *Candida* species in infants receiving fluconazole prophylaxis. Fluconazole prophylaxis for extremely low birth weight neonates may be considered in nurseries with moderate to high rates of invasive candidiasis. Fluconazole can decrease the risk of mucosal (eg, oropharyngeal and esophageal) candidiasis in patients with advanced HIV disease. However, an increased incidence of infections attributable to *C krusei* (which intrinsically is resistant to fluconazole) has been reported in non–HIV-infected patients receiving prophylactic fluconazole. Adults undergoing allogenic hematopoietic stem cell transplantation had significantly fewer *Candida* infections when given fluconazole, but limited data are available for children. Prophylaxis should be considered for children undergoing allogenic hematopoietic stem cell transplantation during the period of neutropenia. Prophylaxis is not recommended routinely for other immunocompromised children, including children with HIV infection.

ISOLATION OF THE HOSPITALIZED PATIENT: Standard precautions are recommended.

CONTROL MEASURES: Prolonged broad-spectrum antimicrobial therapy and use of systemic corticosteroids in susceptible patients promote overgrowth of, and predispose to, invasive infection with *Candida* organisms. Meticulous care of intravascular catheter sites is recommended for any patient requiring long-term intravenous alimentation.

Cat-Scratch Disease
(Bartonella henselae)

CLINICAL MANIFESTATIONS: The predominant manifestation of cat-scratch disease (CSD) in an immunocompetent person is regional lymphadenopathy. Fever and mild systemic symptoms occur in approximately 30% of patients. A skin papule or pustule often is found at the presumed site of bacterial inoculation and usually precedes development of lymphadenopathy by 1 to 2 weeks. Lymphadenopathy involves nodes that drain the site of inoculation—typically axillary, but cervical, submental, epitrochlear, or inguinal nodes can be affected. The skin overlying affected lymph nodes typically is tender, warm, erythematous, and indurated. In approximately 25% of people with CSD, the affected nodes suppurate spontaneously. Occasionally, infection can produce Parinaud oculoglandular syndrome, in which inoculation of the eyelid conjunctiva results in conjunctivitis and ipsilateral preauricular lymphadenopathy. Less common manifestations of CSD (approximately 25%) include encephalopathy, aseptic meningitis, fever of unknown origin, neuroretinitis, osteolytic lesions, hepatitis, granulomata in the liver and spleen, glomerulonephritis, pneumonia, thrombocytopenic purpura, erythema nodosum, and endocarditis.

ETIOLOGY: *Bartonella henselae,* the causative organism of CSD, is a fastidious, slow-growing, gram-negative bacillus that also is the causative agent of bacillary angiomatosis (vascular proliferative lesions of skin and subcutaneous tissue) and bacillary peliosis (reticuloendothelial lesions in visceral organs, primarily the liver). The latter 2 manifestations of infection are reported primarily in patients with human immunodeficiency virus infection. *B henselae* is closely related to *Bartonella quintana,* the agent of louseborne trench fever and a causative agent of bacillary angiomatosis and bacillary peliosis. *B quintana* also can cause endocarditis.

EPIDEMIOLOGY: CSD probably is a common infection, although the true incidence is unknown. Cats are the natural reservoir for *B henselae,* with a seroprevalence of 81% in stray cats and 28% in domestic cats in the United States. Cat-to-cat transmission occurs via the cat flea *(Ctenocephalides felis),* with infection resulting in bacteremia that usually is asymptomatic and lasts weeks to months. Kittens are more likely to be bacteremic than are older cats. Most reported cases occur in people younger than 20 years of age, with more than 90% of patients having a history of recent contact with apparently healthy cats, often kittens. No evidence of person-to-person transmission exists. Infection occurs more often during the autumn and winter. The role of fleas or other arthropods in transmission of *B henselae* to humans is not well established.

The **incubation period** from the time of the scratch to appearance of the primary cutaneous lesion is 7 to 12 days; the period from the appearance of the primary lesion to the appearance of lymphadenopathy is 5 to 50 days (median, 12 days).

DIAGNOSTIC TESTS: The indirect immunofluorescent antibody (IFA) assay for detection of serum antibodies to antigens of *Bartonella* species is useful for diagnosis of CSD. The IFA test is available at many commercial laboratories and through the Centers for Disease Control and Prevention (CDC). Enzyme immunoassays for detection of antibodies to *B henselae* have been developed; however, they have not been demonstrated to be more sensitive or specific than the IFA test. Polymerase chain reaction assays are available in some commercial and research laboratories and at the CDC. If tissue (eg, lymph node) specimens are available, bacilli occasionally may be visualized using Warthin-Starry silver stain; however, this test is not specific for *B henselae*. Early histologic changes in lymph node specimens consist of lymphocytic infiltration with epithelioid granuloma formation. Later changes consist of polymorphonuclear leukocyte infiltration with granulomas that become necrotic and resemble granulomas from patients with tularemia, brucellosis, and mycobacterial infections.

TREATMENT: Management of localized CSD primarily is aimed at relief of symptoms, because the disease usually is self-limited, resolving spontaneously in 2 to 4 months. Painful suppurative nodes can be treated with needle aspiration for relief of symptoms; incision and drainage should be avoided, and surgical excision generally is unnecessary.

Antimicrobial therapy may hasten recovery in acutely or severely ill patients with systemic symptoms, particularly people with hepatic or splenic involvement or painful adenitis, and is recommended for all immunocompromised people. Reports suggest that several oral antimicrobial agents (azithromycin, erythromycin, ciprofloxacin, trimethoprim-sulfamethoxazole, and rifampin) and parenteral gentamicin are effective, but the role of antimicrobial therapy is not clear. The optimal duration of therapy is not known.

Antimicrobial therapy for patients with bacillary angiomatosis and bacillary peliosis has been shown to be beneficial and is recommended. Azithromycin, erythromycin, and doxycycline are effective for treatment of these conditions; therapy should be administered for several months to prevent relapse in immunocompromised people.

ISOLATION OF THE HOSPITALIZED PATIENT: Standard precautions are recommended.

CONTROL MEASURES: People, especially children, should avoid playing roughly with cats and kittens to minimize scratches and bites. Stray cats should not be handled by children. Immunocompromised people should avoid contact with cats that scratch or bite and, when acquiring a new cat, should avoid cats younger than 1 year of age or stray cats. Sites of cat scratches or bites should be washed immediately. Care of cats should include flea control. Testing of cats for *Bartonella* infection is not recommended.

Chancroid

CLINICAL MANIFESTATIONS: Chancroid is an acute ulcerative disease that involves the genitalia. An ulcer begins as a tender erythematous papule, becomes pustular, and erodes over several days, forming a sharply demarcated, somewhat superficial lesion with a serpiginous border. The base of the ulcer is friable and can be covered with a gray or yellow, necrotic, and purulent exudate. Single or multiple ulcers can be present. Unlike a syphilitic chancre, which is painless, the chancroidal ulcer often is painful and nonindurated. The ulcer can be associated with a painful, unilateral inguinal adenitis (bubo), which often is suppurative. Without treatment, ulcer(s) may resolve in several weeks.

In most males, chancroid manifests as a genital ulcer with or without inguinal tenderness and can present less commonly as purulent urethritis; edema of the prepuce is common. In females, most lesions are at the vaginal introitus and symptoms include dysuria, dyspareunia, vaginal discharge, pain on defecation, or anal bleeding. Constitutional symptoms are unusual.

ETIOLOGY: Chancroid is caused by *Haemophilus ducreyi*, which is a gram-negative coccobacillus.

EPIDEMIOLOGY: Chancroid is a sexually transmitted infection associated with poverty, urban prostitution, and illicit drug use. Chancroid is endemic in some areas of the United States and also occurs in discrete outbreaks. Coinfection with syphilis or herpes simplex virus (HSV) occurs in as many as 10% of patients. Chancroid is a well-established cofactor for transmission of human immunodeficiency virus (HIV). Because sexual contact is the only known route of transmission, the diagnosis of chancroid in infants and young children is strong evidence of sexual abuse.

The **incubation period** is 3 to 10 days.

DIAGNOSTIC TESTS: The diagnosis of chancroid usually is based on clinical findings (painful genital ulcer with tender suppurative inguinal adenopathy) with exclusion of other infections associated with genital ulcer disease, such as syphilis, HSV infection, or lymphogranuloma venereum. Direct examination of purulent material using Gram stain may suggest the diagnosis if large numbers of gram-negative coccobacilli are seen. Confirmation can be made by recovery of *H ducreyi* from a genital ulcer or lymph node aspirate. If chancroid is suspected, laboratory personnel should be informed, because special culture media and conditions are required for isolation. Purulent material recovered from intact buboes almost always is sterile. Fluorescent monoclonal antibody stains and polymerase chain reaction assays can provide a specific diagnosis but are not available in most laboratories.

TREATMENT: Recommended regimens include azithromycin or ceftriaxone. Alternatives include erythromycin or ciprofloxacin (see Table 4.3, p 758). Ciprofloxacin is not approved by the US Food and Drug Administration for people younger than 18 years of age for this indication and should not be administered to pregnant or lactating women (see Antimicrobial Agents and Related Therapy, p 737). Patients with HIV infection and uncircumcised males may need prolonged therapy. *H ducreyi* strains with intermediate resistance to ciprofloxacin or erythromycin have been reported worldwide.

Clinical improvement occurs within 3 to 7 days of onset of therapy, and healing is complete in approximately 2 weeks. Adenitis often is slow to resolve and can require needle aspiration or surgical incision. Patients should be reexamined 3 to 7 days after starting therapy to verify that healing is occurring. If healing has not occurred, the diagnosis may be incorrect or the patient may have an additional sexually transmitted infection, and further testing is required. Relapses can occur after initial therapy; however, retreatment with the original regimen usually is effective.

Patients should be evaluated for other sexually transmitted infections, including syphilis, hepatitis B virus infection, *Chlamydia trachomatis* infection, gonorrhea, and HIV infection at the time of diagnosis. Because chancroid is a risk factor for HIV infection and facilitates HIV transmission, if initial HIV or syphilis test results are negative, they should be repeated 3 months after the diagnosis of chancroid is made. All people having sexual contact with patients with chancroid within 10 days before onset of the patient's symptoms need to be examined and treated, even if they are asymptomatic.

ISOLATION OF THE HOSPITALIZED PATIENT: Standard precautions are recommended.

CONTROL MEASURES: Identification, examination, and treatment of sexual partners of patients with chancroid are important control measures. "Partner notification" is used increasingly to identify a treatable reservoir of cases of chancroid during outbreaks, usually occurring among prostitutes. This process can lead to epidemic control. Regular condom use may decrease transmission, and male circumcision is thought to be partially protective.

CHLAMYDIAL INFECTIONS

Chlamydophila (formerly *Chlamydia*) *pneumoniae*

CLINICAL MANIFESTATIONS: Patients may be asymptomatic or mildly to moderately ill with a variety of respiratory tract diseases caused by *Chlamydophila pneumoniae*, including pneumonia, acute bronchitis, prolonged cough, and less commonly, pharyngitis, laryngitis, otitis media, and sinusitis. In some patients, a sore throat precedes the onset of cough by a week or more. Physical examination may reveal nonexudative pharyngitis, pulmonary rales, and bronchospasm. Chest radiography may reveal an infiltrate. Illness is prolonged with cough persisting 2 to 6 weeks and can have a biphasic course culminating in atypical pneumonia.

ETIOLOGY: *C pneumoniae* is an obligate intracellular bacterium. *C pneumoniae* is distinct antigenically, genetically, and morphologically from *Chlamydia* species and, in a reclassification, now is grouped in the genus *Chlamydophila*. All isolates of *C pneumoniae* appear serologically to be related closely.

EPIDEMIOLOGY: *C pneumoniae* infection is assumed to be transmitted from person to person via infected respiratory tract secretions. An animal reservoir is unknown. The disease occurs worldwide, but in tropical and less developed areas, disease occurs earlier in life than in developed countries in temperate climates. In the United States, approximately 50% of adults have *C pneumoniae*-specific serum antibody by 20 years of age, indicating infection by the organism. Initial infection peaks between 5 and 15 years of age. Recurrent infection is common, especially in adults. Clusters of infection have been reported in groups of children and young adults. There is no evidence of seasonality.

The mean **incubation period** is 21 days.

DIAGNOSTIC TESTS: No reliable diagnostic test to identify the organism is available commercially, and none has been approved by the US Food and Drug Administration for use in the United States. Serologic testing has been the primary laboratory means of diagnosis of *C pneumoniae* infection. The microimmunofluorescent antibody test is the most sensitive and specific serologic test for acute infection and is the only endorsed approach. A fourfold increase in immunoglobulin (Ig) G titer or an IgM titer of 16 or greater is evidence of acute infection. Use of a single IgG titer in diagnosis of acute infection is not recommended. In primary infection, IgM antibody appears approximately 2 to 3 weeks after onset of illness, but IgG antibody may not peak until 6 to 8 weeks after onset of illness. In reinfection, IgM may not appear, and IgG increases within 1 to 2 weeks. Early antimicrobial therapy may suppress the antibody response. Past exposure is indicated by a stable IgG titer of 16 or greater. *C pneumoniae* can be isolated from swab specimens obtained from the nasopharynx or oropharynx or from sputum, bronchoalveolar lavage, or tissue biopsy specimens. Specimens are placed into appropriate transport media and held at 4°C (39°F) until inoculated into cell culture; specimens that cannot be processed within 24 hours should be frozen and held at −70°C. A positive culture is confirmed by propagation of the isolate or a positive polymerase chain reaction assay result. Nasopharyngeal shedding can occur for months after acute disease. Immunohistochemistry, used to detect *C pneumoniae* in tissue specimens, requires control antibodies and tissues in addition to skill in recognizing staining artifacts to avoid false-positive results.

TREATMENT: Most respiratory tract infections potentially caused by *C pneumoniae* are treated empirically. For suspected *C pneumoniae* infections, treatment with macrolides, including erythromycin, azithromycin, or clarithromycin, is recommended. Tetracycline or doxycycline may be used but should not be given routinely to children younger than 8 years of age (see Antimicrobial Agents and Related Therapy, p 737). Newer fluoroquinolones (levofloxacin and moxifloxacin) are alternative drugs. In vitro data suggest that *C pneumoniae* is not susceptible to sulfonamides. Although duration of therapy typically is 10 to 14 days for erythromycin, clarithromycin, tetracycline, or doxycycline, a longer course of therapy may be necessary. With azithromycin, the treatment duration typically is 5 days. However, with all of these antimicrobial agents, optimal duration of therapy is not clear.

ISOLATION OF THE HOSPITALIZED PATIENT: Standard precautions are recommended.

CONTROL MEASURES: Recommended prevention measures include minimizing crowding, maintaining personal hygiene, respiratory hygiene (or cough etiquette), and frequent hand hygiene.

Chlamydophila (formerly *Chlamydia*) *psittaci*
(Psittacosis, Ornithosis)

CLINICAL MANIFESTATIONS: Psittacosis (ornithosis) usually is an acute febrile respiratory tract infection with systemic symptoms and signs that often include fever, nonproductive cough, headache, and malaise. Extensive interstitial pneumonia can occur with radiographic changes characteristically more severe than would be expected from physical examination findings. Pericarditis, myocarditis, endocarditis, superficial thrombophlebitis, hepatitis, and encephalopathy are rare complications.

ETIOLOGY: *Chlamydophila psittaci* is an obligate intracellular bacterial pathogen that is distinct antigenically, genetically, and morphologically from *Chlamydia* species and, following reclassification, now is grouped in the genus *Chlamydophila*.

EPIDEMIOLOGY: Birds are the major reservoir of *C psittaci*. The term psittacosis commonly is used, although the term ornithosis more accurately describes the potential for all birds, not just psittacine birds, to spread this infection. Several mammalian species, such as cattle, goats, sheep, and cats, as well as avian species may become infected and develop systemic and debilitating disease. In the United States, psittacine birds (eg, parakeets, parrots, and macaws), pigeons, and turkeys are important sources of human disease.

Importation and illegal trafficking of exotic birds is associated with an increased incidence of disease in humans, because shipping, crowding, and other stress factors may increase shedding of the organism among birds with latent infection. Infected birds, whether asymptomatic or obviously ill, may transmit the organism. Infection usually is acquired by inhaling aerosolized excrement or secretions from the eyes or beaks of birds. Excretion of C psittaci from birds may be intermittent or continuous for weeks or months. Pet owners and workers at poultry slaughter plants, poultry farms, and pet shops are at increased risk of infection. Laboratory personnel working with C psittaci also are at risk. Psittacosis is worldwide in distribution and tends to occur sporadically in any season. Infections are rare in children. Severe illness and abortion have been reported in pregnant women after exposure to infected sheep.

The **incubation period** usually is 5 to 14 days but may be longer.

DIAGNOSTIC TESTS: A confirmed case of psittacosis requires a clinically compatible illness and laboratory confirmation by one of the following: an immunoglobulin (Ig) M antibody titer of 1:16 or greater with microimmunofluorescent (MIF) assay, culture from respiratory tract secretions, or a fourfold or greater increase in either complement fixation (CF) or MIF antibody to a titer of 1:32 or greater in specimens obtained 2 to 3 weeks apart. In the presence of a compatible clinical illness, a single titer of 1:32 or greater by MIF or CF is considered presumptive evidence of infection. CF does not distinguish among infections caused by C psittaci, Chlamydophila pneumoniae, Chlamydia trachomatis, or Chlamydophila pecorum, but MIF is more sensitive and specific for C psittaci. Polymerase chain reaction (PCR) is not available routinely but may distinguish C psittaci from other chlamydial infections. Treatment with antimicrobial agents may suppress the antibody response. Culturing the organism should be attempted only by experienced personnel in laboratories where strict measures to prevent spread of the organism are used during collection and handling of all specimens.

TREATMENT: Tetracycline or doxycycline are the drugs of choice, except for children younger than 8 years of age and pregnant women. Therapy should be administered for 10 to 21 days. Erythromycin and azithromycin are alternative agents and are recommended for younger children and pregnant women.

ISOLATION OF THE HOSPITALIZED PATIENT: Standard precautions are recommended.

CONTROL MEASURES: Reporting cases of human psittacosis to health authorities is mandatory in most states. All birds suspected to be the source of human infection should be seen by a veterinarian for evaluation and management. Birds with C psittaci infection should be isolated and treated with appropriate antimicrobial agents for at least 45 days.[1] Birds suspected of dying from C psittaci infection should be sealed in an impermeable container and transported on dry ice to a veterinary laboratory for testing. All potentially contaminated caging and housing areas should be disinfected thoroughly and aired before reuse to eliminate any infectious organisms. C psittaci is susceptible to most household disinfectants and detergents, including 70% alcohol, 1% Lysol, and a 1:100 dilution of household bleach. People cleaning cages and other bird housing areas should be aware of the potential for infection and avoid scattering the contents. People exposed to common sources of infection should be observed for development of fever or respiratory tract

---

[1]National Association of State Public Health Veterinarians. Compendium of Measures to Control *Chlamydophila psittaci* Infection Among Humans (psittacosis) and Pet Birds (Avian Chlamydiosis), 2008. Available at: **http://www.nasphv.org/Documents/Psittacosis.pdf.**

symptoms; early diagnostic tests should be performed, and therapy should be initiated if symptoms appear.

Chlamydia trachomatis

CLINICAL MANIFESTATIONS: *Chlamydia trachomatis* is associated with a range of clinical manifestations, including neonatal conjunctivitis, trachoma, pneumonia in young infants, genital tract infection, and lymphogranuloma venereum (LGV). **Neonatal chlamydial conjunctivitis** is characterized by ocular congestion, edema, and discharge developing a few days to several weeks after birth and lasting for 1 to 2 weeks and sometimes longer. In contrast to trachoma, scars and pannus formation are rare.

Trachoma is a chronic follicular keratoconjunctivitis with neovascularization of the cornea that results from repeated and chronic infection. Blindness secondary to extensive local scarring and inflammation occurs in 1% to 15% of people with trachoma. Trachoma is rare in the United States.

Pneumonia in young infants usually is an afebrile illness of insidious onset occurring between 2 and 19 weeks after birth. A repetitive staccato cough, tachypnea, and rales are characteristic but not always present. Wheezing is uncommon. Hyperinflation usually accompanies infiltrates seen on chest radiographs. Nasal stuffiness and otitis media may occur. Untreated disease can linger or recur. Severe chlamydial pneumonia has occurred in infants and some immunocompromised adults.

Vaginitis in prepubertal girls; urethritis, cervicitis, endometritis, salpingitis, and perihepatitis (Fitz-Hugh-Curtis syndrome) in postpubertal females; urethritis and epididymitis in males; and Reiter syndrome (arthritis, urethritis, and bilateral conjunctivitis) also can occur. Infection can persist for months to years. Reinfection is common. In postpubertal females, chlamydial infection can progress to acute or chronic pelvic inflammatory disease and result in ectopic pregnancy or infertility.

LGV classically is an invasive lymphatic infection with an initial ulcerative lesion on the genitalia accompanied by tender, suppurative, inguinal, and/or femoral lymphadenopathy that typically is unilateral. However, anorectal infection is associated with anal intercourse and can cause hemorrhagic proctocolitis or stricture among women and men who engage in anal intercourse. The proctocolitis can be moderate to severe and can resemble inflammatory bowel disease.

ETIOLOGY: *C trachomatis* is an obligate intracellular bacterial agent with at least 18 serologic variants (serovars) divided between the following biologic variants (biovars): oculogenital (serovars A–K) and LGV (serovars L1, L2, and L3). Trachoma usually is caused by serovars A through C, and genital and perinatal infections are caused by B and D through K.

EPIDEMIOLOGY: *C trachomatis* is the most common reportable sexually transmitted infection in the United States, with high rates among sexually active adolescents and young adults. Prevalence of the organism consistently is highest among adolescent females. Across 27 states, median prevalence among 15- to 24-year-old females screened in prenatal clinics was 7%, with a range of 2% to 20%. Oculogenital serovars of *C trachomatis* can be transmitted from the genital tract of infected mothers to their newborn infants. Acquisition occurs in approximately 50% of infants born vaginally to infected mothers and in some infants born by cesarean delivery with membranes intact. The risk of conjunctivitis is 25% to 50%, and the risk of pneumonia is 5% to 20% in infants who contract *C trachomatis*. The nasopharynx is the anatomic site most commonly infected.

Genital tract infection in adolescents and adults is transmitted sexually. The possibility of sexual abuse should be considered in prepubertal children beyond infancy who have vaginal, urethral, or rectal chlamydial infection. Asymptomatic infection of the nasopharynx, conjunctivae, vagina, and rectum can be acquired at birth. Nasopharyngeal cultures may remain positive for as long as 28 months, but spontaneous resolution of vaginal and rectal infection occurs by 16 to 18 months of age. Infection is not known to be communicable among infants and children. The degree of contagiousness of pulmonary disease is unknown but seems to be low.

LGV biovars are worldwide in distribution but particularly are prevalent in tropical and subtropical areas. Although disease occurs rarely in the United States, outbreaks of LGV have been reported in Europe, and cases have been reported in the United States in men who have sex with men. Infection often is asymptomatic in women. Perinatal transmission is rare. LGV is infectious during active disease. Little is known about the prevalence or duration of asymptomatic carriage.

The **incubation period** of chlamydial illness is variable, depending on the type of infection, but usually is at least 1 week.

DIAGNOSTIC TESTS: Definitive diagnosis can be made by isolating the organism in tissue culture and by nucleic acid amplification (NAA) testing in selective circumstances.[1] Because *Chlamydia* species are obligate intracellular organisms, culture specimens must contain epithelial cells, not just exudate. NAA tests, such as polymerase chain reaction (PCR), transcription-mediated amplification (TMA) test, and strand-displacement amplification (SDA) test are available. These tests are more sensitive than cell culture, DNA probe, direct fluorescent antibody (DFA) tests, or enzyme immunoassay (EIA), although specificity is variable compared with culture.

Some nonculture tests for detection of *Chlamydia* species, including EIA, DFA tests, DNA probe tests, and NAA tests, are useful for evaluating urethral swab specimens from males, endocervical swab specimens from females, and conjunctival secretion specimens from infants, although not all of these tests have been cleared by the US Food and Drug Administration (FDA) for this use. The PCR, SDA, and TMA assays are useful for evaluating urine specimens from either sex. The FDA has approved TMA for testing vaginal swabs from postmenarcheal adolescents and adults. Nonculture tests are not recommended for detection of *C trachomatis* in urethral swab specimens from females, and only the TMA test is FDA approved for use with vaginal swabs from postmenarcheal adolescents and adults. In addition, NAA testing is not recommended for specimens obtained by rectal or pharyngeal swabs.

If a false-positive test result is likely to have adverse medical, social, or psychological consequences, positive DFA test, EIA, DNA probe test, or NAA test results should be verified by culture, a second nonculture test different from the first, or use of a blocking antibody or competitive probe. When evaluating a child for possible sexual abuse, culture of the organism may be the only acceptable diagnostic test in certain legal jurisdictions. When culture is not available, some experts support using NAA testing if a positive result can be verified by another NAA test. The EIA and DFA test should not be used for testing

---

[1]Centers for Disease Control and Prevention. Screening to detect *Chlamydia trachomatis* and *Neisseria gonorrhoeae* infections—2002. *MMWR Recomm Rep.* 2002;51(RR-15):1–38

rectal, vaginal, or urethral specimens from infants and children because of low sensitivity and specificity.

Serum antibody concentrations are difficult to determine, and only a few clinical laboratories perform this test. In children with pneumonia, an acute microimmunofluorescent serum titer of *C trachomatis*-specific immunoglobulin (Ig) M of 1:32 or greater is diagnostic. Diagnosis of LGV can be supported, but not confirmed, by a positive result (ie, titer greater than 1:64) on a complement fixation test for chlamydiae or a high titer (typically greater than 1:128 but can vary by laboratory) on a microimmunofluorescent serologic test for *C trachomatis*. However, most available serologic tests in the United States are based on EIAs and might not provide a quantitative "titer-based" result.

Diagnosis of genitourinary chlamydial disease in a child, adolescent, or adult should prompt investigation for other sexually transmitted infections, including syphilis, gonorrhea, hepatitis B virus infection, and human immunodeficiency virus infection. In the case of an infant, evaluation of the mother also is advisable.

Diagnosis of ocular trachoma usually is made clinically in countries with endemic infection.

TREATMENT:

- Young infants with **chlamydial conjunctivitis** are treated with oral erythromycin base or ethylsuccinate for 14 days. Oral sulfonamides may be used after the immediate neonatal period for infants who do not tolerate erythromycin. Topical treatment of conjunctivitis is ineffective and unnecessary. Because the efficacy of erythromycin therapy is approximately 80%, a second course may be required, and follow-up of infants is recommended. A diagnosis of *C trachomatis* infection in an infant should prompt treatment of the mother and her sexual partner(s).

  An association between orally administered erythromycin and infantile hypertrophic pyloric stenosis (IHPS) has been reported in infants younger than 6 weeks of age. The risk of IHPS after treatment with other macrolides (eg, azithromycin and clarithromycin) is unknown, although IHPS has been reported after use of azithromycin. Because confirmation of erythromycin as a contributor to cases of IHPS will require additional investigation and because alternative therapies are not as well studied, the American Academy of Pediatrics continues to recommend use of erythromycin for treatment of diseases caused by *C trachomatis*. Physicians who prescribe erythromycin to newborn infants should inform parents about the signs and potential risks of developing IHPS. Cases of pyloric stenosis after use of oral erythromycin or azithromycin should be reported to MedWatch (see MedWatch, p 817).

- **Chlamydial pneumonia** is treated with oral azithromycin for 5 days or erythromycin base or ethylsuccinate for 14 days. Alternative therapies are not well studied for this use. The need for treatment of infants can be avoided by screening pregnant women to detect and treat *C trachomatis* infection before delivery. A diagnosis of *C trachomatis* infection in an infant should prompt treatment of the mother and her sexual partner(s).

- Infants born to mothers known to have untreated chlamydial infection are at high risk of infection; however, prophylactic antimicrobial treatment is not indicated, because the efficacy of such treatment is unknown. Infants should be monitored clinically to ensure appropriate treatment if infection develops. If adequate follow-up cannot be ensured, some experts recommend that preemptive therapy be considered.

- Treatment of **trachoma** is more difficult, and recommendations for therapy differ. The most widely used therapy is topical treatment with erythromycin, tetracycline, or sulfacetamide ointment twice a day for 2 months or twice a day for the first 5 days of the month for 6 consecutive months; or oral erythromycin or doxycycline (for children 8 years of age and older) for 40 days if the infection is severe. However, because of improved adherence and greater efficacy, the World Health Organization encourages use of azithromycin (20 mg/kg, maximum of 1 g) as a single dose or in 3 weekly doses as the first-line antimicrobial agent to treat trachoma.

- For uncomplicated *C trachomatis* **genital tract infection** in adolescents or adults, oral doxycycline (200 mg/day in 2 divided doses) for 7 days or azithromycin in a single 1-g oral dose is recommended. Alternatives include oral erythromycin base (2.0 g/day in 4 divided doses) for 7 days, erythromycin ethyl-succinate (3.2 g/day in 4 divided doses) for 7 days, ofloxacin (600 mg/day in 2 divided doses) for 7 days, or levofloxacin (500 mg, orally, once per day) for 7 days. Erythromycin or azithromycin is the recommended therapy for children between 6 months and 12 years of age; for infants younger than 6 months of age, erythromycin is recommended. Azithromycin (1 g, orally, as a single dose) or amoxicillin (1.5 g/day in 3 divided doses) for 7 days are recommended regimens for pregnant women. Erythromycin base (2 g/day in 4 divided doses) for 7 days is an alternative regimen. Doxycycline, ofloxacin, and levofloxacin are contraindicated during pregnancy. Repeat testing (preferably by culture) is recommended 3 weeks after treatment. Because these regimens for pregnant women may not be highly efficacious, a second course of therapy may be required.

- For **LGV,** doxycycline (200 mg/day in 2 divided doses) for 21 days is the preferred treatment for children 8 years of age and older. Erythromycin base (2 g/day in 4 divided doses) for 21 days is an alternative regimen; azithromycin (1 g once weekly for 3 weeks) is recommended by some experts, although clinical data are lacking.

Follow-up Testing. Nonpregnant patients do not need to be retested for uncomplicated *Chlamydia* infection after completing treatment with doxycycline or azithromycin unless symptoms persist or reinfection is suspected. Retesting for infection using NAA testing should occur no sooner than 4 weeks after completing regimens with erythromycin or amoxicillin. Previously infected adolescents are a high priority for repeat testing for *C trachomatis,* usually 3 to 6 months after initial infection.

ISOLATION OF THE HOSPITALIZED PATIENT: Standard precautions are recommended.

CONTROL MEASURES:

Pregnancy. Identification and treatment of women with *C trachomatis* genital tract infection during pregnancy can prevent disease in the infant. Pregnant women at high risk of *C trachomatis* infection, in particular women younger than 25 years of age and women with new or multiple sexual partners, should be targeted for screening. Some experts advocate routine testing of pregnant women at high risk during the first trimester and again during the third trimester.

Neonatal Chlamydial Conjunctivitis. Recommended topical prophylaxis with erythromycin or tetracycline for all newborn infants for prevention of gonococcal ophthalmia will not prevent neonatal chlamydial conjunctivitis or extraocular infection (see Prevention of Neonatal Ophthalmia, p 827).

Trachoma. Although not seen in the United States for more than 2 decades, trachoma is the second leading cause of blindness worldwide. Trachoma is transmitted by transfer of ocular discharge, and predictors of scarring and blindness for trachoma include increasing age and constant, severe trachoma. The prevention methods recommended by the World Health Organization for global elimination of blindness attributable to trachoma by 2020 include **s**urgery, **a**ntibiotics, **f**ace washing, and **e**nvironmental improvement (SAFE). Azithromycin (20 mg/kg, maximum 1 g) once a year as a single oral dose is used in mass drug administration for trachoma control. Azithromycin typically is given to all the resident population older than 6 months of age, and a 6-week course of topical tetracycline eye ointment is given to infants younger than 6 months of age.

Contacts of Infants With **C** *trachomatis* **Conjunctivitis or Pneumonia.** Mothers of infected infants (and mothers' sexual partners) should be treated for *C trachomatis.*

Gynecologic Examination. Sexually active adolescent females should be tested at least annually for *Chlamydia* infection during preventive health care visits and gynecologic examinations, even if no symptoms are present and even if barrier contraception is reported. Screening of young adult women 20 to 24 years of age also is recommended.

Management of Sexual Partners. All sexual contacts of patients with *C trachomatis* infection (whether symptomatic or asymptomatic), nongonococcal urethritis, mucopurulent cervicitis, epididymitis, or pelvic inflammatory disease should be evaluated and treated for *C trachomatis* infection if the last sexual contact occurred during the 60 days preceding onset of symptoms in the index case. Integrated recommendations for services provided to partners of people with STIs, including *C trachomatis,* are available.[1]

Lymphogranuloma Venereum. Nonspecific preventive measures for LGV are the same as measures for sexually transmitted infections in general and include education, case reporting, condom use, and avoidance of sexual contact with infected people.

CLOSTRIDIAL INFECTIONS

Botulism and Infant Botulism
(Clostridium botulinum)

CLINICAL MANIFESTATIONS: Botulism is a neuroparalytic disorder characterized by an acute, afebrile, symmetric, descending flaccid paralysis. Paralysis is caused by blockade of neurotransmitter at the voluntary motor and autonomic neuromuscular junctions. Three distinct, naturally occurring forms of human botulism exist: foodborne, wound, and infant. Iatrogenic botulism, which results from injection of excess therapeutic botulinum toxin, has been reported. Onset of symptoms occurs abruptly within hours or evolves gradually over several days and includes diplopia, dysphagia, dysphonia, and dysarthria. Cranial nerve palsies are followed by symmetric, descending, flaccid paralysis of somatic musculature in patients who are fully alert. Classic infant botulism, which occurs predominantly in infants younger than 6 months of age (range, 1 day to 12 months), is preceded by or begins with constipation and manifests as decreased movement, loss of facial expression, poor feeding, weak cry, diminished gag reflex, ocular palsies, loss of head control,

---

[1]Centers for Disease Control and Prevention. Recommendations for partner services programs for HIV infection, syphilis, gonorrhea, and chlamydial infection. *MMWR Recomm Rep.* 2008;57(RR-9):1–63

and progressive descending generalized weakness and hypotonia. Sudden infant death can be caused by rapidly progressing botulism.

ETIOLOGY: Botulism results from absorption of botulinum toxins into the circulation from a wound or mucosal surface. Seven antigenic toxin types of *Clostridium botulinum* have been identified. Human botulism is caused by neurotoxins A, B, E, and rarely, F. Non-*botulinum* species of *Clostridium* rarely may produce these neurotoxins and cause disease. Almost all cases of infant botulism are caused by toxin types A and B. A few cases of types E and F have been reported from *Clostridium butyricum* and *Clostridium baritii*, respectively (especially in very young infants). *C botulinum* spores are ubiquitous in soil worldwide.

EPIDEMIOLOGY: Foodborne botulism (28 cases reported in 2007; age range, 13–74 years) results when food contaminated with spores of *C botulinum* is preserved or stored improperly under anaerobic conditions that permit germination, multiplication, and toxin production. Illness follows ingestion of preformed botulinum toxin. Outbreaks have occurred after ingestion of restaurant-prepared foods, home-prepared foods, and commercially canned foods. Immunity to botulinum toxin does not develop in botulism. Botulism is not transmitted from person to person.

Infant botulism (91 laboratory-confirmed cases reported in 2007; age range 1 to 44 weeks; median 15 weeks) results after ingested spores of *C botulinum* or related species germinate, multiply, and produce botulinum toxin in the intestine, probably through a mechanism of transient permissiveness of the intestinal microflora. Most cases occur in breastfed infants at the time of first introduction of nonhuman milk substances; the source of spores usually is not identified. Honey has been identified as an avoidable source. Manufacturers of light and dark corn syrups cannot ensure that any given product will be free of *C botulinum* spores, but no case of infant botulism has been proven to be attributable to consumption of contaminated corn syrup. Rarely, intestinal botulism can occur in older children and adults, usually after intestinal surgery and exposure to antimicrobial agents.

Wound botulism (22 laboratory-confirmed cases reported in 2006; age range 23–58 years) results when *C botulinum* contaminates traumatized tissue, germinates, multiplies, and produces toxin. Gross trauma or crush injury can be a predisposing event. During the last decade, injection of contaminated black tar heroin has been associated with most cases.

The usual **incubation period** for foodborne botulism is 12 to 48 hours (range, 6 hours–8 days). In infant botulism, the **incubation period** is estimated at 3 to 30 days from the time of exposure to the spore-containing material. For wound botulism, the **incubation period** is 4 to 14 days from the time of injury until the onset of symptoms.

DIAGNOSTIC TESTS: A toxin neutralization bioassay in mice[1] is used to identify botulinum toxin in serum, stool, gastric aspirate, or suspect foods. Enriched, selective media is required to isolate *C botulinum* from stool and foods. In infant and wound botulism, the diagnosis is made by demonstrating *C botulinum* toxin or organisms in feces, wound exudate, or tissue specimens. Toxin has been demonstrated in serum in only 1% of US infants with botulism. To increase the likelihood of diagnosis, serum and stool or enema specimens should be obtained from all people with suspected foodborne botulism. In foodborne cases, serum specimens may be positive for toxin as long as 16 days after admission. Stool or enema and gastric aspirates are the best diagnostic specimens for

---

[1] For information, consult your state health department.

culture. A stool or enema specimen for toxin assay and culture is the test of choice for infant botulism. Organisms and toxins can persist in stool for up to 5 months. If obtaining a stool specimen is difficult, a small enema of sterile nonbacteriostatic water should be used. Because results of laboratory testing can be delayed by several days, treatment with antitoxin should be initiated urgently on the basis of clinical suspicion. The most prominent electromyographic finding is an incremental increase of evoked muscle potentials at high-frequency nerve stimulation (20–50 Hz). In addition, a characteristic pattern of brief, small-amplitude, overly abundant motor action potentials (BSAPs) can be seen after stimulation of muscle. This pattern may not be seen in infants, and its absence does not exclude the diagnosis.

TREATMENT:

Meticulous Supportive Care. An important aspect of therapy in all forms of botulism is meticulous supportive care, in particular respiratory and nutritional support.

    Antitoxin for Infant Botulism. Human-derived antitoxin is given urgently. Botulism Immune Globulin for intravenous use (BabyBIG) is licensed by the US Food and Drug Administration for treatment of infant botulism caused by *C botulinum* type A or type B. BabyBIG is made and distributed by the California Department of Public Health (24-hour telephone number: 510-231-7600; **www.infantbotulism.org/**). BabyBIG has been shown to decrease significantly days of mechanical ventilation, days of intensive care unit stay, and overall hospital stays. Equine-derived antitoxin is not used for infant botulism.

    Antitoxin for Foodborne and Wound Botulism. Patients with suspected foodborne and wound botulism should be treated with bivalent equine-derived antitoxin (types A and B) and possibly also monovalent type E antitoxin available from the Centers for Disease Control and Prevention (CDC **[www.cdc.gov/ncidod/dbmd/diseaseinfo/ botulism_g.htm]**) through state health departments. Immediate administration of antitoxin is the key to successful therapy, because antitoxin arrests the progression of paralysis. However, because botulinum neurotoxin binds irreversibly, administration of antitoxin does not reverse the paralysis. Antitoxin should be procured immediately on suspicion of botulism. If contact cannot be made with the state health department, the CDC Emergency Operations Center should be contacted at 770-488-7100 for botulism case consultation and antitoxin. Before administration of equine antitoxin, patients should be tested for hypersensitivity to equine sera (see Antibodies of Animal Origin, p 61). Approximately 9% of people treated with equine antitoxin in an era when larger doses of antitoxin were given experienced some degree of hypersensitivity reaction, but severe reactions are rare.

    Antimicrobial Agents. Antimicrobial therapy is not indicated in infant botulism. Aminoglycoside agents potentiate the paralytic effects of the toxin and should be avoided. Penicillin or metronidazole should be given to patients with wound botulism after antitoxin has been administered.

ISOLATION OF THE HOSPITALIZED PATIENT: Standard precautions are recommended.

CONTROL MEASURES:

- Any case of suspected botulism is required by law to be reported immediately to local and state health departments. Immediate reporting of suspect cases particularly is important because of possible use of botulinum toxin as a bioterrorism weapon.

- Prophylactic equine antitoxin is not recommended for asymptomatic people who have ingested a food known to contain botulinum toxin. Physicians treating a patient who has been exposed to toxin or is suspected of having any type of botulism should contact their state health department immediately. People exposed to toxin who are asymptomatic should have close medical observation in nonsolitary settings.
- Honey should not be given to children younger than 12 months of age.
- An investigational botulinum toxoid vaccine (types A, B, C, D, and E) is available from the CDC for immunization of laboratory workers at high risk of exposure to botulinum toxin.
- Education regarding safe practices in food preparation and home-canning methods should be promoted. Use of a pressure cooker (at 116°C [240.8°F]) is necessary to kill spores of *C botulinum*. Bringing the internal temperature of foods to 85°C (185°F) for 10 minutes will destroy the toxin. Time, temperature, and pressure requirements vary with the product being heated. In addition, food containers that appear to bulge may contain gas produced by *C botulinum* and should be discarded. Other foods that appear to have spoiled should not be eaten or tasted (**www.cdc.gov/botulism/**).

Clostridial Myonecrosis
(Gas Gangrene)

CLINICAL MANIFESTATIONS: Onset is heralded by acute pain at the site of the wound, followed by edema, tenderness, exudate, and progression of pain. Systemic findings initially include tachycardia disproportionate to the degree of fever, pallor, diaphoresis, hypotension, renal failure, and later, alterations in mental status. Crepitus is suggestive but not pathognomonic of *Clostridium* infection and is not always present. Diagnosis is based on clinical manifestations, including the characteristic appearance of necrotic muscle at surgery. Untreated gas gangrene can lead to disseminated myonecrosis, suppurative visceral infection, septicemia, and death within hours.

ETIOLOGY: Clostridial myonecrosis is caused by *Clostridium* species, most often *Clostridium perfringens*, which are large, gram-positive, spore-forming anaerobic bacilli with blunt ends. Other *Clostridium* species (eg, *Clostridium sordellii, Clostridium septicum, Clostridium novyi*) also can be associated with myonecrosis. Disease manifestations are caused by potent clostridial exotoxins. Mixed infection with other gram-positive and gram-negative bacteria is common.

EPIDEMIOLOGY: Clostridial myonecrosis usually results from contamination of open wounds involving muscle. The sources of *Clostridium* species are soil, contaminated objects, and human and animal feces. Dirty surgical or traumatic wounds with significant devitalized tissue and foreign bodies predispose to disease. Nontraumatic gas gangrene occurs occasionally from *Clostridium* organisms in the gastrointestinal tract and in immunocompromised people.

The **incubation period** from the time of injury is 1 to 4 days.

DIAGNOSTIC TESTS: Anaerobic cultures of wound exudate, involved soft tissue and muscle, and blood should be performed. Because *Clostridium* species are ubiquitous, their recovery from a wound is not diagnostic unless typical clinical manifestations are present. A Gram-stained smear of wound discharge demonstrating characteristic gram-positive bacilli and absent or sparse polymorphonuclear leukocytes suggests clostridial infection.

Tissue specimens and aspirates (not swab specimens) are appropriate for anaerobic culture. Because some pathogenic *Clostridium* species are exquisitely oxygen sensitive, care should be taken to optimize anaerobic growth conditions. A radiograph of the affected site can demonstrate gas in the tissue but is a nonspecific finding. Occasionally, blood cultures are positive and are considered diagnostic.

TREATMENT:
- Early and complete surgical excision of necrotic tissue and removal of foreign material is essential.
- Management of shock, fluid and electrolyte imbalance, hemolytic anemia, and other complications is crucial.
- High-dose penicillin G (250 000–400 000 U/kg per day) should be administered intravenously. Clindamycin, metronidazole, imipenem, meropenem, ertapenem, and chloramphenicol can be considered as alternative drugs for penicillin-allergic patients or for treatment of polymicrobial infections. The combination of penicillin G and clindamycin may be superior to penicillin alone because of the theoretical benefit of clindamycin inhibiting toxin synthesis.
- Hyperbaric oxygen may be beneficial, but data from adequately controlled studies on its efficacy are not available.
- Treatment with antitoxin is of no value.

ISOLATION OF THE HOSPITALIZED PATIENT: Standard precautions are recommended.

CONTROL MEASURES: In wound management, prompt and careful débridement, flushing of contaminated wounds, and removal of foreign material should be performed.

Penicillin G (50 000 U/kg per day) or clindamycin (20–30 mg/kg per day) may be of value for prophylaxis in patients with grossly contaminated wounds.

Clostridium difficile

CLINICAL MANIFESTATIONS: Syndromes associated with infections range from asymptomatic carriage to watery diarrhea to pseudomembranous colitis. Pseudomembranous colitis generally is characterized by diarrhea, abdominal cramps, fever, systemic toxicity, and abdominal tenderness. Occasionally, children have marked abdominal tenderness and distention with minimal diarrhea (toxic megacolon). The colonic mucosa often contains 2- to 5-mm, raised, yellowish plaques. Disease characteristically begins while the child is in a hospital receiving antimicrobial therapy but may occur weeks after hospital discharge or after cessation of therapy. Uncommonly, the illness is not associated with antimicrobial therapy or hospitalization. Complications may include toxic megacolon and intestinal perforation. Severe or fatal disease is more likely to occur in neutropenic children with leukemia, in infants with Hirschsprung disease, and in patients with inflammatory bowel disease. Colonization by toxin-producing strains without symptoms is common in newborn infants and in children younger than 1 year of age.

ETIOLOGY: *Clostridium difficile* is a spore-forming, obligate anaerobic, gram-positive bacillus. Disease is related to the action of toxin(s) produced by these organisms. Although other toxins exist, toxins A and B have been associated most strongly with human disease.

EPIDEMIOLOGY: *C difficile* can be isolated from soil and commonly is present in the hospital environment. *C difficile* is acquired from the environment or from stool of other colonized or infected people by the fecal-oral route. Intestinal colonization rates in healthy neonates and young infants can be as high as 50% but usually are less than 5% in children older than 2 years of age and in adults. Hospitals, nursing homes, and child care facilities are major reservoirs for *C difficile*, and therefore, risk factors for acquisition include experiencing prolonged hospitalization, having an infected hospital roommate, and having symptomatically infected patients on the same hospital ward. Risk factors for developing disease include antimicrobial therapy, repeated enemas, prolonged nasogastric tube insertion, underlying bowel disease, gastrointestinal tract surgery, and renal insufficiency. Penicillins, macrolides, clindamycin, cephalosporins, and fluoroquinolones are the antimicrobial drugs most commonly associated with *C difficile* colitis, but colitis has been associated with almost every antimicrobial agent. A previously uncommon strain of *C difficile* with variations in toxin genes has become more resistant to fluoroquinolones and has emerged as a cause of outbreaks in adults and is associated with severe disease.

The **incubation period** is unknown.

DIAGNOSTIC TESTS: Endoscopic findings of pseudomembranes and hyperemic, friable rectal mucosa suggest pseudomembranous colitis. Isolation of *C difficile* from stool is not a useful diagnostic test, because intestinal colonization is not pathogenic in itself. To diagnose *C difficile* disease, stool should be tested for presence of *C difficile* toxins. Commercially available enzyme immunoassays detect toxins A and B, or an enzyme immunoassay for toxin A can be used in conjunction with cell culture cytotoxicity assay, the "gold standard" for toxin B detection. *C difficile* toxin is unstable. The toxin degrades at room temperate and may be undetectable within 2 hours after collection of a stool specimen. Stool specimens that are not tested promptly or maintained at 4°C can yield false-negative results. Latex agglutination tests should not be used. *C difficile* toxin infrequently is identified from stool specimens from healthy adults. Carriage of *C difficile* is common in infants.

TREATMENT:
- Precipitating antimicrobial therapy should be discontinued as soon as possible in patients in whom clinically significant diarrhea or colitis develops.
- Antimicrobial therapy for *C difficile* disease is indicated for patients with severe disease or for patients in whom diarrhea persists after antimicrobial therapy is discontinued.
- Strains of *C difficile* are susceptible to metronidazole and vancomycin. Metronidazole (30 mg/kg per day in 4 divided doses, maximum 2 g/day) is the drug of choice for the initial treatment of most children and adolescents with colitis.
- Oral vancomycin (40 mg/kg per day, orally, in 4 divided doses, to a maximum of 125 mg, orally, 4 times/day) is indicated as initial therapy for patients with severe disease (hospitalized in an intensive care unit, pseudomembranous colitis on endoscopy, underlying intestinal tract disease) and for patients who do not respond to metronidazole.
- Metronidazole is effective when given orally or intravenously; vancomycin is effective only when administered orally or by enema. In severe cases, intravenous metronidazole, with oral or intraluminal vancomycin, is recommended.
- Therapy with either metronidazole or vancomycin should be administered for at least 10 days.
- Up to 25% of patients experience a relapse after discontinuing therapy, but infection usually responds to a second course of the same treatment.
- Drugs that decrease intestinal motility should not be administered.

- Follow-up testing for toxin is not recommended.
- Investigational therapies include other antimicrobial agents (nitazoxanide, rifaximin, tinidazole), Immune Globulin therapy, toxin binders, and restoring intestinal tract flora.

ISOLATION OF THE HOSPITALIZED PATIENT: In addition to standard precautions, contact precautions are recommended for the duration of illness.

CONTROL MEASURES:

- Exercising meticulous hand hygiene, properly handling contaminated waste (including diapers), disinfecting fomites, and limiting use of antimicrobial agents are the best available methods for control of *C difficile* disease. Alcohol-based hand hygiene products do not inactivate *C difficile* spores. Washing hands with soap and water is more effective in removing *C difficile* spores from contaminated hands.
- Thorough cleaning of hospital rooms and bathrooms of patients with *C difficile* colitis is essential. Because *C difficile* forms spores, which are difficult to kill, the organism can resist action of many common hospital disinfectants; many hospitals have instituted cleaning with diluted bleach when outbreaks of *C difficile* diarrhea are not controlled by other measures.
- Children with *C difficile* diarrhea should be excluded from child care settings for the duration of diarrhea, and infection-control measures should be enforced (see Children in Out-of-Home Child Care, p 124).

Clostridium perfringens Food Poisoning

CLINICAL MANIFESTATIONS: *Clostridium perfringens* foodborne illness is characterized by a sudden onset of watery diarrhea and moderate to severe, crampy, midepigastric pain. Vomiting and fever are uncommon. Symptoms usually resolve within 24 hours. The short incubation period, short duration, and absence of fever in most patients differentiates *C perfringens* foodborne disease from shigellosis and salmonellosis, and the infrequency of vomiting and longer incubation period contrast with the clinical features of foodborne disease associated with heavy metals, *Staphylococcus aureus* enterotoxins, and fish and shellfish toxins. Diarrheal illness caused by *Bacillus cereus* enterotoxin can be indistinguishable from that caused by *C perfringens* (see Appendix IX, Clinical Syndromes Associated With Foodborne Diseases, p 860). Enteritis necroticans (known locally as pigbel) is a cause of severe illness and death attributable to *C perfringens* food poisoning among children in Papua, New Guinea. Rare cases have been reported elsewhere.

ETIOLOGY: Food poisoning is caused by a heat-labile toxin produced in vivo by *C perfringens* type A; type C causes enteritis necroticans.

EPIDEMIOLOGY: *C perfringens* is ubiquitous in the environment and commonly is present in raw meat and poultry. At an optimum temperature, *C perfringens* has one of the fastest rates of growth of any bacterium. Spores of *C perfringens* can survive cooking. Spores germinate and multiply during slow cooling and storage at temperatures from 20°C to 60°C (68°C–140°F). Illness results from consumption of food containing high numbers of organisms (greater than 10^5 colony-forming units/g) followed by enterotoxin production in the intestine. Beef, poultry, gravies, and dried or precooked foods are common sources. Infection usually is acquired at banquets or institutions (eg, schools and camps) or from food provided by caterers or restaurants where food is prepared in large quantities and kept warm for prolonged periods. Illness is not transmissible from person-to-person.

The **incubation period** is 6 to 24 hours, usually 8 to 12 hours.

DIAGNOSTIC TESTS: Because the fecal flora of healthy people commonly includes *C perfringens,* counts of *C perfringens* spores of 10^6/g of feces or greater obtained within 48 hours of onset of illness are required to support the diagnosis in ill people. The diagnosis also can be suggested by detection of *C perfringens* enterotoxin in stool by commercially available kits. *C perfringens* can be confirmed as the cause of an outbreak when the concentration of organisms is at least 10^5/g in the epidemiologically implicated food. Although *C perfringens* is an anaerobe, special transport conditions are unnecessary, because the spores are durable. Stool specimens, rather than rectal swab specimens, should be obtained.

TREATMENT: Oral rehydration or, occasionally, intravenous fluid and electrolyte replacement can be indicated to prevent or treat dehydration. Antimicrobial agents are not indicated.

ISOLATION OF THE HOSPITALIZED PATIENT: Standard precautions are recommended.

CONTROL MEASURES: Preventive measures depend on limiting proliferation of *C perfringens* in foods by cooking foods thoroughly and maintaining food at warmer than 60°C (140°F) or cooler than 7°C (45°F). Meat dishes should be served hot shortly after cooking. Foods never should be held at room temperature to cool; they should be refrigerated after removal from warming devices or serving tables. Foods should be reheated to at least 74°C (165.2°F) before serving. Roasts, stews, and similar dishes should be divided into small quantities for cooking and refrigeration.

Coccidioidomycosis

CLINICAL MANIFESTATIONS: The primary infection is acquired by the respiratory route and is asymptomatic or self-limited in 60% of children. Symptomatic disease can resemble influenza or community-acquired pneumonia, with malaise, fever, cough, myalgia, headache, and chest pain. Diffuse erythematous maculopapular rash, erythema multiforme, erythema nodosum, and/or arthralgia commonly occur and can be the only clinical manifestations in some children. Chronic pulmonary lesions are rare, but up to 5% of infected people develop asymptomatic pulmonary radiographic residua (eg, cysts, coin lesions). Nonpulmonary primary infection is rare, usually follows trauma, and includes cutaneous lesions or soft tissue infections with associated regional lymphadenitis.

Disseminated infection is rare, occurring in fewer than 1% of infected people; common sites of dissemination include skin, bones and joints, central nervous system (CNS), and lungs. Dissemination to one or more sites is more common in infants than older children and adults. Meningitis almost invariably is fatal if untreated. Congenital infection is rare.

ETIOLOGY: *Coccidioides* species are dimorphic fungi. In soil, *Coccidioides* organisms exist in hyphal phase. Infectious arthroconidia (ie, spores) produced from hyphae become airborne, infecting the host after inhalation or inoculation. In tissues, arthroconidia enlarge to form spherules; mature spherules release endospores that develop into new spherules and continue the tissue cycle. Using molecular markers, the genus *Coccidioides* is now divided into 2 species: *Coccidioides immitis,* confined geographically mainly to California, and *Coccidioides posadasii,* encompassing the remaining areas of the fungus' distribution within the southwestern United States, northern Mexico, and areas of Central and South America.

EPIDEMIOLOGY: *Coccidioides* species is found in soil extensively and is endemic in the southwestern United States, including California, Arizona, New Mexico, Texas, southern Nevada, and Utah; northern Mexico; and certain areas of Central and South America. People are infected through inhalation of dustborne arthroconidia. In areas with endemic coccidioidomycosis, clusters of cases can follow dust storms, seismic events, archeologic digging, or recreational activities. Exposure need not be extensive to develop infection. Infection is thought to provide lifelong immunity. Person-to-person transmission of coccidioidomycosis does not occur. Preexisting impairment of cellular immunity is a major risk factor for severe primary coccidioidomycosis or relapse of past infection. Black and Filipino people, pregnant women, neonates, elderly people, and immunocompromised people have an increased risk of dissemination and fatal outcome. A small proportion of new cases are identified in people who currently do not reside in regions with endemic infection but previously visited these areas.

The **incubation period** typically is 10 to 16 days; range is less than 1 week to approximately 1 month.

DIAGNOSTIC TESTS: The diagnosis of coccidioidomycosis is best established using serologic, histopathologic, and culture methods. Serologic tests are useful to confirm diagnosis and provide prognostic information. The immunoglobulin (Ig) M response can be detected by latex agglutination test, enzyme immunoassay (EIA), or immunodiffusion. Latex agglutination is a rapid, sensitive test that lacks specificity; hence, positive results should be confirmed by other tests. An IgM response is detectable 1 to 3 weeks after symptoms appear and can be detected in up to 75% of patients with primary disease 3 to 4 months after onset. The IgG response can be detected by immunodiffusion, EIA, or complement fixation test. Complement fixation antibodies in serum usually are of low titer and are transient if the disease is asymptomatic or mild. Persistent high titers (1:32 or greater) occur with severe disease and almost always in disseminated infection. Cerebrospinal fluid (CSF) antibodies also are detectable by complement fixation test. Increasing serum and CSF titers indicate progressive disease, and decreasing titers suggest improvement. Low or nondetectable titers in immunocompromised patients should be interpreted with caution. Because clinical laboratories use different diagnostic test kits, positive results should be confirmed in a reference laboratory.

Spherules are as large as 80 μm in diameter and can be visualized in infected body fluid specimens (eg, pleural fluid, bronchoalveolar lavage) and biopsy specimens of skin lesions or organs. The presence of a mature spherule with endospores is pathognomonic of infection. Culture of the organisms is possible but potentially hazardous to laboratory personnel, because spherules can convert to arthroconidia-bearing mycelia on culture plates. Suspect cultures should be sealed and handled using appropriate safety equipment and procedures. A DNA probe can identify *Coccidioides* species in cultures, thereby decreasing risk of exposure to infectious fungi.

Skin testing may be a useful indicator of exposure and was used for epidemiologic studies. A delayed hypersensitivity reaction to a coccidioidin or spherulin skin test is indicative of past or current infection. A positive skin test result can appear from 10 to 45 days after infection; anergy is common in disseminated disease. Skin tests currently are not available in the United States.

TREATMENT: Antifungal therapy generally is not indicated for uncomplicated primary infection. However, some experts would consider a treatment course with fluconazole or itraconazole for people who are experiencing significant morbidity as evidenced by prolonged duration of symptoms of more than 3 weeks, weight loss of greater than 10%, marked chest pain, or severe malaise.

Amphotericin B deoxycholate is the recommended initial therapy for severe and progressive infection (disseminated infection not involving the CNS) and for immunocompromised patients, including people with human immunodeficiency virus (HIV) infection and pregnant women (see Drugs for Invasive and Other Serious Fungal Infections, Table 4.6, p 772). Fluconazole is the drug of choice for CNS infections in nonpregnant women. Itraconazole and fluconazole also are useful for treatment of less severe disseminated infections. For CNS infections that are unresponsive to fluconazole or associated with severe basilar inflammation, intravenous amphotericin B deoxycholate therapy is augmented by repetitive CSF instillation of this drug. A subcutaneous reservoir can facilitate administration into the cisternal space or lateral ventricle.

The role of lipid formulations of amphotericin B as well as the newer azoles, voriconazole and posaconazole, are not established clearly. These newer agents may be administered in certain clinical settings, such as therapeutic failure in severe coccidioidal disease (eg, meningitis). Lipid formulations of amphotericin B are preferred to amphotericin B deoxycholate when nephrotoxicity is of concern. The newer azoles should be used in consultation with people experienced with their use in treatment of coccidioidomycosis.

Orally administered itraconazole and fluconazole have suppressed coccidioidal meningitis in many patients, but lifelong therapy may be necessary. Itraconazole is preferred for nonmeningeal coccidioidomycosis, including osteomyelitis. Consultation with a specialist for treatment of patients with meningeal disease is recommended.

The duration of antifungal therapy is variable and depends on the site(s) of involvement, clinical response, and mycologic and immunologic test results. In general, therapy is continued until clinical and laboratory evidence indicates that active infection has resolved. The minimum duration of treatment for disseminated coccidioidomycosis is 1 month but may continue for 1 year or longer. The required duration of treatment with azoles is uncertain, except for patients with CNS infection or underlying HIV infection, for whom suppressive therapy is lifelong. Females should be advised to avoid pregnancy while receiving fluconazole, which is teratogenic.

Surgical débridement or excision of lesions in bone, pericardium, and lung has been advocated for localized, symptomatic, persistent, resistant, or progressive lesions. In some localized infections with sinuses, fistulae, or abscesses, amphotericin B has been instilled locally or used for irrigation of wounds.

ISOLATION OF THE HOSPITALIZED PATIENT: Standard precautions are recommended. Care should be taken in handling, changing, and discarding dressings, casts, and similar materials in which arthroconidial contamination could occur.

CONTROL MEASURES: Measures to control dust are recommended in areas with endemic infection, including construction sites, archaeologic project sites, or other locations where activities cause excessive soil disturbance. Immunocompromised people residing in or traveling to areas with endemic infection should be counseled to avoid exposure to activities that may aerosolize spores in contaminated soil.

Coronaviruses, Including SARS

CLINICAL MANIFESTATIONS: Until the outbreak of severe acute respiratory syndrome (SARS) first reported by the World Health Organization in 2003, coronaviruses (CoVs) primarily have been considered to be a frequent cause of the "common cold" or upper respiratory tract illness causing nasal congestion and rhinorrhea. They also have been associated with lower respiratory tract illness, primarily in patients with compromised immune systems, although lower tract disease in previously healthy children has been described. The outbreak of SARS, beginning in China in November 2002, and its link to a novel coronavirus, SARS-CoV, demonstrated that a CoV can cause life-threatening disease. Infection by SARS-CoV should be suspected when a person develops clinical symptoms consistent with those of SARS and has been in an area or been in contact with people who have been in an area where SARS is known or suspected to be occurring. People infected with SARS-CoV first developed systemic symptoms (eg, fever, malaise, and myalgia), often without respiratory tract symptoms. A few days after onset of symptoms, some exposed people developed cough and/or shortness of breath. Many patients had no upper respiratory tract symptoms, and nearly all infected adults developed pneumonia or acute respiratory distress syndrome (ARDS). Twenty-five percent or more of patients with SARS-CoV disease reported diarrhea. SARS was associated with an overall case fatality rate of 10%, which increased to 50% or more in people older than 60 years of age or people with previous medical conditions. In children, particularly children younger than 12 years of age, the clinical course of SARS was shorter and less severe, with less prominent radiographic changes and rare progression to respiratory failure and death.

Additionally, CoV-like particles have been reported in patients with diarrhea, but a link between CoVs and diarrhea, other than in SARS, has not been confirmed. Other CoVs, NL63 and HKU1, have been linked to both upper and lower respiratory tract illness in children and adults.

ETIOLOGY: CoVs are large, enveloped RNA viruses, 80 to 160 nm in diameter, with projections on their surface that, by electron microscopy, give them their characteristic crown-like appearance. Three antigenic groups (groups I, II, and III) of CoVs have been identified. Group I includes a variety of animal CoVs and the human CoVs 229E and NL63; group II includes animal CoVs, the human CoV OC43, and possibly the distantly related SARS-CoV; and group III includes avian CoVs.

EPIDEMIOLOGY: CoV infections are common in many animal species and may provide a reservoir for introduction of new strains to humans. Human CoVs are transmitted primarily by respiratory tract secretions through close contact that probably includes direct person-to-person contact or contact with fomites followed by autoinoculation and inhalation of droplets. Patients with SARS-CoV infection also may have virus in stool, urine, and blood, all of which can provide additional sources of virus for transmission. Patients with SARS-CoV infection are most infectious during the second week of illness, unlike patients with other CoV infections, who are most infectious in the early stages of illness. During the 2003 outbreak, most SARS transmission occurred in hospitals and households.

The human CoVs are distributed worldwide. In temperate climates, CoV outbreaks occur during winter, with young children having the highest infection rate during outbreaks. Presumably, SARS-CoV initially was transmitted to humans from animals in

China—possibly animals sold in wild animal markets in Guangdong Province. Therefore, SARS-CoV may have an animal reservoir in China (eg, horseshoe bats). It is not known whether SARS-CoV is present only in animals within China or if similar viruses are present elsewhere. After the 2003 global outbreak, the only documented SARS cases have been associated with research laboratory exposure among people handling the virus.

The **incubation period** for common CoVs usually is 2 to 5 days. The incubation period for SARS may be longer, typically 2 to 7 days but as long as 10 days.

DIAGNOSTIC TESTS: Diagnostic tests for CoVs generally are not available. Coronaviruses are difficult to grow except with use of special cell lines available in research laboratories. Polymerase chain reaction assays have been developed, and a variety of antibody assays also can be used to detect infection. Viral particles can be visualized by immune electron microscopy. Laboratory diagnosis of SARS should be sought only when there are clinical and epidemiologic factors that suggest SARS-CoV infection. Laboratory guidance is available on the CDC Web site (**www.cdc.gov/ncidod/sars/**).

TREATMENT: There is no proven effective antiviral therapy for CoV infections. Treatment for symptoms of the common cold is appropriate for uncomplicated human CoV infections. There is no recommended treatment for SARS-CoV; several antiviral drugs, including ribavirin and interferon-alpha, have been used, but their efficacy is unknown; steroids have been used to treat SARS-CoV–associated ARDS.

ISOLATION OF THE HOSPITALIZED PATIENT: Standard precautions are recommended for commonly seen CoVs. Airborne, droplet, and contact precautions, in addition to standard precautions, are recommended for patients with SARS-CoV infection.

CONTROL MEASURES: Appropriate hygienic practices, especially hand hygiene, likely will decrease transmission of all CoVs. The severity of illness associated with SARS-CoV infection led to an intense and ultimately very effective public health intervention. The global SARS-CoV outbreak was halted within 4 months. The human impact was mitigated by classic infection control measures, such as aggressive case finding and rapid institution of isolation precautions with appropriate infection control practices, as well as intensive contact tracing, evaluation, monitoring, and appropriate quarantine measures.

Cryptococcus neoformans Infections
(Cryptococcosis)

CLINICAL MANIFESTATIONS: Primary infection is acquired by inhalation of aerosolized fungal elements from contaminated soil and often is asymptomatic or mild. Pulmonary disease, when symptomatic, is characterized by cough, chest pain, and constitutional symptoms. Chest radiographs may reveal a solitary nodule or mass or focal or diffuse infiltrates. Hematogenous dissemination to the central nervous system (CNS), bones, skin, and other sites can occur, but dissemination is rare in children without defects in cell-mediated immunity (eg, children with leukemia, systemic lupus erythematosis, chronic cutaneous candidiasis, congenital immunodeficiency, or acquired immunodeficiency syndrome [AIDS] or people who have undergone solid organ transplantation). Usually, several sites are infected, but manifestations of involvement at one site predominate. Cryptococcal meningitis, the most common and serious form of cryptococcal disease, often follows an indolent course. Symptoms are characteristic of meningitis, meningoencephalitis, or space-occupying lesions but can manifest only as behavioral changes.

Cryptococcal fungemia without apparent organ involvement occurs in patients with human immunodeficiency virus (HIV) infection but is rare in children.

ETIOLOGY: *Cryptococcus neoformans,* an encapsulated yeast that grows at 37°C (98°F), is, with rare exception, the only species of the genus *Cryptococcus* considered to be a human pathogen, except for *Cryptococcus gattii,* which has been reported to cause invasive disease.

EPIDEMIOLOGY: *C neoformans* var *neoformans* and *C neoformans* var *grubii* are isolated primarily from soil contaminated with pigeon or other bird guano and cause most human infections, especially infections in immunocompromised hosts. *C gattii* (formerly *C neoformans* var *gattii*), is associated with several species of eucalyptus as well as other trees and occurs most commonly in tropical and subtropical regions. *C gattii* has emerged as a pathogen being associated with an outbreak of cryptococcosis on Vancouver Island and since has spread to the Pacific Northwest region of the United States. *C gattii* generally causes disease in immunocompetent people. Person-to-person transmission does not occur. *Cryptococcus* species infect 5% to 10% of adults with AIDS, but infection is rare in HIV-infected children.

The **incubation period** is unknown.

DIAGNOSTIC TESTS: Definitive diagnosis requires isolation of the organism from body fluid or tissue specimens. Blood should be cultured by lysis-centrifugation. Media containing cycloheximide, which inhibits growth of *C neoformans,* should not be used. Sabouraud dextrose agar is useful for isolation of *Cryptococcus* from sputum, bronchopulmonary lavage, tissue, or cerebrospinal fluid (CSF) specimens. Use of Niger seed (birdseed) can increase the rate of detection in sputum and urine specimens. Few organisms may be present in the CSF specimen, and a large quantity of CSF may be needed to recover the organism. In children with CNS disease, CSF cell count and protein and glucose concentrations can be normal. The latex agglutination test and enzyme immunoassay for detection of cryptococcal capsular polysaccharide antigen in serum or CSF specimens are excellent rapid diagnostic tests. Antigen is detected in CSF or serum specimens from more than 90% of patients with cryptococcal meningitis. In patients with cryptococcal meningitis, antigen testing can be negative when antigen concentrations are low or very high (prozone effect) or if infection is caused by unencapsulated strains. Polymerase chain reaction assays are investigational. Encapsulated yeast cells can be visualized using India ink or other stains of CSF specimens containing 10^3 or more colony-forming units of yeast per mL.

TREATMENT: Amphotericin B deoxycholate (see Drugs for Invasive and Other Serious Fungal Infections, p 772), in combination with oral flucytosine, is indicated as initial therapy for patients with meningeal and other serious cryptococcal infections. Serum flucytosine concentrations should be maintained between 40 and 60 μg/mL. Patients with meningitis should receive combination therapy for at least 2 weeks followed by consolidation therapy with fluconazole (10 mg/kg per day) for a minimum of 8 to 10 weeks or until CSF culture is sterile. Alternatively, the amphotericin B deoxycholate and flucytosine combination can be continued for 6 to 10 weeks. Lipid formulations of amphotericin B can be substituted for conventional amphotericin B in children with renal impairment. If flucytosine cannot be administered, amphotericin B alone is an acceptable alternative. A lumbar puncture should be performed after 2 weeks of therapy. The 20% to 40% of patients in whom culture is positive at 2 weeks will require a more prolonged treatment course. When infection is refractory to systemic therapy, intrathecal or intraventricular amphotericin B may be required. Patients with less severe disease can be treated with fluconazole or itraconazole, but data on use of these drugs for children with *C neoformans* infection are limited. Another potential treatment option for HIV-infected patients with less severe disease is combination therapy with fluconazole and flucytosine; the toxicity associated with this regimen often limits its usefulness. Increased intracranial pressure occurs frequently despite microbiologic response and often is associated with clinical deterioration. Significant elevation of intracranial pressure should be managed with frequent repeated lumbar punctures or placement of a lumbar drain.

Children with HIV infection who have completed initial therapy for cryptococcosis should receive lifelong suppressive therapy with fluconazole daily. Oral itraconazole daily or amphotericin B deoxycholate 1 to 3 times weekly are alternatives. Data regarding discontinuing this secondary prophylaxis after immune reconstitution as a consequence of highly active antiretroviral therapy are available for adults but not for children.

ISOLATION OF THE HOSPITALIZED PATIENT: Standard precautions are recommended.

CONTROL MEASURES: None.

Cryptosporidiosis

CLINICAL MANIFESTATIONS: Frequent, nonbloody, watery diarrhea is the most common manifestation of cryptosporidiosis, although infection can be asymptomatic. Other symptoms include abdominal cramps, fatigue, fever, vomiting, anorexia, and weight loss. Fever and vomiting can occur among children and often lead to a misdiagnosis of viral gastroenteritis. In infected immunocompetent people, including children, the diarrheal illness is self-limited, usually lasting 1 to 20 days (mean, 10 days). In immunocompromised people, especially people with human immunodeficiency virus (HIV) infection, chronic, severe diarrhea can develop, resulting in malnutrition, dehydration, and death. Pulmonary, biliary tract, or disseminated infection rarely occurs in immunocompromised people.

ETIOLOGY: *Cryptosporidium* species are oocyst-forming coccidian protozoa. Oocysts are excreted in feces and are the infectious form. The most common species causing disease in humans are *Cryptosporidium hominis*, which infects only humans, and *Cryptosporidium parvum*, which infects humans, cattle, and other mammals and is the major species responsible for clinical disease in humans.

EPIDEMIOLOGY: *Cryptosporidium* species have been found in a variety of hosts, including mammals, birds, and reptiles.[1] Extensive waterborne outbreaks have been associated with contamination of municipal water and exposure to contaminated swimming pools. In children, the incidence of cryptosporidiosis is greatest during summer and early fall, corresponding to the outdoor swimming season. Transmission to humans can occur from farm livestock, particularly young animals, including animals found in petting zoos, or pets. Person-to-person transmission occurs and can cause outbreaks in child care centers, with incidences of 30% to 60% reported. *Cryptosporidium* species also causes traveler's diarrhea. Because the oocyst form of the parasite is resistant to chlorine, appropriately functioning water-filtration systems are critical for the safety of public water supplies. Most sand filters used for swimming pools are only partially effective for removing oocysts

---

[1]Centers for Disease Control and Prevention. Cryptosporidiosis surveillance—United States, 2003–2005. *MMWR Surveill Summ.* 2007;56(SS-07):1–10

from contaminated water. As a result, *Cryptosporidium* has become the leading cause of recreational water-associated outbreaks of acute gastroenteritis.[1]

The median **incubation period** is 7 days; the range is 2 to 14 days. In most people, shedding of *C parvum* stops within 2 weeks. In immunocompromised people, the period of oocyst shedding can continue for 2 months.

DIAGNOSTIC TESTS: The detection of oocysts on microscopic examination of stool specimens is diagnostic. Unfortunately, routine laboratory examination of stool for ova and parasites may not detect *Cryptosporidium* species. The formalin ethyl acetate stool concentration method is recommended before staining stool with a modified Kinyoun acid-fast stain. Direct immunofluorescent assay (DFA) for detection of oocysts in stool and enzyme immunoassay (EIA) for detecting antigen in stool are available commercially. With EIA methods, false-positive and false-negative results can occur, and confirmation by microscopy should be considered. Because shedding can be intermittent, at least 3 stool specimens collected on separate days should be examined before considering test results to be negative. Oocysts are small (4–6 μm in diameter) and can be missed in a rapid scan of a slide. Organisms also can be identified in intestinal biopsy tissue or intestinal fluid. Polymerase chain reaction assays are used to identify species and genotype.

TREATMENT: Generally, immunocompetent people need no specific therapy. A 3-day course of nitazoxanide oral suspension has been approved by the US Food and Drug Administration for treatment of immunocompetent children beginning at 12 months of age and adults with diarrhea associated with cryptosporidiosis. Patients with acquired immunodeficiency syndrome with immune reconstitution resulting from highly active antiretroviral therapy frequently will have clearance of *Cryptosporidium* organisms. Paromomycin, alone or with azithromycin, is minimally effective. In immunocompromised patients with cryptosporidiosis, oral administration of human Immune Globulin Intravenous or bovine colostrum has been beneficial. In HIV-infected patients, antiretroviral therapy-associated improvement in CD4+ T-lymphocyte count can improve the course of disease.

ISOLATION OF THE HOSPITALIZED PATIENT: In addition to standard precautions, contact precautions are recommended for diapered or incontinent children.

CONTROL MEASURES: People with diarrhea should not use public recreational waters (eg, swimming pools, lakes, ponds), and people with a diagnosis of cryptosporidiosis should not use recreational waters for 2 weeks after symptoms resolve. There are numerous methods of water purification. Boiling is the most certain way of killing all microorganisms. The time of boiling (1 minute at sea level) will depend on altitude. Because of its thick outer shell, the oocyst is highly resistant to chemical disinfection. Neither chlorine nor iodine is effective. Filtration is the most appropriate alternative to boiling. Filtration devices should have a particle size rating of 1 μm or smaller to remove *Cryptosporidium* species. Backpackers and campers always should have at least one backup method of water purification in case one fails. For additional information, see *Giardia intestinalis* Infections (p 303).

---

[1] Centers for Disease Control and Prevention. Surveillance for waterborne disease and outbreaks associated with recreational water use and other aquatic facility-associated health events—United States, 2005–2006 *MMWR Surveill Summ.* 2008;57(SS-9):1–29

Cutaneous Larva Migrans

CLINICAL MANIFESTATIONS: Nematode larvae produce pruritic, reddish papules at the site of skin entry, a condition referred to as creeping eruption. As the larvae migrate through skin advancing several millimeters to a few centimeters a day, intensely pruritic, serpiginous tracks or bullae are formed. Larval activity can continue for several weeks or months but eventually is self-limiting. An advancing serpiginous tunnel in the skin with an associated intense pruritus virtually is pathognomonic. Rarely, in infections with a large burden of parasites, pneumonitis (Löeffler syndrome), which can be severe, and myositis may follow skin lesions. Occasionally, the larvae reach the intestine and may cause eosinophilic enteritis.

ETIOLOGY: Infective larvae of cat and dog hookworms (ie, *Ancylostoma braziliense* and *Ancylostoma caninum*) are the usual causes. Other skin-penetrating nematodes are occasional causes.

EPIDEMIOLOGY: Cutaneous larva migrans is a disease of children, utility workers, gardeners, sunbathers, and others who come in contact with soil contaminated with cat and dog feces. In the United States, the disease is most prevalent in the Southeast. Most cases in the United States are imported by travelers returning from tropical and subtropical areas.

DIAGNOSTIC TESTS: Because the diagnosis usually is made clinically, biopsies are not indicated. Biopsy specimens typically demonstrate an eosinophilic inflammatory infiltrate, but the migrating parasite is not visualized. Eosinophilia and increased IgE serum concentrations occur in some cases. Larvae have been detected in sputum and gastric washings in patients with the rare complication of pneumonitis. Enzyme immunoassay or Western blot analysis using antigens of *A caninum* have been developed in research laboratories, but these assays are not available for routine diagnostic use.

TREATMENT: The disease usually is self-limited, with spontaneous cure after several weeks or months. Orally administered albendazole or ivermectin is the recommended therapy.

ISOLATION OF THE HOSPITALIZED PATIENT: Standard precautions are recommended.

CONTROL MEASURES: Skin contact with moist soil contaminated with animal feces should be avoided. In warm climates, beaches should be kept free of dog and cat feces.

Cyclosporiasis

CLINICAL MANIFESTATIONS: Profuse, watery diarrhea is the most common symptom of cyclosporiasis, and diarrhea can be profuse and protracted. Nausea, vomiting, anorexia, substantial weight loss, abdominal bloating or cramping, myalgia, and prolonged fatigue also can occur. Low grade fever occurs in approximately 50% of patients. Infection usually is self-limited, but untreated people may have remitting, relapsing symptoms for weeks to months. Asymptomatic infection has been documented most commonly in settings where cyclosporiasis is endemic.

ETIOLOGY: *Cyclospora cayetanensis* is a coccidian protozoan; oocysts are passed in stools.

EPIDEMIOLOGY: *C cayetanensis* is known to be endemic in many resource-limited countries, such as Nepal, Peru, Haiti, Guatemala, and Indonesia and has been reported as a cause of traveler's diarrhea. Both foodborne and waterborne outbreaks have been reported.

Most of the outbreaks in United States and Canada have been associated with consumption of imported fresh produce. Humans are the only known hosts for *C cayetanensis*. Direct person-to-person transmission is unlikely, because excreted oocysts take days to weeks under favorable environmental conditions to sporulate and become infective. The oocysts probably are highly resistant to most disinfectants and can remain viable for prolonged periods in cool, moist environments.

The **incubation period** is approximately 7 days (range, 2–14 days).

DIAGNOSTIC TESTS: Diagnosis is made by identification of oocysts (8–10 μm in diameter) in stool. The oocysts are autofluorescent and variably acid-fast after modified acid-fast staining of stool specimens (ie, oocysts that either have retained or not retained the stain can be visualized). Investigational molecular diagnostic assays (eg, polymerase chain reaction) are available at the Centers for Disease Control and Prevention and some other reference laboratories.

TREATMENT: Trimethoprim-sulfamethoxazole, typically for 7 to 10 days, is the drug of choice. People infected with human immunodeficiency virus may need long-term maintenance therapy (see Drugs for Parasitic Infections, p 783).

ISOLATION OF THE HOSPITALIZED PATIENT: In addition to standard precautions, contact precautions are recommended for diapered or incontinent children.

CONTROL MEASURES: Fresh produce always should be washed thoroughly before it is eaten. This precaution, however, may not eliminate the risk of transmission entirely.

Cytomegalovirus Infection

CLINICAL MANIFESTATIONS: Manifestations of acquired human cytomegalovirus (CMV) infection vary with the age and immunocompetence of the host. Asymptomatic infections are the most common, particularly in children. An infectious mononucleosis-like syndrome with prolonged fever and mild hepatitis, occurring in the absence of heterophil antibody production, may occur in adolescents and adults. Pneumonia, colitis, and retinitis may occur in immunocompromised hosts, including people receiving treatment for malignant neoplasms, people infected with human immunodeficiency virus (HIV), and people receiving immunosuppressive therapy for organ transplantation.

Congenital infection has a spectrum of manifestations but usually is not evident at birth (asymptomatic congenital CMV infection). Approximately 10% of infants with congenital CMV infection have involvement that is evident at birth (symptomatic congenital CMV disease), with manifestations including intrauterine growth retardation, jaundice, purpura, hepatosplenomegaly, microcephaly, intracerebral calcifications, and retinitis; developmental delays are common among these infants as they grow. Sensorineural hearing loss (SNHL) is the most common sequela following congenital CMV infection, with the likelihood of SNHL being higher among infants with symptomatic infection. Congenital CMV infection is the leading nongenetic cause of sensorineural hearing loss in children in the United States. Approximately 21% of all hearing loss at birth is attributable to congenital CMV infection (10% symptomatic and 11% asymptomatic), and 25% of all hearing loss at 4 years of age is attributable to congenital CMV infection. Late-onset and progressive hearing losses occur following congenital CMV infection. Hearing loss following congenital CMV infection may be present at birth or occur later in the first years of life. Approximately 33% to 50% of SNHL attributable to congenital CMV infection is late-onset loss. Approximately 50% of children with SNHL following congenital CMV infection will continue to have further deterioration or progression of their loss. As such, children with congenital CMV infection should be evaluated regularly for early detection and appropriate intervention of suspected hearing losses.

Infection acquired intrapartum from maternal cervical secretions or postpartum from human milk usually is not associated with clinical illness in term babies. In preterm infants, infection resulting from human milk or from transfusion from CMV-seropositive donors has been associated with systemic infections, including lower respiratory tract disease.

ETIOLOGY: Human CMV, a DNA virus, is a member of the herpesvirus group.

EPIDEMIOLOGY: CMV is highly species specific, and only human strains are known to produce human disease. The virus is ubiquitous and has numerous strains. Transmission occurs horizontally (by direct person-to-person contact with virus-containing secretions), vertically (from mother to infant before, during, or after birth), and via transfusions of blood, platelets, and white blood cells from previously infected people (see Blood Safety, p 106). Infections have no seasonal predilection. CMV persists in latent form after a primary infection, and reactivation can occur years later, particularly under conditions of immunosuppression. Reinfection with other strains of CMV occurs in seropositive hosts.

Horizontal transmission probably is the result of salivary contamination, but contact with infected urine also can have a role. Spread of CMV in households and child care centers is well documented. Excretion rates from urine or saliva in children 1 to 3 years of age who attend child care centers usually range from 30% to 40% but can be as high as 70%. Young children can transmit CMV to their parents, including mothers who may be pregnant, and other caregivers, including child care staff (see also Children in Out-of-Home Child Care, p 124). In adolescents and adults, sexual transmission also occurs, as evidenced by detection of virus in seminal and cervical fluids.

Seropositive healthy people have latent CMV in their leukocytes and tissues; hence, blood transfusions and organ transplantation can result in viral transmission. Severe CMV disease following transfusion or organ transplantation is more likely to occur if the recipient is immunosuppressed and seronegative or is a preterm infant. Latent CMV commonly will reactivate in immunosuppressed people and can result in disease if immunosuppression is severe (eg, in patients with acquired immunodeficiency syndrome or solid organ or stem cell transplant recipients).

Vertical transmission of CMV to an infant occurs in one of the following time periods: (1) in utero by transplacental passage of maternal bloodborne virus; (2) at birth by passage through an infected maternal genital tract; or (3) postnatally by ingestion of CMV-positive human milk. Approximately 1% of all live-born infants are infected in utero and excrete CMV at birth, making this the most common congenital viral infection. Congenital infection and associated disabilities can occur no matter in what trimester the mother is infected, but severe sequelae are associated most commonly with primary maternal infection acquired during the first half of gestation. In utero fetal infection can occur in women with no preexisting CMV immunity (maternal primary infection) or in women with preexisting antibody to CMV (maternal nonprimary infection) by means of viral reactivation or acquisition of a different viral strain during pregnancy. Damaging fetal infections following nonprimary maternal infection have been reported, and the role of acquisition of a different viral strain in women with preexisting CMV antibody as a cause of symptomatic infection with sequelae is an area of current research.

Cervical excretion is common among seropositive women, resulting in exposure of many infants to CMV at birth. Cervical excretion rates are highest among young mothers in lower socioeconomic groups. Although interstitial pneumonia caused by CMV can develop during the early months of life, most infected infants remain well. Similarly, although disease can occur in seronegative infants fed CMV-infected human milk, most infants who acquire CMV from ingestion of infected human milk do not develop clinical illness, most likely because of the presence of passively transferred maternal antibody. Among infants who acquire infection from maternal cervical secretions or human milk, preterm infants are at greater risk of CMV illness and possibly sequelae than are full-term infants.

The **incubation period** for horizontally transmitted CMV infections is unknown. Infection usually manifests 3 to 12 weeks after blood transfusions and between 1 and 4 months after tissue transplantation.

DIAGNOSTIC TESTS: The diagnosis of CMV disease is confounded by the ubiquity of the virus, the high rate of asymptomatic excretion, the frequency of reactivated infections, development of serum immunoglobulin (Ig) M CMV-specific antibody in some episodes of reactivation, reinfection with different strains of CMV, and concurrent infection with other pathogens.

Virus can be isolated in cell culture from urine, pharynx, peripheral blood leukocytes, human milk, semen, cervical secretions, and other tissues and body fluids. Recovery of virus from a target organ provides strong evidence that the disease is caused by CMV infection. A presumptive diagnosis can be made on the basis of a fourfold antibody titer increase in paired serum specimens or by demonstration of virus excretion. Techniques for detection of viral DNA in tissues and some fluids, especially cerebrospinal fluid, by polymerase chain reaction assay or hybridization are available. Detection of pp65 antigen in white blood cells is used to detect infection in immunocompromised hosts.

Various immunofluorescent assays, indirect hemagglutination assays, latex agglutination assays, and enzyme immunoassays are preferred for detecting CMV-specific antibodies.

Amniocentesis has been used in several small series of patients to establish the diagnosis of intrauterine infection. Proof of congenital infection requires isolation of CMV from urine, stool, respiratory tract secretions, or CSF obtained within 2 to 4 weeks of birth. Recent findings suggest that congenital CMV infection also might be diagnosed by using polymerase chain reaction assay to detect CMV DNA in newborn dried blood spots, although additional work is needed to define the sensitivity and feasibility of this approach. Differentiation between intrauterine and perinatal infection is difficult later in infancy unless clinical manifestations of the former, such as chorioretinitis or intracranial calcifications, are present. A strongly positive CMV-specific IgM is suggestive during early infancy, but IgM antibody assays vary in accuracy for identification of primary infection.

TREATMENT: Ganciclovir (see Antiviral Drugs, p 777) is approved for both induction and maintenance treatment of retinitis caused by acquired or recurrent CMV infection in immunocompromised patients, including HIV-infected adults, and for prevention of CMV infection in transplant recipients. Ganciclovir also is used to treat CMV infections of other sites (esophagus, colon, lungs) and for preemptive treatment of immunosuppressed adults with CMV antigenemia or viremia. Limited data in children suggest that safety and efficacy are similar to those in adults. Oral ganciclovir no longer is available in the United States, but oral valganciclovir is available in tablet form.

Limited data in neonates with symptomatic congenital CMV disease involving the central nervous system (CNS) suggest possible benefit of 6 weeks of parenteral ganciclovir therapy (6 mg/kg/dose administered intravenously every 12 hours) for protecting against hearing deterioration and potentially in decreasing developmental impairment at 1 to 2 years of age. Therapy is not recommended routinely in this population because of possible toxicities and adverse events associated with prolonged intravenous therapy in young infants with a medication that causes neutropenia in a significant proportion of recipients. If parenteral ganciclovir is used in the management of these patients, its use should be limited to patients with symptomatic congenital CMV disease involving the central nervous system who are able to start treatment within the first month of life. Experts differ in opinion as to whether patients with isolated hearing loss should be classified as symptomatic with CNS involvement; however, patients with such limited involvement are not the group in which therapeutic benefit has been documented. A liquid formulation of valganciclovir is not available commercially, and extemporaneously compounded preparations have not been evaluated sufficiently to ensure the stability and pharmacokinetics of such formulations. A research grade of pharmaceutically produced valganciclovir is being evaluated in clinical trials conducted by the National Institute of Allergy and Infectious Diseases Collaborative Antiviral Study Group.

Preterm infants with perinatally acquired CMV infection can have symptomatic, end-organ disease (eg, pneumonitis, hepatitis, thrombocytopenia). Antiviral treatment has not been studied in this population. If such patients are treated with parenteral ganciclovir, a reasonable approach is to treat for 2 weeks and then reassess responsiveness to therapy. If clinical data suggest benefit of treatment, an additional 1 to 2 weeks of parenteral ganciclovir can be considered if symptoms and signs have not been resolved.

In stem cell transplant recipients, the combination of Immune Globulin Intravenous (or CMV Immune Globulin Intravenous) and ganciclovir administered intravenously has been reported to be synergistic in treatment of CMV pneumonia. Valganciclovir and foscarnet also have been approved for treatment and maintenance of CMV retinitis in adults with acquired immunodeficiency syndrome (AIDS) (see Antiviral Drugs, p 777). Foscarnet is more toxic but may be advantageous for some patients with HIV infection, including people with disease caused by ganciclovir-resistant virus or people who are unable to tolerate ganciclovir. Cidofovir is efficacious for maintenance therapy of CMV retinitis in adults with AIDS and CMV retinitis, but cidofovir has not been studied in children and is nephrotoxic.

As in all human hosts, CMV establishes lifelong latency and, as such, is not eliminated from the body with antiviral treatment of CMV disease. Until immune reconstitution is achieved with highly active antiretroviral therapy (HAART), chronic suppressive therapy should be administered to HIV-infected patients with a history of CMV end-organ disease (eg, retinitis, colitis, pneumonitis) to prevent recurrence. Recognizing limitations of the pediatric data but drawing on the growing experience in adult patients, discontinuing prophylaxis may be considered for pediatric patients 1 to 6 years of age who are receiving HAART therapy and have a sustained (eg, greater than 6 months) increase in CD4+ T-lymphocyte count to greater than 500 cells/mm^3 or CD4+ T-lymphocyte percentage to greater than 15%, and for children older than 6 years of age, an increase in CD4+

T-lymphocyte count to greater than 100 cells/mm^3 or CD4+ T-lymphocyte percentage to greater than 15%. Such decisions should be made in close consultation with an ophthalmologist and should take into account such factors as magnitude and duration of CD4+ T-lymphocyte increase, anatomic location of the retinal lesion, vision in the contralateral eye, and the feasibility of regular ophthalmologic monitoring. All patients who have had anti-CMV maintenance therapy discontinued should continue to undergo regular ophthalmologic monitoring at least 3 to 6 month intervals for early detection of CMV relapse as well as for immune reconstitution uveitis.

ISOLATION OF THE HOSPITALIZED PATIENT: Standard precautions are recommended.

CONTROL MEASURES:

Care of Exposed People. When caring for children, hand hygiene, particularly after changing diapers, is advised to decrease transmission of CMV. Because asymptomatic excretion of CMV is common in people of all ages, a child with congenital CMV infection should not be treated differently from other children.

Although unrecognized exposure to people who are shedding CMV likely is common, concern may arise when immunocompromised patients or nonimmune pregnant women, including health care professionals, are exposed to patients with clinically recognizable CMV infection. Standard precautions should be sufficient to interrupt transmission of CMV (See Infection Control for Hospitalized Children, p 148).

Child Care (also see Children in Out-of-Home Child Care, p 124). Educational programs about the epidemiology of CMV, its potential risks, and appropriate hygienic measures to minimize occupationally acquired infection should be provided for female workers in child care centers. Risk seems to be greatest for child care personnel who provide care for children younger than 2 years of age. Routine serologic screening of staff at child care centers for antibody to CMV is not recommended.

Immunoprophylaxis. Cytomegalovirus Immune Globulin Intravenous has been developed for prophylaxis of disease in seronegative transplant recipients. CMV Immune Globulin Intravenous seems to be moderately effective in kidney and liver transplant recipients. Results of a study of its use in pregnant women to prevent CMV transmission to the fetus were compromised by methodologic difficulties in the conduct of the trial, and use of CMV Immune Globulin Intravenous cannot be recommended for this purpose at the current time. Evaluation of investigational vaccines in healthy volunteers and renal transplant recipients is in progress, and recent data from a phase II trial in pregnant women appear promising.

Prevention of Transmission by Blood Transfusion. Transmission of CMV by blood transfusion to newborn infants or other immune-compromised hosts virtually has been eliminated by use of CMV antibody-negative donors, by freezing red blood cells in glycerol before administration, by removal of the buffy coat, or by filtration to remove white blood cells.

Prevention of Transmission by Human Milk. Pasteurization or freezing of donated human milk can decrease the likelihood of CMV transmission. Holder pasteurization (62.5°C [144.5°F] for 30 minutes) and short-term pasteurization (72°C [161.6°F] for 5 seconds) of milk appear to inactivate CMV; short-term pasteurization may be less harmful to the beneficial constituents of human milk. Freezing milk at −20°C (−4°F) will decrease viral titers but does not eliminate CMV reliably. If fresh donated milk is needed for infants born to CMV antibody-negative mothers, providing these infants with milk from only CMV antibody-negative women should be considered. For further information on human milk banks, see Human Milk (p 118).

Prevention of Transmission in Transplant Recipients. CMV antibody-negative recipients of tissue from CMV-seropositive donors are at high risk of CMV disease. If such circumstances cannot be avoided, administration of antiviral therapy is beneficial for decreasing this risk.

Diphtheria

CLINICAL MANIFESTATIONS: Respiratory diphtheria usually occurs as membranous nasopharyngitis or obstructive laryngotracheitis. Local infections are associated with a low-grade fever and gradual onset of manifestations over 1 to 2 days. Less commonly, diphtheria presents as cutaneous, vaginal, conjunctival, or otic infection. Cutaneous diphtheria is more common in tropical areas and among the urban homeless. Serious complications of diphtheria include severe neck swelling (bull neck) accompanying upper airway obstruction caused by extensive membrane formation, myocarditis, and peripheral neuropathies.

ETIOLOGY: Diphtheria is caused by toxigenic strains of *Corynebacterium diphtheriae;* rarely, a diphtheria-like illness is caused by toxigenic strains of *Corynebacterium ulcerans. C diphtheriae* is an irregularly staining, gram-positive, nonspore-forming, nonmotile, pleomorphic bacillus with 4 biotypes (mitis, intermedius, belfanti, and gravis). All biotypes of *C diphtheriae* may be either toxigenic or nontoxigenic. Toxigenic strains express an exotoxin that consists of an enzymatically active A domain and a binding B domain, which promotes the entry of A into the cell. The toxin gene, *tox,* is carried by a family of related corynebacteria phages. The toxin inhibits protein synthesis in all cells, including myocardial, renal, and peripheral nerve cells, resulting in myocarditis, acute tubular necrosis, and delayed peripheral nerve conduction. Nontoxigenic strains of *C diphtheriae* can cause sore throat and other invasive infections, including endocarditis.

EPIDEMIOLOGY: Humans are the sole reservoir of *C diphtheriae.* The organisms are spread by respiratory tract droplets and by contact with discharges from skin lesions. In untreated people, organisms can be present in discharges from the nose and throat and from eye and skin lesions for 2 to 6 weeks after infection. Patients treated with an appropriate antimicrobial agent usually are communicable for fewer than 4 days. Transmission results from intimate contact with patients or carriers, particularly in people who travel to areas where diphtheria is endemic or people who come into close contact with infected travelers from such areas; rarely, fomites and raw milk or milk products can serve as vehicles of transmission. Severe disease occurs more often in people who are unimmunized or inadequately immunized. Fully immunized people may be asymptomatic carriers or have mild sore throat. The incidence of respiratory diphtheria is greatest during autumn and winter, but summer epidemics can occur in warm climates in which skin infections are prevalent. During the 1990s, epidemic diphtheria occurred throughout the newly independent states of the former Soviet Union, with case-fatality rates ranging from 3% to 23%. Diphtheria remains endemic in these countries as well as in countries in Africa, Latin America, Asia, and the Middle East (**www.cdc.gov/travel/yellowbook**). No locally acquired case of respiratory tract diphtheria has been reported in the United States since 2003. Cases of cutaneous diphtheria likely still occur in the United States, but they are not reportable.

The **incubation period** usually is 2 to 7 days but occasionally is longer.

DIAGNOSTIC TESTS: Specimens for culture should be obtained from the nose or throat or any mucosal or cutaneous lesion. Material should be obtained from beneath the membrane, or a portion of the membrane itself should be submitted for culture. Because special medium is required for isolation (cystine-tellurite blood agar or modified Tinsdale agar), laboratory personnel should be notified that *C diphtheriae* is suspected. In remote areas, specimens collected for culture can be placed in silica gel packs or any transport medium or sterile container and transported to a reference laboratory for culture. When *C diphtheriae* is recovered, the strain should be tested for toxigenicity at a laboratory recommended by state and local authorities. All *C diphtheriae* isolates should be sent through the state health department to the Centers for Disease Control and Prevention (CDC).

TREATMENT:

Antitoxin. Because the condition of patients with diphtheria may deteriorate rapidly, a single dose of equine antitoxin should be administered on the basis of clinical diagnosis, even before culture results are available. To neutralize toxin as rapidly as possible, the preferred route of administration is intravenous. Before intravenous administration of antitoxin, tests for sensitivity to horse serum should be performed, initially with a scratch test of a 1:1000 dilution of antitoxin in saline solution followed by an intradermal test if the scratch test result is negative (see Sensitivity Tests for Reactions to Animal Sera, p 63). If the patient is sensitive to equine antitoxin, desensitization is necessary (see Desensitization to Animal Sera, p 63). Allergic reactions to horse serum can be expected in 5% to 20% of patients. The site and size of the diphtheria membrane, the degree of toxic effects, and the duration of illness are guides for estimating the dose of antitoxin; the presence of soft, diffuse cervical lymphadenitis suggests moderate to severe toxin absorption. Suggested dose ranges are: pharyngeal or laryngeal disease of 48 hours' duration or less, 20 000 to 40 000 U; nasopharyngeal lesions, 40 000 to 60 000 U; extensive disease of 3 or more days' duration or diffuse swelling of the neck, 80 000 to 120 000 U. Antitoxin probably is of no value for cutaneous disease, but some experts recommend 20 000 to 40 000 U of antitoxin, because toxic sequelae have been reported. Antitoxin can be obtained from the CDC (see Directory of Resources, p 831).[1] Although Immune Globulin Intravenous preparations may contain variable amounts of antibodies to diphtheria toxin, use of Immune Globulin Intravenous for therapy of cutaneous or respiratory diphtheria has not been approved or evaluated for efficacy.

Antimicrobial Therapy. Erythromycin given orally or parenterally for 14 days, penicillin G given intramuscularly or intravenously for 14 days, or penicillin G procaine given intramuscularly for 14 days constitute acceptable therapy. Antimicrobial therapy is required to stop toxin production, to eradicate *C diphtheriae,* and to prevent transmission but is not a substitute for antitoxin, which is the primary therapy. Elimination of the organism should be documented 24 hours after completion of treatment by 2 consecutive negative cultures from specimens taken 24 hours apart.

Immunization. Active immunization against diphtheria should be undertaken during convalescence from diphtheria; disease does not necessarily confer immunity.

Cutaneous Diphtheria. Thorough cleansing of the lesion with soap and water and administration of an appropriate antimicrobial agent for 10 days are recommended.

---

[1]See Centers for Disease Control and Prevention. Notice to readers: availability of diphtheria antitoxin through an investigational new drug protocol. *MMWR Morb Mortal Wkly Rep.* 2004;53(19):413 for latest information on obtaining diphtheria antitoxin from the CDC.

Carriers. If not immunized, carriers should receive active immunization promptly, and measures should be taken to ensure completion of the immunization schedule. If a carrier has been immunized previously but has not received a booster of diphtheria toxoid within 5 years, a booster dose of a vaccine containing diphtheria toxoid (DTaP, Tdap, DT, or Td, depending on age) should be given. Carriers should be given oral erythromycin or penicillin G for 10 to 14 days or a single intramuscular dose of penicillin G benzathine (600 000 U for children weighing less than 30 kg and 1.2 million U for children weighing 30 kg or more and adults). Two follow-up cultures should be obtained after completing antimicrobial treatment to ensure detection of relapse, which occurs in as many as 20% of patients treated with erythromycin. The first culture should be obtained 24 hours after completing treatment. If results of cultures are positive, an additional 10-day course of oral erythromycin should be given, and follow-up cultures should be performed again. Erythromycin-resistant strains have been identified, but their epidemiologic significance has not been determined. Fluoroquinolones, rifampin, clarithromycin, and azithromycin have good in vitro activity and may be better tolerated than erythromycin, but they have not been evaluated in clinical infection or in carriers.

ISOLATION OF THE HOSPITALIZED PATIENT: In addition to standard precautions, droplet precautions are recommended for patients and carriers with pharyngeal diphtheria until 2 cultures from both the nose and throat collected 24 hours after completing antimicrobial treatment are negative for *C diphtheriae*. Contact precautions are recommended for patients with cutaneous diphtheria until 2 cultures of skin lesions taken at least 24 hours apart and 24 hours after cessation of antimicrobial therapy are negative.

CONTROL MEASURES:

Care of Exposed People. Whenever diphtheria is suspected strongly or proven, local public health officials should be notified promptly. Management of exposed people is based on individual circumstances, including immunization status and likelihood of adherence to follow-up and prophylaxis. The following are recommended:

- Close contacts of a person suspected to have diphtheria should be identified promptly. Contact tracing should begin in the household and usually can be limited to household members and other people with a history of direct, habitual close contact (including kissing or sexual contacts), health care staff exposed to nasopharyngeal secretions, people sharing utensils or kitchen facilities, and people caring for children.
- For close contacts, *regardless of their immunization status,* the following measures should be taken: (1) surveillance for 7 days for evidence of disease; (2) culture for *C diphtheriae;* and (3) antimicrobial prophylaxis with oral erythromycin (40–50 mg/kg per day for 10 days, maximum 2 g/day) or a single intramuscular injection of penicillin G benzathine (600 000 U for children weighing less than 30 kg and 1.2 million U for children weighing 30 kg or more and adults). The efficacy of antimicrobial prophylaxis is presumed but not proven. Follow-up cultures of pharyngeal specimens should be performed for contacts proven to be carriers after completion of therapy (see Carriers, above). If cultures are positive, an additional 10-day course of erythromycin should be given, and follow-up cultures of pharyngeal specimens should be performed.
- Asymptomatic, previously immunized close contacts should receive a booster dose of an age-appropriate diphtheria toxoid-containing vaccine (DTaP [or DT], Tdap, or Td) if they have not received a booster dose of a diphtheria toxoid-containing vaccine within 5 years (Tdap [10 through 64 years of age] is preferred over Td, if the

adolescent did not previously receive pertussis booster vaccine). Children younger than 7 years of age in need of their fourth dose of DTaP (or DT) should be immunized.

- Asymptomatic close contacts who are not immunized fully (defined as having had fewer than 3 doses of diphtheria toxoid) or people whose immunization status is not known should be immunized with an age-appropriate diphtheria toxoid-containing vaccine (DTaP [or DT], Tdap, or Td).
- Contacts who cannot be kept under surveillance should receive penicillin G benzathine but not erythromycin, because adherence to an oral regimen is less likely, and a dose of DTaP, Tdap, DT, or Td vaccine, depending on the person's age and immunization history.

The use of equine diphtheria antitoxin in unimmunized close contacts is not recommended, because there is no evidence that antitoxin provides additional benefit for contacts who have received antimicrobial prophylaxis.

Immunization. Universal immunization with a diphtheria toxoid-containing vaccine is the only effective control measure. For all indications, diphtheria immunization is administered intramuscularly with tetanus toxoid-containing vaccines and, when indicated, with pertussis-containing vaccines. The schedules for immunization against diphtheria are presented in the chapter on tetanus (see Tetanus, p 655) and in the childhood and adolescent (Fig 1.1–1.3, p 24–28) and adult (**www.cdc.gov/vaccines**) immunization schedules. The value of diphtheria toxoid immunization is proven by the rarity of disease in countries in which high rates of immunization with diphtheria toxoid have been achieved. No locally acquired case has been reported in the United States since 2003. The decreased frequency of endogenous exposure to the organism in countries with high childhood coverage rates implies decreased boosting of immunity. Therefore, ensuring continuing immunity requires regular booster injections of diphtheria toxoid (as Td vaccine) every 10 years after completion of the initial immunization series.

Pneumococcal and meningococcal conjugate vaccines containing diphtheria toxoid or CRM_{197} protein, a nontoxic variant of diphtheria toxin, are not substitutes for diphtheria toxoid immunization.

Immunization of children from 2 months of age to the seventh birthday (see Fig 1.1–1.3) routinely consists of 5 doses of diphtheria and tetanus toxoid-containing vaccines. This typically is accomplished with DTaP vaccine. Immunization against diphtheria and tetanus for children younger than 7 years of age in whom pertussis immunization is contraindicated (see Pertussis, p 504) should be accomplished with DT instead of DTaP vaccine (see Tetanus, p 655).

Other recommendations for diphtheria immunization, including recommendations for older children (7 through 18 years of age) and adults, can be found in the recommended childhood and adolescent (Fig 1.1–1.3, p 24–28) and adult (**www.cdc.gov/ vaccines**) immunization schedules.

- When children and adults require tetanus toxoid for wound management (see Tetanus, p 655), the use of preparations containing diphtheria toxoid (DTaP, Tdap, DT, or Td vaccine as appropriate for age or specific contraindication to pertussis immunization) is preferred to tetanus toxoid and will help to maintain diphtheria and, when appropriate, pertussis immunity.
- Travelers to countries with endemic or epidemic diphtheria should have their diphtheria immunization status reviewed and updated when necessary.

Precautions and Contraindications. See Pertussis (p 504) and Tetanus (p 655).

Ehrlichia and *Anaplasma* Infections
(Human Ehrlichiosis and Anaplasmosis)

CLINICAL MANIFESTATIONS: Previously collectively referred to as ehrlichiosis, 2 distinct names—ehrlichiosis and anaplasmosis—now commonly are used to describe infections caused by *Ehrlichia* species and *Anaplasma* species. In the United States, human infection with *Ehrlichia chaffeensis* causes a disease known as human monocytic ehrlichiosis (HME); another form of ehrlichiosis is attributed to infection with *Ehrlichia ewingii*. Infection with *Anaplasma phagocytophilum* causes a disease known as human granulocytic anaplasmosis (HGA) (Table 3.3, p 285). These 3 infections have similar signs, symptoms, and clinical courses. All are acute, systemic, febrile illnesses that have some clinical similarities to Rocky Mountain spotted fever (RMSF), which often is considered in the differential diagnosis. Common systemic manifestations present in more than 50% of patients include fever, headache, chills, malaise, myalgia, and nausea. More variable symptoms include arthralgia, vomiting, diarrhea, cough, and confusion, usually present in 20% to 50% of patients. For *E chaffeensis*, a rash is reported in approximately 60% of children, although it is reported less commonly in adults; a rash is present in fewer than 10% of people with anaplasmosis. When present, the rash is variable in appearance (usually involving the trunk and sparing the hands and feet) and location and typically develops approximately 1 week after onset of illness. More severe manifestations of these diseases include acute respiratory distress syndrome (ARDS), encephalopathy, meningitis, disseminated intravascular coagulation (DIC), spontaneous hemorrhage, and renal failure. Significant laboratory findings in these diseases may include leukopenia, lymphopenia, thrombocytopenia, and elevated serum hepatic transaminase concentrations. Cerebrospinal fluid abnormalities (ie, pleocytosis with a predominance of lymphocytes and increased total protein concentration) are common. Symptoms typically last 1 to 2 weeks, and recovery generally occurs without sequelae; however, reports suggest the occurrence of neurologic complications in some children after severe disease. Fatal infections have been reported and are reported more commonly for *E chaffeensis* infections (approximately 3% case fatality) than HGA (less than 1% case fatality). Typically, *E chaffeensis* causes more severe disease than does *A phagocytophilum*. Secondary or opportunistic infections may occur in severe illness, resulting in a delay in recognition of ehrlichiosis and the administration of appropriate antimicrobial treatment. People with underlying immunosuppression are at greater risk of severe disease.

ETIOLOGY: In the United States, human ehrlichiosis and anaplasmosis are caused by at least 3 distinct species of obligate intracellular bacteria with a tropism for white blood cells. Ehrlichiosis results from infection with either *E chaffeensis* or *E ewingii*, and anaplasmosis is caused by *A phagocytophilum*. *Ehrlichia* and *Anaplasma* species are gram-negative cocci that measure 0.5 to 1.5 μm in diameter. These agents do not cause the vasculitis or endothelial damage characteristic of other rickettsial diseases such as RMSF.

EPIDEMIOLOGY: Although the reported incidence of *E chaffeensis* and *A phagocytophilum* infections are only 0.6 and 1.4 per million population, respectively, the diseases are underrecognized, and selected active surveillance programs have shown the incidence to be substantially higher in some areas. Recent surveillance data also show that the incidence of reported cases seems to be increasing. Most cases of *E chaffeensis* infection occur in people from the southeastern and south central United States, but a number of cases have been

Table 3.3. Human Ehrlichiosis and Anaplasmosis in the United States

Disease	Causal Agent	Major Target Cell	Tick Vector	Geographic Distribution
Ehrlichiosis caused by *Ehrlichia chaffeensis* (also known as human monocytic ehrlichiosis, or HME)	*E chaffeensis*	Usually monocytes	Lone star tick *(Amblyomma americanum)*	Predominately southeast, south central, and Midwest states
Anaplasmosis (also known as human granulocytic anaplasmosis, or HGA)	*Anaplasma phagocytophilum*	Usually granulocytes	Black-legged or deer tick *(Ixodes scapularis)* or Western black-legged tick *(Ixodes pacificus)*	Northeast and north central states and northern California
Ehrlichiosis caused by *Ehrlichia ewingii*	*E ewingii*	Usually granulocytes	Lone star tick *(A americanum)*	Southeast, south central, and Midwest states

described from other areas. Ehrlichial infections caused by *E chaffeensis* and *E ewingii* are associated with the bite of the lone star tick *(Amblyomma americanum)*. However, the distribution of *A americanum* is expanding, and the geographic range of reported ehrlichiosis may be expected to expand in the future as well. Most cases of human anaplasmosis have been reported in the north central and northeastern United States, particularly Wisconsin, Minnesota, Connecticut, and New York, but cases in many other states, including California, have been reported. *A phagocytophilum* is transmitted by the black-legged or deer tick *(Ixodes scapularis)*, which also is the vector of *Borrelia burgdorferi* (the agent of Lyme disease). In the western United States, *Ixodes pacificus* is the main vector for *A phagocytophilum*. Various mammalian wildlife reservoirs for the agents of human ehrlichiosis have been identified, including white-tailed deer, white-footed mice, and *Neotoma* woodrats. Compared with patients with RMSF (see p 573), reported cases of symptomatic ehrlichiosis characteristically are in older people, with age-specific incidences greatest in those older than 40 years of age. However, recent seroprevalence data indicate that infection with *E chaffeensis* or a closely related bacterium is common in children. Most human infections occur between April and September, and the peak occurrence is from May through July. Coinfections of anaplasmosis with other tickborne diseases, including babesiosis and Lyme disease, have been described.

The **incubation period** of human ehrlichiosis and anaplasmosis typically is 5 to 10 days after a tick bite (median, 9 days).

DIAGNOSTIC TESTS: The Centers for Disease Control and Prevention (CDC) defines a confirmed case of human ehrlichiosis or anaplasmosis as a clinically compatible illness: fever plus one or more of the following: headache, myalgia, anemia, leukopenia, thrombocytopenia, or any elevation of serum hepatic transaminase concentrations plus serologic evidence of a fourfold change in IgG-specific antibody titer by indirect immunofluorescent antibody (IFA) assay between paired serum specimens (one taken in the first week of illness and a second 2–4 weeks later); detection of *Ehrlichia* or *Anaplasma* DNA in a clinical specimen via amplification of a specific target by polymerase chain reaction (PCR) assay; demonstration of *Ehrlichia* or *Anaplasma* antigen in a biopsy/autopsy sample by immunohistochemical methods; or isolation of *Ehrlichia* or *Anaplasma* organisms from a clinical specimen in cell culture. The CDC further defines a probable case as serologic evidence of elevated IgG or IgM antibody reactive with *Ehrlichia* or *Anaplasma* antigen by IFA, enzyme immunosorbent assay (EIA), dot-EIA, or serologic assays in other formats; or identification of morulae in the cytoplasm of monocytes or granulocytes by microscopic examination. Specific antigens are available for the serologic testing of *E chaffeensis* and *A phagocytophilum* infections, although cross-reactivity between the species can make it difficult to interpret the causative agent in areas where geographic distributions overlap. *E ewingii* shares some antigens with *E chaffeensis*, so most cases of *E ewingii* ehrlichiosis can be diagnosed serologically using *E chaffeensis* antigens. These tests are available in reference laboratories, in some commercial laboratories and state health departments, and at the CDC. Examination of peripheral blood smears to detect morulae in peripheral blood monocytes or granulocytes is insensitive. Use of PCR to amplify nucleic acid from peripheral blood of patients in the acute phase of ehrlichiosis seems sensitive, specific, and promising for early diagnosis. Both PCR and isolation can be conducted on appropriate clinical samples sent to specialty research laboratories or the CDC.

TREATMENT: Doxycycline is the drug of choice for treatment of human ehrlichiosis and anaplasmosis, regardless of patient age. The recommended dosage of doxycycline is 4 mg/kg per day, divided every 12 hours, intravenously or orally (maximum 100 mg/dose). Ehrlichiosis and anaplasmosis can be severe or fatal in untreated patients or patients with predisposing conditions, and initiation of therapy early in the course of disease helps minimize complications of illness. Failure to respond to doxycycline within the first 3 days should suggest infection with an agent other than *Ehrlichia* or *Anaplasma* species. Despite concerns regarding dental staining with tetracycline-class antimicrobial agents in young children (see Antimicrobial Agents and Related Therapy, p 737), doxycycline provides superior therapy for this potentially life-threatening disease. Available data suggest that courses of doxycycline less than 14 days do not cause significant discoloration of permanent teeth. Treatment should continue for at least 3 days after defervescence for a minimum total course of 7 days; unequivocal evidence of clinical improvement generally is evident by 1 week, although some symptoms (eg, headache, weakness, malaise) can persist for weeks after adequate therapy. Severe or complicated disease may require longer treatment courses.

The clinical manifestations and geographic distributions of ehrlichiosis, anaplasmosis, and RMSF overlap. As with other rickettsial diseases, when a presumptive diagnosis of ehrlichiosis is made, doxycycline should be started immediately and should not be delayed pending laboratory confirmation of infection.

ISOLATION OF THE HOSPITALIZED PATIENT: Standard precautions are recommended. Human-to-human transmission of ehrlichiosis or anaplasmosis has not been documented.

CONTROL MEASURES: Specific measures focus on limiting exposures to ticks and are similar to those for RMSF and other tickborne diseases (see Prevention of Tickborne Infections, p 191). Prophylactic administration of doxycycline after a tick bite is not indicated because of the low risk of infection. For additional information, see **www.cdc.gov/NCIDOD/DVRD/ehrlichia.** In addition, a collaborative report providing recommendations for "Diagnosis and Management of Tickborne Rickettsial Diseases" is available at **www.cdc.gov/mmwr/pdf/rr/rr5504/pdf.**

Enterovirus (Nonpoliovirus) Infections
(Group A and B Coxsackieviruses, Echoviruses, and Numbered Enteroviruses)

CLINICAL MANIFESTATIONS: Nonpolio enteroviruses are responsible for significant and frequent illnesses in infants and children and result in protean clinical manifestations. The most common manifestation is nonspecific febrile illness, which, in young infants, may lead to evaluation for bacterial sepsis. Other manifestations can include the following: (1) respiratory: coryza, pharyngitis, herpangina, stomatitis, pneumonia, and pleurodynia; (2) skin: exanthem (hand, foot, and mouth); (3) neurologic: aseptic meningitis, encephalitis, and motor paralysis; (4) gastrointestinal/genitourinary: vomiting, diarrhea, abdominal pain, hepatitis, pancreatitis, and orchitis; (5) eye: acute hemorrhagic conjunctivitis and uveitis; (6) heart: myopericarditis; and (7) muscle: myositis, pleurodynia. Neonates, especially those who acquire infection in the absence of serotype-specific maternal antibody, are at risk of severe disease including sepsis, meningoencephalitis, myocarditis, hepatitis, and coagulopathy. Enterovirus 71 infection is associated with hand-foot-and-mouth disease, herpangina, and high rates of neurologic disease, including brainstem encephalomyelitis, paralytic disease, and secondary pulmonary edema/hemorrhage and cardiopulmonary collapse. Other noteworthy, but not exclusive, serotype associations include coxsackievirus A16 with hand-foot-and-mouth disease, coxsackievirus A24 variant and enterovirus 70 with acute hemorrhagic conjunctivitis, and coxsackieviruses B1 through B5 with pleurodynia and myopericarditis.

Patients with humoral and combined immune deficiencies can have persistent central nervous system infections and/or a dermatomyositis-like syndrome. Severe, multisystem disease is reported in stem cell transplant patients.

ETIOLOGY: The enteroviruses are RNA viruses. The nonpolio enteroviruses include more than 90 distinct serotypes formerly subclassified as group A coxsackieviruses, group B coxsackieviruses, echoviruses, and newer, numbered enteroviruses. A new classification system groups these nonpolio enteroviruses into 4 species—human enteroviruses (HEVs) A, B, C, and D—on the basis of genetic similarity, although the traditional serotype names are retained for individual serotypes.[1] Echoviruses 21 and 22 have been reclassified as a new genus (Parechovirus) and are termed human parechoviruses 1 and 2, respectively.

EPIDEMIOLOGY: Humans are the only known reservoir for human enteroviruses, although some primates can become infected. Enterovirus infections are common. They are spread by fecal-oral and respiratory routes and from mother to infant in the peripartum period. Enteroviruses may survive on environmental surfaces for periods long enough to allow transmission from fomites. Hospital nursery and other institutional outbreaks may occur. Infections, clinical attack rates, and disease severity typically are highest in young children, and infections occur more frequently in tropical areas and where poor hygiene and overcrowding are present. In the United States, 78% of enterovirus infections from 1970 through 2005 were detected from June through October, but seasonal patterns are less evident in the tropics. Epidemics of enterovirus 71-associated hand-foot-and-

---

[1]Centers for Disease Control and Prevention. Enterovirus surveillance—United States, 1970-2005. *MMWR Surveill Summ.* 2006;55(SS–8):1–20

mouth disease with neurologic complications, enterovirus 70- and coxsackievirus A24-associated acute hemorrhagic conjunctivitis, and meningitis occur. Fecal viral shedding can continue for several weeks or months after onset of infection, but respiratory tract shedding usually is limited to 1 to 2 weeks or less. Viral shedding can occur without signs of clinical illness.

The usual **incubation period** is 3 to 6 days, except for acute hemorrhagic conjunctivitis, in which the incubation period is 24 to 72 hours.

DIAGNOSTIC TESTS: Polymerase chain reaction (PCR) assays for detection of enterovirus RNA are available at many reference and commercial laboratories for cerebrospinal fluid (CSF) and other specimens. PCR assay is more rapid and more sensitive than cell culture and can detect all enteroviruses, including enteroviruses that are difficult to culture. Patients with enterovirus 71 neurologic disease often have negative CSF PCR results even when they have CSF pleocytosis; in these patients, throat and/or rectal PCR test results are positive. Previously, isolation of enteroviruses in cell culture was the standard diagnostic method. Enteroviruses can be detected by PCR assay and culture from stool, rectal swab, throat specimens, urine, and blood during acute illness and from CSF when meningitis is present. Sensitivity of culture ranges from 0% to 80%, depending on serotype. Many group A coxsackieviruses grow poorly or not at all in vitro. Culture usually requires 3 to 8 days to detect growth, and the serotype of enterovirus isolated in cell culture may be identified with neutralizing antibody or by genomic sequencing at reference laboratories in cases of special clinical interest or for epidemiologic purposes. New methods can combine detection and identification by using PCR assay and genetic sequencing, but these methods currently are limited to some reference laboratories. Although seldom used for diagnosis, acute infection with a known enterovirus serotype can be determined at reference laboratories by demonstration of a change in neutralizing or other serotype-specific antibody titer between acute and convalescent serum specimens or detection of serotype-specific IgM, but these methods relatively are insensitive and expensive; commercially available serologic assays may lack specificity.

TREATMENT: No specific therapy is available. Immune Globulin Intravenous (IGIV) may be beneficial for chronic enteroviral meningoencephalitis in immunodeficient patients. IGIV also has been used in life-threatening neonatal infections, suspected viral myocarditis, and enterovirus 71 neurologic disease, but proof of efficacy for these uses is lacking. The antiviral drug pleconaril has activity against enteroviruses; pleconaril is not available commercially but is being evaluated for use in neonatal disease in clinical trials.

ISOLATION OF THE HOSPITALIZED PATIENT: In addition to standard precautions, contact precautions are indicated for infants and young children for the duration of illness. Cohorting of infected neonates has been effective in controlling nursery outbreaks.

CONTROL MEASURES: Hand hygiene, especially after diaper changing, is important in decreasing spread within families and institutions. Other measures include avoidance of contaminated utensils and fomites and disinfection of surfaces. Recommended chlorination treatment of drinking water and swimming pools may help prevent transmission.

Maintenance administration of IGIV in patients with severe deficits of B-cell function (eg, severe combined immunodeficiency syndrome, X-linked agammaglobulinemia) may prevent chronic enterovirus infection of the central nervous system. Vaccines for virulent serotypes, such as enterovirus 71, are under investigation.

Epstein-Barr Virus Infections
(Infectious Mononucleosis)

CLINICAL MANIFESTATIONS: Infectious mononucleosis manifests typically as fever, exudative pharyngitis, lymphadenopathy, hepatosplenomegaly, and atypical lymphocytosis. The spectrum of diseases is wide, ranging from asymptomatic to fatal infection. Infections commonly are unrecognized in infants and young children. Rash can occur and is more common in patients treated with ampicillin as well as with other penicillins. Central nervous system (CNS) complications include aseptic meningitis, encephalitis, myelitis, optic neuritis, cranial nerve palsies, transverse myelitis, and Guillain-Barré syndrome. Hematologic complications include splenic rupture, thrombocytopenia, agranulocytosis, hemolytic anemia, and hemophagocytic lymphohistiocytosis (HLH, or hemophagocytic syndrome). Pneumonia, orchitis, and myocarditis are observed infrequently. Replication of Epstein-Barr virus (EBV) in B lymphocytes and the resulting lymphoproliferation usually is inhibited by natural killer cells, antibody-dependent cell cytotoxicity, and T-lymphocyte cytotoxic responses. Fatal disseminated infection or B-lymphocyte or T-lymphocyte lymphomas can occur in children with no detectable immunologic abnormality as well as in children with congenital or acquired cellular immune deficiencies.

EBV is associated with several other distinct disorders, including X-linked lymphoproliferative syndrome, post-transplantation lymphoproliferative disorders, Burkitt lymphoma, nasopharyngeal carcinoma, and undifferentiated B- or T-lymphocyte lymphomas of the CNS. X-linked lymphoproliferative syndrome occurs in people with an inherited, maternally derived, recessive genetic defect in signaling lymphocytic activation molecule-associated protein (SAP) and is characterized by several phenotypic expressions, including occurrence of infectious mononucleosis early in life among boys, nodular B-lymphocyte lymphomas often with CNS involvement, and profound hypogammaglobulinemia.

EBV-associated lymphoproliferative disorders result in a number of complex syndromes in patients who are immunocompromised, such as transplant recipients or people infected with human immunodeficiency virus (HIV). The highest incidence of these disorders occurs in liver and heart transplant recipients, in whom the proliferative states range from benign lymph node hypertrophy to monoclonal lymphomas. Other EBV syndromes are of greater importance outside the United States, including Burkitt lymphoma (a B-lymphocyte tumor), found primarily in Central Africa, and nasopharyngeal carcinoma, found in Southeast Asia and the Inuit population. EBV also has been associated with Hodgkin disease (B-lymphocyte tumor), non-Hodgkin lymphomas (B- and T-lymphocyte), gastric carcinoma "lymphoepitheliomas," and a variety of common epithelial malignancies.

Chronic fatigue syndrome is not related specifically to EBV infection; however, fatigue lasting weeks to a few months may follow less than 10% of cases of classic infectious mononucleosis.

ETIOLOGY: EBV is a gammaherpesvirus of the *Lymphocryptovirus* genus and is the most common cause of infectious mononucleosis.

EPIDEMIOLOGY: Humans are the only reservoir of EBV, and approximately 90% of US adults have been infected. Close personal contact usually is required for transmission. The virus is viable in saliva for several hours outside the body, but the role of fomites in transmission is unknown. EBV also may be transmitted by blood transfusion or transplantation. Infection commonly is contracted early in life, particularly among members of lower socioeconomic groups, in which intrafamilial spread is common. Endemic infectious mononucleosis is common in group settings of adolescents, such as in educational institutions. No seasonal pattern has been documented. Intermittent excretion in saliva may be lifelong after infection.

The **incubation period** of infectious mononucleosis is estimated to be 30 to 50 days.

DIAGNOSTIC TESTS: Routine diagnosis depends on serologic testing. Nonspecific tests for heterophil antibody, including the Paul-Bunnell test and slide agglutination reaction test, are available most commonly. The heterophil antibody response primarily is immunoglobulin (Ig) M, which appears during the first 2 weeks of illness and gradually disappears over a 6-month period. The results of heterophil antibody tests often are negative in children younger than 4 years of age with EBV infection, but heterophil antibody tests identify approximately 85% of cases of classic infectious mononucleosis in older children and adults during the second week of illness. An absolute increase in atypical lymphocytes during the second week of illness with infectious mononucleosis is a characteristic but nonspecific finding. However, the finding of greater than 10% atypical lymphocytes together with a positive heterophil antibody test result is considered diagnostic of acute infection.

Multiple specific serologic antibody tests for EBV infection are available in diagnostic virology laboratories (see Table 3.4). The most commonly performed test is for antibody against the viral capsid antigen (VCA). Because IgG antibody against VCA occurs in high titers early after onset of infection and persists for life, testing of acute and convalescent serum specimens for anti-VCA may not be useful for establishing the presence of active infection. Testing for the presence of IgM anti-VCA antibody and the absence of antibodies to Epstein-Barr nuclear antigen (EBNA) is useful for identifying active and recent infections. Because serum antibody against EBNA is not present until several weeks to months after onset of infection, a positive anti-EBNA antibody test excludes an active primary infection. Testing for antibodies against early antigen (EA) is not useful for interpretation of serologic results because of unreliability of the assays that are used. These interpretations are based on quantitative immunofluorescent antibody tests performed during various stages of mononucleosis and its resolution, although detection of antibodies by enzyme immunoassays usually is performed by clinical laboratories. The typical patterns of antibody responses to EBV infection are illustrated in Fig 3.1 (p 291).

Table 3.4. Serum Epstein-Barr Virus (EBV) Antibodies in EBV Infection

Infection	VCA IgG	VCA IgM	EA (D)	EBNA
No previous infection	–	–	–	–
Acute infection	+	+	+/–	–
Recent infection	+	+/–	+/–	+/–
Past infection	+	–	+/–	+

VCA IgG indicates immunoglobulin (Ig) G class antibody to viral capsid antigen; VCA IgM, IgM class antibody to VCA; EA (D), early antigen diffuse staining; and EBNA, EBV nuclear antigen.

Fig 3.1. Schematic representation of the evolution of antibodies to various Epstein-Barr virus antigens in patients with infectious mononucleosis.

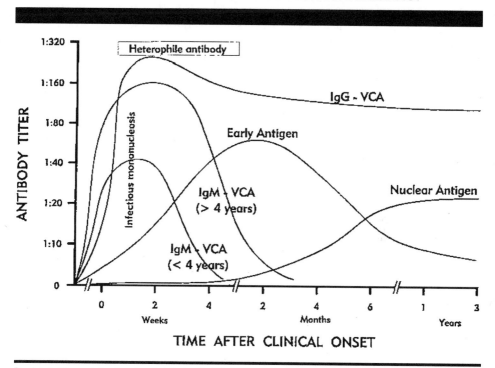

Reprinted with permission from American Society for Microbiology. Manual of Clinical Laboratory Immunology. Rose NR, de Macario EC, Folds JD, eds. Washington, DC: American Society for Microbiology; 1997:Fig 165-7

Serologic tests for EBV are useful particularly for evaluating patients who have heterophil-negative infectious mononucleosis. Testing for other agents, especially cytomegalovirus, toxoplasmosis, and HIV, also may be indicated for some of these patients. Diagnosis of the entire range of EBV-associated illness requires use of molecular and antibody techniques, particularly for patients with immune deficiencies.

Isolation of EBV from oropharyngeal secretions by culture in cord blood cells is possible, but techniques for performing this procedure usually are not available in routine diagnostic laboratories, and viral isolation does not necessarily indicate acute infection. Detection by DNA PCR assay of serum, plasma, and tissue and RNA PCR assay of lymphoid cells or tissue are available commercially and may be useful in evaluation of immunocompromised patients and in complex clinical problems.

TREATMENT: Contact sports should be avoided until the patient is recovered fully from infectious mononucleosis and the spleen no longer is palpable. Patients suspected to have infectious mononucleosis should not be given ampicillin or amoxicillin, which cause nonallergic morbilliform rashes in a high proportion of patients with mononucleosis.

Although therapy with short-course corticosteroids may have a beneficial effect on acute symptoms, because of potential adverse effects, their use should be considered only for patients with marked tonsillar inflammation with impending airway obstruction, massive splenomegaly, myocarditis, hemolytic anemia, or HLH. The dosage of prednisone usually is 1 mg/kg per day, orally (maximum 20 mg/day), for 7 days with subsequent tapering. Life-threatening HLH has been treated with cytotoxic agents and immunomodulators, including cyclosporin and corticosteroids. Although acyclovir has in vitro antiviral activity against EBV, therapy is of no proven value in infectious mononucleosis or in EBV lymphoproliferative syndromes limited to cells with latent viral gene expression. Decreasing immunosuppressive therapy is beneficial for patients with EBV-induced post-transplant lymphoproliferative disorders, whereas an antiviral drug, such as acyclovir, valacyclovir, or ganciclovir, sometimes is used in patients with active replicating EBV infection with or without passive antibody therapy provided by IGIV.

ISOLATION OF THE HOSPITALIZED PATIENT: Standard precautions are recommended.

CONTROL MEASURES: Patients with a recent history of EBV infection or an illness similar to infectious mononucleosis should not donate blood or solid organs.

Escherichia coli and Other Gram-Negative Bacilli
(Septicemia and Meningitis in Neonates)

CLINICAL MANIFESTATIONS: Neonatal septicemia or meningitis caused by *Escherichia coli* and other gram-negative bacilli cannot be differentiated clinically from infections caused by other infectious agents. The first signs of sepsis can be subtle and similar to signs observed in noninfectious processes. Clinical signs of septicemia include fever, temperature instability, heart rate abnormalities, grunting respirations, apnea, cyanosis, lethargy, irritability, anorexia, vomiting, jaundice, abdominal distention, and diarrhea. Meningitis can occur without overt signs suggesting central nervous system involvement. Some gram-negative bacilli, such as *Citrobacter koseri*, *Enterobacter sakazakii*, and *Serratia marcescens*, are associated with brain abscesses in infants with meningitis caused by these organisms.

ETIOLOGY: *E coli* strains with the K1 capsular polysaccharide antigen cause approximately 40% of cases of septicemia and 80% of cases of meningitis. Other important gram-negative bacilli causing neonatal septicemia include non-K1 strains of *E coli* and *Klebsiella* species, *Enterobacter* species, *Proteus* species, *Citrobacter* species, *Salmonella* species, *Pseudomonas* species, and *Serratia* species. Nonencapsulated strains of *Haemophilus influenzae* and anaerobic gram-negative bacilli are rare causes.

EPIDEMIOLOGY: The source of *E coli* and other gram-negative bacterial pathogens in neonatal infections often is the maternal genital tract. The incidence of *E coli* and ampicillin-resistant *E coli* infections has increased during the past decade in very low birth weight but not among term infants. Hospital acquisition of gram-negative organisms through person-to-person transmission from nursery personnel and from nursery environmental sites, such as sinks, countertops, and respiratory therapy equipment, can occur, especially among preterm infants who require prolonged neonatal intensive care management. Predisposing factors in neonatal gram-negative bacterial infections include maternal intrapartum infection, gestation less than 37 weeks, low birth weight, and prolonged rupture of membranes. Metabolic abnormalities (eg, galactosemia), fetal hypoxia, and acidosis have been implicated as predisposing factors. Neonates with defects in the integrity of skin or mucosa (eg, myelomeningocele) or abnormalities of gastrointestinal or genitourinary tracts are at increased risk of gram-negative bacterial infections. In intensive care nurseries, systems for respiratory and metabolic support, invasive or surgical procedures, indwelling vascular lines, and frequent use of antimicrobial agents enable selection and proliferation of strains of gram-negative bacilli that are resistant to multiple antimicrobial agents.

Multiple mechanisms of resistance in gram-negative bacilli can be present simultaneously. Resistance resulting from overproduction of chromosomal or plasmid-derived AmpC beta-lactamase or from plasmid-mediated extended-spectrum beta-lactamases (ESBL), occurring primarily in *E coli* and *Klebsiella* species but reported in many other gram-negative species, has been associated with nursery outbreaks, especially in very low birth weight infants. Organisms that produce ESBL typically are resistant to penicillins, cephalosporins, and monobactams and can be resistant to aminoglycosides.

The **incubation period** is variable; time of onset of infection ranges from birth to several weeks after birth or longer in very low birth weight, preterm infants with prolonged hospitalizations.

DIAGNOSTIC TESTS: The diagnosis is established by growth of *E coli* or other gram-negative bacilli from blood, cerebrospinal fluid (CSF), or other usually sterile sites. Special laboratory procedures are required to recognize ESBL-producing gram-negative organisms.

TREATMENT:

- Initial empiric treatment for suspected gram-negative septicemia in neonates is ampicillin and an aminoglycoside. An alternative regimen of ampicillin and an extended-spectrum cephalosporin (such as cefotaxime) can be used, but rapid emergence of cephalosporin-resistant strains, especially *Enterobacter* species, *Klebsiella* species, and *Serratia* species, can occur when use is routine. Hence, routine use of an extended-spectrum cephalosporin is not recommended unless gram-negative bacterial meningitis is suspected.

- The proportion of *E coli* infections with onset within 72 hours of life that are resistant to ampicillin is high among very low birth weight infants. These *E coli* infections almost invariably are susceptible to gentamicin.

- Once the causative agent and its in vitro antimicrobial susceptibility pattern are known, nonmeningeal infections should be treated with ampicillin, an appropriate aminoglycoside, or an extended-spectrum cephalosporin (such as cefotaxime). Many experts would treat nonmeningeal infections caused by *Enterobacter* species, *Serratia* species, or *Pseudomonas* species and some other less commonly occurring gram-negative bacilli with a beta-lactam antimicrobial agent and an aminoglycoside. For ampicillin-susceptible CSF isolates of *E coli*, meningitis can be treated with ampicillin or an extended-spectrum cephalosporin; meningitis caused by an ampicillin-resistant isolate is treated with an extended-spectrum cephalosporin with or without an aminoglycoside. Combination therapy with beta-lactam and aminoglycoside antimicrobial agents is used for empiric therapy and until CSF is sterile, and some experts continue combination therapy for a longer duration. Expert advice from an infectious disease specialist can be helpful for management of meningitis.

- The empiric drug of choice for treatment of infections caused by ESBL-producing organisms is meropenem, for which there is limited experience in the neonate. Aminoglycosides or cefepime can be used if the organism is susceptible. Expert advice from an infectious disease specialist can help in the management of ESBL-producing gram-negative infections in neonates.
- Duration of therapy is based on clinical and bacteriologic response of the patient and the site(s) of infection; the usual duration of therapy for uncomplicated bacteremia is 10 to 14 days, and for meningitis, the minimum duration is 21 days.
- All infants with meningitis should undergo careful follow-up examinations, including testing for hearing loss, neurologic abnormalities, and developmental delay.

ISOLATION OF THE HOSPITALIZED PATIENT: Standard precautions are recommended. Exceptions include nursery epidemics, infants with *Salmonella* infection, and infants with infection caused by gram-negative bacilli that are resistant to multiple antimicrobial agents, including extended-spectrum beta-lactamase producing strains; in these situations, contact precautions are indicated.

CONTROL MEASURES: Infection-control personnel should be aware of pathogens causing infections in infants so that clusters of infections are recognized and investigated appropriately. Several cases of infection caused by the same genus and species of bacteria occurring in infants in physical proximity or caused by an unusual pathogen indicate the need for an epidemiologic investigation (see Infection Control for Hospitalized Children, p 148). Periodic review of in vitro antimicrobial susceptibility patterns of clinically important bacterial isolates from newborn infants, especially infants in the neonatal intensive care unit, can provide useful epidemiologic and therapeutic information.

Escherichia coli Diarrhea
(Including Hemolytic-Uremic Syndrome)

CLINICAL MANIFESTATIONS: At least 5 pathotypes of diarrhea-producing *Escherichia coli* strains have been identified. Clinical features of disease caused by each pathotype are summarized as follows (also see Table 3.5, p 295):

- Shiga toxin-producing *E coli* (STEC) organisms are associated with diarrhea, hemorrhagic colitis, hemolytic-uremic syndrome (HUS), and postdiarrheal thrombotic thrombocytopenic purpura (TTP). STEC O157:H7 is the prototype and the most virulent member of this *E coli* pathotype. Illness caused by STEC often begins as nonbloody diarrhea but usually progresses to diarrhea with visible or occult blood. Severe abdominal pain is typical; fever occurs in less than one third of cases. Severe infection can result in hemorrhagic colitis.
- Diarrhea caused by enteropathogenic *E coli* (EPEC) is watery and often is severe enough to result in dehydration and even death. Illness occurs almost exclusively in children younger than 2 years of age and predominantly in resource-limited countries, either sporadically or in epidemics. Chronic EPEC diarrhea can result in growth retardation.
- Diarrhea caused by enterotoxigenic *E coli* (ETEC) is a 1- to 5-day self-limited illness of moderate severity, typically with watery stools and abdominal cramps. ETEC is common in infants in resource-limited countries and in travelers to those countries but is uncommon as a cause of diarrhea in the United States.

Table 3.5. Classification of *Escherichia coli* Associated With Diarrhea

E coli Pathotype	Epidemiology	Type of Diarrhea	Mechanism of Pathogenesis
Shiga toxin-producing (STEC)	Hemorrhagic colitis and hemolytic-uremic syndrome in all ages and postdiarrheal thrombotic thrombocytopenic purpura in adults	Bloody or nonbloody	Large bowel adherence and effacement (AE), Shiga toxin production
Enteropathogenic (EPEC)	Acute and chronic endemic and epidemic diarrhea in infants	Watery	Small bowel AE
Enterotoxigenic (ETEC)	Infantile diarrhea in resource-limited countries and travelers' diarrhea in all ages	Watery	Small bowel AE, heat stable/heat labile enterotoxin production
Enteroinvasive (EIEC)	Diarrhea with fever in all ages	Bloody or nonbloody; dysentery	Adherence, mucosal invasion and inflammation of large bowel
Enteroaggregative (EAEC)	Acute and chronic diarrhea in all ages	Watery, occasionally bloody	Small and large bowel adherence, enterotoxin and cytotoxin production

- Diarrhea caused by enteroinvasive *E coli* (EIEC) is similar clinically to diarrhea caused by *Shigella* species. Although dysentery can occur, diarrhea usually is watery without blood or mucus. Patients often are febrile, and stools may contain leukocytes.
- Enteroaggregative *E coli* (EAEC) organisms cause watery diarrhea and are common in people of all ages and in resource-rich as well as resource-limited countries. EAEC has been associated with prolonged diarrhea (14 or more days). Asymptomatic infection can be accompanied by a subclinical inflammatory enteritis, which can cause growth disturbances.

Late Sequelae of STEC Infection. HUS is a serious sequela of STEC enteric infection. In the United States, *E coli* O157:H7 is the STEC serotype most commonly associated with HUS, which is defined by the triad of microangiopathic hemolytic anemia, thrombocytopenia, and acute renal dysfunction. HUS occurs in up to 20% of children with *E coli* O157:H7 diarrhea. The illness is serious and develops during the 2 weeks after onset of diarrhea. Fifty percent of patients require dialysis, and 3% to 5% die. Thrombotic thrombocytopenic purpura occurs in adults, can follow STEC infection, and in addition to the manifestations of HUS, includes neurologic abnormalities and fever, may have a more gradual onset than HUS, and is part of a disease spectrum often designated as TTP-HUS. Children with diarrhea-associated HUS should be observed for diabetes mellitus during their acute illness, and consideration should be given to long-term screening of survivors for diabetes mellitus and abnormal renal function.

ETIOLOGY: Five pathotypes of diarrhea-producing *E coli* have been characterized by their ability to adhere to tissue, toxin production, or type of disease resulting from infection. Each pathotype has a distinct set of somatic (O) and flagellar (H) antigens and pathogenic characteristics.

EPIDEMIOLOGY: Transmission of most diarrhea-associated *E coli* strains is from food or water contaminated with human or animal feces or from infected symptomatic people or carriers. STEC, especially *E coli* O157:H7, is shed in feces of cattle and, to a lesser extent, in feces of sheep, deer, and other ruminants. Human infection is acquired via contaminated food or water or via direct contact with an infected person. STEC can be transmitted via undercooked ground beef, contaminated water or produce, unpasteurized milk, and a wide variety of vehicles contaminated with bovine feces. Contact with animals and their environment and person-to-person or fomite spread are other modes of transmission. Infections caused by *E coli* O157:H7 are detected sporadically or during outbreaks. Outbreaks have been linked to ground beef, exposure to animals in public settings including petting zoos, contaminated apple cider, raw fruits and vegetables, salami, yogurt, drinking water, and ingestion of water in recreational areas. The infectious dose is low, and person-to-person transmission is common during outbreaks. Less is known about the epidemiology of STEC strains other than O157:H7. The non-O157 STEC strains most commonly linked to illness in the United States are O26, O45, O103, O111, O121, and O145.

Most non-STEC pathotypes are associated with disease predominantly in resource-limited countries, where food and water supplies commonly are contaminated and facilities and supplies for hand hygiene are suboptimal. Diarrhea attributable to ETEC occurs in people of all ages but especially is frequent and severe in infants in resource-limited countries. Outbreaks have occurred in adults, usually from ingestion of contaminated food or water. ETEC is a major cause of travelers' diarrhea. EAEC increasingly is recognized as a cause of diarrhea in the United States.

The **incubation period** for most *E coli* strains is 10 hours to 6 days; for *E coli* O157:H7, the incubation period usually is 3 to 4 days (range from 1 to 8 days).

DIAGNOSTIC TESTS: Diagnosis of infection caused by diarrhea-associated *E coli* usually is difficult, because most clinical laboratories cannot differentiate diarrhea-associated *E coli* strains from stool flora *E coli* strains. The exception is *E coli* O157:H7, which can be identified by using MacConkey agar base with sorbitol substituted for lactose. Approximately 90% of human intestinal *E coli* strains rapidly ferment sorbitol, whereas *E coli* O157:H7 strains do not. Sorbitol-negative *E coli* then can be serotyped using commercially available antisera to determine whether they are O157:H7. If a case or outbreak attributable to diarrhea-associated *E coli* is suspected, *E coli* isolates can be sent to the state health laboratory or a reference laboratory for serotyping and identification of pathotypes. Several sensitive, specific, and rapid immunologic assays for detection of Shiga toxin are available commercially.

Strains of STEC should be sought in stool from patients with bloody diarrhea (indicated by history, inspection of stool, or guaiac testing), HUS, and postdiarrheal TTP as well as for contacts of patients with HUS who have any type of diarrhea. People with presumptive diagnoses of intussusception, inflammatory bowel disease, or ischemic colitis sometimes have disease caused by *E coli* O157:H7. Methods of definitive identification of STEC that are used in reference or research laboratories include DNA probes, polymerase chain reaction assay, enzyme immunoassay, and phenotypic testing of strains or stool specimens for Shiga toxin. Serologic diagnosis using enzyme immunoassay to detect serum antibodies to *E coli* O157:H7 lipopolysaccharide is available at the Centers for Disease Control and Prevention for outbreak investigations.

Hemolytic-Uremic Syndrome. For all patients with HUS, stool specimens should be cultured for *E coli* O157:H7 and, if results are negative, for other STEC serotypes. However, the absence of STEC in feces does not preclude the diagnosis of STEC-associated HUS, because HUS typically is diagnosed a week or more after onset of diarrhea, when the organism no longer may be detectable.

TREATMENT: Orally administered solutions usually are adequate to prevent or treat dehydration and electrolyte abnormalities.[1] Antimotility agents should not be administered to children with inflammatory or bloody diarrhea. Careful monitoring of patients with hemorrhagic colitis (including complete blood cell count with smear, blood urea nitrogen, and creatinine concentrations) is recommended to detect changes suggestive of HUS. If patients have no laboratory evidence of hemolysis, thrombocytopenia, or nephropathy 3 days after resolution of diarrhea, their risk of developing HUS is low.

Antimicrobial Therapy. A meta-analysis failed to confirm that children with hemorrhagic colitis caused by STEC have a greater risk of developing HUS if treated with an antimicrobial agent. However, most experts would not treat children with *E coli* O157:H7 enteritis with an antimicrobial agent, because no benefit has been proven and adverse events may occur. For an episode of severe watery diarrhea in a traveler to a resource-limited country, therapy can be provided. Azithromycin or a fluoroquinolone have been the most reliable agents although fluoroquinolones are not approved in people younger than 18 years of age for this indication. Whenever possible, selection of an antimicrobial agent should be based on results of susceptibility testing of the isolate.

ISOLATION OF THE HOSPITALIZED PATIENT: In addition to standard precautions, contact precautions are indicated for patients with all types of *E coli* diarrhea for the duration of illness. For patients with HUS or hemorrhagic colitis attributable to STEC, contact precautions should be continued until diarrhea resolves and results of 2 consecutive stool cultures are negative for *E coli* O157:H7.

CONTROL MEASURES:

Escherichia coli *O157:H7 Infection.* All ground beef should be cooked thoroughly until no pink meat remains and the juices are clear. Raw milk should not be ingested, and only pasteurized apple juice products should be consumed. Because *E coli* O157:H7 potentially is waterborne, people with diarrhea caused by *E coli* O157:H7 should not use recreational water venues (eg, swimming pools, water slides) for 2 weeks after symptoms resolve.

Outbreaks in Child Care Centers. If an outbreak of HUS or diarrhea attributable to *E coli* O157:H7 occurs in a child care center, immediate involvement of public health authorities is critical. Infection caused by *E coli* O157:H7 is reportable, and rapid reporting of cases allows interventions to prevent further disease. Ill children should not be permitted to reenter the child care center until diarrhea has resolved and 2 stool cultures obtained at least 48 hours after antimicrobial therapy has been discontinued are negative for *E coli* O157:H7. Strict attention to hand hygiene is important but can be insufficient to prevent continued transmission. The child care center should be closed to new admissions dur-

---

[1]Centers for Disease Control and Prevention. Managing acute gastroenteritis among children: oral rehydration, maintenance, and nutritional therapy. *MMWR Recomm Rep.* 2003;52(RR-16):1–16

ing an outbreak, and care should be exercised to prevent transfer of exposed children to other centers.

Nursery and Other Institutional Outbreaks. Strict attention to hand hygiene is essential for limiting spread. Exposed patients should be observed closely, their stools should be cultured for the causative organism, and they should be separated from unexposed infants (also see Children in Out-of-Home Child Care, p 124).

Travelers' Diarrhea. Travelers' diarrhea usually is acquired by ingestion of contaminated food or water and is a significant problem for people traveling in resource-limited countries. Diarrhea attributable to STEC is rare in travelers. Travelers should be advised to drink only bottled or canned beverages and boiled or bottled water; travelers should avoid ice, raw produce including salads, and fruit that they have not peeled themselves. Cooked foods should be eaten hot. Antimicrobial agents are not recommended for prevention of travelers' diarrhea. Although several antimicrobial agents, such as trimethoprim-sulfamethoxazole, azithromycin, doxycycline, and ciprofloxacin, can be effective in decreasing the incidence of travelers' diarrhea, the benefit usually is outweighed by the potential risks, including allergic drug reactions, antimicrobial-associated colitis, and the selective pressure of widespread use of antimicrobial agents leading to antimicrobial resistance. If diarrhea occurs, packets of oral rehydration salts can be added to boiled or bottled water and ingested to help maintain fluid balance. If diarrhea in a traveler is moderate or severe or is associated with fever or bloody stools, empiric antimicrobial therapy may be indicated but should be continued for no more than 3 days.

Recreational Water. People with diarrhea caused by these potentially waterborne pathogens should not use recreational water venues (eg, swimming pools, water slides) for 2 weeks after symptoms resolve.

Fungal Diseases

In addition to the mycoses listed by individual agents (aspergillosis, blastomycosis, candidiasis, coccidioidomycosis, cryptococcosis, paracoccidioidomycosis, and sporotrichosis) in Section 3, infants and children with immunosuppression or other underlying conditions can become infected by uncommonly encountered fungi. Children can acquire infection with these fungi through inhalation via the respiratory tract or direct inoculation after traumatic disruption of cutaneous barriers. A list of these fungi and the pertinent underlying host conditions, reservoir or route of entry, clinical manifestations, diagnostic laboratory tests, and treatment for each can be found in Table 3.6 (p 299). Taken as a group, few fungal susceptibility data are available on which to base treatment recommendations for these fungal infections, especially in children. Consultation with a pediatric infectious disease specialist experienced in the diagnosis and treatment of invasive fungal infections should be considered when caring for a child infected with one of these mycoses.

Table 3.6. Additional Fungal Diseases

Disease and Agent	Underlying Host Condition(s)	Reservoir(s) or Route(s) of Entry	Common Clinical Manifestations	Diagnostic Laboratory Test(s)	Treatment
Hyalohyphomycosis					
Fusarium species	Granulocytopenia; stem cell transplantation; severe immunocompromise	Respiratory tract; sinuses; skin	Pulmonary infiltrates; cutaneous lesions; sinusitis; disseminated infection	Culture of blood or tissue specimen	High-dose D-AMB (1–1.5 mg/kg per day)[a,b] or voriconazole[c]
Malassezia species	Immunosuppression; preterm birth; exposure to parenteral nutrition that includes fat emulsions	Skin	Catheter-associated bloodstream infection; interstitial pneumonitis; urinary tract infection; meningitis	Culture of blood, catheter tip, or tissue specimen (requires special laboratory handling)	Removal of catheters and temporary cessation of lipid infusion; D-AMB
Penicilliosis					
Penicillium marneffei	Human immunodeficiency virus infection	Respiratory tract	Pneumonitis; invasive dermatitis; disseminated infection	Culture of blood, bone marrow, or tissue; histopathologic examination of tissue	Itraconazole[d] or D-AMB
Phaeohyphomycosis					
Alternaria species	None or trauma or immunosuppression	Respiratory tract; skin	Sinusitis; cutaneous lesions	Culture and histopathologic examination of tissue	High-dose D-AMB[a,b,c]; Voriconazole[c]
Bipolaris species	None or trauma or immunosuppression	Environment	Sinusitis; disseminated infection	Culture and histopathologic examination of tissue	Itraconazole[d] or D-AMB[a]; surgical excision
Curvularia species	Immunosuppression; altered skin integrity; asthma or nasal polyps; chronic sinusitis	Environment	Allergic fungal sinusitis; invasive dermatitis; disseminated infection	Culture and histopathologic examination of tissue	Allergic fungal sinusitis: surgery and corticosteroids Invasive disease: itraconazole[e] or D-AMB[a]

Table 3.6. Additional Fungal Diseases, continued

Disease and Agent	Underlying Host Condition(s)	Reservoir(s) or Route(s) of Entry	Common Clinical Manifestations	Diagnostic Laboratory Test(s)	Treatment
Exophiala (Wangiella) species, Exserohilum species, or Wangiella species	None or trauma or immunosuppression	Environment	Sinusitis; cutaneous lesions; disseminated infection	Culture and histopathologic examination of tissue	Itraconazole[c]; D-AMB; or voriconazole[f]; surgical excision
Pseudallescheria boydii (Scedosporium apiospermum)	None or trauma or immunosuppression	Environment	Pneumonia; disseminated infection; osteomyelitis or septic arthritis; mycetoma (immunocompetent patients); endocarditis	Culture and histopathologic examination of tissue	Voriconazole[c] or itraconazole[c]; surgical excision for pulmonary infection, as feasible
Trichosporonosis					
Trichosporon species	Immunosuppression; central venous catheter	Normal flora of gastrointestinal tract	Bloodstream infection; endocarditis; pneumonitis	Blood culture; histopathologic examination of tissue	D-AMB[a,b] or voriconazole[c]
Zygomycosis					
Rhizopus; Mucor; Absidia; Rhizomucor species	Immunosuppression; hematologic malignant neoplasm; renal failure; diabetes mellitus; use of nonsterile adhesive dressings	Respiratory tract; skin	Rhinocerebral infection; pulmonary infection; disseminated infection; skin and gastrointestinal tract less commonly	Histopathologic examination of tissue and culture	High dose of D-AMB (1.5 mg/kg per day) or posaconazole[g] and surgical excision, as feasible

D-AMB indicates deoxycholate amphotericin B.

[a] Consider use of a lipid-associated formulation of amphotericin B.

[b] Infection may be refractory to amphotericin B; use of investigational antifungal compounds may be required.

[c] Voriconazole is an alternative agent for adults intolerant of, or with infection refractory to, amphotericin B.

[d] Itraconazole has been shown to be effective for cutaneous disease in adults, but safety and efficacy have not been established in children younger than 12 years of age.

[e] Itraconazole may be the treatment of choice, but data on safety and effectiveness in children are limited.

[f] Voriconazole demonstrates activity in vitro, but no clinical data are available.

[g] Posaconazole demonstrates activity in vitro, but few clinical data are available for children.

Fusobacterium Infections
(Including Lemierre Disease)

CLINICAL MANIFESTATIONS: *Fusobacterium* species may colonize humans and animals. *Fusobacterium necrophorum* and *Fusobacterium nucleatum* can be isolated from oropharyngeal specimens in healthy people, are frequent components of human dental plaque, and may lead to periodontal disease. Invasive disease attributable to *Fusobacterium* species has been reported following otitis media, tonsillitis, gingivitis, and oropharyngeal trauma. Ten percent of published cases of invasive *Fusobacterium* infections are associated with Epstein-Barr virus infection.

Invasive infection with *Fusobacterium* species can lead to life-threatening disease. Otogenic infection is the most frequent primary source in children younger than 5 years of age and can be complicated by meningitis and thrombosis of the dural venous sinuses. Invasive infection following tonsillitis was described in the early 20th century and classically was referred to as postanginal sepsis or Lemierre disease. Lemierre disease occurs most commonly in adolescents and young adults and includes internal jugular vein thrombophlebitis or thrombosis (JVT), evidence of septic embolic lesions in lungs or other sterile sites, and usually isolation of *Fusobacterium* species from blood or other normally sterile sites. Fever and sore throat are followed by severe neck pain (anginal pain) that can be accompanied by unilateral neck swelling, trismus, and dysphagia. People with classic Lemierre disease have a sepsis syndrome with multiple organ dysfunction, disseminated intravascular coagulation, empyema, pyogenic arthritis, or osteomyelitis. Persistent headache or other neurologic signs may indicate the presence of cerebral venous sinus thrombosis (eg, cavernous sinus thrombosis) or meningitis or brain abscess.

JVT can be completely vaso-occlusive. Some children with JVT associated with Lemierre disease have evidence of thrombophilia at diagnosis, which can include presence of antiphospholipid antibodies, abnormal levels of factor VIII, and factor V Leiden. These findings often resolve over several months and may indicate response to the inflammatory, prothrombotic process associated with infection rather than an underlying hypercoagulable state.

ETIOLOGY: *Fusobacterium* species are anaerobic, non–spore-forming, gram-negative bacilli. Human infection usually results from *F necrophorum* subspecies funduliforme, but infections with other species including *F nucleatum*, *Fusobacterium gonidiaformans*, *Fusobacterium naviforme*, *Fusobacterium mortiferum*, and *Fusobacterium varium* have been reported. Infection with *Fusobacterium* species, alone or in combination with other oral anaerobic bacteria, may result in Lemierre disease. Lemierre-like syndromes also have been reported following infection with *Bacteroides* species, anaerobic *Streptococcus* species, other anaerobic bacteria, and methicillin-susceptible and -resistant strains of *Staphylococcus aureus*.

EPIDEMIOLOGY: *Fusobacterium* species commonly are found in soil and in the respiratory tracts of animals, including cattle, dogs, fowl, goats, sheep, and horses, and can be isolated from the oropharynx of healthy people. *Fusobacterium* infections are most common in adolescents and young adults, but infections, including fatal cases of Lemierre disease, have been reported in infants and young children.

DIAGNOSTIC TESTS: *Fusobacterium* species can be isolated using conventional liquid anaerobic blood culture media. However, the organism grows best on semisolid media for fastidious anaerobic organisms or blood agar supplemented with vitamin K, hemin, menadione, and a reducing agent. Colonies are cream to yellow colored, smooth, and round with a narrow zone of hemolysis on blood agar. Many strains fluoresce chartreuse green under ultraviolet light. Most *Fusobacterium* organisms are indole positive. The accurate identification of anaerobes to the species level has become important with the increasing incidence of microorganisms that are resistant to multiple drugs. Sequencing of the16S rRNA gene and phylogenetic analysis can identify anaerobic bacteria to the genus or taxonomic group level and frequently to the species level.

Febrile children and adolescents, especially those with sore throat or neck pain, who are sufficiently ill to warrant a blood culture should have an anaerobic blood culture in addition to aerobic blood culture performed to detect invasive *Fusobacterium* species infection. The imaging modalities of computed tomography and magnetic resonance imaging may be more sensitive than ultrasonography to document thrombosis and thrombophlebitis of the internal jugular vein early in the course of the illness.

TREATMENT: *Fusobacterium* species are susceptible to metronidazole, clindamycin, chloramphenicol, carbapenems, and cefoxitin. Metronidazole is the treatment preferred by many experts, because the drug has excellent activity against all *Fusobacterium* species and good tissue penetration. However, metronidazole lacks activity against microaerophilic streptococci that may coinfect some patients. Clindamycin also is an effective agent. *Fusobacterium* species intrinsically are resistant to gentamicin and fluoroquinolone agents. Tetracyclines have limited activity. Up to 50% of *F nucleatum* and 20% of *F necrophorum* isolates produce beta-lactamases, rendering them resistant to penicillin, ampicillin, and some cephalosporins.

Because *Fusobacterium* infections often are polymicrobial, multiple antimicrobial agents frequently are necessary. Therapy has been advocated with a penicillin/beta-lactamase inhibitor combination (piperacillin-tazobactam or ticarcillin-clavulanate) or a carbapenem (meropenem or imipenem) or combination therapy with metronidazole in addition to other agents active against aerobic oral and respiratory tract pathogens (cefotaxime, ceftriaxone, or cefuroxime). Duration of antimicrobial therapy depends on the anatomic locations and severity of the infection but usually is several weeks. Surgical intervention involving débridement or incision and drainage of abscesses may be necessary. Anticoagulation therapy has been used in both adults and children with JVT and cavernous sinus thrombosis. In cases with extensive thrombosis, anticoagulation therapy may decrease the risk of clot extension and shorten recovery time.

ISOLATION OF THE HOSPITALIZED PATIENT: Standard precautions are recommended. Person-to-person transmission of *Fusobacterium* species has not been documented.

CONTROL MEASURES: Oral hygiene and dental cleanings may reduce density of oral colonization with *Fusobacterium* species, prevent gingivitis and dental caries, and reduce the risk of invasive disease.

Giardia intestinalis Infections
(Giardiasis)

CLINICAL MANIFESTATIONS: Symptomatic infection causes a broad spectrum of clinical manifestations. Children can have occasional days of acute watery diarrhea with abdominal pain, or they may experience a protracted, intermittent, often debilitating disease, which is characterized by passage of foul-smelling stools associated with flatulence, abdominal distention, and anorexia. Anorexia combined with malabsorption can lead to significant weight loss, failure to thrive, and anemia. Asymptomatic infection is common.

ETIOLOGY: *Giardia intestinalis* is a flagellate protozoan that exists in trophozoite and cyst forms; the infective form is the cyst. Infection is limited to the small intestine and biliary tract.

EPIDEMIOLOGY: Giardiasis has a worldwide distribution. Humans are the principal reservoir of infection, but *Giardia* organisms can infect dogs, cats, beavers, and other animals.[1] These animals can contaminate water with feces containing cysts that are infectious for humans. People become infected directly (by hand-to-mouth transfer of cysts from feces of an infected person) or indirectly (by ingestion of fecally contaminated water or food). Many people who become infected with *G intestinalis* remain asymptomatic. Most community-wide epidemics have resulted from a contaminated water supply. Epidemics resulting from person-to-person transmission occur in child care centers and in institutions for people with developmental disabilities. Staff and family members in contact with people in these settings occasionally become infected. Humoral immunodeficiencies predispose to chronic symptomatic *G intestinalis* infections. Surveys conducted in the United States have demonstrated prevalence rates of *Giardia* organisms in stool specimens that range from 1% to 20%, depending on geographic location and age. Duration of cyst excretion is variable but can be months. The disease is communicable for as long as the infected person excretes cysts.

The **incubation period** usually is 1 to 4 weeks.

DIAGNOSTIC TESTS: Identification of trophozoites or cysts in stool specimens, duodenal fluid, or small bowel tissue is performed by direct microscopic examination using staining methods, such as trichrome direct fluorescent antibody assays; by detecting soluble stool antigens using enzyme immunoassay (EIA); or by using polymerase chain reaction technique. Stool usually is collected and preserved in neutral-buffered 10% formalin, but other preservatives can be used, or fresh stool can be examined. A single direct smear examination of stool has a sensitivity of 75% to 95%. Sensitivity is higher for diarrheal stool specimens, because these specimens contain a higher concentration of organisms. Sensitivity is increased by examining 3 or more specimens collected every other day. To enhance detection, microscopic examination of stool specimens or duodenal fluid should be performed soon after collection, or stool should be placed in fixative, concentrated, and examined by wet mount using a permanent stain such as trichrome. Commercially available stool collection kits containing a vial of neutral-buffered 10% formalin and a vial of polyvinyl alcohol fixative in childproof containers are convenient for preserving stool specimens collected at home. Sensitive and specific EIA kits are available commercially. Laboratories can reduce reagent and personnel costs by pooling specimens from

---

[1] Hlavsa MC, Watson JC, Beach MJ, Atlanta Research and Education Foundation. Giardiasis surveillance—United States, 1998–2002. *MMWR Surveill Summ.* 2005;54(SS-1):9–16

patients before evaluation either by microscopy or EIA. The direct fluorescent antibody test kit has the advantage that organisms are visualized. When giardiasis is suspected clinically but the organism is not found on repeated stool examination, examination of duodenal contents obtained by direct aspiration or by using a commercially available string test (Enterotest) may be diagnostic. Rarely, duodenal biopsy is required for diagnosis.

TREATMENT: Dehydration and electrolyte abnormalities should be corrected. Tinidazole, metronidazole, or nitazoxanide are the drugs of choice. A 5- to 7-day course of metronidazole has a cure rate of 80% to 95%. Tinidazole, a nitroimidazole, has a cure rate of 80% to 100% and has the advantage of being administered as a single dose tablet for children 3 years of age and older. A 3-day course of nitazoxanide oral suspension is as effective as metronidazole and has the advantage(s) of treating multiple other intestinal parasites and being approved for use in children 1 year of age and older. Quinacrine and oral suspension of furazolidone are alternatives. Albendazole and mebendazole have been shown to be as effective as metronidazole for treating giardiasis in children and have fewer adverse effects. Paromomycin, a nonabsorbable aminoglycoside that is 50% to 70% effective, is recommended for treatment of symptomatic infection in second and third trimester pregnant women (see Drugs for Parasitic Infections, p 783).

If therapy fails, a course can be repeated with the same drug. Relapse is common in immunocompromised patients who may require prolonged treatment. Some experts recommend combination therapy for giardiasis in immunocompromised patients who are unresponsive to courses of 2 drugs used separately.

Treatment of asymptomatic carriers generally is not recommended. Possible exceptions to prevent transmission are carriers in households of patients with hypogamma-globulinemia or cystic fibrosis.

ISOLATION OF THE HOSPITALIZED PATIENT: In addition to standard precautions, contact precautions for the duration of illness are recommended for diapered and incontinent children.

CONTROL MEASURES:
- In child care centers, improved sanitation and personal hygiene should be emphasized (see also Children in Out-of-Home Child Care, p 124). Hand hygiene by staff and children should be emphasized, especially after toilet use or handling of soiled diapers. When an outbreak is suspected, the local health department should be contacted, and an epidemiologic investigation should be undertaken to identify and treat all symptomatic children, child care workers, and family members infected with *G intestinalis.* People with diarrhea should be excluded from the child care center until they become asymptomatic. Treatment of asymptomatic carriers is not effective for outbreak control. Exclusion of carriers from child care is not recommended.
- Waterborne outbreaks can be prevented by the combination of adequate filtration of water from surface water sources (eg, lakes, rivers, streams), chlorination, and maintenance of water distribution systems.
- People with diarrhea caused by this potentially waterborne pathogen should not use recreational water venues (eg, swimming pools, water slides) for 2 weeks after symptoms resolve. Information about recreational water illness and how to stop transmission of infectious organisms to other people is available at **www.cdc.gov/ healthyswimming.**

Where water might be contaminated, travelers, campers, and hikers should be advised of methods to make water safe for drinking, including boiling, chemical disinfection, and filtration. Boiling is the most reliable method to make water safe for drinking. The time of boiling (1 minute at sea level) will depend on the altitude. Chemical disinfection with iodine is an alternative method of water treatment using either tincture of iodine or tetraglycine hydroperiodide tablets. Chlorine in various forms also can be used for chemical disinfection, but germicidal activity is dependent on several factors, including pH, temperature, and organic content of the water. Commercially available portable water filters provide various degrees of protection. There are many commercially available filters that are marketed as being able to remove *Giardia* and *Cryptosporidium* species from water. Additional information about water purification, including a traveler's guide for buying water filters, can be found at **www.cdc.gov/crypto/factsheets/filters.html.**

Gonococcal Infections

CLINICAL MANIFESTATIONS: Gonococcal infections in children occur in 3 distinct age groups.
- Infection in the **newborn infant** usually involves the eyes. Other types of infection include scalp abscess (which can be associated with fetal monitoring), vaginitis, and disseminated disease with bacteremia, arthritis, or meningitis.
- In children beyond the newborn period, including **prepubertal children,** gonococcal infection may occur in the genital tract and almost always is transmitted sexually. Vaginitis is the most common manifestation. Gonococcal urethritis in the prepubertal male is uncommon. Anorectal and tonsillopharyngeal infection also can occur in prepubertal children.
- In **sexually active adolescents,** as in adults, gonococcal infection of the genital tract in females often is asymptomatic, and common clinical syndromes are vaginitis, urethritis, endocervicitis, and salpingitis. In males, infection often is symptomatic, and the primary site is the urethra. Infection of the rectum and pharynx can occur alone or with genitourinary tract infection in either sex. Rectal and pharyngeal infections often are asymptomatic. Extension from primary genital mucosal sites can lead to epididymitis in males and bartholinitis, pelvic inflammatory disease (PID), and perihepatitis (Fitz-Hugh-Curtis syndrome) in females. Even asymptomatic infection in females can progress to PID, with tubal scarring that can result in ectopic pregnancy or infertility. Infection involving other mucous membranes can produce conjunctivitis, pharyngitis, or proctitis. Hematogenous spread can involve skin and joints (arthritis-dermatitis syndrome) and occurs in up to 3% of untreated people with mucosal gonorrhea. Bacteremia causes a maculopapular rash with necrosis, tenosynovitis, and migratory arthritis. Arthritis may be reactive (sterile) or septic in nature. Meningitis and endocarditis occur rarely. Dissemination is more common in females infected within 1 week of menstruation.

ETIOLOGY: *Neisseria gonorrhoeae* is a gram-negative oxidase-positive diplococcus.

EPIDEMIOLOGY: Gonococcal infections occur only in humans. The source of the organism is exudate and secretions from infected mucosal surfaces; *N gonorrhoeae* is communicable as long as a person harbors the organism. Transmission results from intimate contact, such as sexual acts, parturition, and rarely, household exposure in prepubertal children.

Sexual abuse should be considered strongly when genital, rectal, or pharyngeal colonization or infection are diagnosed in prepubertal children beyond the newborn period. In 2007, there were 355 991 new cases of gonococcal infection reported in the United States. Reported incidence of infection is highest in females 15 through 19 years of age and in males 20 through 24 years of age. Racial disparities are notable: the incidence of infection was 18 times greater among black people, 3.7 times greater among American Indian/Alaska Native people, and 2.1 times greater among Hispanic people than among white people in 2005. Concurrent infection with *Chlamydia trachomatis* is common.

The **incubation period** usually is 2 to 7 days.

DIAGNOSTIC TESTS: Microscopic examination of Gram-stained smears of exudate from the conjunctivae, vagina of prepubertal girls, male urethra, skin lesions, synovial fluid, and when clinically warranted, cerebrospinal fluid (CSF) may be useful in the initial evaluation. Identification of gram-negative intracellular diplococci in these smears can be helpful, particularly if the organism is not recovered in culture. However, because of lower sensitivity, a negative result of Gram stain should not be considered sufficient for ruling out infection.

N gonorrhoeae can be isolated from normally sterile sites, such as blood, CSF, or synovial fluid, using nonselective chocolate agar with incubation in 5% to 10% carbon dioxide. Selective media that inhibit normal flora and nonpathogenic *Neisseria* organisms are used for culture from nonsterile sites, such as the cervix, vagina, rectum, urethra, and pharynx. Specimens for *N gonorrhoeae* culture from mucosal sites should be inoculated immediately onto the appropriate agar, because *N gonorrhoeae* is extremely sensitive to drying and temperature changes.

Caution should be exercised when interpreting the significance of isolation of *Neisseria* organisms, because *N gonorrhoeae* can be confused with other *Neisseria* species that colonize the genitourinary tract or pharynx. At least 2 confirmatory bacteriologic tests involving different principles (eg, biochemical, enzyme substrate, or serologic) should be performed by the laboratory. Interpretation of culture of *N gonorrhoeae* from the pharynx of young children necessitates particular caution because of the high carriage rate of nonpathogenic *Neisseria* species.

Nucleic acid amplification (NAA) tests are highly sensitive and specific when used on male urethral, female endocervical or vaginal swab, and male or female urine specimens.[1] These tests include polymerase chain reaction (PCR), transcription-mediated amplification (TMA), and strand-displacement assays. Only the TMA assay is approved by the US Food and Drug Administration (FDA) for testing vaginal swabs from postmenarcheal females. Other *Neisseria* species may be present in the female genital tract and may result in a false-positive NAA test result. Use of urine specimens increases feasibility of initial testing and follow-up of hard-to-access populations, such as adolescents. These techniques also permit dual testing of urine for *C trachomatis* and *N gonorrhoeae*. Cultures are the most widely used tests for identifying *N gonorrhoeae* from nongenital sites. NAA tests are not approved by the FDA for use on rectal or pharyngeal swabs. Some NAA tests have the potential to cross-react with nongonococcal *Neisseria* that commonly are found in the throat. Some noncommercial laboratories have initiated NAA testing of rectal and pharyngeal swab specimens after establishing the performance of the test to meet

---

[1]Centers for Disease Control and Prevention. Screening to detect *Chlamydia trachomatis* and *Neisseria gonorrhoeae* infections—2002. *MMWR Recomm Rep.* 2002;51(RR-15):1–38

requirements of the Clinical Laboratory Improvement Amendments (CLIA). A limited number of nonculture tests are approved by the FDA for conjunctival specimens. Because nonculture tests cannot provide antimicrobial susceptibility results in cases of persistent gonococcal infection after treatment, clinicians should perform both culture and antimicrobial susceptibility testing.

Sexual Abuse.[1] In all prepubertal children beyond the newborn period and in nonsexually active adolescents who have gonococcal infection, sexual abuse must be considered to have occurred until proven otherwise. Genital, rectal, and pharyngeal secretion cultures should be performed for all patients before antimicrobial treatment is given. All gonococcal isolates from such patients should be preserved. Nonculture gonococcal tests, including Gram stain, DNA probes, enzyme immunoassays, or NAA testing of oropharyngeal, rectal, or genital tract specimens in children, cannot be relied on as the sole method for diagnosis of gonococcal infection for this purpose, because false-positive results can occur. In prepubertal children when culture is not available, some experts support use of NAA testing on vaginal swabs if a positive result can be verified by a different NAA test. When possible, appropriate cultures should be obtained from people who have had contact with a child suspected to have been sexually abused. Children in whom sexual abuse is suspected because of detection of gonorrhea should be evaluated for other sexually transmitted infections, such as *C trachomatis* infection, syphilis, hepatitis B virus infection, and human immunodeficiency virus (HIV) infection.

TREATMENT: Increases in the prevalence of fluoroquinolone resistance among gonococcal isolates in the United States resulted in new treatment recommendations in 2007. Because of the high prevalence of penicillin-, tetracycline-, and quinolone-resistant *N gonorrhoeae*, an extended-spectrum cephalosporin (eg, ceftriaxone, cefixime, or cefotaxime) is recommended as initial therapy for children and adults (see Table 3.7, p 308).[2] Antimicrobial resistance is widespread in many parts of the world, so treatment recommendations may vary depending on where an infection was acquired.

Ceftriaxone is recommended for gonococcal infections of all sites in children and adults. In addition, cefixime is recommended for uncomplicated gonococcal infections of the cervix, urethra, and rectum, and cefotaxime is recommended for gonococcal ophthalmia, scalp abscesses, and disseminated gonococcal infection in newborns.

All patients with presumed or proven gonorrhea should be evaluated for concurrent syphilis, hepatitis B virus, HIV, and *C trachomatis* infections. All patients beyond the neonatal period with gonorrhea should be treated presumptively for *C trachomatis* infection if chlamydial infection has not been ruled out (see *Chlamydia trachomatis*, p 255). A single dose of ceftriaxone, spectinomycin, or azithromycin is not effective treatment for concurrent infection with syphilis (see Syphilis, p 638).

A test-of-cure culture need not be performed in adolescents or adults with uncomplicated gonorrhea who are asymptomatic after being treated with one of the recommended antimicrobial regimens. Children treated with ceftriaxone do not require follow-up cultures unless they remain in an at-risk environment, but if treated with other regimens, follow-up culture is indicated. Patients who have symptoms that persist after treatment or

[1]Kellogg N; American Academy of Pediatrics, Committee on Child Abuse and Neglect. The evaluation of sexual abuse in children. *Pediatrics.* 2005;116(2):506–512

[2]Centers for Disease Control and Prevention. Update to CDC's sexually transmitted disease treatment guidelines, 2006: fluoroquinolones no longer recommended for treatment of gonococcal infections. *MMWR Morb Mortal Wkly Rep.* 2007;56(14):332–336

Table 3.7. Uncomplicated Gonococcal Infection: Treatment of Children Beyond the Newborn Period and Adolescents[a]

Disease[b]	Prepubertal Children Who Weigh Less Than 100 lb (45 kg)	Disease[b]	Patients Who Weigh 100 lb (45 kg) or More and Who Are 8 Years of Age or Older
Uncomplicated vulvovaginitis, cervicitis, urethritis, proctitis, or pharyngitis	Ceftriaxone, 125 mg, IM, in a single dose **OR** Cefixime, 8 mg/kg (maximum 400 mg), orally, in a single dose **OR** Spectinomycin,[b] 40 mg/kg (maximum 2 g), IM, in a single dose **PLUS**[a] Erythromycin base or ethylsuccinate, 50 mg/kg per day (maximum 2 g/day), orally, in 4 divided doses for 14 days **OR** Azithromycin, 20 mg/kg (maximum 1 g), orally, in a single dose	Uncomplicated endocervicitis, urethritis, proctitis, or pharyngitis[c]	Ceftriaxone, 125 mg, IM, in a single dose **OR** Cefixime, 400 mg, orally, in a single dose **OR** Cefpodoxime, 400 mg, orally, in a single dose **OR** Spectinomycin,[b] 2 g, IM, in a single dose **PLUS**[a] Azithromycin, 1 g, orally, in a single dose **OR** Doxycycline, 100 mg, orally, twice a day for 7 days

IM indicates intramuscularly.

[a] In addition to the recommended treatment for gonococcal infection, therapy for *Chlamydia trachomatis* is recommended on the presumption that the patient has concomitant infection.

[b] Spectinomycin is not recommended for treatment of pharyngeal infections; in people who cannot take ceftriaxone or spectinomycin may be used for pharyngitis, but a follow-up culture is necessary. Spectinomycin currently is not available in the United States.

[c] Alternative regimens include spectinomycin (2 g, IM, in a single dose), cefizoxime (500 mg, IM, in a single dose), cefotaxime (500 mg, IM, in a single dose), or cefoxitin (2 g, IM, administered with probenecid, 1 g, orally). Only ceftriaxone is recommended for pharyngitis; in people who cannot take ceftriaxone, spectinomycin may be used, but a follow-up culture is necessary.

whose symptoms recur shortly after treatment should be evaluated by culture for *N gonorrhoeae*, and any gonococci isolated should be tested for antimicrobial susceptibility. Clinicians and laboratory personnel should report treatment failures or resistant gonococcal isolates to their state or local health department. A high prevalence of *N gonorrhoeae* infection is observed in patients who have had gonorrhea in the preceding several months; clinicians should consider advising sexually active adolescents and adults with gonorrhea to be retested 3 months after treatment.

Specific recommendations for management and antimicrobial therapy are as follows:

Neonatal Disease. Infants with clinical evidence of ophthalmia neonatorum, scalp abscess, or disseminated infections should be hospitalized. Cultures of blood, eye discharge, or other sites of infection, such as CSF, should be performed for infants to confirm the diagnosis and determine antimicrobial susceptibility. Tests for concomitant infection with *C trachomatis*, congenital syphilis, and HIV infection should be performed. Results of the maternal test for hepatitis B surface antigen should be confirmed. The mother and her partner(s) also need appropriate examination and management for *N gonorrhoeae*.

Nondisseminated Infections. Recommended antimicrobial therapy, including that for ophthalmia neonatorum, is ceftriaxone (25–50 mg/kg, intravenously or intramuscularly, not to exceed 125 mg) given once. Infants with gonococcal ophthalmia should receive eye irrigations with saline solution immediately and at frequent intervals until the discharge is eliminated. Topical antimicrobial treatment alone is inadequate and is unnecessary when recommended systemic antimicrobial treatment is given. Infants with gonococcal ophthalmia should be hospitalized and evaluated for disseminated infection (sepsis, arthritis, meningitis).

Disseminated Infections. Recommended therapy for arthritis and septicemia is ceftriaxone or cefotaxime for 7 days. Cefotaxime is recommended for infants with hyperbilirubinemia. If meningitis is documented, treatment should be continued for a total of 10 to 14 days.

Gonococcal Infections in Children Beyond the Neonatal Period and in Adolescents. Recommendations for treatment of gonococcal infections, by age and weight, are given in Tables 3.7 (p 308) and 3.8 (p 310).

Special Problems in Treatment of Children (Beyond the Neonatal Period) and Adolescents. Patients with uncomplicated endocervical infection, urethritis, or proctitis who have a history of severe adverse reactions to cephalosporins should be treated with spectinomycin (40 mg/kg, maximum 2 g, given intramuscularly as a single dose) if available. Because data are limited regarding alternative regimens for treating gonorrhea among people who have documented severe cephalosporin allergy, expert infectious disease consultation is recommended. One treatment option is cephalosporin treatment after desensitization. If desensitization is not an option, azithromycin may be considered. Azithromycin (2 g, orally) is effective against uncomplicated gonococcal infection and *C trachomatis* infection, but because of concerns regarding emerging antimicrobial resistance to macrolides, its use should be restricted to limited circumstances.

Patients with uncomplicated pharyngeal gonococcal infection should be treated with ceftriaxone (125 mg, intramuscularly) in a single dose. Spectinomycin is approximately 50% effective for treatment of pharyngeal gonorrhea, so it should be used only in people with a history of severe cephalosporin allergy, and a pharyngeal culture should be obtained 3 to 5 days after treatment to verify eradication. A single

Table 3.8. Complicated Gonococcal Infection: Treatment of Children Beyond the Newborn Period and Adolescents[a]

Disease[b]	Prepubertal Children Who Weigh Less Than 100 lb (45 kg)	Disease[b]	Patients Who Weigh 100 lb (45 kg) or More and Who Are 8 Years of Age or Older
Disseminated gonococcal infection (eg, arthritis-dermatitis syndrome)	Ceftriaxone, 50 mg/kg/day (maximum 1 g/day), IV or IM, once a day for 7 days **PLUS[a]** Erythromycin base or ethylsuccinate 50 mg/kg/day, orally, divided into 4 doses daily for 14 days[c]	Disseminated gonococcal infections[d]	Ceftriaxone, 1 g, IV or IM, given once a day for 7 days[e] **PLUS[a]** Azithromycin 1 g, orally, in a single dose **OR** Doxycycline, 100 mg, orally or IV, twice a day for 7 days
Meningitis or endocarditis	Ceftriaxone, 50 mg/kg/day (maximum 2 g/day), IV or IM, given every 12 h; for meningitis, duration is 10–14 days; for endocarditis, duration is at least 28 days **PLUS[a]** Erythromycin base or ethylsuccinate 50 mg/kg/day, orally, divided into 4 doses daily for 14 days[c]	Meningitis or endocarditis	Ceftriaxone, 1–2 g, IV, every 12 h; for meningitis, duration is 10–14 days; for endocarditis, duration is at least 28 days **PLUS[a]** Azithromycin 1 g, orally, in a single dose **OR** Doxycycline, 100 mg, orally or IV, twice a day for 7 days
Conjunctivitis[f]	Ceftriaxone, 50 mg/kg (maximum 125 mg), IM, in a single dose	Conjunctivitis[f]	Ceftriaxone, 1 g, IM, in a single dose **PLUS[a]** Azithromycin, 1 g, orally, in a single dose **OR** Doxycycline, 100 mg, orally, twice daily for 7 days
		Epididymitis	Ceftriaxone, 250 mg, IM, in a single dose **PLUS[a]** Doxycycline, 100 mg, orally, twice daily for 10 days

Table 3.8. Complicated Gonococcal Infection: Treatment of Children Beyond the Newborn Period and Adolescents,[a] continued

Disease[b]	Prepubertal Children Who Weigh Less Than 100 lb (45 kg)	Patients Who Weigh 100 lb (45 kg) or More and Who Are 8 Years of Age or Older
Pelvic inflammatory disease		See Table 3.43 (p 503)

IV indicates intravenously; IM, intramuscularly.

[a] Concomitant therapy for *Chlamydia trachomatis* is recommended in addition to the recommended treatment for gonococcal infection.

[b] Hospitalization should be considered, especially for people treated as outpatients whose infection has failed to respond and for people who are unlikely to adhere to treatment regimens.

[c] Limited evidence suggests that azithromycin, 20 mg/kg (maximum 1 g), orally, in a single dose, is an alternative treatment for chlamydia in children who weigh less than 45 kg.

[d] An alternative for people who are allergic to beta-lactam drugs is spectinomycin, 2 g, IM, every 12 hours. Spectinomycin treatment requires a follow-up culture if pharyngeal infection exists.

[e] Alternatively, parenteral therapy can be discontinued 24 to 48 hours after improvement occurs, at which time therapy can be switched to an oral regimen (cefixime, 400 mg, orally, twice a day), to complete at least a 7-day course.

[f] Eyes should be lavaged with saline solution to clear accumulated secretions.

Adapted from Centers for Disease Control and Prevention. Sexually transmitted diseases treatment guidelines, 2006. *MMWR Recomm Rep.* 2006;55(RR-11):1–94 (see **www.cdc.gov/std/treatment**).

dose of ceftriaxone is not effective treatment for concurrent infection with syphilis (see Syphilis, p 638). Spectinomycin is not active against *Treponema pallidum*.

Children or adolescents with HIV infection should receive the same treatment for gonococcal infection as children without HIV infection.

Acute PID. *N gonorrhoeae* and *C trachomatis* are implicated in many cases of PID; most cases have a polymicrobial etiology. No reliable clinical criteria distinguish gonococcal from nongonococcal-associated PID. Hence, broad-spectrum treatment regimens are recommended (see Pelvic Inflammatory Disease, p 500).

Acute Epididymitis. Sexually transmitted organisms, such as *N gonorrhoeae* or *C trachomatis*, can cause acute epididymitis in sexually active adolescents and young adults but rarely cause acute epididymitis in prepubertal children. The recommended regimen for sexually transmitted epididymitis is ceftriaxone plus doxycycline or plus erythromycin, depending on the patient's age (see Table 3.8, p 310).

ISOLATION OF THE HOSPITALIZED PATIENT: Standard precautions are recommended, including for newborn infants with ophthalmia.

CONTROL MEASURES:

Neonatal Ophthalmia. For routine prophylaxis of infants immediately after birth, 1% tetracycline ophthalmic ointment or 0.5% erythromycin ophthalmic ointment is instilled into each eye; subsequent irrigation should not be performed (see Prevention of Neonatal Ophthalmia, p 827). Topical antimicrobial agents are less likely to cause a chemical irritation than silver nitrate. Use of povidone iodine has not been studied adequately. Prophylaxis may be delayed for as long as 1 hour after birth to facilitate parent-infant bonding. The efficacy of topical prophylaxis in preventing chlamydial ophthalmia is less clear, likely because colonization of the nasopharynx is not prevented.

Infants Born to Mothers With Gonococcal Infections. When prophylaxis is administered correctly, infants born to mothers with gonococcal infection rarely develop gonococcal ophthalmia. However, because gonococcal ophthalmia or disseminated infection occasionally can occur in this situation, infants born to mothers known to have gonorrhea should receive a single dose of ceftriaxone at a dose of 25 to 50 mg/kg, to a maximum of 125 mg (see Prevention of Neonatal Ophthalmia, p 827).

Children and Adolescents With Sexual Exposure to a Patient Known to Have Gonorrhea. Exposed people should undergo examination, culture, and the same treatment as people known to have gonorrhea.

Pregnancy. All pregnant women at risk of gonorrhea or living in an area in which the prevalence of *N gonorrhoeae* is high should have an endocervical culture for gonococci at the time of their first prenatal visit. A repeat test in the third trimester is recommended for women at continued risk of gonococcal infection. Recommended therapeutic regimens for patients found to be infected are as described previously for gonococcal infection, except that a tetracycline should not be used in pregnant women with PID because of the potential toxic effects on the fetus. Women who are allergic to cephalosporins should be treated with spectinomycin if available, but spectinomycin is unreliable against pharyngeal gonococcal infection. Other options for pregnant women with severe cephalosporin allergy include cephalosporin treatment after desensitization or azithromycin (2 g, orally).

Case Reporting and Management of Sexual Partners. All cases of gonorrhea must be reported to local public health officials (see Appendix V, Nationally Notifiable Infectious Diseases in the United States, p 845). Cases in prepubertal children must be investigated to determine the source of infection. Ensuring that sexual contacts are treated and counseled to use condoms is essential for community control, prevention of reinfection, and prevention of complications in the contact. Recommendations for services provided to partners of people with gonorrhea are available.[1]

For patients with gonorrhea whose partners' treatment cannot be ensured or is unlikely, delivery of antimicrobial therapy (ie, either a prescription or medication) by heterosexual male or female patients to their partners is an option. Use of this approach always should be accompanied by efforts to educate partners about symptoms and to encourage partners to seek clinical evaluation. This approach should not be considered a routine partner management strategy in men who have sex with men because of the high risk of coexisting undiagnosed sexually transmitted infections or HIV infection.

Granuloma Inguinale
(Donovanosis)

CLINICAL MANIFESTATIONS: Initial lesions are single or multiple subcutaneous nodules that progress to form painless, highly vascular, beefy red and friable, granulomatous ulcers without regional adenopathy. Lesions usually involve the genitalia, but anal infections occur in 5% to 10% of patients; lesions at distant sites (eg, face, mouth, or liver) are rare. Subcutaneous extension into the inguinal area results in induration that can mimic inguinal adenopathy (ie, "pseudobubo"). Fibrosis manifests as sinus tracts, adhesions, and lymphedema, resulting in extreme genital deformity. Urethral obstruction can occur.

ETIOLOGY: The disease is caused by *Klebsiella granulomatous* (formerly known as *Calymmatobacterium granulomatis*), an intracellular gram-negative bacillus.

EPIDEMIOLOGY: Indigenous granuloma inguinale occurs only rarely in the United States and most industrialized nations. Donovanosis is endemic in Papua, New Guinea, and parts of India, southern Africa, central Australia, and to a much lesser extent, the Caribbean and parts of South America, most notably Brazil. The highest incidence of disease occurs in tropical and subtropical environments. The incidence of infection seems to correlate strongly with sustained high temperatures and high relative humidity. Infection usually is acquired by sexual intercourse, most commonly with a person with active infection but possibly also from a person with asymptomatic rectal infection. Young children can acquire infection by contact with infected secretions. The period of communicability extends throughout the duration of active lesions or rectal colonization.

The **incubation period** is 8 to 80 days.

DIAGNOSTIC TESTS: The causative organism is difficult to culture, and diagnosis requires microscopic demonstration of dark staining intracytoplasmic Donovan bodies on Wright or Giemsa staining of a crush preparation from subsurface scrapings of a lesion or tissue. The microorganism also can be detected by histologic examination of biopsy specimens. Lesions should be cultured for *Haemophilus ducreyi* to exclude chancroid (pseudogranuloma inguinale). Granuloma inguinale often is misdiagnosed as carcinoma, which can be

---

[1]Centers for Disease Control and Prevention. Recommendations for partner services programs for HIV infection, syphilis, gonorrhea, and chlamydial infection. *MMWR Recomm Rep.* 2008;57(RR-9):1–63

excluded by histologic examination of tissue or by response of the lesion to antimicrobial agents. Diagnosis by polymerase chain reaction assay and serologic testing is available only in research laboratories.

TREATMENT: Doxycycline is the recommended treatment. Doxycycline should not be given to children younger than 8 years of age or pregnant women. Trimethoprim-sulfamethoxazole is an alternative regimen, except in pregnant women. Ciprofloxacin, which is not recommended for use in pregnant or lactating women or children younger than 18 years of age, is effective treatment. Gentamicin can be added if no improvement is evident in several days. Erythromycin or azithromycin are alternative therapies for pregnant women. Antimicrobial therapy is continued for at least 3 weeks or until the lesions have resolved. If antimicrobial therapy is effective, partial healing usually is noted within 7 days. Relapse can occur, especially if the antimicrobial agent is stopped before the primary lesion has healed completely. Complicated or long-standing infection can require surgical intervention.

Patients should be evaluated for other sexually transmitted infections, such as gonorrhea, syphilis, chancroid, and *Chlamydia trachomatis*, hepatitis B virus, and human immunodeficiency virus infections.

ISOLATION OF THE HOSPITALIZED PATIENT: Standard precautions are recommended.

CONTROL MEASURES: Sexual partners should be examined, counseled to use condoms, and offered antimicrobial therapy. The value of therapy in the absence of signs of infection has not been established.

Haemophilus influenzae Infections

CLINICAL MANIFESTATIONS: *Haemophilus influenzae* type b (Hib) causes pneumonia, occult febrile bacteremia, meningitis, epiglottitis, septic arthritis, cellulitis, otitis media, purulent pericarditis, and other less common infections, such as endocarditis, endophthalmitis, osteomyelitis, and peritonitis. Nontype b encapsulated strains occasionally cause invasive disease similar to type b infections. Nontypable strains more commonly cause infections of the respiratory tract (eg, conjunctivitis, otitis media, sinusitis, pneumonia) and, less often, bacteremia, meningitis, chorioamnionitis, and neonatal septicemia.

ETIOLOGY: *H influenzae* is a pleomorphic gram-negative coccobacillus. Encapsulated strains express 1 of 6 antigenically distinct capsular polysaccharides (a through f); non-encapsulated strains fail to react with typing antisera against capsular serotypes a through f and are designated nontypable.

EPIDEMIOLOGY: The natural habitat of the organism is the upper respiratory tract of humans. The mode of transmission is person to person by inhalation of respiratory tract droplets or by direct contact with respiratory tract secretions. In neonates, infection is acquired intrapartum by aspiration of amniotic fluid or by contact with genital tract secretions containing the organism. Asymptomatic colonization by *H influenzae* is common, especially with nontypable and non-type b capsular type strains.

Before introduction of effective Hib conjugate vaccines, Hib was the most common cause of bacterial meningitis in children in the United States. The peak incidence of invasive Hib infections occurred between 6 and 18 months of age. In contrast, the peak age for epiglottitis was 2 to 4 years of age.

Unimmunized children younger than 4 years of age are at increased risk of invasive Hib disease. Factors that predispose to invasive disease include sickle cell disease, asplenia, human immunodeficiency virus (HIV) infection, certain immunodeficiency syndromes, and malignant neoplasms. Historically, invasive Hib was more common in boys; black, Alaska Native, Apache, and Navajo children; child care attendees; children living in crowded conditions; and children who were not breastfed.

Since 1987, when Hib conjugate vaccines were introduced in the United States for children 18 months of age and older (1990 for children 6 weeks of age and older), the incidence of invasive Hib disease has decreased by 99% to fewer than 1 case per 100 000 children younger than 5 years of age. The incidence of invasive infections caused by all other encapsulated and nontypable strains combined also is low. In the United States, invasive Hib disease occurs primarily in underimmunized children and among infants too young to have completed the primary immunization series. Hib remains an important pathogen in resource-limited countries where vaccines are not available routinely.

Nontypable *H influenzae* causes 30% to 52% of episodes of acute otitis media and sinusitis in children. These infections are twice as frequent in boys and peak in the late fall.

The **incubation period** is unknown.

DIAGNOSTIC TESTS: Cerebrospinal fluid (CSF), blood, synovial fluid, pleural fluid, and middle-ear aspirates should be cultured on a medium such as chocolate agar, a medium enriched with factors X and V. Gram stain of an infected body fluid specimen can facilitate presumptive diagnosis. Latex particle agglutination for detection of type b capsular antigen in CSF can be helpful, but a negative test result does not exclude the diagnosis, and false-positive results have been recorded. All *H influenzae* isolates associated with an invasive infection should be serotyped. If serotyping is not available locally, isolates should be submitted to the state health department or to a reference laboratory for testing.

H influenzae otitis media caused by nontypable strains is diagnosed by culture of tympanocentesis fluid; other respiratory tract specimen cultures (eg, throat, ear drainage) are not indicative of middle-ear culture results.

TREATMENT:

- Initial therapy for children with meningitis possibly caused by Hib is cefotaxime or ceftriaxone. Meropenem or the combination of ampicillin and chloramphenicol are alternative empiric regimens. Treatment of other invasive *H influenzae* infections is similar. Therapy is continued at least 10 days by the intravenous route and longer in complicated infections.
- Dexamethasone may be beneficial for treatment of infants and children with Hib meningitis to diminish the risk of neurologic sequelae, including hearing loss, if given before or concurrently with the first dose of antimicrobial agent(s).
- Epiglottitis is a medical emergency. An airway must be established promptly with an endotracheal tube or by tracheostomy.
- Infected synovial, pleural, or pericardial fluid should be removed.
- For empiric treatment of acute otitis media in children younger than 2 years of age or in children 2 years of age or older with severe disease, oral amoxicillin (see details in Pneumococcal Infections, p 524, and Appropriate Use of Antimicrobial Agents, p 740)

is recommended.[1] Duration of therapy is 5 to 10 days. The 5-day course is considered for children 2 years of age and older. In the United States, 30% to 40% of *H influenzae* isolates produce beta-lactamase, necessitating a beta-lactamase–resistant agent, such as amoxicillin-clavulanate; an oral cephalosporin, such as cefuroxime or cefpodoxime; or azithromycin. In vitro susceptibility testing of isolates from middle-ear fluid specimens help guide therapy in complicated or persistent cases.

ISOLATION OF THE HOSPITALIZED PATIENT: In patients with invasive Hib disease, droplet precautions are recommended for 24 hours after initiation of parenteral antimicrobial therapy.

CONTROL MEASURES (FOR INVASIVE HIB DISEASE):
Care of Exposed People. Careful observation of exposed unimmunized or incompletely immunized children who are household, child care, or nursery school contacts of patients with invasive Hib disease is essential. Exposed children in whom febrile illness develops should receive prompt medical evaluation.

   Chemoprophylaxis. The risk of invasive Hib disease is increased among unimmunized household contacts younger than 4 years of age. Rifampin eradicates Hib from the pharynx in approximately 95% of carriers and decreases the risk of secondary invasive illness in exposed household contacts. Nursery and child care center contacts also may be at increased risk of secondary disease. Secondary disease in child care contacts is rare when all contacts are older than 2 years of age.

   Indications and guidelines for chemoprophylaxis in different circumstances are summarized in Table 3.9, (p 317).

- **Household.** Chemoprophylaxis is not recommended for contacts of people with invasive disease caused by nontype b *H influenzae* strains. In households with at least 1 household contact of a person with invasive Hib disease who is younger than 48 months of age and unimmunized or incompletely immunized against Hib, rifampin prophylaxis is recommended for all household contacts. Given that most secondary cases in households occur during the first week after hospitalization of the index case, when indicated, prophylaxis (see Table 3.9, p 317) should be initiated as soon as possible. Because some secondary cases occur later, initiation of prophylaxis 7 days or more after hospitalization of the index patient still may be of some benefit.

- **Child care and nursery school.** When 2 or more cases of invasive disease have occurred within 60 days and unimmunized or incompletely immunized children attend the child care facility or nursery school, rifampin prophylaxis for all attendees and child care providers should be considered. In addition to these recommendations for chemoprophylaxis, unimmunized or incompletely immunized children should receive a dose of vaccine and should be scheduled for completion of the recommended age-specific immunization schedule (see Fig 1.1–1.3, p 24–28).

- **Index case.** Treatment of Hib disease with cefotaxime or ceftriaxone eradicates Hib colonization, eliminating the need for prophylaxis of the index patient. Patients who are treated with meropenem, ampicillin, or chloramphenicol and who are younger than 2 years of age should receive rifampin prophylaxis at the end of therapy for invasive infection.

---

[1] American Academy of Pediatrics, Subcommittee on Management of Acute Otitis Media. Diagnosis and management of acute otitis media. *Pediatrics.* 2004;113(5):1451–1465

Table 3.9. Indications and Guidelines for Rifampin Chemoprophylaxis for Contacts of Index Cases of Invasive *Haemophilus influenzae* Type b (Hib) Disease

Chemoprophylaxis Recommended

- For all household contacts[a] in the following circumstances:
  - ◆ Household with at least 1 contact younger than 4 years of age who is unimmunized or incompletely immunized[b]
  - ◆ Household with a child younger than 12 months of age who has not received the primary series
  - ◆ Household with a contact who is an immunocompromised child, regardless of that child's Hib immunization status
- For nursery school and child care center contacts when 2 or more cases of Hib invasive disease have occurred within 60 days (see text)
- For index patient, if younger than 2 years of age or member of a household with a susceptible contact and treated with a regimen other than cefotaxime or ceftriaxone, chemoprophylaxis usually is provided just before discharge from hospital

Chemoprophylaxis Not Recommended

- For occupants of households with no children younger than 4 years of age other than the index patient
- For occupants of households when all household contacts 12 through 48 months of age have completed their Hib immunization series and when household contacts younger than 12 months of age have completed their primary series of Hib immunizations
- For nursery school and child care contacts of 1 index case, especially people older than 2 years of age
- For pregnant women

[a]Defined as people residing with the index patient or nonresidents who spent 4 or more hours with the index patient for at least 5 of the 7 days preceding the day of hospital admission of the index case.
[b]Complete immunization is defined as having had at least 1 dose of conjugate vaccine at 15 months of age or older; 2 doses between 12 and 14 months of age; or a 2- or 3-dose primary series when younger than 12 months with a booster dose at 12 months of age or older.

- **Dosage.** Rifampin should be given orally once a day for 4 days (in a dose of 20 mg/kg; maximum dose, 600 mg). The dose for infants younger than 1 month of age is not established; some experts recommend lowering the dose to 10 mg/kg. For adults, each dose is 600 mg.

  Immunization. Two single-antigen Hib conjugate vaccine products and 3 combination vaccine products that contain Hib conjugate are available in the United States (see Table 3.10, p 318). The Hib conjugate vaccines consist of the Hib capsular polysaccharide (ie, polyribosylribotol phosphate [PRP] or PRP oligomers) covalently linked to a carrier protein. Protective antibodies are directed against PRP. Conjugate vaccines vary in composition and immunogenicity, and as a result, recommendations for their use differ.

Table 3.10. *Haemophilus influenzae* Type b (Hib) Conjugate Vaccines Licensed for Use in Infants and Children in the United States[a]

Vaccine	Trade Name	Components	Manufacturer
PRP-T	ActHIB	PRP conjugated to tetanus toxoid	Aventis Pasteur, Inc[b]
DTaP/PRP-T[c]	TriHIBit[c]	DTaP vaccine + PRP-T	Aventis Pasteur, Inc[b]
PRP-OMP	PedvaxHIB	PRP conjugated to OMP	Merck & Co, Inc
PRP-OMP-HepB[d]	Comvax	PRP-OMP + hepatitis B vaccine	Merck & Co, Inc
HbOC[e]	HibTITER	PRP conjugated to CRM$_{197}$	Wyeth-Lederle Vaccines
DTaP-IPV/PRP-T[f]	Pentacel	DTaP-IPV + PRP-T	sanofi pasteur

PRP-T indicates polyribosylribotol phosphate-tetanus toxoid; DTaP, diphtheria and tetanus toxoids and acellular pertussis; OMP, outer membrane protein complex from *Neisseria meningitidis;* HepB, hepatitis B vaccine; CRM$_{197}$, a mutant nontoxic diphtheria toxin.

[a] Hib conjugate vaccines may be given in combination products or as reconstituted products, provided the combination or reconstituted vaccine is licensed by the US Food and Drug Administration (FDA) for the child's age and administration of the other vaccine component(s) also is justified.

[b] License holder on product. Parent company is sanofi pasteur.

[c] The DTaP (Tripedia) liquid component is used to reconstitute PRP-T (ActHIB) to form TriHIBit, which is licensed by the FDA only for the fourth dose of the Hib and DTaP series. The DTaP/PRP-T vaccine (TriHiBit) should not be used for primary immunization in infants at 2, 4, or 6 months of age.

[d] The combination *H influenzae* type b (PRP-OMP) and HepB (Recombivax, 5 µg) vaccine is licensed for use at 2, 4, and 12 through 15 months of age (Comvax).

[e] This vaccine no longer is produced in the United States.

[f] The DTaP-IPV liquid component is used to reconstitute a lyophilized ActHIB vaccine component to form Pentacel, which is licensed as a 4-dose series for infants and children at 2, 4, 6, and 15 through 18 months of age.

Depending on the vaccine, the recommended primary series consists of 3 doses given at 2, 4, and 6 months of age or 2 doses given at 2 and 4 months of age (see Recommendations for Immunization, p 320, and Table 3.11, p 319). The recommended doses can be given as a Hib-hepatitis B (HepB) combination or as a diphtheria and tetanus toxoids and acellular pertussis (DTaP)-inactivated poliovirus (IPV)/Hib combination vaccine. The regimens in Table 3.11 (p 319) likely are to be equivalent in protection after completion of the recommended primary series. For health care professionals who serve American Indian/Alaska Native children, it may be prudent to use only PRP-OMP (outer membrane protein complex) Hib vaccine (see American Indian/Alaska Native Children, *Haemophilus influenzae* type b, p 89).

A booster dose of any Hib conjugate vaccine is recommended at 12 through 15 months of age, regardless of which regimen was used for the primary series. This booster dose can be given as a combination vaccine. In periods during which Hib-containing vaccines may be in short supply, interim recommendations include deferral of administration of

Table 3.11. Recommended Regimens for Routine *Haemophilus influenzae* Type b Conjugate Immunization for Children Immunized Beginning at 2 Through 6 Months of Age[a]

Vaccine Product at Initiation	Total No. of Doses To be Administered	Recommended Regimen
PRP-T	4	3 doses at 2-mo intervals initially; fourth dose at 12 through 15 mo of age; any conjugate vaccine for fourth dose[b]
PRP-OMP	3	2 doses 2 months apart; third dose at 12 through 15 mo of age; any conjugate vaccine for third dose[b]

PRP-T indicates polyribosylribotol phosphate-tetanus toxoid; OMP, outer membrane protein complex from *Neisseria meningitidis.*

[a]See text, Table 3.10 (p 318), and Table 1.7 (p 35) for further information about specific vaccines.

[b]The monovalent Hib conjugate vaccines available in the United States are considered interchangeable for primary and booster immunizations. If PRP-OMP is administered only as part of a primary series, the recommended number of doses to complete the series is determined by the other Hib conjugate vaccine.

the routine vaccine booster dose administered at 12 through 15 months of age, except to children in specific groups at high risk.[1] Current status of vaccine shortages and delays can be found at **www.cdc.gov/vaccines/vac-gen/shortages.**

Combination Vaccines. Three combination vaccines that contain Hib are licensed in the United States: DTaP/Hib combination, HepB-Hib combination, and DTaP-IPV/Hib combination (see Table 3.10, p 318) vaccines. The DTaP/Hib combination vaccine is licensed only for the fourth dose of the DTaP and Hib series. The DTaP/Hib combination vaccine is not licensed for use as the primary series at 2, 4, and 6 months of age. The HepB-Hib combination vaccine is licensed for use at 2, 4, and 12 through 15 months of age. The HepB-Hib combination vaccine should not be given to infants younger than 6 weeks of age. The DTaP-IPV/Hib combination vaccine is licensed for children 6 weeks through 4 years of age, given as a 4-dose series at 2, 4, 6, and 15 through 18 months of age. DTaP-IPV/Hib vaccine is not licensed for use in children 5 years of age and older and is not indicated for the booster dose at 4 through 6 years of age. However, DTaP-IPV/Hib that inadvertently is administered to children at 5 through 6 years of age should be counted as a valid dose.

Vaccine Interchangeability. The monovalent Hib conjugate vaccines available in the United States are considered interchangeable for primary and booster immunization. If PRP-OMP vaccine is administered only as part of a primary series, the recommended number of doses to complete the series is determined by the other Hib conjugate vaccine.

Dosage and Route of Administration. The dose of each Hib conjugate vaccine is 0.5 mL, given intramuscularly.

Children With Immunologic Impairment. Children at increased risk of Hib disease may have impaired anti-PRP antibody responses to conjugate vaccines. Examples include children with HIV infection; children with immunoglobulin deficiency; recipients

---

[1]Centers for Disease Control and Prevention. Interim recommendations for the use of *Haemophilus influenzae* type b (Hib) conjugate vaccines related to the recall of certain lots of Hib-containing vaccines (PedvaxHIB® and Comvax®). *MMWR Morb Mortal Wkly Rep.* 2007;56(50):1318–1320

of stem cell transplants; and recipients of chemotherapy for a malignant neoplasm. Some children with immunologic impairment may benefit from more doses of conjugate vaccine than usually indicated (see Recommendations for Immunization, below).

Adverse Reactions. Adverse reactions to the Hib conjugate vaccines are few. Pain, redness, and swelling at the injection site occur in approximately 25% of recipients, but these symptoms typically are mild and last fewer than 24 hours.

Recommendations for Immunization.

Indications and Schedule
- All children should be immunized with an Hib conjugate vaccine beginning at approximately 2 months of age or as soon as possible thereafter (see Table 3.11, p 319). Other general recommendations are as follows:
  - Immunization can be initiated as early as 6 weeks of age.
  - Vaccine can be given during visits for other childhood immunizations (see Simultaneous Administration of Multiple Vaccines, p 33).
- For routine immunization of children younger than 7 months of age, the following guidelines are recommended:
  - **Primary series.** A 3-dose regimen of PRP-T (tetanus toxoid conjugate) or a 2-dose regimen of PRP-OMP should be administered (see Table 3.11, p 319). Doses are given at approximately 2-month intervals. When sequential doses of different vaccine products are given or uncertainty exists about which products previously were administered, 3 doses of any conjugate vaccine are considered sufficient to complete the primary series, regardless of the regimen used.
  - **Booster immunization at 12 through 15 months of age.** For children who have completed a primary series, an additional dose of conjugate vaccine is recommended at 12 through 15 months of age and at least 2 months after the last dose. Any conjugate vaccine or DTaP-Hib combination vaccine is acceptable for this dose. DTaP-IPV/Hib vaccine can be administered as the fourth dose at 15 through 18 months of age after the primary series.
- Children younger than 5 years of age who did not receive Hib conjugate vaccine during the first 6 months of life should be immunized according to the recommended catch-up immunization schedule (see Fig 1.3, p 28). For accelerated immunization in infants younger than 12 months of age, a minimum of a 4-week interval between doses can be used.
- Special circumstances are as follows:
  - **Lapsed immunizations.** Recommendations for children who have had a lapse in the schedule of immunizations are based on limited data. Current recommendations are summarized in Fig 1.3 (p 28).
  - **Preterm infants.** For preterm infants, immunization should be based on chronologic age and should be initiated at 2 months of age according to recommendations in Table 3.11 (p 319).
  - Children with decreased or absent splenic function who have received a primary series of Hib immunizations and a booster dose at 12 months of age or older need not be immunized further. Children who have received a primary series and a booster dose and are undergoing scheduled splenectomy (eg, for Hodgkin disease, spherocytosis, immune thrombocytopenia, or hypersplenism) may benefit from an additional dose of any licensed conjugate vaccine. This dose should be provided at least 7 to

10 days before the procedure. Patients with HIV infection or immunoglobulin (Ig) G2 subclass deficiency and children receiving chemotherapy for malignant neoplasms also are at increased risk of invasive Hib disease. Whether these children will benefit from additional doses after completion of the primary series of immunizations and the booster dose at 12 months of age or later is unknown.

For children 12 through 59 months of age with an underlying condition predisposing to Hib disease who are not immunized or have received only 1 dose of conjugate vaccine before 12 months of age, 2 doses of any conjugate vaccine, separated by 2 months, are recommended. For children in this age group who received 2 doses before 12 months of age, 1 additional dose of conjugate vaccine is recommended.

• Unimmunized children with an underlying disease possibly predisposing to Hib disease who are older than 59 months of age should be immunized with any licensed conjugate vaccine. On the basis of limited data, 2 doses separated by 1 to 2 months are suggested for children with HIV infection or IgG2 deficiency.

• Children with Hib invasive infection younger than 24 months of age can remain at risk of developing a second episode of disease. These children should be immunized according to the age-appropriate schedule for unimmunized children and as if they had received no previous Hib vaccine doses (see Table 3.11, p 319, and Table 1.7, p 35). Immunization should be initiated 1 month after onset of disease or as soon as possible thereafter.

Immunologic evaluation should be performed in children who experience invasive Hib disease despite 2 to 3 doses of vaccine and in children with recurrent invasive disease attributable to type b strains.

Reporting. All cases of *H influenzae* invasive disease, including type b and non-type b, should be reported to the Centers for Disease Control and Prevention through the local or state public health department. Organisms isolated from patients with invasive disease should be sent to the state health department for serotyping.

Hantavirus Pulmonary Syndrome

CLINICAL MANIFESTATIONS: Hantaviruses in humans cause 2 syndromes: hantavirus pulmonary syndrome (HPS), a noncardiogenic pulmonary edema; and hemorrhagic fever with renal syndrome (HFRS) (see Hemorrhagic Fevers and Related Syndromes, p 327). The prodromal illness of HPS is 3 to 7 days and is characterized by fever; chills; headache; myalgia of the shoulders, lower back, and thighs; nausea; vomiting; diarrhea; dizziness; and sometimes cough. Respiratory tract symptoms or signs usually do not occur for the first 3 to 7 days until pulmonary edema and severe hypoxemia appear abruptly after the onset of cough and dyspnea, and then the disease progresses over a few hours. In severe cases, persistent hypotension caused by myocardial dysfunction is present.

The extensive bilateral interstitial and alveolar pulmonary edema and pleural effusions are the result of a diffuse pulmonary capillary leak and appear to be caused by immune responses to hantavirus in endothelial cells of the microvasculature. Intubation and assisted ventilation usually are required for only 2 to 4 days, with resolution heralded by the onset of diuresis and rapid clinical improvement.

The severe myocardial depression is different from that of septic shock; the cardiac indices and the stroke volume index are low, the pulmonary wedge pressure is normal, and systemic vascular resistance is increased. Poor prognostic indicators include persistent hypotension, marked hemoconcentration, a cardiac index of less than 2, and abrupt onset of lactic acidosis with a serum lactate concentration of greater than 4 mmol/L (36 mg/dL).

The mortality rate for patients with HPS in recent years has been 30% to 40%. Asymptomatic and mild forms of disease are rare in adults, but limited information suggests they may be more common in children. Serious sequelae are uncommon.

ETIOLOGY: Hantaviruses are RNA viruses of the Bunyaviridae family. Within the Hantavirus genus, Sin Nombre virus (SNV) is the major cause of HPS in the 4-corners region of the United States. Bayou virus, Black Creek Canal virus, Monongahela virus, and New York virus are responsible for sporadic cases in Louisiana, Texas, Florida, New York, and other areas of the eastern United States. Hantavirus serotypes associated with an HPS syndrome in South America and Panama include Andes virus, Oran virus, Laguna Negra virus, and Choclo virus.

EPIDEMIOLOGY: Rodents, the natural hosts for hantaviruses, acquire a lifelong, asymptomatic, chronic infection with prolonged viruria and virus in saliva, urine, and feces. Humans acquire infection through direct contact with infected rodents, rodent droppings, or nests or inhalation of aerosolized virus particles from rodent urine, droppings, or saliva. Rarely, infection may be acquired from rodent bites or contamination of broken skin with excreta. Person-to-person transmission of hantaviruses has not been demonstrated from patients in the United States. At-risk activities include handling or trapping rodents; cleaning or entering closed, rarely used rodent-infested structures; cleaning feed storage or animal shelter areas; hand plowing; and living in a home with an increased density of mice in or around the home. For backpackers or campers, sleeping in a structure also inhabited by rodents has been associated with HPS. Weather conditions resulting in exceptionally heavy rainfall and improved rodent food supplies can result in a large increase in the rodent population. The increased rodent population results in more frequent contact between humans and infected mice and may account for outbreaks. Most cases occur during spring and summer, and geographic location is determined by the habitat of the rodent carrier.

SNV is transmitted by the deer mouse, *Peromyscus maniculatus;* Black Creek Canal virus is transmitted by the cotton rat, *Sigmodon hispidus;* Bayou virus is transmitted by the rice rat, *Oryzomys palustris;* and New York virus is transmitted by the white-footed mouse, *Peromyscus leucopus.*

The **incubation period** may be 1 to 6 weeks after exposure to infected rodents, their saliva, or excreta but has not been established definitively.

DIAGNOSTIC TESTS: Characteristic laboratory findings include neutrophilic leukocytosis with immature granulocytes, more than 10% immunoblasts (basophilic cytoplasm, prominent nucleoli, and an increased nuclear-cytoplasmic ratio), thrombocytopenia, and increased hematocrit. In fatal cases, SNV has been identified by immunohistochemical staining of capillary endothelial cells in almost every organ in the body. SNV RNA has been detected uniformly by reverse transcriptase-polymerase chain reaction assay of peripheral blood mononuclear cells and other clinical specimens from the first few days of hospitalization up to 10 to 21 days after symptom onset, and the duration of viremia is unknown. Viral RNA is not detected readily in bronchoalveolar lavage fluids.

Hantavirus-specific immunoglobulin (Ig) G and IgM antibodies are present at the onset of clinical disease. A rapid diagnostic test can facilitate immediate appropriate supportive therapy and early transfer to a tertiary care facility. Enzyme immunoassay (available through many state health departments and the Centers for Disease Control and Prevention) and Western blot are assays that use recombinant antigens and have a high degree of specificity for detection of IgG and IgM antibody. Viral culture is not useful for diagnosis and is available only in research laboratories that have specialized facilities to protect laboratory workers. Diagnosis can be made retrospectively by immunohistochemistry assay of tissues obtained from necropsy.

TREATMENT: Patients with suspected HPS should be transferred immediately to a tertiary care facility. Supportive management of pulmonary edema, severe hypoxemia, and hypotension during the first 24 to 48 hours is critical for recovery.

Extracorporeal membrane oxygenation (ECMO) may provide particularly important short-term support for the severe capillary leak syndrome in the lungs.

Ribavirin is active in vitro against hantaviruses including SNV. Two clinical studies (one open-label study and one randomized, placebo-controlled, double-blind study) found that intravenous ribavirin probably is ineffective in treatment of HPS in the cardiopulmonary stage. Steroids are being evaluated in South American trials.

ISOLATION OF THE HOSPITALIZED PATIENT: Standard precautions are recommended. HPS has not been associated with health care-associated or person-to-person transmission in the United States.

CONTROL MEASURES:

Care of Exposed People. Serial clinical examinations should be used to monitor people assessed to be at high risk of infection after a high-risk exposure (see Epidemiology, p 322).

Environmental Control. Hantavirus infections of humans occur primarily in adults and are associated with domestic, occupational, or leisure activities bringing humans into contact with infected rodents, usually in a rural setting. Eradicating the host reservoir is not feasible. The best available approach for disease control and prevention is risk reduction through environmental hygiene practices that discourage rodents from colonizing the home and work environment and that minimize aerosolization and contact with virus in saliva and excreta. Measures to decrease exposure in the home and workplace include eliminating food sources available to rodents in structures used by humans, limiting possible nesting sites, sealing holes and other possible entrances for rodents, and using "snap traps" and rodenticides. Before entering areas with potential rodent infestations, doors and windows should be opened to ventilate the enclosure.

Hantaviruses, because of their lipid envelope, are susceptible to most disinfectants, including diluted bleach solutions, detergents, and most general household disinfectants. Dusty or dirty areas or articles should be moistened with a 10% bleach or other disinfectant solution before being cleaned. Brooms and vacuum cleaners should not be used to clean rodent-infested areas. Use of a 10% bleach solution to disinfect dead rodents and wearing rubber gloves before handling trapped or dead rodents are recommended. Gloves and traps should be disinfected after use. The cleanup of areas potentially infested with hantavirus-infected rodents should be carried out by knowledgeable professionals using appropriate personal protective equipment. Potentially infected material removed should be handled according to local regulations as infectious waste.

Chemoprophylaxis measures or vaccines are not available.

Public Health Reporting. Possible occurrence should be reported immediately to local and state public health authorities.

Helicobacter pylori Infections

CLINICAL MANIFESTATIONS: *Helicobacter pylori* causes chronic active gastritis and increases the risk of duodenal and gastric ulcers; persistent infection with *H pylori* increases the risk of gastric cancer. Acute infection can manifest as epigastric pain, nausea, vomiting, hematemesis, and guaiac-positive stools. Symptoms usually resolve within a few days despite persistence of the organism for years or for life. *H pylori* infection is not associated with autoimmune or chemical gastritis.

ETIOLOGY: *H pylori* is a gram-negative, spiral, curved, or U-shaped microaerophilic bacillus that has 2 to 6 sheathed flagella at one end. It is catalase, oxidase, and urease positive.

EPIDEMIOLOGY: *H pylori* has been isolated from humans and other primates. An animal reservoir for human transmission has not been demonstrated. Organisms are transmitted from infected humans by the fecal-oral and oral-oral routes. Infection rates are low in children in resource-rich countries except in children from lower socioeconomic groups. Most infections are acquired in the first 5 years of life and can reach a prevalence up to 80% in resource-limited countries. Most carriage is asymptomatic, but some people with colonization have histologic findings of chronic gastritis.

The **incubation period** is unknown.

DIAGNOSTIC TESTS: *H pylori* infection can be diagnosed by culture of gastric biopsy tissue on nonselective media (eg, chocolate agar) or selective media (eg, Skirrow agar) at 37°C (98°F) under microaerobic conditions for 2 to 5 days. Organisms usually can be visualized on histologic sections with Warthin-Starry silver, Steiner, Giemsa, or Genta staining. Presence of *H pylori* can be diagnosed but not excluded on the basis of hematoxylin-eosin stains. Because of production of urease by organisms, urease testing of a gastric specimen can give a rapid and specific microbiologic diagnosis. Each of these tests requires endoscopy and biopsy. Noninvasive, commercially available tests include breath tests, which detect labeled carbon dioxide in expired air after oral administration of isotopically labeled urea, and serologic tests for the presence of immunoglobulin G specific for *H pylori*. A stool antigen test also is available commercially. Each of these commercially available tests has a high sensitivity and specificity.

TREATMENT: Treatment is recommended only for infected patients who have peptic ulcer disease (currently or in the past), gastric mucosa-associated lymphoid tissue-type lymphoma, or early gastric cancer. Eradication therapy for *H pylori* consists of at least 7 days of treatment, although eradication rates are higher for regimens of 14 days. Effective treatment regimens include 2 antimicrobial agents (eg, clarithromycin plus either amoxicillin or metronidazole) plus a proton-pump inhibitor (lansoprazole, omeprazole, esomeprazole, rabeprazole, or pantoprazole). These regimens are effective in eliminating the organism, healing the ulcer, and preventing recurrence. Alternate therapies include bismuth subsalicylate plus metronidazole plus tetracycline in people 8 years of age and older plus either a proton-pump inhibitor or an H_2 blocker (cimetidine, famotidine, nizatidine, and ranitidine). Follow-up testing with a breath or stool test can document eradication; some patients require an additional treatment course of 14 days.

ISOLATION OF THE HOSPITALIZED PATIENT: Standard precautions are recommended.

CONTROL MEASURES: Disinfection of gastroscopes prevents transmission of the organism between patients.

Hemorrhagic Fevers Caused by Arenaviruses[1]

CLINICAL MANIFESTATIONS: The arenaviruses include lymphocytic choriomeningitis virus and the agents of 5 hemorrhagic fevers (HFs): Bolivian, Argentine, Brazilian, Venezuelan, and Lassa. The zoonotic diseases associated with these agents range in severity from mild, acute, febrile infections to severe illnesses in which vascular leak, shock, and multiorgan dysfunction are prominent features. Fever, headache, myalgia, conjunctival suffusion, bleeding, and abdominal pain are common early symptoms in all infections. Thrombocytopenia, axillary petechiae, and encephalopathy usually are present in Argentine HF, Bolivian HF, and Venezuelan HF, and exudative pharyngitis often occurs in Lassa fever. Mucosal bleeding occurs in severe cases as a consequence of vascular damage, thrombocytopenia, and platelet dysfunction. Proteinuria is common, but renal failure is unusual. Increased serum concentrations of aspartate transaminase can indicate a severe or fatal outcome of Lassa fever. Shock develops 7 to 9 days after onset of illness in more severely ill patients with these infections. Upper and lower respiratory tract symptoms can develop in people with Lassa fever. Encephalopathic signs such as tremor, alterations in consciousness, and seizures can occur in the South American HFs and in severe cases of Lassa fever.

ETIOLOGY: Arenaviruses are RNA viruses. The major New World arenavirus hemorrhagic fevers occurring in the Western hemisphere are Argentine HF caused by Junin virus, Bolivian HF caused by Machupo virus, and Venezuelan HF caused by Guanarito virus. A fourth arenavirus, Sabia virus, caused 2 unrelated cases of naturally occurring HF in Brazil and 2 laboratory-acquired cases. The Old World complex of arenaviruses includes Lassa virus, which causes Lassa fever, a disease occurring in West Africa, and lymphocytic choriomeningitis (LCM) virus (see Lymphocytic Choriomeningitis, p 437), which produces the least severe infection of the arenaviruses.

EPIDEMIOLOGY: Arenaviruses are maintained in nature by association with specific rodent hosts, in which they produce chronic viremia and viruria. The principal routes of infection are inhalation and contact of mucous membranes and skin (eg, through cuts, scratches, or abrasions) with urine and salivary secretions from these persistently infected rodents. All arenaviruses are infectious as aerosols, and arenaviruses causing hemorrhagic fever should be considered highly hazardous to people working with any of the viruses in the laboratory. The geographic distribution and habitats of the specific rodents that serve as reservoir hosts largely determine the areas with endemic infection and populations at risk. Before a vaccine became available in Argentina, several hundred cases of Argentine HF occurred yearly in agricultural workers and inhabitants of the Argentine pampas. The vaccine is not licensed in the United States. Epidemics of Bolivian HF occurred in small towns between 1962 and 1964; sporadic disease activity in the countryside has continued since then. Venezuelan HF first was identified in 1989 and occurs in rural north-central Venezuela. Lassa fever is endemic in most of West Africa, where rodent hosts live in proximity with humans, causing thousands of infections annually. Lassa fever has been reported in the United States in people who have traveled to West Africa.

The **incubation period**s are from 6 to 17 days.

---

[1]Does not include lymphocytic choriomeningitis virus, which is reviewed on p 437.

DIAGNOSTIC TESTS: Acute infection is diagnosed by demonstrating virus-specific serum immunoglobulin (Ig) M or viral antigen. The IgG antibody response is delayed. Viral nucleic acid also can be detected in acute disease by reverse transcriptase-polymerase chain reaction assay. These viruses may be recovered from blood (collected in a heparin-containing tube) of acutely ill patients as well as from various tissues obtained postmortem, but isolation should be attempted only under Biosafety level-4 conditions. Diagnosis can be made retrospectively by immunohistochemistry assay of tissues obtained from necropsy.

TREATMENT: Intravenous ribavirin decreases the mortality rate significantly in patients with severe Lassa fever, particularly if patients are treated during the first week of illness, and probably is beneficial in treating South American arenavirus infections. Immune plasma has been used as a therapeutic agent in regions of the world where Argentine HF is prevalent.

ISOLATION OF THE HOSPITALIZED PATIENT: In addition to standard precautions, contact and droplet precautions, including careful prevention of needlestick injuries and careful handling of clinical specimens for the duration of illness, are recommended for all hemorrhagic fevers caused by arenaviruses. A negative-pressure ventilation room is recommended for patients with prominent cough or severe disease, and people entering the room should wear personal protection respirators. Additional viral HF-specific isolation precautions have been recommended in the event that a viral HF virus is used as a weapon of biological terrorism.[1]

CONTROL MEASURES:

Care of Exposed People. No specific measures are warranted for exposed people unless direct contamination with blood, excretions, or secretions from an infected patient has occurred. If such contamination has occurred, recording temperature twice daily for 21 days is recommended, with prompt reporting of fever. Immediate therapy with intravenous ribavirin should be considered in patients with Lassa fever at the first sign of disease.

Immunoprophylaxis. An investigational live-attenuated Junin vaccine protects against Argentine HF and probably against Bolivian HF. The vaccine is associated with minimal adverse effects in adults; similar findings have been obtained from limited safety studies in children 4 years of age and older.

Environmental. In town-based outbreaks of Bolivian HF, rodent control has proven successful. Area rodent control is not practical for control of Argentine HF or Venezuelan HF. Intensive rodent control efforts modestly have decreased the rate of peridomestic Lassa virus infection, but rodents eventually reinvade human dwellings, and infection still occurs in rural settings.

Public Health Reporting. Because of the risk of health care-associated transmission, the state health department and the Centers for Disease Control and Prevention should be contacted for specific advice about management and diagnosis of suspected cases.

---

[1] Centers for Disease Control and Prevention. Update: management of patients with suspected viral hemorrhagic fever—United States. *MMWR Morb Mortal Wkly Rep.* 1995;44(25):475–479

Hemorrhagic Fevers and Related Syndromes Caused by Viruses of the Family Bunyaviridae[1]

CLINICAL MANIFESTATIONS: These zoonotic infections are severe febrile diseases in which shock and bleeding can be significant and multisystem involvement can occur. In the United States, one of these infections causes an illness marked by acute respiratory and cardiovascular failure (see Hantavirus Pulmonary Syndrome, p 321).

Hemorrhagic fever with renal syndrome (HFRS) is a complex, multiphasic disease characterized by vascular instability and varying degrees of renal insufficiency. Fever, flushing, conjunctival injection, abdominal pain, and lumbar pain are followed by hypotension, oliguria, and subsequently, polyuria. Petechiae and more serious bleeding manifestations are common. Shock and acute renal insufficiency may occur. Nephropathia epidemica, the clinical syndrome of HFRS in Europe, is a milder disease characterized by an influenza-like illness with abdominal pain and proteinuria. Acute renal dysfunction also occurs, but hypotensive shock or a requirement for dialysis are rare.

Crimean-Congo hemorrhagic fever (CCHF) is a multisystem disease characterized by hepatitis and profuse bleeding. Fever, headache, and myalgia are followed by signs of a diffuse capillary leak syndrome with facial suffusion, conjunctivitis, and proteinuria. Petechiae and purpura often appear on the skin and mucous membranes. A hypotensive crisis often occurs after the appearance of frank hemorrhage from the gastrointestinal tract, nose, mouth, or uterus.

Rift Valley fever (RVF), in most cases, is a self-limited febrile illness. Occasionally, hemorrhagic fever with shock and icterus, encephalitis, or retinitis develops.

ETIOLOGY: Bunyaviridae are segmented, single-stranded RNA viruses with different geographic distributions depending on their vector. Hemorrhagic fever syndromes are associated with viruses from 3 genera: hantaviruses, nairoviruses (CCHF virus), and phleboviruses (RVF and sandfly fever viruses). Old World hantaviruses (Hantaan, Seoul, Dobrava, and Puumala viruses) cause HFRS, and New World hantaviruses (Sin Nombre and related viruses) cause HPS (see Hantavirus Pulmonary Syndrome, p 321).

EPIDEMIOLOGY: The epidemiology of these diseases mainly is a function of the distribution and behavior of their reservoirs and vectors. All genera except hantaviruses are associated with arthropod vectors, and hantavirus infections are associated with exposure to infected rodents.

Classic HFRS occurs throughout much of Asia and Eastern and Western Europe, with up to 100 000 cases per year. The most severe form of the disease is caused by the prototype Hantaan virus and Dobrava viruses in rural Asia and Europe, respectively; Puumala virus is associated with milder disease (nephropathia epidemica) in Europe. Seoul virus is distributed worldwide in association with *Rattus* species and can cause a disease of variable severity. Person-to-person transmission never has been reported with HFRS.

Crimean-Congo hemorrhagic fever occurs in much of sub-Saharan Africa, the Middle East, areas in West and Central Asia, and the Balkans, with a recently described large endemic focus in Turkey. CCHF virus is transmitted by ticks and, occasionally, by contact with viremic animals at slaughter. Health care-associated transmission of CCHF is a serious hazard.

---

[1]Does not include hantavirus pulmonary syndrome, which is reviewed on p 321.

RVF occurs throughout sub-Saharan Africa and has caused epidemics in Egypt in 1977 and 1993–1995, Mauritania in 1987, Saudi Arabia and Yemen in 2000, and Kenya in 1997 and 2006–2007. The virus is arthropodborne and is transmitted from domestic livestock to humans by mosquitoes. The virus also can be transmitted by aerosol and by direct contact with infected aborted tissues or freshly slaughtered infected animal carcasses. Person-to-person transmission has not been reported.

The **incubation period**s for CCHF and RVF range from 2 to 10 days; for HFRS, incubation periods usually are longer, ranging from 7 to 42 days.

DIAGNOSTIC TESTS: CCHF and RVF viruses can be cultivated readily (restricted to Biosafety level-4 laboratories) from blood and tissue specimens of infected patients. Detection of viral antigen by enzyme immunoassay (EIA) is a useful alternative. Serum immunoglobulin (Ig) M and IgG virus-specific antibodies typically develop early in convalescence in CCHF and RVF. In HFRS, at the time of onset of illness or within 48 hours, IgM and IgG antibodies usually are detectable at a time when it is too late for virus isolation and antigen detection. IgM antibodies or rising IgG titers in paired serum specimens, as demonstrated by EIA, are diagnostic; neutralizing antibody tests provide greater virus-strain specificity. Immunofluorescent antibody tests also are used for serologic diagnosis. Polymerase chain reaction assay performed in containment laboratories can be a useful complement to serodiagnostic assays on samples obtained during the acute phase of CCHF, RVF, or HFRS. Diagnosis can be made retrospectively by immunohistochemistry assay of tissues obtained from necropsy.

TREATMENT: Ribavirin given intravenously to patients with HFRS within the first 4 days of illness seems effective in decreasing renal dysfunction, vascular instability, and mortality. Supportive therapy for HFRS should include: (1) avoidance of transporting patients; (2) treatment of shock; (3) monitoring of fluid balance; (4) dialysis for complications of renal failure; (5) control of hypertension during the oliguric phase; and (6) early recognition of possible myocardial failure with appropriate therapy.

Oral and intravenous ribavirin given to patients with CCHF has been associated with milder disease, although no controlled studies have been performed. Experimental animal data also suggest the potential benefit of ribavirin in treatment of hemorrhagic RVF.

ISOLATION OF THE HOSPITALIZED PATIENT: In addition to standard precautions, contact and droplet precautions, including careful prevention of needlestick injuries and management of clinical specimens, are indicated for patients with CCHF for the duration for their illness. Airborne isolation also may be required in certain circumstances when patients undergo procedures that stimulate coughing and promote generation of aerosols. Rift Valley fever and HFRS have not been demonstrated to be contagious, but standard precautions should be followed.

CONTROL MEASURES:

Care of Exposed People. People having direct contact with blood or other secretions from patients with CCHF should be observed closely for 14 days with daily monitoring for fever. Immediate therapy with intravenous ribavirin should be considered at the first sign of disease.

Environmental Immunoprophylaxis. Monitoring of laboratory rat colonies and urban rodent control may be effective for ratborne HFRS.

Crimean-Congo Hemorrhagic Fever. Arachnicides for tick control generally have limited benefit but should be used in stockyard settings. Personal protective measures (eg, physical tick removal and protective clothing with permethrin sprays) may be effective.

Rift Valley Fever. Immunization of domestic animals should have an effect on limiting or preventing RVF outbreaks and protecting humans. Mosquito control usually is not effective.

Public Health Reporting. Because of the risk of health care-associated transmission of CCHF and diagnostic confusion with other viral hemorrhagic fevers, the state health department and the Centers for Disease Control and Prevention should be contacted about any suspected diagnosis of viral hemorrhagic fever and the management plan for the patient.

Hepatitis A

CLINICAL MANIFESTATIONS: Hepatitis A characteristically is an acute, self-limited illness associated with fever, malaise, jaundice, anorexia, and nausea. Symptomatic hepatitis A virus (HAV) infection occurs in approximately 30% of infected children younger than 6 years of age; few of these children will have jaundice. Among older children and adults, infection usually is symptomatic and typically lasts several weeks, with jaundice occurring in 70% or more. Signs and symptoms typically last less than 2 months, although 10% to 15% of symptomatic people have prolonged or relapsing disease lasting as long as 6 months. Fulminant hepatitis is rare but is more common in people with underlying liver disease. Chronic infection does not occur.

ETIOLOGY: HAV is an RNA virus classified as a member of the picornavirus group.

EPIDEMIOLOGY: The most common mode of transmission is person to person, resulting from fecal contamination and oral ingestion (ie, the fecal-oral route). In developing countries, where infection is endemic, most people are infected during the first decade of life. In the United States, hepatitis A was one of the most frequently reported vaccine-preventable diseases in the prevaccine era, but incidence of disease attributable to HAV has declined since hepatitis A vaccine was licensed in 1995. In 2007, 2979 cases were reported to the Centers for Disease Control and Prevention (CDC), compared with 22 000 to 36 000 hepatitis A cases reported annually from 1980 through 1995. These declining rates have been accompanied by a shift in age-specific rates. Historically, the highest rates occurred among children 5 to 14 years of age, and the lowest rates occurred among adults older than 40 years of age. Beginning in the late 1990s, national age-specific rates declined more rapidly among children than among adults; as a result, in recent years, rates have been similar among all age groups. In addition, the previously observed unequal geographic distribution of hepatitis A incidence in the United States, with the highest rates of disease occurring in a limited number of states and communities, has disappeared after introduction of targeted immunization in 1999. Continued surveillance is needed to verify that the decline in incidence is sustained.

Among cases of hepatitis A reported to the CDC, recognized risk factors include close personal contact with a person infected with HAV, international travel, household or personal contact with a child who attends a child care center, a recognized foodborne outbreak, male homosexual activity, and use of illegal drugs. Transmission by blood transfusion or from mother to newborn infant (ie, vertical transmission) is limited to case reports. In approximately 50% of reported cases, the source cannot be determined. Fecal-oral spread from people with asymptomatic infections, particularly young children, likely accounts for many of these cases with an unknown source.

Before availability of vaccine, most HAV infection and illness occurred in the context of community-wide epidemics, in which infection primarily was transmitted in households and extended-family settings. However, community-wide epidemics have not been observed in recent years. Common-source foodborne outbreaks occur; waterborne outbreaks are rare. Health care-associated transmission is unusual, but outbreaks have occurred in neonatal intensive care units from neonates infected through transfused blood who subsequently transmitted HAV to other neonates and staff.

In child care centers, recognized symptomatic (icteric) illness occurs primarily among adult contacts of children. Most infected children younger than 6 years of age are asymptomatic or have nonspecific manifestations. Hence, spread of HAV infection within and outside a child care center often occurs before recognition of the index case(s). Outbreaks have occurred most commonly in large child care centers and specifically in facilities that enroll children in diapers.

Patients infected with HAV are most infectious during the 1 to 2 weeks before onset of jaundice or elevation of liver enzymes, when concentration of virus in the stool is highest. The risk of transmission subsequently diminishes and is minimal by 1 week after onset of jaundice. However, HAV can be detected in stool for longer periods, especially in neonates and young children.

The **incubation period** is 15 to 50 days, with an average of 28 days.

DIAGNOSTIC TESTS: Serologic tests for HAV-specific total (ie, immunoglobulin [Ig] G and IgM) antibody (anti-HAV) are available commercially. The presence of serum IgM anti-HAV indicates current or recent infection, although false-positive results may occur. IgM anti-HAV is detectable in up to 20% of vaccinees when measured 2 weeks after hepatitis A immunization. In most infected people, serum IgM anti-HAV becomes detectable 5 to 10 days before onset of symptoms and declines to undetectable concentrations less than 6 months after infection. However, people who test positive for IgM anti-HAV more than 1 year after infection have been reported. IgG anti-HAV is detectable shortly after the appearance of IgM. A positive total anti-HAV (ie, IgM and IgG) test result and a negative IgM anti-HAV test result indicate past infection and immunity.

TREATMENT: Supportive.

ISOLATION OF THE HOSPITALIZED PATIENT: In addition to standard precautions, contact precautions are recommended for diapered and incontinent patients for at least 1 week after onset of symptoms.

CONTROL MEASURES[1]:

General Measures. The major methods of prevention of HAV infections are improved sanitation (eg, in food preparation and of water sources) and personal hygiene (eg, hand hygiene after diaper changes in child care settings), immunization with hepatitis A vaccine, and administration of Immune Globulin (IG).

---

[1]Centers for Disease Control and Prevention. Prevention of hepatitis A through active or passive immunization: recommendations of the Advisory Committee on Immunization Practices (ACIP). *MMWR Recomm Rep.* 2006;55(RR-7):1–23

Schools, Child Care, and Work. Children and adults with acute HAV infection who work as food handlers or attend or work in child care settings should be excluded for 1 week after onset of the illness.

Immune Globulin. IG for intramuscular administration, when given within 2 weeks after exposure to HAV, is greater than 85% effective in preventing symptomatic infection. When administered for preexposure prophylaxis, 1 dose of 0.02 mL/kg confers protection against hepatitis A for up to 3 months, and a dose of 0.06 mL/kg protects for 3 to 5 months. Recommended preexposure and postexposure IG doses and duration of protection are given in Table 3.12 and Table 3.13 (p 332). Hepatitis A vaccine is preferred for preexposure protection in all populations unless contraindicated and for postexposure prophylaxis for most people 1 through 40 years of age (see Postexposure Prophylaxis, p 335).

Hepatitis A Vaccine. Two inactivated hepatitis A vaccines, Havrix and Vaqta, are available in the United States. The vaccines are prepared from cell culture-adapted HAV, which is propagated in human fibroblasts, purified from cell lysates, formalin inactivated, and adsorbed to an aluminum hydroxide adjuvant. Both hepatitis A vaccines are formulated without a preservative.

Administration, Dosages, and Schedules (see Table 3.14, p 332). Hepatitis A vaccines are licensed for people 12 months of age and older and have pediatric and adult formulations that are administered in a 2-dose schedule. The adult formulations are recommended for people 19 years of age and older. Recommended doses and schedules for these different products and formulations are given in Table 3.14, p 332. A combination hepatitis A/hepatitis B vaccine (Twinrix) is licensed in the United States for people 18 years of age and older and can be administered in a 3-dose schedule or an accelerated 4-dose schedule (see Table 3.14, p 332). All hepatitis A-containing vaccines are administered intramuscularly.

Table 3.12. Recommendations for Preexposure Immunoprophylaxis of Hepatitis A for Travelers

Age	Recommended Prophylaxis	Notes
Younger than 12 mo	IG	0.02 mL/kg[a] protects for up to 3 mo. For trips of 3 mo or longer, 0.06 mL/kg[a] should be given at departure and every 5 mo if exposure to HAV continues.
12 mo through 40 y	Hepatitis A vaccine	
41 y or older	Hepatitis A vaccine with or without IG	If departure is in less than 2 wk, older adults, immunocompromised people, and people with chronic liver disease or other chronic medical conditions can receive IG with the initial dose of hepatitis A vaccine to ensure optimal protection.

IG indicates Immune Globulin; HAV, hepatitis A virus.
[a]IG should be administered deep into a large muscle mass. Ordinarily, no more than 5 mL should be administered in one site in an adult or large child; lesser amounts (maximum 3 mL in one site) should be given to small children and infants.

Table 3.13. Recommendations for Postexposure Immunoprophylaxis of Hepatitis A

Time Since Exposure	Age of Patient	Recommended Prophylaxis
2 wk or less	Younger than 12 mo	IG, 0.02 mL/kg[a]
	12 mo through 40 y	Hepatitis A vaccine[b]
	41 y or older	IG, 0.02 mL/kg,[a] but hepatitis A vaccineb can be used if IG is unavailable[a]
	People of any age who are immunocompromised or have chronic liver disease	IG, 0.02 mL/kg[a]
More than 2 wk	Younger than 12 mo	No prophylaxis
	12 mo or older	No prophylaxis, but hepatitis A vaccine may be indicated for ongoing exposure[b]

IG indicates Immune Globulin.

[a]IG should be administered deep into a large muscle mass. Ordinarily, no more than 5 mL should be administered in one site in an adult or large child; lesser amounts (maximum 3 mL in one site) should be given to small children and infants.

[b]Dosage and schedule of hepatitis A vaccine as recommended according to age in Table 3.14, below.

Table 3.14. Recommended Doses and Schedules for Inactivated Hepatitis A Vaccines[a]

Age	Vaccine	Hepatitis A Antigen Dose	Volume per Dose, mL	No. of Doses	Schedule
12 mo through 18 y	Havrix	720 ELU	0.5	2	Initial and 6–12 mo later
12 mo through 18 y	Vaqta	25 U[b]	0.5	2	Initial and 6–18 mo later
19 y or older	Havrix	1440 ELU	1.0	2	Initial and 6–12 mo later
19 y or older	Vaqta	50 U[b]	1.0	2	Initial and 6–18 mo later
18 y or older	Twinrix[c]	720 ELU	1.0	3 or 4	Initial and 1 and 6 mo later **OR** Initial, 7 and 21–30 days, followed by a dose at 12 mo

ELU indicates enzyme-linked immunosorbent assay units.

[a]Havrix and Twinrix are manufactured by GlaxoSmithKline Biologicals; Vaqta is manufactured and distributed by Merck & Co Inc.

[b]Antigen units (each unit is equivalent to approximately 1 μg of viral protein).

[c]A combination of hepatitis B (Engerix-B, 20 μg) and hepatitis A (Havrix, 720 ELU) vaccine (Twinrix) is licensed for use in people 18 years of age and older in 3-dose and 4-dose schedules.

Immunogenicity. Available hepatitis A vaccines are highly immunogenic when given in their respective recommended schedules and doses. At least 95% of healthy children, adolescents, and adults have protective antibody concentrations when measured 1 month after receipt of the first dose of either single-antigen vaccine. One month after a second dose, more than 99% of healthy children, adolescents, and adults have protective antibody concentrations.

Available data on the immunogenicity of hepatitis A vaccine in infants indicate high rates of seroconversion, but antibody concentrations are lower in infants with passively acquired maternal anti-HAV in comparison with vaccine recipients lacking anti-HAV. By 12 months of age, passively acquired maternal anti-HAV antibody no longer is detectable in most infants. Hepatitis A vaccine is highly immunogenic for children who begin immunization at 12 months of age or older regardless of maternal anti-HAV status.

Efficacy. In double-blind, controlled, randomized trials, the protective efficacy in preventing clinical HAV infection was 94% to 100%.

Efficacy of Postexposure Immunization. A randomized clinical trial conducted among people 2 through 40 years of age comparing postexposure efficacy of IG and hepatitis A vaccine found that the efficacy of a single dose of hepatitis A vaccine was similar to that of IG in preventing symptomatic infection when administered within 14 days after exposure.

Duration of Protection. The need for additional booster doses beyond the 2-dose primary immunization series has not been determined, because long-term efficacy of hepatitis A vaccines has not been established. Detectable antibody persists after a 2-dose series for at least 10 years in adults and 5 to 6 years in children. Kinetic models of antibody decline indicate that protective levels of anti-HAV could be present for 25 years or longer in adults and 14 to 20 years in children.

Vaccine in Immunocompromised Patients. The immune response in immunocompromised people, including people with human immunodeficiency virus infection, may be suboptimal.

Vaccine Interchangeability. The 2 single-antigen hepatitis A vaccines licensed by the US Food and Drug Administration (FDA), when given as recommended, seem to be similarly effective. Studies among adults have found no difference in the immunogenicity of a vaccine series that mixed the 2 currently available vaccines, compared with using the same vaccine throughout the licensed schedule. Therefore, although completion of the immunization regimen with the same product is preferable, immunization with either product is acceptable.

Administration With Other Vaccines. Limited data indicate that hepatitis A vaccine may be administered simultaneously with other vaccines. Vaccines should be given in a separate syringe and at a separate injection site (see Simultaneous Administration of Multiple Vaccines, p 33).

Adverse Events. Adverse reactions are mild and include local pain and, less commonly, induration at the injection site. No serious adverse events attributed definitively to hepatitis A vaccine have been reported.

Precautions and Contraindications. The vaccine should not be administered to people with hypersensitivity to any of the vaccine components. Safety data in pregnant women are not available, but the risk is considered to be low or nonexistent, because the vaccine contains inactivated, purified, virus particles. Because hepatitis A vaccine is inactivated, no special precautions need to be taken when vaccinating immunocompromised people.

Preimmunization Serologic Testing. Preimmunization testing for anti-HAV generally is not recommended for children because of their expected low prevalence of infection. Testing may be cost-effective for people who have a high likelihood of immunity from previous infection, including people whose childhood was spent in a country with high endemicity, people with a history of jaundice potentially caused by HAV, and people older than 50 years of age.

Postimmunization Serologic Testing. Postimmunization testing for anti-HAV is not indicated because of the high seroconversion rates in adults and children. In addition, some commercially available anti-HAV tests may not detect low but protective concentrations of antibody among immunized people.

RECOMMENDATIONS FOR IMMUNOPROPHYLAXIS:

Preexposure Prophylaxis Against HAV Infection (see Tables 3.12, p 331, and 3.14, p 332). Hepatitis A immunization is recommended routinely for children 12 through 23 months of age, for people who are at increased risk of infection, for people who are at increased risk of severe manifestations of hepatitis A if infected, and for any person who wants to obtain immunity.

Children Who Routinely Should Be Immunized or Considered for Immunization.

- All children in the United States should receive hepatitis A vaccine at 12 through 23 months) of age, as recommended in the routine childhood immunization schedule (Fig 1.1, p 24–25). Table 3.14 (p 332) shows FDA-licensed hepatitis A-containing vaccines, doses, and schedules. Children who are not immunized by 2 years of age can be immunized at subsequent visits.

- States, counties, and communities with existing hepatitis A immunization programs for children 2 through 18 years of age are encouraged to maintain these programs. In these areas, new efforts focused on routine immunization of children 12 through 23 months of age should enhance, not replace, ongoing programs directed at a broader population of children.

- In areas without existing hepatitis A immunization programs, catch-up immunization of unimmunized children 2 through 18 years of age can be considered. Such programs might be warranted especially in the context of rising incidence or ongoing outbreaks among children or adolescents.

People at Increased Risk of HAV Infection or Its Consequences Who Routinely Should Be Immunized.

- **People traveling internationally.**[1] All susceptible people traveling to or working in countries that have high or intermediate hepatitis A endemicity should be immunized or receive IG before departure (see Table 3.12, p 331). Travelers to Western Europe, Scandinavia, Australia, Canada, Japan, and New Zealand (ie, countries in which endemicity is low) are at no greater risk of HAV infection than are people living in or traveling to the United States. Hepatitis A vaccine at the appropriate dose is preferred to IG. The first dose of hepatitis A vaccine should be administered as soon

---

[1]Centers for Disease Control and Prevention. Update: prevention of hepatitis A after exposure to hepatitis A virus and in international travelers. Updated recommendations of the Advisory Committee on Immunization Practices (ACIP). *MMWR Morb Mortal Wkly Rep.* 2007;56(41):1080–1084

as travel is considered. On the basis of limited data indicating equivalent postexposure efficacy of vaccine and IG among healthy people 40 years of age or younger, 1 dose of single-antigen vaccine administered at any time before departure can provide adequate protection for most healthy people. However, no data are available for other populations or other hepatitis A vaccine formulations (eg, the combination hepatitis A-hepatitis B vaccine). For optimal protection, older adults, immunocompromised people, and people with chronic liver disease or other chronic medical conditions who are traveling to an area with endemic infection in 2 weeks or less should receive the initial dose of vaccine and simultaneously can receive IG at a separate anatomic site. The vaccine series then should be completed according to the licensed schedule. Travelers who elect not to receive vaccine, are younger than 12 months of age, or are allergic to a vaccine component should receive a single dose of IG (0.02 mL/kg), which provides effective protection for up to 3 months.

- **Homosexual and bisexual men.** Outbreaks of hepatitis A among men who have sex with men have been reported often, including in urban areas in the United States, Canada, and Australia. Therefore, men (adolescents and adults) who have sex with men should be immunized. Preimmunization serologic testing may be cost-effective for older people in this group.
- **Users of injection and noninjection drugs.** Periodic outbreaks among injection and noninjection drug users have been reported in many parts of the United States and in Europe. Adolescents and adults who use illegal drugs should be immunized. Preimmunization serologic testing may be cost-effective for older people in this group.
- **Patients with clotting-factor disorders.** Reported outbreaks of hepatitis A in patients with hemophilia receiving solvent-detergent–treated factor VIII and factor IX concentrates were identified during the 1990s, primarily in Europe, although 1 case in the United States was reported. Therefore, susceptible patients who receive clotting-factor concentrates, especially people receiving solvent-detergent–treated preparations, should be immunized. Preimmunization testing for anti-HAV may be cost-effective for older people in this group.
- **People at risk of occupational exposure (eg, handlers of nonhuman primates and people working with HAV in a research laboratory setting).** Outbreaks of hepatitis A have been reported among people working with non-human primates. Infected primates were born in the wild, not primates that had been born and raised in captivity. People working with HAV-infected primates or with HAV in a research laboratory setting should be immunized.
- **People with chronic liver disease.** Because people with chronic liver disease are at increased risk of fulminant hepatitis A, susceptible patients with chronic liver disease should be immunized. Susceptible people who are awaiting or have received liver transplants should be immunized.

Postexposure Prophylaxis (see Table 3.13, p 332).[1] People who have been exposed to HAV and previously have not received hepatitis A vaccine should receive a single dose of single-antigen hepatitis A vaccine or IG as soon as possible (see Table 3.13 for prophylaxis guidance and dosages). The efficacy of IG or vaccine for postexposure prophylaxis when administered more than 2 weeks after exposure has not been established.

---

[1]Centers for Disease Control and Prevention. Update: prevention of hepatitis A after exposure to hepatitis A virus and in international travelers. Updated recommendations of the Advisory Committee on Immunization Practices (ACIP). *MMWR Morb Mortal Wkly Rep.* 2007;56(41):1080–1084

Information about the relative efficacy of vaccine compared with IG postexposure is limited, and no data are available for people older than 40 years of age or people with underlying medical conditions. For healthy people 12 months through 40 years of age, hepatitis A vaccine at the age-appropriate dose is preferred to IG because of vaccine advantages, including long-term protection and ease of administration. For people older than 40 years of age, IG is preferred because of the absence of data regarding vaccine performance in this age group and the increased risk of severe manifestations of hepatitis A with increasing age. However, vaccine can be used if IG is unavailable. The magnitude of risk of HAV transmission should be considered in decisions to use IG or vaccine. IG should be used for children younger than 12 months of age, immunocompromised people, people with chronic liver disease, and people for whom vaccine is contraindicated. People who are given IG and for whom hepatitis A vaccine also is recommended for other reasons should receive a dose of vaccine simultaneously with IG. For people who receive vaccine, the second dose should be given according to the licensed schedule to complete the series.

- **Household and sexual contacts.** All previously unimmunized people with close personal contact with a person with serologically confirmed HAV infection, such as household and sexual contacts, should receive vaccine or IG within 2 weeks after the most recent exposure (Table 3.13, p 332). Serologic testing of contacts is not recommended, because testing adds unnecessary cost and may delay administration of postexposure prophylaxis.
- **Newborn infants of HAV-infected mothers.** Perinatal transmission of HAV is rare. Some experts advise giving IG (0.02 mL/kg) to the infant if the mother's symptoms began between 2 weeks before and 1 week after delivery. Efficacy in this circumstance has not been established. Severe disease in healthy infants is rare.
- **Child care center staff, employees, and children and their household contacts.** Outbreaks of HAV infection at child care centers have been recognized since the 1970s, but their frequency has decreased as hepatitis A immunization rates in children have increased and as hepatitis A incidence among children has declined. Because infections in children usually are mild or asymptomatic, outbreaks often are identified only when adult contacts (eg, parents) become ill. Serologic testing to confirm HAV infection in suspected cases is indicated.

Vaccine or IG (Table 3.13, p 332) should be administered to all previously unimmunized staff members and attendees of child care centers or homes if (1) 1 or more cases of hepatitis A are recognized in children or staff members; or (2) cases are recognized in 2 or more households of center attendees. In centers that provide care only to children who do not wear diapers, vaccine or IG need be given only to classroom contacts of an index-case patient. When an outbreak occurs (ie, hepatitis A cases in 2 or more families), vaccine or IG also should be considered for members of households that have children (center attendees) in diapers.

Children and adults with hepatitis A should be excluded from the center until 1 week after onset of illness, until the postexposure prophylaxis program has been completed in the center, or until directed by the health department. Although precise data concerning the onset of protection after postexposure prophylaxis are not available, allowing prophylaxis recipients to return to the child care center setting immediately after receipt of the vaccine or IG dose seems reasonable.

- **Schools.** Schoolroom exposure generally does not pose an appreciable risk of infection, and postexposure prophylaxis is not indicated when a single case occurs and the source of infection is outside the school. However, hepatitis A vaccine or IG could be used for unimmunized people who have close contact with the index patient if transmission within the school setting is documented.
- **Hospitals.** Usually, health care-associated hepatitis A in hospital personnel has occurred through spread from patients with acute HAV infection in whom the diagnosis was not recognized. Careful hygienic practices should be emphasized when a patient with jaundice or known or suspected hepatitis A is admitted to the hospital. When outbreaks occur, hepatitis A vaccine or IG is recommended for people in close contact with infected patients (Table 3.13, p 332). Routine preexposure use of hepatitis A vaccine for hospital personnel is not recommended.
- **Exposure to an infected food handler.** If a food handler is diagnosed with hepatitis A, vaccine or IG should be provided to other food handlers at the same establishment (Table 3.13, p 332). Food handlers with acute HAV infection should be excluded for 1 week after onset of illness. Because common-source transmission to patrons is unlikely, postexposure prophylaxis with vaccine or IG typically is not indicated but may be considered if the food handler directly handled food during the time when the food handler likely was infectious and had diarrhea or poor hygiene practices, and prophylaxis can be provided within 2 weeks of exposure. Routine hepatitis A immunization of food handlers is not recommended.
- **Common-source exposure.** Postexposure prophylaxis usually is not recommended, because these outbreaks commonly are recognized too late for prophylaxis to be effective in preventing HAV infection in exposed people. Hepatitis A vaccine or IG can be considered if it can be administered to exposed people within 2 weeks of an exposure to the HAV-contaminated water or food.

Hepatitis B

CLINICAL MANIFESTATIONS: People acutely infected with hepatitis B virus (HBV) may be asymptomatic or symptomatic. The likelihood of developing symptoms of acute hepatitis is age dependent: less than 1% of infants younger than 1 year of age, 5% to 15% of children 1 to 5 years of age, and 30% to 50% of people older than 5 years of age are symptomatic. Among people with symptomatic HBV infection, the spectrum of signs and symptoms is varied and includes subacute illness with nonspecific symptoms (eg, anorexia, nausea, or malaise), clinical hepatitis with jaundice, or fulminant hepatitis. Extrahepatic manifestations, such as arthralgia, arthritis, macular rashes, thrombocytopenia, or papular acrodermatitis (Gianotti-Crosti syndrome), can occur early in the course of the illness and may precede jaundice. Acute HBV infection cannot be distinguished from other forms of acute viral hepatitis on the basis of clinical signs and symptoms or nonspecific laboratory findings.

Chronic HBV infection is defined as presence of hepatitis B surface antigen (HBsAg) in serum for at least 6 months or by the presence of HBsAg in a person who tests negative for antibody of the immunoglobulin (Ig) M subclass to hepatitis B core antigen (IgM anti-HBc).

Age at the time of acute infection is the primary determinant of the risk of progressing to chronic infection. More than 90% of infants infected perinatally will develop chronic HBV infection. Between 25% and 50% of children infected between 1 and 5 years of age become chronically infected, whereas only 2% to 6% of acutely infected older children and adults develop chronic HBV infections. Patients who develop acute HBV infection while immunosuppressed or with an underlying chronic illness have an increased risk of developing chronic infection. In the absence of treatment, up to 25% of infants and children who acquire chronic HBV infection will die prematurely from HBV-related hepatocellular carcinoma or cirrhosis.

The clinical course of untreated chronic HBV infection varies according to the population studied, reflecting differences in the age at acquisition, the rate of loss of hepatitis B e antigen (HBeAg), and possibly, HBV genotype. Perinatally infected children usually have normal alanine transaminase (ALT) concentrations and minimal or mild liver histologic abnormalities for years to decades after initial infection ("immune tolerant phase"). Chronic HBV infection acquired during later childhood or adolescence usually is accompanied by more active liver disease and increased serum transaminase concentrations. Patients with detectable HBeAg *(HBeAg-positive chronic hepatitis B)* usually have high concentrations of HBV DNA and HBsAg in serum and are more likely to transmit infection. Because HBV-associated liver injury is thought to be immune-mediated, in people coinfected with human immunodeficiency virus (HIV) and HBV, the return of immune competence with antiretroviral treatment of HIV infection may lead to a reactivation of HBV-related liver inflammation and damage. Over time (years to decades), HBeAg becomes undetectable in many chronically infected people. This transition often is accompanied by development of antibody to HBeAg (anti-HBe) and decreases in serum HBV DNA and serum transaminase concentrations and may be preceded by a temporary exacerbation of liver disease. These patients have *inactive chronic infection* but still may have exacerbations of hepatitis. Serologic reversion (reappearance of HBeAg) is more common if loss of HBeAg is not accompanied by development of anti-HBe; reversion with loss of anti-HBe also can occur.

Some patients who lose HBeAg may continue to have ongoing histologic evidence of liver damage and moderate to high concentrations of HBV DNA *(HBeAg-negative chronic hepatitis B)*. Patients with histologic evidence of chronic HBV infection, regardless of HBeAg status, remain at higher risk of death attributable to liver failure compared with HBV-infected people with no histologic evidence of liver inflammation and fibrosis. Other factors that may influence natural history of chronic infection include gender, race, alcohol use, and coinfection with hepatitis C or hepatitis D viruses.

Resolved hepatitis B is defined as clearance of HBsAg, normalization of serum transaminase concentrations, and development of antibody to HBsAg (anti-HBs). Chronically infected adults clear HBsAg and develop anti-HBs at the rate of 1% to 2% annually; during childhood, the annual clearance rate is less than 1%. Reactivation of resolved chronic infection is possible if these patients become immunosuppressed.

ETIOLOGY: Hepatitis B virus is a DNA-containing, 42-nm-diameter hepadnavirus. Important components of the viral particle include an outer lipoprotein envelope containing HBsAg and an inner nucleocapsid consisting of hepatitis B core antigen. Antibody to HBsAg (anti-HBs) provides protection from HBV infection. The viral polymerase can be detected in preparations of plasma containing HBV.

EPIDEMIOLOGY: HBV is transmitted through infected blood or body fluids. Although HBsAg has been detected in multiple body fluids, only serum, semen, and saliva have been demonstrated to be infectious. People with chronic HBV infection are the primary reservoirs for infection. Common modes of transmission include percutaneous and permucosal exposure to infectious body fluids, sharing or using nonsterilized needles or syringes, sexual contact with an infected person, and perinatal exposure to an infected mother. Transmission by transfusion of contaminated blood or blood products is rare in the United States because of routine screening of blood donors and viral inactivation of certain blood products (see Blood Safety, p 106).

Perinatal transmission of HBV is highly efficient and usually occurs from blood exposures during labor and delivery. In utero transmission of HBV is rare, accounting for less than 2% of perinatal infections in most studies. The risk of an infant acquiring HBV from an infected mother as a result of perinatal exposure is 70% to 90% for infants born to mothers who are HBsAg and HBeAg positive; the risk is 5% to 20% for infants born to HBsAg-positive but HBeAg-negative mothers.

Person-to-person spread of HBV can occur in settings involving interpersonal contact over extended periods, such as in a household with a person with chronic HBV infection. In regions of the world with a high prevalence of chronic HBV infection, horizontal transmission between children in household settings may account for a substantial amount of transmission. The precise mechanisms of transmission from child to child are unknown; however, frequent interpersonal contact of nonintact skin or mucous membranes with blood-containing secretions or, perhaps, saliva probably are the most likely means of transmission. Transmission from sharing inanimate objects, such as razors or toothbrushes, also may occur. HBV can survive in the environment for 1 week or longer but is inactivated by commonly used disinfectants, including household bleach diluted 1:10 with water. HBV is not transmitted by the fecal-oral route.

Transmission among children in the United States is unusual because of high coverage with hepatitis B vaccine. Unimmunized children living in immigrant families from countries where HBV infection is endemic (eg, Southeast Asia, China, Africa) are at risk of infection. Other children at increased risk of infection include residents of institutions for people with developmental disabilities and patients undergoing hemodialysis. Person-to-person transmission has been reported in child care settings, but risk of transmission in child care facilities in the United States has become negligible as a result of high infant hepatitis B immunization rates.

Acute HBV infection occurs most commonly among adolescents and adults in the United States. Since 1990, the incidence of acute hepatitis B has declined in all age categories, with the largest declines occurring in children younger than 15 years of age (98%) and young adults 15 through 24 years of age (90%). Groups at highest risk include users of injection drugs, people with multiple heterosexual partners, and men who have sex with men. Others at increased risk include people with occupational exposure to blood or body fluids, staff of institutions and nonresidential child care programs for children with developmental disabilities, patients undergoing hemodialysis, and sexual or household contacts of people with an acute or chronic infection. Approximately 15% of infected people do not have a readily identifiable risk characteristic. HBV infection in adolescents and adults is associated with other sexually transmitted infections, including syphilis and human immunodeficiency virus (HIV).

The prevalence of HBV infection and patterns of transmission vary markedly throughout the world (see Table 3.15). Approximately 45% of people worldwide live in regions of high HBV endemicity, where the prevalence of chronic HBV infection is greater than 8%. Historically in these regions, most new infections occurred as a result of perinatal or early childhood infections. In regions of intermediate HBV endemicity, where the prevalence of HBV infection is 2% to 7%, multiple modes of transmission (ie, perinatal, household, sexual, injection drug use, and health care-associated) contribute to the burden of infection. In countries of low endemicity, where chronic HBV infection prevalence is less than 2% (including the United States), most new infections occur among adolescents and adults and are attributable to sexual and injection drug use exposures. However, many people born in countries with high endemicity live in the United States. Infant immunization programs in many countries with high and intermediate endemicity have reduced greatly the seroprevalence of HBsAg among immunized children. For example, among Alaska Native people in a region where 16% of unimmunized people 11 through 30 years of age were infected chronically, none of the children 10 years of age or younger were found to be infected chronically after implementation of a routine hepatitis B immunization program.

The **incubation period** for acute infection is 45 to 160 days, with an average of 90 days.

DIAGNOSTIC TESTS: Serologic antigen tests are available commercially to detect HBsAg and HBeAg. Serologic assays also are available for detection of anti-HBs, anti-HBc, IgM anti-HBc, and anti-HBe (see Table 3.16, p 341). In addition, hybridization assays, nucleic acid amplification testing, and gene-amplification techniques (eg, polymerase

Table 3.15. Estimated International HBsAg Prevalence[a]

Region	Estimated HBsAg Prevalence
North America	0.1%
Mexico and Central America	0.3%
Caribbean (except Haiti)	1.0%
Haiti	5.6%
South America	0.7%
Western Europe	0.7%
Eastern Europe and North Asia	2.8%
Africa	9.3%
Middle East	3.2%
East Asia	7.4%
Southeast Asia	9.1%
South Asia	2.8%
Australia and New Zealand	0.9%
Pacific Islands	12.0%

HBsAg indicates hepatitis B surface antigen.
[a]Centers for Disease Control and Prevention. A comprehensive immunization strategy to eliminate transmission of hepatitis B virus infection in the United States. Recommendations of the Advisory Committee on Immunization Practices (ACIP). Part II: immunization of adults. *MMWR Recomm Rep.* 2006;55(RR-16):1–33.

Table 3.16. Diagnostic Tests for Hepatitis B Virus (HBV) Antigens and Antibodies

Factors To Be Tested	HBV Antigen or Antibody	Use
HBsAg	Hepatitis B surface antigen	Detection of acutely or chronically infected people; antigen used in hepatitis B vaccine
Anti-HBs	Antibody to HBsAg	Identification of people who have resolved infections with HBV; determination of immunity after immunization
HBeAg	Hepatitis B e antigen	Identification of infected people at increased risk of transmitting HBV
Anti-HBe	Antibody to HBeAg	Identification of infected people with lower risk of transmitting HBV
Anti-HBc	Antibody to HBcAg[a]	Identification of people with acute, resolved, or chronic HBV infection (not present after immunization)
IgM anti-HBc	IgM antibody to HBcAg	Identification of people with acute or recent HBV infections (including HBsAg-negative people during the "window" phase of infection)

HBcAg indicates hepatitis B core antigen; IgM, immunoglobulin M.
[a]No test is available commercially to measure HBcAg.

chain reaction, branched DNA methods) are available to detect and quantify HBV DNA. HBsAg is detectable during acute infection. If infection is self-limited, HBsAg disappears in most patients within a few weeks to several months after infection, followed by appearance of anti-HBs. The brief time between disappearance of HBsAg and appearance of anti-HBs is termed the *window period* of infection. During the window period, the only marker of acute infection is IgM anti-HBc, which is highly specific for establishing the diagnosis of acute infection. However, IgM anti-HBc usually is not present in infants infected perinatally. People with chronic HBV infection have circulating HBsAg and anti-HBc; on rare occasions, anti-HBs also is present. Both anti-HBs and anti-HBc are detected in people with resolved infection, whereas anti-HBs alone is present in people immunized with hepatitis B vaccine. The presence of HBeAg in serum correlates with higher concentrations of HBV and greater infectivity. Tests for HBeAg and HBV DNA are useful in the selection of candidates to receive antiviral therapy and to monitor the response to therapy.

TREATMENT: No specific therapy for acute HBV infection is available. Hepatitis B Immune Globulin (HBIG) and corticosteroids are not effective.

Current indications for treatment of chronic HBV infection include evidence of ongoing HBV viral replication, as indicated by the presence for longer than 6 months of serum HBV DNA greater than 20 000 IU/mL with or without HBeAg positivity and either serum alanine aminotransferase (ALT) concentrations at least twice the upper limit of normal for longer than 6 months or evidence of chronic hepatitis on liver biopsy.

Children without necroinflammatory liver disease usually do not warrant antiviral therapy. Treatment is not recommended for children with immunotolerant chronic HBV infection (ie, normal serum transaminase concentrations despite HBV DNA presence). There are few large randomized controlled trials of antiviral therapies for chronic hepatitis B in childhood. Chronic HBV infection in children can be treated with the following US Food and Drug Administration (FDA)-approved drugs: interferon-alfa (interferon alfa-2b and pegylated interferon alfa-2a) and lamivudine. The optimal agent and duration of therapy for chronic hepatitis B in children remain unclear. Studies indicate that approximately 24% to 30% of children with increased transaminase concentrations who are treated with interferon alfa-2b for 6 months lose HBeAg, compared with approximately 10% of untreated controls. Interferon-alfa is less effective for chronic infections acquired during early childhood, especially if transaminase concentrations are normal. Children with chronic HBV infection who were treated with lamivudine had higher rates of virologic response (loss of detectable HBV DNA and loss of HBeAg) after 1 year of treatment than did children who received placebo (23% vs 13%). Although resistance to lamivudine develops quickly, therapy is continued. Children coinfected with HIV and HBV should receive the lamivudine dose approved for treatment of HIV. Consultation with health care professionals with expertise in treating chronic hepatitis B in children is recommended.

The FDA has approved nucleoside analogues (ie, lamivudine, entecavir, and telbivudine) and a nucleotide analogue (adefovir) for treatment of chronic HBV infection in adults, but safety and effectiveness for children have not been established. Other nucleoside analogs are being developed.

Children and adolescents who have chronic HBV infection are at risk of developing serious liver disease, including primary hepatocellular carcinoma (HCC), with advancing age. Although the peak incidence of primary HCC attributable to HBV infection is in the fifth decade of life, HCC occasionally occurs in children who become infected perinatally or in early childhood. Children with chronic HBV infection should be screened periodically for hepatic complications using serum liver transaminase tests, alpha-fetoprotein concentration, and abdominal ultrasonography. Definitive recommendations on the frequency and indications for specific tests are not yet available because of a lack of data on their reliability in predicting sequelae. Patients with persistently elevated serum ALT concentrations (exceeding twice the upper limit of normal) and patients with an increased serum alpha-fetoprotein concentration or abnormal findings on abdominal ultrasonography should be referred to a specialist in management of chronic HBV infection for further management. All patients with chronic HBV infection who are not immune to hepatitis A should receive hepatitis A vaccine.

ISOLATION OF THE HOSPITALIZED PATIENT: Standard precautions are indicated for patients with acute or chronic HBV infection. For infants born to HBsAg-positive mothers, no special care in addition to standard precautions, other than removal of maternal blood by a gloved attendant, is necessary.

CONTROL MEASURES:

Strategy for Prevention of HBV Infection. The primary goal of hepatitis B prevention programs is decreasing the rates of chronic HBV infection and HBV-related chronic liver disease. A secondary goal is prevention of acute HBV infection. In the United States over the past 2 decades, a comprehensive immunization strategy to eliminate HBV transmission has been implemented progressively and now includes the following 4 components[1,2]: (1) universal immunization of infants beginning at birth; (2) prevention of perinatal HBV infection through routine screening of all pregnant women and appropriate immunoprophylaxis of infants born to HBsAg-positive women and infants born to women with unknown HBsAg status; (3) routine immunization of children and adolescents who previously have not been immunized; and (4) immunization of previously unimmunized adults at increased risk of infection.

Hepatitis B Immunoprophylaxis. Two types of products are available for immunoprophylaxis. Hepatitis B Immune Globulin (HBIG) provides short-term protection (3–6 months) and is indicated only in specific postexposure circumstances (see Care of Exposed People, p 352). Hepatitis B vaccine is used for preexposure and postexposure protection and provides long-term protection. Preexposure immunization with hepatitis B vaccine is the most effective means to prevent HBV transmission. Accordingly, hepatitis B immunization is recommended for all infants, children, and adolescents through 18 years of age. Infants should be immunized as part of the routine childhood immunization schedule. All children 11 through 12 years of age should have a review of their immunization records and should complete the vaccine series if they have not received the vaccine or are immunized incompletely.

Postexposure immunoprophylaxis with either hepatitis B vaccine and HBIG or hepatitis B vaccine alone effectively prevents infection after exposure to HBV. Effectiveness of postexposure immunoprophylaxis is related directly to the time elapsed between exposure and administration. Immunoprophylaxis is most effective if given within 12 to 24 hours of exposure. Serologic testing of all pregnant women for HBsAg is essential for identifying women whose infants will require postexposure immunoprophylaxis beginning at birth (see Care of Exposed People, p 352).

Hepatitis B Immune Globulin.[3] HBIG is prepared from hyperimmunized donors whose plasma is known to contain a high concentration of anti-HBs, to be negative for antibodies to HIV and hepatitis C virus (HCV), and to be negative for HCV RNA. The process used to prepare HBIG inactivates or eliminates HBV, HIV, and HCV. Standard Immune Globulin is not effective for postexposure prophylaxis against HBV infection, because concentrations of anti-HBs are too low.

Hepatitis B Vaccine. Highly effective and safe hepatitis B vaccines produced by recombinant DNA technology are licensed in the United States in single-antigen formulations and as components of combination vaccines. Plasma-derived hepatitis B vaccines no longer are available in the United States but are used successfully in some countries. The recombinant vaccines contain 10 to 40 µg of HBsAg protein/mL. Pediatric formulations contain no thimerosal or only trace amounts. Although the concentration of recombinant

[1]Centers for Disease Control and Prevention. A comprehensive immunization strategy to eliminate transmission of hepatitis B virus infection in the United States: recommendations of the Advisory Committee on Immunization Practices (ACIP) part 1: immunization of infants, children, and adolescents. *MMWR Recomm Rep.* 2005;54(RR-16):1–31

[2]Centers for Disease Control and Prevention. A comprehensive immunization strategy to eliminate transmission of hepatitis B virus infection in the United States: recommendations of the Advisory Committee on Immunization Practices (ACIP) part II: immunization of adults. *MMWR Recomm Rep.* 2006;55(RR-16):1–33

[3]Dosages recommended for postexposure prophylaxis are for products licensed in the United States. Because concentration of anti-HBs in other products may vary, different dosages may be recommended in other countries.

HBsAg protein differs among vaccine products, rates of seroconversion are equivalent when given to immunocompetent infants, children, adolescents, or young adults in the doses recommended (see Table 3.17).

Hepatitis B vaccine can be given concurrently with other vaccines (see Simultaneous Administration of Multiple Vaccines, p 33).

Vaccine Interchangeability. In general, the various brands of age-appropriate hepatitis B vaccines are interchangeable within an immunization series. The immune response using 1 or 2 doses of a vaccine produced by one manufacturer followed by 1 or more subsequent doses from a different manufacturer is comparable to a full course of immunization with a single product. However, until additional data supporting inter-changeability of acellular pertussis-containing hepatitis B combination vaccines are available, vaccines from the same manufacturer should be used, whenever feasible, for at least

Table 3.17. Recommended Dosages of Hepatitis B Vaccines

Patients	Vaccine[a]		Combination Vaccine
	Recombivax HB[b] Dose, μg (mL)	Engerix-B[c] Dose, μg (mL)	Twinrix[d]
Infants of HBsAg-negative mothers and children and adolescents younger than 20 y of age	5 (0.5)	10 (0.5)	Not applicable
Infants of HBsAg-positive mothers (HBIG [0.5 mL] also is recommended)	5 (0.5)	10 (0.5)	Not applicable
Adults 20 y of age or older	10 (1.0)	20 (1.0)	20 (1.0)
Adults undergoing dialysis and other immunosuppressed adults	40 (1.0)[e]	40 (2.0)[f]	Not applicable

HBsAg indicates hepatitis B surface antigen; HBIG, Hepatitis B Immune Globulin.

[a]Both vaccines are administered in a 3-dose schedule; 4 doses may be administered if a birth dose is given and a combination vaccine is used to complete the series. Only single-antigen hepatitis B vaccine can be used for the birth dose. Single-antigen or combination vaccine containing hepatitis B vaccine may be used to complete the series.

[b]Available from Merck & Co Inc.
- A 2-dose schedule, administered at 0 months and then 4 to 6 months later, is licensed for adolescents 11 through 15 years of age using the adult formulation of Recombivax HB (10 μg).
- A combination of hepatitis B (Recombivax, 5 μg) and *Haemophilus influenzae* type b (PRP-OMP) vaccine is recommended for use at 2, 4, and 12 through 15 months of age (Comvax). This vaccine should not be administered at birth, before 6 weeks of age, or after 71 months of age. For additional information, see *Haemophilus influenzae* Infections (p 314).

[c]Available from GlaxoSmithKline Biologicals. The US Food and Drug Administration also has licensed this vaccine for use in an optional 4-dose schedule at 0, 1, 2, and 12 months for all age groups. A 0-, 12-, and 24-month schedule is licensed for children 5 through 16 years of age, and a 0-, 1-, and 6-month schedule is licensed for adolescents 11 through 16 years of age.
- A combination of diphtheria and tetanus toxoids and acellular pertussis (DTaP), inactivated poliovirus (IPV), and hepatitis B (Engerix-B 10 μg) is recommended for use at 2, 4, and 6 months of age (Pediarix). This vaccine should not be administered at birth, before 6 weeks of age, or at 7 years of age or older. For additional information, see Pertussis (p 504).

[d]A combination of hepatitis B (Engerix-B, 20 μg) and hepatitis A (Havrix, 720 enzyme-linked immunosorbent assay units [ELU]) vaccine (Twinrix) is licensed for use in people 18 years of age and older in a 3-dose schedule administered at 0 mo, 1 mo, and 6 or more months later. Alternately, a 4-dose schedule at days 0, 7, and 21 to 30 followed by a booster dose at 12 months may be used.

[e]Special formulation for adult dialysis patients given at 0, 1, 2, and 6 months.

[f]Two 1.0-mL doses given in 1 or 2 injections in a 4-dose schedule at 0, 1, 2, and 6 months of age.

the first 3 doses in the pertussis series (see Pertussis, p 504). In addition, a 2-dose schedule for adolescents 11 through 15 years of age is licensed only for Recombivax HB.

Routes of Administration. Vaccine is administered intramuscularly in the antero-lateral thigh or deltoid area, depending on the age and size of the recipient (see Vaccine Administration, p 17). Administration in the buttocks or intradermally has been associated with decreased immunogenicity and is not recommended at any age.

Efficacy and Duration of Protection. Hepatitis B vaccines licensed in the United States have a 90% to 95% efficacy for preventing HBV infection and clinical HBV infection among susceptible children and adults. Long-term studies of immunocompetent adults and children indicate that immune memory remains intact for up to 2 decades and protects against symptomatic acute infections and chronic HBV infection, even though anti-HBs concentrations may become low or undetectable over time. Breakthrough infections (detected by presence of anti-HBc or HBV DNA) have occurred in a limited number of immunized people, but these infections typically are transient and asymptomatic. Chronic HBV infection in immunized people has been documented in dialysis patients whose anti-HBs concentrations fell below 10 mIU/mL and rarely in infants born to HBsAg-positive mothers.

Booster Doses. For children and adults with normal immune status, routine booster doses of vaccine are not recommended. For hemodialysis patients and other immuno-compromised people at continued risk of infection, the need for booster doses should be assessed by annual anti-HBs testing, and a booster dose should be given when the anti-HBs concentration is less than 10 mIU/mL.

Adverse Reactions. The adverse effects most commonly reported in adults and children are pain at the injection site, reported by 3% to 29% of recipients, and a temperature greater than 37.7°C (99.8°F), reported by 1% to 6% of recipients. Anaphylaxis is uncommon, occurring in approximately 1 in 600 000 recipients, according to vaccine adverse events passive reporting surveillance systems. Large, controlled epidemiologic studies show no association between hepatitis B vaccine and sudden infant death syndrome, diabetes mellitus, or demyelinating disease, including multiple sclerosis.

Immunization During Pregnancy or Lactation. No adverse effect on the developing fetus has been observed when pregnant women have been immunized. Because HBV infection may result in severe disease in the mother and chronic infection in the newborn infant, pregnancy is not a contraindication to immunization. Lactation is not a contraindication to immunization.

Serologic Testing. Susceptibility testing before immunization is not indicated routinely for children or adolescents. Testing for previous infection may be considered for people in risk groups with high rates of HBV infection, such as people born in countries with intermediate and high HBV endemicity, users of injection drugs, homosexually or bisexually active men, and household contacts of HBsAg-positive people, provided testing does not delay or impede immunization efforts.

Routine postimmunization testing for anti-HBs is not necessary but is recommended 1 to 2 months after the third vaccine dose for the following specific groups: (1) hemodialysis patients; (2) people with HIV infection; (3) people at occupational risk of exposure from needlestick injuries (certain health care and public safety workers); (4) immunocompromised patients at risk of exposure to HBV; and (5) regular sexual contacts of HBsAg-positive people. Infants born to HBsAg-positive mothers should have postimmunization testing for HBsAg and anti-HBs performed at 9 to 18 months of age, generally at the next well-child visit after completion of the vaccine series (see Prevention of Perinatal HBV Infection, p 352).

Management of Nonresponders. Vaccine recipients who do not develop a serum anti-HBs response (10 mIU/mL or greater) after a primary vaccine series should be reimmunized (unless they are determined to be HBsAg positive) with an additional 3-dose series. People who remain anti-HBs negative 1 to 2 months after a reimmunization series are unlikely to respond to additional doses of vaccine.

Altered Doses and Schedules. Larger vaccine doses are required to induce protective anti-HBs concentrations in adult hemodialysis patients and for immunocompromised adults, including HIV-seropositive people (see Table 3.17, p 344). Humoral immune response to hepatitis B vaccine also may be reduced in children and adolescents who are receiving hemodialysis or are immunocompromised. However, few data exist concerning the response to higher doses of vaccine in children and adolescents, and no specific recommendations can be made. For people with progressive chronic renal failure, hepatitis B vaccine is recommended early in the disease course to provide protection and potentially decrease the need for larger doses once dialysis is initiated. A 2-dose schedule of the adult formulation of Recombivax is licensed for 11- through 15-year-olds; the second dose is given 4 to 6 months after the first dose (see Table 3.17, p 344).

Preexposure Universal Immunization of Infants, Children, and Adolescents. Hepatitis B immunization is recommended for all infants, children, and adolescents through 18 years of age. Delivery hospitals should develop policies and procedures that ensure administration of a birth dose as part of the routine care of all medically stable infants weighing 2000 g or more at birth, unless there is a physician's order to defer immunization and a report of the serologic status of the mother is in the infant's medical record. The hepatitis B vaccine series (3 or 4 doses; see discussion about birth dose in next paragraph) for infants born to HBsAg-negative mothers should be completed by 6 to 18 months of age. All children and adolescents who have not been immunized against HBV should begin the series during any visit.

High seroconversion rates and protective concentrations of anti-HBs (10 mIU/mL or greater) are achieved when hepatitis B vaccine is administered in any of the various recommended schedules, including schedules begun soon after birth in term infants. Only single-antigen hepatitis B vaccine can be used for doses given between birth and 6 weeks of age. Single-antigen or combination vaccine may be used to complete the series; 4 doses of vaccine may be administered if a birth dose is given and a combination vaccine containing a hepatitis B component is used to complete the series.[1] For guidelines for minimum scheduling time between vaccine doses for infants, see Table 1.5 (p 22). The schedule should be chosen to facilitate a high rate of adherence to the primary vaccine series. For immunization of older children and adolescents, doses may be given in a schedule of 0, 1, and 6 months; of 0, 1, and 4 months; or of 0, 2, and 4 months. For older children and adolescents, spacing at 0, 12, and 24 months results in equivalent immunogenicity and can be used when an extended administration schedule is acceptable on the basis of risk of exposure. A 2-dose schedule for one vaccine formulation is licensed for people 11 through 15 years of age; the schedule is 0 and then 4 to 6 months later (see Table 3.17, p 344).

---

[1] Centers for Disease Control and Prevention. General recommendations of the Advisory Committee on Immunization Practices (ACIP). *MMWR Recomm Rep.* 2009; in press

The recommended schedule for routine hepatitis B immunization of infants born to HBsAg-negative mothers is given in Fig 1.1 (p 24–25). Age-specific vaccine dosages are given in Table 3.17 (p 344). Combination products containing hepatitis B vaccine may be given in the United States, provided they are licensed by the US Food and Drug Administration for the child's current age and administration of the other vaccine component(s) also is indicated. Children and adolescents who previously have not received hepatitis B vaccine should be immunized routinely at any age with the age-appropriate doses and schedule. Selection of a vaccine schedule should consider the need to achieve completion of the vaccine series. In all settings, immunization should be initiated even though completion of the vaccine series might not be ensured.

Preexposure Immunization of Adults.[1]

- Hepatitis B immunization is recommended as a 3-dose series for all unimmunized adults at risk of HBV infection (see Table 3.18, p 348) and for all adults seeking protection from HBV infection. Acknowledgment of a specific risk factor is not a requirement for immunization.

- In settings where a high proportion of adults are likely to have risk factors for HBV infection, all unimmunized adults should be assumed to be at risk and should receive hepatitis B immunization. These settings include (1) sexually transmitted infection treatment facilities; (2) HIV testing and treatment facilities; (3) facilities providing drug abuse treatment and prevention services; (4) health care settings targeting services to injection drug users; (5) correctional facilities; (6) health care settings serving men who have sex with men; (7) chronic hemodialysis facilities and end-stage renal disease programs; and (8) institutions and nonresidential care facilities for people with developmental disabilities.

- Standing orders should be implemented to identify and immunize eligible adults in primary care and specialty medical settings. If ascertainment of risk for HBV infection is a barrier to immunization in these settings, health care professionals may use alternative immunization strategies, such as offering hepatitis B vaccine to all unimmunized adults in age groups with highest risk of infection (eg, younger than 45 years of age).

Lapsed Immunizations. For infants, children, adolescents, and adults with lapsed immunizations (ie, the interval between doses is longer than that in one of the recommended schedules), the vaccine series can be completed, regardless of the interval from the last dose of vaccine (see Lapsed Immunizations, p 34).

SPECIAL CONSIDERATIONS:

Preterm Infants. Studies demonstrate that decreased seroconversion rates might occur among certain preterm infants with low birth weight (ie, less than 2000 g) after administration of hepatitis B vaccine at birth. However, by the chronologic age of 1 month, all medically stable preterm infants (see Preterm and Low Birth Weight Infants, p 68), regardless of initial birth weight or gestational age, are as likely to respond to hepatitis B immunization as are term and larger infants.

All preterm infants who are born to an HBsAg-positive mother should receive immunoprophylaxis with hepatitis B vaccine and HBIG within 12 hours after birth, followed by the remaining doses in the series as recommended and postimmunization testing

[1]Centers for Disease Control and Prevention. A comprehensive immunization strategy to eliminate transmission of hepatitis B virus infection in the United States: recommendations of the Advisory Committee on Immunization Practices (ACIP) part II: immunization of adults. *MMWR Recomm Rep.* 2006;55(RR-16):1–33

Table 3.18. Adults Recommended to Receive Hepatitis B Immunization[a]

People at Risk of Infection by Sexual Exposure
- Sex partners of hepatitis B surface antigen (HBsAg)-positive people
- Sexually active people who are not in a long-term, mutually monogamous relationship (eg, people with more than 1 sex partner during the previous 6 months)
- People seeking evaluation or treatment for a sexually transmitted infection
- Men who have sex with men

People at Risk of Infection by Percutaneous or Mucosal Exposure to Blood
- Current or recent injection-drug users
- Household contacts of HBsAg-positive people
- Residents and staff of facilities for people with developmental disabilities
- Health-care and public safety workers with reasonably anticipated risk of exposure to blood or blood-contaminated body fluids
- People with end-stage renal disease, including predialysis, hemodialysis, peritoneal dialysis, and home dialysis patients

Others
- International travelers to regions with high or intermediate levels (HBsAg prevalence of 2% or greater) of endemic HBV infection (see Table 3.15, p 340)
- People with chronic liver disease
- People with human immunodeficiency (HIV) infection
- All other people seeking protection from HBV infection

[a]Centers for Disease Control and Prevention. A comprehensive immunization strategy to eliminate transmission of hepatitis B virus infection in the United States: recommendations of the Advisory Committee on Immunization Practices (ACIP) Part II: immunization of adults. *MMWR Recomm Rep.* 2006;55(RR-16):1–33

appropriate for term infants (see Table 3.19, p 349 and Table 3.20, p 351). If the preterm infant born to an HBsAg-positive mother weighs less than 2000 g at birth, the birth dose of hepatitis B vaccine should not be counted toward completion of the hepatitis B vaccine series, and 3 additional doses of hepatitis B vaccine should be administered beginning when the infant is 1 month of age (see Table 3.19, p 349). Only monovalent hepatitis B vaccines should be used from birth to 6 weeks of age.

If maternal HBsAg status is unknown at birth, the preterm infant should receive hepatitis B vaccine within 12 hours of birth. For preterm infants weighing greater than 2000 g at birth, the mother's HBsAg status should be determined as quickly as possible and if positive, HBIG should be given as soon as possible, but within 7 days of birth, at a separate site from the hepatitis B vaccine. If the infant's birth weight is less than 2000 g and the maternal HBsAg status cannot be determined within 12 hours of life, HBIG should be given, because the less reliable immune response in preterm infants weighing less than 2000 g precludes the option of the 7-day waiting period acceptable for term and larger preterm infants. Only monovalent hepatitis B vaccine should be used from birth through 6 weeks of life.

All preterm infants of HBsAg-negative mothers with a birth weight of less than 2000 g can receive the first dose of hepatitis B vaccine series starting at 1 month of chronologic age or at hospital discharge if before 1 month of chronologic age. Preterm infants weighing more than 2000 g and low birth weight infants who are medically stable and showing consistent weight gain when discharged from the hospital before 1 month of age

Table 3.19. Hepatitis B Immunoprophylaxis Scheme by Infant Birth Weight[a]

Maternal Status	Infant Birth Weight 2000 g or More	Infant Birth Weight Less Than 2000 g
HBsAg positive	Hepatitis B vaccine + HBIG (within 12 h of birth)	Hepatitis B vaccine + HBIG (within 12 h of birth)
	Continue vaccine series beginning at 1–2 mo of age according to recommended schedule for infants born to HBsAg-positive mothers (see Table 3.20)	Continue vaccine series beginning at 1–2 mo of age according to recommended schedule for infants born to HBsAg-positive mothers (see Table 3.20)
		Immunize with 4 vaccine doses; do not count birth dose as part of vaccine series
	Check anti-HBs and HBsAg after completion of vaccine series[b]	Check anti-HBs and HBsAg after completion of vaccine series[b]
	HBsAg-negative infants with anti-HBs levels 10 mIU/mL or greater are protected and need no further medical management	HBsAg-negative infants with anti-HBs levels 10 mIU/mL or greater are protected and need no further medical management
	HBsAg-negative infants with anti-HBs levels less than 10 mIU/mL should be reimmunized with 3 doses at 2-mo intervals and retested	HBsAg-negative infants with anti-HBs levels less than 10 mIU/mL should be reimmunized with 3 doses at 2-mo intervals and retested
	Infants who are HBsAg positive should receive appropriate follow-up, including medical evaluation for chronic liver disease	Infants who are HBsAg positive should receive appropriate follow-up, including medical evaluation for chronic liver disease
HBsAg status unknown	Test mother for HBsAg immediately after admission for delivery	Test mother for HBsAg immediately after admission for delivery
	Hepatitis B vaccine (within 12h of birth)	Hepatitis B vaccine (within 12h of birth)
	Administer HBIG (within 7 days) if mother tests HBsAg positive; if mother's HBsAg status remains unknown, some experts would administer HBIG (within 7 days)	Administer HBIG if mother tests HBsAg positive or if mother's HBsAg result is not available within 12 h of birth
	Continue vaccine series beginning at 1–2 mo of age according to recommended schedule based on mother's HBsAg result (see Table 3.20)	Continue vaccine series beginning at 1–2 mo of age according to recommended schedule based on mother's HBsAg result (see Table 3.20)
		Immunize with 4 vaccine doses; do not count birth dose as part of vaccine series

Table 3.19. Hepatitis B Immunoprophylaxis Scheme by Infant Birth Weight,[a] continued

Maternal Status	Infant Birth Weight 2000 g or More	Infant Birth Weight Less Than 2000 g
HBsAg negative	Hepatitis B vaccine at birth[c]	Hepatitis B vaccine dose 1 at 30 days of chronologic age if medically stable, or at hospital discharge if before 30 days of chronologic age
	Continue vaccine series beginning at 1–2 mo of age (see Table 3.20)	Continue vaccine series beginning at 1–2 mo of age (see Table 3.20)
	Follow-up anti-HBs and HBsAg testing not needed	Follow-up anti-HBs and HBsAg testing not needed

HBsAg indicates hepatitis B surface antigen; HBIG, hepatitis B Immune Globulin; anti-HBs, antibody to HBsAg.
[a]Extremes of gestational age and birth weight no longer are a consideration for timing of hepatitis B vaccine doses.
[b]Test at 9 to 18 months of age, generally at the next well-child visit after completion of the primary series. Use testing method that allows determination of a protective concentration of anti-HBs (10 mIU/mL or greater).
[c]The first dose may be delayed until after hospital discharge for an infant who weighs 2000 g or greater and whose mother is HBsAg negative, but only if a physician's order to withhold the birth dose and a copy of the mother's original HBsAg-negative laboratory report are documented in the infant's medical record.

may receive the first dose of hepatitis B vaccine at the time of discharge. Infants born to HBsAg-negative mothers do not need to have postimmunization serologic testing for anti-HBs. Table 3.19 provides a summary of the recommendations for immunization of preterm and low birth weight infants on the basis of maternal hepatitis B status and infant birth weight. For information on use of combination vaccines containing hepatitis B as a component to complete the series, see Table 3.20 (p 351).

Considerations for High-Risk Groups:
Health Care Professionals and Others With Occupational Exposure to Blood.
The risk of HBV exposure to a health care professional depends on the tasks the person performs. Health care professionals who have contact with blood or other potentially infectious body fluids should be immunized. Because the risks of occupational HBV infection often are highest during the training of health care professionals, immunization should be initiated as early as possible before or during training and before contact with blood.

Patients Undergoing Hemodialysis. Immunization is recommended for susceptible patients undergoing hemodialysis. Immunization early in the course of renal disease is encouraged, because response is better than in advanced disease. Specific dosage recommendations have not been made for children undergoing hemodialysis. Some experts recommend increased doses of hepatitis B vaccine for children receiving hemodialysis to increase immunogenicity.

People Born in Countries Where the Prevalence of Chronic HBV Infection Is 2% or Greater. Foreign-born people (including immigrants, refugees, asylum seekers, and internationally adopted children) from countries where the prevalence of chronic HBV infection is 2% or greater (see Table 3.15, p 340) should be screened for HBsAg regardless of immunization status. Previously unimmunized family members and other household contacts should be immunized if a household member is found to be

Table 3.20. Hepatitis B Vaccine Schedules for Infants by Maternal Hepatitis B Surface Antigen (HBsAg) Status[a,b]

Maternal HBsAg Status	Single-Antigen Vaccine		Single-Antigen + Combination	
	Dose	Age	Dose	Age
Positive	1[c]	Birth (12 h or less)	1[c]	Birth (12 h or less)
	HBIG[d]	Birth (12 h or less)	HBIG[d]	Birth (12 h or less)
	2	1 through 2 mo	2	2 mo
	3[e]	6 mo	3	4 mo
			4[e]	6 mo (Pediarix) or 12 through 15 mo (Comvax)
Unknown[f]	1[c]	Birth (12 h or less)	1[c]	Birth (12 h or less)
	2	1 through 2 mo	2	2 mo
	3[e]	6 mo	3	4 mo
			4[e]	6 mo (Pediarix) or 12 through 15 mo (Comvax)
Negative	1[c,g]	Birth before discharge)	1[c,g]	Birth (before discharge)
	2	1 through 2 mo	2	2 mo
	3[e]	6 through 18 mo	3	4 mo
			4[e]	6 mo (Pediarix) or 12 through 15 mo (Comvax)

HBIG indicates Hepatitis B Immune Globulin.

[a] Centers for Disease Control and Prevention. A comprehensive immunization strategy to eliminate transmission of hepatitis B virus infection in the United States: recommendations of the Advisory Committee on Immunization Practices (ACIP) part 1: immunization of infants, children, and adolescents. *MMWR Recomm Rep.* 2005;54(RR-16):1–31.

[b] See Table 3.19 for vaccine schedules for preterm infants weighing less than 2000 g.

[c] Recombivax HB or Engerix-B should be used for the birth dose. Comvax and Pediarix cannot be administered at birth or before 6 weeks of age.

[d] HBIG (0.5 mL) administered intramuscularly in a separate site from vaccine.

[e] The final dose in the vaccine series should not be administered before 24 weeks (164 days) of age.

[f] Mothers should have blood drawn and tested for HBsAg as soon as possible after admission for delivery; if the mother is found to be HBsAg positive, the infant should receive HBIG as soon as possible but no later than 7 days of age.

[g] On a case-by-case basis and only in rare circumstances, the first dose may be delayed until after hospital discharge for an infant who weighs 2000 g or more and whose mother is HBsAg negative, but only if a physician's order to withhold the birth dose and a copy of the mother's original HBsAg-negative laboratory report are documented in the infant's medical record.

HBsAg positive. In addition, HBsAg-positive people should be reported to the local health department and receive medical management to reduce their risk of chronic liver disease.

Inmates in Juvenile Detention and Other Correctional Facilities. Previously unimmunized or underimmunized people in juvenile and adult facilities, including jails, should be immunized appropriately. If the length of stay is not sufficient to complete the immunization series, the series should be initiated and follow-up mechanisms with a health care facility should be established to ensure completion of the series (see Hepatitis and Youth in Correctional Settings, p 172).

International Travelers. People traveling to areas where the prevalence of chronic HBV infection is 2% or greater (see Table 3.15, p 340) should be immunized. Immunization should begin at least 4 to 6 months before travel so that a 3-dose regimen can be completed (see Preexposure Universal Immunization, p 346). If immunization is initiated fewer than 4 months before departure, the alternative 4-dose schedule of 0, 1, 2, and 12 months, licensed for one vaccine (see Table 3.17, p 344), should provide protection if the first 3 doses can be administered before travel. Individual clinicians may choose to use an accelerated schedule (eg, doses at days 0, 7, and 21) for travelers who will depart before an approved immunization schedule can be completed. The FDA has not licensed schedules that involve immunization at more than one time point during a single month for hepatitis B vaccine licensed in the United States. People who receive immunization on an accelerated schedule that is not FDA licensed also should receive a booster dose at 12 months after initiation of the series to promote long-term immunity.

Care of Exposed People (Postexposure Immunoprophylaxis) (Also See Table 3.21, p 353).
Prevention of Perinatal HBV Infection. Transmission of perinatal HBV infection can be prevented in approximately 95% of infants born to HBsAg-positive mothers by early active and passive immunoprophylaxis of the infant (ie, immunization and HBIG administration). Immunization subsequently should be completed during the first 6 months of life. Hepatitis B immunization alone, initiated at or shortly after birth, also is highly effective for preventing perinatal HBV infections.

Serologic Screening of Pregnant Women. Prenatal HBsAg testing of all pregnant women is recommended to identify newborn infants who require immediate postexposure prophylaxis. All pregnant women should be tested during an early prenatal visit with every pregnancy. Testing should be repeated at the time of admission to the hospital for delivery for HBsAg-negative women who are at high risk of HBV infection or who have had clinical HBV infection. Women who are HBsAg-positive should be reported to local health departments for appropriate case management to ensure follow-up of their infants and immunization of sexual and household contacts. In populations where HBsAg testing of pregnant women is not feasible (eg, in remote areas without access to a laboratory), all infants should receive hepatitis B vaccine within 12 hours of birth, the second dose by 2 months of age, and the third dose at 6 months of age.

Management of Infants Born to HBsAg-Positive Women. Infants born to HBsAg-positive mothers, including preterm and low birth weight infants, should receive the initial dose of hepatitis B vaccine within 12 hours of birth (see Table 3.17, p 344, for appropriate dosages), and HBIG (0.5 mL) should be given concurrently but at a different anatomic site. The effectiveness of HBIG diminishes the longer after exposure that it is initiated. The interval of effectiveness is unlikely to exceed 7 days. Subsequent doses of vaccine should be given as recommended in Table 3.19 (p 349) and Table 3.20 (p 351). For preterm infants who weigh less than 2000 g at birth, the initial vaccine dose should not be counted in the required 3-dose schedule (a total of 4 doses of hepatitis B vaccine should be administered), and the subsequent 3 doses should be given in accordance with the schedule for immunization of preterm infants (see Preterm and Low Birth Weight Infants, p 68).

Infants born to HBsAg-positive women should be tested for anti-HBs and HBsAg after completion of the immunization series, at 9 to 18 months of age (generally at the next well-child visit). Testing should not be performed before 9 months of age to avoid detection of anti-HBs from HBIG administered during infancy and to maximize the

Table 3.21. Guide to Postexposure Immunoprophylaxis of Unimmunized People to Prevent Hepatitis B Virus Infection

Type of Exposure	Immunoprophylaxis[a]
Household contact of HBsAg-positive person	Administer hepatitis B vaccine series
Discrete exposure to an HBsAg-positive source[b]:	
• Percutaneous (eg, bite, needlestick) or mucosal exposure to HBsAg-positive blood or body fluids that contain blood	Administer hepatitis B vaccine + HBIG; complete vaccine series
• Sexual contact or needle sharing with an HBsAg-positive person	Administer hepatitis B vaccine + HBIG; complete vaccine series
• Victim of sexual assault/abuse by a perpetrator who is HBsAg positive	Administer hepatitis B vaccine + HBIG; complete vaccine series
Discrete exposure to a source with unknown HBsAg status:	
• Percutaneous (eg, bite, needlestick) or mucosal exposure to blood or body fluids that contain blood with unknown HBsAg status	Administer hepatitis B vaccine series
• Victim of sexual assault/abuse by a perpetrator with unknown HBsAg status	Administer hepatitis B vaccine series

HBsAg indicates hepatitis B surface antigen; HBIG, Hepatitis B Immune Globulin.

[a]Immunoprophylaxis should be administered as soon as possible, preferably within 24 hours after exposure. Studies are limited on the maximum interval after exposure during which postexposure prophylaxis is effective, but the interval is unlikely to exceed 7 days for percutaneous exposures and 14 days for sexual exposures.

[b]If person previously was immunized with hepatitis B vaccine series, administer hepatitis B vaccine booster dose.

likelihood of detecting late HBV infections. Testing for HBsAg will identify infants who become infected chronically despite immunization (because of intrauterine infection or vaccine failure) and will aid in their long-term medical management. Testing for IgM anti-HBc is unreliable for infants. Infants with anti-HBs concentrations less than 10 mIU/mL and who are HBsAg negative should receive 3 additional doses of vaccine (see Table 3.19) followed by testing for anti-HBs 1 month after the third dose. Alternatively, 1 to 3 additional doses of vaccine can be administered, followed by testing for anti-HBs 1 month after each dose, to determine whether subsequent doses are needed.

Term Infants Born to Mothers Not Tested During Pregnancy for HBsAg. Pregnant women whose HBsAg status is unknown at delivery should undergo blood testing as soon as possible to determine their HBsAg status. While awaiting results, the infant should receive the first hepatitis B vaccine dose within 12 hours of birth in the dose recommended for infants born to HBsAg-positive mothers (see Table 3.17, p 344). Because hepatitis B vaccine, when given at birth, is highly effective for preventing perinatal infection in term infants, the possible added value and the cost of HBIG do not warrant its immediate use in term infants when the mother's HBsAg status is not known. If the woman is found to be HBsAg positive, term infants should receive HBIG (0.5 mL) as soon as possible, but within 7 days of birth, and should complete the hepatitis B immunization series as recommended (see Tables 3.17, p 344, and 3.19, p 349). If HBIG is unavailable, the infant still should receive the 2 subsequent doses of hepatitis B vaccine at 1 to 2 and 6 months of age. If the mother is found to be HBsAg negative, hepatitis B immunization in the dose and schedule recommended for term infants born to HBsAg-negative mothers should be completed (see Table 3.17, p 344). If the mother's HBsAg status remains unknown, some experts would administer HBIG within 7 days of birth and complete the hepatitis B immunization series as recommended for infants born to mothers who are HBsAg positive (Table 3.19, p 349).

Preterm Infants Born to Mothers Not Tested During Pregnancy for HBsAg. Maternal HBsAg status should be determined as soon as possible. Preterm infants born to mothers whose HBsAg status is unknown should receive hepatitis B vaccine within the first 12 hours of life. Preterm infants weighing more than 2000 g at birth who are born to mothers whose HBsAg status is unknown should follow recommendations for term infants. Preterm infants weighing less than 2000 g at birth who are born to mothers whose HBsAg status is unknown should receive HBIG (0.5 mL) if the mother's HBsAg status cannot be determined within the initial 12 hours of birth because of the potentially decreased immunogenicity of vaccine in these infants. In these infants, the initial vaccine dose should not be counted toward the 3 doses of hepatitis B vaccine required to complete the immunization series. The subsequent 3 doses (for a total of 4 doses) are given in accordance with recommendations for immunization of preterm infants with a birth weight less than 2000 g according to the HBsAg status of the mother (see Table 3.19, p 349). Follow-up testing on completion of the immunization series is recommended for all preterm infants of HBsAg-positive mothers (see Management of Infants Born to HBsAg-Positive Women, p 352).

Breastfeeding. Breastfeeding of the infant by an HBsAg-positive mother poses no additional risk of acquisition of HBV infection by the infant with appropriate administration of hepatitis B vaccine and HBIG (see Human Milk, p 118).

Household Contacts and Sexual Partners of HBsAg-Positive People. Household and sexual contacts of HBsAg-positive people (acute or chronic HBV infection) identified through prenatal screening, blood donor screening, or diagnostic or other serologic testing should be immunized.

Infants (ie, younger than 12 months of age) who have close contact with primary caregivers with acute HBV infection require immunoprophylaxis. If, at the time of exposure, the infant has been immunized fully or has received at least 2 doses of vaccine, the infant should be presumed protected, and HBIG is not required. If only 1 dose of vaccine has been administered, the second dose should be administered if the interval is appropriate, or HBIG should be administered if immunization is not yet due. If immunization has not been initiated, the infant should receive HBIG (0.5 mL), and hepatitis B vaccine should be given in accordance with the routinely recommended 3-dose schedule (see Preexposure Universal Immunization, p 346).

Prophylaxis with HBIG for other unimmunized household contacts of HBsAg-positive people is not indicated unless they have a discrete, identifiable exposure to the index patient (see next paragraph).

Postexposure Prophylaxis for People With Discrete Identifiable Exposures to Blood or Body Fluids That Contain Blood. Management of people with a discrete, identifiable percutaneous (eg, needlestick, laceration, or bite) or mucosal (eg, ocular or mucous membrane) exposure to blood or body fluids that contain blood includes consideration of whether the HBsAg status of the person who was the source of exposure is known and the hepatitis B immunization and response status of the exposed person (also see Table 3.22, p 355). Immunization is recommended for any person who was exposed but not previously immunized. If possible, a blood specimen from the person who was the

Table 3.22. Recommendations for Hepatitis B Prophylaxis After Percutaneous Exposure to Blood That Contains or Might Contain HBsAg[a]

| Exposed Person | Treatment When Source Is | | |
	HBsAg Positive	HBsAg Negative	Unknown or Not Tested
Unimmunized	Administer HBIG[b] (1 dose) and initiate hepatitis B vaccine series	Initiate hepatitis B vaccine series	Initiate hepatitis B vaccine series
Previously immunized			
Known responder	No treatment	No treatment	No treatment
Known nonresponder	HBIG (1 dose) and initiate reimmunization[c] or HBIG (2 doses)	No treatment	If known high-risk source, treat as if source were HBsAg positive
Response unknown	Test exposed person for anti-HBs[d] and administer vaccine booster dose[e]	No treatment	Test exposed person for anti-HBs[d] • If inadequate, vaccine booster dose[e] • If inadequate, no treatment

HBsAg indicates hepatitis B surface antigen; HBIG, Hepatitis B Immune Globulin; anti-HBs, antibody to HBsAg.
[a]Centers for Disease Control and Prevention. Updated US Public Health Service guidelines for the management of occupational exposures to HBV, HCV, and HIV and recommendations for postexposure prophylaxis. *MMWR Recomm Rep.* 2001;50(RR-11):1–52.
[b]Dose of HBIG, 0.06 mL/kg, intramuscularly.
[c]The option of giving 1 dose of HBIG (0.06 mL/kg) and reinitiating the vaccine series is preferred for nonresponders who have not completed a second 3-dose vaccine series. For people who previously completed a second vaccine series but failed to respond, 2 doses of HBIG (0.06 mL/kg) are preferred, 1 dose as soon as possible after exposure and the second 1 month later.
[d]Adequate anti-HBs is ≥10 mIU/mL.
[e]The person should be evaluated for antibody response after the vaccine booster dose. For people who receive HBIG, anti-HBs testing should be performed when passively acquired antibody from HBIG no longer is detectable (eg, 4–6 months); for people who did not receive HBIG, anti-HBs testing should be performed 1 to 2 months after the vaccine booster dose. If anti-HBs is inadequate (less than 10 mIU/mL) after the vaccine booster dose, 2 additional doses should be administered to complete a 3-dose reimmunization series.

source of the exposure should be tested for HBsAg, and appropriate prophylaxis should be administered according to the hepatitis B immunization status and anti-HBs response status (if known) of the exposed person (see Table 3.22 and Injuries From Discarded Needles in the Community, p 184). Detailed guidelines for management of health care professionals and other people exposed to blood that is or might be HBsAg-positive is provided in the recommendations of the Advisory Committee on Immunization Practices of the Centers for Disease Control and Prevention (CDC).[1]

---

[1]Centers for Disease Control and Prevention. A comprehensive immunization strategy to eliminate transmission of hepatitis B virus infection in the United States: recommendations of the Advisory Committee on Immunization Practices (ACIP) part 1: immunization of infants, children, and adolescents. *MMWR Recomm Rep.* 2005;54(RR-16):1–31

HBsAg-Positive Source. If the source is HBsAg positive, unimmunized people should receive both HBIG and hepatitis B vaccine as soon as possible after exposure, preferably within 24 hours (see Table 3.22, p 355). The vaccine series should be completed using an age-appropriate dose and schedule. People who are in the process of being immunized but who have not completed the vaccine series should receive the appropriate dose of HBIG and should complete the vaccine series. Children and adolescents who have written documentation of a complete hepatitis B vaccine series and who did not receive postimmunization testing should receive a single vaccine booster dose.

Source With Unknown HBsAg Status. If the HBsAg status of the source is unknown, unimmunized people should receive the hepatitis B vaccine series with the first dose initiated as soon as possible after exposure, preferably within 24 hours (see Table 3.22, p 355). The vaccine series should be completed using an age-appropriate dose and schedule. Children and adolescents with written documentation of a complete hepatitis B vaccine series require no further treatment.

Victims of Sexual Assault or Abuse. For unimmunized victims of sexual assault or abuse, active postexposure prophylaxis (ie, vaccine alone) should be initiated, with the first dose of vaccine given as part of the initial clinical evaluation. If the offender is known to be HBsAg positive, HBIG also should be administered. The vaccine series should be completed using an age-appropriate dose and schedule. (For discussion of management of previously immunized people, see Postexposure Prophylaxis for People With Discrete Identifiable Exposures to Blood or Body Fluids That Contain Blood, p 354.)

Child Care. All children, including children in child care, should receive hepatitis B vaccine as part of their routine immunization schedule. Immunization not only will decrease the potential for transmission after bites but also will allay anxiety about transmission from attendees who may be HBsAg positive.

Children who are HBsAg positive and who have no behavioral or medical risk factors, such as unusually aggressive behavior (eg, frequent biting), generalized dermatitis, or a bleeding problem, should be admitted to child care without restrictions. Under these circumstances, the risk of HBV transmission in child care settings is negligible, and routine screening for HBsAg is not warranted. Admission of HBsAg-positive children with behavioral or medical risk factors should be assessed on an individual basis by the child's physician, the program director, and public health authorities (for further discussion, see Children in Out-of-Home Child Care, p 124).

Effectiveness of Hepatitis B Prevention Programs. Routine hepatitis B immunization programs have resulted in significant decreases in the prevalence of chronic HBV infection among children in populations with a high incidence of HBV infection. There is an association between higher coverage with hepatitis B vaccine and larger decreases in HBsAg prevalence. The incidence of acute HBV infection among US children younger than 15 years of age decreased by 98% between 1990 and 2007.

Although the long-term sequelae of chronic HBV infection usually are not recognized until adulthood, cirrhosis and HCC do occur in children. In Taiwan, the average annual incidence of HCC among children 6 to 14 years of age decreased significantly within 10 years of routine infant hepatitis B immunization. Worldwide, routine infant immunization programs are expected to decrease significantly the incidence of death from cirrhosis and HCC attributable to HBV infection over the next 30 to 50 years.

The Division of Viral Hepatitis at the CDC maintains a Web site (**www.cdc.gov/hepatitis**) with information on hepatitis for health care professionals and the public.

Hepatitis C

CLINICAL MANIFESTATIONS: Signs and symptoms of hepatitis C virus (HCV) infection are indistinguishable from signs of hepatitis A or hepatitis B virus infections. Acute disease tends to be mild and insidious in onset, and most infections are asymptomatic. Jaundice occurs in fewer than 20% of patients, and abnormalities in liver transaminase concentrations generally are less pronounced than those in patients with hepatitis B virus infection. Persistent infection with HCV occurs in 50% to 60% of infected children, even in the absence of biochemical evidence of liver disease. Most children with chronic infection are asymptomatic. Although chronic hepatitis develops in approximately 70% to 80% of infected adults, limited data indicate that chronic hepatitis and cirrhosis occur less commonly in children. Infection with HCV is the leading indication for liver transplantation among adults in the United States.

ETIOLOGY: HCV is a small, single-stranded RNA virus and is a member of the Flavivirus family. Multiple HCV genotypes and subtypes exist.

EPIDEMIOLOGY: The incidence of acute symptomatic HCV infection in the United States was 0.2 per 100 000 in 2005; after asymptomatic infection and underreporting were considered, approximately 20 000 new cases were estimated to have occurred. For all age groups, the incidence of HCV infection decreased in the United States during the 1990s and has remained low and stable since then. Nevertheless, a substantial burden of disease still exists in the United States because of the propensity of HCV to establish chronic infection and the high incidence of acute HCV infection through the 1980s. The prevalence of HCV infection in the general population of the United States is estimated at 1.3%, equating to an estimated 3.2 million people in the United States who have chronic HCV infection. Seroprevalences vary among populations according to their associated risk factors.

HCV primarily is spread by parenteral exposure to blood of HCV-infected people. The most common risk factors for acquiring infection are injection drug use, having multiple sexual partners, or having received blood products before 1992. The current risk of HCV infection after blood transfusion in the United States is estimated to be 1 per 2 million units transfused because of exclusion of high-risk donors and of HCV-positive units after antibody testing and screening of pools of blood units by some form of nucleic acid amplification (NAA) test (see Blood Safety, p 106). All intravenous and intramuscular Immune Globulin products available commercially in the United States undergo an inactivation procedure for HCV or are documented to be HCV RNA negative before release.

Seventy-five percent or more of chronic HCV cases reported to public health authorities are in injection drug users who have shared needles or injection paraphernalia and, to a lesser extent, in people who received transfusions before 1992, when routine screening of donor blood for HCV began; almost all of these infected people are outside the pediatric age range. Data from recent multicenter, population-based cohort studies indicate that approximately one third of young injection drug users 18 to 30 years of age are infected with HCV. Approximately 1% to 10% of cases appear to be in people with multiple sexual partners, with increasing risk associated with the number of partners, and in people with sporadic percutaneous exposures, such as health care professionals (approximately 1% of cases). Approximately half of the 18 000 people with hemophilia (almost all male) who received transfusions before adoption of heat treatment of clotting factors in 1987 are HCV seropositive. All of these patients should be older than 18 years of age at this time. Prevalence is moderately high among people with frequent but smaller direct percutaneous exposures, such as patients receiving hemodialysis (10%–20%).

Any body fluid contaminated with infected blood can be a source of infection. However, sexual transmission among monogamous couples is uncommon, with infection found only in 1.5% of spouses without other risk factors. Transmission among family contacts also is uncommon but can occur from direct or inapparent percutaneous or mucosal exposure to blood.

Seroprevalence among pregnant women in the United States has been estimated at 1% to 2%. The risk of perinatal transmission averages 5% to 6%, and transmission occurs only from women who are HCV RNA positive at the time of delivery. Maternal coinfection with human immunodeficiency virus (HIV) has been associated with increased risk of perinatal transmission of HCV, which depends in part on the serologic concentration of HCV RNA in the mother. Serum antibody to HCV (anti-HCV) and HCV RNA have been detected in colostrum, but the risk of HCV transmission is similar in breastfed and bottle-fed infants.

All people with HCV-RNA in their blood are considered to be infectious.

The **incubation period** for HCV disease averages 6 to 7 weeks, with a range of 2 weeks to 6 months. The time from exposure to development of viremia generally is 1 to 2 weeks.

DIAGNOSTIC TESTS: The 2 major types of tests available for laboratory diagnosis of HCV infections are immunoglobulin (Ig) G antibody enzyme immunoassays for HCV and NAA tests to detect HCV RNA. Assays for IgM to detect early or acute infection are not available. The third-generation enzyme immunoassays are at least 97% sensitive and more than 99% specific. False-negative results early in the course of acute infection can result from the prolonged interval between exposure and onset of illness and seroconversion. Within 15 weeks after exposure and within 5 to 6 weeks after onset of hepatitis, 80% of patients will have positive test results for serum anti-HCV antibody. Among infants born to anti-HCV–positive mothers, passively acquired maternal antibody may persist for up to 18 months.

Food and Drug Administration (FDA)-licensed diagnostic NAA tests for qualitative detection of HCV RNA are available. HCV RNA can be detected in serum or plasma within 1 to 2 weeks after exposure to the virus and weeks before onset of liver enzyme abnormalities or appearance of anti-HCV. Assays for detection of HCV RNA are used commonly in clinical practice to identify anti-HCV–positive patients who have HCV infection, for identifying infection in infants early in life (ie, perinatal transmission) when maternal antibody interferes with ability to detect antibody produced by the infant, and for monitoring patients receiving antiviral therapy. However, false-positive and false-negative results can occur from improper handling, storage, and contamination of test specimens. Viral RNA may be detected intermittently, and thus, a single negative assay result is not conclusive. Quantitative assays for measuring the concentration of HCV RNA are available but are less sensitive than qualitative assays. The clinical value of these quantitative assays appears to be primarily as a prognostic indicator for patients undergoing or about to undergo antiviral therapy.

TREATMENT: Therapy is aimed at inhibiting HCV replication, eradicating infection, and improving the natural history of disease. Therapies are expensive, can cause significant adverse reactions, and are effective in approximately half of people treated. Interferon-alfa or peginterferon-alfa alone and peginterferon-alfa in combination with ribavirin are approved by the FDA for treatment of chronic HCV infection in adults. Response to treatment varies depending on the genotype with which the person is infected. Combination therapy with pegylated interferon-alfa and ribavirin results in sustained virologic response, defined as undectable HCV RNA concentrations 12 or more months after treatment cessation, in approximately 50% of adult patients infected with genotype 1 and approximately 80% in patients with genotypes 2 or 3. The FDA has approved use of (nonpegylated) interferon-alfa–2b in combination with ribavirin for treatment of HCV infection in children 3 to 17 years of age. The few studies of combination therapy in children suggest that children have increased sustained virologic response rates and fewer adverse events compared with adults. Children with severe disease or histologically advanced pathologic features (bridging necrosis or active cirrhosis) should be referred to a specialist in the management of chronic HCV infection. All treatment regimens are associated with adverse events. Major adverse effects of combination therapy include influenza-like symptoms, hematologic abnormalities, and neuropsychiatric symptoms. Education of patients, their family members, and caregivers about adverse effects and their prospective management is an integral aspect of treatment.

All patients with chronic HCV infection should be immunized against hepatitis A and hepatitis B because of the very high rate of severe hepatitis in patients with chronic liver disease from HCV who then get hepatitis A or B infections.

Management of Chronic HCV Infection. With advancing age, people who have chronic HCV infection are at risk of developing chronic hepatitis and its complications, including cirrhosis and primary hepatocellular carcinoma (HCC). Factors associated with more severe disease in most studies include older age at acquisition, HIV infection, excessive alcohol consumption, and male gender. Among children, liver disease progression appears to be accelerated when comorbid conditions, including childhood cancer, iron overload, thalassemia, or HIV coinfection are present. Pediatricians need to be alert to concomitant infections and alcohol abuse and careful in prescription of drugs, such as acetaminophen and some antiretroviral agents (such as stavudine), in patients with HCV infection. Children with chronic infection should be followed closely, including sequential monitoring of serum hepatic transaminases, because of potential long-term risk of chronic liver disease. Definitive recommendations on frequency of screening have not been established. Children in whom a diagnosis of HCV infection is made should be referred to a specialist in management of HCV for further care. The need for screening tests for HCC in children has not been determined.

ISOLATION OF THE HOSPITALIZED PATIENT: Standard precautions are recommended.

CONTROL MEASURES:

Care of Exposed People.

Immunoprophylaxis. On the basis of lack of clinical efficacy in humans and data from studies using animals, use of Immune Globulin for postexposure prophylaxis against HCV infection is not recommended.

Breastfeeding. Mothers infected with HCV should be advised that transmission of HCV by breastfeeding has not been documented. According to guidelines of the Centers for Disease Control and Prevention (CDC) and the American Academy of Pediatrics, maternal HCV infection is not a contraindication to breastfeeding. Mothers who are

HCV positive and choose to breastfeed should consider abstaining if their nipples are cracked or bleeding.

Child Care. Exclusion of children with HCV infection from out-of-home child care is not indicated.

Serologic Testing for HCV Infection.

People Who Have Risk Factors for HCV Infection. Routine serologic testing is recommended for current or former injection drug users, recipients of one or more units of blood or blood products before July 1992, recipients of a solid organ transplant before July 1992, patients receiving long-term hemodialysis, people who received clotting-factor concentrates produced before 1987, people with persistently abnormal alanine transaminase (ALT) concentrations, and people in settings with documented high HCV infection prevalence and where risk-factor ascertainment is poor (eg, inmates of correctional facilities).

Pregnant Women. Routine serologic testing of pregnant women for HCV infection is not recommended.

Children Born to Women With HCV Infection. Children born to women previously identified to be HCV infected should be tested for HCV infection, because approximately 5% of these children will acquire the infection. The duration of presence of passive maternal antibody in infants can be as long as 18 months. Therefore, testing for anti-HCV should not be performed until after 18 months of age. If earlier diagnosis is desired, NAA testing to detect HCV RNA may be performed at or after the infant's first well-child visit at 1 to 2 months of age.

Adoptees. Routine serologic testing of adoptees, either domestic or international, is not recommended. See Medical Evaluation of Internationally Adopted Children for Infectious Diseases (p 177) for specific situations when serologic testing is warranted.

Counseling of Patients With HCV Infection.
All people with HCV infection should be considered infectious, should be informed of the possibility of transmission to others, and should refrain from donating blood, organs, tissues, or semen and from sharing toothbrushes and razors.

Infected people should be counseled to avoid hepatotoxic agents, including medications, and should be informed of the risks of excessive alcohol ingestion. All patients with chronic HCV infection should be immunized against hepatitis A and hepatitis B.

Changes in sexual practices of infected people with a steady partner are not recommended; however, they should be informed of the possible risks and use of precautions to prevent transmission. People with multiple sexual partners should be advised to decrease the number of partners and to use condoms to prevent transmission. No data exist to support counseling a woman against pregnancy.

The Division of Viral Hepatitis at the CDC has a toll-free telephone number for information on viral hepatitis (1–888–4HEPCDC) and maintains a Web site (**www.cdc.gov/hepatitis**) with information on hepatitis for health care professionals and the public, which includes specific information for people who have received blood transfusions before 1992. Information also can be obtained from the National Institutes of Health Web site (**http://digestive.niddk.nih.gov/ddiseases/pubs/chronichepc/index.htm**).

Practice guidelines for diagnosis, management, and treatment of hepatitis C are available from the American Association for the Study of Liver Disease (**www.aasld.org/practiceguidelines/Pages/ViralHepatitis.aspx**).

Hepatitis D

CLINICAL MANIFESTATIONS: Hepatitis D virus (HDV) causes infection only in people with acute or chronic hepatitis B virus (HBV) infection; HDV requires HBV as a helper virus and cannot produce infection in the absence of HBV. The importance of HDV infection lies in its ability to convert an asymptomatic or mild chronic HBV infection into fulminant or more severe or rapidly progressive disease. Acute coinfection with HBV and HDV usually causes an acute illness indistinguishable from acute HBV infection alone, except that the likelihood of fulminant hepatitis can be as high as 5%.

ETIOLOGY: HDV measures 36 to 43 nm in diameter and consists of an RNA genome and a delta protein antigen, both of which are coated with hepatitis B surface antigen (HBsAg).

EPIDEMIOLOGY: HDV can cause an infection at the same time as the initial HBV infection (coinfection), or it can infect a person already chronically infected with HBV (superinfection). Acquisition of HDV is by parenteral, percutaneous, or mucous membrane inoculation. HDV can be acquired from blood or blood products, through injection drug use, or by sexual contact, but only if HBV also is present. Transmission from mother to newborn infant is uncommon. Intrafamilial spread can occur among people with chronic HBV infection. High-prevalence areas include southern Italy and parts of Eastern Europe, South America, Africa, and the Middle East. In contrast to HBV infection, HDV infection is uncommon in the Far East. In the United States, HDV infection is found most commonly in people who abuse injection drugs, people with hemophilia, and people who have emigrated from areas with endemic infection.

The **incubation period** for HDV superinfection is approximately 2 to 8 weeks. When HBV and HDV viruses infect simultaneously, the incubation period is similar to that of HBV (45–160 days; average, 90 days).

DIAGNOSTIC TESTS: Enzyme immunoassay for antibody to HDV (anti-HDV) is available commercially. Anti-HDV may not be present until several weeks after onset of illness, and acute and convalescent sera may be required to confirm the diagnosis. Absence of immunoglobulin (Ig) M hepatitis B core antibody (anti-HBc), which is indicative of early HBV infection, suggests that the person has both chronic HBV infection and superinfection with HDV. Testing for IgM anti-HDV response is not useful for distinguishing acute from chronic HDV infection, because IgM anti-HDV persists during chronic infection. Tests for IgM anti-HDV, hepatitis D antigen, and HDV RNA are research procedures.

TREATMENT: HDV has proven difficult to treat. However, data suggest pegylated interferon-alpha may result in up to 40% of patients having a sustained response to treatment. Further study of pegylated interferon monotherapy or as combination therapy with lamivudine need to be performed before treatment of HDV can be advised routinely.

ISOLATION OF THE HOSPITALIZED PATIENT: Standard precautions are recommended.

CONTROL MEASURES: The same control and preventive measures used for HBV infection are indicated. Because HDV cannot be transmitted in the absence of HBV infection, hepatitis B immunization protects against HDV infection. People with chronic HBV infection should take extreme care to avoid exposure to HDV.

Hepatitis E

CLINICAL MANIFESTATIONS: Hepatitis E virus (HEV) infection is an acute illness with symptoms including jaundice, malaise, anorexia, fever, abdominal pain, and arthralgia. Subclinical infection also occurs. Disease is more common among adults than among children and is more severe in pregnant women, in whom mortality rates can approach 10%. Chronic HEV infection has not been reported.

ETIOLOGY: HEV is a spherical, nonenveloped, positive-strand RNA virus. Hepatitis E virus formerly was classified in the family Caliciviridae, genus Calicivirus, but now is classified in the genus Hepevirus of the family Hepeviridae. There are 4 major recognized genotypes with a single known serotype.

EPIDEMIOLOGY: Transmission of HEV is by the fecal-oral route. Unlike the other agents of viral hepatitis, certain HEV strains also have zoonotic hosts, such as swine. Person-to-person transmission appears to be much less efficient than with hepatitis A virus. Sporadic HEV infection has been reported in much of the developing world and is common on the Indian subcontinent, where some studies have shown HEV to be the most common etiology of acute viral hepatitis. Large, often waterborne outbreaks also have been reported in developing countries, including one outbreak in Mexico in 1986. In the United States, HEV infection is uncommon and generally occurs in travelers returning from countries with endemic infection. Several cases of domestically acquired HEV infection have been reported in the United States, all with viruses that are phylogenetically similar to HEV isolated from US swine.

DIAGNOSTIC TESTS: Testing for IgM and IgG anti-HEV is available through commercial reference laboratories. Because anti-HEV assays are not approved by the US Food and Drug Administration and their performance characteristics are not well characterized, results should be interpreted with caution, particularly in cases lacking a discrete onset of illness associated with jaundice or with no recent history of travel to a country with endemic infection. Definitive diagnosis may be made by demonstrating viral RNA in serum or stool by means of reverse transcriptase-polymerase chain reaction assay, which is available only in research settings (eg, with prior approval through the Centers for Disease Control and Prevention).

TREATMENT: Supportive.

ISOLATION OF THE HOSPITALIZED PATIENT: In addition to standard precautions, contact precautions are recommended for diapered and incontinent patients for the duration of illness.

CONTROL MEASURES: Provision of safe water is the most effective prevention measure. A recombinant HEV vaccine was evaluated in a phase II clinical trial and was demonstrated to be effective in preventing disease but is not available outside the research setting.

Herpes Simplex

CLINICAL MANIFESTATIONS:

Neonatal. In newborn infants, herpes simplex virus (HSV) infection can manifest as the following: (1) disseminated disease involving multiple organs, most prominently liver and lungs, but in 60% to 75% of cases also involving the central nervous system; (2) localized central nervous system (CNS) disease, with or without skin involvement (CNS disease); or (3) disease localized to the skin, eyes, and mouth (SEM disease). Approximately 20% of cases of neonatal HSV manifest as disseminated disease, one third manifest as CNS disease, and 40% to 45% manifest as SEM disease. Approximately 60% of neonates with disseminated disease or CNS disease have skin lesions, and approximately 80% to 85% of neonates with SEM disease will have skin involvement. In the absence of skin lesions, the diagnosis of neonatal HSV infection is difficult. Disseminated infection should be considered in neonates with sepsis syndrome, negative bacteriologic culture results, and severe liver dysfunction. HSV also should be considered as a causative agent in neonates with fever, irritability, and abnormal cerebrospinal fluid (CSF) findings, especially in the presence of seizures or during a time of year when enteroviruses are not circulating in the community. Although asymptomatic HSV infection is common in older children, it rarely, if ever, occurs in neonates.

Neonatal herpetic infections often are severe, with attendant high mortality and morbidity rates, even when antiviral therapy is administered. Recurrent skin lesions are common in surviving infants and may be associated with CNS sequelae if skin lesions occur frequently during the first 6 months of life.

Initial signs of HSV infection can occur anytime between birth and approximately 6 weeks of age, although most infected infants develop clinical disease within the first month of life. Infants with disseminated disease and SEM disease have an earlier age of onset, typically presenting between the first and second weeks of life; infants with CNS disease usually present with illness between the second and third weeks of life.

Children Beyond the Neonatal Period and Adolescents. Most primary HSV infections during the period of childhood beyond the neonatal period are asymptomatic. Gingivostomatitis, which is the most common clinical manifestation of HSV during childhood, is caused by HSV type 1 (HSV-1) and is characterized by fever, irritability, tender submandibular adenopathy, and an ulcerative enanthem involving the gingiva and mucous membranes of the mouth, often with perioral vesicular lesions.

Genital herpes, which is the most common manifestation of primary HSV infection in adolescents and adults, is characterized by vesicular or ulcerative lesions of the male or female genital organs, perineum, or both. Genital herpes usually is caused by HSV type 2 (HSV-2), but at least 20% of genital herpes is caused by HSV-1. Most cases of primary genital herpes infection are not recognized as such by the infected person or diagnosed by a health care professional.

Eczema herpeticum with vesicular lesions concentrated in the areas of eczematous involvement can develop in patients with dermatitis who are infected with HSV.

In immunocompromised patients, severe local lesions and, less commonly, disseminated HSV infection with generalized vesicular skin lesions and visceral involvement can occur.

After primary infection, HSV persists for life in a latent form. The site of latency for virus causing herpes labialis is the trigeminal ganglion, and the usual site of latency for genital herpes is the sacral dorsal root ganglia, although any of the sensory ganglia can be involved, depending on the site of primary infection. Reactivation of latent virus most commonly is asymptomatic. When symptomatic, recurrent herpes labialis HSV-1 manifests as single or grouped vesicles in the perioral region, usually on the vermilion border of the lips (typically called "cold sores" or "fever blisters"). Symptomatic recurrent genital herpes manifests as vesicular lesions on the penis, scrotum, vulva, cervix, buttocks, perianal areas, thighs, or back. Recurrences may be heralded by a prodrome of burning or itching at the site of an incipient recurrence, identification of which can be useful in instituting antiviral therapy early.

Conjunctivitis and keratitis can result from primary or recurrent HSV infection. Herpetic whitlow consists of single or multiple vesicular lesions on the distal parts of fingers. HSV infection also can be a precipitating factor in erythema multiforme.

HSV encephalitis (HSE) occurs in children beyond the neonatal period or in adolescents and adults and can result from primary or recurrent HSV-1 infection. Symptoms and signs usually include fever, alterations in the state of consciousness, personality changes, seizures, and focal neurologic findings. Encephalitis commonly has an acute onset with a fulminant course, leading to coma and death in untreated patients. HSE usually involves the temporal lobe; thus, temporal lobe abnormalities on imaging studies or encephalography in the context of a consistent clinical picture should increase the suspicion for HSE. Cerebrospinal fluid pleocytosis with a predominance of lymphocytes and some erythrocytes is usual. HSV infection also can cause meningitis with nonspecific clinical manifestations that usually are mild and self-limited. Such episodes of meningitis usually are associated with genital HSV-2 infection. A number of unusual CNS manifestations of HSV have been described, including Bell palsy, atypical pain syndromes, trigeminal neuralgia, ascending myelitis, postinfectious encephalomyelitis, and Mollaret meningitis.

ETIOLOGY: HSVs are enveloped, double-stranded, DNA viruses. Two distinct HSV species exist: HSV-1 and HSV-2. Infections with HSV-1 usually involve the face and skin above the waist; however, an increasing number of genital herpes cases are attributable to HSV-1. Infections with HSV-2 usually involve the genitalia and skin below the waist in sexually active adolescents and adults. However, either type of virus can be found in either area. HSV-2 is the most common cause of herpes disease in neonates (75% of cases). As with all human herpesviruses, HSV-1 and HSV-2 establish latency following primary infection, with periodic symptomatic or asymptomatic reactivation from latency to cause recurrent infection or disease.

EPIDEMIOLOGY: HSV infections are ubiquitous and can be transmitted from people who are symptomatic or asymptomatic with primary or recurrent infections.

Neonatal. The incidence of neonatal HSV infection is estimated to range from 1 in 3000 to 1 in 20 000 live births. HSV is transmitted to a neonate most often during birth through an infected maternal genital tract but can be caused by an ascending infection through ruptured or apparently intact amniotic membranes. Intrauterine infections causing congenital malformations have been implicated in rare cases. Other less common sources of neonatal infection include postnatal transmission from a parent or other caregiver, most often from a nongenital infection (eg, mouth or hands) or from another infected infant or caregiver in the nursery, probably via the hands of health care professionals attending to the infants.

The risk of HSV transmission to a neonate born to a mother with primary genital infection is estimated to be 25% to 60%. In contrast, the risk to a neonate born to a mother shedding HSV as a result of reactivated infection is 2%. Distinguishing between primary and recurrent HSV infections in women by history or physical examination may be impossible, because primary and recurrent genital infections may be asymptomatic or associated with nonspecific findings (eg, vaginal discharge, genital pain, or shallow ulcers). More than three quarters of infants who contract HSV infection have been born to women who had no history or clinical findings suggestive of genital HSV infection during or preceding pregnancy.

Children Beyond the Neonatal Period and Adolescents. Patients with primary gingivostomatitis or genital herpes usually shed virus for at least 1 week and occasionally for several weeks. Patients with recurrent infection shed virus for a shorter period, typically 3 to 4 days. Intermittent asymptomatic reactivation of oral and genital herpes is common and occurs throughout the remainder of a person's life, occurring on approximately 1% of days among people previously infected. The greatest concentration of virus is shed during symptomatic primary infections and the lowest concentration of virus is shed during asymptomatic recurrent infections.

Infections with HSV-1 usually result from direct contact with infected oral secretions or lesions. Infections with HSV-2 usually result from direct contact with infected genital secretions or lesions through sexual activity. Genital infections caused by HSV-1 in children can result from autoinoculation of virus from the mouth, but sexual abuse always should be considered in prepubertal children with genital HSV-2 infections. Therefore, genital HSV isolates from children should be typed to differentiate between HSV-1 and HSV-2.

The incidence of HSV-2 infection correlates with the number of sexual partners and with acquisition of other sexually transmitted infections. After primary genital infection, which often is asymptomatic, some people experience frequent clinical recurrences, and others have no clinically apparent recurrences. Genital HSV-2 infection is more likely to recur than is genital HSV-1 infection.

Inoculation of skin occurs from direct contact with HSV-containing oral or genital secretions. This contact can result in herpes gladiatorum among wrestlers, herpes rugbiaforum among rugby players, or herpetic whitlow of the fingers in any exposed person.

The **incubation period** for HSV infection occurring beyond the neonatal period ranges from 2 days to 2 weeks.

DIAGNOSTIC TESTS: Herpes simplex virus grows readily in cell culture. Special transport media are available that allow transport to local or regional laboratories for culture. Cytopathogenic effects typical of HSV infection usually are observed 1 to 3 days after inoculation. Methods of culture confirmation include fluorescent antibody staining and enzyme immunoassays. Cultures that remain negative by day 15 likely will continue to remain negative. Polymerase chain reaction (PCR) assay often can detect HSV DNA in CSF from patients with CNS infection during the neonatal period (neonatal HSV CNS disease) and with HSE in older children and adults and is the diagnostic method of choice for CNS HSV involvement. Histologic examination and viral culture of a brain tissue biopsy specimen is the most definitive method of confirming the diagnosis of HSE. Cultures of CSF from a patient with HSE usually are negative.

For diagnosis of neonatal HSV infection, swabs of the mouth, nasopharynx, conjunctivae, and rectum and specimens of skin vesicles, blood, and CSF should be obtained for culture ("surface cultures"). Positive cultures obtained from any of these sites more than 12 to 24 hours after birth indicate viral replication and, therefore, are suggestive of infant infection rather than merely contamination after intrapartum exposure. Rapid diagnostic techniques also are available, such as direct fluorescent antibody (DFA) staining of vesicle scrapings or enzyme immunoassay detection of HSV antigens. These techniques are as specific but slightly less sensitive than culture. Typing HSV strains differentiates between HSV-1 and HSV-2 isolates. PCR assay is a sensitive method for detecting HSV DNA and is of particular value for evaluating CSF specimens from neonates with suspected HSV CNS disease. As with any PCR assay, false-negative and false-positive results can occur. Blood PCR may be of benefit in the diagnosis of neonatal HSV disease, but its use should not supplant the standard work-up of such patients (which includes surface cultures and CSF PCR); no data exist to support use of serial blood PCR assay to monitor response to therapy. Radiographs and clinical manifestations can suggest HSV pneumonitis, and elevated transaminase values can suggest HSV hepatitis; both are seen commonly in neonatal HSV disseminated disease. Histologic examination of lesions for the presence of multinucleated giant cells and eosinophilic intranuclear inclusions typical of HSV (eg, with Tzanck test) has low sensitivity.

Both type-specific and type-common antibodies to HSV develop during the first several weeks after infection and persist indefinitely. Although type-specific HSV-2 antibody usually indicates previous anogenital infection, the presence of HSV-1 antibody does not distinguish anogenital from orolabial infection reliably, because at least 20% of initial genital infections are caused by HSV-1. Type-specific serologic tests can be useful in confirming a clinical diagnosis of genital herpes. Additionally, these serologic tests can be used to diagnose people with unrecognized infection and to manage sexual partners of people with genital herpes. There is growing evidence that type-specific antibody avidity testing may prove useful for evaluating risk of neonatal infection. The presence of low-avidity HSV-2 immunoglobulin (Ig) G in serum of near-term pregnant women has been correlated with an elevated risk of neonatal infection. Serologic testing is not useful in neonates.

Several glycoprotein G (gG)-based type-specific assays have been approved by the US Food and Drug Administration (FDA), including at least one that can be used as a point-of-care test. The sensitivities and specificities of these tests for detection of HSV-2 IgG antibody vary from 90% to 100%; false-negative results may occur, especially early after infection, and false-positive results can occur, especially in patients with low likelihood of HSV infection. Therefore, repeat testing or a confirmatory test (eg, an immunoblot assay if the initial test was an enzyme-linked immunosorbent assay) may be indicated in some settings.

TREATMENT: For recommended antiviral dosages and duration of therapy with systemic acyclovir, valacyclovir, and famciclovir and with topical penciclovir for different HSV infections, see Antiviral Drugs (p 777). Valacyclovir is an L-valyl ester of acyclovir that is metabolized to acyclovir after oral administration, resulting in higher serum concentrations than are achieved with oral acyclovir and similar serum concentrations as are achieved with intravenous administration of acyclovir. Famciclovir is converted rapidly to penciclovir after oral administration. Table 3.23 (p 367) shows drugs for HSV by type of infection. Neither valacyclovir nor famciclovir is approved by the FDA for use in children.

Table 3.23. Recommended Therapy for Herpes Simplex Virus Infections[a]

Infection	Drug[b]
Neonatal	Parenteral acyclovir
Keratoconjunctivitis	Trifluridine[c] **OR** Iododeoxyuridine **OR** Vidarabine
Genital	Acyclovir **OR** Famciclovir **OR** Valacyclovir
Mucocutaneous (immunocompromised or primary gingivostomatitis)	Acyclovir **OR** Famciclovir **OR** Valacyclovir
Acyclovir-resistant (severe infections, immunocompromised)	Parenteral foscarnet
Encephalitis	Parenteral acyclovir

[a]See text and Table 4.8 (p 777) for details.
[b]Famciclovir and valacyclovir are approved for treatment of adults.
[c]Treatment of herpes simplex virus ocular infection should involve an ophthalmologist.

Neonatal. Parenteral acyclovir is the treatment of choice for neonatal HSV infections. Acyclovir should be administered to all neonates with HSV infection, regardless of manifestations and clinical findings. The best outcome in terms of morbidity and mortality is observed among infants with SEM disease. Although most neonates treated for HSV CNS disease survive, most survivors suffer substantial neurologic sequelae. Approximately 20% of neonates with disseminated disease die despite antiviral therapy. The dosage of acyclovir is 60 mg/kg per day in 3 divided doses, given intravenously for 14 days in SEM disease and for 21 days in CNS disease or disseminated disease. Approximately 50% of infants surviving neonatal HSV experience cutaneous recurrences, but optimal management of these recurrences is not established. The value of long-term suppressive or intermittent acyclovir therapy for neonates surviving neonatal HSV disease is not known and continues to be evaluated.

Infants with ocular involvement attributable to HSV infection should receive a topical ophthalmic drug (1% trifluridine, 0.1% iododeoxyuridine, or 3% vidarabine) as well as parenteral antiviral therapy.

Genital Infection.

Primary. Many patients with first-episode herpes initially have mild clinical manifestations but may go on to develop severe or prolonged symptoms. Therefore, most patients with initial genital herpes should receive antiviral therapy. In adults, acyclovir and valacyclovir decrease the duration of symptoms and viral shedding in primary genital herpes. Oral acyclovir therapy (400 mg, orally, 3 times/day for 7–10 days; or 200 mg, orally, 5 times/day for 7–10 days), initiated within 6 days of onset of disease, shortens the duration of illness and viral shedding by 3 to 5 days. Valacyclovir and famciclovir do not seem to be more effective than acyclovir, but they offer the advantage of less frequent dosing (famciclovir, 250 mg, orally, 3 times/day for 7–10 days; valacyclovir, 1 g, orally, 2 times/day for 7–10 days). No pediatric formulations of valacyclovir or famciclovir are available. Intravenous acyclovir is indicated for patients with a severe or complicated primary infection that requires hospitalization. Topical acyclovir (5%) ointment for primary genital herpes infection is not recommended. Systemic or topical treatment of primary herpetic lesions does not affect the subsequent frequency or severity of recurrences.

Recurrent. Antiviral therapy for recurrent genital herpes can be administered either episodically to ameliorate or shorten the duration of lesions or continuously as suppressive therapy to decrease the frequency of recurrences. Many patients benefit from antiviral therapy; therefore, options for treatment should be discussed with all patients. Oral acyclovir therapy initiated within 1 day of lesion onset or during the prodrome that precedes some outbreaks shortens the mean clinical course by approximately 1 day. If episodic therapy is used, a prescription for the medication should be provided with instructions to initiate treatment immediately when symptoms begin. Valacyclovir and famciclovir are licensed for treatment of adults with recurrent genital herpes; however, no data exist for treatment of pediatric disease.

In adults with frequent genital HSV recurrences (6 or more episodes per year), daily oral acyclovir suppressive therapy is effective for decreasing the frequency of symptomatic recurrences. After approximately 1 year of continuous daily therapy, acyclovir should be discontinued and the recurrence rate should be assessed. If recurrences are observed, additional suppressive therapy should be considered. Acyclovir appears to be safe for adults receiving the drug for more than 15 years, but longer-term effects are unknown. Data also support suppressive therapy in adults with valacyclovir or famciclovir.

Data on use of valacyclovir or famciclovir for suppressive therapy in children are not available. The safety of systemic valacyclovir and famciclovir therapy in pregnant women has not been established. Available data do not indicate an increased risk of major birth defects in comparison with the general population in women treated with acyclovir during the first trimester. Acyclovir may be administered orally to pregnant women with first-episode genital herpes or severe recurrent herpes and should be given intravenously to pregnant women with severe HSV infection. Counseling and education of infected adolescents/adults and their sexual partners, especially on the potential for recurrent episodes and how to reduce transmission to partners, is a critical part of management. Pregnant women or women of childbearing age with genital herpes should be encouraged to inform their health care professionals and those who will care for the newborn infant.

Mucocutaneous.

Immunocompromised Hosts. Intravenous acyclovir is effective for treatment and prevention of mucocutaneous HSV infections. Topical acyclovir also may accelerate healing of lesions in immunocompromised patients. Acyclovir-resistant strains of HSV have been isolated from immunocompromised people receiving prolonged treatment with acyclovir. Under these circumstances, progressive disease may be observed despite acyclovir therapy. Foscarnet is the drug of choice for disease caused by acyclovir-resistant HSV isolates.

Immunocompetent Hosts. Limited data are available on the effects of acyclovir on the course of primary or recurrent nongenital mucocutaneous HSV infections in immunocompetent hosts. Therapeutic benefit has been noted in a limited number of children with primary gingivostomatitis treated with oral acyclovir. Slight therapeutic benefit of oral acyclovir therapy has been demonstrated among adults with recurrent herpes labialis. When used as treatment for HSV orolabial disease, a dose of 80 mg/kg per day in 4 divided doses should be used, with a maximum of 3200 mg/day. Topical acyclovir is ineffective. A topical formulation of penciclovir (Denavir) and another drug, docosanol (Abreva), have only limited activity for therapy of herpes labialis and are not recommended.

In a small controlled study in adults with recurrent herpes labialis (6 or more episodes per year), prophylactic acyclovir given in a dosage of 400 mg, twice a day, was effective for decreasing the frequency of recurrent episodes. Although no studies of prophylactic therapy have been performed in children, those with frequent recurrences may benefit from continuous oral acyclovir therapy, with reevaluation being performed after 6 months to 1 year of continuous therapy; a dose of 30 mg/kg per day in 3 divided doses with a maximum 1000 mg/day is reasonable to begin as suppressive therapy in children. Valacyclovir has been approved for suppression of genital herpes in immunocompetent adults.

Other HSV Infections.

Central Nervous System. Patients with HSE should be treated for 21 days with intravenous acyclovir. Therapy is less effective in older adults than in children. Patients who are comatose or semicomatose at initiation of therapy also have a poorer outcome. For people with Bell palsy, the combination of acyclovir and prednisone may be considered.

Ocular. Treatment of eye lesions should be undertaken in consultation with an ophthalmologist. Several topical drugs, such as 1% trifluridine, 0.1% iododeoxyuridine, and 3% vidarabine, have proven efficacy for superficial keratitis. Topical corticosteroids by themselves are contraindicated in suspected HSV conjunctivitis; however, ophthalmologists may choose to use corticosteroids in conjunction with antiviral drugs to treat locally invasive infections. For children with recurrent ocular lesions, oral suppressive therapy with acyclovir (30 mg/kg per day in 3 divided doses; maximum 1000 mg/day) may be of benefit.

ISOLATION OF THE HOSPITALIZED PATIENT: In addition to standard precautions, the following recommendations should be followed.

Neonates With HSV Infection. Neonates with HSV infection should be hospitalized and managed with contact precautions if mucocutaneous lesions are present.

Neonates Exposed to HSV During Delivery. Infants born to women with active HSV lesions should be managed with contact precautions during the incubation period. Some experts believe that contact precautions are unnecessary if exposed infants were born by cesarean delivery, provided membranes were ruptured for less than 4 hours. The risk of HSV infection in infants born to mothers with a history of recurrent genital herpes who have no genital lesions at delivery is low, and special precautions are not necessary.

One method of infection control for neonates with documented perinatal exposure to HSV is continuous rooming-in with the mother in a private room.

Women in Labor and Postpartum Women With HSV Infection. Women with active HSV lesions should be managed with contact precautions during labor, delivery, and the postpartum period. These women should be instructed about the importance of careful hand hygiene before and after caring for their infants. The mother may wear a clean covering gown to help avoid contact of the infant with lesions or infectious secretions. A mother with herpes labialis or stomatitis should wear a disposable surgical mask when touching her newborn infant until the lesions have crusted and dried. She should not kiss or nuzzle her newborn until lesions have cleared. Herpetic lesions on other skin sites should be covered.

Breastfeeding is acceptable if no lesions are present on the breasts and if active lesions elsewhere on the mother are covered (see Human Milk, p 118).

Children With Mucocutaneous HSV Infection. Contact precautions are recommended for patients with severe mucocutaneous HSV infection. Patients with localized recurrent lesions should be managed with standard precautions.

Patients With HSV Infection of the CNS. Standard precautions are recommended for patients with infection limited to the CNS.

CONTROL MEASURES:

Prevention of Neonatal Infection. Surveillance genital cultures for HSV obtained weekly during pregnancy are not recommended. Women with a history of recurrent genital HSV infection are recognized to be at low risk of transmitting HSV to their infants (see Epidemiology, p 364).

Management of infants exposed to HSV during delivery differs according to the status of the mother's infection, mode of delivery, and expert opinion (see Care of Newborn Infants Whose Mothers Have Active Genital Lesions, below). Current recommendations for management of pregnant women for prevention of HSV infection include the following:

- **During pregnancy.** During prenatal evaluations, all pregnant women should be asked about past or current signs and symptoms consistent with genital herpes infection in themselves and their sexual partners.
- Although antiviral therapy for women with a history of genital HSV infection is recommended by some obstetricians during the final weeks of pregnancy to suppress maternal recurrence of viral shedding, the safety of antiviral therapy for the fetus and its efficacy in preventing viral shedding, rate of cesarean delivery, or neonatal infection have not been established. Cases of neonatal HSV disease have occurred among women who received antiviral prophylaxis during the latter weeks of pregnancy.
- **Women in labor.** During labor, all women should be asked about recent and current signs and symptoms consistent with genital herpes infection, and they should be examined carefully for evidence of genital infection. Suspicious lesions should be cultured to assist in subsequent management of the newborn. Cesarean delivery for women who have clinically apparent HSV infection decreases the risk of neonatal HSV infection. In the absence of genital lesions, a maternal history of genital HSV is not an indication for cesarean delivery. Fetal scalp monitors should be avoided when possible in infants of women suspected of having active genital herpes infection during labor.

Care of Newborn Infants Whose Mothers Have Active Genital Lesions at Delivery. Because the risk to infants exposed to HSV lesions during delivery varies in different circumstances (from 2% for recurrent genital HSV to 25% to 60% for first-episode genital HSV), management of the asymptomatic, exposed neonate is controversial. For neonates born vaginally or by cesarean delivery whose mothers have active genital HSV lesions, HSV cultures should be obtained at 12 to 24 hours of life; sites for HSV culture should include swabs of the mouth, nasopharynx, conjunctivae, and rectum (see Diagnostic Tests, p 365).

For infants born vaginally to mothers with a first-episode genital infection, some experts recommend empiric parenteral acyclovir treatment. Timing of initiation of acyclovir in such a situation could be after HSV cultures are obtained at 12 to 24 hours of life or earlier; if it is the latter, HSV cultures still should be obtained before starting antiviral therapy, even though it is less than 12 hours after delivery. Most experts would not administer acyclovir as empiric therapy to neonates born to women with active recurrent genital HSV lesions. The infant's parents or caregivers, however, should be educated about the signs and symptoms of neonatal HSV infection during the first 6 weeks of life.

If the neonate's HSV cultures obtained at 12 to 24 hours of life subsequently grow HSV, HSV infection is confirmed and the infant then should be evaluated for HSV disease. Evaluation should include lumbar puncture for CSF indices and HSV PCR and determination of serum hepatic transaminases. An infant with no evidence of HSV disease should be treated empirically with intravenous acyclovir for 14 days in hopes of preventing the HSV infection from progressing to HSV disease. An infant with evidence of SEM disease, CNS disease, or disseminated disease should be managed as described in Treatment, Neonatal (p 367).

If, within the first 6 weeks of life, a neonate born to a woman with active HSV lesions develops clinical findings suggestive of HSV infection, such as skin or scalp rashes (especially vesicular lesions) or unexplained manifestations (such as those of sepsis), cultures and rapid diagnostic tests (eg, PCR or CSF analysis) should be performed, and acyclovir therapy should be initiated immediately. The sensitivity of viral cultures for detecting neonatal infection in infants whose mothers were treated with antiviral medication during pregnancy is not known.

Differentiating primary genital infection from recurrent HSV infection in the mother would be helpful for assessing the risk of HSV infection for the exposed infant, but the distinction may be difficult. First-episode clinical infections are not always primary infections. Often, primary infections are asymptomatic, in which case the first symptomatic episode will represent a reactivated recurrent infection. In selected instances, serologic testing can be useful. For example, if a woman with herpetic lesions has no detectable HSV antibodies, she is experiencing a primary infection. Assessment of seropositive women necessitates differentiation of HSV-1 from HSV-2 antibodies using commercially available type-specific serologic assays such as the HerpeSelect Test.

Care of Newborn Infants Whose Mothers Have a History of Genital Herpes But No Active Genital Lesions at Delivery. An infant whose mother has known, recurrent genital infection but no genital lesions at delivery should be observed for signs of infection (eg, vesicular lesions of the skin, respiratory distress, seizures, or signs of sepsis) but should not have specimens for surface cultures for HSV obtained at 12 to 24 hours of life and should not receive empiric parenteral acyclovir. Education of parents and caregivers about the signs and symptoms of neonatal HSV infection during the first 6 weeks of life is prudent.

An infant born to a woman with a history of genital herpes but no lesions at delivery who presents within the first 6 weeks of life with fever and irritability or other symptoms compatible with HSV infection should be evaluated immediately for possible HSV infection (as well as for bacterial infection) (see Diagnostic Tests, p 365). Acyclovir therapy should be initiated if any of the culture or PCR results are positive, CSF indices are abnormal, or HSV infection otherwise is suspected.

Infected Hospital Personnel. Transmission of HSV in newborn nurseries from infected personnel to newborn infants rarely has been documented. The risk of transmission to infants by personnel who have herpes labialis or who are asymptomatic oral shedders of virus is low. Compromising patient care by excluding personnel with cold sores who are essential for the operation of the nursery must be weighed against the potential risk of newborn infants becoming infected. Personnel with cold sores who have contact with infants should cover and not touch their lesions and should comply with hand hygiene policies. Transmission of HSV infection from personnel with genital lesions is not likely as long as personnel comply with hand hygiene policies. Personnel with an active herpetic whitlow should not have responsibility for direct care of neonates or immunocompromised patients and should wear gloves and use hand hygiene during direct care of other patients.

Infected Household, Family, and Other Close Contacts of Newborn Infants. Intrafamilial transmission of HSV to newborn infants has been described but is rare. Household members with herpetic skin lesions (eg, herpes labialis or herpetic whitlow) should be counseled about the risk and should avoid contact of their lesions with newborn infants by taking the same measures as recommended for infected hospital personnel as well as avoiding kissing and nuzzling the infant while they have active lip lesions or touching the infant while they have herpetic whitlow. Cases of possible HSV transmission to the genitalia of male neonates have been reported following ritual circumcision involving mouth suction of the site by the performer of the circumcision.

Care of People With Extensive Dermatitis. Patients with dermatitis are at risk of developing eczema herpeticum. If these patients are hospitalized, special care should be taken to avoid exposure to HSV. These patients should not be kissed by people with cold sores or touched by people with herpetic whitlow.

Care of Children With Mucocutaneous Infections Who Are in Child Care or School. Oral HSV infections are common among children who are in child care or school. Most of these infections are asymptomatic, with shedding of virus in saliva occurring in the absence of clinical disease. Only children with HSV gingivostomatitis (ie, primary infection) who do not have control of oral secretions should be excluded from child care. Exclusion of children with cold sores (ie, recurrent infection) from child care or school is not indicated.

Children with uncovered lesions on exposed surfaces pose a small potential risk to contacts. If children are certified by a physician to have recurrent HSV infection, covering the active lesions with clothing, a bandage, or an appropriate dressing when they attend child care or school is sufficient.

HSV Infections Among Wrestlers and Rugby Players. Infection with HSV-1 has been transmitted during athletic competition involving close physical contact and frequent skin abrasions, such as wrestling (herpes gladiatorum) and rugby (herpes rugbiaforum or scrum pox). Competitors often do not recognize or may deny possible infection. Transmission of these infections can be limited or prevented by the following: (1) examination of wrestlers and rugby players for vesicular or ulcerative lesions on exposed areas of their bodies and around their mouths or eyes before practice or competition by a person familiar with the appearance of mucocutaneous infections (including HSV, herpes zoster, and impetigo); (2) exclusion of athletes with these conditions from competition or practice until healing occurs or a physician's written statement declaring their condition noninfectious is obtained; and (3) cleaning wrestling mats with a freshly prepared solution of household bleach (one quarter cup of bleach in 1 gallon of water) applied for a minimum contact time of 15 seconds at least daily and, preferably, between matches. Despite these precautions, HSV spread during wrestling and other sports involving close personal contact still can occur through contact with asymptomatic infected people.

Histoplasmosis

CLINICAL MANIFESTATIONS: *Histoplasma capsulatum* causes symptoms in fewer than 5% of infected people. Clinical manifestations are classified according to site (pulmonary or disseminated), duration (acute or chronic), and pattern (primary or reactivation) of infection. Most symptomatic patients have acute pulmonary histoplasmosis, an influenza-like illness with nonpleuritic chest pain, hilar adenopathy, and mild pulmonary infiltrates; symptoms persist for 2 days to 2 weeks. Intense exposure to spores can cause severe respiratory tract symptoms and diffuse nodular pulmonary infiltrates, prolonged fever, fatigue, and weight loss. Erythema nodosum can occur in adolescents. Primary cutaneous infections after trauma are rare.

Progressive disseminated histoplasmosis (PDH) can develop in otherwise healthy infants and children younger than 2 years of age. Early manifestations include prolonged fever, failure to thrive, and hepatosplenomegaly; if untreated, malnutrition, diffuse adenopathy, pneumonia, mucosal ulceration, pancytopenia, disseminated intravascular coagulopathy, and gastrointestinal tract bleeding can ensue. Central nervous system involvement is common. Cellular immune dysfunction caused by primary immunodeficiency disorders, human immunodeficiency virus (HIV) infection, or immunosuppressive therapy (including tumor necrosis factor-alpha inhibitors) may predispose patients with acute histoplasmosis to develop PDH. An early sign is fever with no apparent focus. Later, diffuse pneumonitis, skin lesions, meningitis, lymphadenopathy, hepatosplenomegaly, pancytopenia, and coagulopathy occur.

ETIOLOGY: *H capsulatum var capsulatum* is a dimorphic fungus. It grows in the environment as a microconidia-bearing mold but converts to the yeast phase at body temperature.

EPIDEMIOLOGY: *H capsulatum* is encountered in many parts of the world and is endemic in the eastern and central United States, particularly the Mississippi, Ohio, and Missouri River valleys. Infections occur sporadically; in outbreaks when weather conditions predispose to spread of spores; or in point-source epidemics after exposure to gardening activities, playing in barns, hollow trees, caves, or bird roosts, or excavation, demolition, cleaning, or renovation of contaminated buildings. The mold form is found in moist soil and its growth is facilitated by bat, bird, and chicken droppings. Spores are spread in dry and windy conditions or when occupational or recreational activities disturb contaminated sites. Infection is acquired when microconidia are inhaled. The inoculum size, strain virulence, and immune status of the host affect severity of illness. Reinfection is possible but requires a large inoculum. Person-to-person transmission does not occur.

The **incubation period** is variable but usually is 1 to 3 weeks.

DIAGNOSTIC TESTS: Culture is the definitive method of diagnosis. *H capsulatum* from bone marrow, blood, sputum, and tissue specimens grows on standard mycologic media in 1 to 6 weeks. The lysis-centrifugation method is preferred for blood cultures. A DNA probe for *H capsulatum* permits rapid identification.

Demonstration of typical intracellular yeast forms by examination with Gomori methenamine silver or other stains of tissue, blood, bone marrow, or bronchoalveolar lavage specimens strongly supports the diagnosis of histoplasmosis when clinical, epidemiologic, and other laboratory studies are compatible.

Detection of *H capsulatum* galactomannan antigen in serum, urine, a bronchoalveolar lavage specimen, or cerebrospinal fluid using a quantitative enzyme immunoassay is possible using a rapid, commercially available diagnostic test. Antigen detection is most sensitive for severe, acute pulmonary infections and for progressive disseminated infections. Results often are transiently positive early in the course of acute, self-limited pulmonary infections. A negative test result does not exclude infection. If the result initially is positive, the antigen test also is useful in monitoring treatment response and, after treatment, identifying relapse. Cross-reactions occur in patients with blastomycosis, coccidioidomycosis, paracoccidioidomycosis, and *Penicillium marneffei* infection; clinical and epidemiologic circumstances assist in differentiating these infections.

Both mycelial-phase (histoplasmin) and yeast-phase antigens are used in serologic testing for complement-fixing antibodies to *H capsulatum*. A fourfold increase in either yeast-phase or mycelial-phase titers or a single titer of 1:32 or greater in either test is presumptive evidence of active or recent infection. Cross-reacting antibodies can result from *Blastomyces dermatitidis* and *Coccidioides immitis* infections. In the immunodiffusion test, H bands, although infrequently encountered, are highly suggestive of acute infection; M bands also occur in acute or recent infection. The immunodiffusion test is more specific than the complement fixation test, but the complement fixation test is more sensitive.

TREATMENT: Immunocompetent children with uncomplicated, primary pulmonary histoplasmosis rarely require antifungal therapy. Indications for therapy include PDH in infants, serious illness after intense exposures, and acute infection in immunocompromised patients.

Amphotericin B is recommended for disseminated disease and other serious infections (see Drugs for Invasive and Other Serious Fungal Infections, p 772), because most experts believe clinical improvement occurs more rapidly with amphotericin B than with the azoles. In mild to moderate disease in which antifungal therapy is warranted, itraconazole is preferred by most experts and, when used in adults, is more effective, has fewer adverse effects, and is less likely to induce resistance than is fluconazole. Monotherapy with itraconazole also has proven effective in treatment of mild to moderate disseminated histoplasmosis in HIV-infected patients, and although the safety and efficacy of itraconazole for use in children have not been established, anecdotal experience has found it to be well tolerated and effective.

Treatment is indicated for severe pulmonary infections, usually following intense exposure, that are accompanied by diffuse infiltrates and respiratory distress. Amphotericin B is recommended for 1 to 2 weeks, and after clinical improvement, itraconazole is recommended for an additional 12 weeks. Methylprednisolone during the first 1 to 2 weeks of antifungal therapy is used if respiratory complications develop. Less severe primary pulmonary infections that are associated with fever, malaise, and weight loss lasting longer than 4 weeks may benefit from oral itraconazole given for 6 to 12 weeks, although the effectiveness of this treatment is not well documented. Mediastinal adenitis that causes obstruction of the bronchus or another mediastinal structure may improve with a brief course of corticosteroids. In these instances, itraconazole should be used concurrently and continued for 6 to 12 weeks to prevent dissemination.

If monotherapy with amphotericin B is used to treat PDH in a nonimmunocompromised infant or child, the recommended duration of therapy is 4 to 6 weeks. An alternative regimen uses induction with amphotericin B therapy for 2 to 4 weeks and, when there has been substantial clinical improvement and a decline in the serum concentration of histoplasmosis antigen, then oral itraconazole for 12 weeks. Longer periods of therapy may be required for patients with severe disease, primary immunodeficiency syndromes, or acquired immunodeficiency that cannot be reversed or patients who experience relapse despite appropriate therapy. After completion of treatment for PDH, urine antigen concentrations should be monitored for 12 months. Stable, low concentrations of urine antigen that are not accompanied by signs of active infection may not necessarily require prolongation or resumption of treatment.

Erythema nodosum, arthritis syndromes, and pericarditis do not necessitate antifungal therapy. Pericarditis is treated with indomethacin. Dense fibrosis of mediastinal structures without an associated granulomatous inflammatory component does not respond to antifungal therapy.

ISOLATION OF THE HOSPITALIZED PATIENT: Standard precautions are recommended.

CONTROL MEASURES: In outbreaks, investigation for a common source of infection is indicated. Exposure to soil and dust from areas with significant accumulations of bird and bat droppings should be avoided, especially by immunocompromised people, or, if unavoidable, controlled through use of appropriate respiratory protection (eg, N95 respirator), gloves, and disposable clothing. Guidelines for preventing histoplasmosis designed for health and safety professionals, environmental consultants, and people supervising workers involved in activities in which contaminated materials are disturbed are available. Additional information about the guidelines is available from the National Institute for Occupational Safety and Health (NIOSH; publication No. 2005-109, available from Publications Dissemination, 4676 Columbia Parkway, Cincinnati, OH 45226-1998; telephone 800-356-4674); the National Center for Zoonotic, Vectorborne, and Enteric Diseases of the Centers for Disease Control and Prevention (telephone 404-639-3158); and the NIOSH Web site (**www.cdc.gov/niosh/docs/2005-109/pdfs/2005-109.pdf**).

Hookworm Infections
(*Ancylostoma duodenale* and *Necator americanus*)

CLINICAL MANIFESTATIONS: Patients with hookworm infection often are asymptomatic; however, chronic hookworm infection is a common cause of moderate and severe hypochromic microcytic anemia in people living in tropical developing countries, and heavy infection can cause hypoproteinemia with edema. Chronic hookworm infection in children may lead to physical growth delay, deficits in cognition, and developmental delay. After contact with contaminated soil, initial skin penetration of larvae, usually involving the feet, can cause a stinging or burning sensation followed by pruritus and a papulovesicular rash that may persist for 1 to 2 weeks. Pneumonitis associated with migrating larvae is uncommon and usually mild, except in heavy infections. Colicky abdominal pain, nausea, and/or diarrhea and marked eosinophilia can develop 4 to 6 weeks after exposure. Blood loss secondary to hookworm infection develops 10 to 12 weeks after infection and symptoms related to serious iron-deficiency anemia can develop in long-standing moderate or heavy hookworm infections. After oral ingestion of infectious *Ancylostoma duodenale larvae,* disease can manifest with pharyngeal itching, hoarseness, nausea, and vomiting shortly after ingestion.

ETIOLOGY: *Necator americanus* is the major cause of hookworm infection worldwide, although *A duodenale* also is an important hookworm in some regions. Mixed infections are common. Both are roundworms (nematodes) with similar life cycles.

EPIDEMIOLOGY: Humans are the only reservoir. Hookworms are prominent in rural, tropical, and subtropical areas where soil contamination with human feces is common. Although both hookworm species are equally prevalent in many areas, *A duodenale* is the predominant species in the Mediterranean region, northern Asia, and the west coast of South America. *N americanus* is predominant in the Western hemisphere, sub-Saharan Africa, Southeast Asia, and a number of Pacific islands. Larvae and eggs survive in loose, sandy, moist, shady, well-aerated, warm soil (optimal temperature 23°C–33°C [73°F–91°F]). Hookworm eggs from stool hatch in soil in 1 to 2 days as rhabditiform larvae. These larvae develop into infective filariform larvae in soil within 5 to 7 days and can persist for weeks to months. Percutaneous infection occurs after exposure to infectious larvae. *A duodenale* transmission can occur by oral ingestion and possibly through human milk. Untreated infected patients can harbor worms for 5 years or longer.

The time from exposure to development of noncutaneous symptoms is 4 to 12 weeks.

DIAGNOSTIC TESTS: Microscopic demonstration of hookworm eggs in feces is diagnostic. Adult worms or larvae rarely are seen. Approximately 5 to 8 weeks are required after infection for eggs to appear in feces. A direct stool smear with saline solution or potassium iodide saturated with iodine is adequate for diagnosis of heavy hookworm infection; light infections require concentration techniques. Quantification techniques (eg, Kato-Katz, Beaver direct smear, or Stoll egg-counting techniques) to determine the clinical significance of infection and the response to treatment may be available from state or reference laboratories.

TREATMENT: Albendazole, mebendazole, and pyrantel pamoate all are effective treatments (see Drugs for Parasitic Infections, p 783). In children 1 to 2 years of age in whom experience with these drugs is limited, the World Health Organization (WHO) recommends reducing the albendazole dose to half of that given to older children and adults. The dose of pyrantel pamoate is determined by weight. A repeat stool examination, using a concentration technique, should be performed 2 weeks after treatment, and if the result is positive, repeating therapy is indicated. Nutritional supplementation, including iron, is important when anemia is present. Severely affected children may require blood transfusion.

ISOLATION OF THE HOSPITALIZED PATIENT: Only standard precautions are recommended, because there is no direct person-to-person transmission.

CONTROL MEASURES: Sanitary disposal of feces to prevent contamination of soil is necessary in areas with endemic infection. Treatment of all known infected people and screening of high-risk groups (ie, children and agricultural workers) in areas with endemic infection can help decrease environmental contamination. Wearing shoes also may be helpful, but children frequently are exposed to hookworm larvae over their entire body surface. Despite relatively rapid reinfection, periodic deworming treatments targeting school-aged children have been advocated to prevent morbidity associated with heavy intestinal helminth infections. A hookworm vaccine is being developed.

Human Bocavirus

CLINICAL MANIFESTATIONS: Human bocavirus (HBoV) was first identified in 2005 from a cohort of children with acute respiratory tract symptoms. Cough, rhinorrhea, and fever are the most prominent symptoms reported in most preschool children in whom HBoV is detected as the sole pathogen. HBoV is found more frequently in children with acute respiratory tract infections than in asymptomatic children and also has been associated with episodes of wheezing. HBoV has been identified in 5% to 10% of all children with acute respiratory tract infections in various inpatient and outpatient settings using many different criteria to identify children for testing. The role of HBoV as a pathogen in human infection is confounded by simultaneous detection of other viral pathogens in patients from whom HBoV is identified, with coinfection rates as high as 80%. Support for the role of HBoV as a true pathogen comes from finding the virus in the respiratory tract, blood, and stool of some ill children and the finding of seroconversion after symptomatic disease. The role of HBoV in gastrointestinal tract disease remains defined poorly. Infection with HBoV appears to be ubiquitous, as nearly all children develop serologic evidence of previous HBoV infection by 5 years of age.

ETIOLOGY: HBoV is a nonenveloped, single-stranded DNA virus classified in the family *Parvoviridae* on the basis of its genetic similarity to the closely related **bo**vine parvovirus 1 and **ca**nine minute virus, from which the name "**boca**virus" was derived. Two distinct genotypes have been described, although there are no data regarding antigenic variation or distinct serotypes.

EPIDEMIOLOGY: Detection of HBoV has been described only in humans. Transmission is presumed to be from respiratory tract secretions, although fecal-oral transmission may be possible on the basis of the finding of HBoV in stools of children, including symptomatic children with diarrhea.

The frequent codetection of other viral pathogens of the respiratory tract in association with HBoV has led to speculation about the role played by HBoV; it may be a true copathogen, it may be shed for long periods after primary infection, or it may reactivate during subsequent viral infections. A prospective analysis of the duration of shedding in infected children has not been described.

HBoV circulates worldwide and throughout the year. In temperate climates, seasonal clustering in the spring associated with increased transmission of other respiratory tract viruses has been reported.

DIAGNOSTIC TESTS: No commercial test is available to diagnose HBoV infection. HBoV polymerase chain reaction and detection of HBoV-specific antibody are used by research laboratories to detect the presence of virus and infection, respectively.

TREATMENT: No specific therapy is available.

ISOLATION OF THE HOSPITALIZED PATIENT: The presence of virus in respiratory tract secretions and stool suggests that, in addition to standard precautions, contact precautions should be effective in limiting the spread of infection for the duration of the symptomatic illness in infants and young children. However, prolonged shedding of virus in respiratory tract secretions and in stool may occur after resolution of symptoms, particularly in immune-compromised hosts.

CONTROL MEASURES: Although possible health care-associated transmission of HBoV has been described, investigations on transmissibility of HBoV in the community or hospital settings have not been published. Appropriate hand hygiene, particularly when handling respiratory tract secretions or the diapers of ill children, is recommended. The presence of HBoV in serum also raises the possibility of transmission by transfusion, although this mode of transmission has not been documented.

Human Herpesvirus 6 (Including Roseola) and 7

CLINICAL MANIFESTATIONS: Clinical manifestations of primary infection with human herpesvirus 6 (HHV-6) include roseola (exanthem subitum) in approximately 20% of infected children, undifferentiated febrile illness without rash or localizing signs, and other acute febrile illnesses (febrile seizures, encephalitis and other neurologic disorders, and mononucleosis-like syndromes), often accompanied by cervical and postoccipital lymphadenopathy, gastrointestinal tract or respiratory tract signs, and inflamed tympanic membranes. Fever characteristically is high (temperature greater than 39.5°C [103.0°F]) and persists for 3 to 7 days. Approximately 20% of all emergency department visits for febrile children 6 through 12 months of age are attributable to HHV-6. In roseola, an erythematous maculopapular rash lasting hours to days is noted once fever resolves. Febrile seizures occur during the febrile period in approximately 10% to 15% of primary infections. A bulging anterior fontanelle occurs occasionally in patients with roseola. HHV6 and HHV7 may cause neurologic disease, including encephalitis. The virus persists and may reactivate. The clinical circumstances and manifestations of reactivation in healthy people are not known. Illness associated with reactivation, primarily in immunocompromised hosts, has been described in association with manifestations such as fever, rash, hepatitis, bone marrow suppression, pneumonia, and encephalitis.

Recognition of the varied clinical manifestations of human herpesvirus 7 (HHV-7) infection is evolving. Many, if not most, primary infections with HHV-7 may be asymptomatic or mild; some may present as typical roseola and may account for second or recurrent cases of roseola. Febrile illnesses associated with seizures also have been reported. Some investigators suggest that the association of HHV-7 with these clinical manifestations results from the ability of HHV-7 to reactivate HHV-6 from latency.

ETIOLOGY: HHV-6 and HHV-7 are lymphotropic agents that are closely related members of the Herpesviridae family. Strains of HHV-6 belong to 1 of 2 major groups, variants A and B. Almost all primary infections in children are caused by variant B strains except infections in some parts of Africa.

EPIDEMIOLOGY: Humans are the only known natural host for HHV-6 and HHV-7. Transmission of HHV-6 to an infant most likely results from asymptomatic shedding of virus in secretions of a family member, caregiver, or other close contact with persistent infection. During the febrile phase of primary infection, HHV-6 can be isolated from peripheral blood lymphocytes and saliva and may be detected in cerebrospinal fluid by polymerase chain reaction assay. Virus-specific maternal antibody is present uniformly in the serum of infants at birth and provides transient protection. As the concentration of maternal antibody decreases during the first year of life, the rate of infection increases rapidly, peaking between 6 and 24 months of age. Essentially all children acquire primary HHV-6 infection and are seropositive before 4 years of age. Infections occur throughout the year without a seasonal pattern. Secondary cases rarely are identified. Occasional outbreaks of roseola have been reported. HHV-6 can integrate into host chromosomes, and therefore, hereditary transmission of integrated viral DNA is possible, resulting in lifetime persistence of viral DNA in host cells, including blood and lymphocytes.

HHV-7 infection occurs somewhat later in life than HHV-6. By adulthood, the seroprevalence of HHV-7 is approximately 85%. Lifelong latent infection with HHV-6 and HHV-7 is established after primary infection. Infectious HHV-7 is present in more than 75% of saliva specimens obtained from healthy adults. Transmission of HHV-6 and HHV-7 to young children is likely to occur from contact with infected respiratory tract secretions of healthy contacts.

The mean **incubation period** for HHV-6 may be 9 to 10 days, and for HHV-7, the incubation period is not known.

DIAGNOSTIC TESTS: A fourfold increase in serum antibody concentration alone does not necessarily indicate new infection, because an increase in titer also may occur with reactivation and in association with other infections. However, seroconversion from negative to positive in paired sera is good evidence of recent primary infection. Detection of specific immunoglobulin (Ig) M antibody also is not reliable, because IgM antibodies to HHV-6 may be present in some asymptomatic previously infected people. Commercial assays for antibody detection can detect HHV-6–specific IgG, but these assays do not distinguish between primary infection and viral persistence or reactivation. Nearly all children older than 2 years of age have an antibody titer to HHV-6.

Reference laboratories offer diagnostic testing by the polymerase chain reaction (PCR) for HHV-6 DNA in blood and cerebrospinal fluid (CSF) specimens. However, chromosomal integration of HHV-6 DNA always will result in a positive PCR test result with a high viral load, potentially confounding the interpretation of a positive test result. Chromosomal integration has been reported in 0.8% of adult blood donors. The diagnosis of active HHV-6 infection should not be made without first excluding chromosomal integration by measuring DNA load in serum or CSF and comparing it with the DNA load in whole blood.

Diagnostic tests for HHV-7 also are limited to research laboratories, and reliable differentiation between primary infection and reactivation is problematic. Serodiagnosis of HHV-7 is confounded by serologic cross-reactivity with HHV-6 and by the potential ability of HHV-6 to be reactivated by HHV-7 and possibly other infections. For both HHV-6 and HHV-7, measurements of specific IgG antibody avidity are under investigation as tools by which primary infection versus viral reactivation/reinfection can be distinguished.

TREATMENT: Supportive. A few anecdotal reports suggest that use of ganciclovir may be beneficial for immunocompromised patients with serious HHV-6 disease.

ISOLATION OF THE HOSPITALIZED PATIENT: Standard precautions are recommended.

CONTROL MEASURES: None.

Human Herpesvirus 8

CLINICAL MANIFESTATIONS: Human herpesvirus (HHV-8) is the etiologic agent associated with Kaposi sarcoma (KS), primary effusion lymphoma, and multicentric Castleman disease (MCD). A primary infection syndrome consisting of fever and rash has been described in regions with endemic infection (the Mediterranean, Middle East, and Africa). Pediatric KS is a common cancer in many parts of Africa among patients with and without human immunodeficiency virus (HIV) infection but is extremely rare in the United States. KS is an important cause of cancer-related death among immunosuppressed patients and organ transplant recipients. In the United States, KS most commonly is seen in people with severe immunocompromise resulting from HIV infection. Primary effusion lymphoma also is exceedingly uncommon in children. MCD has been described in adolescents, but the proportion of cases attributable to infection with HHV-8 is unknown.

ETIOLOGY: HHV-8 is a member of the family Herpesviridae, the gammaherpesvirus subfamily, closely related to herpesvirus saimiri of monkeys and Epstein-Barr virus.

EPIDEMIOLOGY: Increasing virologic and epidemiologic evidence suggests that HHV-8 is transmitted and acquired through the oral cavity; virus is shed frequently in saliva of infected people and is latent in peripheral blood mononuclear cells and lymphoid tissue. Blood transfusion has been associated with acquisition of HHV-8 in regions with endemic infection. In the United States, infection with HHV-8 is uncommon among children (less than 5%), although pockets of higher prevalence (approximately 25%) have been reported in specific geographic regions and among adolescents with or at high risk of acquiring HIV. In areas of the world where HHV-8 is endemic, HHV-8 frequently is acquired before puberty, likely through contact with maternal or sibling saliva.

The **incubation period** of HHV-8 is unknown.

DIAGNOSTIC TESTS: Both serologic and nucleic acid amplification tests for HHV-8 are available, but no HHV-8 screening method has been approved by the Food and Drug Administration. Screening for HHV-8 may be advisable for blood transfusion and organ transplantation procedures once a suitable method is available, but existing diagnostic tests are of limited clinical utility. The detection of HHV-8 DNA in peripheral blood may help establish a diagnosis of MCD and follow response to treatment.

TREATMENT: No effective antiviral treatment is known for HHV-8.

ISOLATION OF THE HOSPITALIZED PATIENT: Standard precautions are recommended.

CONTROL MEASURES: None.

Human Immunodeficiency Virus Infection[1]

CLINICAL MANIFESTATIONS: Human immunodeficiency virus (HIV) infection results in a wide array of clinical manifestations and varied natural history. HIV type 1 (HIV-1) is much more common in the United States than is HIV type 2 (HIV-2). This chapter, therefore, addresses HIV-1 infection, unless otherwise specified. Acquired immunodeficiency syndrome (AIDS) is the name given to the most advanced stage of HIV-1 infection. The Centers for Disease Control and Prevention (CDC) has devised a case definition

---

[1] For a complete listing of current policy statements from the American Academy of Pediatrics regarding human immunodeficiency virus and acquired immunodeficiency syndrome, see **http://aappolicy.aappublications.org/.**

that comprises AIDS-defining conditions that are used for surveillance (Table 3.24). The CDC classifies all infected children younger than 13 years of age by varying degrees of clinical expression of disease (Table 3.25, p 382) and immunologic status (Table 3.26, p 384).[1,2] This pediatric classification system emphasizes the importance of the CD4+ T-lymphocyte count and percentage as critical immunologic parameters and as markers of prognosis. Data regarding plasma HIV-1 RNA concentration (viral load) are not included in this classification.

Table 3.24. 1993 Revised Case Definition of AIDS-Defining Conditions for Adults and Adolescents 13 Years of Age and Older[a]

- Candidiasis of bronchi, trachea, or lungs
- Candidiasis, esophageal
- Cervical cancer, invasive
- Coccidioidomycosis, disseminated or extrapulmonary
- Cryptococcosis, extrapulmonary
- Cryptosporidiosis, chronic intestinal (greater than 1 mo duration)
- Cytomegalovirus disease (other than liver, spleen, or nodes)
- Cytomegalovirus retinitis (with loss of vision)
- Encephalopathy, HIV related
- Herpes simplex: chronic ulcer(s) (greater than 1 mo duration) or bronchitis, pneumonitis, or esophagitis
- Histoplasmosis, disseminated or extrapulmonary
- Isosporiasis, chronic intestinal (greater than 1 mo duration)
- Kaposi sarcoma
- Lymphoma, Burkitt (or equivalent term)
- Lymphoma, immunoblastic (or equivalent term)
- Lymphoma, primary or brain
- *Mycobacterium avium* complex or *Mycobacterium kansasii* infection, disseminated or extrapulmonary
- *Mycobacterium tuberculosis* infection, any site, pulmonary or extrapulmonary
- *Mycobacterium,* other species or unidentified species infection, disseminated or extrapulmonary
- *Pneumocystis jirovecii* pneumonia
- Pneumonia, recurrent
- Progressive multifocal leukoencephalopathy
- *Salmonella* septicemia, recurrent
- Toxoplasmosis of brain
- Wasting syndrome attributable to HIV
- CD4+ T-lymphocyte count less than 200/μL (0.20 x 10^9/L) or CD4+ T-lymphocyte percentage less than 15%

AIDS indicates acquired immunodeficiency syndrome; HIV, human immunodeficiency virus.
[a]Modified from Centers for Disease Control and Prevention. 1993 revised classification system for HIV infection and expanded surveillance case definition for AIDS among adolescents and adults. *MMWR Recomm Rep.* 1992;41(RR–17):1–19.

---

[1]Centers for Disease Control and Prevention. 1993 revised classification system for HIV infection and expanded surveillance case definition for AIDS among adolescents and adults. *MMWR Recomm Rep.*1992;41(RR–17):1–19
[2]Centers for Disease Control and Prevention. 1994 revised classification system for human immunodeficiency virus infection in children less than 13 years of age. Official authorized addenda: human immunodeficiency virus infection codes and official guidelines for coding and reporting ICD-9-CM. *MMWR Recomm Rep.* 1994;43(RR-12):1–19

Table 3.25. Clinical Categories for Children Younger Than 13 Years of Age With Human Immunodeficiency Virus (HIV) Infection[a]

Category N: Not Symptomatic

Children who have no signs or symptoms considered to be the result of HIV infection or have only 1 of the conditions listed in Category A.

Category A: Mildly Symptomatic

- Children with 2 or more of the conditions listed but none of the conditions listed in categories B and C.
- Lymphadenopathy (≥0.5 cm at more than 2 sites; bilateral at 1 site)
- Hepatomegaly
- Splenomegaly
- Dermatitis
- Parotitis
- Recurrent or persistent upper respiratory tract infection, sinusitis, or otitis media

Category B: Moderately Symptomatic

- Children who have symptomatic conditions other than those listed for category A or C that are attributed to HIV infection.
- Anemia (hemoglobin, <8 g/dL [<80 g/L]), neutropenia (white blood cell count, <1000/μL [<1.0 × 10⁹/L]), and/or thrombocytopenia (platelet count, <100 × 10³/μL [<100 × 10⁹/L]) persisting for ≥30 days
- Bacterial meningitis, pneumonia, or sepsis (single episode)
- Candidiasis, oropharyngeal (thrush), persisting (>2 mo) in children older than 6 mo of age
- Cardiomyopathy
- Cytomegalovirus infection, with onset before 1 mo of age
- Diarrhea, recurrent or chronic
- Hepatitis
- Herpes simplex virus (HSV) stomatitis, recurrent (>2 episodes within 1 year)
- HSV bronchitis, pneumonitis, or esophagitis with onset before 1 mo of age
- Herpes zoster (shingles) involving at least 2 distinct episodes or more than 1 dermatome
- Leiomyosarcoma
- Lymphoid interstitial pneumonia or pulmonary lymphoid hyperplasia complex
- Nephropathy
- Nocardiosis
- Persistent fever (lasting >1 mo)
- Toxoplasmosis, onset before 1 mo of age
- Varicella, disseminated (complicated chickenpox)

Category C: Severely Symptomatic

- Serious bacterial infections, multiple or recurrent (ie, any combination of at least 2 culture-confirmed infections within a 2-y period), of the following types: septicemia, pneumonia, meningitis, bone or joint infection, or abscess of an internal organ or body cavity (excluding otitis media, superficial skin or mucosal abscesses, and indwelling catheter-related infections)
- Candidiasis, esophageal or pulmonary (bronchi, trachea, lungs)
- Coccidioidomycosis, disseminated (at site other than or in addition to lungs or cervical or hilar lymph nodes) Cryptococcosis, extrapulmonary
- Cryptosporidiosis or isosporiasis with diarrhea persisting >1 mo
- Cytomegalovirus disease with onset of symptoms after 1 mo of age (at a site other than liver, spleen, or lymph nodes)
- Encephalopathy (at least 1 of the following progressive findings present for at least 2 mo in the absence of a concurrent illness other than HIV infection that could explain the findings): (1) failure to attain or loss of developmental milestones or loss of intellectual ability, verified by standard developmental scale or neuropsychologic tests; (2) impaired brain growth or acquired microcephaly demonstrated by head circumference measurements or brain atrophy demonstrated by computed tomography or magnetic resonance imaging (serial imaging required for children younger than 2 y of age); (3) acquired symmetric motor deficit manifested by 2 or more of the following: paresis, pathologic reflexes, ataxia, or gait disturbance
- HSV infection causing a mucocutaneous ulcer that persists for greater than 1 mo or bronchitis, pneumonitis, or esophagitis for any duration affecting a child older than 1 mo of age

- Histoplasmosis, disseminated (at a site other than or in addition to lungs or cervical or hilar lymph nodes)
- Kaposi sarcoma
- Lymphoma, primary, in brain
- Lymphoma, small, noncleaved cell (Burkitt), or immunoblastic; or large-cell lymphoma of B-lymphocyte or unknown immunologic phenotype
- *Mycobacterium tuberculosis*, disseminated or extrapulmonary
- *Mycobacterium*, other species or unidentified species infection, disseminated (at a site other than or in addition to lungs, skin, or cervical or hilar lymph nodes)
- *Pneumocystis jiroveci* pneumonia
- Progressive multifocal leukoencephalopathy
- *Salmonella* (nontyphoid) septicemia, recurrent
- Toxoplasmosis of the brain with onset at after 1 mo of age
- Wasting syndrome in the absence of a concurrent illness other than HIV infection that could explain the following findings: (1) persistent weight loss >10% of baseline; (2) downward crossing of at least 2 of the following percentile lines on the weight-for-age chart (eg, 95th, 75th, 50th, 25th, 5th) in a child 1 y of age or older; OR (3) <5th percentile on weight-for-height chart on 2 consecutive measurements, ≥30 days apart; PLUS (1) chronic diarrhea (ie, at least 2 loose stools per day for >30 days); OR (2) documented fever (for >30 days, intermittent or constant)

ᵃModified from Centers for Disease Control and Prevention. 1994 revised classification system for human immunodeficiency virus infection in children less than 13 years of age. Official authorized addenda: human immunodeficiency virus infection codes and official guidelines for coding and reporting ICD-9-CM. *MMWR Recomm Rep.* 1994;43(RR-12):1–19

Table 3.26. Pediatric Human Immunodeficiency Virus (HIV) Classification for Children Younger Than 13 Years of Age[a]

Immunologic Definitions	Immunologic Categories Age-Specific CD4+ T-Lymphocyte Count and Percentage of Total Lymphocytes[b]						Clinical Classifications[c]			
	Younger Than 12 mo		1 Through 5 y		6 Through 12 y		N: No Signs or Symptoms	A: Mild Signs and Symptoms	B: Moderate Signs and Symptoms[d]	C: Severe Signs and Symptoms[d]
	µL	%	µL	%	µL	%				
1: No evidence of suppression	≥1500	≥25	≥1000	≥25	≥500	≥25	N1	A1	B1	C1
2: Evidence of moderate suppression	750–1499	15–24	500–999	15–24	200–499	15–24	N2	A2	B2	C2
3: Severe suppression	<750	<15	<500	<15	<200	<15	N3	A3	B3	C3

[a]Modified from Centers for Disease Control and Prevention. 1994 revised classification system for human immunodeficiency virus infection in children less than 13 years of age. Official authorized addenda: human immunodeficiency virus infection codes and official guidelines for coding and reporting ICD-9-CM. *MMWR Recomm Rep.* 1994;43(RR-12):1–19

[b]To convert values in µL to Système International units (x 10⁹/L), multiply by 0.001.

[c]Children whose HIV infection status is not confirmed are classified by using this grid with a letter E (for perinatally exposed) placed before the appropriate classification code (eg, EN2).

[d]Lymphoid interstitial pneumonitis in category B or any condition in category C is reportable to state and local health departments as acquired immunodeficiency syndrome (AIDS-defining conditions) (see Table 3.25, p 382, for further definition of clinical categories).

Early manifestations of pediatric HIV infection include unexplained fevers, generalized lymphadenopathy, hepatomegaly, splenomegaly, failure to thrive, persistent or recurrent oral and diaper candidiasis, recurrent diarrhea, parotitis, hepatitis, central nervous system (CNS) disease (eg, hyperreflexia, hypertonia, floppiness, developmental delay), lymphoid interstitial pneumonia, recurrent invasive bacterial infections, and other opportunistic infections (eg, viral and fungal).[1] With timely diagnostic testing and appropriate treatment, clinical manifestations of HIV-1 and occurrence of AIDS-defining illnesses are rare among children in industrialized nations.

The frequency of infections attributable to different opportunistic pathogens in the era before highly active antiretroviral therapy (HAART) varied by age, pathogen, previous infection history, and immunologic status. In the pre-HAART era, the most common opportunistic infections observed among children in the United States were infections caused by invasive encapsulated bacteria, *Pneumocystis jirovecii* (previously known as *Pneumocystis carinii*), varicella-zoster virus, cytomegalovirus, herpes simplex virus, *Mycobacterium avium* complex (MAC), and *Candida* species. Less commonly observed opportunistic pathogens included Epstein-Barr virus, *Mycobacterium tuberculosis*, *Cryptosporidium* species, *Isospora* species, other enteric pathogens, *Aspergillus* species, and *Toxoplasma gondii*. In the HAART era, there has been a substantial decrease in frequency of all opportunistic infections.

Malignant neoplasms in children with HIV-1 infection are relatively uncommon, but leiomyosarcomas and non-Hodgkin B-cell lymphomas of the Burkitt type (including some that arise in the CNS), occur more commonly in children with HIV-1 infection than in immunocompetent children. Kaposi sarcoma is rare in children in the United States.

Development of an opportunistic infection, particularly *P jirovecii* pneumonia (PCP), progressive neurologic disease, and severe wasting, are associated with a poor prognosis. In the absence of treatment, prognosis for survival also is poor in infants who were infected perinatally and who have high viral loads (ie, greater than 100 000 copies/mL), markedly decreased CD4+ T-lymphocyte counts (see Table 3.27, p 386, for age-specific CD+ T-lymphocyte count ranges) and percentages (less than 15%), and symptoms developing during the first 6 months of life. When HAART regimens are begun early, prognosis and survival rates improve dramatically. Although median survival to 9 years of age was reported before more potent combinations of antiretroviral (ARV) drugs became available, recent studies in the United States and Europe show greater than 95% survival to 16 years of age or older and preservation of reasonable immune system function, especially in children and adolescents who adhere to their medical regimens.

ETIOLOGY: Two types of HIV cause disease in humans: HIV-1 and HIV-2. These viruses are cytopathic lentiviruses belonging to the family Retroviridae, and they are related closely to the simian immunodeficiency viruses (SIVs), agents that occur naturally among African green monkeys and sooty mangabeys. Three distinct genetic groups of HIV-1 exist worldwide: M (major), O (outlier), and N (new). Group M viruses are the most prevalent worldwide and comprise 8 genetic subtypes, or clades, known as A through H. The HIV-1 genome is 10 kb in length and has both conserved and highly variable domains.

---

[1]Centers for Disease Control and Prevention. Guidelines for prevention and treatment of opportunistic infections among HIV-exposed and HIV-infected children. Recommendations from CDC, the National Institutes of Health, the HIV Medicine Association of the Infectious Diseases Society of America, the Pediatric Infectious Diseases Society, and the American Academy of Pediatrics. *MMWR*. 2009; in press. Available at: **http://aidsinfo.nih.gov/Guidelines/GuidelineDetail.aspx?GuidelineID=14**

Table 3.27. Laboratory Diagnosis of HIV Infection[a]

Test	Comment
HIV DNA PCR	Preferred test to diagnose HIV-1 subtype B infection in infants and children younger than 18 months of age; highly sensitive and specific by 2 weeks of age and available; performed on peripheral blood mononuclear cells. False-negative results can occur in non-B subtype HIV-1 infections.
HIV p24 Ag	Less sensitive, false-positive results during first month of life, variable results; not recommended.
ICD p24 Ag	Negative test result does not rule out infection; not recommended
HIV culture	Expensive, not easily available, requires up to 4 weeks to do test; not recommended.
HIV RNA PCR	Not recommended for routine testing of infants and children younger than 18 months of age, because a negative result cannot be used to exclude HIV infection definitively. Preferred test to identify non-B subtype HIV-1 infections.

[a]HIV indicates human immunodeficiency virus; PCR, polymerase chain reaction; Ag, antigen; and ICD, immune complex dissociated.

Three principal genes—*gag, pol,* and *env*—encode the major structural and enzymatic proteins, and 6 accessory genes regulate gene expression and aid in assembly and release of infectious virions. The *env* glycoprotein attaches to receptors on the host cell membrane and is the site of action of neutralizing antibody. *Env* particularly is prone to mutational change. HIV-1 is an RNA virus that requires the activity of a viral enzyme, reverse transcriptase, to convert the viral RNA to DNA. A double-stranded DNA copy of the viral genome then can incorporate into the host cell genome, where it persists as a provirus and is essentially invisible to the immune system.

HIV-2, the second AIDS-causing virus, predominantly is found in the French-speaking countries of West Africa, with the highest rates of infection in Guinea-Bissau. The prevalence of HIV-2 in the United States is extremely low. HIV-2 is thought to have a milder disease course with a longer time to development of AIDS than is HIV-1. Nonnucleoside reverse-transcriptase inhibitors (NNRTIs) are not effective against HIV-2, whereas nucleoside reverse transcriptase inhibitors (NRTIs) and protease inhibitors have varying efficacy against HIV-2. CDC guidelines state that HIV-2 serologic testing should be performed in patients who: (1) are from areas of high prevalence, mainly Western Africa; (2) share needles or have sex partners known to be infected with HIV-2 or from areas with endemic infection; (3) received transfusions or other nonsterile medical care in areas with endemic infection; or (4) are children of women with risk factors for HIV-2 infection. The identification of HIV-2 represents a diagnostic dilemma in the United States, because screening enzyme immunoassays, including the newer rapid tests, may not detect HIV-2. Routine Western blots are specific mainly for HIV-1 antibodies, although indeterminate Western blots (ie, detection of only 1 antigen, usually the p24 antigen) may suggest infection with HIV-2. Enzyme immunoassays (EIAs) approved by the US Food and Drug Administration (FDA) for detection of antibody to HIV-2 are Abbott HIVAB HIV-1/2 (rDNA) EIA, Genetic Systems HIV-1/2 Peptide EIA, and Genetic Systems HIV-2 EIA. No assays are approved by the FDA for determination of HIV-2 viral load in the United States.

EPIDEMIOLOGY: Humans are the only known reservoir for HIV-1 and HIV-2. Latent virus persists in peripheral blood mononuclear cells and in cells of the brain, bone marrow, and genital tract even when plasma viral load is undetectable. Only blood, semen, cervicovaginal secretions, and human milk have been implicated epidemiologically in transmission of infection.

Established modes of HIV-1 transmission are the following: (1) sexual contact (vaginal, anal, or orogenital); (2) percutaneous blood exposure (from contaminated needles or other sharp instruments); (3) mucous membrane exposure to contaminated blood or other body fluids; (4) mother-to-child transmission during pregnancy, around the time of labor and delivery, and postnatally through breastfeeding; and (5) transfusion with contaminated blood products. As a result of highly effective screening methods, blood, blood components, and clotting factor virtually have been eliminated as a cause of HIV-1 transmission in the United States. In the United States in the absence of documented sexual contact or parenteral or mucous membrane contact with blood-containing body fluids and mother-to-child transmission, transmission of HIV-1 rarely occurs in families or households or as a result of routine care in hospitals or clinics. Moreover, transmission of HIV-1 has not been documented in schools or child care settings in the United States.

Cases of AIDS in children have accounted for less than 1% of all reported cases in the United States. Since the mid 1990s, the number of reported cases of AIDS in children decreased significantly as a result of a dramatic decrease in the rate of mother-to-child transmission of HIV-1 with recommendations for antenatal HIV-1 testing and with implementation of efficacious interventions for prevention of such transmission, including complete avoidance of breastfeeding, ARV prophylaxis, and cesarean delivery before onset of labor and before rupture of membranes. Combination ARV regimens during pregnancy have been associated with lower rates of mother-to-child transmission than has zidovudine alone. Currently in the United States, most HIV-1–infected pregnant women receive 3-drug combination ARV regimens either for treatment if required for their own health or for prophylaxis of transmission (in which case the drugs are stopped after delivery). The CDC estimates that each year, 100 to 200 infants with HIV-1 infection are born in the United States. Mother-to-child transmission of HIV-1 accounts for virtually all new infections in preadolescent children. In industrialized nations, less than 1% of cases of HIV-1 infection in children result from sexual abuse by an HIV-1–seropositive person, from receipt of contaminated blood or blood products, or from accidental exposure to contaminated syringes or sharp objects.

The rate of acquisition of HIV-1 during adolescence continues to increase and contributes to the large number of cases in young adults. HIV-1 infection in adolescents occurs disproportionately in youths of minority race or ethnicity. Transmission of HIV-1 among adolescents is attributable primarily to sexual exposure and relatively little to illicit intravenous drug use. Young men of minority race or ethnicity who have sex with men particularly are at high risk of acquiring HIV-1 infection, whereas infection among young women primarily is acquired heterosexually. In 2005, approximately 14% of newly diagnosed HIV-1 infections in the United States were estimated to occur among people 13 to 24 years of age. Among adolescents, the incidence of HIV-1 infection in females 13 to 15 years of age exceeds that in males; for adolescents 16 to 19 years of age, the prevalence is equal between females and males. Most HIV-1–infected adolescents are asymptomatic, and without testing, they remain unaware that they are infected.

The risk of infection for an infant born to an HIV-1–seropositive mother who did not receive interventions to prevent transmission is estimated to range from 12% to 40%. Studies on timing of mother-to-child transmission of HIV-1 suggest that less than half of all transmission events occur in utero. The greatest numbers of transmissions occur at the time of delivery. Transmission also occurs postnatally as a result of breastfeeding. Maternal viral load is a critical factor affecting the likelihood of mother-to-child transmission of HIV-1, although transmission has been observed across the entire range of maternal plasma viral loads. The risk of transmission particularly is high for women with a primary HIV-1 infection during the last trimester of pregnancy. Such women are more likely to have higher viral loads and are less likely to have mounted an immune response. Other factors associated with an increased risk of transmission include a low maternal CD4+ T-lymphocyte count, advanced maternal illness, intrapartum events resulting in increased exposure of the fetus to maternal blood, chorioamnionitis, mother-infant *HLA* concordance, preterm delivery, and prolonged labor. Prolonged rupture of fetal membranes is associated with an increased risk of transmission and must be considered when evaluating the need for special obstetric interventions. Cesarean delivery performed before onset of labor and before rupture of membranes has been shown to reduce mother-to-child intrapartum transmission; current US guidelines recommend cesarean delivery before onset of labor and before rupture of membranes for HIV-1–infected women with a viral load greater than 1000 copies/mL near the time of delivery.

Postnatal transmission to neonates and young infants occurs mainly as a result of breastfeeding.[1] Worldwide, an estimated one third to one half of cases of mother-to-child HIV-1 transmission events occur as a result of breastfeeding. HIV-1 genomes have been detected in cellular and cell-free fractions of human milk. In the United States, HIV-1–infected mothers are advised not to breastfeed, because safe alternatives to human milk are available readily. Because human milk cell-associated HIV-1 can be detected even in women receiving HAART, replacement feeding continues to be recommended for US mothers on HAART. In resource-limited countries where replacement feeding is not affordable, feasible, acceptable, sustainable, and safe, exclusive breastfeeding for the first 6 months of life is recommended, with continued breastfeeding with additional nutritional supplementation after 6 months if these criteria still are not met. In addition to breastfeeding, premastication of food for teething infants has been linked to late HIV-1 transmissions in 3 infants in the United States categorized originally as HIV-1–uninfected, with documentation of bleeding gums or oral sores in 2 of the 3 caregivers at the time of premastication.

INCUBATION PERIOD: Although the onset of symptoms is approximately 12 through 18 months of age for untreated, perinatally infected infants in the United States, some become ill in the first few months of life, whereas others remain asymptomatic for more than 5 years and, rarely, until early adolescence. Without therapy, 2 patterns of symptomatic infection have been recognized: 15% to 20% of untreated children in the United States die before 4 years of age, with a median age at death of 11 months (termed rapid progressors), and 80% to 85% of untreated children have delayed onset of milder symptoms and survive beyond 5 years of age (termed slow progressors).

[1]Read JS; American Academy of Pediatrics, Committee on Pediatric AIDS. Human milk, breastfeeding, and transmission of human immunodeficiency virus type 1 in the United States. *Pediatrics*. 2003;112(5):1196–1205

DIAGNOSTIC TESTS[1]: Laboratory diagnosis of HIV-1 infection during infancy is based on detection of virus or viral nucleic acid (Table 3.27, p 386). Because most infants born to HIV-1–seropositive mothers have acquired maternal antibodies passively, antibody assays cannot be used for diagnosis of infection in neonates or young infants. However, in children 18 months of age and older, HIV-1 antibody assays can be used for diagnosis.

In the United States, the preferred test for diagnosis of HIV-1 infection in infants is the HIV-1 DNA polymerase chain reaction (PCR) assay. Approximately 30% to 40% of HIV-1–infected infants will have a positive DNA PCR assay result in samples obtained before 48 hours of age. A positive result by 48 hours of age suggests in utero transmission. The DNA PCR assay routinely can detect 1 to 10 DNA copies of proviral DNA in peripheral blood mononuclear cells. Approximately 93% of infected infants have detectable HIV-1 DNA by 2 weeks of age, and approximately 95% of HIV-1–infected infants have a positive HIV-1 DNA PCR assay result by 1 month of age. A single HIV-1 DNA PCR assay has a sensitivity of 95% and a specificity of 97% for samples collected from infected infants 1 to 36 months of age.

Virus isolation by culture is less sensitive than the DNA PCR assay, is expensive, and is available in few diagnostic laboratories; definitive results may take up to 28 days. This test no longer is recommended for routine diagnosis.

Detection of the p24 antigen (including immune complex dissociated) is substantially less sensitive than the HIV-1 DNA PCR assay or culture. An additional drawback is the occurrence of false-positive test results in samples obtained from infants younger than 1 month of age. This test generally should not be used, although newer assays have been reported to have sensitivities similar to HIV-1 DNA PCR assays.

Plasma HIV-1 RNA assays may be used to diagnose HIV-1 infection. However, a false-negative test result may occur in neonates receiving ARV prophylaxis. Although use of HAART can reduce plasma viral loads to undetectable levels, results of DNA PCR, which detects cell-associated integrated HIV-1 DNA, remain positive even in people with undetectable viral loads. In the absence of therapy, plasma viral loads among infants with perinatally acquired HIV-1 infection increase rapidly to very high levels (from several hundred thousand to more than 1 million copies/mL) after birth, decreasing only slowly to a "set point" by approximately 2 years of age. This contrasts to infection in adults, in whom a viral load "set point" occurs approximately 6 months after acquisition of infection. An HIV-1 RNA assay with only low-level viral copy number in an HIV-1–exposed infant may yield a false-positive result, reinforcing the importance of repeating any positive assay result to confirm the diagnosis of HIV-1 infection in infancy. Like the DNA PCR, the sensitivity of HIV-1 RNA assays for diagnosing infections in the first week of life is low (25%–40%). The test is licensed by the FDA only in a quantitative format and currently is used for quantifying virus as a predictor of disease progression rather than for routine diagnosis of HIV-1 infection in infants. RNA assays are used to monitor changes in viral load in the course of ARV therapy.

Diagnostic testing with HIV-1 DNA or RNA assays is recommended at 14 to 21 days of age, and if results are negative, repeated at 1 to 2 months of age and again at 4 to 6 months of age. Viral diagnostic testing in the first few days of life (eg, less than 48 hours of age) is recommended by some experts to allow for the early identification of infants

---

[1]Read JS; American Academy of Pediatrics, Committee on Pediatric AIDS. Diagnosis of HIV-1 infection in children younger than 18 months in the United States. *Pediatrics.* 2008;120(6):e1547–e1562. Available at: **http://pediatrics.aappublications.org/cgi/content/full/120/6/e1547**

with infection acquired in utero. If testing is performed at birth, umbilical cord blood should not be used because of possible contamination with maternal blood. Obtaining the sample as early as 14 days of age may facilitate decisions about initiating ARV therapy for infants found to be HIV-1 infected, because such children still would be receiving their 6-week course of zidovudine prophylaxis. An infant is considered infected if 2 separate samples test positive by DNA PCR.[1,2,3]

In nonbreastfeeding infants younger than 18 months of age with no positive HIV-1 virologic test results, *presumptive* exclusion of HIV-1 infection is based on:
- Two negative HIV-1 DNA or RNA virologic tests, from separate specimens, both of which were obtained at 2 weeks of age or older and 1 of which was obtained at 4 weeks of age or older; or
- One negative HIV-1 DNA or RNA virologic test from a specimen obtained at 8 weeks of age or older; or
- One negative HIV-1 antibody test obtained at 6 months of age or older;

AND

- No other laboratory or clinical evidence of HIV-1 infection (ie, no subsequent positive results from virologic tests if tests were performed and no AIDS-defining condition for which there is no other underlying condition of immunosuppression).

In nonbreastfeeding infants younger than 18 months of age with no positive HIV-1 virologic test results, *definitive* exclusion of HIV-1 is based on:
- At least 2 negative HIV-1 DNA or RNA virologic tests, both of which were obtained at 1 month of age or older and 1 of which was obtained at 4 months of age or older;
- At least 2 negative HIV-1 antibody tests from separate specimens obtained at 6 months of age or older; and
- No other laboratory or clinical evidence of HIV-1 infection (ie, no subsequent positive results from virologic tests if tests were performed, and no AIDS-defining condition for which there is no other underlying condition of immunosuppression).

In infants with 2 negative HIV-1 DNA PCR test results, many clinicians will confirm the absence of antibody (ie, loss of passively acquired natural antibody) to HIV-1 on testing at 12 through 18 months of age ("seroreversion"). An infant with 2 antibody-negative blood samples drawn at least 1 month apart and obtained after 6 months of age is considered uninfected.

EIAs are used widely as the initial test for serum HIV-1 antibody. These tests are highly sensitive and specific. Repeated EIA testing of initially reactive specimens is common practice and is followed by Western blot analysis to confirm the presence of antibody specific to HIV-1. A positive HIV-1 antibody test result (EIA followed by Western

---

[1]Centers for Disease Control and Prevention. Revised surveillance case definitions for HIV infection among adults, adolescents, and children aged <18 months and for HIV infection and AIDS among children aged 18 months to <13 years—United States, 2008. *MMWR Recomm Rep.* 2008;57(RR-10):1–12
[2]Centers for Disease Control and Prevention. Guidelines for prevention and treatment of opportunistic infections among HIV-exposed and HIV-infected children. Recommendations from CDC, the National Institutes of Health, the HIV Medicine Association of the Infectious Diseases Society of America, the Pediatric Infectious Diseases Society, and the American Academy of Pediatrics. *MMWR.* 2009; in press. Available at: **http://aidsinfo.nih.gov /Guidelines/GuidelineDetail.aspx?GuidelineID=14**
[3]Havens PL, Mofenson LM; American Academy of Pediatrics, Committee on Pediatric AIDS. Evaluation and management of the infant exposed to HIV-1 in the United States. *Pediatrics.* 2009;123(1):175–187

blot analysis) in a child 18 months of age or older almost always indicates infection,[1] although passively acquired maternal antibody rarely can persist beyond 18 months of age. An HIV-1 antibody test can be performed on samples of blood or oral fluid. Rapid tests for HIV-1 antibodies have been licensed for use in the United States; these tests are used widely throughout the world, particularly to screen mothers of undocumented serostatus in maternity settings; as with standard EIA tests, confirmatory testing is required for a positive rapid test. Results from rapid testing are available within 20 minutes; however, confirmatory Western blot analysis results may be delayed for 1 to 2 weeks in some settings.

Perinatally infected infants commonly have high viral loads. As infection progresses, there is a gradual depletion of cell-mediated immune function. The peripheral blood lymphocyte count at birth and during the first years of infection can be normal for age, but eventually lymphopenia develops, resulting from a decrease in the total number of circulating CD4+ T lymphocytes. Although immune activation results in an elevation in CD8+ T lymphocytes with initial HIV-1 infection, eventual depletion of CD8+ T lymphocytes also occurs. Sometimes, lymphocyte counts do not decrease until late in the course of infection. Changes in cell populations frequently result in a decrease in the normal CD4+ to CD8+ T-lymphocyte ratio of 1.0 or greater. This nonspecific finding, although characteristic of HIV-1 infection, also occurs with other acute viral infections, including infections caused by cytomegalovirus (CMV) and Epstein-Barr virus. Risk of opportunistic infections correlates with the CD4+ T-lymphocyte percentage and count. The normal values for peripheral CD4+ T-lymphocyte counts are age related, and the lower limits of normal are provided in Table 3.26 (p 384).

Although B-lymphocyte counts remain normal or somewhat increased, humoral immune dysfunction may precede and accompany cellular dysfunction. Increased serum immunoglobulin (Ig) concentrations of all isotypes, particularly IgG and IgA, are manifestations of the humoral immune dysfunction, but they are not necessarily directed at specific pathogens of childhood. Specific antibody responses to antigens to which the patient previously has not been exposed usually are abnormal; later in disease, recall antibody responses, including those to vaccine-associated antigens, are slow and diminish in magnitude. A small proportion (less than 10%) of patients will develop panhypogammaglobulinemia. Such patients have a particularly poor prognosis.

Consent for Diagnostic Testing. The CDC recommends that diagnostic HIV-1 testing and opt-out HIV-1 screening be part of routine clinical care in all health-care settings for patients 13 through 64 years of age while also preserving the patient's option to decline HIV-1 testing and ensuring a provider-patient relationship conducive to optimal clinical and preventive care. Patients or people responsible for the patient's care should be notified orally that testing is planned, advised of the indication for testing and the implications of positive and negative test results, and offered an opportunity to ask questions and to decline testing. With such notification, the patient's general consent for medical care is considered sufficient for diagnostic HIV-1 testing. Although parental involvement in an adolescent's health care usually is desirable, it typically is not required when the adolescent consents to HIV-1 testing. However, laws concerning consent and confidentiality for HIV-1 care differ among states. Public health statutes and legal precedents allow for

[1] Centers for Disease Control and Prevention. Revised surveillance case definitions for HIV infection among adults, adolescents, and children aged <18 months and for HIV infection and AIDS among children aged 18 months to <13 years—United States, 2008. *MMWR Recomm Rep.* 2008;57(RR-10):1–12

evaluation and treatment of minors for sexually transmitted infections without parental knowledge or consent, but not every state has defined HIV-1 infection explicitly as a condition for which testing or treatment may proceed without parental consent. Health care professionals should endeavor to respect an adolescent's request for privacy. HIV-1 screening should be discussed with all adolescents and encouraged for adolescents who are sexually active. Repeat HIV-1 antibody testing should be performed for adolescents who remain at risk of HIV-1 infection. Providing information regarding HIV-1 infection, diagnostic testing, transmission, and implications of infection should be regarded as an essential component of the anticipatory guidance provided to all adolescents as part of primary care.

Access to clinical care, preventive counseling, and support services is essential for people with positive HIV-1 test results.

TREATMENT: Primary care physicians are encouraged to participate actively in the care of HIV-1–infected patients. Because HIV-1 infection is an area of medicine that is changing rapidly, a pediatric HIV-1 expert should be consulted in the care of HIV-1–infected infants, children, and adolescents. Current treatment recommendations for HIV-1–infected children are available online **(http://aidsinfo.nih.gov).** When possible, enrollment of HIV-1–infected children in clinical trials should be encouraged. Information about trials for adolescents and children can be obtained by contacting the AIDS Clinical Trials Information Service.[1]

ARV therapy is indicated for most HIV-1–infected children. The principal objectives of therapy are to suppress viral replication maximally, to restore and preserve immune function, to reduce HIV-associated morbidity and mortality, to minimize drug toxicity, to maintain normal growth and development, and to improve quality of life. Initiation of ARV therapy depends on the age of the child and on a combination of virologic, immunologic, and clinical criteria.[2] Because HIV-1 treatment options and recommendations change with time and vary with the occurrence of ARV drug resistance and reports of adverse reactions, consultation with an expert in pediatric HIV-1 infection is recommended. Initiation of ARV therapy is recommended for all HIV-1–infected infants as soon as infection is confirmed, regardless of clinical, immunologic, or virologic parameters. Aggressive therapy is warranted in the youngest children who are at greatest risk of rapid disease progression. Data from both observational studies and clinical trials indicate that very early initiation of therapy reduces morbidity and mortality compared with starting treatment when clinically or immunologically symptomatic. It is assumed that early therapy will keep the viral load low, reduce viral mutation and evolution, and control widespread dissemination of virus to sites where virus can persist.

Initiation of ARV therapy is recommended as follows[2]: (1) HIV-1–infected infants should receive ARV therapy irrespective of clinical symptoms, immune status, or viral load; (2) children 1 year of age and older should receive ARV therapy if they have AIDS or significant HIV-related symptoms (clinical category C or most clinical category B conditions), regardless of CD4+ T-lymphocyte counts or plasma viral load values; (3) children

---

[1]See Appendix I, Directory of Resources, p 831: AIDS Clinical Trials Information Service (available at **http://aidsinfo.nih.gov**)

[2]Centers for Disease Control and Prevention. Guidelines for the use of antiretroviral agents in pediatric HIV infection. *MMWR Recomm Rep.* 1998;47(RR-4):1–31. See **http://aidsinfo.nih.gov** for updates of new drugs and new treatment recommendations.

1 through 4 years of age should begin ARV therapy if they have a CD4+ T-lymphocyte percentage less than 25%, and children 5 years of age or older should begin ARV therapy if they have a CD4+ T-lymphocyte count less than 350 cells/mm³, regardless of symptoms or plasma viral load.

Starting ARV therapy should be considered[1] for HIV-1-infected children 1 year of age or older who are asymptomatic or have mild symptoms (clinical category N and A or the following clinical category B conditions: single episode of serious bacterial infection or lymphoid interstitial pneumonitis) and have the following CD4+ T-lymphocyte and plasma viral load values: (1) children 1 through 4 years of age: CD4+ T-lymphocyte percentage of 25% or greater and plasma viral load of 100 000 copies/mL or more; (2) children 5 years of age or older: CD4+ T-lymphocyte count of 350 cells/mm³ or more and plasma viral load of 100 000 copies/mL or more.

ARV therapy may be deferred[1] for HIV-1-infected children 1 year of age and older who are asymptomatic or have mild symptoms and have the following CD4+ T-lymphocyte and plasma viral load values: (1) children 1 through 4 years of age: CD4+ T-lymphocyte percentage of 25% or greater and plasma viral load less than 100 000 copies/mL; (2) children 5 years of age or older: CD4+ T-lymphocyte count of 350 cells/mm³ or more and plasma viral load less than 100 000 copies/mL.

The child and the child's primary health care professional must be able to adhere to the prescribed regimen. Initiation of treatment of adolescents[2] generally follows guidelines for adults, for whom treatment is recommended if an AIDS-defining illness is present or if the CD4+ T-lymphocyte count is less than 350 cells/mm³. Dosages of medications for adolescents in early puberty are administered according to pediatric schedules, whereas those in late puberty are administered according to adult schedules.

In general, combination ARV therapy with at least 3 drugs is recommended for all HIV-1-infected people requiring ARV therapy. Drug regimens most often include 2 nucleoside analogue reverse-transcriptase inhibitors (NRTIs) plus either a protease inhibitor or a nonnucleoside reverse-transcriptase inhibitor (NNRTI) (**http://aidsinfo.nih.gov**). ARV resistance testing (viral genotyping) is recommended before starting treatment, because infected infants may acquire resistant virus from their mothers. Suppression of virus to undetectable levels is the desired goal. A change in ARV therapy should be considered if there is evidence of disease progression (virologic, immunologic, or clinical), toxic effects or intolerance to drugs, development of resistance, or availability of data suggesting the possibility of a superior regimen.

Immune Globulin Intravenous (IGIV) therapy has been used in combination with ARV agents for HIV-1-infected children with hypogammaglobulinemia (IgG less than 400 mg/dL [4.0 g/L]) and could be considered for HIV-1-infected children who have recurrent, serious bacterial infections, such as bacteremia, meningitis, or pneumonia. Trimethoprim-sulfamethoxazole prophylaxis may provide comparable protec-

---

[1] Centers for Disease Control and Prevention. Guidelines for the use of antiretroviral agents in pediatric HIV infection. *MMWR Recomm Rep.* 1998;47(RR-4):1–31. See **http://aidsinfo.nih.gov** for updates of new drugs and new treatment recommendations.

[2] Centers for Disease Control and Prevention. Guidelines for using antiretroviral agents among HIV-infected adults and adolescents. Recommendations of the Panel on Clinical Practice for Treatment of HIV. *MMWR Recomm Rep.* 2002;51(RR-7):1–56. See **http://aidsinfo.nih.gov** for periodic updates of new drugs and new treatment recommendations.

tion. Typically, neither form of prophylaxis is necessary for patients receiving effective ARV therapy.

Early prophylaxis, diagnosis, and aggressive treatment of opportunistic infections may prolong survival.[1,2] This particularly is true for PCP, which accounts for approximately one third of pediatric AIDS diagnoses overall and may occur early in the first year of life. Because mortality rates are high, chemoprophylaxis should be given to all HIV-exposed infants with indeterminate HIV-1 infection status starting at 4 to 6 weeks of age. Prophylaxis is not recommended for infants who meet criteria for presumptive or definitive HIV-1–uninfected status. Thus, for infants with negative HIV-1 viral test results at 2 and 4 weeks of age (and no positive tests or clinical symptoms and who are, therefore, presumptively not infected with HIV-1), PCP prophylaxis would not need to be initiated. If PCP prophylaxis is started at 4 to 6 weeks of age in an HIV-1–exposed infant with indeterminate HIV-1 infection status, prophylaxis can be stopped if the child subsequently meets criteria for presumptive or definitive lack of HIV-1 infection. All infants with HIV-1 infection should receive PCP prophylaxis through 1 year of age regardless of immune status. The need for PCP prophylaxis for HIV-1–infected children 1 year of age and older is determined by the degree of immunocompromise, as determined by CD4+ T-lymphocyte counts (see *Pneumocystis jirovecii* Infections, p 536).

Guidelines for prevention and treatment of opportunistic infections in children, adolescents, and adults provide indications for administration of drugs for infection with MAC, CMV, *T gondii*, and other organisms.[1,2] Successful suppression of HIV-1 replication in the blood to undetectable levels by HAART has resulted in relatively normal CD4+ and CD8+ T-lymphocyte counts, leading to a dramatic decrease in the occurrence of most opportunistic infections, such as PCP, disseminated and localized CMV infection, and those caused by atypical mycobacteria and invasive bacteria. Limited data on the safety of discontinuing prophylaxis in HIV-1–infected children receiving HAART are available. Prophylaxis should not be discontinued in HIV-1–infected infants. For older children, many experts consider discontinuing PCP prophylaxis for HIV-1–infected children who have received at least 6 months of HAART on the basis of CD4+ lymphocyte results[1]: (1) for children 1 through 5 years of age: CD4+ T-lymphocyte percentage of at least 15% or CD4+ T-lymphocyte absolute count of at least 500 cells/mm^3 for more than 3 consecutive months; (2) for children 6 years of age or older: CD4+ T-lymphocyte percentage of at least 15% or the CD4+ T-lymphocyte absolute count of at least 200 cells/mm^3 for more than 3 consecutive months. Subsequently, the CD4+ T-lymphocyte absolute count or percentage should be reevaluated at least every 3 months. Prophylaxis should be reinstituted if the original criteria for prophylaxis are reached again.

Immunization Recommendations (see also Immunization in Special Clinical Circumstances, p 68, and Table 1.14, p 74).

[1]Centers for Disease Control and Prevention. Guidelines for prevention and treatment of opportunistic infections among HIV-exposed and HIV-infected children. Recommendations from CDC, the National Institutes of Health, the HIV Medicine Association of the Infectious Diseases Society of America, the Pediatric Infectious Diseases Society, and the American Academy of Pediatrics. *MMWR.* 2009; in press. Available at: **http://aidsinfo.nih.gov/contentfiles/Pediatric_OI.pdf.**

[2]Centers for Disease Control and Prevention. Guidelines for prevention and treatment of opportunistic infections in HIV-infected adults and adolescents. Recommendations from CDC, the National Institutes of Health, and the HIV Medicine Association of the Infectious Diseases Society of America. *MMWR Early Release.* 2009;58(March 24, 2009):1–207. Available at: **http://www.cdc.gov/mmwr/pdf/rr/rr58e324.pdf.**

All routine infant immunizations should be given to HIV-1–exposed infants. If HIV-1 infection is confirmed, then guidelines for the HIV-1–infected child should be followed. Children with HIV-1 infection should be immunized as soon as is age appropriate with inactivated vaccines. Trivalent inactivated influenza vaccine (TIV) should be given annually. Additionally, live virus-containing MMR and varicella vaccines should be given to asymptomatic HIV-1–infected children and adolescents with appropriate CD4 percentages (ie, CD4+ T-lymphocyte count greater than 15% in children). Measles-mumps-rubella-varicella (MMRV) vaccine should not be administered to HIV-infected infants. Rotavirus vaccine may be given to HIV-1–exposed and HIV-1–infected infants. The suggested schedule for administration of these vaccines is provided in the recommended childhood and adolescent immunization schedule (Fig 1.1–1.3, p 24–28). The immunologic response to these vaccines in HIV-1–infected children may be less robust and less persistent than in immunologically normal children.

Children Who Are HIV-1 Seronegative Residing in the Household of a Patient With Symptomatic HIV-1 Infection. Members of households in which an adult or child has HIV-1 infection can receive MMR vaccine, because these vaccine viruses are not transmitted person to person. To decrease the risk of transmission of influenza to patients with symptomatic HIV-1 infection, all household members 6 months of age or older should receive yearly influenza immunization (see Influenza, p 400). Immunization with varicella vaccine of siblings and susceptible adult caregivers of patients with HIV-1 infection is encouraged to prevent acquisition of wild-type varicella-zoster virus infection, which can cause severe disease in immunocompromised hosts. Transmission of varicella vaccine virus from an immunocompetent host to a household contact is uncommon.

Passive Immunization of Children With HIV-1 Infection.

- **Measles** (see Measles, p 444). Symptomatic HIV-1–infected children who are exposed to measles should receive intramuscular Immune Globulin (IG) prophylaxis (0.5 mL/kg, maximum 15 mL), regardless of immunization status, and exposed, asymptomatic HIV-1–infected patients also should receive intramuscular IG but at a lower dose (0.25 mL/kg). Children who have received IGIV within 2 weeks of exposure do not require additional passive immunization.

- **Tetanus.** Children with HIV-1 infection who sustain wounds classified as tetanus prone (see Tetanus, p 655, and Table 3.77, p 657) should receive Tetanus Immune Globulin regardless of immunization status.

- **Varicella.** HIV-1–infected children without a history of previous chickenpox or children who have not received 2 doses of varicella vaccine should receive VariZIG or, if not available, IGIV within 96 hours of close contact with a person who has chickenpox or shingles (see Varicella-Zoster Infections, p 714). Similar postexposure prophylaxis regimens have been recommended for children with moderate to severe immune compromise who previously have been immunized with varicella vaccine. An alternative to VariZIG for passive immunization is IGIV, 400 mg/kg, administered once within 96 hours after exposure. Children who have received IGIV within 2 weeks of exposure do not require additional passive immunization.

ISOLATION OF THE HOSPITALIZED PATIENT: Standard precautions should be followed by all health care personnel. The risk to health care personnel of acquiring HIV-1 infection from a patient is minimal, even after accidental exposure from a needlestick injury (see Epidemiology, p 387). Nevertheless, every effort should be made to avoid exposures to blood and other body fluids that could contain HIV-1.

CONTROL MEASURES:

Interruption of Mother-to-Child Transmission of HIV. A number of prophylactic pharmacologic regimens and specific obstetric interventions used in concert have resulted in a marked decrease in the occurrence of perinatally acquired HIV-1 infection in the United States. Recommendations of the US Public Health Service, the American Academy of Pediatrics (AAP), and the American College of Obstetricians and Gynecologists include the following.[1,2,3,4]

The AAP and CDC recommend documented, routine HIV-1 testing for all pregnant women in the United States after notifying the patient that testing will be performed, unless the patient declines HIV-1 testing ("opt-out" consent or "right of refusal"). For women in labor with undocumented HIV-1 infection status during the current pregnancy, immediate maternal HIV-1 testing with opt-out consent, using a rapid HIV-1 antibody test, is recommended. In some states, routinely offering HIV-1 testing during pregnancy is mandated by law. Routine education about HIV-1 infection and testing should be part of a comprehensive program of health care for all women during their childbearing years.

The decrease in the rate of mother-to-child transmission of HIV-1 observed in the United States over the past several years is attributable to development and implementation of 3 efficacious interventions: complete avoidance of breastfeeding, ARV prophylaxis, and cesarean delivery before onset of labor and before rupture of membranes.[4] Additionally, in resource-limited countries where complete avoidance of breastfeeding (replacement feeding) often is not safe, exclusive breastfeeding is associated with a lower risk of postnatal transmission than is mixed feeding, although postnatal transmission of HIV-1 still occurs with either mode of feeding. The goal should be to diagnose HIV-1 infection early in pregnancy to allow antenatal implementation of interventions to prevent transmission (ARV prophylaxis and cesarean delivery before onset of labor and before rupture of membranes) as well as appropriate care and treatment of the HIV-1–infected mother.

The first clinical trial of ARV prophylaxis for prevention of mother-to-child transmission assessed oral administration of zidovudine to pregnant women with HIV-1 infection beginning at 14 to 34 weeks' gestation and continuing throughout pregnancy, intravenous administration of zidovudine during labor until delivery (ie, intrapartum), and oral administration of zidovudine to the infant for the first 6 weeks of life. This intervention decreased mother-to-child transmission of HIV-1 by two thirds (see Table 3.28, p 397). Observational studies suggest that use of combination ARV regimens during pregnancy is associated with a lower risk of mother-to-child transmission of HIV-1 than is zidovudine alone. Currently in the United States, most HIV-1–infected pregnant women receive combination ARV regimens either for treatment of their HIV disease (in which case drugs are continued by the mother postpartum, with the exception of

---

[1]For complete listing of current policy statements from the American Academy of Pediatrics regarding human immunodeficiency virus and acquired immunodeficiency syndrome, see **http://aappolicy.aappublications. org/.**

[2]American Academy of Pediatrics, American College of Obstetricians and Gynecologists. Human immunodeficiency virus screening. Joint Statement of the American Academy of Pediatrics and the American College of Obstetricians and Gynecologists. *Pediatrics.* 1999;104(1 Pt 1):128 (Reaffirmed May 2005)

[3]Havens PL, Mofenson LM; American Academy of Pediatrics, Committee on Pediatric AIDS. Evaluation and management of the infant exposed to HIV-1 in the United States. *Pediatrics.* 2009;123(1):175–187

[4]American Academy of Pediatrics, Committee on Pediatric AIDS. HIV testing and prophylaxis to prevent mother-to-child transmission in the United States. *Pediatrics.* 2008;122(5):1127–1134

Table 3.28. Zidovudine Regimen for Decreasing the Rate of Perinatal Transmission of Human Immunodeficiency Virus (HIV)[a]

Period of Time	Route	Dosage
During pregnancy, initiate anytime after wk 14 of gestation and continue throughout pregnancy[b]	Oral	200 mg, 3 times per day or 300 mg, 2 times per day
During labor and delivery[c]	Intravenous	2 mg/kg during the first hour, then 1 mg/kg per hour until delivery
For the newborn infant, as soon as possible after birth[d]	Oral	2 mg/kg, 4 times per day, for the first 6 wk of life

[a]US Public Health Service. Public Health Service Task Force Recommendations for Use of Antiretroviral Drugs in Pregnant HIV-1-Infected Women for Maternal Health and for Interventions to Reduce Perinatal HIV-1 Transmission in the United States. Rockville, MD: AIDSInfo, Department of Health and Human Services; 2008 (available at **http://aidsinfo.nih.gov/contentfiles/PerinatalGL.pdf**).Information about other antiretroviral drugs for decreasing the rate of perinatal transmission of HIV can be found online (**http://aidsinfo.nih.gov**).

[b]Most women in industrialized countries are treated with potent combinations of 3 antiretroviral agents (highly active antiretroviral therapy [HAART]) started after the first trimester (unless treatment is required for maternal health reasons, in which case the benefit of starting during the first trimester outweighs potential risk to the infant) and continuing to delivery. Oral zidovudine may be used as part of that therapy.

[c]Recommended even for women treated with other antiretroviral agents during pregnancy. Intravenous zidovudine is administered for 3 hours before cesarean delivery.

[d]The effectiveness of antiretroviral agents for prevention of perinatal HIV-1 transmission decreases with delay in initiation after birth. Initiation of postexposure prophylaxis after the first 48 hours of life is not likely to be efficacious in preventing transmission.

efavirenz, which is teratogenic) or for prophylaxis of transmission (in which case drugs often are discontinued postpartum). Intravenous zidovudine is given during labor along with other drugs in the antepartum regimen, and the infant subsequently receives 6 weeks of zidovudine prophylaxis.

Health care professionals who treat HIV-1–infected pregnant women and their newborn infants should report instances of prenatal exposure to ARV drugs (either alone or in combination) to the Antiretroviral Pregnancy Registry (1-800-258-4263 or **www.apregistry.com**). Long-term follow-up is recommended for all infants born to women who have received ARV drugs during pregnancy.

Intrapartum management of HIV-1–infected women and the immediate postpartum care of their newborn infants are multifaceted. The woman's regular HIV-1 health care professional should be contacted to announce the impending delivery and to review the patient's current and postpartum ARV regimen. For women in labor with undocumented HIV-1 infection status, a rapid HIV-1 test should be performed as soon as possible. The HIV-1–infected woman should be started on intravenous zidovudine immediately (regardless of whether she has been taking ARV drugs before and/or during pregnancy; see Table 3.28). Her routine oral ARV drugs should be continued on schedule (with the exception of stavudine [d4T, Zerit], which should not be coadministered with zidovudine). Any procedures that compromise the integrity of fetal skin during labor and delivery (eg, fetal electrodes) or that increase the occurrence of maternal bleeding (eg, instrumented vaginal delivery, episiotomy, vaginal tears) should be avoided when possible. Prolonged rupture of membranes has been shown to increase the risk of mother-to-infant transmission of HIV, whereas elective caesarean delivery before the onset of labor and before rupture of membranes has been shown to reduce the risk of mother-to-infant transmission and is recommended for women with plasma viral loads greater than 1000 copies/mL and women with unknown plasma viral loads around the time of delivery. The newborn infant should be bathed and cleaned of maternal secretions (especially bloody secretions) as soon as possible after birth. Newborn infants should begin ARV prophylaxis as soon as possible after birth, preferably within 12 hours after birth. In the United States, neonatal prophylaxis generally consists of zidovudine for 6 weeks. Additional ARV medications sometimes are used in combination in high-risk situations, such as lack of antepartum or intrapartum maternal ARV prophylaxis and/or incomplete maternal viral suppression. Detailed guidance is available.[1] Both the mother and the infant should have prescriptions for the HIV-1 drugs when they leave the hospital, and the infant should have an appointment for a postpartum visit at 2 to 4 weeks of age to monitor medication adherence.

For a newborn infant whose mother's HIV-1 serostatus is unknown, the newborn infant's health care professional should perform rapid HIV-1 antibody testing on the mother or the infant, with appropriate consent as required by state and local law. Test results should be reported to health care professionals quickly enough to allow effective ARV prophylaxis to be administered to the infant as soon after birth as possible. In some states, rapid testing of the neonate is required by law if the mother has refused to be tested. Because infant ARV prophylaxis should be initiated before 12 hours of age, rapid return of the test result to the health care professional is critical to allow the infant to start prophylaxis in a timely manner.

The newborn infant's health care professional should be informed of the mother's serostatus so that appropriate care and follow-up of the infant can be accomplished. A mother who is HIV positive and her infant should be referred to a facility that provides HIV-related services for both adults and children.

Breastfeeding (also see Human Milk, p 118). Transmission of HIV-1 by breastfeeding has been demonstrated, especially from mothers who acquire HIV-1 infection late in pregnancy or during the postpartum period. The rate of late postnatal HIV-1 transmission (after 4 weeks of age) in sub-Saharan African countries is approximately 9 transmissions per 100 child-years of breastfeeding (0.7% transmission/month of breastfeeding) and is relatively constant. Late postnatal transmission is associated with reduced maternal CD4+ T-lymphocyte count, plasma and human milk viral load, mastitis/breast abscess, and infant oral lesions (eg, oral thrush). In countries where safe alternative sources of infant feeding are readily available, affordable, and culturally accepted, such as the United States, HIV-1–infected women should be counseled not to breastfeed their infants or donate to human milk banks.

In general, women who are known to be HIV-1 seronegative should be encouraged to breastfeed. However, women who are HIV-1 seronegative and who are known to have HIV-1–infected sex partners or to be active injection drug users should be counseled about the potential risk of transmitting HIV-1 through human milk and about methods to decrease the risk of acquiring HIV-1 infection either late in pregnancy or postpartum.

---

[1]US Public Health Service. Public Health Service Task Force Recommendations for Use of Antiretroviral Drugs in Pregnant HIV-1-Infected Women for Maternal Health and for Interventions to Reduce Perinatal HIV-1 Transmission in the United States. Rockville, MD: AIDSInfo, Department of Health and Human Services; 2005. Available at: **www.aidsinfo.nih.gov/guidelines/default_db2.usp?id66**

Premastication. Possible transmission of HIV-1 by caregivers who premasticate food for infants has been described in 3 cases in the United States. In 2 of the cases, the caregivers had bleeding gums or sores in their mouths during the time they premasticated the food. Phylogenetic testing was conducted and documented matches of the viral strains in 2 of the caregiver-infant dyads. It is hypothesized that the transmission was via bloodborne virus rather than via salivary virus. The CDC recommends that in the United States, where safe alternative methods of feeding are available, HIV-1–infected caregivers should be asked about whether they practice premastication and counseled not to premasticate food for infants.

HIV-1 in the Athletic Setting. Athletes and staff of athletic programs can be exposed to blood during athletic activity. Recommendations have been developed by the AAP for prevention of transmission of HIV-1 and other bloodborne pathogens in the athletic setting (see School Health, Infections Spread by Blood and Body Fluids, p 146).

Sexual Abuse. In cases of sexual abuse, the child should be tested serologically as soon as possible and then periodically for 6 months (eg, at 4–6 weeks, 12 weeks, and 6 months after sexual contact) (see Sexually Transmitted Infections, p 162). Serologic evaluation of the perpetrator for HIV-1 infection should be attempted soon after the incident but usually cannot be performed until indictment has occurred. Counseling of the child and family needs to be provided (see Sexually Transmitted Infections, p 162).

Postexposure Prophylaxis for Possible Sexual or Other Nonoccupational Exposure to HIV-1.[1] Decisions to provide ARV agents to people after possible nonoccupational (ie, community) exposure to HIV-1 must balance the potential benefits and risks. Decisions regarding the need for ARV prophylaxis in such instances are predicated on the probability that the source is infected or contaminated with HIV-1, the likelihood of transmission by the particular exposure, and the interval between exposure and the initiation of therapy balanced against the expected adverse effects associated with the regimen of drugs.

The risk of transmission of HIV-1 from a puncture wound attributable to a needle found in the community is lower than 0.3%. The actual risks of HIV infection in an infant or child after a needlestick injury or sexual abuse are unknown. To date, there are no confirmed transmissions of HIV from accidental nonoccupational needlestick injuries (needles found in the community). The estimated risk of HIV transmission per episode of receptive penile-anal sexual exposure is 50 per 10 000 exposures; whereas the estimated risk per episode of receptive vaginal exposure is 10 per 10 000 exposures.

All ARV agents are associated with adverse effects. In HIV-1–infected adults receiving combination therapy for treatment of HIV, an estimated 24% to 36% discontinue the drugs because of adverse effects. Adverse effects also are reported by a significant proportion of adults without HIV infection receiving ARV drugs for postexposure prophylaxis. Use of daily nevirapine for postexposure prophylaxis is not recommended because of the high incidence of severe (and rarely fatal) adverse effects in adults with normal CD4+ T-lymphocyte counts; such adverse effects have not been reported with single-dose intrapartum/infant nevirapine used for prevention of mother-to-child transmission.

---

[1] US Department of Health and Human Services. Antiretroviral postexposure prophylaxis after sexual, injection-drug use, or other nonoccupational exposure to HIV in the United States: recommendations from the U.S. Department of Health and Human Services. *MMWR Recomm Rep.* 2005;54(RR-2):1–20

ARV agents generally should not be used if the risk of transmission is low (eg, trivial needlestick injury with a drug needle from an unknown nonoccupational source) or if care is sought more than 72 hours after the reported exposure.[1] The benefits of post-exposure prophylaxis are greatest when risk of infection is high, intervention is prompt, and adherence is likely. Consultation with an experienced pediatric HIV-1 health care professional is essential.

Transition of Adolescents to Adult HIV-1 Health Care Settings. In industrialized nations, it increasingly has become likely that HIV-1–infected children will survive (and thrive) well into adolescence and young adulthood. Therefore, pediatric and adult HIV programs may benefit from establishment of transition programs to introduce adolescents to the adult health care setting. Successful transition requires careful proactive planning by caregivers in both pediatric and adult venues and a multifaceted, deliberate exercise that pays heed to the medical, psychosocial, life-skills, educational, and family-centered needs of the patient.

The transition period is a convenient time to review the ARV regimen with the adolescent, to recalculate dosages if necessary, and to stress repeatedly the need for adherence. It also is an ideal time to teach about contraception, prevention of sexually transmitted infections, and safer sex practices.

Influenza

CLINICAL MANIFESTATIONS: Influenza typically begins with the sudden onset of fever, often accompanied by chills or rigors, headache, malaise, diffuse myalgia, and nonproductive cough. Subsequently, respiratory tract signs including sore throat, nasal congestion, rhinitis, and cough become more prominent. Conjunctival injection, abdominal pain, nausea, vomiting, and diarrhea less commonly are associated with influenza illness. In some children, influenza can appear as an upper respiratory tract infection or as a febrile illness with few respiratory tract signs. Influenza is an important cause of otitis media. Acute myositis characterized by calf tenderness and refusal to walk has been described. In infants, influenza can produce a sepsis-like picture and occasionally can cause croup, bronchiolitis, or pneumonia. Although the large majority of children with influenza recover fully after 3 to 7 days, previously healthy children can have severe symptoms and complications. Neurologic complications associated with influenza range from febrile seizures to severe encephalopathy and encephalitis with status epilepticus, with resulting neurologic sequelae or death. Reye syndrome has been associated with influenza infection. Death from influenza-associated myocarditis has been reported. Invasive secondary infections or coinfections with group A streptococcus, *Staphylococcus* aureus (including methicillin-resistant *S aureus* [MRSA]), *Streptococcus pneumoniae,* or other bacterial pathogens can result in severe disease and death.

ETIOLOGY: Influenza viruses are orthomyxoviruses of 3 genera or types (A, B, and C). Epidemic disease is caused by influenza virus types A and B, and both influenza A and B virus antigens are included in influenza vaccines. Type C influenza viruses cause sporadic mild influenza-like illness in children, and type C antigens are not included in influenza vaccines. Influenza A viruses are subclassified into subtypes by 2 surface antigens,

[1]Havens PL; American Academy of Pediatrics, Committee on Pediatric AIDS. Postexposure prophylaxis in children and adolescents for nonoccupational exposure to human immunodeficiency virus. *Pediatrics.* 2003;111(6):1475–1489 (Reaffirmed January 2007)

hemagglutinin (HA) and neuraminidase (NA). Currently circulating human influenza A subtypes include H1N1, H1N2, and H3N2 viruses. Specific antibodies to these various antigens, especially to hemagglutinin, are important determinants of immunity. Minor antigenic variation within the same influenza B type or influenza A subtypes is called *antigenic drift*. Antigenic drift occurs continuously and results in new strains of influenza A and B viruses, leading to seasonal epidemics. *Antigenic shifts* are major changes in influenza A viruses that result in new infectious subtypes that contain a new HA alone or with a new NA. Antigenic shift occurs only with influenza A viruses and can lead to pandemics if a strain can infect humans and be transmitted efficiently from person to person in a sustained manner in the setting of little or no preexisting immunity; 3 such pandemics occurred in the 20th century.

Humans, including children, occasionally are infected with influenza A viruses of swine or avian origin. Human infections with swine viruses identified in the United States have manifested as typical influenza-like illness, and confirmation of infection caused by an influenza virus of swine origin has been discovered retrospectively during routine typing of human influenza isolates. Rare but severe infections with influenza A subtype H5N1 viruses have been identified since 1997 in Asia, Africa, Europe, and the Middle East, areas where these viruses are present in domestic or wild birds. Other influenza subtypes of avian origin, including H7, also are identified occasionally in humans. Infection with a novel influenza A virus now is a nationally reportable disease and should be reported to the Centers for Disease Control and Prevention (CDC) through state health departments.

EPIDEMIOLOGY: Influenza is spread from person to person primarily by respiratory droplets created by coughing or sneezing. Contact with respiratory droplet-contaminated surfaces is another possible mode of transmission. During community outbreaks of influenza, the highest attack rates occur among school-aged children. Secondary spread to adults and other children within a family is common. Incidence and disease severity depend, in part, on immunity developed as a result of previous experience (by natural disease) or recent influenza immunization with the circulating strain or a related strain. Antigenic drift in the circulating strain(s) is associated with seasonal epidemics. In temperate climates, seasonal epidemics usually occur during winter months. Peak influenza activity in the United States can occur anytime from November to May but most commonly occurs in January and February. Community outbreaks can last 4 to 8 weeks or longer. Circulation of 2 or 3 influenza virus strains in a community may be associated with a prolonged influenza season of 3 months or more and bimodal peaks in activity. Influenza is highly contagious, especially among semienclosed institutionalized populations. Patients may become infectious during the 24 hours before onset of symptoms. Viral shedding in nasal secretions usually peaks during the first 3 days of illness and ceases within 7 days but can be prolonged in young children and immunodeficient patients. Viral shedding is correlated directly with degree of fever.

Attack rates in healthy children generally have been found to be 10% to 40% each year, but illness rates as low as 3% also have been reported. Children younger than 5 years of age visit clinics or emergency departments for influenza illness at the rate of 1 to 2 children per 100 annually. Influenza and its complications have been reported to result in a 10% to 30% increase in the number of courses of antimicrobial agents prescribed to children during the influenza season. These medical care encounters for children with influenza result in considerable costs and likely are an important cause of inappropriate antimicrobial use.

Hospitalization rates among children younger than 2 years of age are similar to hospitalization rates among people 65 years of age and older. Rates vary among studies (190–480 per 100 000 population) because of differences in methodology and severity of influenza seasons. However, children younger than 24 months of age consistently are at substantially higher risk of hospitalization than are older children, and the risk of hospitalization attributable to influenza infection is highest in the youngest children. Antecedent influenza infection sometimes is associated with development of pneumococcal or staphylococcal pneumonia in children. Methicillin-resistant staphylococcal community-acquired pneumonia, with a rapid clinical progression and a high fatality rate, has been reported in previously healthy children and adults with concomitant influenza infection. Rates of hospitalization and morbidity attributable to complications, such as bronchitis and pneumonia, are even greater in children with high-risk conditions, including hemoglobinopathies, bronchopulmonary dysplasia, asthma, cystic fibrosis, malignancy, diabetes mellitus, chronic renal disease, and congenital heart disease. Influenza virus infection in neonates also has been associated with considerable morbidity, including a sepsis-like syndrome, apnea, and lower respiratory tract disease.

Fatal outcomes, including sudden death, have been reported in both chronically ill and previously healthy children. Of 153 laboratory-confirmed influenza-related pediatric deaths reported from 40 states during the 2003-2004 influenza season, 96 (63%) were children younger than 5 years of age and 61 (40%) were children younger than 2 years of age. Among the 149 children who died and for whom information on underlying health status was available, 100 (67%) did not have an underlying medical condition that was an indication for immunization at that time. In the following 3 seasons, the number of deaths among children reported annually ranged from 46 to 71. In California during the 2003-2004 and 2004-2005 influenza seasons, 51% of children with laboratory-confirmed influenza who died and 40% of children who required admission to an intensive care unit had no underlying medical conditions. Of the 53 pediatric patients 6 years of age or older who died in 2006-2007 and for whom immunization status was known, 50 (94%) had not been immunized against influenza. Bacterial coinfections with a variety of pathogens, including both methicillin-susceptible *S aureus* and MRSA, have been noted in reported deaths among children. These data indicate that although deaths are more frequent among children with risk factors for influenza complications, most pediatric deaths occur among children with no known high-risk conditions. All influenza-associated pediatric deaths are nationally notifiable and should be reported to the CDC through state health departments.

The **incubation period** usually is 1 to 4 days, with a mean of 2 days.

Influenza Pandemics. A pandemic is defined by the emergence and global spread of a new influenza A virus subtype to which the population has little or no immunity and that spreads rapidly from human to human. Pandemics, therefore, can lead substantially to increased morbidity and mortality rates compared with seasonal influenza. During the 20th century, there were 3 influenza pandemics, in 1918 (H1N1), 1957 (H2N2), and 1968 (H3N2). The pandemic in 1918 killed at least 20 million people in the United States and perhaps as many as 50 million people worldwide. A severe pandemic could overwhelm the health care system and disrupt critical societal functions. Pediatric health care professionals should be familiar with national, state, and institutional pandemic plans, including recommendations for vaccine and antiviral drug use, health care surge capacity, and personal protective strategies that can be communicated to patients and families. Public health authorities have developed plans for pandemic preparedness and response to a pandemic in the United States. Current status on aspects of pandemic influenza can be found at **www.pandemicflu.gov.**

DIAGNOSTIC TESTS: Specimens for viral culture, immunofluorescent, or rapid diagnostic tests should be obtained if possible during the first 72 hours of illness, because the quantity of virus shed decreases rapidly as illness progresses beyond that point. Specimens of nasopharyngeal secretions obtained by swab, aspirate, or wash should be placed in appropriate transport media for culture. After inoculation into eggs or cell culture, virus usually can be isolated within 2 to 6 days. Rapid diagnostic tests for identification of influenza A and B antigens in respiratory tract specimens are available commercially, although their reported sensitivity (44%–97%) and specificity (76%–100%) compared with viral culture are variable and differ by test and specimen type. Direct fluorescent antibody (DFA) and indirect immunofluorescent antibody (IFA) staining for detection of influenza A and B antigens in nasopharyngeal or nasal specimens are available at most hospital-based laboratories and can yield results in 3 to 4 hours. Results of immunofluorescent and rapid diagnostic tests should be interpreted in the context of the clinical findings and local community influenza activity, because the prevalence of circulating influenza viruses influences the positive and negative predictive values of these influenza screening tests. False-positive results are more likely to occur during periods of low influenza activity; false-negative results are more likely to occur during periods of peak influenza activity. Serologic diagnosis can be established retrospectively by a fourfold or greater increase in antibody titer in serum specimens obtained during the acute and convalescent stages of illness, as determined by hemagglutination inhibition testing, complement fixation testing, neutralization testing, or enzyme immunoassay (EIA); however, serologic testing rarely is useful in patient management, because 2 serum samples collected 10 to 14 days apart are required. Reverse transcriptase-polymerase chain reaction (RT-PCR) testing of respiratory tract specimens may be available at some institutions and offers potential for high sensitivity and specificity.

TREATMENT: Influenza A viruses, including 2 subtypes (H1N1 and H3N2), and influenza B viruses, circulate worldwide, but the prevalence of each can vary among communities and within a single community over the course of an influenza season. In the United States, 2 classes of antiviral medications currently are available for treatment or prophylaxis of influenza infections: neuraminidase inhibitors (oseltamivir and zanamivir) and adamantanes (amantadine and rimantadine). Guidelines for the use of these 4 antiviral agents are summarized in Table 3.29 (p 404). No antiviral agent currently is approved for use in infants younger than 12 months of age.

Since 2005, all H3N2 strains in the United States have been resistant to adamantanes. Influenza B viruses intrinsically are resistant to adamantanes. Since January 2006, the neuraminidase inhibitors (oseltamivir, zanamivir) have been the only recommended influenza antiviral drugs because of this widespread resistance to the adamantanes and the activity of neuraminidase inhibitors against influenza A and B viruses. In 2007–2008, a significant increase in oseltamivir resistance was reported among influenza A (H1N1) viruses worldwide. During the 2007–2008 influenza season, 11% of H1N1 viruses tested in the United States were resistant to oseltamivir. During the 2008–2009 influenza season,

Table 3.29. Antiviral Drugs for Influenza

Drug (Trade Name)	Virus	Administration	Treatment Indications[a]	Prophylaxis Indications[a]	Adverse Effects
Oseltamivir[b] (Tamiflu)	A and B	Oral	1 y of age or older	1 y of age or older	Nausea, vomiting
Zanamivir (Relenza)	A and B	Inhalation	7 y of age or older	5 y of age or older	Bronchospasm
Amantadine[c] (Symmetrel)	A	Oral	1 y of age or older	1 y of age or older	Central nervous system, anxiety, gastrointestinal
Rimantadine[c] (Flumadine)	A	Oral	13 y of age or older	1 y of age or older	Central nervous system, anxiety, gastrointestinal

[a]US Food and Drug Administration (FDA)-approved ages.
[b]High prevalence of resistance among H1N1 influenza strains.
[c]High prevalence of adamantane resistance among H3N2 and B influenza strains.

See **www.cdc.gov/flu/professionals/antivirals/index.htm** or **www.aapredbook.org/flu** for current information for use of antiviral drugs for treatment or chemoprophylaxis against influenza.

virtually all H1N1 influenza strains were resistant to oseltamivir but remained susceptible to zanamivir, amantadine, and rimantadine. Data indicate that oseltamivir-resistant influenza A (H1N1) viruses do not cause different or more severe symptoms compared with oseltamivir-susceptible influenza A (H1N1) viruses. Influenza A (H3N2) and B viruses remain susceptible to oseltamivir. The proportion of influenza A (H1N1) viruses among all influenza A and B viruses that will circulate during any influenza season cannot be predicted and likely will vary geographically among communities throughout the season.

These resistance patterns among circulating influenza A virus strains present challenges in selecting antiviral medications for treatment and chemoprophylaxis of influenza and provide additional reasons for clinicians to test patients for influenza virus infection and to consult surveillance data in their community when evaluating people with acute respiratory tract illnesses during the influenza season. Enhanced surveillance for influenza antiviral resistance is ongoing at the CDC in collaboration with local and state health departments. Each year, options for treatment or chemoprophylaxis of influenza in the United States will depend on influenza strain resistance patterns. Recommendations for influenza chemoprophylaxis and treatment can be found at **www.cdc.gov/flu/professionals/antivirals/index.htm** or **www.aapredbook.org/flu.**

Therapy for influenza virus infection should be considered for (1) patients in whom shortening or ameliorating clinical signs and symptoms particularly may be beneficial, such as children at increased risk of severe or complicated influenza infection; (2) healthy children with moderate to severe illness; and (3) people with special environmental, family, or social situations for which ongoing illness would be detrimental. Children with severe influenza should be evaluated carefully for possible coinfection with bacterial pathogens (eg, *Staphylococcus aureus*) that might require antimicrobial therapy. Clinicians who want to have influenza isolates tested for susceptibility should contact their state health department.

If antiviral therapy is prescribed, treatment should be started as soon after illness onset as possible, because benefit is greatest when treatment is initiated within 48 hours of onset of symptoms.[1,2] Treatment should be discontinued approximately 24 to 48 hours after symptoms resolve. The duration of treatment studied was 5 days for both the neuraminidase inhibitors (oseltamivir and zanamivir) and the adamantanes (amantadine and rimantadine). Recommended dosages for drugs approved for treatment and prophylaxis of influenza are given in Table 4.8 (p 777). Patients with any degree of renal insufficiency should be monitored for adverse events. Only zanamivir, which is administered by inhalation, does not require adjustment for people with severe renal insufficiency.

The most common adverse effects of oseltamivir are nausea and vomiting. Postmarketing reports, mostly from Japan, have noted self-injury and delirium with use of oseltamivir among pediatric patients, but recent data suggest that these occurrences were related to influenza disease itself rather than antiviral therapy. Nevertheless, cautioning parents and patients regarding abnormal behavior is advised. Zanamivir use has been associated with bronchospasm in some people and is not recommended for use in patients with underlying airway disease. Both amantadine and rimantadine, but especially amantadine, may cause the central nervous system symptom of agitation, which resolves with discontinuation of the drug. An increased incidence of seizures has been reported in children with epilepsy who receive amantadine and, to a lesser extent, in children who receive rimantadine. Because of a lower incidence of adverse events, rimantadine generally is preferred over amantadine for both prophylaxis and treatment.

Control of fever with acetaminophen or other appropriate antipyretic agents may be important in young children, because fever and other symptoms of influenza could exacerbate underlying chronic conditions. Children and adolescents with influenza should not receive aspirin or any salicylate-containing products because of the resulting increased risk of developing Reye syndrome.

ISOLATION OF THE HOSPITALIZED PATIENT: In addition to standard precautions, droplet precautions are recommended for children hospitalized with influenza or an influenza-like illness for the duration of the illness. Respiratory tract secretions should be considered infectious, and strict hand hygiene procedures should be used.

CONTROL MEASURES:

Influenza Vaccine. Trivalent inactivated influenza vaccine (TIV) and live-attenuated influenza vaccine (LAIV) are multivalent vaccines containing 3 virus strains (one each of A [H3N2], A [H1N1], and B). Typically, 1 or more strains are changed each year in anticipation of the predominant influenza strains expected to circulate in the United States in the upcoming influenza season. Because viruses for both vaccines are grown in eggs, neither should be administered to anyone with known severe allergic reactions (eg, hives, angioedema, allergic asthma, and systemic anaphylaxis) to chicken, egg proteins, or any other component of the vaccines. Less severe or local manifestations of allergy to egg or feathers are not contraindications to administration of influenza vaccine.

---

[1] American Academy of Pediatrics, Committee on Infectious Diseases. Prevention of influenza: recommendations for influenza immunization of children, 2008–2009. *Pediatrics.* 2008;122(5):1135–1141

[2] Centers for Disease Control and Prevention. Prevention and control of influenza: recommendations of the Advisory Committee on Immunization Practices (ACIP), 2009. *MMWR Recomm Rep.* 2009; in press

TIV distributed in the United States is either subvirion vaccine, prepared by disrupting the lipid-containing membrane of the virus, or purified surface-antigen vaccine. TIV is licensed for use in people 6 months of age or older and is administered via intramuscular injection. Not all influenza vaccines are licensed for use in children as young as 6 months of age. LAIV is cold adapted, developed by passaging the viruses at successively lower temperatures in tissue culture, so that replication occurs only in the upper respiratory tract. LAIV is licensed for people 2 through 49 years of age and is administered via intranasal spray.

Immunogenicity in Children. Children 6 months through 9 years of age who previously have not been immunized against influenza require 2 doses of TIV or LAIV administered at least 1 month apart to produce a satisfactory antibody response (see Table 3.30 and Table 3.31, p 407). If a child younger than 9 years of age receives only 1 dose of either TIV or LAIV in their first season of being immunized, then 2 doses should be given the following influenza season. In subsequent seasons, children younger than 9 years of age should receive a single annual dose, regardless of the number of doses previously given. Children 9 years of age or older require only 1 dose, regardless of their influenza immunization history.

Vaccine Efficacy and Effectiveness. The efficacy (ie, prevention of illness among vaccine recipients in controlled trials) and effectiveness (ie, prevention of illness in populations receiving vaccine) of influenza vaccines depend primarily on the age and immunocompetence of vaccine recipients, the degree of similarity between the viruses in the vaccine and those in circulation, and the outcome being measured. Protection against virologically confirmed influenza illness after immunization with TIV in healthy children older than 2 years of age usually is 70% to 80%, with a range of 50% to 95% depending on the closeness of vaccine strain match to the circulating wild strain. Efficacy of LAIV was 86% to 96% against virologically confirmed influenza A (H3N2) virus infection in a large clinical pediatric trial during 1 year. Efficacy of TIV in children 6 through 23 months of age is lower than in older children, although data are limited. Several recent randomized controlled trials have shown that, among young children, LAIV has a 32% to 55% greater relative efficacy in preventing laboratory-confirmed influenza compared with TIV; however, additional experience over multiple influenza seasons is needed to determine optimal

Table 3.30. Schedule for Trivalent Inactivated Influenza Vaccine (TIV) Dosage by Age[a]

Age	Dose, mL[b]	No. of Doses	Route[c]
6 through 35 mo	0.25	1–2[d]	Intramuscular
3 through 8 y	0.5	1–2[d]	Intramuscular
9 y or older	0.5	1	Intramuscular

[a]Manufacturers include sanofi pasteur (Fluzone, split-virus vaccine licensed for people 6 months of age or older), Novartis Vaccine (Fluvirin, purified surface antigen, licensed for people 4 years of age or older), CSL Biotherapies (Afluria, split-virus vaccine licensed for people 18 years of age or older), and GlaxoSmithKline Biologicals (Fluarix and FluLaval, split-virus vaccines licensed for people 18 years of age or older).

[b]Dosages are those recommended in recent years. Physicians should refer to the product circular each year to ensure that the appropriate dosage is given.

[c]For adults and older children, the recommended site of immunization is the deltoid muscle. For infants and young children, the preferred site is the anterolateral aspect of the thigh.

[d]Two doses administered at least 4 weeks apart are recommended for children younger than 9 years of age who are receiving inactivated trivalent influenza vaccine for the first time. If possible, the second dose should be administered before December.

Table 3.31 Schedule for Live-Attenuated Influenza Vaccine (LAIV)[a]

Age	Dose, mL[b]	No. of Doses	Route
2 through 8 y	0.2	1–2[c]	Intranasal
9 y or older	0.2	1	Intranasal

[a]Manufacturer: MedImmune Vaccines, Inc (FluMist).
[b]Dosage is the one recommended in recent years. Physicians should refer to the product circular each year to ensure that the appropriate dosage is given.
[c]Two doses administered at least 4 weeks apart are recommended for children younger than 9 years of age who are receiving LAIV for the first time. If possible, the second dose should be administered before December.

utilization of these 2 vaccines in children. The effectiveness of influenza immunization on acute respiratory tract illness is less evident in pediatric than in adult populations because of the frequency of upper respiratory tract infections and influenza-like illness caused by other viral agents in young children. The duration of protection is approximately 1 year.

Coadministration With Other Vaccines. TIV can be administered simultaneously with other live and inactivated vaccines. Although information on how concurrent administration of LAIV with other vaccines affects the safety or efficacy of either LAIV or the simultaneously administered vaccine has not been well studied, it generally is recommended that inactivated or live vaccines be administered simultaneously with LAIV. After administration of a live vaccine, at least 4 weeks should pass before another live vaccine is administered.

Recommendations for Influenza Immunization.[1,2] Annual influenza immunization, beginning in September or when vaccine becomes available and extending into February and beyond, is recommended for (1) all children 6 months through 18 years of age; (2) household contacts and out-of-home caregivers of children 0 through 59 months of age and adults 50 years of age and older; and (3) household contacts and caregivers of people with medical conditions that place them at higher risk of severe complications from influenza.

The following people from 19 through 49 years of age who are at increased risk of severe complications from influenza should receive annual immunization:

- Asthma or other chronic pulmonary diseases, such as cystic fibrosis
- Hemodynamically significant cardiac disease
- Immunosuppressive disorders or therapy (see Special Considerations, p 408)
- Human immunodeficiency virus (HIV) infection (see Human Immunodeficiency Virus Infection, p 380)
- Sickle cell anemia and other hemoglobinopathies
- Diseases requiring long-term salicylate therapy, such as rheumatoid arthritis or Kawasaki disease, which may increase the risk of developing Reye syndrome after influenza illness
- Chronic renal dysfunction
- Chronic metabolic disease, including diabetes mellitus

---

[1]Centers for Disease Control and Prevention. Prevention and control of influenza: recommendations of the Advisory Committee on Immunization Practices (ACIP), 2009. *MMWR Recomm Rep.* 2009; in press (for updates, see **www.cdc.gov/flu**)

[2]American Academy of Pediatrics, Committee on Infectious Diseases. Prevention of influenza: recommendations for influenza immunization for children, 2008-2009. *Pediatrics.* 2008;122(5):1135–1141 (for updates, see **www.aap.org**)

- People with any condition (eg, cognitive dysfunction, spinal cord injuries, seizure disorders, or other neuromuscular disorders) that can compromise respiratory function or handling of respiratory tract secretions or that can increase the risk of aspiration.

LAIV Indications. LAIV is indicated for healthy nonpregnant people 2 through 49 years of age who want to be protected against influenza or who are contacts of people with an age or medical indication for immunization. TIV is preferred for close contacts of very severely immunosuppressed people (ie, those requiring care in a protective environment).

People should not receive LAIV if they received other live vaccines within the last 4 weeks, have a moderate to severe febrile illness, are receiving salicylates, have a known or suspected immune deficiency, have a history of Guillain-Barré syndrome (GBS), have a history of anaphylactic reaction to egg protein, or have reactive airway disease or other conditions that traditionally would place them in a high-risk category for severe influenza (chronic pulmonary disorders or cardiac disorders, pregnancy, chronic metabolic disease, renal dysfunction, hemoglobinopathies, or immunosuppressive therapy).

Special Considerations, LAIV. Clinicians and immunization programs should screen for possible reactive airways diseases when considering use of LAIV for children 2 through 4 years of age and avoid use in children with asthma or a recent wheezing episode. Health care professionals should consult the patient's medical record, when available, to identify children 2 through 4 years of age with asthma or recurrent wheezing that might indicate asthma. Some children 2 through 4 years of age have a history of wheezing with respiratory tract illnesses but have not been diagnosed with asthma. Therefore, to identify children who might be at higher risk of asthma and possibly at increased risk of wheezing after receiving LAIV, people administering LAIV should also ask parents/guardians of children 2 through 4 years of age: "In the past 12 months, has a health care professional ever told you that your child had wheezing or asthma?" LAIV is not recommended for children whose parent or guardian answers yes to this question or for children who had a wheezing episode or asthma diagnosis noted in his or her medical record within the past 12 months. Precaution also should be taken when considering LAIV administration to people with minor acute illness, such as a mild upper respiratory tract infection with or without fever. Although the vaccine most likely can be given in this case, LAIV should not be delivered if nasal congestion will impede delivery of the vaccine to the nasopharyngeal mucosa, until the congestion-inducing illness is resolved.

Special Considerations, TIV. Consideration should be given to the potential risks and benefits of administering influenza vaccine to any child with known or suspected immunodeficiency. In children receiving immunosuppressive chemotherapy, influenza immunization may result in a less robust response than in immunocompetent children. The optimal time to immunize children with malignant neoplasms who must undergo chemotherapy is more than 3 weeks after chemotherapy has been discontinued, when the peripheral granulocyte and lymphocyte counts are greater than $1000/\mu L$ (1.0×10^9/L). Children who no longer are receiving chemotherapy generally have high rates of seroconversion. TIV is the influenza vaccine of choice for any child living with a family member or household contact who is immunocompromised severely (ie, in a protected environment). The preference of TIV over LAIV for such people is because of the theoretical risk of infection in an immunocompromised contact of a LAIV-immunized child. As a precautionary measure, people recently immunized with LAIV should restrict contact with severely immunocompromised (ie, in a protected environment) patients for 7 days after LAIV immunization, even though there have been no reports of LAIV transmission between these 2 groups.

Children with hemodynamically unstable cardiac disease constitute a large group potentially at high risk of complications of influenza. The immune response and safety of TIV in these children are comparable to the immune response and safety in healthy children.

Corticosteroids administered for brief periods or every other day seem to have a minimal effect on antibody response to influenza vaccine. Prolonged administration of high doses of corticosteroids (ie, a dose of prednisone of either 2 mg/kg or greater or a total of 20 mg/day or greater or an equivalent) may impair antibody response. Influenza immunization can be deferred temporarily during the time of receipt of high-dose corticosteroids, provided deferral does not compromise the likelihood of immunization before the start of influenza season (see Vaccine Administration, p 17).

Pregnancy. Women, including adolescents, who will be pregnant during influenza season should receive TIV during the autumn, because pregnancy increases the risk of complications and hospitalization from influenza. Because the currently available intramuscularly administered TIV is not a live-virus vaccine and rarely is associated with major systemic reactions, most experts consider the vaccine safe during any stage of pregnancy. LAIV is contraindicated during pregnancy.

Close Contacts of High-Risk Patients. Immunization of people who are in close contact with children with high-risk conditions or with any child younger than 60 months (5 years) of age is an important means of protection for these children. In addition, immunization of pregnant women may benefit their unborn infants, because transplacentally acquired antibody may protect infants from infection with influenza virus. Immunization is recommended for the following people:
- All health care professionals in contact with pediatric patients in hospitals, outpatient care settings, and chronic care facilities[1]
- Household contacts, including siblings and primary caregivers, of high-risk children of any age and all healthy children 0 through 59 months of age
- Children who are members of households with high-risk adults (ie, adults with underlying medical conditions that predispose them to severe influenza infection or adults 50 years of age or older), any children younger than 60 months (5 years) of age, and children with HIV infection
- Providers of home care to children 0 through 59 months of age and to other high-risk groups of children and adolescents
- Close contacts of infants younger than 6 months of age (see Recommendations for Influenza Immunization, p 407), because this high-risk group cannot be protected directly by immunization or antiviral prophylaxis.

Breastfeeding. Breastfeeding is not a contraindication for immunization with either TIV or LAIV.

Timing of Vaccine Administration. Influenza vaccine should be administered as soon as available each year, preferably before the start of influenza season, at the time specified in the yearly recommendations of the CDC Advisory Committee on Immunization Practices (**www.cdc.gov/flu**). Traditionally, the recommended time ranges from

---

[1]Centers for Disease Control and Prevention. Influenza vaccination of health-care personnel. Recommendations of the Healthcare Infection Control Practices Advisory Committee (HICPAC) and the Advisory Committee on Immunization Practices (ACIP). *MMWR Recomm Rep.* 2006;55(RR-2):1–16

the beginning of October to the end of January, unless vaccine supplies are available and sufficient to immunize people earlier in September. Influenza vaccine administration throughout the entire season now is recommended, because the influenza season extends into March and April. Immunization throughout the season may protect some people against late outbreaks of influenza. In addition, there may be more than 1 peak of activity during an influenza season, so later immunization still may help protect from a later peak caused by a different strain of influenza virus that same season. The recommended vaccine dose and schedule for different age groups are given in Tables 3.30 (p 406) and 3.31 (p 407).

Annual influenza immunization is recommended, because immunity can decrease during the year after immunization and because in most years, at least one of the vaccine antigens is changed to match ongoing antigenic changes in circulating strains. Strategies to maximize immunization levels include using reminder/recall systems and programs for standing orders. Missed opportunities to provide influenza vaccine can be reduced by administering vaccine before and during the influenza season to people during hospitalizations, routine health-care visits, or most any other health care encounter.

Reactions, Adverse Effects, and Contraindications

Inactivated Influenza Vaccine. TIV contains only killed, noninfectious viruses and, therefore, cannot produce an active influenza infection. The most common symptoms associated with TIV administration are soreness at the injection site and fever. Usually occurring 6 to 24 hours after immunization, fever affects approximately 10% to 35% of children younger than 2 years. Mild systemic symptoms, such as nausea, lethargy, headache, muscle aches, and chills, also can occur with TIV injection. In children 13 years of age or older, local reactions occur in approximately 10% of recipients.

Although a very slight increase in the number of cases of GBS was reported during the "swine flu" vaccine program of 1976, obtaining strong epidemiologic evidence for a possible limited increase in risk for a rare condition with multiple causes is difficult. GBS has an annual incidence of 10 to 20 cases per 1 million adults, and during the 1976 swine influenza vaccine program, 1 case of GBS was reported per 100 000 people immunized. The risk of influenza vaccine-associated GBS was higher among people 25 years of age or older than among people younger than 25 years of age. If there is an association between seasonal influenza vaccine and GBS, the risk is rare, at no more than 1 to 2 cases per million doses. Whether influenza immunization specifically might increase the risk of recurrence of GBS is unknown. However, avoiding immunizing people who are not at high risk of severe influenza complications and who are known to have experienced GBS within 6 weeks after a previous influenza vaccine dose is prudent. Immunization of children who have asthma or cystic fibrosis with available TIV is not associated with a detectable increase in adverse events or exacerbations. Because past reports are conflicting, the issue of safety of TIV immunization for children and adults with HIV infection is uncertain. However, experts generally believe that the benefits of immunization with TIV for children with HIV infection far outweigh risks.

Children with known severe allergic reactions (eg, hives, angioedema, allergic asthma, or systemic anaphylaxis) to chicken or egg proteins should not receive these vaccines, because both TIV and LAIV are developed with embryonated hen eggs. Although TIV has been administered safely to such children after skin testing and, when appropriate, desensitization, these children should not receive either TIV or LAIV because of their risk of reactions, the likely need for yearly immunization, and availability of chemoprophylaxis against influenza infection. Less severe or local manifestations of allergy to egg or feathers are not contraindications to administration of influenza vaccine.

Live-Attenuated Influenza Vaccine. No statistically significant differences were observed in clinical studies between placebo and LAIV recipients in rates of fever, rhinitis, or nasal congestion. A retrospective analysis of a large pediatric trial in Northern California revealed a statistically significant increase in asthma events among children 12 through 59 months of age after dose 1 of LAIV (relative risk: 3.53; 90% confidence interval: 1.1–15.7). There was no clustering of wheezing events. In a randomized controlled trial conducted among children 6 through 59 months of age, rates of medically significant wheezing were higher among children 6 through 23 months of age who received LAIV (5.9%) compared with those who received TIV (3.8%), and rates of hospitalizations attributable to any cause also were significantly higher among LAIV recipients. However, similar low rates of medically significant wheezing and hospitalizations were observed in children 24 through 59 months of age regardless of the influenza vaccine given.

LAIV should not be administered to people with asthma or children younger than 5 years of age with recurrent wheezing. The risk, if any, of wheezing caused by LAIV among children 2 through 4 years of age with a history of asthma or wheezing is unknown.

LAIV shedding can occur after immunization, although the amount of detectable virus is less than occurs during natural influenza infection. The proposed explanation for the low incidence of transmission is that the vaccine virus is shed for a shorter duration and in a much smaller quantity than are wild-type strains. In the rare instance when shed vaccine virus is transmitted to a nonimmunized contact, illness has not occurred. Further evaluation of transmission of LAIV is being conducted.

Chemoprophylaxis: An Adjunct Method of Protecting Children Against Influenza. Chemoprophylaxis should not be considered a substitute for immunization in most cases. However, the influenza antiviral drugs currently licensed are important adjuncts to influenza immunization for control and prevention of influenza disease. Because of high rates of resistance of influenza A (H3N2) and B strains to amantadine or rimantadine and of influenza A (H1N1) to oseltamivir, recommendations for use of these drugs for chemoprophylaxis may vary by location and season, depending on susceptibility patterns. For current recommendations about chemoprophylaxis against influenza, see **www.cdc. gov/flu/professionals/antivirals/index.htm** or **www.aapredbook.org/flu**.

Indications for Chemoprophylaxis. Chemoprophylaxis may be considered for the following situations:

- Protection of unimmunized high-risk children or children who were immunized less than 2 weeks before influenza circulation, because adequate immune response develops 2 weeks after immunization
- Protection of children at increased risk of severe infection or complications, such as high-risk children for whom the vaccine is contraindicated (ie, children with a history of anaphylactic reaction to eggs)
- Protection of unimmunized close contacts of high-risk children
- Protection of immunocompromised children who may not respond to vaccine
- Control of influenza outbreaks in a closed setting, such as an institution with unimmunized high-risk children
- Protection of immunized high-risk children if the vaccine strain poorly matches circulating influenza strains

Chemoprophylaxis does not interfere with the immune response to TIV; however, people immunized with LAIV should not receive antiviral prophylaxis for 14 days after receipt of LAIV, because the vaccine strains are susceptible to antiviral drugs.

Information about influenza surveillance is available through the CDC Voice Information System (influenza update, 888-232-3228) or through **www.cdc.gov/flu**.

Isosporiasis

CLINICAL MANIFESTATIONS: Watery diarrhea is the most common symptom and can be profuse and protracted, even in immunocompetent people. Manifestations are similar to those caused by *Cryptosporidium* species and *Cyclospora* species and can include abdominal pain, cramping, anorexia, nausea, vomiting, weight loss, and low-grade fever. The proportion of infected people who are asymptomatic is unknown. Severity of infection ranges from self-limiting in immunocompetent hosts to debilitating and life threatening in immunocompromised patients, particularly people infected with human immunodeficiency virus (HIV).

ETIOLOGY: *Isospora belli* is a spore-forming coccidian protozoan; oocysts are passed in stools.

EPIDEMIOLOGY: Infection occurs predominately in tropical and subtropical regions of the world and can cause traveler's diarrhea. Infection results from ingestion of sporulated oocysts (eg, in contaminated food and water). Humans are the only known host for *I belli* and shed mature (noninfective) oocysts in feces. These oocysts must mature (sporulate) outside the host, in the environment, to become infective. Under favorable conditions, sporulation can be completed in 1 to 2 days. Oocysts are resistant to most disinfectants and can remain viable for prolonged periods in a cool, moist environment.

The **incubation period** is approximately 7 days.

DIAGNOSTIC TESTS: Identification of oocysts in feces or in duodenal aspirates or finding developmental stages of the parasite in biopsy specimens of the small intestine is diagnostic. Oocysts in stool are 5 times larger than *Cryptosporidium* organisms and are elongate and ellipsoidal. Oocysts can be shed in low numbers, even by people with profuse diarrhea. This constraint underscores the utility of repeated stool examinations, sensitive recovery methods (eg, concentration methods) and detection methods that highlight the organism (eg, oocysts stain bright red with modified acid-fast techniques and they autofluoresce when viewed by ultraviolet fluorescent microscopy).

TREATMENT: Trimethoprim-sulfamethoxazole for 7 to 10 days is the drug of choice (see Drugs for Parasitic Infections, p 783). Immunocompromised patients may need higher doses and longer duration of therapy. Pyrimethamine is an alternative treatment for people who cannot tolerate trimethoprim-sulfamethoxazole. Ciprofloxacin is less effective than trimethoprim-sulfamethoxazole. Ciprofloxacin is not approved for this use in people younger than 18 years of age. Maintenance therapy to prevent recurrent disease may be indicated for people infected with HIV.

ISOLATION OF THE HOSPITALIZED PATIENT: In addition to standard precautions, contact precautions are recommended for diapered and incontinent people.

CONTROL MEASURES: Preventive measures include avoiding fecal exposure (eg, food, water, skin, and fomites contaminated with stool) and practicing hand and personal hygiene.

Kawasaki Disease

CLINICAL MANIFESTATIONS: Kawasaki disease is a febrile, exanthematous, multisystem vasculitis of importance, because approximately 20% of untreated children will develop coronary artery abnormalities. Most cases of Kawasaki disease occur in children younger than 12 years of age. The illness is characterized by fever and the following clinical features: (1) bilateral bulbar conjunctival injection without exudate; (2) erythematous mouth and pharynx, strawberry tongue, and red, cracked lips; (3) a polymorphous, generalized, erythematous rash that can be morbilliform, maculopapular, or scarlatiniform or may resemble erythema multiforme; (4) changes in the peripheral extremities consisting of induration of the hands and feet with erythematous palms and soles, often with later periungual desquamation; and (5) acute, nonsuppurative, usually unilateral, cervical lymphadenopathy with at least one node 1.5 cm in diameter. For diagnosis of classic Kawasaki disease, patients should have fever for at least 4 days and at least 4 of these 5 features without alternative explanation for the findings. The epidemiologic case definition also allows diagnosis of Kawasaki disease when a person has fewer than 4 principal clinical criteria in the presence of coronary artery aneurysms. Irritability, abdominal pain, diarrhea, and vomiting commonly are associated features. Other findings include urethritis with sterile pyuria (70% of cases), mild anterior uveitis (25%–50%), mild hepatic dysfunction (40%), arthritis or arthralgia (10%–20%), meningismus with cerebrospinal fluid pleocytosis (25%), pericardial effusion of at least 1 mm (less than 5%), gallbladder hydrops (less than 10%), and myocarditis manifested by congestive heart failure (less than 5%). Fine desquamation in the groin area can occur in the acute phase of disease.[1]

Incomplete Kawasaki disease can be diagnosed in febrile patients when fever plus fewer than 4 of the characteristic features are present. Patients with fewer than 4 of the characteristic features and who have additional findings not listed above (eg, purulent conjunctivitis) should not be considered to have incomplete Kawasaki disease. Incomplete Kawasaki disease is more common in infants younger than 12 months of age than in older children. Infants with Kawasaki disease also have a higher risk of developing coronary artery aneurysms than do older children, making diagnosis and timely treatment especially important in this age group. The laboratory findings of incomplete cases are similar to findings of classic cases. Therefore, although laboratory findings in Kawasaki disease are nonspecific, they may prove useful in increasing or decreasing the likelihood of incomplete Kawasaki disease. If coronary artery ectasia or dilatation is evident, the diagnosis is confirmed. A normal early echocardiographic study does not exclude the diagnosis but may be useful in evaluation of patients with suspected incomplete Kawasaki disease. Incomplete Kawasaki disease should be considered in any child with unexplained fever for 5 days or longer in association with 2 or more of the principal features of this illness and supportive laboratory data (eg, erythrocyte sedimentation rate [ESR] 40 mm/hour or greater or C-reactive protein [CRP] concentration 3.0 mg/dL or greater). Fig 3.2 shows the American Heart Association algorithm for diagnosis and treatment of suspected incomplete Kawasaki disease.

---

[1]For further information on the diagnosis of this disease, see Newburger JW, Takahashi M, Gerber MA, et al. Diagnosis, treatment and long-term management of Kawasaki disease: a statement for health professionals from the Committee on Rheumatic Fever, Endocarditis and Kawasaki Disease, Council on Cardiovascular Disease in the Young, American Heart Association. *Circulation.* 2004;110(17):2747–2771 (also in *Pediatrics.* 2004;114[6]:1708–1733)

Without aspirin and Immune Globulin Intravenous (IGIV) therapy, fever can last 2 weeks or longer. After fever resolves, patients can remain anorectic and/or irritable for 2 to 3 weeks. During this phase, desquamation of the groin, fingers, and toes and fine desquamation of other areas may occur. Recurrent disease occurring months to years later develops in approximately 2% of patients.

Coronary artery abnormalities can be demonstrated with 2-dimensional echocardiography in 20% to 25% of patients who are not treated within 10 days of onset of fever. Increased risk of developing coronary artery aneurysms is associated with male sex; age younger than 12 months or older than 8 years; fever for more than 10 days; high baseline neutrophil (greater than 30 000 cells/mm^3) and band count; low hemoglobin concentration (less than 10 g/dL); hypoalbuminemia, hyponatremia, or thrombocytopenia at presentation; fever persisting after IGIV administration; and persistence of elevated ESR or CRP for more than 30 days or recurrent elevations. Hispanic ethnicity also has been associated with high risk of coronary artery aneurysms, which may be related to delayed diagnosis and treatment. Aneurysms of the coronary arteries have been demonstrated by echocardiography as early as 5 to 7 days after onset of illness but more typically occur between 1 and 4 weeks after onset of illness; their initial appearance later than 6 weeks is uncommon. Giant coronary artery aneurysms (diameter 8 mm or greater) are likely to be associated with long-term complications. Aneurysms occurring in other medium-sized arteries (eg, iliac, femoral, renal, and axillary vessels) are uncommon and generally do not occur in the absence of significant coronary abnormalities. In addition to coronary artery disease, carditis can involve the pericardium, myocardium, or endocardium, and mitral or aortic regurgitation or both can develop. Carditis generally resolves when fever resolves.

In children with mild coronary artery dilation or ectasia, coronary artery dimensions often return to baseline within 6 to 8 weeks after onset of disease. Approximately 50% of coronary aneurysms (fewer giant aneurysms) regress to normal luminal size within 1 to 2 years, although this process can be accompanied by development of coronary stenosis. In addition, regression of aneurysm(s) may result in a poorly compliant, fibrotic vessel wall.

The current case-fatality rate in the United States and Japan is less than 0.1% to 0.2%. The principal cause of death is myocardial infarction resulting from coronary artery occlusion attributable to thrombosis or progressive stenosis. Rarely, a large coronary artery aneurysm may rupture. The relative risk of mortality is highest within 6 weeks of onset of symptoms, but myocardial infarction and sudden death can occur months to years after the acute episode. There is hypothetical concern that the vasculitis of Kawasaki disease may predispose to premature coronary artery disease.

ETIOLOGY: The cause is unknown. Epidemiologic and clinical features suggest an infectious cause.

EPIDEMIOLOGY: Peak age of occurrence in the United States is between 18 and 24 months. Fifty percent of patients are younger than 2 years of age, and 80% are younger than 5 years of age; children older than 8 years of age less commonly develop the disease. In children younger than 6 months of age, the diagnosis often is delayed, because the symptom complex of Kawasaki disease is incomplete. The prevalence of coronary artery abnormalities is higher when diagnosis and treatment are delayed beyond the 10th day of illness. The male-to-female ratio is approximately 1.5:1. In the United States, 3000 to 5000 cases are estimated to occur each year; the incidence is highest in

FIG 3.2. EVALUATION OF SUSPECTED INCOMPLETE KAWASAKI DISEASE (KD).[a]

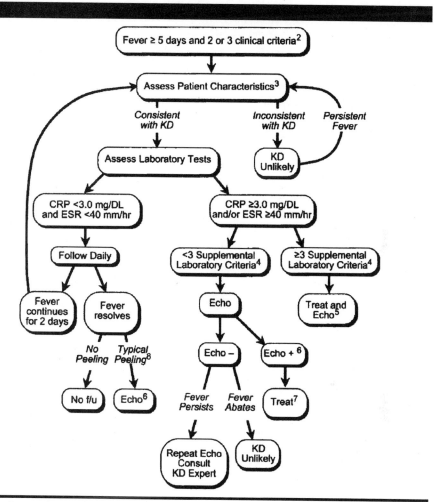

Evaluation of suspected incomplete Kawasaki disease. (1) In the absence of gold standard for diagnosis, this algorithm cannot be evidence based but rather represents the informed opinion of the expert committee. Consultation with an expert should be sought anytime assistance is needed. (2) Infants ≤6 months old on day ≥7 of fever without other explanation should undergo laboratory testing and, if evidence of systemic inflammation is found, an echocardiogram, even if the infants have no clinical criteria. (3) Patient characteristics suggesting Kawasaki disease are provided in text. Characteristics suggesting disease other than Kawasaki disease include exudative conjunctivitis, exudative pharyngitis, discrete intraoral lesions, bullous or vesicular rash, or generalized adenopathy. Consider alternative diagnoses. (4) Supplemental laboratory criteria include albumin ≤3.0 g/dL, anemia for age, elevation of alanine aminotransferase, platelets after 7 d ≥450 000/mm³, white blood cell count ≥15 000/mm³, and urine ≥10 white blood cells/high-power field. (5) Can treat before performing echocardiogram. (6) Echocardiogram is considered positive for purposes of this algorithm if any of 3 conditions are met: z score of LAD or RCA ≥2.5, coronary arteries meet Japanese Ministry of Health criteria for aneurysms, or ≥3 other suggestive features exist, including perivascular brightness, lack of tapering, decreased LV function, mitral regurgitation, pericardial effusion, or z scores in LAD or RCA of 2–2.5. (7) If the echocardiogram is positive, treatment should be given to children within 10 d of fever onset and those beyond day 10 with clinical and laboratory signs (CRP, ESR) of ongoing inflammation. (8) Typical peeling begins under nail bed of fingers and then toes.

[a]Used with permission from Newburger JW, Takahashi M, Gerber MA, et al. Diagnosis, treatment and long-term management of Kawasaki disease: a statement for health professionals from the Committee on Rheumatic Fever, Endocarditis and Kawasaki Disease, Council on Cardiovascular Disease in the Young, American Heart Association. *Circulation.* 2004;110(17):2747–2771

those of Asian background. Kawasaki disease first was described in Japan, where a pattern of endemic occurrence with superimposed epidemic outbreaks was recognized. A similar pattern of steady or increasing endemic disease with occasional sharply defined community-wide epidemics has been recognized in North America and Hawaii. Clusters generally occur during winter and spring. No evidence indicates person-to-person or common-source spread, although the incidence is slightly higher in siblings of children with the disease.

The **incubation period** is unknown.

DIAGNOSTIC TESTS: No specific diagnostic test is available. The diagnosis is established by fulfillment of the clinical criteria (see Clinical Manifestations, p 413) and clinical or laboratory exclusion of other possible illnesses, such as measles, parvovirus B19 infection, adenovirus or enterovirus infections, staphylococcal or streptococcal toxin-mediated disease, rickettsial exanthems, drug reactions (eg, Stevens-Johnson syndrome), leptospirosis, systemic onset juvenile idiopathic arthritis, and reactive arthritis. A greatly increased ESR and serum CRP concentration during the first 2 weeks of illness and an increased platelet count (greater than $450\,000/mm^3$) on days 10 to 21 of illness are almost universal laboratory features. ESR and platelet count usually are normal within 6 to 8 weeks; CRP concentration returns to normal much sooner.

TREATMENT: Management during the acute phase is directed at decreasing inflammation of the myocardium and coronary artery wall and providing supportive care. Therapy should be initiated when the diagnosis is established or strongly suspected, optimally within the first 10 days of illness. Once the acute phase has passed, therapy is directed at prevention of coronary artery thrombosis. Specific recommendations for therapy include the following measures.

Immune Globulin Intravenous. Therapy with high-dose IGIV and aspirin initiated within 10 days of the onset of fever substantially decreases progression to coronary artery dilation and aneurysms, compared with treatment with aspirin alone, and results in more rapid resolution of fever and other clinical and laboratory indicators of acute inflammation. Therapy with IGIV should be initiated as soon as possible; its efficacy when initiated later than the 10th day of illness or after detection of aneurysms has been evaluated in only one controlled trial. However, therapy with IGIV and aspirin should be provided for patients diagnosed after day 10 who have manifestations of continuing inflammation (eg, fever or elevated ESR or CRP concentration) or of evolving coronary artery disease. Despite prompt treatment with IGIV and aspirin, 2% to 4% of patients develop coronary artery abnormalities.

Dose. A dose of 2 g/kg as a single dose, given over 10 to 12 hours, has been proven to reduce the risk of coronary artery aneurysm from 17% to 4%. Few complications occur from this regimen.

Retreatment. Up to 20% of patients who receive IGIV and aspirin therapy have persistent fever after IGIV or recurrence of fever after an initial period of being afebrile. In these situations, retreatment with IGIV (2 g/kg) within 24 to 48 hours of persistent or recrudescent fever and continued aspirin therapy generally is given. Persistent or recrudescent fever is associated with high concentrations of proinflammatory cytokines and an increased risk of coronary artery abnormalities. The benefit and possible detriment of use of systemic corticosteroids in treatment of Kawasaki disease are controversial. Corticosteroids are not beneficial for primary therapy. For the limited number of patients who are refractory to at least 2 doses of IGIV, rescue therapy of intravenous methylprednisolone (usually 30 mg/kg/day for 1 to 3 days) or infliximab (5 mg/kg as one infusion) may be administered in attempt to reduce inflammation and improve coronary artery outcomes. Lack of data on use of these modalities precludes definitive recommendations.

Aspirin. Aspirin is used for anti-inflammatory and antithrombotic actions, although aspirin alone does not decrease risk of coronary artery abnormalities. The optimal dose or duration of aspirin treatment is unknown. Aspirin is administered in doses of 80 to 100 mg/kg per day in 4 divided doses once the diagnosis is made. Children with acute Kawasaki disease have decreased aspirin absorption and increased clearance and rarely achieve therapeutic serum concentrations. In most children, it is not necessary to monitor aspirin concentrations. After fever is controlled for 48 hours (usually around the 14th day of illness), the aspirin dose is decreased to 3 to 5 mg/kg per day for antithrombotic activity. Aspirin is discontinued if no coronary artery abnormalities have been detected by 6 to 8 weeks after onset of illness. Low-dose aspirin therapy should be continued indefinitely for people in whom coronary artery abnormalities are present. Because of the theoretical risk of Reye syndrome in patients with influenza or varicella receiving salicylates, parents of children receiving aspirin should be instructed to contact their child's physician promptly if the child develops symptoms of or is exposed to either disease. In general, ibuprofen should be avoided in children with coronary aneurysms taking aspirin for its antiplatelet effects, because ibuprofen antagonizes the platelet inhibition that is induced by aspirin. The child and household contacts should be given influenza vaccine at diagnosis of Kawasaki disease according to seasonal recommendations.

Cardiac Care.[1] An echocardiogram should be obtained at the time of diagnosis and then 1 to 2 and 6 to 8 weeks after onset. Children at higher risk—for example, those with persistent or recrudescent fever after initial IGIV or baseline coronary abnormalities—should have more frequent echocardiograms to guide the need for additional therapies. Children also should be assessed during this time for arrhythmias, congestive heart failure, and valvular regurgitation. The care of patients with significant cardiac abnormalities should involve a pediatric cardiologist experienced in management of patients with Kawasaki disease and in assessing echocardiographic studies of coronary arteries in children. Long-term management of Kawasaki disease should be based on the extent of coronary artery involvement. In patients with persistent moderately large coronary artery abnormalities that are not large enough to require anticoagulation, prolonged low-dose aspirin and clopidogrel (1 mg/kg/day) are recommended in combination. Development of giant coronary artery aneurysms (diameter 8 mm or larger) usually requires addition of anticoagulant therapy, such as warfarin or low-molecular weight heparin, to prevent thrombosis. Anticoagulation also sometimes is used in young infants with coronary artery aneurysms measuring less than 8 mm in diameter but for whom the size is equivalent to giant aneurysms when body surface area is considered. For example, a 3-month-old infant with coronary arteries 6 or 7 mm in diameter often would be a candidate for anticoagulation.

---

[1]Newburger JW, Takahashi M, Gerber MA, et al. Diagnosis, treatment and long-term management of Kawasaki disease: a statement for health professionals from the Committee on Rheumatic Fever, Endocarditis and Kawasaki Disease, Council on Cardiovascular Disease in the Young, American Heart Association. *Circulation.* 2004;110(17):2747–2771 (also in *Pediatrics.* 2004;114[6]:1708–1733)

Subsequent Immunization. Measles and varicella-containing vaccines should be deferred for 11 months after high-dose IGIV for treatment of Kawasaki disease. If the child's risk of exposure to measles or varicella is high, the child should be immunized and then reimmunized at least 11 months after administration of IGIV (see Measles, p 444). The schedule for administration of inactivated childhood vaccines should not be interrupted.

ISOLATION OF THE HOSPITALIZED PATIENT: Standard precautions are indicated.

CONTROL MEASURES: None.

Kingella kingae Infections

CLINICAL MANIFESTATIONS: The most common infections associated with *Kingella kingae* are suppurative arthritis and osteomyelitis. Almost all of these infections occur in children younger than 5 years of age. *K kingae* may be a major cause of skeletal infections in children younger than 3 years of age. Pyogenic arthritis caused by *K kingae* generally is monoarticular, most commonly involving the knee, followed in frequency by the hip or ankle. Clinical manifestations of pyogenic arthritis are similar to manifestations associated with infection attributable to other bacterial pathogens in immunocompetent children, although a subacute course may be more common. Osteomyelitis caused by *K kingae* has clinical manifestations similar to *Staphylococcus aureus* osteomyelitis, but epiphyseal infection and a subacute course may be more common. The distal femur is the most common site of osteomyelitis. *K kingae* also has been associated with diskitis, endocarditis in children with underlying heart disease (HACEK group of organisms), meningitis, occult bacteremia, and pneumonia.

ETIOLOGY: *Kingella* organisms are fastidious, gram-negative coccobacilli previously classified as *Moraxella*. Of the 4 species in the genus *Kingella*, *K kingae* is the species most commonly associated with infection.

EPIDEMIOLOGY: The human oropharynx is the usual habitat of *K kingae*. The organism more frequently colonizes the respiratory tracts of children than adults and can be transmitted among children in child care centers, generally without causing disease. Infection may be associated with preceding or concomitant stomatitis or upper respiratory tract illness.

The **incubation period** is variable.

DIAGNOSTIC TESTS: *K kingae* can be isolated from blood, synovial fluid, bone exudate, cerebrospinal fluid, respiratory tract secretions, and other sites of infection. Organisms grow better in aerobic conditions with enhanced carbon dioxide. In patients with pyogenic arthritis and osteomyelitis, blood cultures often are negative for *K kingae*. *K kingae* is difficult to isolate on routinely used solid media. Synovial fluid and bone aspirates from patients with suspected *K kingae* infection should be inoculated into Bactec, BacT/Alert, or similar blood culture systems and held for at least 7 days to maximize recovery. *K kingae* should be suspected in young children with culture-negative skeletal infections.

TREATMENT: Penicillin is the drug of choice for treatment of invasive infections attributable to beta-lactamase–negative strains of *K kingae*. Other beta-lactam agents also are effective. Strains generally are susceptible to aminoglycosides, ciprofloxacin, erythromycin, chloramphenicol, and oxacillin and are resistant to trimethoprim, clindamycin, and vancomycin. Gentamicin in combination with penicillin can be useful for the initial treatment of endocarditis. The third-generation cephalosporins cefotaxime or ceftriaxone also may be used to treat endocarditis.

ISOLATION OF THE HOSPITALIZED PATIENT: Standard precautions are recommended.

CONTROL MEASURES: None.

Legionella pneumophila Infections

CLINICAL MANIFESTATIONS: Legionellosis is associated with 2 clinically and epidemiologically distinct illnesses: Legionnaires disease and Pontiac fever. **Legionnaires disease** varies in severity from mild to severe pneumonia characterized by fever, cough, and progressive respiratory distress. Legionnaires disease can be associated with chills, myalgia, gastrointestinal tract, central nervous system, and renal manifestations. Respiratory failure and death can occur. **Pontiac fever** is a milder febrile illness without pneumonia that occurs in epidemics and is characterized by an abrupt onset and a self-limited, influenza-like illness.

ETIOLOGY: *Legionella* species are fastidious aerobic bacilli that stain gram negative after recovery on buffered charcoal yeast extract (BCYE) media. At least 20 different species have been implicated in human disease, but most documented *Legionella* infections in the United States are caused by *Legionella pneumophila* serogroup 1.

EPIDEMIOLOGY: Legionnaires disease is acquired through inhalation of aerosolized water contaminated with *L pneumophila*. Person-to-person transmission has not been demonstrated. More than 80% of cases are sporadic; the sources of infection can be related to exposure to *L pneumophila*-contaminated water in the home, workplace, or hospitals or other medical facilities or to aerosol-producing devices in public places. Outbreaks have been ascribed to common-source exposure to contaminated cooling towers, evaporative condensers, potable water systems, whirlpool spas, humidifiers, and respiratory therapy equipment. Outbreaks have occurred in hospitals, hotels, and other large buildings as well as on cruise ships. Health care-associated infections can occur and often are related to contamination of the hot water supply. Legionnaires disease occurs most commonly in people who are elderly, are immunocompromised, or have underlying lung disease. Infection in children is rare and usually is asymptomatic or mild and unrecognized. Severe disease has occurred in children with malignant neoplasms, severe combined immunodeficiency, chronic granulomatous disease, organ transplantation, end-stage renal disease, underlying pulmonary disease, and immunosuppression; in children receiving systemic corticosteroids; and as a health care-associated infection in newborn infants.

The **incubation period** for Legionnaires disease (pneumonia) is 2 to 10 days; for Pontiac fever, the incubation period is 1 to 2 days.

DIAGNOSTIC TESTS: Recovery of *L pneumophila* from respiratory tract secretions, lung tissue, pleural fluid, or other normally sterile fluid specimens by using BCYE media provides definitive evidence of infection, but the sensitivity of culture is laboratory dependent. Detection of *Legionella* antigen in urine by commercially available immunoassays is highly specific. Such tests are sensitive for *L pneumophila* serogroup 1, but these tests rarely detect antigen in patients infected with other *L pneumophila* serogroups or other *Legionella* species. The bacterium can be demonstrated in specimens by direct immunofluorescent assay, but this test is less sensitive and the specificity is technician dependent and lower than culture or urine immunoassay. For serologic diagnosis, a fourfold increase in titer of antibodies to *L pneumophila* serogroup 1, measured by indirect immunofluorescent antibody (IFA) assay, confirms a recent infection. Convalescent serum samples should be obtained 3 to 4 weeks after onset of symptoms; however, an antibody titer increase can be delayed for 8 to 12 weeks. The positive predictive value of a single titer of 1:256 or greater is low and does not provide definitive evidence of infection. Antibodies to several gram-negative organisms, including *Pseudomonas* species, *Bacteroides fragilis,* and *Campylobacter jejuni,* can cause false-positive IFA test results. Newer serologic assays, such as enzyme immunoassay or tests using *Legionella* antigens other than serogroup 1, are available commercially but have not been standardized adequately.

TREATMENT: Intravenous azithromycin has replaced intravenous erythromycin as the drug of choice. Once the condition of a patient is improving, oral therapy can be substituted. Addition of rifampin should be considered for patients with confirmed disease who are severely ill or immunocompromised or in whom the infection does not respond promptly to intravenous azithromycin. Fluoroquinolones, including ciprofloxacin, levofloxacin, and moxifloxacin, are bactericidal and effective but are not approved for this indication in children younger than 18 years of age. Doxycycline and trimethoprim-sulfamethoxazole are alternative drugs. Doxycycline should not be used for pregnant women or children younger than 8 years of age because of the risk of dental staining. Duration of therapy is 5 to 10 days for azithromycin and 14 to 21 days for other drugs; longer courses are recommended for patients who are immunocompromised or who have severe disease.

ISOLATION OF THE HOSPITALIZED PATIENT: Standard precautions are recommended.

CONTROL MEASURES: Monochloramine (rather than free chlorine) treatment of municipal water supplies has been associated with a decrease in health care-associated Legionnaires disease. Hospitals should maintain hot water at the highest temperature allowable by state regulations or codes, preferably 60°C (140°F) or greater, and maintain cold water temperature at less than 20°C (68°F) to minimize waterborne *Legionella* contamination. Occurrence of even a single laboratory-confirmed health care-associated case of legionellosis warrants consideration of an epidemiologic and environmental investigation. Hospitals with transplantation programs (solid organ or stem cell) should maintain a high index of suspicion of legionellosis, use sterile water for the filling and terminal rinsing of nebulization devices, and consider performing periodic culturing for *Legionella* species in the potable water supply of the transplant unit. Some hospitals may choose to perform periodic, routine culturing of water samples from the hospital's potable water system to detect *Legionella* species.

The usual methods for decontaminating potable water supplies to prevent health care-associated cases are hyperchlorination often followed by maintenance of a 1- to 2-mg/L (1- to 2-ppm) free residual chlorine concentration in the heated water, superheating (to 66°C [150°F] or greater) followed by maintenance of a hot water temperature at the faucet of greater than 50°C (122°F).

Leishmaniasis

CLINICAL MANIFESTATIONS: The 3 major clinical syndromes are as follows:

- ***Cutaneous leishmaniasis.*** After inoculation by the bite of an infected female phlebotomine sand fly (approximately 2–3 mm long), parasites proliferate locally in mononuclear phagocytes, leading to an erythematous papule, which typically evolves to become a nodule and then a shallow ulcerative lesion with raised borders. Lesions can, however, persist as nodules or papules. Lesions commonly are located on exposed areas of the body (eg, face and extremities) and may be accompanied by satellite lesions, which appear as sporotrichoid-like nodules, and regional adenopathy. Clinical manifestations of Old World and New World (American) cutaneous leishmaniasis are similar. Spontaneous resolution of lesions may take weeks to years and usually results in a flat atrophic (cigarette paper) scar.

- ***Mucosal leishmaniasis (espundia).*** Mucosal infection may become clinically evident from months to years after the cutaneous lesions heal; sometimes mucosal and cutaneous lesions are noted simultaneously. Parasites may disseminate to the naso-oropharyngeal mucosa. In some patients, granulomatous ulceration and necrosis follows, leading to facial disfigurement, secondary infection, and mucosal perforation, which may occur months to years after the initial cutaneous lesion heals.

- ***Visceral leishmaniasis (kala-azar).*** After cutaneous inoculation of parasites, organisms spread throughout the mononuclear macrophage system to the spleen, liver, and bone marrow. The resulting clinical illness typically manifests as fever, anorexia, weight loss, splenomegaly, hepatomegaly, lymphadenopathy (in some geographic areas), anemia, leukopenia, thrombocytopenia sometimes associated with hemorrhage, hypo-albuminemia, and hypergammaglobulinemia. Secondary gram-negative enteric and mycobacterial infections are common (eg, tuberculosis). Untreated clinically manifested visceral infection (ie, visceral leishmaniasis) nearly always is fatal. Reactivation of latent visceral infection can occur in patients who become immunocompromised, including people with concurrent human immunodeficiency virus (HIV) infection and recipients of stem cell or solid organ transplants.

ETIOLOGY: In the human host, *Leishmania* species are obligate intracellular parasites of mononuclear phagocytes. Cutaneous leishmaniasis typically is caused by *Leishmania tropica*, *Leishmania major*, and *Leishmania aethiopica* (Old World species) and by *Leishmania mexicana*, *Leishmania amazonensis*, *Leishmania braziliensis*, *Leishmania panamensis*, *Leishmania guyanensis*, and *Leishmania peruviana* (New World species). Mucosal leishmaniasis typically is caused by *L braziliensis*, *L panamensis*, and *L guyanensis*. Visceral leishmaniasis is caused by *Leishmania donovani*, *Leishmania infantum*, and *Leishmania chagasi*, which also can cause cutaneous leishmaniasis. However, people with typical cutaneous leishmaniasis caused by these organisms rarely develop visceral leishmaniasis.

EPIDEMIOLOGY: Leishmaniasis typically is a zoonosis with a variety of mammalian reservoir hosts, including canines and rodents. Vectors are female phlebotomine sand flies. Leishmaniasis is endemic in 88 countries, from northern Argentina to southern Texas (not including Uruguay or Chile), in southern Europe, Asia (not southeast Asia), the Middle East, and Africa (particularly East and North Africa, with sporadic cases elsewhere) but not in Australia or Oceania. More than 90% of cases worldwide occur in Bangladesh, northeastern India (particularly Bihar State), Nepal, and Sudan (Old World) and in north-eastern Brazil (New World). The estimated annual number of new cases of cutaneous leishmaniasis is approximately 1.5 million; more than 90% of these new worldwide cases are in Afghanistan, Algeria, Iran, Iraq, Saudi Arabia, and Syria (Old World) and in Brazil and Peru (New World). Geographic distribution of cases evaluated in the developed world reflects travel and immigration patterns. The number of cases has increased as a result of increased travel to areas with endemic infection; for example, with ecotourism activities in South America and military activities in Iraq and Afghanistan, the number of imported cases within North America has increased.

The **incubation periods** for the different forms of leishmaniasis range from several days to several years but usually are in the range of several weeks to 6 months. In cutaneous leishmaniasis, primary skin lesions typically appear several weeks after parasite inoculation. In visceral infection, the incubation period typically ranges from 2 to 6 months.

DIAGNOSTIC TESTS: Definitive diagnosis is made by demonstration of the presence of the parasite. A common way of identifying the parasite is by microscopic identification of intracellular leishmanial organisms on Wright- or Giemsa-stained smears or histologic sections of infected tissues. In cutaneous disease, tissue can be obtained by a 3-mm punch biopsy, by lesion scrapings, or by needle aspiration of the raised nonnecrotic edge of the lesion. In visceral leishmaniasis, the organisms can be identified in the spleen and, less commonly, in bone marrow and the liver. The sensitivity is highest for splenic aspiration, but so is the risk. In East Africa in patients with lymphadenopathy, the organisms also can be identified in lymph nodes. Blood cultures, especially of buffy-coat preparations, have been positive in some patients, and organisms sometimes may be observed in blood smears or observed in or cultured from buffy-coat preparations in HIV-infected patients. Isolation of parasites by culture of appropriate tissue specimens in specialized media should be attempted when possible. Culture media and further information can be provided by the Centers for Disease Control and Prevention (CDC) (**www.cdc.gov/travel**). Investigational polymerase chain reaction assays are available at some reference laboratories.

The diagnosis of some forms of leishmaniasis can be aided by performance of serologic testing, which is available at the CDC. Serologic test results usually are positive in cases of visceral and mucosal leishmaniasis if the patient is immunocompetent but often are negative in cutaneous leishmaniasis. False-positive results may occur in patients with other infectious diseases, especially American trypanosomiasis.

TREATMENT: The decision whether to treat people with leishmaniasis should be made on an individual basis, with the assistance of infectious disease experts or consultation from the CDC Drug Service (404-639-3670). Treatment always is indicated for patients with mucosal or visceral leishmaniasis. Liposomal amphotericin B is the only treatment approved by the US Food and Drug Administration for visceral leishmaniasis and is the most efficacious and least toxic of the antileishmanial drugs available in the United States. Sodium stibogluconate, available through the CDC under an investigational new drug protocol, generally has high efficacy but carries the risk of cardiac and other toxicity. Because of the high prevalence of primary antimonial resistance in India and Nepal, sodium stibogluconate should not be used for visceral leishmaniasis patients infected in South Asia; liposomal amphotericin B or conventional amphotericin B desoxycholate should be used instead. Treatment of cutaneous leishmaniasis should be considered, especially if skin lesions are or could become disfiguring (eg, facial lesions or disabling lesions near joints), are persistent, or are known to be or might be caused by leishmanial species that can disseminate to the naso-oropharyngeal mucosa (see Drugs for Parasitic Infections, p 783).

ISOLATION OF THE HOSPITALIZED PATIENT: Standard precautions are recommended.

CONTROL MEASURES: The best way for travelers to prevent leishmaniasis is by protecting themselves from sand-fly bites. Vaccines and drugs for preventing infection are not available. To decrease risk of being bitten, travelers should:
- Stay in well-screened or air-conditioned areas when feasible. Avoid outdoor activities, especially from dusk to dawn, when sand flies are most active.
- When outside, wear long-sleeved shirts, long pants, and socks.
- Apply insect repellent on uncovered skin and under the ends of sleeves and pant legs. Follow instructions on the label of the repellent. The most effective repellents are those that contain the chemical diethyltoluamide (DEET) (see Prevention of Mosquitoborne Infections, p 193).
- Spray clothing with permethrin-containing insecticides. The insecticide should be reapplied after every 5 washings.
- Spray living and sleeping areas with an insecticide.
- If not sleeping in an area that is well screened or air conditioned, a bed net tucked under the mattress is recommended. If possible, a bed net that has been soaked in or sprayed with permethrin should be used. The permethrin will be effective for several months if the bed net is not washed. Sand flies are smaller than mosquitoes and, therefore, can get through smaller holes. Fine-mesh netting (at least 18 holes to the inch) is needed for an effective barrier against sand flies. This particularly is important if the bed net has not been treated with permethrin. However, sleeping under such a closely woven bed net in hot weather can be uncomfortable.
- Bed nets, repellents containing DEET, and permethrin should be purchased before traveling.

Leprosy

CLINICAL MANIFESTATIONS: Leprosy (Hansen disease) is a curable infection involving skin, peripheral nerves, mucosa of the upper respiratory tract, and testes. The clinical forms of leprosy reflect the cellular immune response to *Mycobacterium leprae* and the organism's unique tropism for peripheral nerves. Leprosy manifests as tuberculoid and lepromatous forms. Characteristic features are the following:
- ***Indeterminate.*** This is the earliest clinically detectable form of leprosy found in 10% to 20% of infected people. One to 3 hypopigmented macules, 2 to 4 cm in diameter, with a poorly defined border but no erythema or induration occur. Anesthesia is minimal or absent. Histopathologic examination often is inconclusive; granulomas can be present but bacilli rarely are found. Most lesions heal spontaneously; the remainder can progress to one of the classic forms.
- ***Tuberculoid.*** One or a few well-demarcated, hypopigmented or erythematous, hypoesthetic or anesthetic skin lesions, often with raised, active, spreading edges and central clearing, occur. The superficial nerve closest to the lesion(s) is thickened. Cell-mediated immune responses are intact.
- ***Borderline.*** The lesions clinically and histologically are less well defined than are the 2 polar categories (tuberculoid and lepromatous). In borderline tuberculoid (BT) variety, lesions are greater in number but smaller in size than those of tuberculoid, and

the margins are less distinct, with thickening of superficial nerves commonly noted. In borderline lepromatous (BL) variety, a large number of asymmetrically distributed lesions with macules, papules, plaques, and nodules can present with mild anesthesia. Superficial nerve trunks are spared.

- **Lepromatous.** Initially, numerous, ill-defined, hypopigmented, or erythematous macules are noted that progress to papules, nodules, or plaques; hypoesthesia occurs late. Dermal infiltration of the face, hands, and feet in a bilateral and symmetric distribution can occur without preceding maculopapular lesions. *M leprae*-specific, cell-mediated immunity is diminished greatly, but serum antibody responses to *M leprae*-derived antigens can occur, or titers of nonspecific antibodies (such as rheumatoid factor or nontreponemal tests for syphilis) can be increased.

The cell-mediated immunity of most patients and their clinical presentation occur between the 2 extremes of tuberculoid and lepromatous forms. Leprosy lesions usually do not itch or hurt; they lack sensation to heat, touch, and pain. The classic presentation of the "leonine facies" and loss of lateral eyebrows (madarosis) occurs in patients with end-stage lepromatous leprosy. A simplified scheme introduced by the World Health Organization classifies leprosy involving 1 to 5 patches of skin as paucibacillary and leprosy involving more than 5 patches as multibacillary.

Serious consequences of leprosy occur from immune reactions and nerve involvement with resulting anesthesia, which can lead to repeated unrecognized trauma, ulcerations, fractures, and bone resorption. A diagnosis of leprosy should be considered in any patient with hypoesthetic or anesthetic skin rash.

Leprosy Reactions: Acute clinical exacerbations reflect abrupt changes in immunological balance, especially common during initial years of treatment. Two major types are seen: type 1 (reversal reaction) predominantly is observed in borderline leprosy from a sudden increase in effective cell-mediated immunity. Acute tenderness and swelling at the site of cutaneous and neural lesions with development of new lesions are the major manifestations. Ulcerations can occur. Fever and systemic toxicity are uncommon. Type 2 (erythema nodosum leprosum) occurs in borderline and lepromatous forms as a systemic inflammatory response. Tender, red dermal papules or nodules resembling erythema nodosum along with high fever, migrating polyarthralgia, painful swelling of lymph nodes and spleen, iridocyclitis, and rarely, nephritis can occur.

ETIOLOGY: Leprosy is caused by *M leprae,* an obligate intracellular, acid-fast bacillus that can have variable results on Gram stain.

EPIDEMIOLOGY: Leprosy primarily is a disease of poverty and rural residency. Approximately 5% of people are susceptible genetically to infection with *M leprae.* Accordingly, spouses of leprosy patients are not likely to develop leprosy, but biologic parents, children, and siblings who are household contacts of untreated patients with leprosy are at increased risk. The major source of infectious material probably is nasal secretions from patients with untreated or drug-resistant infection. Little shedding of *M leprae* from involved intact skin occurs. People with human immunodeficiency virus (HIV) infection are not at increased risk of becoming infected with *M leprae.* Concomitant HIV infection and leprosy can result in worsening of symptoms of leprosy during HIV treatment as a result of immune reconstitution inflammatory syndrome. In 2007, 101 new cases of leprosy were reported in the United States. Native-born US citizens with leprosy predominantly were from Hawaii, California, Texas, Louisiana, New York, and Massachusetts.

Foreign-born patients with leprosy (more than 75% of reported cases) were immigrants predominantly from Mexico, India, the Dominican Republic, Brazil, and the Philippines. More than 60% of the world's leprosy patients reside in Southeast Asia, the majority of those in India. The infectivity of lepromatous patients probably ceases after treatment is instituted, often within a few days or weeks of initiating rifampin therapy or approximately 3 months after initiating therapy with dapsone or clofazimine.

The **incubation period** ranges from 1 to many years but usually is 3 to 5 years. The incubation period of the tuberculoid form tends to be shorter than that for the lepromatous form.

DIAGNOSTIC TESTS: Histopathologic examination of skin biopsy by an experienced pathologist is the best method of establishing the diagnosis and is the basis for classification of leprosy. Acid-fast bacilli can be found in slit-smears or biopsy specimens of skin lesions but rarely from patients with the tuberculoid and indeterminate forms of disease. Organisms have not been cultured successfully in vitro. Drug resistance is tested by the mouse footpad inoculation test, which is performed only in specialized laboratories.

A polymerase chain reaction (PCR) test for *M leprae* is available on a limited basis after consultation with the National Hansen's Disease (Leprosy) Program (800-642-2477; **www.hrsa.gov/hansens**). For early diagnosis, clinical suspicion is vital. Recent studies from India in early cases indicate that in situ hybridization and in situ PCR techniques are promising and have shown comparable results with in vitro PCR; both allow concomitant histopathologic examination.

TREATMENT: Therapy for patients with leprosy should be undertaken in consultation with an expert in leprosy. The National Hansen's Disease (Leprosy) Program (800-642-2477 or 225-578-9841) provides consultation on clinical and pathologic issues and can provide information about local Hansen disease clinics and clinicians who have experience with the disease.

Leprosy is curable. The primary goal of therapy is prevention of permanent nerve damage, which can be accomplished by early diagnosis and treatment. Combination antimicrobial therapy called multidrug therapy (MDT) can be obtained free of charge in the United States from the National Hansen's Disease (Leprosy) Program. It is important to treat *M leprae* infections with more than 1 antimicrobial agent to minimize development of antimicrobial-resistant organisms. Adults are treated with dapsone, rifampin, and clofazimine.

Treatment Regimens Recommended by the National Hansen's Disease (Leprosy) Program.
Multibacillary leprosy (6 patches or more):
1. Dapsone, 100 mg/day, orally, for 24 months. Pediatric dose: 1 mg/kg, orally, every 24 hours. Maximum dose: 100 mg/day for 24 months; **and**
2. Rifampin, 600 mg/day, orally, for 24 months. Pediatric dose: 10 mg/kg per day for 24 months; **and**
3. Clofazimine, 50 mg/day, orally, for 24 months (for nonpregnant adults only).

Paucibacillary leprosy (1–5 patches):
1. Dapsone, 100 mg/day, orally, for 12 months. Pediatric dose: 1 to 2 mg/kg, orally, every 24 hours. Maximum dose: 100 mg/day for 12 months; **and**
2. Rifampin, 600 mg/day, orally, for 24 months. Pediatric dose: 10 to 20 mg/kg per day, orally, for 12 months.

Before beginning antimicrobial therapy, patients should be tested for glucose-6-phosphate dehydrogenase deficiency, have baseline complete blood cell counts and liver function test results documented, and be evaluated for any evidence of tuberculosis infection, especially if the patient is infected with HIV. This consideration is important to avoid monotherapy of active tuberculosis with rifampin while treating active Hansen disease.

Adverse reactions of MDT commonly include darkening of skin caused by daily clofazimine therapy. This will resolve within several months of completing the clofazimine therapy.

Reactions should be treated aggressively to prevent peripheral nerve damage. Treatment with prednisone, 1 mg/kg per day, orally, can be initiated. The severe type 2 reaction, known as erythema nodosum leprosum (ENL), occurs in patients with multibacillary leprosy. Treatment with thalidomide is available for ENL under the Calgene S.T.E.P.S. Program (888-771-0141) and is used under strict supervision because of its teratogenicity. Thalidomide is not approved for use in children younger than 12 years of age. Most patients can be treated as outpatients. Rehabilitative measures, including surgery and physical therapy, may be necessary for some patients.

All patients with Hansen disease should be educated about signs and symptoms of neuritis and cautioned to report signs and symptoms of neuritis immediately so that corticosteroid therapy can be instituted.

Relapse of disease after completing MDT is rare (0.01%–0.14% of patients with Hansen disease) and can present as new skin patches with loss of skin sensation. Relapse usually is attributable to reactivation of drug-susceptible organisms. People with relapses of disease require another course of MDT.

ISOLATION OF THE HOSPITALIZED PATIENT: Standard precautions are indicated.

CONTROL MEASURES: Hand hygiene is recommended for all people in contact with a patient with lepromatous leprosy. Disinfection of nasal secretions, handkerchiefs, and other fomites should be considered until treatment is established. Household contacts, particularly contacts of patients with multibacillary disease, should be examined initially and then annually for 5 years. Postnatal transmission can occur during breastfeeding. Chemoprophylaxis is not recommended. Local public health department regulations for leprosy vary and should be consulted.

A single bacille Calmette-Guérin (BCG) immunization is reported to be approximately 50% protective against leprosy. The first commercially available leprosy vaccine was approved in India in January 1998. This vaccine was approved as an immunotherapeutic adjuvant to be used with multidrug therapy; this vaccine is not available in the United States. Neither BCG nor the heat-killed leprosy vaccine is recommended for use in household contacts of people with leprosy in the United States.

Newly diagnosed or suspected cases of leprosy in the United States should be reported to local and state public health departments, the Centers for Disease Control and Prevention, and the National Hansen's Disease (Leprosy) Program.

Leptospirosis

CLINICAL MANIFESTATIONS: Leptospirosis is an acute febrile disease with varied manifestations characterized by vasculitis. The severity of disease ranges from asymptomatic or subclinical to self-limited systemic illness (approximately 90% of patients) to life-threatening illness with jaundice, renal failure, and hemorrhagic pneumonitis. The clinical presentation typically is biphasic, with an acute septicemia phase usually lasting 1 week, which is followed by a second immune-mediated phase. Regardless of its severity, the acute phase is characterized by nonspecific symptoms, including fever, chills, headache, nausea, vomiting, and a transient rash. The most distinct clinical findings are conjunctival suffusion without purulent discharge (30%–99% of cases) and myalgias of the calf and lumbar regions (40% to 100% of cases). In some patients, the 2 phases are separated by a short-lived abatement of fever (3–4 days). Findings commonly associated with the immune-mediated phase include fever, aseptic meningitis, conjunctival suffusion, uveitis, muscle tenderness, adenopathy, and purpuric rash. Approximately 10% of patients have severe illness, including jaundice and renal dysfunction (Weil syndrome), hemorrhagic pneumonitis, cardiac arrhythmias, or circulatory collapse associated with a case-fatality rate of 5% to 15%. The overall duration of symptoms for both phases of disease varies from less than 1 week to several months. Asymptomatic or subclinical infection is frequent, and seroconversion can occur, especially in settings of endemic infection.

ETIOLOGY: Leptospirosis is caused by pathogenic spirochetes of the genus *Leptospira*. Leptospires previously were classified into 2 serologically determined species, then subdivided into antigenically defined serovars. Current genotypic classification divides the genus into 24 named species.

EPIDEMIOLOGY: The reservoirs for *Leptospira* species include a wide range of wild and domestic animals that may remain asymptomatic shedders for years. *Leptospira* organisms excreted in animal urine, amniotic fluid, or placental tissue may remain viable in moist soil or water for weeks to months in warm climates. Humans usually become infected via entry of leptospires through contact of mucosal surfaces or abraded skin with contaminated soil, water, or animal tissues. Infection may be acquired through direct contact with infected animals or their tissues or through contact with infective urine or fluids from carrier animals or urine-contaminated soil or water. People who are predisposed by occupation include abattoir and sewer workers, miners, veterinarians, farmers, and military personnel. Recreational exposures and clusters of disease have been associated with wading, swimming (especially swallowing water), or boating in contaminated water, particularly during flooding. Person-to-person transmission is rare.

The **incubation period** usually is 5 to 14 days, range 2 to 20 days.

DIAGNOSTIC TESTS: *Leptospira* organisms can be isolated from blood or cerebrospinal fluid specimens during the early septicemic phase of illness and from urine specimens after day 7 to 10 of illness. However, isolation of the organism may be difficult, requiring special media and techniques and incubation for up to 16 weeks. In addition, the sensitivity of culture for diagnosis is low. For these reasons, serum specimens always should be obtained to facilitate diagnosis. Antibodies usually develop during the second week of illness and can be measured by commercially available immunoassays; however, increases in antibody titer can be transient, delayed, or absent in some patients. Microscopic agglutination, the confirmatory serologic test, is performed only in reference laboratories and requires acute and convalescent specimens. Immunohistochemical techniques can detect leptospiral antigens in infected tissues. Polymerase chain reaction assays for detection of *Leptospira* organisms have been developed but are available only in research laboratories.

TREATMENT: Intravenous penicillin is the drug of choice for patients with severe infection requiring hospitalization. Penicillin G decreases the duration of systemic symptoms and the persistence of associated laboratory abnormalities and may prevent development of leptospiruria. As with other spirochete infections, a Jarisch-Herxheimer reaction (an acute febrile reaction accompanied by headache, myalgia, and an aggravated clinical picture lasting less than 24 hours) can develop after initiation of penicillin therapy. Parenteral cefotaxime, doxycycline, or ceftriaxone has been demonstrated in randomized clinical trials to be equal in efficacy to penicillin G for treatment of severe leptospirosis. For patients with mild disease, oral doxycycline has been shown to shorten the course of illness and decrease the occurrence of leptospiruria. Doxycycline should not be used in pregnant women or children younger than 8 years of age because of the risk of dental staining.

ISOLATION OF THE HOSPITALIZED PATIENT: In addition to standard precautions, contact precautions are recommended for contact with urine.

CONTROL MEASURES:

- Immunization of animals can prevent clinical disease attributable to infecting serovars contained within the vaccine. However, immunization may not prevent animals from shedding leptospires in their urine and, thus, contaminating environments with which humans may come in contact.
- In areas with known endemic infection, reservoir-control programs may be useful.
- Swimmers should attempt to avoid immersion or swallowing water in potentially contaminated fresh water.
- Protective clothing, boots, and gloves should be worn to decrease risk to people with occupational exposure.
- Doxycycline, 200 mg, given orally once a week to adults, may provide effective prophylaxis against clinical disease and could be considered for high-risk occupational groups with short-term exposure. However, indications for prophylactic doxycycline use for children have not been established.

Listeria monocytogenes Infections
(Listeriosis)

CLINICAL MANIFESTATIONS: Listeriosis is a severe but relatively uncommon infection caused by *Listeria monocytogenes*. Listeriosis primarily is foodborne and occurs most frequently among pregnant women and their fetuses or newborn infants, people of advanced age, or immunocompromised people. Infections are categorized as maternal, neonatal, or childhood with or without associated predisposing conditions. Maternal infections can be asymptomatic or can be associated with an influenza-like illness, fever, malaise, headache, gastrointestinal tract symptoms, and back pain. Approximately 65% of women experience a prodromal illness before the diagnosis of listeriosis in their fetus or newborn infant. Amnionitis during labor, brown staining of amniotic fluid, or asymptomatic perinatal infection can occur. Neonatal illnesses have early-onset and late-onset syndromes similar to those of group B streptococcal infections. Preterm birth, pneumonia, and septicemia are common in early-onset disease. An erythematous rash with small, pale papules characterized histologically by granulomas can occur in severe newborn infection and is termed "granulomatosis infantisepticum." Late-onset infections occur after the first week of life and usually result in meningitis. Clinical features characteristic of listeriosis outside the neonatal period or pregnancy are meningitis with or without parenchymal brain involvement in: (1) immunocompromised hosts, including people with organ transplantation, acquired immunodeficiency syndrome, hematologic malignancies, or immunosuppression attributable to corticosteroids; (2) people older than 50 years of age; or (3) people for whom reports from the laboratory indicate "diphtheroids" on Gram stain or culture. *L monocytogenes* also can cause rhombencephalitis (brain stem encephalitis), brain abscess, and endocarditis. Outbreaks caused by contaminated food usually are characterized clinically by fever and diarrhea.

ETIOLOGY: *L monocytogenes* is an aerobic, nonspore-forming, motile, gram-positive bacillus that produces a narrow zone of hemolysis on blood agar medium.

EPIDEMIOLOGY: *L monocytogenes* causes an estimated 2500 serious illnesses and 500 deaths annually in the United States. The organism is distributed widely in the environment and is an important cause of zoonoses, especially in herd animals. Foodborne transmission causes outbreaks and sporadic infections. Incriminated foods include unpasteurized milk and soft cheeses; prepared ready-to-eat meats, such as hot dogs, deli meat, and pâté; undercooked poultry; humus; and unwashed raw vegetables. The incidence of listeriosis has decreased substantially since 1989, when US regulatory agencies began enforcing rigorous screening guidelines for *L monocytogenes* in ready-to-eat foods. Fetal infection most likely results from transplacental transmission following maternal bacteremia, although some infections occur through ascending spread from vaginal colonization. Maternal infection is associated with abortion, preterm delivery, neonatal infection, and fetal death. Late-onset neonatal infection can result from acquisition of the organism during passage through the birth canal or from environmental sources, followed by hematogenous invasion of the organism from intestine. Health care-associated nursery outbreaks also have been reported.

The **incubation period** is variable, ranging from 1 day to more than 3 weeks.

DIAGNOSTIC TESTS: The organism can be recovered on blood agar media from cultures of blood, cerebrospinal fluid (CSF), meconium, gastric washings, placental tissue, amniotic fluid, and other infected tissue specimens, including joint, pleural, or pericardial fluid. Gram stain of gastric aspirate material, placental tissue, biopsy specimens of the rash of early-onset infection, or CSF from an infected patient may demonstrate the organism. *L monocytogenes* can be mistaken for a contaminant or saprophyte because of its morphologic similarity to diphtheroids and streptococci.

TREATMENT:

- Initial therapy with intravenous ampicillin and an aminoglycoside, usually gentamicin, is recommended for severe infections. This combination is more effective than ampicillin alone in vitro and in animal models of *L monocytogenes* infection. In immunocompetent hosts, ampicillin alone can be given once a favorable clinical response has occurred or for patients with mild infections. For penicillin-allergic patients, some experts recommend alternative regimens using trimethoprim-sulfamethoxazole or high-dose vancomycin. Cephalosporins are not active against *L monocytogenes.*

- For invasive infections without associated meningitis, treatment for 10 to 14 days usually is sufficient. For *L monocytogenes* meningitis, most experts recommend 14 to 21 days of treatment. Longer courses are needed for patients who are severely ill or who have endocarditis or rhombencephalitis. Diagnostic imaging of the brain near the end of anticipated therapy allows determination of parenchymal involvement of the brain and the need for prolonged therapy.

ISOLATION OF THE HOSPITALIZED PATIENT: Standard precautions are recommended.

CONTROL MEASURES:

- Antimicrobial therapy for infection diagnosed during pregnancy may prevent fetal or perinatal infection and its consequences.
- General guidelines for preventing listeriosis are similar to those for preventing other foodborne illnesses: (1) thoroughly cook raw foods from animal sources; (2) wash raw vegetables; (3) keep uncooked meats separate from vegetables, uncooked foods, and ready-to-eat foods; (4) avoid unpasteurized dairy products; and (5) wash hands, knives, and cutting boards after exposure to uncooked foods. In addition, people at high risk of listeriosis (pregnant women and immunocompromised people) should follow the dietary recommendations in Table 3.32.
- Listerosis is a nationally notifiable disease in the United States; cases should be reported to the regional health department to facilitate early recognition and control of common-source outbreaks.

Table 3.32. Dietary Recommendations for People at High Risk of Listeriosis[a]

- Avoid soft cheeses (eg, feta, Brie, Camembert, blue-veined, and Mexican queso fresco cheese). Hard cheeses; processed cheeses, including sliced cheese, cream cheese, cheese spreads, and cottage cheese; and yogurt need not be avoided.
- Cook leftover foods or ready-to-eat foods (eg, hot dogs) until steaming hot before eating.
- Avoid foods from delicatessen counters (eg, prepared salads, meats, cheeses) or heat/reheat these foods until steaming before eating.
- Avoid refrigerated pâtés and other meat spreads or heat/reheat these foods before eating; canned or shelf-stable pâté and meat spreads need not be avoided.
- Avoid raw or unpasteurized milk, including goat's milk, or milk products or foods that contain unpasteurized milk or milk products.

[a]Pregnant women and people who are immunocompromised by illness or therapy.

Lyme Disease[1]
(Lyme Borreliosis, Borrelia burgdorferi Infection)

CLINICAL MANIFESTATIONS: Clinical manifestations of Lyme disease are divided into 3 stages: early localized, early disseminated, and late disease. Early localized disease is characterized by a distinctive rash, *erythema migrans,* at the site of a recent tick bite.

[1]Wormser GP, Dattwyler RJ, Shapiro ED, et al. The clinical assessment, treatment, and prevention of Lyme disease, human granulocytic anaplasmosis, and babesiosis: clinical practice guidelines by the Infectious Diseases Society of America. *Clin Infect Dis.* 2006;43(9):1089–1134

Erythema migrans is the most common manifestation of Lyme disease in children; only a small proportion of children are diagnosed with early disseminated or late Lyme disease without a history of erythema migrans. Erythema migrans begins as a red macule or papule that usually expands over days to weeks to form a large, annular, erythematous lesion that typically increases in size to 5 cm or more in diameter, sometimes with partial central clearing. The lesion usually is painless and not pruritic. Localized erythema migrans can vary greatly in size and shape and may have vesicular or necrotic areas in its center and can be confused with cellulitis. Fever, malaise, headache, mild neck stiffness, myalgia, and arthralgia often accompany the rash of early localized disease.

Approximately 15% of patients with Lyme disease come to medical attention with early disseminated disease, most commonly multiple erythema migrans. This rash usually occurs several weeks after an infective tick bite and consists of secondary annular, erythematous lesions similar to, but usually smaller than, the primary lesion. These lesions reflect spirochetemia with cutaneous dissemination. Other common manifestations of early disseminated illness (that may occur with or without rash) are palsies of the cranial nerves (especially cranial nerve VII), lymphocytic meningitis, and conjunctivitis. Systemic symptoms, such as arthralgia, myalgia, headache, and fatigue, also are common during the early disseminated stage. Carditis, which usually manifests as various degrees of heart block, occurs rarely in children. Occasionally, people with early Lyme disease have concurrent human granulocytic anaplasmosis or babesiosis, transmitted by the same tick, which may contribute to symptomatology.

Late disease is characterized most commonly by relapsing arthritis that usually is pauciarticular and affects large joints, particularly knees. Arthritis can occur without a history of earlier stages of illness (including erythema migrans). Peripheral neuropathy and central nervous system manifestations also can occur rarely during late disease. Children who are treated with antimicrobial agents in the early stage of disease almost never develop late disease.

Because congenital infection occurs with other spirochetal infections, there has been concern that an infected pregnant woman could transmit *Borrelia burgdorferi* to her fetus. No causal relationship between maternal Lyme disease and abnormalities of pregnancy or congenital disease caused by *B burgdorferi* has been documented conclusively. No evidence exists that Lyme disease can be transmitted via human milk.

ETIOLOGY: In the United States, infection is caused by the spirochete *B burgdorferi* sensu stricto.

EPIDEMIOLOGY: Lyme disease occurs primarily in 3 distinct geographic regions of the United States. Most cases occur in southern New England and in the eastern mid-Atlantic states. The disease also occurs, but with lower frequency, in the upper Midwest, especially Wisconsin and Minnesota, and less commonly on the West Coast, especially northern California. The occurrence of cases in the United States correlates with the distribution and frequency of infected tick vectors—*Ixodes scapularis* in the east and Midwest and *Ixodes pacificus* in the west. Reported cases from states without known enzootic risks may have been acquired in states with endemic infection or may be misdiagnoses resulting from false-positive serologic test results. Rash similar to erythema migrans has been reported in states without endemic infection; however, the etiology of this condition remains unknown. Most cases of early disease occur between April and October; more than 50% of cases occur during June and July. People of all ages may be affected, but incidence in the United States is highest among children 5 through 9 years of age and adults 45 through 54 years of age.

The **incubation period** from tick bite to appearance of single or multiple erythema migrans lesions ranges from 1 to 32 days with a median of 11 days. Late manifestations can occur months to years after the tick bite.

Endemic Lyme disease transmitted by ixodid ticks occurs in Canada, Europe, states of the former Soviet Union, China, and Japan. The primary tick vector in Europe is *Ixodes ricinus,* and the primary tick vector in Asia is *Ixodes persulcatus.* Clinical manifestations of infection vary somewhat from manifestations seen in the United States, probably because of different genomospecies of *Borrelia.*

DIAGNOSTIC TESTS: During the early stages of Lyme disease, the diagnosis is best made clinically by recognizing the characteristic rash, a singular lesion of erythema migrans, because antibodies against *B burgdorferi* are not detectable in most people within the first few weeks after infection. During the first 4 weeks of infection, serodiagnostic tests are insensitive and are not recommended generally. Although cultures of a biopsy specimen of the perimeter of the skin lesion often yield the organism, cultures of *Borrelia* species (which require special media) are not available commercially and are not recommended. Diagnosis in patients with early disseminated disease who have multiple lesions of erythema migrans also is made clinically. Diagnosis of early disseminated disease without rash or late Lyme disease should be made on the basis of clinical findings and serologic test results. Some patients who are treated with antimicrobial agents for early Lyme disease never develop antibodies against *B burgdorferi;* they are cured and are not at risk of late disease. Most patients with early disseminated disease and virtually all patients with late disease have antibodies against *B burgdorferi.* Once such antibodies develop, they persist for many years and perhaps for life. Consequently, tests for antibodies should not be used to assess the success of treatment. The results of serologic tests for Lyme disease should be interpreted with careful consideration of the clinical setting and the quality of the testing laboratory.

A 2-step approach is recommended for serologic diagnosis of *B burgdorferi.* First, a quantitative screening test for serum antibodies should be performed using a sensitive enzyme immunoassay (EIA) or immunofluorescent antibody assay (IFA). Serum specimens that yield positive or equivocal results then should be tested by a standardized Western immunoblot for presence of antibodies to *B burgdorferi;* serum specimens that yield negative results by EIA or IFA should not be tested further by immunoblot. Immunoblot test should not be performed if EIA test result is negative or instead of an EIA; positive immunoblot results likely would not be attributable to Lyme disease. When testing to confirm early disseminated disease without rash, immunoglobulin (Ig) G and IgM immunoblot assays should be performed. To confirm late disease, only an IgG immunoblot assay should be performed, because false-positive results may occur with the IgM immunoblot. In people with symptoms lasting longer than 1 month, a positive IgM test result alone (ie, negative IgG test) is likely to represent a false-positive result and should not be the basis on which to diagnose Lyme disease. A positive result of an IgG immunoblot test requires detection of antibody ("bands") to 5 or more of the following: 18, 23/24, 28, 30, 39, 41, 45, 60, 66, and 93 kDa polypeptides. A positive test result of IgM immunoblot requires detection of antibody to at least 2 of the 23/24, 39, and 41 kDa polypeptides. Two-step testing is needed, because EIA and IFA may yield false-positive results because of the presence of antibodies directed against spirochetes in normal oral flora that cross-react with antigens of *B burgdorferi* or to cross-reactive antibodies in patients with other spirochetal infections (eg, syphilis, leptospirosis, relapsing fever), certain viral infections (eg, varicella, Epstein-Barr virus), or certain autoimmune diseases (eg, systemic lupus erythematosus).

A licensed serologic test that detects antibody to a peptide of the immunodominant conserved region of the variable surface antigen vlsE of *B burgdorferi* appears to have equivalent specificity and sensitivity compared with the 2-step protocol. Polymerase chain reaction (PCR) testing (using a laboratory with excellent quality procedures) has been used to detect *B burgdorferi* DNA in joint fluid. Urinary antigen detection has no role in diagnosis.

Suspected central nervous system Lyme disease can be confirmed by demonstration of intrathecal production of antibodies against *B burgdorferi*. However, interpretation of results of antibody tests of cerebrospinal fluid is complex, and physicians should seek the advice of a specialist experienced in management of patients with Lyme disease to assist in interpreting results.

The widespread practice of ordering serologic tests for patients with nonspecific symptoms, such as fatigue or arthralgia, who have a low probability of having Lyme disease or because of parental pressure, is discouraged. Almost all positive serologic test results in these patients are false-positive results. In areas with endemic infection, subclinical infection and seroconversion also can occur, and the patient's symptoms merely are coincidental. Patients with acute Lyme disease almost always have objective signs of infection (eg, erythema migrans, facial nerve palsy, arthritis). Nonspecific symptoms commonly accompany these specific signs but almost never are the only evidence of Lyme disease.

TREATMENT: Consensus practice guidelines for assessment, treatment, and prevention of Lyme disease have been published by the Infectious Diseases Society of America. Care of children should follow recommendations in Table 3.33, p 434. Antimicrobial therapy for nonspecific symptoms or for asymptomatic seropositivity or by routes of administration or durations not specified in Table 3.33 is discouraged. Use of alternative diagnostic approaches or therapies recommended by other groups or people also is discouraged.

Early Localized Disease. Doxycycline is the drug of choice for children 8 years of age and older and, unlike amoxicillin, also treats patients with anaplasmosis. For children younger than 8 years of age, amoxicillin is recommended. For patients who are allergic to penicillin, the alternative drug is cefuroxime. Erythromycin and azithromycin are less effective. Most experts treat people with early Lyme disease for 14 to 21 days.

Treatment of erythema migrans almost always prevents development of later stages of Lyme disease. Erythema migrans usually resolves within several days of initiating treatment, but other signs and symptoms may persist for several weeks, even in successfully treated patients.

Early Disseminated and Late Disease. Orally administered antimicrobial agents are recommended for treating multiple erythema migrans and uncomplicated Lyme arthritis. Oral agents also are appropriate for treatment of facial nerve palsy without clinical manifestations of meningitis; lumbar puncture is not indicated. If symptoms or signs of other central nervous system involvement, such as meningitis or raised intracranial pressure, are present, lumbar puncture is performed. If cerebrospinal fluid pleocytosis is found, parenterally administered antimicrobial therapy is indicated. Up to one third of patients with arthritis have persistence of synovitis and joint swelling at the conclusion of antimicrobial therapy, which almost always resolves without repeating the course of antimicrobial

Table 3.33. Recommended Treatment of Lyme Disease in Children

Disease Category	Drug(s) and Dose[a]
Early localized disease[a]	
8 y of age or older	Doxycycline, 100 mg, orally, twice a day for 14–21 days[b]
Younger than 8 y of age or unable to tolerate doxycycline	Amoxicillin, 50 mg/kg per day, orally, divided into 3 doses (maximum 1.5 g/day) for 14–21 days **OR** Cefuroxime, 30 mg/kg per day in 2 divided doses (maximum 1000 mg/day) or 1.0 g/day for 14–21 days
Early disseminated and late disease	
Multiple erythema migrans	Same oral regimen as for early localized disease, but for 21 days
Isolated facial palsy	Same oral regimen as for early localized disease, but for 21–28 days[c,d]
Arthritis	Same oral regimen as for early localized disease, but for 28 days
Persistent or recurrent arthritis[e]	Ceftriaxone sodium, 75–100 mg/kg, IV or IM, once a day (maximum 2 g/day) for 14–28 days **OR** Penicillin, 300 000 U/kg per day, IV, given in divided doses every 4 h (maximum 20 million U/day) for 14–28 days **OR** Same oral regimen as for early disease
Carditis	Ceftriaxone or penicillin: see persistent or recurrent arthritis
Meningitis or encephalitis	Ceftriaxone[f] or penicillin: see persistent or recurrent arthritis, but for 14–28 days

IV indicates intravenously; IM, intramuscularly.
[a] For patients who are allergic to penicillin, cefuroxime and erythromycin are alternative drugs.
[b] Tetracyclines are contraindicated in pregnancy.
[c] Corticosteroids should not be given.
[d] Treatment has no effect on the resolution of facial nerve palsy; its purpose is to prevent late disease.
[e] Arthritis is not considered persistent or recurrent unless objective evidence of synovitis exists at least 2 months after treatment is initiated. Some experts administer a second course of an oral agent before using an IV-administered antimicrobial agent.
[f] Ceftriaxone should be administered IV for treatment of meningitis or encephalitis.

therapy. Some experts would treat a patient who has recurrent or persistent arthritis after treatment with one course of oral antimicrobial therapy with another course of oral antimicrobial therapy. Central nervous system infection should be treated with parenterally administered antimicrobial therapy. The optimal duration of therapy for manifestations of early disseminated or late disease is not well established, but there is no evidence that children with any manifestation of Lyme disease benefit from prolonged courses of orally or parenterally administered antimicrobial agents. Accordingly, the maximum duration of a single course of therapy is 4 weeks (see Table 3.33).

The Jarisch-Herxheimer reaction (an acute febrile reaction accompanied by headache, myalgia, and an aggravated clinical picture lasting less than 24 hours) can occur when therapy is initiated. Nonsteroidal anti-inflammatory agents may be beneficial, and the antimicrobial agent should be continued.

Pregnancy. Tetracyclines are contraindicated. Otherwise, therapy is the same as recommended for nonpregnant people.

ISOLATION OF THE HOSPITALIZED PATIENT: Standard precautions are recommended.

CONTROL MEASURES:

Ticks. See Prevention of Tickborne Infections (p 191).

Chemoprophylaxis. Many people who seek medical attention for a tick bite have been bitten by a species of tick that does not transmit Lyme disease, or the recovered material is not a tick. The overall risk of infection with *B burgdorferi* after a recognized deer tick bite is less than 1% and, even in areas with highly endemic rates of infection, is sufficiently low that prophylactic antimicrobial treatment is not indicated routinely for most people. People bitten by an ixodid tick in areas with low incidence of Lyme disease should not receive chemoprophylaxis. The risk is extremely low after attachment (eg, a flat, nonengorged deer tick is found) and is higher after engorgement, especially if a nymphal deer tick has been attached for at least 72 hours. Analysis of the tick for spirochete infection has a poor predictive value and is not recommended. On the basis of a study of doxycycline for prevention of Lyme disease after a deer tick bite, some experts recommend a single 200-mg dose (4.4 mg/kg for body weight less than 45 kg) of doxycycline for people 8 years of age and older who have been bitten in an area with hyperendemic infection (ie, local rate of infection of these ticks with *B burgdorferi* is 20% or greater) who have found an engorged deer tick, especially if the suspected duration of attachment is 72 hours or longer and prophylaxis can be started within 72 hours after the tick was removed. Data are insufficient to recommend amoxicillin prophylaxis.

Blood Donation. Patients with active disease should not donate blood, because spirochetemia occurs in early Lyme disease. Patients who have been treated for Lyme disease can be considered for blood donation.

Vaccines. A Lyme disease vaccine was licensed by the US Food and Drug Administration on December 21, 1998, for people 15 to 70 years of age but was withdrawn in early 2002 and no longer is available.

Lymphatic Filariasis
(Bancroftian, Malayan, and Timorian)

CLINICAL MANIFESTATIONS: Most filarial infections are asymptomatic. Even in asymptomatic people, adult filarial worms commonly cause subclinical lymphatic dilatation and dysfunction. Lymphadenopathy is the most common clinical sign of lymphatic filariasis in children, most frequently of the inguinal, crural, and axillary lymph nodes, in association with living adult worms. Death of the adult worm triggers an acute inflammatory response, which progresses distally (retrograde) along the affected lymphatic vessel, usually in the limbs. If present, systemic symptoms, such as headache or fever, generally are mild. In postpubertal males, adult *Wuchereria bancrofti* organisms are found most commonly in the intrascrotal lymphatic vessels; thus, inflammation resulting from adult worm death may present as funiculitis, epididymitis, or orchitis. A tender granulomatous nodule may be palpable at the site of the dead adult worms. The chronic manifestations of lymphedema and hydrocele rarely occur in children. Recurrent secondary bacterial infections hasten the progression of lymphedema to its advanced stage, known as elephantiasis. Chyluria can occur as a manifestation of bancroftian filariasis. Cough, fever, marked eosinophilia, and high serum immunoglobulin E concentrations are manifestations of the tropical pulmonary eosinophilia (TPE) syndrome.

ETIOLOGY: Filariasis is caused by 3 filarial nematodes: *W bancrofti, Brugia malayi,* and *Brugia timori.*

EPIDEMIOLOGY: The parasite is transmitted by the bite of infected species of various genera of mosquitoes, including *Culex, Aedes, Anopheles,* and *Mansonia. W bancrofti,* the most prevalent cause of lymphatic filariasis, is found in Haiti, the Dominican Republic, Guyana, northeast Brazil, sub-Saharan and North Africa, and Asia, extending from India through the Indonesian archipelago to the western Pacific islands. Humans are the only definitive host for the parasite. *B malayi* is found mostly in Southeast Asia and parts of India. *B timori* is restricted to certain islands at the eastern end of the Indonesian archipelago. Live adult worms release microfilariae into the bloodstream, and because adult worms live on average for 5 to 8 years and reinfection is common, microfilariae infective for mosquitoes may remain in the patient's blood for decades; individual microfilaria have a lifespan up to 1.5 years. The adult worm is not transmissible from person to person or by blood transfusion, but microfilariae may be transmitted by transfusion.

The **incubation period** is not well established; the period from acquisition to the appearance of microfilariae in blood can be 3 to 12 months, depending on the species of parasite.

DIAGNOSTIC TESTS: Microfilariae generally can be detected microscopically on blood smears obtained at night (10 PM−4 AM), although variations in the periodicity of microfilaremia have been described depending on the parasite and the geographic location of the host. Adult worms or microfilariae can be identified in tissue specimens obtained at biopsy. Serologic enzyme immunoassays are available, but interpretation of results is affected by cross-reactions of filarial antibodies with antibodies against other helminths. Assays for circulating parasite antigen of *W bancrofti* are available commercially but are not licensed by the US Food and Drug Administration. Ultrasonography can be used to visualize adult worms. Lymphatic filariasis often must be diagnosed clinically, because dependable serologic assays are not available uniformly, and in patients with lymphedema, microfilariae no longer may be present.

TREATMENT: The main goal of treatment of an infected person is to kill the adult worm. Diethylcarbamazine citrate (DEC), which is both microfilaricidal and active against the adult worm, is the drug of choice for lymphatic filariasis (see Drugs for Parasitic Infections, p 783). Once lymphedema is established (the late phase of chronic disease), the disease is not affected by chemotherapy. Ivermectin is effective against the microfilariae of *W bancrofti* but has no effect on the adult parasite. In some studies, combination therapy with single-dose DEC-albendazole or ivermectin-albendazole has been shown to be more effective than any one drug alone in suppressing microfilaremia.

Complex decongestive physiotherapy may be effective for treating lymphedema. Chyluria originating in the bladder responds to fulguration; chyluria originating in the kidney usually cannot be corrected. Prompt identification and treatment of bacterial superinfections, particularly streptococcal and staphylococcal infections, and careful treatment of intertriginous and ungual fungal infections are important aspects of therapy for lymphedema.

ISOLATION OF THE HOSPITALIZED PATIENT: Standard precautions are recommended.

CONTROL MEASURES: Control measures have been instituted on the basis of annual community-wide combinations of DEC and albendazole (worldwide except Africa) or albendazole and ivermectin (in Africa) to decrease or possibly eliminate transmission. No vaccine is available for filariasis.

Lymphocytic Choriomeningitis

CLINICAL MANIFESTATIONS: Postnatal infection is asymptomatic in approximately one third of cases. Symptomatic infection may result in a mild to severe influenza-like illness, which includes fever, malaise, myalgia, retro-orbital headache, photophobia, anorexia, and nausea. Fever usually lasts 1 to 3 weeks, and rash is rare. A biphasic febrile course is common; after a few days without symptoms, the second phase may occur in up to half of symptomatic patients, consisting of neurologic manifestations that vary from aseptic meningitis to severe encephalitis. From 10% to 15% of all cases of aseptic meningitis are caused by lymphocytic choriomeningitis (LCM) virus, and it can be the most common cause of aseptic meningitis during winter months. Arthralgia or arthritis, respiratory tract symptoms, orchitis, and leukopenia develop occasionally. Recovery without sequelae is the usual outcome. Infection during pregnancy has been associated with spontaneous abortion. Congenital infection may cause severe abnormalities, including hydrocephalus, chorioretinitis, intracranial calcifications, microcephaly, and mental retardation. Congenital LCM may be difficult to differentiate from congenital infection attributable to cytomegalovirus (CMV), toxoplasmosis, or rubella. Patients with immune abnormalities may experience severe or fatal illness, as observed in patients receiving organs from LCM virus-infected donors.

ETIOLOGY: LCM virus is an arenavirus.

EPIDEMIOLOGY: LCM is a chronic infection of common house mice, which often are infected asymptomatically and chronically shed virus in urine and other excretions. In addition, pet hamsters, laboratory mice, guinea pigs, and colonized golden hamsters can have chronic infection and can be sources of human infection. Humans are infected by aerosol or by ingestion of dust or food contaminated with the virus from the urine, feces, blood, or nasopharyngeal secretions of infected rodents. The disease is most prevalent in young adults. LCM virus has not been associated with human-to-human transmission except by transplacental passage of the virus and via organ transplantation from an acutely infected, undiagnosed, LCM virus-infected organ donor. The source of the virus in one organ donor was traced to a pet hamster purchased by the donor.

The **incubation period** usually is 6 to 13 days and occasionally is as long as 3 weeks.

DIAGNOSTIC TESTS: In patients with central nervous system disease, mononuclear pleocytosis occasionally exceeding several thousand cells is present in the cerebrospinal fluid (CSF). Hypoglycorrhachia also can occur. LCM virus can be isolated from blood, CSF, urine, and rarely, nasopharyngeal secretion specimens. Reverse transcriptase-polymerase chain reaction assays can be used on CSF. Acute and convalescent serum specimens can be tested for increases in antibody titers by immunofluorescent or enzyme immunoassay.

Demonstration of virus-specific immunoglobulin M antibodies in serum or CSF specimens is useful. In congenital infections, diagnosis usually is suspected at the sequela phase, and diagnosis usually is made by serologic testing. Diagnosis can be made retrospectively by immunohistochemistry assay of tissues obtained from necropsy.

TREATMENT: Supportive.

ISOLATION OF THE HOSPITALIZED PATIENT: Standard precautions are recommended.

CONTROL MEASURES: Infection can be controlled by preventing rodent infestation in animal and food storage areas. Because the virus is excreted for long periods of time by rodent hosts, attempts should be made to monitor laboratory and wholesale colonies of mice and hamsters for infection. Pet rodents or wild mice in a patient's home should be considered likely sources of infection. Although the risk for LCM virus infection from pet rodents is low, pregnant women should avoid exposure to wild or pet rodents and their aerosolized excreta. Guidelines for minimizing risk of human LCM virus infection associated with rodents are available[1] (also see Diseases Transmitted by Animals, p 198).

Malaria

CLINICAL MANIFESTATIONS: The classic symptoms of malaria are high fever with chills, rigor, sweats, and headache, which may be paroxysmal. If appropriate treatment is not administered, fever and paroxysms may occur in a cyclic pattern. Depending on the infecting species, fever classically appears every other or every third day. Other manifestations can include nausea, vomiting, diarrhea, cough, tachypnea, arthralgia, myalgia, and abdominal and back pain. Anemia and thrombocytopenia are common, and pallor and jaundice caused by hemolysis may occur. Hepatosplenomegaly may be present. More severe disease occurs in people without previous exposure, young children, and people who are pregnant or immunocompromised.

Infection with *Plasmodium falciparum,* one of the 4 *Plasmodium* species that infects humans, potentially is fatal and most commonly manifests as a febrile nonspecific illness without localizing signs. Severe *P falciparum* disease may manifest as one of the following clinical syndromes, all of which are medical emergencies and may be fatal unless treated:

- **Cerebral malaria,** which may have variable neurologic manifestations, including generalized seizures, signs of increased intracranial pressure, confusion, and progression to stupor, coma, and death;
- **Hypoglycemia,** which may occur with metabolic acidosis and hypotension associated with hyperparasitemia or be associated with quinine treatment;
- **Noncardiogenic pulmonary edema;**
- **Renal failure** caused by acute tubular necrosis (rare in children younger than 8 years of age);
- **Respiratory failure and metabolic acidosis,** without pulmonary edema;
- **Severe anemia** attributable to high parasitemia sequestration and hemolysis associated with hypersplenism; or

---

[1]Centers for Disease Control and Prevention. Update: interim guidance for minimizing risk for human lymphocytic choriomeningitis virus infection associated with pet rodents. *MMWR Morb Mortal Wkly Rep.* 2005;54(32):799–801

- **Vascular collapse and shock** associated with hypothermia and adrenal insufficiency People with asplenia who become infected may be at increased risk of more severe illness and death.

Syndromes primarily associated with *Plasmodium vivax* and *Plasmodium ovale* infection are as follows:
- **Anemia** attributable to acute parasitemia;
- **Hypersplenism** with danger of late splenic rupture; and
- **Relapse,** for as long as 3 to 5 years after the primary infection, attributable to latent hepatic stages.

Syndromes associated with *Plasmodium malariae* infection include:
- **Chronic asymptomatic parasitemia** for as long as several years after the last exposure; and
- **Nephrotic syndrome** from deposition of immune complexes in the kidney.

Congenital malaria secondary to perinatal transmission rarely may occur. Most congenital cases have been caused by *P vivax* and *P falciparum; P malariae* and *P ovale* account for fewer than 20% of such cases. Manifestations can resemble those of neonatal sepsis, including fever and nonspecific symptoms of poor appetite, irritability, and lethargy.

ETIOLOGY: The genus *Plasmodium* includes species of intraerythrocytic parasites that infect a wide range of mammals, birds, and reptiles. The 4 species that frequently infect humans are *P falciparum, P vivax, P ovale,* and *P malariae. Plasmodium knowlesi,* misdiagnosed as *P malariae,* has been shown to infect humans in Malaysia.

EPIDEMIOLOGY: Malaria is endemic throughout the tropical areas of the world and is acquired from the bite of the female nocturnal-feeding *Anopheles* species of mosquito. One half of the world's population lives in areas where transmission occurs. Worldwide, 300 to 500 million cases and an estimated 1 million deaths occur each year. Most deaths occur in young children. Malarial infection poses substantial risks to pregnant women and their fetuses and may result in spontaneous abortion and stillbirth. The risk of malaria is highest, but variable, for travelers to sub-Saharan Africa, Papua New Guinea, the Solomon Islands, and Vanuatu; the risk is intermediate on the Indian subcontinent and is low in most of Southeast Asia and Latin America. The potential for malaria transmission is ongoing in areas with previous elimination if infected people return and the mosquito vector is still present. These conditions have resulted in recent cases in travelers to areas such as Jamaica, the Dominican Republic, and the Bahamas. Health care professionals should check an up-to-date source (**wwwn.cdc.gov/travel**) to determine malaria risk when providing pretravel malaria advice or evaluating a febrile returned traveler. Transmission is possible in more temperate climates, including areas of the United States where *Anopheles* species mosquitoes are present. Nearly all of the approximately 1500 annual reported cases in the United States result from infection acquired abroad.[1] Rarely, mosquitoes in airplanes flying from tropical climates have been the source of cases in people working or residing near international airports. Uncommon modes of malaria transmission are congenital, through transfusions, or through the use of contaminated needles or syringes.

---

[1] Centers for Disease Control and Prevention. Malaria surveillance—United States, 2006. *MMWR Surveill Summ.* 2008;57(SS–5):24–39

P vivax and *P falciparum* are the most common species worldwide. *P vivax* malaria is prevalent on the Indian subcontinent and in Central America. *P falciparum* malaria is prevalent in Africa and Papua New Guinea. *P vivax* and *P falciparum* species are the most common malaria species in southern and Southeast Asia, Oceania, and South America. *P malariae*, although much less common, has a wide distribution. *P ovale* malaria occurs most often in West Africa but has been reported in other areas.

Relapses may occur in *P vivax* and *P ovale* malaria because of a persistent hepatic (hypnozoite) stage of infection. Recrudescence of *P falciparum* and *P malariae* infection occurs when a persistent low-concentration parasitemia causes recurrence of symptoms of the disease. In areas of Africa and Asia with hyperendemic infection, reinfection in people with partial immunity results in a high prevalence of asymptomatic parasitemia.

The spread of chloroquine-resistant *P falciparum* strains throughout the world is of increasing importance. Resistance to other antimalarial drugs now is occurring in many areas where the drugs are used widely. Resistance to sulfadoxine-pyrimethamine is common throughout Africa, and mefloquine resistance has been documented in Myanmar (Burma), Thailand, Cambodia, Vietnam, and China. Chloroquine-resistant *P vivax* has been reported in Indonesia, Papua New Guinea, the Solomon Islands, Myanmar, India, and Guyana. Malaria symptoms can develop as soon as 7 days after exposure in an area with endemic malaria to as late as several months after departure. More than 80% of cases diagnosed in the United States have onset of symptoms after their return to the United States.

DIAGNOSTIC TESTS: Definitive diagnosis relies on identification of the parasite microscopically on stained blood films. Both thick and thin blood films should be examined. The thick film allows for concentration of the blood to find parasites that may be present in small numbers, whereas the thin film is most useful for species identification and determination of the degree of parasitemia (the percentage of erythrocytes harboring parasites). If initial blood smears test negative for *Plasmodium* species but malaria remains a possibility, the smear should be repeated every 12 to 24 hours during a 72-hour period.

In areas with hyperendemic infection, the presence of malaria on a blood smear is not conclusive evidence of malaria as a cause of the manifesting illness, because other infections often are superimposed on low-concentration parasitemia in children and adults with partial immunity.

Confirmation and identification of the species of malaria parasites on the blood smear is important in guiding therapy. Serologic testing generally is not helpful, except in epidemiologic surveys. Polymerase chain reaction (PCR) assay is available in reference laboratories and some state health departments. DNA probes and malarial ribosomal RNA testing may provide rapid and accurate diagnosis in the future but currently are used in experimental studies only. A new US Food and Drug Administration (FDA)-approved test for antigen detection (a rapid diagnostic test) is available in the United States. It is the only antigen-detection kit available and is approved for use by hospitals and commercial laboratories. All rapid diagnostic tests are recommended to be conducted in parallel with routine microscopy to provide further information needed for patient treatment, such as the percentage of erythrocytes harboring parasites. A negative rapid diagnostic test result should be confirmed by microscopic examination, because low-level parasitemia may not be detected. Also, information about the sensitivity of rapid diagnostic tests for the 2 less common species of malaria, *P ovale* and *P malariae*, is limited. More information about rapid diagnostic testing for malaria is available at **www.cdc.gov/ malaria/diagnosis_treatment/diagnosis.htm.**

TREATMENT: The choice of malaria chemotherapy is based on the infecting species, possible drug resistance, and the severity of disease (see Drugs for Parasitic Infections, p 783). Severe malaria is defined as any one or more of the following: parasitemia greater than 5% of red blood cells, signs of central nervous system or other end-organ involvement, shock, acidosis, and/or hypoglycemia. Patients with severe malaria require intensive care and parenteral treatment until the parasite density decreases to less than 1% and they are able to tolerate oral therapy. Exchange transfusion may be warranted when parasitemia exceeds 10% or if there is evidence of complications (eg, cerebral malaria or renal failure) at lower parasite densities. For patients with severe malaria in the United States, intravenous artesunate has become available through a joint FDA-Centers for Disease Control and Prevention (CDC) investigational new drug protocol. Clinicians may contact the physician on call through the CDC malaria hotline (770-488-7788, Monday–Friday, 8:00 am–4:30 pm Eastern Time; or 777-488-7100 at all other times) for additional information and release of the drug.[1] For patients with *P falciparum* malaria, sequential blood smears to determine percentage of erythrocytes harboring parasites are indicated to monitor treatment. Assistance with management of malaria is available 24 hours a day through the CDC Malaria Hotline (770-488-7788).

ISOLATION OF THE HOSPITALIZED PATIENT: Standard precautions are recommended.

CONTROL MEASURES: Control of the *Anopheles* species mosquito population, protection against mosquito bites, treatment of infected people, and chemoprophylaxis of travelers to areas with endemic infection are effective. Measures to prevent contact with mosquitoes, especially from dusk to dawn (because of the nocturnal biting habits of the female *Anopheles* mosquito), through use of bed nets impregnated with insecticide, mosquito repellents containing diethyltoluamide (DEET) (see Prevention of Mosquitoborne Infections, p 193), and protective clothing also are beneficial and should be optimized. The most current information on country-specific risks, drug resistance, and resulting recommendations for travelers can be obtained by contacting the CDC (**www.cdc.gov/ malaria/** or the Malaria Hotline at 770-488-7788).

Chemoprophylaxis for Travelers to Areas With Endemic Malaria.[2] More than 80% of malaria-infected patients reported in the United States did not follow a CDC-recommended prophylaxis regimen. The appropriate chemoprophylactic regimen is determined by the traveler's risk of acquiring malaria in the area(s) to be visited and by the risk of exposure to chloroquine- or mefloquine-resistant *P falciparum* or chloroquine-resistant *P vivax.* Indications for prophylaxis for children are identical to those for adults. Pediatric dosages should be calculated on the basis of the child's current weight; children's dosages never should exceed adult dosages. The drugs used for malaria chemoprophylaxis generally are well tolerated. However, adverse reactions can occur. Minor adverse reactions do not

---

[1]Centers for Disease Control and Prevention. Notice to readers: new medication for severe malaria available under an investigational new drug protocol. *MMWR Morb Mortal Wkly Rep.* 2007;56(30):769–770

[2]For further information on prevention of malaria in travelers, see the annual publication of the US Public Health Service, *Health Information for International Travel,* 2008. Atlanta, GA: US Department of Health and Human Services, Public Health Service, Centers for Disease Control and Prevention, National Center for Infectious Diseases, Division of Quarantine; 2008. Available at: **wwwn.cdc.gov/travel/ contentYellowBook.aspx**

require stopping the drug. Travelers with serious adverse reactions should be advised to contact their health care professional.

Chemoprophylaxis should begin before arrival in the area with endemic infection (starting 1 week before for mefloquine and chloroquine and 1–2 days before for doxycycline and atovaquone-proguanil), allowing time to develop blood concentrations of the drug. If there is desire to ensure tolerance of the antimalarial drug to be used for prophylaxis, then the drug should be started earlier so that there is time to assess any adverse events before departure and time to change to another effective drug if needed. For example, if there is concern about individual tolerance with mefloquine, then prophylaxis can be started 3 weeks before travel. Most adverse events will occur during the first 3 doses, and if the individual does not tolerate mefloquine, then there is still time to prescribe alternative therapy before travel.

Travelers to areas where chloroquine-resistant malaria species have not been reported should take chloroquine, once weekly, starting 1 week before exposure for the duration of exposure and for 4 weeks after departure from the area with endemic malaria. Adverse reactions that can occur include gastrointestinal tract disturbance, headache, dizziness, blurred vision, insomnia, and pruritus, but these generally are mild and do not require discontinuation of the drug. Travelers to areas without reported chloroquine-resistance also may choose to take one of the 3 drug regimens described below.

Three drugs with similar efficacy are available in the United States for prevention of chloroquine-resistant malaria. Travelers to areas where chloroquine-resistant *P falciparum* exists should take atovaquone-proguanil, doxycycline, or mefloquine.

- A fixed-dose combination of atovaquone-proguanil is approved for prevention and treatment of chloroquine-resistant *P falciparum* malaria. Atovaquone-proguanil is taken daily, starting 1 day before exposure and continuing for the duration of exposure and for 1 week after departure from the area with endemic malaria. A pediatric formulation is available in the United States but is not approved for prophylaxis in children weighing less than 11 kg. However, recommendations of the CDC suggest that atovaquone-proguanil can be used in children weighing 5 kg or more, when travel to areas where chloroquine-resistant *P falciparum* exists cannot be avoided. Atovaquone-proguanil is contraindicated for pregnant women. The rare adverse effects reported by people using atovaquone-proguanil for chemoprophylaxis are abdominal pain, nausea, vomiting, mouth ulcers, and headache.
- Doxycycline is taken daily, starting 1 to 2 days before exposure, for the duration of exposure and for 4 weeks after departure from the area with endemic malaria. Travelers taking doxycycline should be advised of the need for strict adherence to daily dosing; the advisability of always taking the drug on a full stomach; and the possible adverse effects, including diarrhea, photosensitivity, and increased risk of monilial vaginitis. Doxycycline also can decrease the effectiveness of oral contraceptives in women of childbearing age. Use of doxycycline should be avoided for pregnant women and for children younger than 8 years of age because of the risk of dental staining (see Antimicrobial Agents and Related Therapy, p 737).
- Mefloquine is taken once weekly, starting 1 week before travel, continuing weekly during travel, and for 4 weeks after travel has concluded (see Drugs for Parasitic Infections, p 783). Mefloquine is not approved by the FDA for children who weigh less than 5 kg or are younger than 6 months of age. However, recommendations of the CDC suggest that mefloquine be considered for use in children, regardless of weight or age

restrictions, when travel to areas where chloroquine-resistant *P falciparum* exists and cannot be avoided. However, parents should be advised not to travel to countries with endemic malaria with children weighing less than 5 kg or younger than 6 weeks of age because of the risks associated with infection (septicemia or malaria) in young infants. The most common central nervous system abnormalities associated with mefloquine are dizziness, headache, insomnia, and disturbing dreams. Mefloquine has been associated with rare serious adverse events (including psychoses or seizures) at prophylactic doses; these reactions are more common with the higher doses used for treatment. Other adverse events that occur with prophylactic doses include gastrointestinal tract disturbances, headache, depression, and anxiety disorders. Mefloquine is contraindicated for use in travelers with a known hypersensitivity to mefloquine; people with active depression or a history of depression; people with general anxiety disorders, psychosis, schizophrenia, or other major psychiatric disturbances; people with a history of seizures (not including febrile seizures); and people with a history of cardiac conduction abnormalities. Although a warning about concurrent use with beta-blockers is given in the product labeling, a review of available data suggests that mefloquine may be used by people concurrently receiving beta-blockers if they have no underlying arrhythmia. Caution should be advised for travelers involved in tasks requiring fine motor coordination and spatial discrimination. Patients in whom mefloquine prophylaxis fails should be monitored closely if they are treated with quinidine or quinine sulfate, because either drug may exacerbate the known adverse effects of mefloquine.

Children should avoid travel to areas where chloroquine-resistant *P falciparum* exists unless they can take a highly effective drug, such as atovaquone-proguanil, doxycycline, or mefloquine. If other antimalarial drugs cannot be used, **in consultation with local malaria experts or experts at the CDC (CDC Malaria Hotline, 770-488-7788),** primaquine may be used to prevent malaria while the traveler is in the area with a risk of malaria. NOTE: Travelers must be tested for glucose-6-phosphate dehydrogenase (G6PD) deficiency and have a documented G6PD in the normal range before primaquine use. Primary primaquine prophylaxis should begin 1 to 2 days before departure to the area with risk of malaria and should be continued once a day while in the area with risk of malaria and daily for 7 days after leaving the area. The drug should not be used during pregnancy.

Prophylaxis During Pregnancy and Lactation. Malaria in pregnancy carries significant risks of morbidity and mortality for both the mother and fetus. Malaria may increase the risk of adverse outcomes in pregnancy, including abortion, preterm birth, and stillbirth. For these reasons and because no chemoprophylactic regimen is completely effective, women who are pregnant or likely to become pregnant should try to avoid travel to areas where they could contract malaria. Women traveling to areas where drug-resistant *P falciparum* has not been reported may take chloroquine prophylaxis. Harmful effects on the fetus have not been demonstrated when chloroquine is given in the recommended doses for malaria prophylaxis. Pregnancy and lactation, therefore, are not contraindications for malaria prophylaxis with chloroquine.

For pregnant women who travel to areas where chloroquine-resistant *P falciparum* exists, mefloquine should be recommended for chemoprophylaxis during the second and third trimesters. For women in their first trimester, most evidence suggests that use of mefloquine is not associated with adverse fetal or pregnancy outcomes, such as spontaneous abortions, stillbirths, and birth defects, when taken in prophylactic doses, but more data are necessary to make conclusive statements about its safety in early pregnancy. Consequently, mefloquine is the drug of choice for prophylactic use for women who are pregnant or likely to become pregnant when exposure to chloroquine-resistant *P falciparum* is unavoidable. Lactating mothers of infants weighing more than 5 kg may also use atovaquone-proguanil for prophylaxis when exposure to chloroquine-resistant *P falciparum* is unavoidable.

Self-Treatment of Malaria. Malaria can be treated effectively early in the course of disease, but delay of appropriate treatment can have serious or even fatal consequences. Travelers who do not take an antimalarial drug for prophylaxis or who are on a less-than-effective regimen or who may be in very remote areas can be given a self-treatment course of atovaquone-proguanil. Travelers should be advised that self-treatment is not considered a replacement for seeking prompt medical help. A self-treatment regimen should be discussed with a physician expert in travel medicine before departure.

Travelers taking atovaquone-proguanil as their antimalarial drug regimen should not take atovaquone-proguanil as their self-treatment drug and should use an alternative treatment regimen; the CDC Malaria Hotline (770-488-7788) provides advice on management of travelers who cannot use atovaquone-proguanil for self-treatment.

Travelers should be advised that any fever or influenza-like illness that develops within 3 months of departure from an area with endemic malaria requires immediate medical evaluation, including blood films to rule out malaria.

Prevention of Relapses. To prevent relapses of *P vivax* or *P ovale* infection after departure from areas where these species are primaquine resistant or tolerant, use of high-dose primaquine should be considered. Primaquine can cause hemolysis in patients with G6PD deficiency; thus, all patients should be screened for this condition before primaquine therapy is initiated.

Personal Protective Measures. All travelers to areas where malaria is endemic should be advised to use personal protective measures, including the following: (1) using insecticide-impregnated mosquito nets while sleeping; (2) remaining in well-screened areas; (3) wearing protective clothing; and (4) using mosquito repellents containing DEET. To be effective, most repellents require frequent reapplications (see Prevention of Mosquitoborne Infections, p 193, for recommendations regarding prevention of mosquitoborne infections and use of insect repellents).

Measles

CLINICAL MANIFESTATIONS: Measles is an acute viral disease characterized by fever, cough, coryza, conjunctivitis, an erythematous maculopapular rash, and a pathognomonic enanthema (Koplik spots). Complications including otitis media, bronchopneumonia, laryngotracheobronchitis (croup), and diarrhea occur commonly in young children. Acute encephalitis, which often results in permanent brain damage, occurs in approximately 1 of every 1000 cases. Death, predominantly resulting from respiratory and neurologic complications, occurs in 1 to 3 of every 1000 cases reported in the United States. Case fatality rates are increased in children younger than 5 years of age and immunocompromised children, including children with leukemia, human immunodeficiency virus (HIV) infection, and severe malnutrition. Sometimes the characteristic rash does not develop in immunocompromised patients.

Subacute sclerosing panencephalitis (SSPE) is a rare degenerative central nervous system disease characterized by behavioral and intellectual deterioration and seizures that occurs 7 to 10 years after wild-type measles virus infection. Widespread measles immunization has led to the virtual disappearance of SSPE in the United States.

ETIOLOGY: Measles virus is an RNA virus with 1 serotype, classified as a member of the genus Morbillivirus in the Paramyxoviridae family.

EPIDEMIOLOGY: The only natural hosts of measles virus are humans. Measles is transmitted by direct contact with infectious droplets or, less commonly, by airborne spread. Measles is one of the most highly communicable of all infectious diseases. In temperate areas, the peak incidence of infection usually occurs during late winter and spring. In the prevaccine era, most cases of measles in the United States occurred in preschool and young school-aged children, and few people remained susceptible by 20 years of age. The childhood and adolescent immunization program in the United States has resulted in a greater than 99% decrease in the reported incidence of measles since measles vaccine first was licensed in 1963.

From 1989 to 1991, the incidence of measles in the United States increased because of low immunization rates in preschool-aged children, especially in urban areas. From 1997 through 2007, the incidence of measles in the United States has been low (37–116 cases reported per year), consistent with an absence of endemic transmission. In 2000, an independent panel of internationally recognized experts reviewed available data and unanimously agreed that measles no longer is endemic in the United States. Cases of measles continue to occur, however, as a result of importation of the virus from other countries. Cases are considered international importations if the rash onset occurs within 18 days after entering the United States. During the first 7 months of 2008, 131 cases of measles were reported to the Centers for Disease Control and Prevention (CDC) from 15 states.[1] Seventeen of the 131 cases were importations from 10 countries. Of the cases, 91% were in people who were unimmunized or of unknown immunization status, 76% were in people younger than 20 years of age, and 16 episodes were in infants. This increase was not the result of a greater number of imported cases, but was the result of greater viral transmission after importation into the United States.

Vaccine failure occurs in as many as 5% of people who have received a single dose of vaccine at 12 months of age or older. Although waning immunity after immunization may be a factor in some cases, most cases of measles in previously immunized children seem to occur in people in whom response to the vaccine was inadequate (ie, primary vaccine failures).

Patients are contagious from 1 to 2 days before onset of symptoms (3–5 days before the rash) to 4 days after appearance of the rash. Immunocompromised patients who may have prolonged excretion of the virus in respiratory tract secretions can be contagious for the duration of the illness. Patients with SSPE are not contagious.

The **incubation period** generally is 8 to 12 days from exposure to onset of symptoms. In family studies, the average interval between appearance of rash in the index case and subsequent cases is 14 days, with a range of 7 to 18 days. In SSPE, the mean incubation period of 84 cases reported between 1976 and 1983 was 10.8 years.

---

[1]Centers for Disease Control and Prevention. Update: measles—United States, January–July 2008. *MMWR Morb Mortal Wkly Rep.* 2008;57(33):893–896

DIAGNOSTIC TESTS: Measles virus infection can be diagnosed by a positive serologic test result for measles immunoglobulin (Ig) M antibody, a significant increase in measles IgG antibody concentration in paired acute and convalescent serum specimens by any standard serologic assay, or isolation of measles virus or identification of measles RNA (by reverse transcriptase-polymerase chain reaction assay) from clinical specimens, such as urine, blood, throat, or nasopharyngeal secretions. The state public health laboratory or the CDC Measles Laboratory will process these viral specimens. The simplest method of establishing the diagnosis of measles is testing for IgM antibody on a single serum specimen obtained during the first encounter with a person suspected of having disease. The sensitivity of measles IgM assays varies and may be diminished during the first 72 hours after rash onset. If the result is negative for measles IgM and the patient has a generalized rash lasting more than 72 hours, a second serum specimen should be obtained and the measles IgM test should be repeated. Measles IgM is detectable for at least 1 month after rash onset in unimmunized people but might be absent or present only transiently in people immunized with 2 vaccine doses. People with febrile rash illness who are seronegative for measles IgM should be tested for rubella using the same specimens. Genotyping of viral isolates allows determination of patterns of importation and transmission, and genome sequencing can be used to differentiate between wild-type and vaccine virus infection. All cases of suspected measles should be reported immediately to the local or state health department without waiting for results of diagnostic tests.

TREATMENT: No specific antiviral therapy is available. Measles virus is susceptible in vitro to ribavirin, which has been given by the intravenous and aerosol routes to treat severely affected and immunocompromised children with measles. However, no controlled trials have been conducted, and ribavirin is not approved by the US Food and Drug Administration for treatment of measles.

Vitamin A. Vitamin A treatment of children with measles in developing countries has been associated with decreased morbidity and mortality rates. Low serum concentrations of vitamin A also have been found in children in the United States, and children with more severe measles illness have lower vitamin A concentrations. A 2005 Cochrane review[1] of vitamin A for treating measles in children found an association between using 2 doses of vitamin A on 2 consecutive days with a reduced risk of measles mortality in children younger than 2 years of age; a reduction in measles mortality was not seen after only 1 dose of vitamin A. The World Health Organization currently recommends vitamin A for all children with acute measles, regardless of their country of residence. Vitamin A for treatment of measles is administered once daily for 2 days, at the following doses:
- 200 000 IU for children 12 months of age or older;
- 100 000 IU for infants 6 through 11 months of age; and
- 50 000 IU for infants younger than 6 months of age.

Parenteral and oral formulations of vitamin A are available in the United States. An additional (ie, a third) age-specific dose should be given 2 through 4 weeks later to children with clinical signs and symptoms of vitamin A deficiency.

ISOLATION OF THE HOSPITALIZED PATIENT: In addition to standard precautions, airborne transmission precautions are indicated for 4 days after the onset of rash in otherwise healthy children and for the duration of illness in immunocompromised patients.

---

[1]Huiming Y, Chaomin W, Meng M. Vitamin A for treating measles in children. *Cochrane Database Syst Rev.* 2005;(4):CD001479

CONTROL MEASURES:
Care of Exposed People.
Use of Vaccine. Exposure to measles is not a contraindication to immunization. Available data suggest that measles vaccine, if given within 72 hours of measles exposure, will provide protection in some cases. If the exposure does not result in infection, the vaccine should induce protection against subsequent measles exposures. Immunization is the intervention of choice for control of measles outbreaks in schools and child care centers.

Use of Immune Globulin. Immune Globulin (IG) can be given intramuscularly to prevent or modify measles in a susceptible person within 6 days of exposure. The usual recommended dose is 0.25 mL/kg given intramuscularly; immunocompromised children should receive 0.5 mL/kg intramuscularly (the maximum dose in either instance is 15 mL). IG is indicated for susceptible household or other close contacts of patients with measles, particularly contacts younger than 1 year of age, pregnant women, and immunocompromised people for whom the risk of complications is highest or other people for whom measles vaccine is contraindicated. IG is not indicated for household or other close contacts who have received 1 dose of vaccine at 12 months of age or older unless they are immunocompromised.

Immune Globulin Intravenous (IGIV) preparations generally contain measles antibodies at approximately the same concentration per gram of protein as IG, although the concentration may vary by lot and manufacturer. For patients who receive IGIV regularly, the usual dose of 400 mg/kg should be adequate for measles prophylaxis after exposures occurring within 3 weeks of receiving IGIV.

For children who receive IG for modification or prevention of measles after exposure, measles vaccine (if not contraindicated) should be given 5 months (if the dose was 0.25 mL/kg) or 6 months (if the dose was 0.5 mL/kg) after IG administration, provided that the child is at least 12 months of age. Intervals between administration of IGIV or other biological products and measles-containing vaccines vary (see Table 3.34, p 448).

HIV Infection. All children and adolescents with HIV infection and children of unknown HIV infection status born to HIV-infected women who are exposed to wild-type measles should receive IG prophylaxis (0.5 mL/kg, intramuscularly; maximum dose 15 mL), regardless of their measles immunization status (see Human Immunodeficiency Virus Infection, p 380). An exception is the patient receiving IGIV (400 mg/kg) at regular intervals whose last dose was received within 3 weeks of exposure. Because of the rapid metabolism of IGIV, some experts recommend administration of an additional dose of IGIV if exposure to measles occurs 2 or more weeks after the last regular dose of IGIV.

Hospital Personnel. To decrease health care-associated infection, immunization programs should be established to ensure that all people who work or volunteer in health care facilities who may be in contact with patients with measles are immune to measles (see Health Care Personnel, p 94).

Measles Vaccine. The only measles vaccine licensed in the United States is a live further-attenuated strain prepared in chicken embryo cell culture. Measles vaccines provided through the Expanded Programme on Immunization in developing countries meet the World Health Organization standards and usually are comparable to the vaccine available in the United States. Measles vaccine is available in combination formulations, which include measles-mumps-rubella (MMR) and measles-mumps-rubella-varicella (MMRV) vaccines. Single-antigen measles vaccine currently is not produced in the United States. Measles-containing vaccine in a dose of 0.5 mL is given subcutaneously. Measles-

Table 3.34. Suggested Intervals Between Immune Globulin Administration and Measles Immunization (MMR, MMRV, or Monovalent Measles Vaccine)

Indications or Product	Route	Dose U or mL	Dose mg IgG/kg	Interval, mo[a]
Tetanus prophylaxis (as TIG)	IM	250 U	10	3
Hepatitis A prophylaxis (as IG)				
Contact prophylaxis	IM	0.02 mL/kg	3.3	3
International travel	IM	0.06 mL/kg	10	3
Hepatitis B prophylaxis (as HBIG)	IM	0.06 mL/kg	10	3
Rabies prophylaxis (as RIG)	IM	20 IU/kg	22	4
Varicella prophylaxis (as VariZIG)	IM	125 U/10 kg (maximum 625 U)	20–40	5
Measles prophylaxis (as IG)				
Standard	IM	0.25 mL/kg	40	5
Immunocompromised host	IM	0.50 mL/kg	80	6
RSV prophylaxis (palivizumab monoclonal antibody)[b]	IM	...	15 mg/kg (monoclonal)	None
Cytomegalovirus Immune Globulin	IV	3 mL/kg	150	6
Blood transfusion				
Washed RBCs	IV	10 mL/kg	Negligible	0
RBCs, adenine-saline added	IV	10 mL/kg	10	3
Packed RBCs	IV	10 mL/kg	20–60	5
Whole blood	IV	10 mL/kg	80–100	6
Plasma or platelet products	IV	10 mL/kg	160	7
Replacement (or therapy) of immune deficiencies (as IGIV)	IV	...	300–400	8
ITP (as IGIV)	IV	...	400	8
ITP	IV	...	1000	10
ITP for Kawasaki disease	IV	...	1600–2000	11

MMR indicates measles-mumps-rubella; MMRV, measles-mumps-rubella-varicella; IgG, immunoglobulin G; TIG, Tetanus Immune Globulin; IG, Immune Globulin; IM, intramuscular; HBIG, Hepatitis B IG; RIG, Rabies IG; VariZIG, Varicella-Zoster Immune Globulin; RSV, respiratory syncytial virus; IV, intravenous; RBCs, Red Blood Cells; IGIV, IG intravenous; ITP, immune (formerly termed "idiopathic") thrombocytopenic purpura.

[a]These intervals should provide sufficient time for decreases in passive antibodies in all children to allow for an adequate response to measles vaccine. Physicians should not assume that children are fully protected against measles during these intervals. Additional doses of IG or measles vaccine may be indicated after exposure to measles (see text).

[b]Monoclonal antibodies, such as palivizumab, and tumor necrosis factor (TNF) inhibitors do not interfere with response to vaccines.

containing vaccines can be given simultaneously with other immunizations in a separate syringe at a separate site (see Simultaneous Administration of Multiple Vaccines, p 33).

Serum measles antibodies develop in approximately 95% of children immunized at 12 months of age and 98% of children immunized at 15 months of age. Protection conferred by a single dose is durable in most people. However, a small proportion (5% or less) of immunized people may lose protection after several years. More than 99% of people who receive 2 doses separated by at least 4 weeks, with the first dose administered on or after their first birthday, develop serologic evidence of measles immunity. Immunization is not deleterious for people who already are immune.

Improperly stored vaccine may fail to protect against measles. Since 1979, an improved stabilizer has been added to the vaccine that makes it more resistant to heat inactivation. For recommended storage of MMR and MMRV vaccines, see the manufacturers' package labels.

Vaccine Recommendations (see Table 3.35, p 450, for summary).

Age of Routine Immunization. The first dose of measles vaccine should be given at 12 through 15 months of age. Delays in administering the first dose contributed to large outbreaks in the United States from 1989 to 1991. Initial immunization at 12 months of age is recommended for preschool-aged children in high-risk areas, especially large urban areas. The second dose is recommended routinely at school entry (ie, 4 through 6 years of age) but can be given at any earlier age (eg, during an outbreak or before international travel), provided the interval between the first and second doses is at least 28 days. Children who were not reimmunized at school entry should receive the second dose by 11 through 12 years of age. If a child receives a dose of measles vaccine before 12 months of age, 2 additional doses are required beginning at 12 through 15 months of age and separated by at least 4 weeks.

Use of MMRV Vaccine.[1]

• MMRV vaccine is indicated for simultaneous immunization against measles, mumps, rubella, and varicella among children 12 months through 12 years of age; MMRV vaccine is not indicated for people outside this age group.

• MMRV vaccine may be administered with the other vaccines recommended at 12 through 15 months of age and at 4 through 6 years of age (see Fig 1.1, p 24–25).

• At least 28 days should elapse between a dose of measles-containing vaccine, such as MMR vaccine, and a dose of MMRV vaccine.

• Because of concern for increased risk of febrile seizures among children 12 through 23 months of age after administration of MMRV vaccine, the Advisory Committee on Immunization Practices of the CDC removed the previous preference for administering combination MMRV vaccine over separate injections of equivalent component vaccines (MMR and varicella vaccines).[2] Data are being evaluated for consideration of future policy options for use of MMRV (see **www.cdc.gov/vaccines** for updates).

• Children with HIV infection should not receive MMRV.

High School Students and Adults. Because of the occurrence of measles cases in older children and young adults, emphasis must be placed on identifying and appropriately immunizing potentially susceptible adolescents and young adults in high school, college, and health care settings. People should be considered susceptible unless they have documentation of at least 2 doses of measles vaccine administered at least 28 days apart, physician-diagnosed measles, or laboratory evidence of immunity to measles or were born before 1957. A parental report of immunization is not considered adequate documenta-

---

[1]Centers for Disease Control and Prevention. Notice to readers: licensure of a combined live attenuated measles, mumps, rubella, and varicella vaccine. *MMWR Morb Mortal Wkly Rep.* 2005;54(47):1212–1214
[2]Centers for Disease Control and Prevention. Update: recommendations from the Advisory Committee on Immunization Practices (ACIP) regarding administration of combination MMRV vaccine. *MMWR Morb Mortal Wkly Rep.* 2008;57(10):258–260

Table 3.35. Recommendations for Measles Immunization[a]

Category	Recommendations
Unimmunized, no history of measles (12 through 15 mo of age)	MMR vaccine is recommended at 12 through 15 mo of age; a second dose is recommended at least 28 days after the first dose and usually is given at 4 through 6 y of age
Children 6 through 11 mo of age in epidemic situations[b] or before international travel	Immunize with MMR vaccine; reimmunization with MMR vaccine at 12 through 15 mo of age is necessary, and a third dose is indicated at 4 through 6 y of age
Children 4 through 12 y of age who have received 1 dose of measles vaccine at 12 mo of age or older	Reimmunize (1 dose)
Students in college and other post-high school institutions who have received 1 dose of measles vaccine at 12 mo of age or older	Reimmunize (1 dose)
History of immunization before the first birthday	Consider susceptible and immunize (2 doses)
History of receipt of inactivated measles vaccine or unknown type of vaccine, 1963–1967	Consider susceptible and immunize (2 doses)
Further attenuated or unknown vaccine given with IG	Consider susceptible and immunize (2 doses)
Allergy to eggs	Immunize; no reactions likely (see text for details)
Neomycin allergy, nonanaphylactic	Immunize; no reactions likely (see text for details)
Severe hypersensitivity (anaphylaxis) to neomycin or gelatin	Avoid immunization
Tuberculosis	Immunize (see Tuberculosis, p 680); if patient has untreated tuberculosis disease, start antituberculosis therapy before immunizing
Measles exposure	Immunize and/or give IG, depending on circumstances (see text, p 447)
HIV infected	Immunize (2 doses) unless severely immunocompromised (see text, p 453), and give IG if exposed to measles
Personal or family history of seizures	Immunize; advise parents of slightly increased risk of seizures
Immunoglobulin or blood recipient	Immunize at the appropriate interval (see Table 3.34, p 448)

MMR indicates measles-mumps-rubella vaccine; MMRV, measles-mumps-rubella-varicella vaccine; IG, Immune Globulin; HIV, human immunodeficiency virus.
[a]See text for details and recommendations for use of MMRV vaccine.
[b]See Outbreak Control (p 454).

tion. Physicians should provide an immunization record for patients only if they have administered the vaccine or have seen a record documenting immunization.

Colleges and Other Institutions for Education Beyond High School. Colleges and other institutions should require that all entering students have documentation of physician-diagnosed measles, serologic evidence of immunity, or receipt of 2 doses of measles-containing vaccines. Students without documentation of any measles immunization or immunity should receive MMR or another measles-containing vaccine on entry, followed by a second dose 4 weeks later, if not contraindicated.

Immunization During an Outbreak. During an outbreak, MMR vaccine may be given to infants as young as 6 months of age (see Outbreak Control, p 454). However, seroconversion rates after MMR immunization are significantly lower in children immunized before the first birthday than are seroconversion rates in children immunized after the first birthday. Therefore, children immunized before their first birthday should be immunized with MMR or MMRV vaccine at 12 through 15 months of age (at least 28 days after the initial measles immunization) and again at school entry (4 through 6 years of age).

International Travel. People traveling internationally should be immune to measles. For young children traveling internationally, the age for initial measles immunization may need to be lowered. Infants 6 through 11 months of age should receive 1 dose of MMR vaccine before departure, and then they should receive a measles-containing vaccine at 12 through 15 months of age (at least 28 days after the initial measles immunization) and again at 4 through 6 years of age. Children 12 through 15 months of age should be given their first dose of MMR vaccine before departure and again by 4 through 6 years of age. Children 12 months of age or older who have received 1 dose and are traveling to areas where measles is endemic or epidemic should receive their second dose before departure, provided the interval between doses is 28 days or more.

International Adoptees. The US Department of State requires that internationally adopted children 10 years of age and older receive several vaccines, including MMR, before entry into the United States. Internationally adopted children who are younger than 10 years of age are exempt from Immigration and Nationality Act regulations pertaining to immunization of immigrants before arrival in the United States (see Refugees and Immigrants, p 97); adoptive parents are required to sign a waiver indicating their intention to comply with US-recommended immunizations after their child's arrival in the United States.

Health Care Facilities. Physician-diagnosed natural measles infection, evidence of measles immunity, or receipt of 2 doses of measles vaccine is recommended before beginning employment for all health care professionals born in 1957 or after (see Health Care Personnel, p 94). For recommendations during an outbreak, see Outbreak Control (p 454).

Adverse Events. A temperature of 39.4°C (103°F) or higher develops in approximately 5% to 15% of vaccine recipients, usually between 6 and 12 days after receipt of MMR vaccine; fever generally lasts 1 to 2 days but may last as long as 5 days. Most people with fever otherwise are asymptomatic. Transient rashes have been reported in approximately 5% of vaccine recipients. Transient thrombocytopenia occurs in 1 in 25 000 to 1 in 2 million people after administration of measles-containing vaccines, specifically MMR (see Thrombocytopenia, p 453).

Rates of most local and systemic adverse events for children immunized with MMRV vaccine were comparable to rates for children immunized with MMR and varicella vaccines administered concomitantly. However, recipients of MMRV vaccine had a significantly greater rate of fever 102°F (38.9°C) or higher than did recipients of MMR and varicella administered concomitantly (22% vs 15%, respectively), and measles-like rash was observed in 3% of recipients of MMRV vaccine and 2% of recipients of MMR and varicella vaccines administered concomitantly.

The reported frequency of central nervous system conditions, such as encephalitis and encephalopathy, after measles immunization is less than 1 per million doses administered in the United States. Because the incidence of encephalitis or encephalopathy after measles immunization in the United States is lower than the observed incidence of encephalitis of unknown cause, some or most of the rare reported severe neurologic disorders may be related coincidentally, rather than causally, to measles immunization. Febrile seizures are known to occur 8 to 14 days after administration of the first dose of MMR vaccine. Approximately 1 additional febrile seizure occurs for every 3000 to 4000 children who receive MMR vaccine. Preliminary results of a CDC postlicensure MMRV safety study suggest that the rate of febrile seizures 7 to 10 days after immunization was approximately 2 times higher in children 12 through 23 months of age who received MMRV vaccine (9 per 10 000 children immunized) compared with children who received MMR and varicella vaccines at separate injection sites at the same visit (4 per 10 000 children immunized),[1] which is consistent with previously documented increased rates of fever following MMRV immunization. Multiple studies, as well as an Institute of Medicine Vaccine Safety Review, refute a causal relationship between autism and MMR vaccine or between inflammatory bowel disease and MMR vaccine. After reimmunization, reactions are expected to be similar clinically but much less frequent, because most of the vaccine recipients are immune.

Seizures. Children predisposed to febrile seizures may experience seizures after measles immunization. Children with histories of seizures or children whose first-degree relatives have histories of seizures may be at a slightly increased risk of a seizure but should be immunized, because the benefits greatly outweigh the risks.

Subacute Sclerosing Panencephalitis. Measles vaccine, by protecting against measles, decreases significantly the possibility of developing SSPE.

Precautions and Contraindications (also see Table 3.34, p 448).

Febrile Illnesses. Children with minor illnesses, such as upper respiratory tract infections, may be immunized (see Vaccine Safety and Contraindications, p 40). Fever is not a contraindication to immunization. However, if other manifestations suggest a more serious illness, the child should not be immunized until recovered.

Allergic Reactions. Hypersensitivity reactions occur rarely and usually are minor, consisting of wheal and flare reactions or urticaria at the injection site. Reactions have been attributed to trace amounts of neomycin or gelatin or some other component in the vaccine formulation. Anaphylaxis is rare. Measles vaccine is produced in chicken embryo cell culture and does not contain significant amounts of egg white (ovalbumin) cross-reacting proteins. Children with egg allergy are at low risk of anaphylactic reactions to measles-containing vaccines (including MMR and MMRV). Skin testing of children

[1]Centers for Disease Control and Prevention. Update: recommendations from the Advisory Committee on Immunization Practices (ACIP) regarding administration of combination MMRV vaccine. *MMWR Morb Mortal Wkly Rep.* 2008;57(10):258–260

for egg allergy is not predictive of reactions to MMR vaccine and is not required before administering MMR or other measles-containing vaccines. People with allergies to chickens or feathers are not at increased risk of reaction to the vaccine.

People who have had a significant hypersensitivity reaction after the first dose of measles vaccine should: (1) be tested for measles immunity, and if immune, should not be given a second dose; or (2) receive evaluation and possible skin testing before receiving a second dose. People who have had an immediate anaphylactic reaction to previous measles immunization should not be reimmunized but require testing to determine whether they are immune.

People who have experienced anaphylactic reactions to gelatin or topically or systemically administered neomycin should receive measles vaccine only in settings where such reactions could be managed and after consultation with an allergist or immunologist. Most often, however, neomycin allergy manifests as contact dermatitis, which is not a contraindication to receiving measles vaccine.

Thrombocytopenia. Rarely, MMR vaccine can be associated with thrombocytopenia within 2 months of immunization, with a temporal clustering 2 to 3 weeks after immunization. On the basis of case reports, the risk of vaccine-associated thrombocytopenia may be higher for people who previously experienced thrombocytopenia, especially when it occurred in temporal association with earlier MMR immunization. The decision to immunize these children should be based on assessment of immunity after the first dose and the benefits of protection against measles, mumps, and rubella in comparison with the risks of recurrence of thrombocytopenia after immunization. The risk of thrombocytopenia is higher after the first dose of vaccine than after the second dose. There have been no reported cases of thrombocytopenia associated with receipt of MMR vaccine that have resulted in death in otherwise healthy people.

Recent Administration of IG. IG preparations interfere with the serologic response to measles vaccine for variable periods, depending on the dose of IG administered. Suggested intervals between IG or blood-product administration and measles immunization are given in Table 3.34 (p 448). If vaccine is given at intervals shorter than those indicated, as may be warranted if the risk of exposure to measles is imminent, the child should be reimmunized at or after the appropriate interval for immunization (and at least 4 weeks after the earlier immunization) unless serologic testing indicates that measles-specific antibodies were produced.

If IG is to be administered in preparation for international travel, administration of vaccine should precede receipt of IG by at least 2 weeks to preclude interference with replication of the vaccine virus.

Tuberculosis. Tuberculin skin testing is not a prerequisite for measles immunization. Antituberculosis therapy should be initiated before administering MMR vaccine to people with untreated tuberculosis infection or disease. Tuberculin skin testing, if otherwise indicated, can be performed on the day of immunization. Otherwise, testing should be postponed for 4 to 6 weeks, because measles immunization temporarily may suppress tuberculin skin test reactivity.

Altered Immunity. Immunocompromised patients with disorders associated with increased severity of viral infections should not be given live measles virus vaccine (except for those with HIV infection; see Immunocompromised Children, p 72, and HIV Infection, below). The risk of exposure to measles for immunocompromised patients can be decreased by immunizing their close susceptible contacts. Management of immunodeficient and immunosuppressed patients exposed to measles can be facilitated by previous knowledge of their immune status. Susceptible patients with immunodeficiencies should receive IG after measles exposure (see Care of Exposed People, p 447).

Corticosteroids. For patients who have received high doses of corticosteroids (2 mg/kg or greater or greater than 20 mg/day of prednisone or its equivalent) for 14 days or more and who are not otherwise immunocompromised, the recommended interval before immunization is at least 1 month (see Immunocompromised Children, p 72). In general, inhaled steroids do not cause immunosuppression and are not a contraindication to measles immunization.

HIV Infection. Measles immunization (given as MMR vaccine) is recommended at the usual ages for people with asymptomatic HIV infection and for people with symptomatic infection who are not severely immunocompromised, because measles can be severe and often fatal in patients with HIV infection (see Human Immunodeficiency Virus Infection, p 380). Severely immunocompromised HIV-infected infants, children, adolescents, and young adults, as defined by low CD4+ T-lymphocyte counts or percentage of total lymphocytes, should not receive measles virus-containing vaccine, because vaccine-related pneumonia has been reported (see Human Immunodeficiency Virus Infection, p 380). All members of the household of an HIV-infected person should receive MMR *unless* they are HIV infected and severely immunosuppressed, were born before 1957, have had physician-diagnosed measles, have laboratory evidence of measles immunity, have had age-appropriate immunizations, or have a contraindication to measles vaccine. Because measles vaccine virus is not shed after immunization, HIV-infected people are not at risk of measles vaccine virus infection if household members are immunized.

Regardless of immunization status, symptomatic HIV-infected patients who are exposed to measles should receive IG prophylaxis, because immunization may not provide protection (see Care of Exposed People, p 447).

Personal or Family History of Seizures. Children with a personal or family history of seizures should be immunized after parents or guardians are advised that the risk of seizures after measles immunization is increased slightly. Because fever induced by measles vaccine usually occurs between 6 and 12 days after immunization, prevention of vaccine-related febrile seizures is difficult. Children receiving anticonvulsants should continue such therapy after measles immunization.

Pregnancy. A measles-containing vaccine should not be given to women known to be pregnant. Women who are given MMR should not become pregnant for at least 28 days. This precaution is based on the theoretical risk of fetal infection, which applies to administration of any live-virus vaccine to women who might be pregnant or who might become pregnant shortly after immunization. No evidence, however, substantiates this theoretical risk. In the immunization of adolescents and young adults against measles, asking women if they are pregnant, excluding women who are, and explaining the theoretical risks to others are recommended precautions.

Outbreak Control. Every suspected measles case should be reported immediately to the local health department, and every effort must be made to verify that the illness is measles, especially if the illness may be the first case in the community. Subsequent prevention of the spread of measles depends on prompt immunization of people at risk of exposure or people already exposed who cannot provide documentation of measles immunity readily, including the date of immunization. People who have not been immunized within

72 hours of exposure or who have been exempted from measles immunization for medical, religious, or other reasons should be excluded from school, child care, and health care settings until at least 2 weeks after the onset of rash in the last case of measles.

Schools and Child Care Facilities. During measles outbreaks in child care facilities, schools, and colleges and other institutions of higher education, all students, their siblings, and personnel born in 1957 or after who cannot provide documentation that they received 2 doses of measles-containing vaccine on or after their first birthday or other evidence of measles immunity should be immunized. People receiving their second dose, as well as unimmunized people receiving their first dose before or within 72 hours of exposure as part of the outbreak control program, may be readmitted immediately to the school or child care facility.

Health Care Facilities. If an outbreak occurs in an area served by a hospital or within a hospital, all employees, volunteers, and other personnel with direct patient contact who were born in 1957 or after who cannot provide documentation that they have received 2 doses of measles vaccine on or after their first birthday or other evidence of immunity to measles should receive a dose of measles vaccine. Because some health care professionals born before 1957 have acquired measles in health care facilities, immunization of older employees who may have occupational exposure to measles also should be considered. Susceptible personnel who have been exposed should be relieved of direct patient contact from the fifth to the 21st day after exposure, regardless of whether they received vaccine or IG after the exposure. Personnel who become ill should be relieved of patient contact for 4 days after rash develops.

Meningococcal Infections

CLINICAL MANIFESTATIONS: Invasive infection usually results in meningococcemia, meningitis, or both. Onset often is abrupt in meningococcemia, with fever, chills, malaise, myalgia, limb pain, prostration, and a rash that initially can be macular, maculopapular, petechial, or purpuric. The maculopapular and petechial rash is indistinguishable from the rash caused by viral infections, and the purpuric rash may occur in severe sepsis as a result of other bacterial pathogens, including *Streptococcus pneumoniae*. The progression of disease often is rapid. In fulminant cases, purpura, limb ischemia, coagulopathy, pulmonary edema, shock (characterized by tachycardia, tachypnea, oliguria, and poor peripheral perfusion, with confusion and hypotension late in the disease), coma, and death can ensue in hours despite appropriate therapy. Signs and symptoms of meningococcal meningitis are indistinguishable from signs and symptoms of acute meningitis caused by *S pneumoniae* or other meningeal pathogens. In severe and fatal cases of meningococcal meningitis, raised intracranial pressure is a predominant presenting feature. The case-fatality rate for meningococcal disease is 10%, and death is associated with young age, absence of meningitis, coma, hypotension, leukopenia, and thrombocytopenia. Less common manifestations include pneumonia, febrile occult bacteremia, conjunctivitis, septic arthritis, and chronic meningococcemia. Invasive meningococcal infections can be complicated by arthritis, myocarditis, pericarditis, and endophthalmitis. A self-limiting postinfectious inflammatory syndrome occurs in less than 10% of cases 4 or more days after onset of meningococcal infection and most commonly presents as fever and arthritis or vasculitis. Iritis, scleritis, pericarditis, and polyserositis are less common manifestations.

Sequelae associated with meningococcal disease occur in 11% to 19% of patients and include hearing loss, neurologic disability, digit or limb amputations, and skin scarring.

ETIOLOGY: *Neisseria meningitidis* is a gram-negative diplococcus with at least 13 serogroups based on capsule type.

EPIDEMIOLOGY: Strains belonging to groups A, B, C, Y, and W-135 are implicated most commonly in invasive disease worldwide. Serogroup A has been associated frequently with epidemics outside the United States, primarily in sub-Saharan Africa. An increase in cases of serogroup W-135 meningococcal disease has been associated with the Hajj pilgrimage in Saudi Arabia. Since 2002, serogroup W-135 meningococcal disease has been reported in sub-Saharan African countries during epidemic seasons. An unprecedented increase in cases of serogroup X meningococcal disease was observed in Niger in 2006. Recent prolonged outbreaks of serogroup B meningococcal disease have occurred in New Zealand, France, and Oregon.

The distribution of meningococcal serogroups in the United States has shifted in the past 2 decades. Serogroups B, C, and Y each account for approximately 30% of reported cases, but serogroup distribution varies by age, location, and time. Approximately three quarters of cases among adolescents and young adults are caused by serogroups C, Y, or W-135 and potentially are preventable with available vaccines. In infants, more than 50% of cases are caused by serogroup B and are not preventable with vaccines available in the United States.

Since introduction in the United States of *Haemophilus influenzae* type b and pneumococcal polysaccharide-protein conjugate vaccines for infants, *N meningitidis* has become the leading cause of bacterial meningitis in children and remains an important cause of septicemia. Disease most often occurs in children 2 years of age or younger; the peak attack rate occurs in children younger than 1 year of age. Another peak occurs in adolescents 15 through 18 years of age. Freshman college students who live in dormitories and military recruits in boot camp have a higher rate of disease compared with people who are the same age and are not living in such accommodations. Close contacts of patients with meningococcal disease are at increased risk of becoming infected. Patients with deficiency of a terminal complement component (C5–C9), C3 or properdin deficiencies, hypogammaglobulinemia, or anatomic or functional asplenia are at increased risk of invasive and recurrent meningococcal disease. Patients are considered capable of transmitting the organism for up to 24 hours after initiation of effective antimicrobial treatment. Asymptomatic colonization of the upper respiratory tract provides the source from which the organism is spread. Transmission occurs from person to person through droplets from the respiratory tract and requires close contact.

Outbreaks have occurred in communities and institutions, including child care centers, schools, colleges, and military recruit camps. An increased number of meningococcal outbreaks in the United States were reported during the 1990s. However, most cases of meningococcal disease are endemic, with fewer than 5% associated with outbreaks. Outbreaks often are heralded by a shift in the distribution of cases to an older age group. Serologic typing, multilocus sequence typing, multilocus enzyme electrophoresis, and pulsed-field gel electrophoresis of enzyme-restricted DNA fragments can be useful epidemiologic tools during a suspected outbreak to detect concordance among invasive strains.

The **incubation period** is 1 to 10 days, usually less than 4 days.

DIAGNOSTIC TESTS: Cultures of blood and cerebrospinal fluid (CSF) are indicated for patients with suspected invasive meningococcal disease. Cultures of a petechial or purpuric lesion scraping, synovial fluid, and other usually sterile body fluid specimens yield the organism in some patients. A Gram stain of a petechial or purpuric scraping, CSF, and buffy coat smear of blood can be helpful. Because *N meningitidis* can be a component of the nasopharyngeal flora, isolation of *N meningitidis* from this site is not helpful diagnostically. Bacterial antigen detection in CSF supports the diagnosis of a probable case if the clinical illness is consistent with meningococcal disease. A serogroup-specific polymerase chain reaction (PCR) test to detect *N meningitidis* from clinical specimens is used routinely in the United Kingdom, where up to 56% of cases are confirmed by PCR testing alone. This test particularly is useful in patients who receive antimicrobial therapy before cultures are obtained. In the United States, PCR-based assays are available in some research and public health laboratories.

Case definitions for invasive meningococcal disease are given in Table 3.36.

SUSCEPTIBILITY TESTING: *N meningitidis* isolates with decreased susceptibility to penicillin have been identified sporadically from several regions of the United States and widely from Spain, Italy, and parts of Africa. Resistant meningococcal isolates for which the minimum inhibitory concentration to penicillin is more than 1 μg/mL are rare. Most reported isolates are moderately susceptible, with a minimum inhibitory concentration to penicillin of between 0.12 μg/mL and 1.0 μg/mL. Treatment with high-dose penicillin is effective against moderately susceptible strains. Cefotaxime and ceftriaxone show a high degree of in vitro activity against moderately penicillin-susceptible meningococci. In 2007 and 2008, the first ciprofloxacin-resistant strains of *N meningitidis*-causing disease were detected in certain areas of the United States. Laboratories are encouraged to conduct surveillance for antimicrobial-resistant isolates of meningococcal disease, especially serogroup B isolates. State and local health departments should notify the Centers for

Table 3.36. Surveillance Case Definitions for Invasive Meningococcal Disease

Confirmed

A clinically compatible case and isolation of *Neisseria meningitidis* from a usually sterile site, for example:
- Blood
- Cerebrospinal fluid
- Synovial fluid
- Pleural fluid
- Pericardial fluid
- Isolation from skin scraping of petechial or purpuric lesions

Probable

A clinically compatible case with either a positive result of antigen test or immunohistochemistry of formalin-fixed tissue or a positive polymerase chain reaction test of blood or cerebrospinal fluid without a positive sterile site culture

Suspect

- A clinically compatible case and gram-negative diplococci in any sterile fluid, such as cerebrospinal fluid, synovial fluid, or scraping from a petechial or purpuric lesion
- Clinical purpura fulminans without a positive blood culture

Disease Control and Prevention (CDC) if resistance to ciprofloxacin or other agents used for prophylaxis is detected.

TREATMENT: The priority in management of meningococcal disease is the treatment of shock in meningococcemia and of raised intracranial pressure in severe cases of meningitis. Empiric therapy with cefotaxime or ceftriaxone is recommended, because both meningococcemia and meningococcal meningitis are indistinguishable clinically from disease caused by other bacterial pathogens, including S pneumoniae. Once the microbiologic diagnosis is established, penicillin G is the drug of choice and should be administered intravenously (250 000–300 000 U/kg/day; maximum, 12 million U/day, divided every 4–6 hours) for patients with invasive meningococcal disease, including meningitis (see Chemoprophylaxis). Cefotaxime, ceftriaxone, and ampicillin are acceptable alternatives. Ceftriaxone is the most cost-effective agent (reduced nursing time and single daily dose), clears CSF rapidly, clears nasopharyngeal carriage effectively after 1 dose, and allows outpatient management for completion of therapy when appropriate. In a patient with a serious penicillin allergy characterized by anaphylaxis, chloramphenicol is recommended, if available. For travelers from areas such as Spain, where penicillin resistance has been reported, cefotaxime, ceftriaxone, or chloramphenicol is recommended. Five to 7 days of antimicrobial therapy is adequate. In meningococcemia presenting with shock, early and rapid fluid resuscitation and consideration of inotropic and ventilatory support may reduce mortality. In view of the lack of evidence in pediatric populations, adjuvant therapies are not recommended. The postinfectious inflammatory syndromes associated with meningococcal disease often respond to nonsteroidal anti-inflammatory drugs.

ISOLATION OF THE HOSPITALIZED PATIENT: In addition to standard precautions, droplet precautions are recommended until 24 hours after initiation of effective antimicrobial therapy.

CONTROL MEASURES:
Care of Exposed People.

Chemoprophylaxis. Close contacts of all people with invasive meningococcal disease (see Table 3.37, p 459), whether endemic or in an outbreak situation, are at high risk and should receive chemoprophylaxis. The attack rate for household contacts is 500 to 800 times the rate for the general population. The decision to give chemoprophylaxis to contacts of people with meningococcal disease is based on risk of contracting invasive disease. Throat and nasopharyngeal cultures are of no value in deciding who should receive chemoprophylaxis and are not recommended.

Chemoprophylaxis is warranted for people who have been exposed directly to a patient's oral secretions through close social contact, such as kissing or sharing of toothbrushes or eating utensils as well as child care and preschool contacts during the 7 days before onset of disease in the index case. In addition, people who frequently slept in the same dwelling as the infected person within this period should receive chemoprophylaxis. For airline travel lasting more than 8 hours, passengers who are seated directly next to an infected person should receive prophylaxis. Routine prophylaxis is not recommended for health care professionals (Table 3.37, p 459) unless they have had intimate exposure to respiratory secretions, such as occurs with unprotected mouth-to-mouth resuscitation, intubation, or suctioning before or less than 24 hours after antimicrobial therapy was initiated. Chemoprophylaxis ideally should be initiated within 24 hours after the index patient is identified; prophylaxis given more than 2 weeks after exposure has little value.

Table 3.37. Disease Risk for Contacts of People With Meningococcal Disease

High risk: chemoprophylaxis recommended (close contacts)
- Household contact, especially children younger than 2 years of age
- Child care or pre-school contact at any time during 7 days before onset of illness
- Direct exposure to index patient's secretions through kissing or through sharing toothbrushes or eating utensils, markers of close social contact, at any time during 7 days before onset of illness
- Mouth-to-mouth resuscitation, unprotected contact during endotracheal intubation at any time 7 days before onset of illness
- Frequently slept in same dwelling as index patient during 7 days before onset of illness
- Passengers seated directly next to the index case during airline flights lasting more than 8 hours

Low risk: chemoprophylaxis not recommended
- Casual contact: no history of direct exposure to index patient's oral secretions (eg, school or work)
- Indirect contact: only contact is with a high-risk contact, no direct contact with the index patient
- Health care professionals without direct exposure to patient's oral secretions

In outbreak or cluster
- Chemoprophylaxis for people other than people at high risk should be administered only after consultation with local public health authorities

Antimicrobial Regimens for Prophylaxis (see Table 3.38, p 460). Rifampin, ceftriaxone, ciprofloxacin, and azithromycin are appropriate drugs for chemoprophylaxis in adults. The drug of choice for most children is rifampin (Table 3.38, p 460). If antimicrobial agents other than ceftriaxone or cefotaxime (both of which will eradicate nasopharyngeal carriage) are used for treatment of invasive meningococcal disease, the child should receive chemoprophylaxis before hospital discharge to eradicate nasopharyngeal carriage of *N meningitidis*.

Ceftriaxone, given in a single intramuscular dose, has been demonstrated to be as effective as oral rifampin in eradicating pharyngeal carriage of group A meningococci. The efficacy of ceftriaxone has been confirmed only for serogroup A strains, but its effect likely is similar for other serogroups. Ceftriaxone has the advantage of ease of administration, which increases adherence, and is safe for use during pregnancy. Rifampin is not recommended for pregnant women.

Ciprofloxacin, administered to adults in a single oral dose, also is effective in eradicating meningococcal carriage (see Table 3.38, p 460). Ciprofloxacin is not routinely recommended for people younger than 18 years of age or for pregnant women; its use in infants and children may be justified after careful assessment of the risks and benefits for the individual patient (see Antimicrobial Agents and Related Therapy, p 737). In areas of the United States where ciprofloxacin-resistant strains of *N meningitidis* have been detected, ciprofloxacin should not be used for chemoprophylaxis. Ciprofloxacin resistance is being monitored, and updates for chemoprophylaxis will be made as needed. Use of azithromycin as a single oral dose has been shown to be effective for eradication of nasopharyngeal carriage and can be used on a limited basis where ciprofloxacin resistance has been detected.

Postexposure Immunoprophylaxis. Because secondary cases can occur several weeks or more after onset of disease in the index case, meningococcal vaccine is an adjunct to chemoprophylaxis when an outbreak is caused by a serogroup prevented by

Table 3.38. Recommended Chemoprophylaxis Regimens for High-Risk Contacts and People With Invasive Meningococcal Disease

Age of Infants, Children, and Adults	Dose	Duration	Efficacy, %	Cautions
Rifampin[a]				
<1 mo	5 mg/kg, orally, every 12 h	2 days		
≥1 mo	10 mg/kg (maximum 600 mg), orally, every 12 h	2 days	90–95	Can interfere with efficacy of oral contraceptives and some seizure and anticoagulant medications; can stain soft contact lenses
Ceftriaxone				
<15 y	125 mg, intramuscularly	Single dose	90–95	To decrease pain at injection site, dilute with 1% lidocaine
≥15 y	250 mg, intramuscularly	Single dose	90–95	To decrease pain at injection site, dilute with 1% lidocaine
Ciprofloxacin[a,b]				
≥1 mo	20 mg/kg (maximum 500 mg), orally	Single dose	90–95	Not recommended routinely for people younger than 18 years of age; use may be justified after assessment of risks and benefits for the individual patient
Azithromycin	10 mg/kg (maximum 500 mg)	Single dose	90	Not recommended routinely. Equivalent to rifampin for eradication of *Neisseria meningitidis* from nasopharynx in one study.

[a]Not recommended for use in pregnant women.
[b]Use only if fluoroquinolone-resistant strains of *N meningitidis* have not been identified in the community; Centers for Disease Control and Prevention. Emergence of fluoroquinolone-resistant *Neisseria meningitidis*—Minnesota and North Dakota, 2007–2008. *MMWR Morb Mortal Wkly Rep.* 2008;57(7):173–175.

the vaccine. For control of meningococcal outbreaks caused by vaccine-preventable serogroups (A, C, Y, and W-135), the preferred vaccine in adults and children older than 2 years of age is tetravalent meningococcal (A, C, Y, and W-135) conjugate vaccine (MCV4), but the tetravalent meningococcal (A, C, Y, and W-135) polysaccharide vaccine (MPSV4) is acceptable. Meningococcal vaccines are being studied for use in children younger than age 2 years of age, and clinical trials of several serogroup B vaccines are underway.

Meningococcal Vaccines. There are 2 meningococcal vaccines licensed in the United States for use in children and adults against serotypes A, C, Y, and W-135, with a third being considered for licensure by the Food and Drug Administration. MPSV4 was licensed in 1981 for use in children 2 years of age and older. MPSV4 is administered subcutaneously as a single 0.5-mL dose and can be given concurrently with other vaccines but at different anatomic sites. The second vaccine, MCV4, was licensed in 2005 for use in people 11 through 55 years of age and in 2007 for children 2 through 10 years of age. MCV4 is administered intramuscularly as a single 0.5-mL dose and also can be given concurrently with other recommended vaccines. No vaccine is available in the United States for prevention of serogroup B meningococcal disease.

Serogroup A meningococcal polysaccharide vaccine, given as MPSV4, is immunogenic in children as young as 3 months of age, although the immune response in young children is not comparable to that seen in adults. For children younger than 18 months of age, 2 doses administered 3 months apart have been given for control of epidemics, although data regarding the efficacy of this schedule are not available. Serogroup A is a rare cause of invasive disease in the United States. Response to the other polysaccharides when MPSV4 is administered to infants younger than 24 months of age is poor.

In children 2 through 5 years of age, measurable concentrations of antibodies against group A and C polysaccharides decrease substantially during the first 3 years after a single dose of MPSV4. In school-aged children and adults, MPSV4-induced protection persists for at least 3 to 5 years.

Indications for Use of Meningococcal Vaccines (Table 3.39, p 462).
Routine childhood immunization with MCV4 is not recommended for children 2 through 10 years of age, because the infection rate is low in children in this age group, the immune response is poor in children 2 through 3 years of age, and the duration of immunity is not known. However, MCV4 is recommended for children 2 through 10 years of age who are in high-risk groups.

Recommendations for use of MCV4 are as follows:
- Adolescents 11 through 18 years of age should be immunized routinely with a single dose of MCV4.
- Adolescents should be immunized routinely at the 11- through 12-year health care visit, when immunization status (see Fig 1.2, p 26–27) and other preventive services can be addressed. Subsequent annual visits throughout adolescence also are recommended.
- People at increased risk of meningococcal disease should be immunized with MCV4 if they are at least 2 years of age. These people include:
  - Children or adolescents who have terminal complement or properdin deficiencies or those who have anatomic or functional asplenia (see Children With Asplenia, p 84).
  - Children or adolescents who travel to or reside in countries where *N meningitidis* is hyperendemic or epidemic (CDC Travelers' Health Hotline 877-FYI-TRIP or online at **www.cdc.gov/travel**).
  - College freshmen living in dormitories.
  - Military recruits.
- Because people with human immunodeficiency virus (HIV) infection are likely to be at higher risk of meningococcal disease, although not to the extent that they are at risk of invasive *S pneumoniae* infection, they may elect to be immunized with MCV4 if they are at least 2 years of age.

Table 3.39. Recommended Meningococcal Vaccines in Previously Unimmunized People to Prevent Invasive Meningococcal Disease Caused by Serogroups A, C, Y, and W-135

Population Group	Younger Than 2 y of Age	2 Through 10 y of Age	11 Through 18 y of Age	19 Through 55 y of Age
General population	NR	NR	MCV4, intramuscularly, at 11 through 18 y of age	NR
At increased risk: • College freshmen living in dormitories[a] • Certain travelers[a] • Outbreaks of A, C, Y, or W-135 disease • People with increased susceptibility[b]	NR	MCV4, intramuscularly, or MPSV4, subcutaneously	MCV4, intramuscularly, preferred (MPSV4 acceptable)	MCV4 intramuscularly preferred (MPSV4 acceptable)

NR indicates not recommended; MCV4, tetravalent meningococcal (A, C, Y, and W-135) conjugate vaccine; MPSV4, tetravalent meningococcal (A, C, Y, and W-135) polysaccharide vaccine.
[a]See text.
[b]People with anatomic or functional asplenia, terminal complement component (C5-C9) or properdin deficiencies, military recruits, and microbiologists routinely exposed to *Neisseria meningitidis.*

- People, including parents of children who wish to decrease their risk of meningococcal disease, may elect to receive MCV4 if they are 2 years of age or older.
- For control of meningococcal outbreaks caused by vaccine-preventable serogroups (A, C, Y, or W-135), MCV4 should be used for people 2 through 55 years of age, but MPSV4 is acceptable if MCV4 is not available.
- Immunization with MCV4 is preferred for children previously immunized with MPSV4 if at least 3 years have elapsed since receiving MPSV4.
- MCV4 is given to all military recruits in the United States.

Reimmunization. Appropriate reimmunization intervals after MCV4 have yet to be determined. In children 2 years of age and older and adults, concentrations of bactericidal antibodies against serogroups A, C, Y, and W-135 3 years after a single dose of MCV4 are equal to or greater than bactericidal antibodies of people given MPSV4 6 months after immunization.

Adverse Reactions and Precautions. Frequent adverse reactions after MPSV4 and MCV4 immunization include localized pain, irritability, headache, and fatigue. Most reactions are mild and resolve 3 days after immunization. Pain, induration, swelling, and redness at the injection site in 2- through 18-year-olds are slightly greater after administration of MCV4 compared with MPSV4. Fever is reported by 2% to 5% of adolescents who receive either MPSV4 or MCV4. Meningococcal immunization recommendations should not be altered because of pregnancy if a woman is at increased risk of meningococcal disease. Guillain-Barré syndrome (GBS) was reported in 22 adolescents aged 11 through 19 years who received MCV4 between June 2005 and October 2007.[1] The temporal association provoked a recommendation that MCV4 should not be given to adolescents or adults with a history of GBS. The available data cannot determine with certainty whether MCV4 increases the risk for GBS and do not affect immunization recommendations. However, cases of GBS or other clinically significant adverse events after MCV4 should be reported to the Vaccine Adverse Event Reporting System (**www. vaers.hhs.gov**). MPSV4 may be an acceptable alternative to MCV4 for people with a history of GBS.

Reporting. All confirmed, presumptive, and probable cases of invasive meningococcal disease must be reported to the appropriate health department (see Table 3.36, p 457). Timely reporting can facilitate early recognition of outbreaks and serogrouping of isolates so that appropriate prevention recommendations can be implemented rapidly.

Counseling and Public Education. When a case of invasive meningococcal disease is detected, the physician should provide accurate and timely information about meningococcal disease and the risk of transmission to families and contacts of the infected person. Some experts recommend that patients with invasive meningococcal disease be evaluated for a terminal complement deficiency, and if a deficiency is detected, patients should receive MCV4 if 2 or more years of age, and patients and parents should be counseled about the risk of recurrent invasive meningococcal disease. Public health questions, such as whether a mass immunization program is needed, should be referred to the local health department. In appropriate situations, early provision of information in collaboration with the local health department to schools or other groups at increased risk and to the media may help minimize public anxiety and unrealistic or inappropriate demands for intervention.

Human Metapneumovirus

CLINICAL MANIFESTATIONS: Since discovery in 2001, human metapneumovirus (hMPV) has been shown to cause acute respiratory tract illness in patients of all ages. Human metapneumovirus is one of the leading causes of bronchiolitis in infants and also causes pneumonia, asthma exacerbations, croup, and upper respiratory tract infections (URIs) with concomitant acute otitis media in children. Otherwise healthy young children infected with hMPV usually have mild or moderate symptoms, but some young children have severe disease requiring hospitalization. Patients from whom hMPV is isolated may have concurrent infection with other viral agents. Risk factors for severe hMPV infection include immunodeficiency disease or therapy causing immunosuppression at any age; fatalities from hMPV infection have been reported in stem cell or lung transplant recipients. Preterm birth and underlying cardiopulmonary disease likely are risk factors, but the degree of risk associated with these conditions is not defined fully.

Serologic studies suggest that all children are infected at least once by 5 years of age. Recurrent infection occurs throughout life and, in healthy people, usually is mild or asymptomatic.

---

[1]Centers for Disease Control and Prevention. Update: Guillain-Barré syndrome among recipients of Menactra meningococcal conjugate vaccine—United States, June 2005–September 2006. *MMWR Morb Mortal Wkly Rep.* 2006;55(41):1120–1124

ETIOLOGY: hMPV is an enveloped single-stranded negative-sense RNA virus of the family Paramyxoviridae. Four major genotypes of virus have been identified, and these viruses fall into 2 major antigenic subgroups (designated A and B), which usually circulate simultaneously each year but in varying proportions. Whether the 2 subgroups exhibit pathogenic differences is unknown.

EPIDEMIOLOGY: Humans are the only source of infection. Formal transmission studies have not been reported, but transmission is likely to occur by direct or close contact with contaminated secretions. Health care-associated infections have been reported.

hMPV infections usually occur in annual epidemics during late winter and early spring in temperate climates. The hMPV season in a community generally coincides with or overlaps the respiratory syncytial virus season. During this overlapping period, bronchiolitis may be caused by either or both viruses. Sporadic infection may occur throughout the year. In otherwise healthy infants, the duration of viral shedding is 1 to 2 weeks. Prolonged shedding (weeks to months) has been reported in severely immunocompromised hosts.

The **incubation period** is estimated to be 3 to 5 days in most cases.

DIAGNOSTIC TESTS: Rapid diagnostic immunofluorescent assays based on hMPV antigen detection by monoclonal antibodies are available commercially. The assays for hMPV developed and used by research laboratories include reverse transcriptase-polymerase chain reaction (RT-PCR) amplification of viral genes (both conventional and real time) and viral isolation from nasopharyngeal secretions using cell culture. Viral isolation requires trypsin and specialized cell cultures of LLC-MK2, Vero, or primary monkey kidney cells. Approximately half of nasopharyngeal cultures that have positive results for hMPV by RT-PCR assay yield cultivable virus by current techniques but require prolonged incubation. Serologic testing of acute and convalescent serum specimens can be used to confirm the first episode of infection.

TREATMENT: Treatment is supportive and includes hydration, careful clinical assessment of respiratory status, including measurement of oxygen saturation, use of supplemental oxygen, and if necessary, mechanical ventilation. hMPV is susceptible to ribavirin in vitro, but no controlled clinical data are available to assess therapeutic benefit in people (eg, immunocompromised patients with severe hMPV disease).

Antimicrobial Agents. The rate of bacterial lung infection or bacteremia associated with hMPV infection is not defined, but is suspected to be low. Therefore, antimicrobial agents are not indicated in treatment of infants hospitalized with hMPV bronchiolitis or pneumonia unless evidence exists for the presence of a bacterial infection.

Isolation of the Hospitalized Patient: In addition to standard precautions, contact precautions are recommended for the duration of hMPV-associated illness among infants and young children. Patients with known hMPV infection should be cared for in single rooms or placed in a cohort of hMPV-infected patients.

CONTROL MEASURES: Control of health care-associated hMPV infection depends on adherence to contact precautions. Exposure to hMPV-infected people, including other patients, staff, and family members, may not be recognized, because illness in contacts may be mild.

Preventive measures include limiting exposure to settings where exposure to hMPV may occur (eg, child care centers) and emphasis on hand hygiene in all settings, including the home, especially when contacts of high-risk children have respiratory tract infections.

Microsporidia Infections
(Microsporidiosis)

CLINICAL MANIFESTATIONS: Patients with intestinal infection have watery, nonbloody diarrhea, generally without fever, although asymptomatic infection may be more common than originally suspected. Intestinal infection is most common in immunocompromised people, especially people who are infected with human immunodeficiency virus (HIV), in whom infection often results in chronic diarrhea. The clinical course can be complicated by malnutrition and progressive weight loss. Chronic infection in immunocompetent people is rare. Other clinical syndromes that can occur in HIV-infected and immuno-compromised patients include keratoconjunctivitis, sinusitis, myositis, nephritis, hepatitis, cholangitis, peritonitis, prostatitis, cystitis, disseminated disease, and wasting syndrome.

ETIOLOGY: Microsporidia are obligate intracellular, spore-forming parasites. They have been reclassified from protozoa to fungi. The genera *Encephalitozoon, Enterocytozoon, Nosema, Pleistophora, Trachipleistophora, Brachiola,* and *Vittaforma* and *Microsporidium* have been implicated in human infection, as have unclassified species. *Enterocytozoon bieneusi* and *Encephalitozoon (Septata) intestinalis* are causes of chronic diarrhea in HIV-infected people.

EPIDEMIOLOGY: Most microsporidian infections are transmitted by oral ingestion of spores. Microsporidium spores commonly are found in surface water, and human strains have been identified in municipal water supplies and ground water. Several studies indicate that waterborne transmission occurs. Person-to-person spread by the fecal-oral route also occurs. Spores also have been detected in other body fluids, but their role in transmission is unknown. Data suggest the possibility of zoonotic transmission.

The **incubation period** is unknown.

DIAGNOSTIC TESTS: Infection with gastrointestinal *Microsporidia* species can be documented by identification of organisms in biopsy specimens from the small intestine. *Microsporidia* species spores also can be detected in formalin-fixed stool specimens or duodenal aspirates stained with a chromotrope-based stain (a modification of the trichrome stain) and examined by an experienced microscopist. Gram, acid-fast, periodic acid-Schiff, and Giemsa stains also can be used to detect organisms in tissue sections. The organisms often are not noticed, because they are small, stain poorly, and evoke minimal inflammatory response. Use of stool concentration techniques does not seem to improve the ability to detect *E bieneusi* spores. Polymerase chain reaction assay also can be used for diagnosis. Identification for classification purposes and diagnostic confirmation of species requires electron microscopy or molecular techniques.

TREATMENT: Restoration of immune function can be critical in control of any microsporidian infection. For a limited number of patients, albendazole, metronidazole, atovaquone, nitazoxanide, and fumagillin have been reported to decrease diarrhea but without eradication of the organism. Albendazole is the drug of choice for infections caused by *E intestinalis* but is not effective for *E bieneusi* infections, which may respond to fumagillin. Recurrence of diarrhea is common after therapy is discontinued. In HIV-infected patients, highly active antiretroviral therapy-associated improvement in CD4+ T-lymphocyte cell count can favorably modify the course of disease.

ISOLATION OF THE HOSPITALIZED PATIENT: In addition to standard precautions, contact precautions are recommended for diapered and incontinent children for the duration of illness.

CONTROL MEASURES: None have been documented. In HIV-infected and other immunocompromised people, decreased exposure may result from attention to hand hygiene, drinking bottled or boiled water, and avoiding unpeeled fruits and vegetables.

Molluscum Contagiosum

CLINICAL MANIFESTATIONS: Molluscum contagiosum is a benign, usually asymptomatic viral infection of the skin with no systemic manifestations. It usually is characterized by 2 to 20 discrete, 5-mm-diameter, flesh-colored to translucent, dome-shaped papules, some with central umbilication. Lesions commonly occur on the trunk, face, and extremities but rarely are generalized. Molluscum contagiosum is a self-limited infection that usually resolves spontaneously in 6 to 12 months but may take as long as 4 years to completely disappear. An eczematous reaction encircles lesions in approximately 10% of patients. People with eczema, immunocompromising conditions, and human immunodeficiency virus infection tend to have more widespread and prolonged eruptions.

ETIOLOGY: The cause is a poxvirus, which is the sole member of the genus *Molluscipoxvirus*. DNA subtypes can be differentiated, but subtype is not significant in pathogenesis.

EPIDEMIOLOGY: Humans are the only known source of the virus, which is spread by direct contact, including sexual contact, or by fomites. Lesions can be disseminated by autoinoculation. Infectivity generally is low, but occasional outbreaks have been reported, including outbreaks in child care centers. The period of communicability is unknown.

The **incubation period** seems to vary between 2 and 7 weeks but may be as long as 6 months.

DIAGNOSTIC TESTS: The diagnosis usually can be made clinically from the characteristic appearance of the lesions. Wright or Giemsa staining of cells expressed from the central core of a lesion reveals characteristic intracytoplasmic inclusions. Electron microscopic examination of these cells identifies typical poxvirus particles. Adolescents and young adults with genital molluscum contagiosum should have screening tests for other sexually transmitted infections.

TREATMENT: There is no consensus on the management of molluscum contagiosum in children and adolescents. Genital lesions should be treated to prevent spread to sexual contacts. Treatment of nongenital lesions is only for cosmetic reasons. Lesions in healthy people typically are self-limited, and treatment may not be necessary. However, therapy may be warranted to: (1) alleviate discomfort, including itching; (2) reduce autoinoculation; (3) limit transmission of the virus to close contacts; (4) reduce cosmetic concerns; and (5) prevent scarring and secondary infection. Physical destruction of the lesions is the most rapid and effective means of curing molluscum contagiosum lesions. Modalities available for physical destruction include: curettage, cryotherapy with liquid nitrogen, electrodesiccation, and chemical agents designed to initiate a local inflammatory response (podophyllin, tretinoin, cantharidin, 25% to 50% trichloroacetic acid, liquefied phenol, silver nitrate, tincture of iodine, or potassium hydroxide). Most data available for any of these modalities are anecdotal, and randomized trials usually are limited because of small sample sizes. Because physical destruction of the lesions is painful, appropriate local anesthesia is required. Systemic therapy with cimetidine has been tried because of its systemic immunomodulatory effects. However, available data have not supported a benefit. Cidofovir is a cytosine nucleotide analogue with in vitro activity against molluscum contagiosum; successful intravenous treatment of immunocompromised adults with severe lesions has been reported. Cidofovir is an antiviral agent with significant toxicity. Genital lesions in children are not acquired frequently by sexual transmission, but other signs of sexual abuse should be sought.

ISOLATION OF THE HOSPITALIZED PATIENT: Standard precautions are recommended.

CONTROL MEASURES: No control measures are known for isolated cases. For outbreaks, which are common in the tropics, restricting direct person-to-person contact and sharing of potentially contaminated fomites may decrease spread. Molluscum contagiosum should not prevent a child from attending child care or school or from swimming in public pools. When possible, lesions not covered by clothing should be covered by a watertight bandage. The bandage should be changed daily or when soiled.

Moraxella catarrhalis Infections

CLINICAL MANIFESTATIONS: Common infections include acute otitis media and sinusitis. Bronchopulmonary infection occurs predominantly among patients with chronic lung disease or impaired host defenses. The role of *Moraxella catarrhalis* in children with persistent cough is controversial. Rare manifestations are bacteremia (sometimes associated with focal infections, such as preseptal cellulitis, osteomyelitis, septic arthritis, abscesses, or a rash indistinguishable from that observed in meningococcemia) and conjunctivitis or meningitis in neonates. Other unusual manifestations include endocarditis and shunt-associated ventriculitis.

ETIOLOGY: *M catarrhalis* is a gram-negative aerobic diplococcus. Almost 100% of strains produce beta-lactamase that mediates resistance to penicillins.

EPIDEMIOLOGY: *M catarrhalis* is part of the normal flora of the upper respiratory tract of humans. The mode of transmission is presumed to be direct contact with contaminated respiratory tract secretions or droplet spread. Infection is most common in infants and young children but occurs at all ages. The duration of carriage by infected and colonized children and the period of communicability are unknown.

The **incubation period** is unknown.

DIAGNOSTIC TESTS: The organism can be isolated on blood or chocolate agar culture media after incubation in air or with increased carbon dioxide. Culture of middle ear or sinus aspirates is indicated for patients with unusually severe infection, patients with infection that fails to respond to treatment, and immunocompromised children. Concomitant recovery of *M catarrhalis* with other pathogens (*Streptococcus pneumoniae* or *Haemophilus influenzae*) may indicate mixed infection.

TREATMENT: Although most strains of *Moraxella* species produce beta-lactamase and are resistant to amoxicillin in vitro, this agent remains effective as empiric therapy for otitis media and other respiratory tract infections. When *M catarrhalis* is isolated from appropriately obtained specimens (middle ear fluid, sinus aspirates, or lower respiratory tract secretions) or when initial therapy has been unsuccessful, appropriate antimicrobial agents include amoxicillin-clavulanate, cefuroxime, cefdinir, cefpodoxime, erythromycin, clarithromycin, azithromycin, trimethoprim-sulfamethoxazole, or, in people 18 years of age or older, a fluoroquinolone. If parenteral antimicrobial therapy is needed to treat *M catarrhalis* infection, in vitro data indicate that cefotaxime, ceftriaxone, and ceftazidime are effective.

ISOLATION OF THE HOSPITALIZED PATIENT: Standard precautions are recommended.

CONTROL MEASURES: None.

Mumps

CLINICAL MANIFESTATIONS: Mumps is a systemic disease characterized by swelling of one or more of the salivary glands, usually the parotid glands. Approximately one third of infections do not cause clinically apparent salivary gland swelling and may manifest primarily as respiratory tract infection. More than 50% of people with mumps have cerebrospinal fluid pleocytosis, but fewer than 10% have symptoms of central nervous system infection. Orchitis is a common complication after puberty, but sterility rarely occurs. Other rare complications include arthritis, thyroiditis, mastitis, glomerulonephritis, myocarditis, endocardial fibroelastosis, thrombocytopenia, cerebellar ataxia, transverse myelitis, ascending polyradiculitis, pancreatitis, oophoritis, and hearing impairment. In the absence of an immunization program, mumps typically occurs during childhood. Infection occurring among adults is more likely to be severe, and death resulting from mumps and its complications, although rare, occurs most often in adults. Mumps during the first trimester of pregnancy is associated with an increased rate of spontaneous abortion. Although mumps virus can cross the placenta, no evidence exists that this results in congenital malformation.

ETIOLOGY: Mumps is caused by an RNA virus classified as a Rubulavirus in the Paramyxoviridae family. Other causes of parotitis include infection with cytomegalovirus, parainfluenza virus types 1 and 3, influenza A virus, coxsackieviruses and other enteroviruses, lymphocytic choriomeningitis virus, human immunodeficiency virus (HIV), *Staphylococcus aureus*, nontuberculous mycobacterium, and less often, other gram-positive and gram-negative bacteria; salivary duct calculi; starch ingestion; drug reactions (eg, phenylbutazone, thiouracil, iodides); and metabolic disorders (diabetes mellitus, cirrhosis, and malnutrition).

EPIDEMIOLOGY: Mumps occurs worldwide, and humans are the only known natural hosts. The virus is spread by contact with infected respiratory tract secretions. Mumps virus is the only cause of epidemic parotitis. Historically, the peak incidence was between January and May and among children younger than 10 years of age. Mumps vaccine was licensed in the United States in 1967 and recommended for routine childhood immunization in 1977. After implementation of the 1-dose mumps vaccine program, the incidence of mumps in the United States declined to very low levels. Mumps outbreaks occurred between 1986 and 1991, however, affecting both unimmunized adolescents and young adults and also highly immunized middle and high school populations. After implementation of the 2-dose MMR vaccine policy, recommended in 1989 for measles control, mumps again declined to extremely low levels. From 2000 to 2005, seasonality was no longer evident, and there were fewer than 300 reported cases per year. In 2006, a large-scale mumps outbreak occurred in the United States, with 6584 reported cases. Many of the cases occurred among people 18 through 24 years of age, many of whom were college students who had received 2 doses of mumps vaccine. Because 2 doses of mumps-containing vaccine are not 100% effective in a setting with high immunization coverage such as the United States, most mumps cases likely will occur in people who have received 2 doses.[1] The period of maximum communicability is 1 to 2 days before onset of parotid swelling to 5 days after onset of parotid swelling. Virus has been isolated from saliva from 7 days before through 9 days after onset of swelling.

The **incubation period** usually is 16 to 18 days, but cases may occur from 12 to 25 days after exposure.

DIAGNOSTIC TESTS: Despite the outbreak in 2006, mumps is an uncommon infection in the United States, and parotitis has other etiologies, including other infectious agents. People with parotitis lasting 2 days or more without other apparent cause should undergo diagnostic testing to confirm mumps virus as the cause or to diagnose other etiologies (eg, influenza A virus, parainfluenza viruses 1 and 3, and bacterial causes). Mumps can be confirmed by isolating the virus in cell culture inoculated with buccal swab (Stenson duct exudates), throat washing, saliva, or spinal fluid specimens; by detection of mumps virus nucleic acid in those specimens by reverse transcriptase-polymerase chain reaction; by detection of mumps-specific immunoglobulin (Ig) M antibody; or by a significant increase between acute and convalescent titers in serum mumps IgG antibody titer determined by standard quantitative or semi-quantitative serologic assay (most commonly, semi-quantitative enzyme immunoassay). If the initial IgM test result is negative, a second (convalescent) serum specimen obtained 2 to 3 weeks after onset of signs or symptoms may test positive. A delayed IgM response has been observed in people with confirmed mumps, especially in immunized populations.

Confirming the diagnosis of mumps in highly immunized populations may be challenging because the IgM response may be absent or short lived; acute IgG titers might already be high, so no significant increase can be detected between acute and convalescent specimens; and mumps virus might be present in clinical specimens only during the first few days after illness onset. Emphasis should be placed on obtaining clinical specimens within 1 to 3 days after onset of symptoms (usually parotitis). In the case of specimens for virus culture or PCR assay, immediately place specimens in a cold storage container and transport to the laboratory.

TREATMENT: Supportive.

ISOLATION OF THE HOSPITALIZED PATIENT: In addition to standard precautions, droplet precautions are recommended until 5 days after onset of parotid swelling.

CONTROL MEASURES:
School and Child Care. Children should be excluded for 5 days from onset of parotid gland swelling. For control measures during an outbreak, see Outbreak Control, p 472.

Care of Exposed People. Mumps vaccine has not been demonstrated to be effective in preventing infection after exposure. However, a mumps-containing vaccine can be given after exposure, because immunization will provide protection against subsequent exposures. Immunization during the incubation period presents no increased risk. The routine use of mumps vaccine is not recommended for people born before 1957, because most of these people are immune. For health care professionals born before 1957, however, immunization with 1 dose of a mumps-containing vaccine should be considered routinely for

---

[1]Centers for Disease Control and Prevention (CDC). Brief report: update: mumps activity—United States, January 1–October 7, 2006. *MMWR Morb Mortal Wkly Rep.* 2006;55(42):1152–1153

people without evidence of immunity, and 2 doses should be considered during an outbreak. Immune Globulin (IG) and Mumps Immune Globulin are not effective as postexposure prophylaxis. Mumps Immune Globulin no longer is available in the United States.

Mumps Vaccine. Live-attenuated mumps vaccine has been licensed in the United States since 1967. Vaccine is administered by subcutaneous injection of 0.5 mL of measles-mumps-rubella (MMR) vaccine (licensed for people 12 months of age or older) or measles-mumps-rubella-varicella (MMRV) vaccine (licensed for children 12 months through 12 years of age). Monovalent mumps vaccine no longer is produced in the United States. Protective efficacy of the vaccine in clinical trials is estimated to be greater than 95% with a single dose. Postlicensure data, however, indicate that the effectiveness of 1 dose of mumps vaccine has been approximately 80% (range 64%–95%), and on the basis of fewer studies globally, 2-dose vaccine effectiveness has been approximately 90% (range 88%–95%). Some studies and investigations conducted during the mumps outbreaks in the late 1980s and during the 2006 outbreak indicate that vaccine-induced immunity might wane. Additional studies are underway, and long-term monitoring of vaccine immunity is planned.

Vaccine Recommendations:

- Mumps vaccine should be given as MMR or MMRV routinely to children at 12 through 15 months of age, with a second dose of MMR typically administered at 4 through 6 years of age. The second dose of MMR may be administered before 4 years of age provided at least 28 days have elapsed since the first dose. The second dose of mumps vaccine provides an additional safeguard against primary and secondary vaccine failure, although the 2006 mumps outbreak highlighted the potential for limited mumps outbreaks in populations highly immunized with 2 doses. Administration of MMR is not harmful if given to a person already immune to one or more of the viruses (from previous infection or immunization).

- Mumps immunization is of particular importance for children approaching puberty, adolescents, and adults who have not had mumps or mumps vaccine. At office visits of prepubertal children and adolescents, the status of immunity to mumps should be assessed. People should be immunized unless they have documentation of adequate immunization, physician-diagnosed mumps, or serologic evidence of immunity or were born before 1957. Adequate immunization is 2 doses of mumps-containing vaccine for school-aged children and adults at high risk (ie, health care professionals, students at post-high school educational institutions, and international travelers), and a single dose of mumps-containing vaccine for other adults born in or after 1957. Additionally, health care professionals born before 1957 without other evidence of immunity should consider receiving 1 dose of mumps-containing vaccine routinely and, in an outbreak setting, they strongly should consider receiving 2 doses.

- Children 12 months of age or older, adolescents, and adults born during or after 1957 without evidence of immunity should be offered mumps-containing vaccine according to vaccine policy (see above) before beginning travel, because mumps is endemic throughout most of the world. Children younger than 12 months of age need not be given mumps vaccine before travel, but they may receive it as MMR vaccine if measles immunization is indicated.

- A mumps-containing vaccine may be given with other vaccines at different injection sites and with separate syringes (see Simultaneous Administration of Multiple Vaccines, p 33).

Adverse Reactions. Adverse reactions associated with mumps vaccine are rare. Orchitis, parotitis, and low-grade fever have been reported rarely after immunization. Temporally related reactions, including febrile seizures, nerve deafness, aseptic meningitis, encephalitis, rash, pruritus, and purpura, may follow immunization rarely; however, causality has not been established. Allergic reactions also are rare (see Measles, Precautions and Contraindications [p 452], and Rubella, Precautions and Contraindications [p 583]). Other reactions that occur after immunization with MMR or MMRV vaccine may be attributable to other components of the vaccines (see Measles, p 444, Rubella, p 579, and Varicella-Zoster Infections, p 714).

Reimmunization with mumps vaccine as MMR is not associated with an increased incidence of reactions, and postlicensure data on MMRV vaccine are limited.

Precautions and Contraindications. See Measles, p 444, Rubella, p 579, and Varicella-Zoster Infections, p 714, if MMRV is used.

Febrile Illness. Children with minor illnesses with or without fever, such as upper respiratory tract infections, may be immunized (see Vaccine Safety and Contraindications, p 40). Fever is not a contraindication to immunization. However, if other manifestations suggest a more serious illness, the child should not be immunized until recovered.

Allergies. Hypersensitivity reactions occur rarely and usually are minor, consisting of wheal and flare reactions or urticaria at the injection site. Reactions have been attributed to trace amounts of neomycin or gelatin or some other component in the vaccine formulation. Anaphylaxis is rare; MMR and MMRV vaccines are produced in chicken embryo cell culture and do not contain significant amounts of egg white (ovalbumin) cross-reacting proteins. Children with egg allergy are at low risk of anaphylactic reactions to MMR or MMRV vaccine. Skin testing of children for egg allergy is not predictive of reactions to MMR or MMRV vaccine and is not required before administering MMR or other mumps-containing vaccines. People with allergies to chickens or feathers are not at increased risk of reaction to the vaccine. People who have experienced anaphylactic reactions to gelatin or topically or systemically administered neomycin should receive mumps vaccine only in settings where such reactions could be managed and after consultation with an allergist or immunologist. Most often, however, neomycin allergy manifests as contact dermatitis, which is not a contraindication to receiving mumps vaccine (see Measles, p 444).

Recent Administration of IG. Although the effect of IG administration on the immune response to mumps vaccine is unknown, mumps vaccine should be given at least 2 weeks before or 3 months after administration of IG or blood transfusion because of the theoretical possibility that antibody will neutralize vaccine virus and interfere with successful immunization. Because high doses of IG (such as doses given for treatment of Kawasaki disease) can inhibit the response to measles vaccine for longer intervals, MMR and MMRV immunization should be deferred for a longer period after administration of IG (see Measles, p 444).

Altered Immunity. Patients with immunodeficiency diseases and people receiving immunosuppressive therapy (eg, patients with leukemia, lymphoma, or generalized malignant disease), including high doses of systemically administered corticosteroids, alkylating agents, antimetabolites, or radiation, or people who otherwise are immunocompromised should not receive mumps vaccine (see Immunocompromised Children, p 72). Exceptions are patients with HIV infection who are not immunocompromised severely (age-specific CD4+ T-lymphocyte counts of 15% or greater); these patients should be immunized against mumps with MMR vaccine (see Human Immunodeficiency Virus Infection, p 380). The risk of mumps exposure for patients with altered immunity can be decreased by immunizing their close susceptible contacts. Immunized people do not transmit mumps vaccine virus.

After cessation of immunosuppressive therapy, mumps immunization should be deferred for at least 3 months (with the exception of corticosteroid recipients [see the next paragraph]). This interval is based on the assumptions that immunologic responsiveness will have been restored in 3 months and the underlying disease for which immunosuppressive therapy was given is in remission or under control. However, because the interval can vary with the intensity and type of immunosuppressive therapy, radiation therapy, underlying disease, and other factors, a definitive recommendation for an interval after cessation of immunosuppressive therapy when mumps vaccine can be administered safely and effectively often is not possible.

Corticosteroids. For patients who have received high doses of corticosteroids (2 mg/kg/day or greater or greater than 20 mg/day of prednisone or equivalent) for 14 days or more and who otherwise are not immunocompromised, the recommended interval is at least 1 month, after corticosteroids are discontinued (see Immunocompromised Children, p 72).

Pregnancy. Conception should be avoided for 28 days after mumps immunization because of the theoretical risk associated with live-virus vaccine. Susceptible postpubertal females should not be immunized if they are known to be pregnant. Live-attenuated mumps virus vaccine can infect the placenta, although the virus has not been isolated from fetal tissues from susceptible females who received vaccine and underwent elective abortions. Mumps immunization during pregnancy has not been associated with congenital malformations (see Measles, p 444, and Rubella, p 579).

Outbreak Control. When determining means to control outbreaks, immunization or exclusion of students without evidence of immunity who refuse immunization from affected schools and schools judged by local public health authorities to be at risk of transmission should be considered. Excluded students can be readmitted immediately after immunization. Students who continue to be exempted from mumps immunization because of medical, religious, or other reasons should be excluded until at least 26 days after the onset of parotitis in the last person with mumps in the affected school. Experience with outbreak control for other vaccine-preventable diseases indicates that this strategy is effective. During an outbreak, a second dose of live mumps vaccine should be offered to the following groups: (1) children and adults for whom 1 dose routinely is recommended (preschool-aged children and low-risk adults), if these age groups are affected by the outbreak; (2) inadequately immunized people for whom 2 doses routinely are recommended (school and college students, health care professionals, international travelers); and (3) health care professionals born before 1957 without other evidence of immunity who previously have received 1 dose of mumps vaccine.

Mycoplasma pneumoniae and Other Mycoplasma Species Infections

CLINICAL MANIFESTATIONS: The most common clinical syndromes are acute bronchitis and upper respiratory tract infections, including pharyngitis and, occasionally, otitis media or myringitis, which may be bullous. Coryza, sinusitis, and croup are rare. Malaise, fever, and occasionally, headache are nonspecific manifestations of infection. In approximately 10% of school-aged children, pneumonia with cough and widespread rales on physical examination develops within a few days and lasts for 3 to 4 weeks. The cough often initially is nonproductive but later can become productive. Approximately 10% of children with pneumonia exhibit a rash, which most often is maculopapular. Radiographic abnormalities are variable, but bilateral, diffuse infiltrates are common, and focal abnormalities, such as consolidation, effusion, and hilar adenopathy, may occur.

Unusual manifestations include nervous system disease (eg, aseptic meningitis, encephalitis, acute disseminated encephalomyelitis, cerebellar ataxia, transverse myelitis, peripheral neuropathy) as well as myocarditis, pericarditis, polymorphous mucocutaneous eruptions (including Stevens-Johnson syndrome), hemolytic anemia, and arthritis. In patients with sickle cell disease, Down syndrome, immunodeficiencies, and chronic cardiorespiratory disease, severe pneumonia with pleural effusion may develop. A substantial proportion of acute chest syndrome and pneumonia associated with sickle cell disease appears to be attributable to *M pneumoniae*. *M pneumoniae* also has been associated with exacerbations of asthma.

Multiple other *Mycoplasma* species colonize mucosal surfaces of humans and can produce disease in children. *Mycoplasma hominis* infection has been reported in neonates and children (both immunocompetent and immunocompromised). Intra-abdominal abscesses, septic arthritis, endocarditis, pneumonia, meningoencephalitis, brain abscess, and surgical wound infections all have been reported. The diagnosis should be considered in children with a bacterial culture-negative purulent infection.

ETIOLOGY: Mycoplasmas, including *M pneumoniae*, lack a cell wall and are pleomorphic. Mycoplasmas cannot be detected using light microscopy.

EPIDEMIOLOGY: Mycoplasmas are ubiquitous in animals and plants, but *M pneumoniae* causes disease only in humans. *M pneumoniae* is transmissible by respiratory droplets during close contact with a symptomatic person. Outbreaks have been described in hospitals, military bases, colleges, and summer camps. Occasionally *M pneumoniae* causes ventilator-associated pneumonia. *M pneumoniae* is a leading cause of pneumonia in school-aged children and young adults and less frequently causes pneumonia in children younger than 5 years of age. Infections occur throughout the world, in any season, and in all geographic settings. Community-wide epidemics occur every 4 to 7 years. Rates of secondary infection are high within households of people with *M pneumoniae* infection. In family studies, approximately 30% of household contacts develop pneumonia. Asymptomatic carriage after infection may occur for weeks to months. Immunity after infection is not long lasting.

The **incubation period** usually is 2 to 3 weeks (range, 1–4 weeks).

DIAGNOSTIC TESTS: *M pneumoniae* can be grown in special enriched broth or agar media, but most clinical facilities lack the capacity to perform this culture. Isolation takes up to 21 days. *M pneumoniae* colonizes the respiratory tract for several weeks after acute infection despite appropriate therapy. Polymerase chain reaction (PCR) tests for *M pneumoniae* increasingly are available and have been used as the diagnostic tests at many medical centers and some reference laboratories. Where available, PCR has replaced other tests, because PCR enables more rapid diagnosis in acutely ill patients. Identification of *M pneumoniae* by PCR or in culture from a patient with compatible clinical manifestations suggests causation. No PCR kits are available commercially in the United States, and tests prepared at different institutions use different primer sequences and target different genes, which precludes generalizations about sensitivity and specificity.

Commercially available immunofluorescent tests and enzyme immunoassays detect *M pneumoniae*-specific immunoglobulin (Ig) M and IgG antibodies. IgM antibodies generally are not detectable within the first 7 days after onset of symptoms. Although the presence of IgM antibodies indicates recent *M pneumoniae* infection, antibodies persist in serum for several months and may not indicate current infection; false-positive test results also occur. Serologic diagnosis also can be made with the complement-fixation assay by demonstrating a fourfold or greater increase in antibody titer between acute and convalescent serum specimens. Complement-fixation assay results should be interpreted cautiously, because the assay is both less sensitive and less specific than is immunofluorescent assay or enzyme immunoassay. IgM antibody titer peaks at approximately 3 to 6 weeks and persists for 2 to 3 months after infection.

Serum cold hemagglutinin titers traditionally were considered a marker of *M pneumoniae* infection but are positive in only 50% of patients with pneumonia caused by *M pneumoniae*. Serum cold hemagglutinin titers also are nonspecific, because titers can be increased in adenovirus, Epstein-Barr virus, and measles infections. The diagnosis of mycoplasma-associated central nervous system disease (acute or postinfectious) is controversial. No single test has adequate sensitivity or specificity to establish this diagnosis.

The organism can be recognized in clinical laboratories by noting growth on blood agar plates of translucent colonies noted after 2 to 3 days of incubation. When Gram stain of the colonies is performed, no bacteria are noted. PCR assay of body fluids for *Mycoplasma hominis* is available at reference laboratories and may be helpful diagnostically.

TREATMENT: Acute bronchitis and upper respiratory tract illness caused by *M pneumoniae* generally are mild and self-limited. No evidence supports routine testing or antimicrobial therapy for these syndromes. Observational data indicate that children with pneumonia attributable to *M pneumoniae* have shorter duration of symptoms and fewer relapses when treated with an antimicrobial agent active against *M pneumoniae*. There is no evidence that treatment of nonrespiratory tract disease with antimicrobial agents alters the course of illness. Routine antimycoplasma therapy for asthma is inappropriate unless specific findings of pneumonia are present. Because mycoplasmas lack a cell wall, they inherently are resistant to beta-lactam agents. Macrolides, including erythromycin, azithromycin, and clarithromycin, are the preferred antimicrobial agents for treatment of pneumonia in children younger than 8 years of age. Tetracycline and doxycycline also are effective and may be used for children 8 years of age and older. Fluoroquinolones are effective but are not recommended as first-line agents for children.

M hominis usually is resistant to erythromycin and azithromycin but generally is susceptible to clindamycin, tetracyclines, and fluoroquinolones.

ISOLATION OF THE HOSPITALIZED PATIENT: In addition to standard precautions, droplet precautions are recommended for the duration of symptomatic illness.

CONTROL MEASURES: Hand hygiene lowers household transmission of respiratory pathogens and should be encouraged.

Tetracycline or azithromycin prophylaxis for close contacts has been shown to limit transmission in family and institutional outbreaks. However, antimicrobial prophylaxis for asymptomatic exposed contacts is not recommended routinely, because most secondary illnesses will be mild and self-limited. Prophylaxis with a macrolide or tetracycline can be considered for people at increased risk of severe illness with *M pneumoniae*, such as children with sickle cell disease who are close contacts of a person who is acutely ill with *M pneumoniae*.

Household contacts who have symptoms of cough and fever should be monitored for development of pneumonia. The administration of antimicrobial agents for symptomatic household contacts who do not have pneumonia has not been evaluated systematically.

Nocardiosis

CLINICAL MANIFESTATIONS: Immunocompetent children typically develop cutaneous or lymphocutaneous disease with pustular or ulcerative lesions that remain localized after soil contamination of a skin injury. Invasive disease occurs most commonly in immunocompromised patients, particularly people with chronic granulomatous disease, organ transplantation, human immunodeficiency virus infection, or disease requiring long-term systemic corticosteroid therapy. In these children, infection characteristically begins in the lungs, and illness can be acute, subacute, or chronic. Pulmonary disease commonly manifests as rounded nodular infiltrates that can undergo cavitation. Hematogenous spread may occur from the lungs to the brain (single or multiple abscesses), in skin (pustules, pyoderma, abscesses, mycetoma), or occasionally in other organs. *Nocardia* organisms can be recovered from patients with cystic fibrosis, but their role as a lung pathogen is not clear.

ETIOLOGY: *Nocardia* species are aerobic actinomycetes, a large and diverse group of gram-positive bacteria, which include *Actinomyces israelii* (the cause of actinomycosis), *Rhodococcus equi*, and *Tropheryma whippelii* (Whipple disease). Pulmonary or disseminated disease most commonly is caused by the *Nocardia asteroides* complex, which includes *Nocardia farcinica* and *Nocardia nova*. Primary cutaneous disease most commonly is caused by *Nocardia brasiliensis*. *Nocardia pseudobrasiliensis* is associated with pulmonary, central nervous system (CNS), or systemic nocardiosis. Other pathogenic species include *Nocardia abscessus*, *Nocardia otitidiscaviarum*, *Nocardia transvalensis*, *Nocardia veterana*, *Nocardia cyriacigeorgica*, and *Nocardia paucivarans*.

EPIDEMIOLOGY: Found worldwide, *Nocardia* species are ubiquitous environmental saprophytes living in soil, organic matter, and water. Lungs are the portals of entry for pulmonary or disseminated disease. Direct skin inoculation occurs, often as the result of contact with contaminated soil after trauma. Person-to-person and animal-to-human transmission do not occur.

The **incubation period** for pulmonary disease is unknown.

DIAGNOSTIC TESTS: Isolation of *Nocardia* organisms from body fluid, abscess material, or tissue specimens provides a definitive diagnosis. Stained smears of sputum, body fluids, or pus demonstrating beaded, branched, weakly gram-positive, variably acid-fast rods suggest the diagnosis. Brown and Brenn and methenamine silver stains are recommended to demonstrate microorganisms in tissue specimens. *Nocardia* organisms are slow growing but grow readily on blood and chocolate agar in 3 to 5 days. Cultures from normally sterile sites should be maintained for 3 weeks in an appropriate liquid medium. Serologic tests for *Nocardia* species are not useful.

TREATMENT: Trimethoprim-sulfamethoxazole or a sulfonamide alone (eg, sulfisoxazole or sulfamethoxazole) has been the drug of choice. Preparations that are less urine soluble, such as sulfadiazine, should be avoided. In some areas, sulfonamide resistance has led to the use of carbapenems in severely ill patients. Immunocompetent patients with primary lymphocutaneous disease usually respond after 6 to 12 weeks of therapy. Drainage of abscesses is beneficial. Immunocompromised patients and patients with invasive disease should be treated for 6 to 12 months and for at least 3 months after apparent cure because of the tendency for relapse. Patients with acquired immunodeficiency syndrome may need even longer therapy. For patients with CNS disease, disseminated disease, or overwhelming infection, amikacin plus ceftriaxone (on the basis of in vitro susceptibility testing) should be included for the first 4 to 12 weeks of treatment or until the patient's condition is improved clinically. Patients with meningitis or brain abscess should be monitored with serial neuroimaging studies. If infection does not respond to trimethoprim-sulfamethoxazole, other agents, such as clarithromycin *(N nova)*, amoxicillin-clavulanate *(N brasiliensis* and *N abscessus)*, imipenem, or meropenem may be beneficial. Linezolid is highly active against all *Nocardia* species in vitro; case series including a small number of patients demonstrate that linezolid may be effective for treatment of invasive infections. Drug susceptibility testing is recommended by the Clinical and Laboratory Standards Institute for isolates from patients with invasive disease and patients who are unable to tolerate a sulfonamide.

ISOLATION OF THE HOSPITALIZED PATIENT: Standard precautions are recommended.

CONTROL MEASURES: None.

Onchocerciasis
(River Blindness, Filariasis)

CLINICAL MANIFESTATIONS: The disease involves skin, subcutaneous tissues, lymphatic vessels, and eyes. Subcutaneous, nontender nodules of varying sizes containing adult worms develop 6 to 12 months after initial infection. In patients in Africa, nodules tend to be found on the lower torso, pelvis, and lower extremities, whereas in patients in Central and South America, the nodules more often are located on the upper body (the head and trunk) but may occur on the extremities. After the worms mature, microfilariae are produced that migrate to the tissues and may cause a chronic, pruritic, papular dermatitis. After a period of years, skin can become lichenified and hypo- or hyperpigmented. The presence of living or dead microfilariae in the ocular structures leads to photophobia and inflammation of the cornea, iris, ciliary body, retina, choroid, and optic nerve. Loss of visual acuity and blindness can result if the disease is untreated.

ETIOLOGY: *Onchocerca volvulus* is a filarial nematode.

EPIDEMIOLOGY: *O volvulus* has no significant animal reservoir. Microfilariae in skin infect *Simulium* species flies when they take a blood meal and then in 10 to 14 days develop into infectious larvae that are transmitted with subsequent bites. Black flies breed in fast-flowing streams and rivers (hence the colloquial name of the disease, "river blindness"). The disease occurs primarily in equatorial Africa, but small foci are found in southern Mexico, Guatemala, northern South America, and Yemen. Prevalence is greatest among people who live near vector breeding sites. The infection is not transmissible by person-to-person contact or blood transfusion.

The **incubation period** from larval inoculation to microfilariae in the skin usually is 6 to 12 months but can be as long as 3 years.

DIAGNOSTIC TESTS: Direct examination of a 1- to 2-mg shaving or biopsy specimen of the epidermis and upper dermis (taken from the iliac crest area) can reveal microfilariae. Microfilariae are not found in blood. Adult worms may be demonstrated in excised nodules that have been sectioned and stained. A slit-lamp examination of the anterior chamber of an involved eye may reveal motile microfilariae or "snowflake" corneal lesions. Eosinophilia is common. Specific serologic tests and polymerase chain reaction techniques for detection of microfilariae in skin are available only in research laboratories.

TREATMENT: Ivermectin, a microfilaricidal agent, is the drug of choice for treatment of onchocerciasis. Treatment decreases dermatitis and the risk of developing severe ocular disease but does not kill the adult worms (which can live for more than a decade) and, thus, is not curative. One single oral dose of ivermectin (150 µg/kg) should be given every 6 to 12 months until asymptomatic. Adverse reactions to treatment are caused by the death of microfilariae and can include rash, edema, fever, myalgia, and rarely, asthma exacerbation and hypotension. Precautions to ivermectin treatment include pregnancy, breastfeeding (in the first week), central nervous system disorders, and high levels of circulating *Loa loa* microfilariaemia. Safety and effectiveness in pediatric patients weighing less than 15 kg have not been established. A 6-week course of doxycycline has been demonstrated to render adult female worms sterile for long periods of time and may be considered as adjunctive therapy for children 8 years of age or older and nonpregnant adults. Diethylcarbamazine is contraindicated, as it may cause adverse ocular reactions.

ISOLATION OF THE HOSPITALIZED PATIENT: Standard precautions are recommended.

CONTROL MEASURES: Repellents and protective clothing (long sleeves and pants) can decrease exposure to bites from black flies, which bite by day. Treatment of vector breeding sites with larvicides has been effective for controlling black fly populations, particularly in West Africa. A highly successful initiative being led by the World Health Organization has mass distributed hundreds of millions of ivermectin treatments (which is donated by the drug manufacturer for this purpose) to communities with severe endemic disease from onchocerciasis. There is no vaccine available for onchocerciasis.

Human Papillomaviruses

CLINICAL MANIFESTATIONS: Most human papillomavirus (HPV) infections produce no lesions and are inapparent clinically. However, HPVs can produce benign epithelial proliferation (warts) of the skin and mucous membranes and are associated with anogenital dysplasias and cancers. Cutaneous nongenital warts include common skin warts, plantar warts, flat warts, thread-like (filiform) warts, and epidermodysplasia verruciformis. Warts also occur on the mucous membranes, including the anogenital, oral, nasal, and conjunctival areas and the respiratory tract, where respiratory papillomatosis occurs.

Common **skin warts** are dome-shaped with conical projections that give the surface a rough appearance. They usually are painless and multiple, occurring commonly on the hands and around or under the nails. When small dermal vessels become thrombosed, black dots appear in the warts. Plantar warts on the foot may be painful and are characterized by marked hyperkeratosis, sometimes with black dots.

Flat warts ("juvenile warts") commonly are found on the face and extremities of children and adolescents. They usually are small, multiple, and flat topped; seldom exhibit papillomatosis; and rarely cause pain. Filiform warts occur on the face and neck. Cutaneous warts are benign.

Anogenital warts, also called **condylomata acuminata,** are skin-colored warts with a cauliflower-like surface that range in size from a few millimeters to several centimeters. In males, these warts may be found on the penis, scrotum, or anal and perianal area. In females, these lesions may occur on the vulva or perianal areas and less commonly in the vagina or on the cervix. Anogenital warts often are multiple and attract attention because of their appearance. Warts usually are painless, although they may cause itching, burning, local pain, or bleeding.

Persistent anogenital HPV infection may be associated with clinically apparent dysplastic lesions, particularly in the female genital tract (cervix and vagina). Abnormal cells associated with these lesions often are detected during Pap smear testing of the cervix and are classified morphologically as representing low- or high-grade squamous intraepithelial lesions (L-SIL or H-SIL, respectively). On biopsy, these precursor lesions are classified as low-grade cervical intraepithelial neoplasia (CIN 1) or high-grade cervical intraepithelial neoplasia (CIN 2 or 3). Over 1 to 2 decades, persistent HPV infection with high-risk HPV types can undergo neoplastic progression and lead to invasive cancers of the cervix, vagina, or vulva. In addition, HPV is the causal agent of many anal, penile, and oropharyngeal cancers.

Juvenile recurrent respiratory papillomatosis is a rare condition character-ized by recurring papillomas in the larynx or other areas of the upper respiratory tract. This condition is diagnosed most commonly in children between 2 and 5 years of age and manifests as a voice change, stridor, or abnormal cry. Respiratory papillomas have been associated with respiratory tract obstruction in young children. Adult onset also has been described.

Epidermodysplasia verruciformis is a rare, lifelong, severe papillomavirus infection believed to be a consequence of an inherited deficiency of cell-mediated immu-nity. Lesions may resemble flat warts but often are similar to tinea versicolor, covering the torso and upper extremities. Most appear during the first decade of life, but malignant transformation, which occurs in approximately one third of affected people, usually is delayed until adulthood.

ETIOLOGY: Human papillomaviruses are members of the *Papillomavirus* family and are DNA viruses. More than 100 types have been identified. These viruses are grouped into cutaneous and mucosal types on the basis of their tendency to infect particular types of epithelium. Most often, HPV types found in nongenital warts will be cutaneous types, and those in respiratory papillomatosis, anogenital warts, dysplasias, or cancers will be mucosal types. More than 40 HPV types can infect the genital tract. On the basis of their epidemiologic association with cancers, mucosal HPVs are divided into low-risk and high-risk types. More than 18 high-risk types are recognized, with types 16, 18, 31, and 45 most frequently being associated with cervical cancer, and types 16 and 18 most frequently being associated with oropharyngeal cancers. Types 6 and 11 frequently are associated with condylomata acuminata, recurrent respiratory papillomatosis, and con-junctival papillomas and carcinomas.

EPIDEMIOLOGY: Papillomaviruses are distributed widely among mammals and are species-specific. Cutaneous warts occur commonly among school-aged children; the prevalence rate is as high as 50%. HPV infections are transmitted from person to person by close contact. Nongenital warts are acquired through contact with HPV and minor trauma to the skin. An increase in the incidence of plantar warts has been associated with swimming in public pools. The intense and often widespread appearance of warts in patients with compromised cellular immunity (particularly patients who have undergone transplantation and people with human immunodeficiency virus infection) suggests that alterations in immunity predispose to reactivation of latent intraepithelial infection.

Anogenital HPV infection is the most common sexually transmitted infection in the United States. Most infections are transient and clear spontaneously. Anogenital HPV infections are transmitted primarily by sexual contact and most are subclinical. Persistent infection with high-risk types of HPV is associated with development of cervical cancer, with more than 10 000 new cases and 3700 deaths attributed to HPV annually, and with vulvar and vaginal cancers.

Rarely, infection is transmitted to a child through the birth canal during delivery or transmitted from nongenital sites. Respiratory papillomatosis is believed to be acquired by aspiration of infectious secretions during passage through an infected birth canal. When anogenital warts are found in a child who is beyond infancy but is prepubertal, sexual abuse must be considered.

The **incubation period** is unknown but is estimated to range from 3 months to several years. Papillomavirus acquired by a neonate at the time of birth may never cause clinical disease or may become apparent over several years (eg, respiratory papillomatosis). Anogenital and pharyngeal malignant neoplasias are rare long-term sequelae of chronic persistent infection, usually occurring more than 10 years after infection.

DIAGNOSTIC TESTS: Most cutaneous and anogenital warts are diagnosed through clinical inspection. Respiratory papillomatosis is diagnosed using endoscopy and biopsy. Cervical dysplasias may be detected via (1) cytologic examination of exfoliated cells in a Papanicolaou (Pap) test, either by conventional or liquid-based cytology; or (2) histologic examination of cervical tissue biopsy. Cervical biopsy can show HPV-associated lesions such as warts, dysplasias, and carcinomas. Although characteristic cytologic and histologic changes may suggest the presence of HPV, diagnosing infection requires a molecular test.

Although HPV can be propagated under special laboratory conditions, it cannot be cultured from patient samples; therefore, a definitive diagnosis of HPV infection is based on detection of viral nucleic acid (DNA or RNA) or capsid protein. A test that detects high-risk types of HPV DNA in exfoliated cells obtained from the cervix is available for clinical use (Hybrid Capture 2 [Digene]). The test detects any of 13 high-risk types, and the result is reported as negative or positive. The test is recommended for use in combination with Pap testing in specific circumstances to help determine whether further assessments, such as colposcopy, are necessary.

TREATMENT[1]**:** Treatment of HPV infection is directed toward eliminating lesions that result from the infection rather than HPV itself. Most nongenital warts eventually regress spontaneously but may persist for months or years. The optimal treatment for warts that do not resolve spontaneously has not been identified. Most methods of treatment use

---

[1]Centers for Disease Control and Prevention. Sexually transmitted diseases treatment guidelines—2006. *MMWR Recomm Rep.* 2006;55(RR-11):1–94

chemical or physical destruction of the infected epithelium, such as application of salicylic acid products, cryotherapy with liquid nitrogen, or laser or surgical removal of warts. Daily treatment with tretinoin has been useful for widespread flat warts in children. Care must be taken to avoid a deleterious cosmetic result with therapy. Pharmacologic treatments for refractory warts, including cimetidine, have been used with varied success.

The optimal treatment for anogenital warts has not been identified. Spontaneous regression occurs within months in some cases. Treatments are characterized as patient applied or administered by a health care professional and include destructional/excisional treatments, antiproliferative methods, and immune-modulating therapy. Many of the agents used for treatment have not been tested for safety and efficacy in children, and some agents are contraindicated in pregnancy. Although most forms of therapy are successful for initial removal of warts, treatment may not eradicate HPV infection from the surrounding tissue. Recurrences are common and probably attributable to reactivation rather than reinfection. Patients should be followed-up during and after treatment for genital warts, because many treatments can result in local symptoms or adverse effects.

HPV infection of the cervix is common in sexually active adolescents and can be associated with epithelial dysplasia, commonly low-grade lesions. Routinely scheduled Pap screening of cervical cells should be initiated within 3 years of the onset of consensual or nonconsensual sexual activity or by 21 years of age, whichever occurs first. HPV testing should not be used routinely in females younger than 20 years of age. Adolescents with cervical dysplasia should be cared for by a physician who is knowledgeable in management of cervical dysplasia. The American Society for Colposcopy and Cervical Pathology's 2006 Consensus Guidelines for the Management of Women with Abnormal Cervical Cancer Screening Tests can be viewed at **www.asccp.org/consensus/ cytological.shtml.**

Respiratory papillomatosis is difficult to treat and is best managed by an otolaryngologist. Local recurrence is common, and repeated surgical procedures for removal often are necessary. Extension or dissemination of respiratory papillomas from the larynx into the trachea, bronchi, or lung parenchyma can result in increased morbidity and mortality. Intralesional interferon, indole-3-carbinole, photodynamic therapy, and intralesional cidofovir have been used as investigational treatments and may be of benefit for patients with frequent recurrences.

Oral warts can be removed through cryotherapy, electrocautery, or surgical excision.

ISOLATION OF THE HOSPITALIZED PATIENT: Standard precautions are recommended.

CONTROL MEASURES AND CARE OF EXPOSED PEOPLE: Suspected child abuse should be reported to the appropriate local agency if anogenital warts are found in a child who is beyond infancy but prepubertal.

Sexual abstinence, monogamous relationships, delayed sexual debut, and minimizing the number of sex partners are modes of reducing risk of anogenital HPV infection. Consistent and correct use of latex condoms can decrease risk of anogenital HPV infection when the infected areas are covered or protected by the condom. In addition, use of latex condoms has been associated with a decrease in the risk of genital warts and cervical cancer. The degree and duration of contagiousness in patients with a history of genital infection is unknown.

Sex partners of people with genital warts may benefit from examination to assess for the presence of anogenital warts or other sexually transmitted infections. Cervical cancer screening guidelines are available from the American Cancer Society (**http://caonline.amcancersoc.org/cgi/content/short/52/6/342**) and the US Preventive Services Task Force (**www.ahrq.gov/clinic/uspstf/uspscerv.htm**).

Although infection with HPV types 6 and 11 leading to respiratory papillomatosis is believed to be acquired during passage through the birth canal, this condition has occurred in infants born by cesarean delivery. Because the preventive value of cesarean delivery is unknown, it should not be performed solely to prevent transmission of HPV to the newborn infant.

HPV Vaccines. A quadrivalent (HPV4 [types 6, 11, 16 and 18]) vaccine (Gardasil [Merck & Co Inc]) was licensed for use in the United States by the US Food and Drug Administration (FDA) in June, 2006. An application for FDA licensure for a bivalent (HPV2 [types 16 and 18]) vaccine (Cervarix [GlaxoSmithKline]) was submitted to the FDA in March 2007. Both vaccines have been found to be highly effective in preventing infection and disease associated with types included in the vaccines. The Advisory Committee on Immunization Practices (ACIP) and the AAP recommended HPV4 vaccine for routine immunization of females 11 through 12 years of age (although the series can be started at 9 years of age) and catch-up immunization of females 13 through 26 years of age. Recommendations will be developed for HPV2 vaccine when the vaccine is licensed by the FDA. HPV2 vaccine is available in several other countries. Although a successful immunization program holds particular promise for reduction in the incidence of cervical cancer, women who have received an HPV vaccine must continue to have regular Pap testing, because the vaccine does not provide protection against all HPV types associated with development of cervical cancer or infection acquired before immunization.

Vaccine Recommendations.[1,2] Antigens in HPV4 vaccine are the L1 major capsid proteins of HPV types 6, 11, 16, and 18, expressed in *Saccharomyces cerevisiae* (baker's yeast). These proteins self-assemble into immunogenic virus-like particles (VLPs), which contain no infectious material. After purification, VLPs are absorbed on an aluminum-containing adjuvant.

Dosage and Administration. The recommended dose of HPV4 vaccine is 0.5 mL, administered to females by intramuscular administration in 3 doses. The second dose should be administered 2 months after the first dose, and the third dose should be administered 6 months after the first dose.

- The minimal interval between doses 1 and 2 is 4 weeks.
- The minimal interval between doses 2 and 3 is 12 weeks (and at least 24 weeks after the first dose).
- If the vaccine schedule is interrupted, the vaccine series does not need to be restarted.
- Doses of vaccine received after a shorter-than-recommended interval should be readministered.

---

[1] Centers for Disease Control and Prevention. Quadrivalent human papillomavirus vaccine: recommendations of the Advisory Committee on Immunization Practices (ACIP). *MMWR Recomm Rep.* 2007;56(RR-2):1–24. Available at: **http://www.cdc.gov/mmwr/PDF/rr/rr5602.pdf**

[2] American Academy of Pediatrics, Committee on Infectious Diseases. Prevention of human papillomavirus infection: provisional recommendations for immunization of girls and women with quadrivalent human papillomavirus vaccine. *Pediatrics.* 2007;120(3):666–668

- Vaccine recipients should be seated and observed for 15 minutes after immunization because of the risk of syncope in adolescents receiving injections.

The vaccine is available in single-dose vials and prefilled syringes and contains no antimicrobial agents or thimerosal. The vaccine should be stored at 2°C to 8°C (36°F–46°F) and not frozen. Recommendations for use of HPV4 vaccine are as follows:

- Routine immunization of females 11 through 12 years of age; the series can be started as young as 9 years of age.
- Immunization of females 13 through 26 years of age who have not been immunized previously with the complete series.

Females with evidence of current HPV infection, such as cervical dysplasia, a positive HPV DNA test result, or anogenital warts should receive immunization, because infection with all 4 vaccine HPV types is unlikely and the vaccine could provide protection against HPV infection with types not already acquired.

The vaccine currently is not licensed for use in males or in females younger than 9 years of age or older than 26 years of age. Studies are ongoing to assess efficacy of vaccine use in males and in females 27 through 45 years of age.

Efficacy. Studies of HPV4 vaccine among 15- through 26-year-old females who were naive to all 4 HPV vaccine types demonstrated efficacy against cervical, vulvar, and vaginal cancers caused by HPV types 16 and 18; genital warts caused by HPV types 6 and 11; and precancerous dysplastic lesions caused by types 6, 11, 16, and 18.

The vaccine offers no protection against cervical cancer caused by high-risk HPV acquired before immunization. Females infected with one or more of the HPV types contained in the vaccine before immunization are, when immunized, are protected against disease caused by the other vaccine types. Studies through 5 years have shown no waning of protection.

Immunogenicity. In immunogenicity studies, more than 99% or more of healthy vaccine recipients develop antibodies against the virus-like particles in the vaccine 1 month after receipt of the third dose. Antibody responses in young adolescent females 9 through 15 years of age were higher than in antibody responses in females 16 through 26 years of age. Antibody titers decrease over time after the third dose but plateau by 18 through 24 months after receipt of the third dose. At 5 years, antibody titers remained well above those associated with naturally acquired HPV infection. A serologic correlate of immunity is not established for HPV vaccine.

Precautions and Contraindications.

- HPV vaccine can be administered to people with minor acute illnesses.
- Immunization of people with moderate or severe acute illnesses should be deferred until after the patient improves.
- HPV vaccine is contraindicated in people with a history of immediate hypersensitivity to yeast or to any vaccine component.
- The vaccine is not recommended for use during pregnancy. The practitioner should inquire about pregnancy in sexually active patients, but a pregnancy test is not required before starting the immunization series. If a vaccine recipient becomes pregnant, subsequent doses should be postponed until the postpartum period. Limited data show no adverse effect of HPV vaccine on pregnancy. For a pregnant woman who inadvertently receives the HPV vaccine, a vaccine-in-pregnancy registry has been established (1-800-986-8999) to monitor outcomes of exposure during pregnancy.

- The vaccine may be administered to lactating women.
- HPV may be administered to immunocompromised females, but the immune response and vaccine efficacy may be reduced in such recipients.

Paracoccidioidomycosis
(South American Blastomycosis)

CLINICAL MANIFESTATIONS: Disease occurs primarily in adults and is rare in children. The site of initial infection is the lungs. Clinical patterns are categorized as an acute-subacute form that predominates in childhood and a chronic form that is the typical clinical pattern in adults. In both forms, constitutional symptoms, such as fever, malaise, and weight loss, are common. In the more common acute-subacute form, symptoms are related to the extensive involvement of the reticuloendothelial system with enlarged lymph nodes and involvement of liver, spleen, bone marrow, and bones as well as joints, skin, and mucous membranes. Occasionally, enlarged lymph nodes coalesce and form abscesses or fistulas. The chronic form of the illness can be localized to the lungs or can disseminate. Oral, upper respiratory tract, and gastrointestinal tract granulomatous or ulcerative mucosal lesions are a less common manifestation of disease in children than in adults. Infection can be latent for years before causing illness.

ETIOLOGY: *Paracoccidioides brasiliensis* is a dimorphic fungus with a yeast and a mycelial phase.

EPIDEMIOLOGY: The infection occurs in Latin America, from Mexico to Argentina. The natural reservoir is unknown, although soil is suspected. The mode of transmission is unknown; person-to-person transmission does not occur.

The **incubation period** is highly variable, ranging from 1 month to many years.

DIAGNOSTIC TESTS: Round, multiple-budding cells with a distinguishing pilot's wheel appearance can be seen in 10% potassium hydroxide preparations of sputum specimens, bronchoalveolar lavage specimens, scrapings from ulcers, and material from lesions or in tissue biopsy specimens. The organism can be cultured on most enriched media, including blood agar at 37°C (98°F) and Sabouraud dextrose agar (with cycloheximide) at 24°C (75°F). Complement fixation, enzyme immunoassay, and immunodiffusion methods are useful for detecting specific antibodies.

TREATMENT: Amphotericin B is preferred by many experts for treatment of people with severe paracoccidioidomycosis, but amphotericin B is not curative (see Drugs for Invasive and Other Serious Fungal Infections, p 772). Itraconazole is the drug of choice for less severe or localized infection and to complete treatment when amphotericin B is used initially. Prolonged therapy for at least 6 months is necessary to minimize the relapse rate. Itraconazole is associated with fewer adverse effects and has a lower relapse rate (3%–5%) than does ketoconazole, which is an alternative drug. A sulfonamide (trimethoprim-sulfamethoxazole) can be used in resource-limited countries, but maintenance treatment must be continued for 3 to 5 years to lessen the risk of relapse, which occurs in 10% to 15% of optimally treated patients. Voriconazole and itraconazole may be alternatives, but data for their use in children with paracoccidioidomycosis are not available.

ISOLATION OF THE HOSPITALIZED PATIENT: Standard precautions are recommended.

CONTROL MEASURES: None.

Paragonimiasis

CLINICAL MANIFESTATIONS: There are 2 major forms of paragonimiasis: 1) disease attributable to *Paragonimus westermani* and *Paragonimus heterotremus*, causing primary pulmonary disease with or without extrapulmonary manifestations; and 2) disease attributable to other species of *Paragonimus*, for which humans are accidental hosts and manifestations generally are extrapulmonary, resulting in a larva migrans syndrome. The disease has an insidious onset and a chronic course. Pulmonary disease is associated with chronic cough and dyspnea, but most infections probably are inapparent or result in mild symptoms. Heavy infestations cause paroxysms of coughing, which often produce blood-tinged sputum that is brown because of the presence of *Paragonimus* species eggs. Hemoptysis can be severe. Pleural effusion, pneumothorax, bronchiectasis, and pulmonary fibrosis with clubbing can develop. Extrapulmonary manifestations also may involve liver, spleen, abdominal cavity, intestinal wall, intra-abdominal lymph nodes, skin, and central nervous system, with meningoencephalitis, seizures, and space-occupying tumors attributable to invasion of the brain by adult flukes, usually occurring within a year of pulmonary infection. Symptoms tend to subside after approximately 5 years but can persist for as many as 20 years.

Extrapulmonary paragonimiasis is associated with migratory allergic subcutaneous nodules containing juvenile worms. Pleural effusion is common, as is invasion of the brain.

ETIOLOGY: In Asia, classical paragonimiasis is caused by *P westermani* and *P heterotremus* adult flukes and their eggs. The adult flukes of *P westermani* are up to 12 mm long and 7 mm wide and occur throughout the Far East. A triploid parthenogenetic form of *P westermani*, which is larger, produces more eggs and elicits greater disease, has been described in Japan, Korea, Taiwan, and parts of eastern China. *P heterotremus* occurs in Southeast Asia and adjacent parts of China. Extrapulmonary paragonimiasis is caused by larval stages of *Paragonimus skrjabini* and *Paragonimus miyazakii*. The worms rarely mature. *P skrjabini* occurs in China, and *P miyazakii* occurs in Japan. African forms causing extrapulmonary paragonimiasis include *Paragonimus africanus* (Nigeria, Cameroon) and *Paragonimus uterobilateralis* (Liberia, Guinea, Nigeria, Gabon). *Paragonimus mexicanus* and *Paragonimus ecuadoriensis* occur in Mexico, Costa Rica, Ecuador, and Peru. *Paragonimus kellicotti*, a lung fluke of mink and opossums in the United States, also can cause a zoonotic infection in humans.

EPIDEMIOLOGY: Transmission occurs when raw or undercooked freshwater crabs or crayfish containing larvae (metacercariae) are ingested. The metacercariae excyst in the small intestine and penetrate the abdominal cavity, where they remain for a few days before migrating to the lungs. *P westermani* and *P heterotremus* mature within the lungs over 6 to 10 weeks, when they then begin egg production. Eggs escape from pulmonary capsules into the bronchi and exit from the human host in sputum or feces. Eggs hatch in freshwater within 3 weeks, giving rise to miracidia. Miracidia penetrate freshwater snails and emerge several weeks later as cercariae, which encyst within the muscles and viscera of freshwater crustaceans before maturing into infective metacercariae. Transmission also occurs when humans ingest raw pork, usually from wild pigs, containing the juvenile stages of *Paragonimus* species (described as occurring in Japan).

Humans are accidental ("dead-end") hosts for *P skrjabini* and *P miyazakii*. These flukes cannot mature in humans and, hence, do not produce eggs.

Paragonimus species also infect a variety of other mammals, such as canids, mustelids, felids, and rodents, which can serve as animal reservoir hosts.

The **incubation period** is variable; egg production begins approximately 8 weeks after ingestion of *P westermani* metacercariae.

DIAGNOSTIC TESTS: Microscopic examination of stool, sputum, pleural effusion, cerebrospinal fluid, and other tissue specimens may reveal eggs. A Western blot serologic antibody test, available at the Centers for Disease Control and Prevention (CDC), is sensitive and specific; antibody levels detected by immunoblot decrease slowly after the infection is cured by treatment. Charcot-Leyden crystals and eosinophils in sputum are useful diagnostic elements. Chest radiographs may appear normal or resemble radiographs from patients with tuberculosis. Misdiagnosis is likely unless paragonimiasis is suspected.

TREATMENT: Praziquantel in a 2-day course is the treatment of choice and is associated with high cure rates as demonstrated by disappearance of egg production and radiographic lesions in the lungs. The drug also is effective for some extrapulmonary manifestations. Bithionol, available from the CDC, is an alternative drug (see Drugs for Parasitic Infections, p 783).

ISOLATION OF THE HOSPITALIZED PATIENT: Standard precautions are recommended.

CONTROL MEASURES: Cooking of crabs and crayfish for several minutes until the meat has congealed and turned opaque kills metacercariae. Similarly, meat from wild pigs should be well cooked before eating. Control of animal reservoirs is not possible.

Parainfluenza Viral Infections

CLINICAL MANIFESTATIONS: Parainfluenza viruses are the major cause of laryngotracheobronchitis (croup), but they also commonly cause upper respiratory tract infection, pneumonia, and/or bronchiolitis.[1] Parainfluenza virus types 1 and 2 are the most common pathogens associated with croup, and parainfluenza virus type 3 most commonly is associated with bronchiolitis and pneumonia in infants and young children. Rarely, parotitis, aseptic meningitis, and encephalitis have been associated with type 3 infections. Parainfluenza virus infections can exacerbate symptoms of chronic lung disease in children and adults. Infections particularly can be severe and persistent in immunodeficient children and are associated most commonly with type 3 virus. Infections with type 4 virus are not as well characterized, but studies using reverse transcriptase-polymerase chain reaction assays suggest that they may be more common than previously appreciated. Parainfluenza infections do not confer complete protective immunity; therefore, reinfections can occur with all serotypes and at any age, but reinfections usually cause a mild illness limited to the upper respiratory tract.

ETIOLOGY: Parainfluenza viruses are enveloped RNA viruses classified as paramyxoviruses. Four antigenically distinct types—1, 2, 3, and 4 (with 2 subtypes, 4A and 4B)—have been identified.

EPIDEMIOLOGY: Parainfluenza viruses are transmitted from person to person by direct contact and exposure to contaminated nasopharyngeal secretions through respiratory tract droplets and fomites. Parainfluenza viral infections produce sporadic infections as

---

[1] American Academy of Pediatrics Subcommittee on Diagnosis and Management of Bronchiolitis. Diagnosis and management of bronchiolitis. *Pediatrics.* 2006;118(4):1774–1793

well as epidemics of disease. Seasonal patterns of infection are distinctive, predictable, and cyclic. Different serotypes have distinct epidemiologic patterns. Type 1 virus tends to produce outbreaks of respiratory tract illness, usually croup, in the autumn of every other year. A major increase in the number of cases of croup in the autumn usually indicates a parainfluenza type 1 outbreak. Type 2 virus also can cause outbreaks of respiratory tract illness in the autumn, often in conjunction with type 1 outbreaks, but type 2 outbreaks tend to be less severe, irregular, and less common. Parainfluenza type 3 virus usually is prominent during spring and summer in temperate climates but often continues into autumn, especially in years when autumn outbreaks of parainfluenza virus types 1 or 2 are absent. Infections with type 4 virus are recognized less commonly and can be associated with mild to severe illnesses.

The age of primary infection varies with serotype. Primary infection with all types usually occurs by 5 years of age. Infection with type 3 virus more often occurs in infants and is a prominent cause of lower respiratory tract illnesses. By 12 months of age, 50% of infants have acquired type 3 infection. Infections between 1 and 5 years of age are associated most commonly with type 1 virus and less so with type 2 virus. Age at acquisition of type 4 infection is not as well understood.

Immunocompetent children with primary parainfluenza infection may shed virus for up to 1 week before onset of clinical symptoms and until 1 to 3 weeks after symptoms have disappeared, depending on serotype. Severe lower respiratory tract disease with prolonged shedding of the virus can develop in immunodeficient people. In these patients, infection may spread beyond the respiratory tract to the liver and lymph nodes.

The **incubation period** ranges from 2 to 6 days.

DIAGNOSTIC TESTS: Rapid antigen identification techniques, including immunofluorescent assays, enzyme immunoassays, and fluoroimmunoassays, can be used to detect the virus in nasopharyngeal secretions, but the sensitivities of the tests vary. Virus may be isolated from nasopharyngeal secretions usually within 4 to 7 days of culture inoculation or earlier by using centrifugation of a specimen onto a monolayer of susceptible cells with subsequent staining for viral antigen (shell viral assay). Confirmation is made by rapid antigen detection, usually immunofluorescent. Reverse transcriptase-polymerase chain reaction assays, with high sensitivity and specificity, are available for detection and differentiation of parainfluenza viruses. Serologic diagnosis, made retrospectively by a significant increase in antibody titer between serum specimens obtained during acute infection and convalescence, is less useful, because infection may not always be accompanied by a significant homotypic antibody response.

TREATMENT: Specific antiviral therapy is not available. Most infections are self-limited and require no treatment. Monitoring for hypoxia and hypercapnia in more severely affected children with lower respiratory tract disease may be helpful. The following treatment recommendations apply to laryngotracheobronchitis. Racemic epinephrine aerosol commonly is given to severely affected, hospitalized patients with laryngotracheobronchitis to decrease airway obstruction. Parenteral dexamethasone in high doses, oral dexamethasone, and nebulized corticosteroids have been demonstrated to lessen the severity and duration of symptoms and hospitalization in patients with moderate to severe laryngotracheobronchitis. Oral dexamethasone also is effective for outpatients with less severe croup. Management otherwise is supportive. Antimicrobial agents should be reserved for documented secondary bacterial infections.

ISOLATION OF THE HOSPITALIZED PATIENT: In addition to standard precautions, contact precautions are recommended for hospitalized infants and young children for the duration of illness. Strict adherence to infection-control procedures, including prevention of environmental contamination by respiratory tract secretions and careful hand hygiene, should control health care-associated spread. Immunocompromised patients with type 3 infection should be isolated to prevent health care-associated spread.

CONTROL MEASURES: Efforts should be aimed at decreasing health care-associated infection. Hand hygiene should be emphasized.

Parasitic Diseases

Many parasitic diseases traditionally have been considered exotic and, therefore, frequently are not included in differential diagnoses of patients in the United States, Canada, and Europe. Nevertheless, a number of these organisms are endemic in industrialized countries, and overall, parasites are among the most common causes of morbidity and mortality in various and diverse geographic locations worldwide. Outside the tropics and subtropics, parasitic diseases particularly are common among tourists returning to their own countries, immigrants from areas with highly endemic infection, and immunocompromised people. Physicians and clinical laboratory personnel need to be aware of where these infections may be acquired, their clinical presentations, and methods of diagnosis and should advise travelers how to prevent infection. Table 3.40 (p 488) gives details on some infrequently encountered parasitic diseases.

Consultation and assistance in diagnosis and management of parasitic diseases are available from the Centers for Disease Control and Prevention (CDC), state health departments, and university departments or divisions of geographic medicine, tropical medicine, pediatric infectious disease, international health, and public health.

The CDC distributes several drugs that are not available commercially in the United States for treatment of parasitic diseases. These drugs are indicated by footnotes in Table 4.11, Manufacturers of Some Antiparasitic Drugs (p 814). To request these drugs, a physician must contact the CDC Drug Service (see Appendix I, Directory of Resources, p 831) and provide the following information: (1) the physician's name, address, and telephone number; (2) the type of infection to be treated and the method by which the infection was diagnosed; (3) the patient's name, age, weight, sex, and if the patient is female, whether she is pregnant; and (4) basic demographic, clinical, and epidemiologic information. Consultation with a medical officer from the CDC is required before a drug is distributed.

Important human parasitic infections are discussed in individual chapters in section 3; the diseases are arranged alphabetically, and the discussions include recommendations for drug treatment. Tables 4.9 (p 784), 4.10 (p 811), and 4.11 (p 814), reproduced from *The Medical Letter* (see Drugs for Parasitic Infections, p 783), provide dosage recommendations and other relevant information for specific antiparasitic drugs. Although the recommendations for administration of these drugs given in the disease-specific chapters are similar, they may not be identical in all instances because of differences of opinion among experts. Both sources should be consulted.

Table 3.40. Additional Parasitic Diseases[a]

Disease and/or Agent	Where Infection May Be Acquired	Definitive Host	Intermediate Host	Modes of Human Infection	Directly Communicable (Person to Person)	Diagnostic Laboratory Tests in Humans	Causative Form of Parasite	Manifestations in Humans
Angiostrongylus cantonensis	Widespread in the tropics, particularly Pacific Islands, Southeast Asia, and Central America	Rats	Snails and slugs	Eating improperly cooked infected mollusks or, potentially, food contaminated by mollusk secretions containing larvae	No	Eosinophils in CSF; rarely, identification of larvae in CSF or at autopsy; serologic test	Larval worms	Eosinophilia, meningoencephalitis
Angiostrongylus costaricensis	Central and South America	Rodents	Snails and slugs	Eating poorly cooked infected mollusks or, potentially, food contaminated by mollusk secretions containing larvae	No	Gel diffusion; identification of larvae and eggs in tissue	Larval worms	Abdominal pain, eosinophilia
Anisakiasis	Cosmopolitan, mainly Japan	Marine mammals	Certain saltwater fish, squid, and octopus	Eating uncooked infected fish	No	Identification of recovered larvae in granulomas or vomitus	Larval worms	Acute gastrointestinal disease

Table 3.40. Additional Parasitic Diseases,ᵃ continued

Disease and/ or Agent	Where Infection May Be Acquired	Definitive Host	Intermediate Host	Modes of Human Infection	Directly Communicable (Person to Person)	Diagnostic Laboratory Tests in Humans	Causative Form of Parasite	Manifestations in Humans
Clonorchis sinensis, Opisthorchis viverrini, Opisthorchis felineus (flukes)	Far East, Eastern Europe, Russian Federation	Humans, cats, dogs, other mammals	Certain freshwater snails	Eating uncooked infected freshwater fish	No	Eggs in stool or duodenal fluid	Larvae and mature flukes	Abdominal pain; hepatobiliary disease
Dracunculiasis (Dracunculus medinensis) (guinea worm)	Foci in Africa	Humans	Crustacea (copepods)	Drinking infested water	No	Identification of emerging or adult worm in subcutaneous tissues	Adult female worm	Emerging roundworm; inflammatory response; systemic and local blister or ulcer in skin
Fasciolopsiasis (Fasciolopsis buski)	Far East	Humans, pigs, dogs	Certain freshwater snails, plants	Eating uncooked infected plants	No	Eggs or worm in feces or duodenal fluid	Larvae and mature worms	Diarrhea, constipation, vomiting, anorexia, edema of face and legs, ascites

Table 3.40. Additional Parasitic Diseases,[a] continued

Disease and/ or Agent	Where Infection May Be Acquired	Definitive Host	Intermediate Host	Modes of Human Infection	Directly Communicable (Person to Person)	Diagnostic Laboratory Tests in Humans	Causative Form of Parasite	Manifestations in Humans
Intestinal capillariasis (*Capillaria philippinensis*)	Philippines, Thailand	Humans, fish-eating birds	Fish	Ingestion of uncooked infected fish	Uncertain	Eggs and parasite in feces	Larvae and mature worms	Protein-losing enteropathy, diarrhea, malabsorption, ascites, emaciation

CSF indicates cerebrospinal fluid.

[a] For recommended drug treatment, see Drugs for Parasitic Infections (p 783).

Parvovirus B19
(Erythema Infectiosum, Fifth Disease)

CLINICAL MANIFESTATIONS: Infection with parvovirus B19 is recognized most often as erythema infectiosum (EI), which is characterized by a distinctive rash that may be preceded by mild systemic symptoms, including fever in 15% to 30% of patients. The facial rash can be intensely red with a "slapped cheek" appearance that often is accompanied by circumoral pallor. A symmetric, maculopapular, lace-like, and often pruritic rash also occurs on the trunk, moving peripherally to involve the arms, buttocks, and thighs. The rash can fluctuate in intensity and recur with environmental changes, such as temperature and exposure to sunlight, for weeks to months. A brief, mild, nonspecific illness consisting of fever, malaise, myalgia, and headache often precedes the characteristic exanthema by approximately 7 to 10 days. Arthralgia and arthritis occur in less than 10% of infected children but commonly among adults, especially women. Knees are involved most commonly in children, but a symmetric polyarthropathy of knees, fingers, and other joints is common in adults.

Human parvovirus B19 also can cause other manifestations (Table 3.41, p 492), including asymptomatic infection, a mild respiratory tract illness with no rash, a rash atypical for EI that may be rubelliform or petechial, papulopurpuric gloves-and-socks syndrome (PPGSS; painful and pruritic papules, petechiae, and purpura of hands and feet, often with fever and enanthem), polyarthropathy syndrome (arthralgia and arthritis in adults in the absence of other manifestations of EI), chronic erythroid hypoplasia with severe anemia in immunodeficient patients (eg, HIV-infected patients, patients receiving immune suppressive therapy, etc), and transient aplastic crisis lasting 7 to 10 days in patients with hemolytic anemias (eg, sickle cell disease and autoimmune hemolytic anemia) and other conditions associated with low hemoglobin concentrations, including hemorrhage, severe anemia, and thalassemia. Patients with transient aplastic crisis may have a prodromal illness with fever, malaise, and myalgia, but rash usually is absent. The B-19–associated red blood cell aplasia is related to lytic infection in erythrocyte precursors. In addition, parvovirus B19 infection sometimes has been associated with decreases in numbers of platelets, lymphocytes, and neutrophils.

Parvovirus B19 infection occurring during pregnancy can cause fetal hydrops, intrauterine growth retardation, isolated pleural and pericardial effusions, and death but is not a proven cause of congenital anomalies. The risk of fetal death is between 2% and 6% when infection occurs during pregnancy. The greatest risk appears to occur during the first half of pregnancy.

ETIOLOGY: Human parvovirus B19 is a nonenveloped, single-stranded DNA virus that replicates only in human erythrocyte precursors.

EPIDEMIOLOGY: Parvovirus B19 is distributed worldwide and is a common cause of infection in humans, who are the only known hosts. Modes of transmission include contact with respiratory tract secretions, percutaneous exposure to blood or blood products, and vertical transmission from mother to fetus. Since 2002, plasma derivatives have been screened using quantitative DNA measurement to decrease the risk of parvovirus B19 transmission. Parvovirus B19 infections are ubiquitous, and cases of EI can occur sporadically or in outbreaks in elementary or junior high schools during late winter and early spring. Secondary spread among susceptible household members is common, with infection occurring in approximately 50% of susceptible contacts in some studies. The

Table 3.41. Clinical Manifestations of Human Parvovirus B19 Infection

Conditions	Usual Hosts
Erythema infectiosum (fifth disease)	Immunocompetent children
Polyarthropathy syndrome	Immunocompetent adults (more common in women)
Chronic anemia/pure red cell aplasia	Immunocompromised hosts
Transient aplastic crisis	People with hemolytic anemia (ie, sickle cell anemia)
Hydrops fetalis/congenital anemia	Fetus (first 20 weeks of pregnancy)
Persistent anemia	Immunocompromised people

transmission rate in schools is less, but infection can be an occupational risk for school and child care personnel, with approximately 20% of susceptible contacts becoming infected. In young children, antibody seroprevalence generally is 5% to 10%. In most communities, approximately 50% of young adults and often more than 90% of elderly people are seropositive. The annual seroconversion rate in women of childbearing age has been reported to be approximately 1.5%. The timing of the presence of parvovirus B19 DNA in serum and respiratory tract secretions indicates that people with EI are most infectious before onset of the rash and are unlikely to be infectious after onset of the rash and/or joint symptoms. In contrast, patients with aplastic crises are contagious from before the onset of symptoms through at least the week after onset. Symptoms of the PPGSS occur in association with viremia and before development of antibody response, and affected patients should be considered infectious.

The **incubation period** from acquisition of parvovirus B19 to onset of initial symptoms usually is between 4 and 14 days but can be as long as 21 days. Rash and joint symptoms occur 2 to 3 weeks after infection.

DIAGNOSTIC TESTS: In the immunocompetent host, detection of serum parvovirus B19-specific immunoglobulin (Ig) M antibody is the preferred diagnostic test. A positive IgM test result indicates that infection probably occurred within the previous 2 to 4 months. On the basis of radioimmunoassay or enzyme immunoassay results, antibody may be detected in 90% or more of patients at the time of the EI rash and by the third day of illness in patients with transient aplastic crisis. Serum IgG antibody appears by approximately day 7 of EI and persists for life; therefore, presence of parvovirus B19 IgG is not necessarily indicative of acute infection. These assays are available through commercial laboratories and through some state health department and research laboratories. However, their sensitivity and specificity may vary, particularly for IgM antibody. The optimal method for detecting chronic infection in the immunocompromised patient is demonstration of virus by nucleic acid hybridization or polymerase chain reaction (PCR) assays, because parvovirus B19 antibody is present variably in persistent infection. Because parvovirus B19 DNA can be detected at low levels by PCR assay in serum for up to 9 months after the acute viremic phase, detection of parvovirus B19 DNA by PCR assay does not necessarily indicate acute infection. Less-sensitive nucleic acid hybridization assay results usually are positive for only 2 to 4 days after onset of illness. For immunocompromised patients with severe anemia associated with chronic infection, dot blot hybridization of serum specimens may have adequate sensitivity. Parvovirus B19 has not been grown in standard cell culture.

TREATMENT: For most patients, only supportive care is indicated. Patients with aplastic crises may require transfusion. For treatment of chronic infection in immunodeficient patients, Immune Globulin Intravenous (IGIV) therapy often is effective and should be considered. Some cases of parvovirus B19 infection concurrent with hydrops fetalis have been treated successfully with intrauterine blood transfusions.

ISOLATION OF THE HOSPITALIZED PATIENT: In addition to standard precautions, droplet precautions are recommended for hospitalized children with aplastic crises, children with PPGSS, or immunosuppressed patients with chronic infection and anemia for the duration of hospitalization. For patients with transient aplastic or erythrocyte crisis, these precautions should be maintained for 7 days.

Pregnant health care professionals should be informed of the potential risks to the fetus from parvovirus B19 infections and about preventive measures that may decrease these risks, for example, attention to strict infection control procedures and not caring for immunocompromised patients with chronic parvovirus infection or patients with parvovirus B19-associated aplastic crises, because patients in both groups are likely to be contagious.

CONTROL MEASURES:
- Women who are exposed to children at home or at work (eg, teachers or child care providers) are at increased risk of infection with parvovirus B19. However, because school or child care center outbreaks often indicate wider spread in the community, including inapparent infection, women are at some degree of risk of exposure from other sources at home or in the community. In view of the high prevalence of parvovirus B19 infection, the low incidence of ill effects on the fetus, and the fact that avoidance of child care or classroom teaching can decrease but not eliminate the risk of exposure, routine exclusion of pregnant women from the workplace where EI is occurring is not recommended. Women of childbearing age who are concerned can undergo serologic testing for IgG antibody to parvovirus B19 to determine their susceptibility to infection.
- Pregnant women who discover that they have been in contact with children who were in the incubation period of EI or with children who were in aplastic crisis should have the relatively low potential risk of infection explained to them, and the option of serologic testing should be offered. Fetal ultrasonography may prove useful in these situations.
- Children with EI may attend child care or school, because they no longer are contagious once the rash appears.
- Transmission of parvovirus B19 is likely to be decreased through use of routine infection-control practices, including hand hygiene and proper disposal of used facial tissues.

Pasteurella Infections

CLINICAL MANIFESTATIONS: The most common manifestation in children is cellulitis at the site of a scratch or bite of a cat, dog, or other animal. Cellulitis typically develops within 24 hours of the injury and includes swelling, erythema, tenderness, and serous or sanguinopurulent discharge at the site. Regional lymphadenopathy, chills, and fever can occur. Local complications, such as septic arthritis, osteomyelitis, and tenosynovitis, are common. Less common manifestations of infection include septicemia, meningitis, endocarditis, respiratory tract infections (eg, pneumonia, pulmonary abscesses, pleural empyema), appendicitis, hepatic abscess, peritonitis, urinary tract infection, and ocular infections (eg, conjunctivitis, corneal ulcer, endophthalmitis). People with liver disease or underlying host defense abnormalities are predisposed to bacteremia attributable to *Pasteurella multocida*.

ETIOLOGY: Species of the genus *Pasteurella* are nonmotile, facultative anaerobic, gram-negative coccobacilli or rods that are primary pathogens in animals. The most common human pathogen is *P multocida*. Most human infections are caused by the following species or subspecies: *P multocida* subspecies *multocida*, *P multocida* subspecies *septica*, *Pasteurella canis*, *Pasteurella stomatis*, *Pasteurella dagmatis*, and *Pasteurella haemolytica*.

EPIDEMIOLOGY: *Pasteurella* species are found in the oral flora of 70% to 90% of cats, 25% to 50% of dogs, and many other animals. Transmission can occur from the bite or scratch of a cat or dog or, less commonly, from another animal. Respiratory tract spread from animals to humans also occurs. In a significant proportion of cases, no animal exposure can be identified. Human-to-human spread has not been documented.

The **incubation period** usually is less than 24 hours.

DIAGNOSTIC TESTS: The isolation of *Pasteurella* species from skin lesion drainage or other sites of infection (eg, blood, joint fluid, cerebrospinal fluid, sputum, pleural fluid, or suppurative lymph nodes) is diagnostic. Although *Pasteurella* species resemble several other organisms morphologically and grow on many culture media at 37°C (98°F), laboratory differentiation is not difficult.

TREATMENT: The drug of choice is penicillin. Other effective oral agents include ampicillin, amoxicillin-clavulanate, cefuroxime, cefpodoxime, doxycycline, and fluoro-quinolones. For patients allergic to beta-lactam agents, azithromycin or trimethoprim-sulfamethoxazole are alternative choices, but clinical experience with these agents is limited. Doxycycline is effective but should be avoided in children younger than 8 years of age whenever possible. Fluoroquinolones are effective but are not recommended for this use in patients younger than 18 years of age. For suspected polymicrobial infection, oral amoxicillin-clavulanate or, for severe infection, intravenous ampicillin-sulbactam, ticarcillin-clavulanate, or piperacillin-tazobactam can be given. The duration of therapy usually is 7 to 10 days for local infections and 10 to 14 days for more severe infections. Antimicrobial therapy should be continued for 4 to 6 weeks for bone and joint infections. Wound drainage or débridement may be necessary.

ISOLATION OF THE HOSPITALIZED PATIENT: Standard precautions are recommended.

CONTROL MEASURES: Limiting contact with wild animals and education about appropriate contact with domestic animals can help to prevent *Pasteurella* infections (see Bite Wounds, p 187). Animal bites and scratches should be irrigated, cleansed, and débrided promptly. Antimicrobial prophylaxis for children with an animal bite wound should be initiated according to the recommendations in Table 2.18, p 189.

Pediculosis Capitis[1]
(Head Lice)

CLINICAL MANIFESTATIONS: Itching is the most common symptom of head lice infestation, but many children are asymptomatic. Adult lice or eggs (nits) are found on the hair and are most readily apparent behind the ears and near the nape of the neck. Excoriations and crusting caused by secondary bacterial infection may occur and often are associated with regional lymphadenopathy. Head lice usually deposit their eggs on a hair shaft 4 mm or less from the scalp. Because hair grows at a rate of approximately 1 cm per month, the duration of infestation can be estimated by the distance of the nit from the scalp.

ETIOLOGY: *Pediculus humanus capitis* is the head louse. Both nymphs and adult lice feed on human blood.

EPIDEMIOLOGY: In the United States, head lice infestation is most common in children attending child care and elementary school. Head lice are not a sign of poor hygiene, and all socioeconomic groups are affected. In the United States, infestations are less common in African-American children than in children of other races. Head lice infestation is not influenced by hair length or frequency of shampooing or brushing. Head lice are not a health hazard, because they are not responsible for spread of any disease. Transmission occurs mainly by direct head-to-head contact with hair of infested people. Transmission by contact with personal belongings, such as combs, hair brushes, and hats, is uncommon. Away from the scalp, head lice survive less than 2 days at room temperature, and their eggs generally become nonviable within a week and cannot hatch at a lower ambient temperature than that near the scalp.

The **incubation period** from the laying of eggs to the hatching of the first nymph is usually about 8 to 9 days but can vary from 7 to 12 days, being somewhat shorter in hot climates and longer in cold climates. Lice mature to the adult stage approximately 9 to 12 days later. Adult females then may lay eggs (nits), but these will develop only if the female has mated.

DIAGNOSTIC TESTS: Identification of eggs (nits), nymphs, and lice with the naked eye is possible; the diagnosis can be confirmed by using a hand lens or microscope. Nymphal and adult lice shun light and move rapidly and conceal themselves. It is important to differentiate nits from dandruff, benign hair casts (a layer of follicular cells that may slide easily off the hair shaft), plugs of desquamated cells, external hair debris, and fungal infections of the hair. Because nits remain firmly affixed to the hair, even if dead or hatched, the mere presence of nits is not a sign of an active infestation.

TREATMENT: The following agents can be effective for treating head lice (see Drugs for Parasitic Infections, p 783). Therapy could be started with over-the-counter 1% permethrin, but resistance approaching 50% in the United States has been documented. For treatment failures with permethrin or pyrethrins, malathion should be used. When lice are resistant to all topical agents, ivermectin may be used, although it is not approved by the Food and Drug Administration (FDA) as a pediculicide. No drug is truly ovicidal, but of the available topical agents, only malathion has ovicidal activity. Drugs that leave a

---

[1]American Academy of Pediatrics, Committee on School Health and Committee on Infectious Diseases. Head lice. *Pediatrics.* In press

residual may kill nymphs as they emerge from eggs. Safety is a major concern with pediculicides, because the infestation itself does not present a risk to the host. Pediculicides should be used only as directed and with care. Instructions on proper use of any product should be explained carefully. Pediculicides usually require more than one application. Ideally, retreatment should occur after the eggs that are present at the time of initial treatment have hatched, but before any new eggs have been produced.

- **Malathion (0.5%).** This organophosphate pesticide that is both pediculicidal and partially ovicidal is available only by prescription as a lotion and is highly effective as formulated in the United States. The safety and effectiveness of malathion lotion have not been assessed by the FDA in children younger than 6 years of age. Malathion lotion is applied to dry hair, left to dry naturally, and then removed 8 to 12 hours later by washing and rinsing the hair. The product should be reapplied 7 to 9 days later only if live lice still are present at that time. The alcohol base of the lotion is flammable; therefore, do not expose the lotion or wet hair to lighted cigarettes, open flames, or electric heat sources, such as hair dryers or curling irons, during treatment. The product, if ingested, can cause severe respiratory distress. Malathion is contraindicated in children younger than 2 years of age because of the possibility of increased scalp permeability and absorption.
- **Permethrin (1%).** Permethrin is available without a prescription in a 1% lotion that is applied to the scalp and hair for 10 minutes after shampooing with a nonconditioning shampoo and towel drying the hair. Permethrin has advantages over other pediculicides: a low potential for toxic effects and a high cure rate. Although activity of permethrin can continue for 2 weeks or more after application, some experts advise a second treatment 9 to 10 days after the first one, especially if hair is washed within a week after the first treatment.
- **Pyrethrin-based products.** Pyrethrins are natural extracts from the chrysanthemum and are available (usually formulated with the synergist piperonyl butoxide) without a prescription as shampoos or mousse preparations (both to be applied to dry hair). Pyrethrins have no residual activity, and repeated application 9 to 10 days later is necessary to kill newly hatched lice. Resistance to permethrin renders pyrethrin-based products ineffective. Pyrethrins are contraindicated in people who are allergic to chrysanthemums or ragweed.
- **Permethrin (5%).** A 5% permethrin cream is available by prescription that usually is applied overnight for scabies (as young as 2 months of age). Anecdotally, it has been used for the treatment of head lice that appear to be recalcitrant to other treatments, but lice resistant to over-the-counter formulation (ie, 1% permethrin) likely will not succumb to the prescription formulation. The 5% permethrin cream is applied to the scalp and left on for several hours or overnight and then rinsed off. Treatment may be repeated 9 to 10 days later.
- **Crotamiton (10%).** Crotamiton has not been evaluated for safety and effectiveness in children or evaluated by the FDA as a pediculicide. Crotamiton (10%) lotion is used to treat scabies, and limited studies have shown it to be effective against head lice when applied to the scalp and left on for 24 hours before rinsing out.
- **Oral trimethoprim-sulfamethoxazole.** Oral trimethoprim-sulfamethoxazole has not been evaluated by the FDA as a pediculicide. Although some data suggest a 10-day course of this antimicrobial agent is effective against head lice, the use of trimethoprim-sulfamethoxazole to treat lice is controversial. Oral trimethoprim-sulfamethoxazole

plus topical 1% permethrin lotion may be more effective but should be reserved for treatment failures. Rare but severe allergic reactions (Stevens-Johnson syndrome) to trimethoprim-sulfamethoxazole make it less desirable if alternative therapies exist.

- **Oral ivermectin.** Oral ivermectin has not been evaluated by the FDA as a pediculicide. Ivermectin is an anthelmintic agent that may be effective against head lice if sufficient concentration is present in the blood at the time a louse feeds. It has been given as a single oral dose of 200 μg/kg, with a second dose given after 9 to 10 days. Because it blocks essential neural transmission if it crosses the blood-brain barrier and young children may be at higher risk of this adverse drug reaction, currently, ivermectin should not be used in children weighing less than 15 kg (33 pounds).

Data are lacking to determine whether suffocation of lice by application of some occlusive agents, such as petroleum jelly, olive oil, butter, or fat-containing mayonnaise, is effective as a method of treatment. Because pediculicides kill lice shortly after application, detection of living lice on scalp inspection 24 hours or more after treatment suggests incorrect use of pediculicide, hatching of lice after treatment, reinfestation, or resistance to therapy. In such situations, after excluding incorrect use, immediate retreatment with a different pediculicide followed by a second application 9 to 10 days later is recommended. Itching or mild burning of the scalp caused by inflammation of the skin in response to topical therapeutic agents can persist for many days after lice are killed and is not a reason for retreatment. Topical corticosteroid and oral antihistamine agents may be beneficial for relieving these signs and symptoms. Manual removal of nits after successful treatment with a pediculicide is helpful, because none of the pediculicides are 100% ovicidal. Fine-toothed nit combs designed for this purpose are available. Removal of nits is tedious and time consuming but may be attempted for aesthetic reasons, to decrease diagnostic confusion, or to decrease the chance of self-reinfestation.

ISOLATION OF THE HOSPITALIZED PATIENT: In addition to standard precautions, contact precautions are recommended until the patient has been treated with an appropriate pediculicide.

CONTROL MEASURES: Household and other close contacts should be examined and treated if infested. Bedmates of infested people should be treated prophylactically at the same time as the infested household members and contacts. Prophylactic treatment of other noninfested people is not recommended. Children should not be excluded or sent home early from school because of head lice. Parents of infested (ie, with at least 1 live, crawling louse) children should be notified and informed that their child should be treated. The presence of nits alone does not justify treatment.

"No-nit" policies requiring that children be free of nits before they return to a child care facility or school have not been effective in controlling head lice transmission and are not recommended. Egg cases further from the scalp are easier to discover, but these tend to be empty (hatched) or nonviable and, thus, are of no consequence.

Supplemental measures generally are not required to eliminate an infestation. Head lice are only rarely transferred via fomites from shared headgear, clothing, combs, or bedding. Special handling of such items is not likely to be useful. Environmental insecticide sprays increase chemical exposure of household members and have not been helpful in the control of head lice. Treatment of dogs, cats, or other pets is not indicated, because they do not play a role in the transmission of human head lice.

Pediculosis Corporis
(Body Lice)

CLINICAL MANIFESTATIONS: Intense itching, particularly at night, is common with body lice infestations. Bites from these lice manifest as small erythematous macules, papules, and excoriations primarily on the trunk. Body lice live in clothes or bedding and lay their eggs on or near the seams of clothing. Rarely, a louse can be seen feeding on the skin. Secondary bacterial infection of the skin caused by scratching is common.

ETIOLOGY: *Pediculus humanus corporis* (or *humanus*) is the body louse. Nymphs and adult lice feed on human blood.

EPIDEMIOLOGY: Body lice generally are restricted to people with poor hygiene living with others under poor conditions (refugee camps, poorly run prisons, conditions of destitute or "street" people) or who share clothes or bedding with other infested people. Unlike head lice, fomites have a role in transmission of body lice. Body lice cannot survive away from a blood source for longer than approximately 5 to 7 days at room temperature. In contrast with head lice, body lice are well-recognized vectors of disease (eg, epidemic typhus, trench fever, and epidemic relapsing fever).

The **incubation period** from laying eggs to hatching of the first nymph is approximately 1 to 2 weeks, depending on temperature. Lice mature and are capable of reproducing 9 to 19 days after hatching depending on whether infested clothing is removed for sleeping.

DIAGNOSTIC TESTS: Identification of eggs, nymphs, and lice with the naked eye is possible; the diagnosis can be confirmed by using a hand lens or microscope. Adult and nymphal body lice seldom are seen on the body, because they generally are sequestered in clothing.

TREATMENT: Treatment consists of improving hygiene and cleaning clothes and bedding. Infested materials can be decontaminated by washing in hot water, by machine drying at hot temperatures, by dry cleaning, or by pressing with a hot iron. Temperatures exceeding 53.5°C (128.3°F) for 5 minutes are lethal to lice and eggs. Pediculicides usually are not necessary if materials are laundered at least weekly (see Drugs for Parasitic Infections, p 783). Some people with much body hair may require full-body treatment with a pediculicide, because lice and eggs may adhere to body hair.

ISOLATION OF THE HOSPITALIZED PATIENT: In addition to standard precautions, contact precautions are recommended until the patient has been treated.

CONTROL MEASURES: The most important factor in the control of body lice infestation is the ability to change and wash clothing. Close contacts should be examined and treated appropriately; clothing and bedding should be laundered.

Pediculosis Pubis
(Pubic Lice, Crab Lice)

CLINICAL MANIFESTATIONS: Pruritus of the anogenital area is a common symptom in pubic lice infestations ("crabs" or "pthiriasis"). The parasite most frequently is found in the pubic region but also can infest on the eyelashes, eyebrows, beard, axilla, perianal area, and rarely, the scalp. A characteristic sign of heavy pubic lice infestation is the presence of bluish or slate-colored macules (maculae ceruleae) on the chest, abdomen, or thighs.

ETIOLOGY: *Pthirus pubis* is the pubic or crab louse. Nymphs and adult lice feed on human blood.

EPIDEMIOLOGY: Pubic lice infestations are more prevalent in adults and usually are transmitted through sexual contact. Transmission by contaminated items, such as towels, would be uncommon. Pubic lice on the eyelashes of children may be evidence of sexual abuse, although other modes of transmission are possible. Infested people should be examined for other sexually transmitted infections, including syphilis and infection with *Neisseria gonorrhoeae*, *Chlamydia trachomatis*, hepatitis B virus, and human immunodeficiency virus. Adult pubic lice can survive off a host for up to 36 hours, and their eggs can remain viable for up to 10 days under suitable environmental conditions.

The **incubation period** from the laying of eggs to the hatching of the first nymph is approximately 6 to 10 days. Adult lice capable of reproducing do not appear until approximately 2 to 3 weeks after hatching.

DIAGNOSTIC TESTS: Identification of eggs (nits), nymphs, and lice with the naked eye is possible; the diagnosis can be confirmed by using a hand lens or microscope.

TREATMENT: All hairy areas of the body should be examined for evidence of pubic lice. Lice and their eggs can be removed manually, or the hairs can be shaved to eliminate immediately the infestation. Caution should be used when inspecting, removing or treating lice on or near the eyelashes. The pediculicides used to treat other kinds of louse infestations are effective for treatment of pubic lice (see Pediculosis Capitis, p 495). Retreatment is recommended as for head lice. Topical pediculicides should not be used for infestation of eyelashes by pubic lice; petrolatum ointment applied to the eyelashes 2 to 4 times daily for 8 to 10 days is effective.

ISOLATION OF THE HOSPITALIZED PATIENT: In addition to standard precautions, contact precautions are recommended until the patient has been treated with an appropriate pediculicide.

CONTROL MEASURES: All sexual contacts should be examined and treated, as needed. Patients should be advised to avoid sexual contact until they and their sex partner have been treated successfully. Bedding, towels, and clothing can be decontaminated by laundering in hot water and machine drying using a hot cycle or by dry cleaning.

Pelvic Inflammatory Disease[1]

CLINICAL MANIFESTATIONS: Pelvic inflammatory disease (PID) comprises a spectrum of inflammatory disorders of the female upper genital tract, including any combination of endometritis, parametritis, salpingitis, oophoritis, tubo-ovarian abscess, and pelvic peritonitis. PID typically manifests as dull, continuous, unilateral or bilateral lower abdominal or pelvic pain that may range from indolent to severe. Additional symptoms may include fever, vomiting, an abnormal vaginal discharge, and irregular vaginal bleeding (signaling endometritis). Some patients have sharp right upper abdominal quadrant pain as a result of perihepatitis. Symptoms often begin within a week after the onset of menses, depending on the etiologic agent.

Examination findings vary but may include fever, lower abdominal tenderness, tenderness on lateral motion of the cervix, unilateral or bilateral adnexal tenderness, and adnexal fullness. Leukocytosis, an elevated erythrocyte sedimentation rate, elevated C-reactive protein concentration, and/or an adnexal mass demonstrated by abdominal or transvaginal ultrasonography may be laboratory or imaging findings useful to support the diagnosis.

No single symptom, sign, or laboratory finding is sensitive and specific for the diagnosis of acute PID. Adnexal tenderness in a patient who has been sexually active has been described as the most sensitive finding for PID. Many episodes of PID go unrecognized by patients and/or health care professionals, because patients may be relatively asymptomatic ("silent PID") and do not seek care or because symptoms are mild and nonspecific. The diagnostic criteria recommended currently by the Centers for Disease Control and Prevention (CDC) are presented in Table 3.42 (p 501).

Complications of PID may include perihepatitis (Fitz-Hugh-Curtis syndrome) and tubo-ovarian abscess. Important long-term sequelae are recurrent infection, chronic pelvic pain, a sevenfold increase in incidence of ectopic pregnancy, and infertility resulting from tubal occlusion. Risk of tubal infertility is estimated to be 12% after a single episode of PID and more than 50% after 3 or more episodes. Factors that may increase the likelihood of infertility are delay in diagnosis, older age at time of infection, chlamydial disease, PID determined to be severe by laparoscopic examination, and delayed antimicrobial therapy.

ETIOLOGY: Sexually transmitted organisms, especially *Neisseria gonorrhoeae* and *Chlamydia trachomatis*, are implicated in most cases of PID. However, other organisms, such as anaerobes, including *Bacteroides* species and *Peptostreptococcus* species; facultative anaerobes, including *Gardnerella vaginalis, Haemophilus influenzae, Streptococcus* species, and enteric gram-negative bacilli; genital tract mycoplasmas, including *Mycoplasma hominis* and *Ureaplasma urealyticum;* and cytomegalovirus, also are associated with PID. Polymicrobial infection is common.

EPIDEMIOLOGY: As is true for other sexually transmitted infections (STIs), the incidence of PID is highest among adolescents and young adults. Bacterial vaginosis (see Bacterial Vaginosis, p 228) is present in many cases of PID. Risk factors for PID include numerous sexual partners, use of an intrauterine device in the presence of an existing infection or

---

[1]Centers for Disease Control and Prevention. Sexually transmitted infections treatment guidelines—2006. *MMWR Recomm Rep.* 2006;55(RR-11):1–94

Table 3.42. Criteria for Clinical Diagnosis of Pelvic Inflammatory Disease (PID)

Minimum Criteria

Empiric treatment of PID should be initiated in sexually active young women and others at risk of STIs if the following **minimum criteria** are present and no other cause(s) for the illness can be identified:

• Uterine or adnexal tenderness

Additional Criteria

More elaborate diagnostic evaluation often is needed, because incorrect diagnosis and management might cause unnecessary morbidity. These additional criteria may be used to enhance the specificity of the minimum criteria listed previously. Additional criteria that support a diagnosis of PID include the following:

• Oral temperature greater than 38.3°C (101°F)
• Mucopurulent cervical or vaginal discharge
• Presence of white blood cells (WBCs) on saline microscopy of vaginal secretions
• Increased erythrocyte sedimentation rate
• Increased C-reactive protein concentration
• Laboratory documentation of cervical infection with *Neisseria gonorrhoeae* or *Chlamydia trachomatis*

Most women with PID have mucopurulent cervical discharge **OR** evidence of WBCs on a microscopic evaluation of a saline preparation of vaginal fluid. If the cervical discharge appears normal AND no WBCs are found on the wet preparation, the diagnosis of PID is unlikely, and alternative causes of pain should be sought.

The **most specific criteria** for diagnosing PID include the following:

• Endometrial biopsy with histopathologic evidence of endometritis
• Transvaginal ultrasonography or magnetic resonance imaging techniques showing thickened, fluid-filled tubes with or without free pelvic fluid or tubo-ovarian complex
• Laparoscopic abnormalities consistent with PID

A diagnostic evaluation that includes some of these more extensive studies may be warranted in selected cases.

STIs indicates sexually transmitted infections.

Adapted from the Centers for Disease Control and Prevention. Sexually transmitted infections treatment guidelines—2006. *MMWR Recomm Rep.* 2006; 55(RR-11):1-94 (see **www.cdc.gov/std/treatment**)

multiple sexual partners, douching, and previous episodes of PID. Latex condoms may reduce the risk of PID. Other barrier contraceptive methods, such as the contraceptive sponge and diaphragm, also have been shown to be effective in preventing transmission of STIs. Oral contraceptive pills decrease the likelihood of PID in the face of gonococcal cervicitis. Ascending pelvic infection rarely, if ever, occurs as a complication of gonococcal vaginitis in prepubertal girls.

An **incubation period** for PID is undefined. In women with gonococcal cervicitis, symptoms of PID generally appear during the first half of the menstrual cycle.

DIAGNOSTIC TESTS: The diagnosis of PID usually is made on the basis of clinical findings (see Table 3.42) and can be supported by findings of a preponderance of leukocytes in cervical secretions, leukocytosis, an increased C-reactive protein concentration or erythrocyte sedimentation rate, identification of *N gonorrhoeae* in an endocervical culture, or presence of *C trachomatis* as a coexistent infection (see Gonococcal Infections, p 305, and *Chlamydia trachomatis*, p 255). Samples for *N gonorrhoeae* and *C trachomatis* should be obtained before treatment is begun, but treatment should not be delayed pending results of tests if suspicion is high for PID. Ultrasonography and laparoscopy are useful when appendicitis, ruptured ovarian cyst, or ectopic pregnancy are possible differential diagnoses. Laparoscopy also permits bacteriologic specimens to be obtained directly from tubal exudate or the cul-de-sac. However, laparoscopy cannot detect endometritis and is not indicated for diagnosis in most cases of PID. Because PID and ectopic pregnancy both can produce abdominal pain and irregular bleeding, a pregnancy test is indicated in the diagnostic evaluation of the adolescent with suspected PID or lower abdominal pain regardless of menstrual history.

TREATMENT: Because the clinical diagnosis of PID, even in the most experienced hands, is imprecise and because the consequences of untreated infection are substantial, most experts provide antimicrobial therapy to patients who fulfill minimum criteria rather than limiting therapy to patients who fulfill additional criteria for the diagnosis of PID (Table 3.42, p 501). To minimize the risks of progressive infection and subsequent infertility, treatment should be instituted as soon as the clinical diagnosis is made and before results of culture are available. All people who are diagnosed with PID should be tested for *N gonorrhoeae* and *C trachomatis;* however, other organisms that can be present in the vaginal flora have been associated with PID.

Observation and treatment in the hospital are suggested in the following circumstances: (1) a surgical emergency, such as ectopic pregnancy or appendicitis, cannot be excluded; (2) adherence to or tolerance of an outpatient treatment regimen and follow-up within 72 hours cannot be ensured; (3) the patient's illness is severe (eg, nausea, vomiting, severe pain, overt peritonitis, or high fever); (4) a tubo-ovarian abscess is present; (5) the patient is pregnant; (6) the patient has failed to respond clinically to outpatient therapy; or (7) another serious condition cannot be excluded. Although in the past, many experts have recommended hospitalization for all adolescent patients with PID, data to support this recommendation are lacking. Current data are insufficient to determine whether more aggressive interventions are indicated for women with PID and human immunodeficiency virus (HIV) infection.

An antimicrobial regimen for treatment of PID should be empiric and broad spectrum and should provide coverage directed against the most common causative agents. Antimicrobial regimens consistent with those recommended by the CDC are summarized in Table 3.43 (p 503). Clinical outcome data are limited regarding the use of cephalosporins other than cefotetan and cefoxitin (such as ceftriaxone, cefotaxime, or ceftizoxime). Some experts believe that these agents can be used to replace cefoxitin or cefotetan for inpatient treatment of PID; however, cefoxitin and cefotetan are more active against anaerobic bacteria. Consideration should be given to selecting an antimicrobial regimen that is effective against *N gonorrhoeae* and *C trachomatis.* Because of antimicrobial resistance, a fluoroquinolone no longer is recommended for treatment of *N gonorrhoeae*.[1] Empiric therapy for anaerobic pathogens should be provided for patients with tubo-ovarian abscess, recurrent PID, or recent pelvic surgery. If the patient has an intrauterine device in place, the device should be removed immediately. In patients treated orally or

---

[1]Centers for Disease Control and Prevention. Update to CDC's sexually transmitted disease treatment guidelines, 2006: fluoroquinolones no longer recommended for treatment of gonococcal infections. *MMWR Morb Mortal Wkly Rep.* 2007;56(14):332–336

Table 3.43. Recommended Treatment of Pelvic Inflammatory Disease (PID)[a]

Parenteral: Regimen A[b]

Cefotetan, 2 g, IV, every 12 h

OR

Cefoxitin, 2 g, IV, every 6 h

PLUS

Doxycycline, 100 mg, orally or IV, every 12 h to complete 14 days

OR

Parenteral: Regimen B[c]

Clindamycin, 900 mg, IV, every 8 h

PLUS

Gentamicin: loading dose, IV or IM (2 mg/kg), followed by maintenance dose (1.5 mg/kg) every 8 h. Single daily dosing may be substituted.

NOTE

Parenteral therapy may be discontinued 24 hours after a patient improves clinically; continuing oral therapy should consist of doxycycline (100 mg, orally, twice a day) or clindamycin (450 mg, orally, 4 times a day) to complete a total of 14 days of therapy.

Ambulatory: Regimen[d]

Ceftriaxone, 250 mg, IM, once

OR

Cefoxitin, 2 g, IM, and probenecid, 1 g, orally, in a single dose concurrently, once

OR

Other parenteral third-generation cephalosporin[e] (eg, ceftizoxime or cefotaxine),

PLUS

Doxycycline, 100 mg, orally, twice a day for 14 days

WITH or WITHOUT

Metronidazole, 500 mg, orally, twice a day for 14 days

Alternative Ambulatory Regimens

If parenteral cephalosporin therapy is not feasible, use of fluoroquinolones may be considered if community prevalence and individual risk of gonorrhea is low (see www.cdc.gov/std/treatment). Tests for gonorrhea must be performed before instituting therapy and management as follows if the test is positive:

- GC NAA test positive: parenteral cephalosporin recommended
- GC culture positive: treatment based on susceptibility results
- GC isolate: quinolone resistant or susceptibility cannot be assessed, parenteral cephalosporin recommended

IV indicates intravenous; IM, intramuscular; NAA, nucleic acid amplification; GC, gonococcal.

[a] For further alternative treatment regimens, see Centers for Disease Control and Prevention. Sexually transmitted infections treatment guidelines—2006. *MMWR Recomm Rep.* 2006;55(RR-11) (see www.cdc.gov/std/treatment for updated treatment regimens)

[b] Hospitalization is recommended for severe illness, pregnancy, or unable to tolerate or follow ambulatory regimens.

[c] Alternative parenteral regimens include ampicillin-sulbactam plus doxycycline.

[d] Patients with inadequate response to outpatient therapy after 72 hours should be reevaluated for possible misdiagnosis and should receive parenteral therapy. Because of widespread fluoroquinolone-resistant gonococci, fluoroquinolones are not recommended for PID in the United States.

[e] Data to indicate whether expanded-spectrum cephalosporins (ceftizoxime, cefotaxime, ceftriaxone) can replace cefoxitin or cefotetan are limited. Many authorities believe they also are effective therapy for PID, but they are less active against anaerobes.

parenterally, clinical improvement can be expected within 72 hours after initiation of treatment. Accordingly, outpatients should be reevaluated routinely on the third or fourth day of treatment.

ISOLATION OF THE HOSPITALIZED PATIENT: Standard precautions are recommended.

CONTROL MEASURES[1]:

- Male sexual partners of patients with PID should receive diagnostic evaluation for gonococcal and chlamydial urethritis and then should be treated presumptively for both infections if they had sexual contact with the patient during the 60 days preceding onset of symptoms in the patient. A large proportion of these males will be asymptomatic.
- The patient should abstain from sexual intercourse until she and her partner(s) have completed treatment.
- The patient and her partner(s) should be encouraged to use condoms consistently.
- The patient should be tested for syphilis and HIV infection, and a Papanicolaou test should be performed if appropriate (see CDC guidelines[2]).
- Unimmunized or incompletely immunized patients should begin or complete human papillomavirus and hepatitis B immunization (see Recommended Childhood and Adolescent Immunization Schedule, p 24–28).
- Because of the high risk of reinfection, some experts recommend that patients with PID whose initial test for *N gonorrhoeae* and *C trachomatis* was positive be retested 3 months after completing treatment.
- The diagnosis of PID provides an opportune time to educate the adolescent about prevention of STIs, including abstinence, consistent use of barrier methods of protection, and the importance of receiving periodic screening for STIs.

Pertussis (Whooping Cough)

CLINICAL MANIFESTATIONS: Pertussis begins with mild upper respiratory tract symptoms similar to the common cold (catarrhal stage) and progresses to cough and then usually to paroxysms of cough (paroxysmal stage) characterized by inspiratory whoop and commonly followed by vomiting. Fever is absent or minimal. Symptoms wane gradually over weeks to months (convalescent stage). Disease in infants younger than 6 months of age can be atypical with a short catarrhal stage, gagging, gasping, or apnea as prominent early manifestations; absence of whoop; and prolonged convalescence. Sudden unexpected death can be caused by pertussis. Cough illness in immunized children and adults can be mild and unrecognized. The duration of classic pertussis is 6 to 10 weeks. Approximately one half of adolescents with pertussis cough for 10 weeks or longer. Complications among adolescents and adults include syncope, sleep disturbance, incontinence, rib fractures, and pneumonia. Pertussis is most severe when it occurs during the first 6 months of life, particularly in preterm and unimmunized infants. Complications among infants include pneumonia (22%), seizures (2%), encephalopathy (less than 0.5%), and death. Case-fatality rates are approximately 1% in infants younger than 2 months of age and less than 0.5% in infants 2 through 11 months of age.

[1]Centers for Disease Control and Prevention. Recommendations for partner services programs for HIV infection, syphilis, gonorrhea, and chlamydial infection. *MMWR Recomm Rep.* 2008;57(RR-9):1–63
[2]Centers for Disease Control and Prevention. Sexually transmitted infections treatment guidelines—2006. *MMWR Recomm Rep.* 2006;55(RR-11):1–94

ETIOLOGY: Pertussis is caused by a fastidious, gram-negative, pleomorphic bacillus, *Bordetella pertussis.* Other causes of sporadic prolonged cough illness include *Bordetella parapertussis, Mycoplasma pneumoniae, Chlamydia trachomatis, Chlamydophila pneumoniae, Bordetella bronchiseptica,* and certain respiratory tract viruses, particularly adenoviruses and respiratory syncytial viruses.

EPIDEMIOLOGY: Humans are the only known hosts of *B pertussis.* Transmission occurs by close contact with cases via aerosolized droplets. Neither infection nor immunization provides lifelong immunity. Lack of natural booster events and waning immunity since childhood immunization were responsible for the increase in cases of pertussis in people older than 10 years of age noted before use of the adolescent booster immunization. Additionally, waning immunity and reduced transplacental antibody led to increase in pertussis in very young infants. As many as 80% of immunized household contacts of symptomatic cases acquire infection, mainly because of waning immunity, with varying degrees of cough illness. Older siblings (including adolescents) and adults with mild or unrecognized atypical disease are important sources of pertussis for infants and young children. Infected people are most contagious during the catarrhal stage and the first 2 weeks after cough onset. Factors affecting the length of communicability include age, immunization status or previous episode of pertussis, and appropriate antimicrobial therapy.

The **incubation period** is 7 to 10 days, with a range of 5 to 21 days.

DIAGNOSTIC TESTS: Culture is considered the "gold standard" for laboratory diagnosis of pertussis. Although culture is 100% specific, *B pertussis* is a fastidious organism. Culture requires collection of an appropriate nasopharyngeal specimen, obtained either by aspiration or with Dacron (polyethylene terephthalate) or calcium alginate swabs. Specimens must be placed into special transport media (Regan-Lowe) immediately and not allowed to dry and transported promptly to the laboratory. Culture can be negative if taken from a previously immunized person, if antimicrobial therapy has been started, if more than 3 weeks has elapsed since cough onset, or if the specimen is not handled appropriately. A negative culture does not exclude the diagnosis of pertussis.

Polymerase chain reaction (PCR) assay increasingly is used for detection of *B pertussis* because of its improved sensitivity and more rapid result. The PCR test requires collection of an adequate nasopharyngeal specimen using a Dacron swab or nasal wash. Calcium alginate swabs are inhibitory to PCR and should not be used for PCR tests. The PCR test lacks sensitivity in previously immunized people but still may be superior to culture. Unacceptably high rates of false-positive results are reported from some laboratories. No Food and Drug Administration (FDA)-licensed PCR test is available, and there are no widely accepted standardized protocols, reagents, or reporting formats. Direct fluorescent antibody (DFA) testing no longer is recommended.

In the absence of immunization within 2 years, an elevated serum immunoglobulin (Ig) G antibody to pertussis toxin (PT) after 3 to 4 weeks of onset of cough is suggestive of recent *B pertussis* infection. An increasing titer or a single IgG anti-PT value 100 EU/mL or greater can be used for diagnosis. Although commercial serologic tests for pertussis infection exist, none is licensed by the FDA for diagnostic use. Cutoff points for diagnostic values of PT IgG have not been established by the FDA, and IgA and IgM assays lack adequate sensitivity and specificity.

An increased absolute white blood cell count with an absolute lymphocytosis often is present in infants and young children but not in adolescents with pertussis.

TREATMENT:
Antimicrobial agents administered during the catarrhal stage may ameliorate the disease. After the cough is established, antimicrobial agents have no discernible effect on the course of illness but are recommended to limit the spread of organisms to others. Macrolides are the drugs of choice for infected people and their contacts. Azithromycin, erythromycin, or clarithromycin are appropriate first-line agents for treatment and prophylaxis (see Table 3.44, p 507).[1] Resistance of *B pertussis* to macrolide antimicrobial agents has been reported rarely. Penicillins and cephalosporins are not effective against *B pertussis.*

Antimicrobial agents for infants younger than 6 months of age require special consideration. The FDA has not approved azithromycin or clarithromycin for use in infants younger than 6 months of age. An association between orally administered erythromycin and infantile hypertrophic pyloric stenosis (IHPS) has been reported in infants younger than 1 month of age. Although substantial use of azithromycin in infants younger than 1 month of age without IHPS has been reported, IHPS following azithromycin has been reported. Until additional information is available, azithromycin is the drug of choice for treatment or prophylaxis of pertussis in infants younger than 1 month of age. All infants younger than 1 month of age (and preterm infants until a similar postconception age) who receive any macrolide should be monitored for development of IHPS during and for 1 month after completing the course (see Table 3.44, p 507). Cases of pyloric stenosis should be reported to MedWatch (see MedWatch, p 817). For infants younger than 1 month of age, the risk of developing severe pertussis and life-threatening complications outweighs the potential risk of IHPS that has been associated with azithromycin.

Trimethoprim-sulfamethoxazole is an alternative for patients older than 2 months of age who cannot tolerate macrolides or who are infected with a macrolide-resistant strain. Studies evaluating trimethoprim-sulfamethoxazole as treatment for pertussis are limited.

ISOLATION OF THE HOSPITALIZED PATIENT: In addition to standard precautions, droplet precautions are recommended for 5 days after initiation of effective therapy, or if appropriate antimicrobial therapy is not given in older people, until 3 weeks after the onset of cough.

CONTROL MEASURES:
Care of Exposed People.

Household and Other Close Contacts. Close contacts younger than 7 years of age or older than 10 years of age who are unimmunized or underimmunized should have pertussis immunization initiated or continued using age-appropriate products according to the recommended schedule (see Table 3.45, p 508).

Chemoprophylaxis is recommended for all household contacts and other close contacts, including those in child care, regardless of age and immunization status. Early use of chemoprophylaxis in household contacts may limit secondary transmission. If 21 days have elapsed since onset of cough in the index case, chemoprophylaxis has limited value but should be considered for households with high-risk contacts (eg, young infants, preg-

---

[1] Centers for Disease Control and Prevention. Recommended antimicrobial agents for the treatment and postexposure prophylaxis of pertussis: 2005 CDC guidelines. *MMWR Recomm Rep.* 2005;54(RR–14):1–16

Table 3.44. Recommended Antimicrobial Therapy and Postexposure Prophylaxis for Pertussis in Infants, Children, Adolescents, and Adults[a]

| Age | Recommended Drugs | | | Alternative |
	Azithromycin	Erythromycin	Clarithromycin	TMP-SMX
Younger than 1 mo	10 mg/kg/day as a single dose for 5 days[b]	40 mg/kg/day in 4 divided doses for 14 days	Not recommended	Contraindicated at younger than 2 mo of age
1 through 5 mo	See above	See above	15 mg/kg per day in 2 divided doses for 7 days	2 mo of age or older; TMP, 8 mg/kg/day; SMX, 40 mg/kg/day in 2 doses for 14 days
6 mo or older and children	10 mg/kg as a single dose on day 1 (maximum 500 mg); then 5 mg/kg/day as a single dose on days 2 through 5 (maximum 250 mg/day)	40 mg/kg/day in 4 divided doses for 14 days (maximum 2 g/day)	15 mg/kg/day in 2 divided doses for 7 days (maximum 1 g/day)	See above
Adolescents and adults	500 mg as a single dose on day 1, then 250 mg as a single dose on days 2 through 5	2 g/day in 4 divided doses for 14 days	1 g/day in 2 divided doses for 7 days	TMP, 200 mg/day; SMX, 1600 mg/day in 2 divided doses for 14 days

TMP indicates trimethoprim; SMX, sulfamethoxazole.

[a]Centers for Disease Control and Prevention. Recommended antimicrobial agents for the treatment and postexposure prophylaxis of pertussis: 2005 CDC guidelines. *MMWR Recommen Rep.* 2005;54(**RR**-14):1–16

[b]Preferred macrolide for this age because of risk of idiopathic hypertrophic pyloric stenosis associated with erythromycin.

Table 3.45. Composition and Recommended Use of Vaccines With Tetanus Toxoid, Diphtheria Toxoid, and Acellular Pertussis Components Licensed in the United States[a]

Pharmaceutical[b,c]	Manufacturer	Pertussis Antigens	Recommended Use
DTaP Vaccine for Children Younger Than 7 Years of Age			
DTaP (Tripedia)	sanofi pasteur	PT, FHA	**All 5 doses**, children 6 wk through 6 y of age
DTaP (Infanrix)	GlaxoSmithKline Biologicals	PT, FHA, pertactin	**All 5 doses**, children 6 wk through 6 y of age
DTaP/Hib (TriHIBit)[c]	sanofi pasteur	PT, FHA	**Fourth dose only;** TriHIBit can be used for the fourth dose at 15 through 18 mo of age after 3 doses of DTaP and a primary series of any Hib vaccine
DTaP (Daptacel)	sanofi pasteur	PT, FHA, pertactin, fimbriae types 2 and 3	**All 5 doses**, children 6 wk through 6 y of age
DTaP-hepatitis B-IPV (Pediarix)	GlaxoSmithKline Biologicals	PT, FHA, pertactin	**First 3 doses** at 6- to 8-wk intervals beginning at 2 mo of age; then 2 doses of DTaP are needed to complete the 5-dose series before 7 y of age
DTaP-IPV/Hib (Pentacel)	sanofi pasteur	PT, FHA, pertactin, fimbriae types 2 and 3	**First 4 doses** at 2, 4, 6, and 15 through 18 mo of age
DTaP-IPV (Kinrix)	GlaxoSmithKline Biologicals	PT, FHA, pertactin	Booster dose for **fifth dose** of DTaP and **fourth dose** of IPV at 4 through 6 y of age
Tdap Vaccines for Adolescents			
Tdap (Boostrix)	GlaxoSmithKline Biologicals	PT, FHA, pertactin	Single dose at 11 through 12 y of age instead of Td (see text for additional recommendations)
Tdap (Adacel)	sanofi pasteur	PT, FHA, pertactin, fimbriae types 2 and 3	Single dose at 11 through 12 y of age instead of Td (see text for additional recommendations)

DTaP indicates pediatric formulation of diphtheria and tetanus toxoids and acellular pertussis vaccines; PT, pertussis toxoid; FHA, filamentous hemagglutinin; Hib, *Haemophilus influenzae* type b vaccine; IPV, inactivated poliovirus; Tdap, adolescent/adult formulation of tetanus toxoid, reduced diphtheria toxoid, and acellular pertussis vaccine; Td, tetanus and reduced diphtheria toxoids (for children 7 years of age or older and adults).

[a] DTaP recommended schedule is 2, 4, 6, and 15 through 18 months and 4 through 6 years of age. The fourth dose can be given as early as 12 months of age, provided 6 months have elapsed since the third dose was given. The fifth dose is not necessary if the fourth dose was given on or after the fourth birthday. Refer to manufacturers' package inserts for comprehensive product information regarding indications and use of the vaccines listed.

[b] ACEL-IMUNE and Certiva no longer are distributed.

[c] TriHIBit is ActHIB (lyophilized) reconstituted with Tripedia; Pentacel is ActHIB (lyophilized) reconstituted with sanofi pasteur DTaP-IPV.

nant women, and people who have contact with infants). The agents, doses, and duration of prophylaxis are the same as for treatment of pertussis (see Table 3.44, p 507).

People who have been in contact with an infected person should be monitored closely for respiratory tract symptoms for 21 days after last contact with the infected person. Close contacts with cough should be evaluated and treated for pertussis when appropriate.

Child Care. Pertussis immunization and chemoprophylaxis should be given as recommended for household and other close contacts. Child care providers and exposed children, especially incompletely immunized children, should be observed for respiratory tract symptoms for 21 days after contact has been terminated. Children and child care providers who are symptomatic or who have confirmed pertussis should be excluded from child care pending physician evaluation and completion of 5 days of the recommended course of antimicrobial therapy if pertussis is suspected. Untreated adults should be excluded until 21 days have elapsed from cough onset.

Schools. Students and staff members with pertussis should be excluded from school until they have completed 5 days of the recommended course of antimicrobial therapy. People who do not receive appropriate antimicrobial therapy should be excluded from school for 21 days after onset of symptoms. Public health officials should be consulted for further recommendations to control pertussis transmission in schools. The immunization status of children should be reviewed, and age-appropriate vaccine should be given, if indicated, as for household and other close contacts. Parents and employees should be notified about possible exposures to pertussis. Exclusion of exposed people with cough illness should be considered pending evaluation by a physician.

Health Care Settings. All health care professionals should observe standard precautions and wear a respiratory mask when examining a patient with a cough illness suspected or confirmed to be pertussis. Exposed, unprotected people should be given prophylaxis promptly. Macrolide prophylaxis is targeted broadly to all potentially exposed people and health care professionals to interrupt successfully the first generation of transmission. Control measures should be implemented even when one case of pertussis is recognized in a hospital, institution, outpatient clinic, or other health care setting. Confirmed and suspected cases should be reported to local health departments, and their involvement should be sought in control measures. Further guidance for evaluation and management of pertussis exposure in health care settings is available (**www.cdc.mmwr/pdf/ RR/RR5303.pdf**).

People (patients, health care personnel, caregivers) defined as close contacts or high-risk contacts of a patient or health care professional with pertussis should be given chemoprophylaxis (and immunization when indicated) as recommended for household contacts (see Table 3.44, p 507). Health care personnel with symptoms of pertussis should be excluded from work for at least the first 5 days of the recommended course of antimicrobial therapy. Health care personnel with symptoms of pertussis who cannot take, or who object to, antimicrobial therapy should be excluded from work for 21 days from onset of cough. Use of a respiratory mask is not sufficient protection during this time. Preexposure immunization of health care personnel with tetanus toxoid, reduced diphtheria toxoid, and acellular pertussis (Tdap) vaccine is recommended (see Health Care Personnel, p 94).

Immunization. Universal immunization with pertussis vaccine is recommended for children younger than 7 years of age and for adolescents 11 through 18 years of age and into adulthood. The pertussis vaccines used in the United States are acellular vaccines in combination with diphtheria and tetanus toxoids (pediatric DTaP and Tdap formulated for use in adolescents and adults). Recommendations for use of DTaP for children younger than 7 years of age are shown in Fig 1.1 (p 24–25). Tdap vaccines contain reduced quantities of diphtheria toxoid and some pertussis antigens; immunization as a single dose is recommended for people 11 years of age and older. One Tdap product is licensed to be given beginning at 10 years of age. Acellular vaccines are adsorbed onto an aluminum salt and must be administered intramuscularly. Acellular pertussis vaccines marketed in the United States contain 2 or more immunogens derived from *B pertussis* organisms: inactivated pertussis toxin (toxoid), filamentous hemagglutinin, fimbrial proteins (agglutinogens), and pertactin (an outer membrane 69-kd protein). All DTaP and Tdap vaccines contain pertussis toxoid (see Table 3.45 for products). Although licensed vaccines differ in their formulation of pertussis antigens, their efficacy is similar.

Dose and Route. Each 0.5-mL dose of DTaP and Tdap is given intramuscularly. Use of a decreased volume of individual doses of pertussis vaccines or multiple doses of decreased-volume (fractional) doses is not recommended.

Interchangeability of Acellular Pertussis Vaccines. Insufficient data exist on the safety, immunogenicity, and efficacy of different DTaP vaccines when administered interchangeably in the primary series (eg, first 4 doses in the routine series) to make recommendations. In circumstances in which the type of DTaP product(s) received previously is not known or the previously administered product(s) is not readily available, any DTaP vaccine licensed for use in the primary series may be used. There is no need to match Tdap vaccine manufacturer with DTaP vaccine manufacturer used for earlier doses.

Recommendations for Routine Childhood Immunization With DTaP Vaccine. Six doses of pertussis-containing vaccine are recommended: 4 primary doses and 1 booster dose of DTaP before school entry and a dose of Tdap at 11 years of age. The first dose of DTaP is given at 2 months of age, followed by 2 additional doses at intervals of approximately 2 months. The fourth dose of DTaP vaccine is recommended at 15 through 18 months of age, and the fifth dose of DTaP vaccine is given before school entry (kindergarten or elementary school) at 4 through 6 years of age. If the fourth dose of pertussis vaccine is delayed until after the fourth birthday, the fifth dose is not indicated.

Other recommendations are as follows:

- For the fourth dose, DTaP may be administered as early as 12 months of age if the interval between the third and fourth doses is at least 6 months.
- Simultaneous administration of DTaP and other recommended vaccines is acceptable. Vaccines should not be mixed in the same syringe unless the specific combination is licensed by the FDA (see Simultaneous Administration of Multiple Vaccines, p 33, and *Haemophilus influenzae* Infections, p 314).
- If pertussis is prevalent in the community, immunization can be started as early as 6 weeks of age, and doses 2 and 3 in the primary series can be given at intervals of 4 weeks.
- DTaP is not licensed or recommended for people 7 years of age or older. Tdap is licensed beginning at 10 (Boostrix) or 11 (Adacel) years of age.
- Children younger than 7 years of age who have begun but not completed their primary immunization schedule with DTP (eg, outside the United States) should receive DTaP to complete the pertussis immunization schedule.

- Children who have a contraindication to pertussis immunization should receive no further doses of a pertussis-containing vaccine (see Contraindications and Precautions to DTaP Immunization, p 513).
  Combined Vaccines. Several combination vaccines are licensed for use (see Table 3.45, p 508) and may be used when feasible and when any components are indicated.

Recommendations for Scheduling Pertussis Immunization for Children Younger Than 7 Years of Age in Special Circumstances.

- For the child whose pertussis immunization schedule is resumed after deferral or interruption of the recommended schedule, the next dose in the sequence should be given, regardless of the interval since the last dose—that is, the schedule is not reinitiated (see Lapsed Immunizations, p 34).
- For children who have received fewer than the recommended number of doses of pertussis vaccine but who have received the recommended number of diphtheria and tetanus toxoid (DT) vaccine doses for their age (ie, children started on DT, then given DTaP), DTaP should be given to complete the recommended pertussis immunization schedule. However, the total number of doses of diphtheria and tetanus toxoids (as DT, DTaP, or DTP) should not exceed 6 before the seventh birthday.
- Although well-documented pertussis confers short-term protection against infection, the duration of protection is unknown. DTaP (or Tdap in older people) should be given to complete the immunization series.
  Medical Records. Charts of children for whom pertussis immunization has been deferred should be flagged, and the immunization status of these children should be assessed periodically to ensure that they are immunized appropriately.

Adverse Events After DTaP Immunization in Children Younger Than 7 Years of Age.

- **Local and febrile reactions.** Reactions to DTaP most commonly include redness, edema, induration, and tenderness at the injection site; drowsiness; fretfulness; anorexia; vomiting; crying; and slight to moderate fever. These local and systemic manifestations after pertussis immunization occur within several hours of immunization and subside spontaneously without sequelae. Swelling involving the entire thigh or upper arm has been reported in 2% to 3% of vaccinees after administration of the fourth and fifth doses of a variety of acellular pertussis vaccines. Limb swelling may be accompanied by erythema, pain, and fever. Although thigh swelling may interfere with walking, most children have no limitation of activity; the condition resolves and has no sequelae. The pathogenesis is unknown.

  Entire limb swelling after a fourth dose of DTaP does not portend an increased risk of this reaction after the fifth dose and is not a contraindication to further immunization. It may be helpful to inform parents preemptively of the increase in reactogenicity that has been reported after the fourth and fifth doses of DTaP vaccine.

  A review by the Institute of Medicine (IOM) based on case-series reports found evidence of a causal relationship between receipt of tetanus toxoid-containing vaccines and brachial neuritis. However, the frequency of this event has not been determined.[1] Brachial neuritis is listed in the Vaccine Injury Table.

---

[1]Institute of Medicine, Vaccine Safety Committee. *Adverse Events Associated with Childhood Vaccines. Evidence Bearing on Causality.* Stratton KR, Howe CJ, Johnston RB, eds. Washington, DC: National Academies Press; 1994

Bacterial or sterile abscesses at the site of the injection are rare. Bacterial abscesses indicate contamination of the product or nonsterile technique and should be reported (see Reporting of Adverse Events, p 42). Sterile abscesses probably are hypersensitivity reactions. Their occurrence does not contraindicate further doses of DTaP vaccine.

- **Allergic reactions.** The rate of anaphylaxis to DTP was estimated to be approximately 2 cases per 100 000 injections; the incidence of allergic reactions after immunization with DTaP is unknown. Severe anaphylactic reactions and resulting deaths, if any, are rare after pertussis immunization. Transient urticarial rashes that occur occasionally after pertussis immunization, unless appearing immediately (ie, within minutes), are unlikely to be anaphylactic (IgE-mediated) in origin.

- **Seizures.** The incidence of seizures occurring within 48 hours of administration of DTP was estimated to be 1 case per 1750 doses administered. Seizures have been reported substantially less often after DTaP vaccine. Seizures associated with pertussis-containing vaccines usually are febrile seizures. These seizures have not been demonstrated to result in subsequent development of recurrent afebrile seizures (ie, epilepsy) or other neurologic sequelae. Predisposing factors to seizures occurring within 48 hours after administration of DTP were underlying convulsive disorder, personal history of seizures, and family history of seizures (see Children With a Personal or Family History of Seizures, p 86).

- **Hypotonic-hyporesponsive episodes.** These episodes (also termed "collapse" or "shock-like state") were reported to occur at a frequency of 1 per 1750 doses of DTP administered, although reported rates varied widely. These episodes occur significantly less often after immunization with DTaP. A follow-up study of a group of children who experienced a hypotonic-hyporesponsive episode (HHE) after immunization with DTP vaccine demonstrated no evidence of subsequent serious neurologic damage or intellectual impairment.

- **Temperature 40.5°C (104.8°F) or higher.** After administration of DTP, approximately 0.3% of recipients were reported to develop temperature of 40.5°C (104.8°F) or higher within 48 hours. The rate after administration of DTaP is significantly less.

- **Prolonged crying.** Persistent, severe, inconsolable screaming or crying for 3 or more hours was observed in up to 1% of infants within 48 hours of immunization with DTP. The frequency of inconsolable crying for 3 or more hours is significantly less after immunization with DTaP. The significance of persistent crying is unknown. It has been noted after receipt of immunizations other than pertussis vaccine and is not known to be associated with sequelae.

Evaluation of Adverse Events Temporally Associated With Pertussis Immunization. Appropriate diagnostic studies should be undertaken to establish the cause of serious adverse events occurring temporally with immunization rather than assuming that they are caused by the vaccine. The Centers for Disease Control and Prevention has established independent Clinical Immunization Safety Assessment (CISA) centers to assess people with selected adverse events and offer recommendations for management. Nonetheless, the cause of events temporally related to immunization, even when unrelated to the immunization received, cannot always be established after extensive diagnostic and investigative studies.

The preponderance of evidence does not support a causal relationship between immunization with DTP and sudden infant death syndrome, infantile spasms, or serious acute neurologic illness resulting in permanent neurologic injury. Active surveillance performed by the IMPACT network of Canadian pediatric centers screening more than 12 000 admissions for neurologic disorders between 1993 and 2002 found no case of encephalopathy attributable to DTaP after administration of more than 6.5 million doses.

Contraindications and Precautions to DTaP Immunization. Adverse events that occurred in temporal association with pertussis immunization that are contraindications or precautions for further administration of DTaP are listed in Table 3.46, p 514. A contraindication specifies that the vaccine should not be administered. A precaution specifies a situation in which a vaccine may be indicated if, after careful assessment, the benefit of the vaccine for the person is judged to outweigh the risk of complications.[1]

Children in the first year of life with neurologic disorders that necessitate temporary deferral of DTaP should not receive DT, because in the United States, the risk of acquiring diphtheria or tetanus by children younger than 1 year of age is remote. At or before the first birthday, the decision to give DTaP or DT should be made to ensure that the child is at least completely immunized against diphtheria and tetanus; as children become ambulatory, their risk of tetanus-prone wounds increases. For children who begin deferral of DTaP after 1 year of age, DT immunization should be completed according to the recommended schedule (see Diphtheria, p 280, and/or Tetanus, p 655).

Preterm Birth. Preterm birth is not a reason to defer immunization (see Preterm and Low Birth Weight Infants, p 68). Preterm birth is associated with increased risk of complications and death from pertussis in infancy.

Family History of Seizures (see also Children With a Personal or Family History of Seizures, p 86). Children with a family history of a seizure disorder or adverse events after receipt of a pertussis-containing vaccine in a family member should receive pertussis immunization on schedule.

Recommendations for Routine Adolescent Booster Immunization With Tdap[2,3]

- Adolescents 11 through 18 years of age should receive a single dose of Tdap instead of Td for booster immunization against tetanus, diphtheria, and pertussis. The preferred age for Tdap immunizations is 11 through 12 years of age.
- Adolescents 11 through 18 years of age who received Td but not Tdap are encouraged to receive a single dose of Tdap to provide protection against pertussis. An interval of 2 years between Td and Tdap immunization is suggested. However, Tdap can be given at shorter intervals in settings of increased risk of pertussis (eg, close contact of a case, outbreak setting, close contact of a young infant), because benefits of protection from pertussis outweigh the risk of possible increased local and systemic reactions.

[1]Centers for Disease Control and Prevention. General recommendations on immunization: recommendations of the Advisory Committee on Immunization Practices (ACIP). *MMWR Recomm Rep.* 2009; in press

[2]American Academy of Pediatrics, Committee on Infectious Diseases. Prevention of pertussis among adolescents: recommendations for use of tetanus toxoid, reduced diphtheria toxoid, and acellular pertussis (Tdap) vaccine. *Pediatrics.* 2006;117(3):965–978

[3]Centers for Disease Control and Prevention. Preventing tetanus, diphtheria, and pertussis among adolescents: use of tetanus toxoid, reduced diphtheria toxoid and acellular pertussis vaccines: recommendations of the Advisory Committee on Immunization Practices (ACIP). *MMWR Recomm Rep.* 2006;55(RR-3):1–34

Table 3.46. Contraindications and Precautions for Administration of DTaP in Children

Contraindications
- An immediate anaphylactic reaction after receipt of DTaP[a]
- Encephalopathy within 7 days after receipt of DTaP[b]
- Progressive neurologic disorder[c]

Precautions
- Seizure with or without fever, occurring within 3 days of immunization with DTP or DTaP vaccine
- Persistent, severe, inconsolable screaming or crying for 3 or more hours within 48 hours of immunization
- Collapse or shock-like state (HHE) within 48 hours of immunization
- Temperature of 40.5°C (105°F) or greater, unexplained by another cause, within 48 hours of immunization
- Guillain-Barré syndrome within 6 weeks after a previous dose of tetanus toxoid-containing vaccine

DTaP indicates diphtheria and tetanus toxoids and acellular pertussis vaccine; DTP, diphtheria and tetanus toxoids and whole-cell pertussis vaccine.

[a]Further immunization with any of the 3 components in DTaP vaccine should be deferred because of uncertainty about which antigen may be responsible. People who experience anaphylactic reactions may be referred to an allergist for evaluation and desensitization if a specific allergen can be demonstrated.

[b]This syndrome has been defined as a severe, acute central nervous system disorder unexplained by another cause, which may be manifested by major alterations of consciousness or by generalized or focal seizures that persist for more than a few hours without recovery within 24 hours. Prudence justifies considering such an illness occurring within 7 days of receipt of pertussis-containing vaccine as a contraindication to additional doses of pertussis vaccine, and DT vaccine should be substituted for each of the recommended subsequent doses of diphtheria and tetanus toxoid.

[c]To avoid confusion regarding causation, DTaP immunization should be deferred in children with a progressive neurologic disorder (including infantile spasms, uncontrolled epilepsy, progressive encephalopathy) until neurologic status is stabilized and clarified. Stable neurologic conditions (including developmental delay, cerebral palsy, history of previous seizures) are not a contraindication for DTaP immunization. Efforts also should be undertaken to ensure pertussis immunization of children attending child care centers, special clinics, or residential care institutions.

- Adolescents 11 through 18 years of age for whom Tdap and tetravalent meningococcal conjugate vaccine (MCV4) are indicated should be given both vaccines during the same visit. If immunization on the same day is not feasible, a minimum interval of 1 month between Tdap and MCV4 should occur.

Recommendations for Adolescent Booster Immunization With Tdap Vaccine in Special Situations (see Table 3.47, p 515). Special situations are highlighted below. Only one dose of Tdap should be administered to an adolescent.

- **Pregnancy and postpartum period.** Both the AAP and the CDC Advisory Committee on Immunization Practices (ACIP) state that pregnancy is not a contraindication to Tdap (or Td) immunization. Because the risk of acquiring pertussis in adolescence and the association of pertussis in very young infants with a mother with cough illness, the AAP recommends that pregnant adolescents be given the same considerations for immunization as nonpregnant adolescents. AAP recommendations for use of Tdap in pregnancy differ from those of the ACIP. ACIP prefers postpartum immunization of mothers as soon as possible, as well as the infant's contacts, the so-called "cocoon strategy." The AAP and ACIP recommend that immunization status of household contacts of newborn infants should be evaluated, and those who are eligible

Table 3.47. Special Situation Recommendations for Use of a Single Dose of Tdap in 11- Through 18-Year-Old Adolescents

Situation	Recommendations
Tetanus prophylaxis indicated for wound management	Should receive Tdap (if not previously given) instead of Td. Should administer Tdap concurrently with MCV4 (Menactra), if feasible, in people not previously immunized. Do not defer giving a tetanus-containing vaccine when indicated if Tdap, MCV4, or both are not available.
Lack of availability of Tdap or MCV4	The available vaccine generally should be administered and the other administered when missed vaccine becomes available (also see below).
Use of Td when Tdap is not available	Should receive Td when Tdap is indicated but not available if the last DTP/DTaP/DT/Td was administered at least 10 y previously. If vaccine was administered less than 10 y previously, immunization can be deferred temporarily (awaiting Tdap) if follow-up is likely.
History of pertussis	Should receive Tdap.
History of receipt of DT or Td but incomplete pertussis immunization	Should receive catch-up dose of Tdap; a 2-y interval generally is used (also see above).
History of no DTP/DTaP/ DT or Td immunization	Should receive catch-up doses of 3 Td-containing vaccines, one of which is Tdap.
History of receipt of DTP/ DTaP/DT or Td but incomplete records	Consider serologic testing. If tetanus or diphtheria antibody concentrations are 0.1 IU/mL or greater, presume previous immunization and administer a single dose of Tdap (to be considered the adolescent booster dose).
Pregnancy	Pregnancy is not a contraindication to Tdap (or Td) immunization. Pregnant adolescents should be given the same considerations for immunization as nonpregnant adolescents (see text).
Postpartum	Mothers of newborn infants should be given a dose of Tdap as soon as is feasible if they previously have not received Tdap. Household contacts should have immunization status evaluated and should be given DTaP or Tdap if indicated as soon as is feasible.[a]

Table 3.47. Special Situation Recommendations for Use of a Single Dose of Tdap in 11- Through 18-Year-Old Adolescents, continued

Children 7 through 10 y of age with history of incomplete childhood DTP/DTaP immunization	Neither Tdap vaccine is licensed for use in children younger than 10 y of age. Required series of Td should be given, with a single adolescent booster dose of Tdap. Boostrix could be substituted for one dose of Td in children who are 10 y of age.
People older than 18 y of age	The safety and immunogenicity of Tdap as a single booster dose has been demonstrated for people 19 through 64 y of age. Recommendations for use are available.[b]

Tdap indicates tetanus toxoid, reduced diphtheria toxoid and acellular pertussis vaccine; Td, diphtheria and tetanus toxoids (for children 7 years of age or older and adults); MCV4, tetravalent meningococcal conjugate vaccine; DTP, diphtheria and tetanus toxoids and whole-cell pertussis vaccine; DT, diphtheria and tetanus toxoids vaccine (for children younger than 7 years of age).

[a] Infants younger than 12 months of age are at highest risk of pertussis-related complications and hospitalizations compared with older age groups; young infants have the highest risk of death from pertussis.

[b] Centers for Disease Control and Prevention. Preventing tetanus, diphtheria and pertussis among adults: use of tetanus toxoid, reduced diphtheria toxoid, and acellular pertussis vaccines. Recommendations of the Advisory Committee on Immunization Practices (ACIP). *MMWR Recomm Rep.* 2006;55(RR–3):1–34

for DTaP or Tdap should be immunized as soon as feasible. Protection against pertussis may develop 7 to 10 days after immunization.

If Tdap or Td is indicated, administration in the second or third trimester (and before 36 weeks of gestation) is preferred to minimize a perception of an association of immunization with adverse pregnancy outcomes, which are more common during the first trimester. No evidence exists of a risk of immunizing pregnant women with inactivated bacterial vaccines or toxoids or inactivated viral vaccines. Both Tdap and Td are categorized as pregnancy category C agents by the FDA. Well-controlled human studies and animal reproduction studies acceptable by the FDA have not been conducted for Tdap. Because of lack of data on use of Tdap in pregnant women, both Tdap manufacturers have established pregnancy registries for women immunized with Tdap during pregnancy. Health care professionals are encouraged to report Tdap immunization during pregnancy to the following registries: Boostrix, to GlaxoSmithKline Biologicals at 1-888-825-5249; and Adacel, to sanofi pasteur at 1-800-822-2463.

- **Inadvertent administration of Tdap or pediatric DTaP.** Tdap is not indicated for children younger than 10 years of age. If Tdap is administered inadvertently instead of DTaP to a child younger than 7 years of age as the first, second, or third dose of the immunization series, the Tdap dose should not be counted and DTaP should be given on the same day or as soon as possible, to keep the child on schedule for all vaccines. The remaining doses of the DTaP series should be administered on the usual schedule with at least a 4-week interval between the replacement dose of DTaP and the next dose of DTaP. If Tdap is administered inadvertently instead of DTaP to a child younger than 7 years of age as the fourth or fifth dose in the series, the dose should be counted as valid. If Tdap was administered as the fourth dose, the child should receive a fifth dose of the series using DTaP on the usual schedule. The routine recommendations for adolescent Tdap immunization would apply to children who inadvertently received Tdap instead of DTaP at younger than 7 years of age.

  If Tdap is administered inadvertently instead of Td to a child 7 to 9 years of age, the Tdap dose should be counted as the adolescent Tdap booster. The child should receive a vaccine containing tetanus and diphtheria toxoids 10 years after the inadvertent Tdap dose.

  DTaP is not indicated for people 7 years of age or older. If DTaP is administered inadvertently to a child 7 years of age or older or to an adolescent, the dose should be counted as the adolescent Tdap booster.

- **Recommendations for booster immunization with Tdap for adolescents older than 18 years of age and adults.** The safety and immunogenicity of one Tdap dose as a single booster immunization against tetanus, diphtheria, and pertussis has been demonstrated for people 19 through 64 years of age. The CDC recommends a single dose of Tdap vaccine in people older than 18 years of age to replace 1 decennial Td booster, if they previously have not received Tdap.[1]

Adverse Events After Administration of Tdap in Adolescents. Local adverse events after administration of Tdap or Td in adolescents are common (any pain, 71%–78%; any redness, 20%–23%; any swelling, 18%–21%), and any pain was more common after Tdap versus

[1]Centers for Disease Control and Prevention. Preventing tetanus, diphtheria and pertussis among adults: use of tetanus toxoid, reduced diphtheria toxoid, and acellular pertussis vaccines. Recommendations of the Advisory Committee on Immunization Practices (ACIP). *MMWR Recomm Rep.* 2006;55(RR-3):1–34

Td during prelicensure trials in the United States but not in studies in Canada and Europe. Rates of severe pain (1%–4%), severe redness (2%–6%), or severe swelling (2%–6%) after administration of Tdap versus Td were similar in prelicensure trials. A few adolescents in prelicensure studies had extensive arm swelling after administration of Tdap or Td, which was self-limited. Attention to proper immunization technique and use of standard routes of administration (ie, intramuscular for Tdap and Td) may minimize the risk of local adverse events and optimize immunogenicity.

Systemic adverse events after administration of Tdap or Td in adolescents are common (any fever, 3%–14%; any headache, 40%–44%; tiredness, 27%–37%) and may be slightly more common after Tdap versus Td. Fever greater than 38.9°C (102.0°F), severe headache, or severe tiredness occurred in less than 4% of adolescents after Tdap or Td administration in prelicensure trials. Mild gastrointestinal tract symptoms, sore joints, and generalized body aches are not uncommon after administration of Tdap or Td.

Syncope can occur after immunization, is more common among adolescents and young adults, and can result in serious injury. Vaccinees should be observed for 15 minutes after immunization. If syncope occurs, patients should be observed until symptoms resolve.

Contraindications and Precautions for Use of Tdap in Adolescents. Contraindications and Precautions to administration of Tdap are shown in Table 3.48, p 519.

Deferral of Administration of Tdap. If there is a history of severe Arthus hypersensitivity reaction after a previous dose of a tetanus toxoid-containing and/or a diphtheria toxoid-containing vaccine (including MCV4, which contains diphtheria toxoid as a carrier protein) administered less than 10 years previously, Tdap or Td immunization should be deferred for at least 10 years after administration of the tetanus or diphtheria toxoid-containing vaccine.

Conditions That Are Not Contraindications or Precautions to Administration of Tdap. The following conditions are NOT contraindications or precautions for Tdap. Adolescents with these conditions can receive a dose of Tdap if otherwise indicated. The first 4 bulleted conditions are precautions for administration of pediatric DTP/DTaP but are NOT contraindications or precautions for Tdap immunization in adolescents.

- Temperature 105°F (40.5°C) or greater within 48 hours after DTP/DTaP immunization not attributable to another cause.
- Collapse or shock-like state (HHE) within 48 hours after DTP/DTaP immunization.
- Persistent crying lasting 3 hours or longer, occurring within 48 hours after DTP/DTaP immunization.
- Convulsions with or without fever, occurring within 3 days after DTP/DTaP immunization.
- History of an extensive limb-swelling reaction after pediatric DTP/DTaP or Td immunization that was not an Arthus hypersensitivity reaction.
- Stable neurologic disorder, including well-controlled seizures, a history of seizure disorder, and cerebral palsy.
- Brachial neuritis.

Table 3.48. Contraindications and Precautions for Administration of Tdap in Adolescents

Contraindications
- History of immediate anaphylactic reaction[a] after any component of the vaccine
- History of encephalopathy[b] within 7 days after a pertussis vaccine

Precautions
- History of Guillain-Barré syndrome within 6 weeks of a dose of a tetanus toxoid vaccine[c]
- Progressive neurologic disorder, uncontrolled epilepsy, or progressive encephalopathy until the condition has stabilized[d]

[a]Because of the importance of tetanus immunization, people with a history of anaphylaxis to components should be referred to an allergist to determine whether they have a specific allergy to tetanus toxoid, can be desensitized to tetanus toxoid, and safely can receive tetanus toxoid (TT) immunization.
[b]See footnote b in Table 3.46 for definition.
[c]If decision is made to continue tetanus toxoid, Tdap is preferred if indicated.
[d]This condition is a contraindication for DTaP but a precaution for Tdap. The precaution is for the pertussis component. If decision is made to withhold pertussis immunization, Td may be used.

- Latex allergy other than anaphylactic allergies (eg, a history of contact to latex gloves). The tip and rubber plunger of the Boostrix needleless syringe contain latex. This Boostrix product should not be administered to adolescents with a history of a severe (anaphylactic) allergy to latex but may be administered to people with less severe allergies (eg, contact allergy to latex gloves). The Boostrix single-dose vial and Adacel preparations do not contain latex.
- Breastfeeding.
- Immunosuppression, including people with HIV infection. Tdap poses no known safety concern for immunosuppressed people. The immunogenicity of Tdap in people with immunosuppression has not been studied and could be suboptimal.

Pinworm Infection
(Enterobius vermicularis)

CLINICAL MANIFESTATIONS: Although some people are asymptomatic, pinworm infection (enterobiasis) may cause pruritus ani and, rarely, pruritus vulvae. Pinworms have been found in the lumen of the appendix, but most evidence indicates that they do not cause acute appendicitis. Many clinical findings, such as grinding of the teeth at night, weight loss, and enuresis, have been attributed to pinworm infections, but proof of a causal relationship has not been established. Urethritis, vaginitis, salpingitis, or pelvic peritonitis may occur from aberrant migration of an adult worm from the perineum.

ETIOLOGY: *Enterobius vermicularis* is a nematode or roundworm.

EPIDEMIOLOGY: Enterobiasis occurs worldwide and commonly clusters within families. Prevalence rates are higher in preschool- and school-aged children, in primary caregivers for infected children, and in institutionalized people; up to 50% of these populations may be infected.

Egg transmission occurs by the fecal-oral route either directly or indirectly via contaminated hands or fomites such as shared toys, bedding, clothing, toilet seats, and baths. Female pinworms usually die after depositing eggs on the perianal skin. Reinfection occurs either by autoinfection or by infection following ingestion of eggs from another person. A person remains infectious as long as female nematodes are discharging eggs on perianal skin. Eggs remain infective in an indoor environment usually for 2 to 3 weeks. Humans are the only known natural hosts; dogs and cats do not harbor *E vermicularis*.

The **incubation period** from ingestion of an egg until an adult gravid female migrates to the perianal region is 1 to 2 months or longer.

DIAGNOSTIC TESTS: Diagnosis is made when adult worms are visualized in the perianal region, which is best examined 2 to 3 hours after the child is asleep. Very few ova are present in stool; therefore, examination of stool specimens for ova and parasites is not recommended. Alternatively, diagnosis is made by touching the perianal skin with transparent (not translucent) adhesive tape to collect any eggs that may be present; the tape is then applied to a glass slide and examined under a low-power microscopic lens. Specimens should be obtained on 3 consecutive mornings when the patient first awakens, before washing. Eosinophilia is unusual and should not be attributed to pinworm infection. Serologic testing is not available or useful for diagnosis.

TREATMENT: The drugs of choice are mebendazole, pyrantel pamoate, and albendazole, all of which are given in a single dose and repeated in 2 weeks. Pyrantel pamoate is available without prescription. For children younger than 2 years of age, in whom experience with these drugs is limited, risks and benefits should be considered before drug administration. Reinfection with pinworms occurs easily; prevention should be discussed when treatment is given. Infected people should bathe in the morning; bathing removes a large proportion of eggs. Frequently changing the infected person's underclothes, bedclothes, and bed sheets may decrease the egg contamination of the local environment and risk of reinfection. Specific personal hygiene measures (eg, exercising hand hygiene before eating or preparing food, keeping fingernails short, avoiding scratching of the perianal region, and avoiding nail biting) may decrease risk of autoinfection and continued transmission. Repeated infections should be treated by the same method as the first infection. All household members should be treated as a group in situations in which multiple or repeated symptomatic infections occur. Vaginitis is self-limited and does not require separate treatment.

ISOLATION OF THE HOSPITALIZED PATIENT: Standard precautions are indicated.

CONTROL MEASURES: Control is difficult in child care centers and schools, because the rate of reinfection is high. In institutions, mass and simultaneous treatment, repeated in 2 weeks, can be effective. Hand hygiene is the most effective method of prevention. Bed linen and underclothing of infected children should be handled carefully, should not be shaken (to avoid spreading ova into the air), and should be laundered promptly.

Pityriasis Versicolor
(Tinea Versicolor)

CLINICAL MANIFESTATIONS: Pityriasis versicolor (formerly tinea versicolor) is a common superficial yeast infection of the skin characterized by multiple scaling, oval, and patchy macular lesions usually distributed over upper portions of the trunk, proximal areas of the arms, and neck. Facial involvement particularly is common in children. Lesions may be hypopigmented or hyperpigmented (fawn colored or brown). Lesions fail to tan during the summer and during the winter are relatively darker, hence the term *versicolor*. Common conditions confused with this disorder include pityriasis alba, postinflammatory hypopigmentation, vitiligo, melasma, seborrheic dermatitis, pityriasis rosea, and dermatologic manifestations of secondary syphilis.

ETIOLOGY: The cause of pityriasis versicolor is *Malassezia* species, a group of lipid-dependent yeasts that exist on healthy skin in yeast phase and cause clinical lesions only when substantial growth of hyphae occurs. Moist heat and lipid-containing sebaceous secretions encourage rapid overgrowth.

EPIDEMIOLOGY: Pityriasis versicolor occurs worldwide but is more prevalent in tropical and subtropical areas. Although primarily a disorder of adolescents and young adults, pityriasis versicolor also may occur in prepubertal children and infants. *Malassezia* species commonly colonize the skin in the first year of life and usually are harmless commensals. *Malassezia* can be associated with bloodstream infections, especially in neonates receiving total parenteral nutrition with lipids.

The **incubation period** is unknown.

DIAGNOSIS: The clinical appearance usually is diagnostic. Involved areas are fluorescent yellow under Wood light examination. Skin scrapings examined microscopically in a potassium hydroxide wet mount preparation or stained with methylene blue or May-Grünwald-Giemsa stain disclose the pathognomonic clusters of yeast cells and hyphae ("spaghetti and meatball" appearance). Growth of this yeast on culture requires a source of long-chain fatty acids, which may be provided by overlaying Sabouraud dextrose agar medium with sterile olive oil.

TREATMENT: Topical treatment with selenium sulfide as 2.5% lotion or 1% shampoo has been the traditional treatment of choice. These preparations are applied in a thin layer covering the body surface from the face to the knees for 30 minutes daily for a week, followed by monthly applications for 3 months to help prevent recurrences. In adults, topical ketoconazole 2% shampoo used as a single application daily for 5 days is an effective alternative. Other topical preparations with therapeutic efficacy include sodium hyposulfite or thiosulfate in 15% to 25% concentrations (eg, Tinver lotion) applied twice a day for 2 to 4 weeks. Small focal infections may be treated with topical antifungal agents, such as ciclopirox, clotrimazole, econazole, ketoconazole, miconazole, oxiconazole, or naftifine (see Topical Drugs for Superficial Fungal Infections, p 773). Because *Malassezia* species are part of normal flora, relapses are common. Multiple topical treatments may be necessary.

Oral antifungal therapy has advantages over topical therapy, including ease of administration and shorter duration of treatment, but oral therapy is more expensive and associated with a greater risk of adverse reactions. A single dose of ketoconazole (400 mg orally) or fluconazole (400 mg orally) or a 5-day course of itraconazole (200 mg orally, once a day) has been effective in adults. Some experts recommend that children receive 3 days of ketoconazole therapy rather than the single dose given to adults. For pediatric dosage recommendations for ketoconazole, fluconazole, and itraconazole, see Recommended Doses of Parenteral and Oral Antifungal Drugs, p 768. These drugs have not been studied extensively in children for this purpose and are not approved by the US Food and Drug Administration for this indication. Exercise to increase sweating and skin concentrations of medication may enhance the effectiveness of systemic therapy. Patients should be advised that repigmentation may not occur for several months after successful treatment.

ISOLATION OF THE HOSPITALIZED PATIENT: Standard precautions are recommended.

CONTROL MEASURES: Infected people should be treated.

Plague

CLINICAL MANIFESTATIONS: Naturally acquired plague most commonly manifests in the **bubonic** form, with acute onset of fever and painful swollen regional lymph nodes (buboes). Buboes develop most commonly in the inguinal region but also occur in axillary or cervical areas. Less commonly, plague manifests in the **septicemic** form (hypotension, acute respiratory distress, purpuric skin lesions, intravascular coagulopathy, organ failure) or as **pneumonic** plague (cough, fever, dyspnea, and hemoptysis) and rarely as meningeal, pharyngeal, ocular, or gastrointestinal plague. Abrupt onset of fever, chills, headache, and malaise are characteristic in all cases. Occasionally, patients have symptoms of mild lymphadenitis or prominent gastrointestinal tract symptoms, which may obscure the correct diagnosis. When left untreated, plague often will progress to overwhelming sepsis with renal failure, acute respiratory distress syndrome, hemodynamic instability, diffuse intravascular coagulation, necrosis of distal extremities, and death. Plague has been referred to as black death or blackwater fever.

ETIOLOGY: Plague is caused by *Yersinia pestis*, a pleomorphic, bipolar-staining, gram-negative coccobacillus.

EPIDEMIOLOGY: Plague is a zoonotic infection primarily maintained in rodents and fleas that occurs in many areas of the world, especially Africa. Plague has been reported throughout the western United States, with most human cases (approximately 85%) occurring in New Mexico, Arizona, California, and Colorado as isolated cases or in small clusters. More cases occur during summers that follow mild, wet winters and wet springs with cooler summer temperatures. In the United States, human plague is a rural disease usually associated with epizootic infections in ground squirrels, prairie dogs, and other wild rodents. Bubonic or primary septicemic plague usually occurs from the bites of infected rodent fleas or by direct contact with tissues and fluids of infected rodents or other mammals, including domestic cats. Secondary pneumonic plague arises from hematogenous seeding of the lungs with *Y pestis* in patients with bubonic or septicemic plague. Primary pneumonic plague is acquired by inhalation of respiratory tract droplets from a human or animal with pneumonic plague. Only the pneumonic form has been shown to be transmitted person-to-person, and the last known case of person-to-person transmission in the United States occurred in 1924. However, humans rarely can develop primary pneumonic plague following exposure to domestic cats with respiratory tract plague infections. Epidemics of human plague usually occur as a consequence of epizootics in domestic rodents or after exposures to pneumonic plague.

The **incubation period** is 2 to 8 days for bubonic plague and 1 to 6 days for primary pneumonic plague.

DIAGNOSTIC TESTS: The diagnosis of plague usually is confirmed by culture of *Y pestis* from blood, bubo aspirate, or another clinical specimen. The organism has a bipolar (safety-pin) appearance when viewed with Wayson or Gram stains. A positive fluorescent antibody test result for the presence of *Y pestis* in direct smears or cultures of a bubo aspirate, sputum, cerebrospinal fluid, or blood specimen provides presumptive evidence of *Y pestis* infection. The organism can be detected in fixed tissues by monoclonal antibody-based histochemical analysis methods at the Centers for Disease Control and Prevention (CDC). A single positive serologic test result by passive hemagglutination assay or enzyme immunoassay in an unimmunized patient who previously has not had plague also provides presumptive evidence of infection. Seroconversion and/or a fourfold difference in antibody titer between 2 serum specimens obtained 4 weeks to 3 months apart also confirms the diagnosis of plague. Polymerase chain reaction assay and immunohistochemical staining for rapid diagnosis of *Y pestis* are available in some reference or public health laboratories. Isolates suspected as *Y pestis* should be reported immediately to the state health department and submitted to the Division of Vector-Borne Infectious Diseases of the CDC. Genotyping, performed at the CDC, should be performed on all isolates, particularly for pneumonic cases, to determine whether the isolate is endemic to the area or suspicious for an engineered or imported strain of *Y pestis*.

TREATMENT: For children, streptomycin is the treatment of choice in most cases. Gentamicin in standard doses for age given intramuscularly or intravenously appears to be an equally effective alternative to streptomycin. Tetracycline, doxycycline, chloramphenicol, trimethoprim-sulfamethoxazole, and ciprofloxacin are alternative drugs. Chloramphenicol is the preferred treatment for plague meningitis. Trimethoprim-sulfamethoxazole should not be considered a first-line treatment option when treating bubonic plague and should not be used as monotherapy to treat pneumonic or septicemic plague, because some studies have shown higher treatment failure rates and delayed treatment responses. Fluoroquinolones also have been found to be effective in some cases of plague but currently are not approved by the US Food and Drug Administration for this indication. The usual duration of antimicrobial treatment is 7 to 10 days or until several days after lysis of fever.

Drainage of abscessed buboes may be necessary; drainage material is infectious until effective antimicrobial therapy has been administered.

ISOLATION OF THE HOSPITALIZED PATIENT: For patients with bubonic plague, standard precautions are recommended. For patients with suspected pneumonic plague, respiratory droplet precautions should be initiated immediately and continued for 48 hours after initiation of effective antimicrobial treatment.

CONTROL MEASURES: Plague is controlled in humans by suppression of rodent reservoir hosts and their fleas and by early detection and treatment of people with disease.

Care of Exposed People. All people with exposure to a known or suspected plague source, such as *Y pestis*-infected fleas or infectious tissues, in the previous 6 days should be offered antimicrobial prophylaxis or be cautioned to report fever greater than 38.5°C (101.0°F) or other illness to their physician. People with close exposure (less than 2 m) to a patient with pneumonic plague should receive antimicrobial prophylaxis, but isolation of asymptomatic people is not recommended. For people 8 years of age or older, doxycycline or ciprofloxacin is recommended. For children younger than 8 years of age, doxycycline, tetracycline, chloramphenicol, or trimethoprim-sulfamethoxazole are alternative drugs. Trimethoprim-sulfamethoxazole efficacy is unknown. The risk of prophylactic treatment with chloramphenicol includes aplastic anemia. The risk of prophylactic treatment with doxycycline or tetracycline includes dental staining. The possible benefit of prophylactic therapy should be weighed against these risks. Prophylaxis is given for 7 days from the time of last exposure and in the usual therapeutic doses.

Other Measures. State public health authorities should be notified immediately of any suspected cases of human plague. The public should be educated about risk factors for plague, measures to prevent disease, and signs and symptoms of infection. People living in areas with endemic infection should be informed about the role of dogs and cats in bringing plague-infected rodent fleas into peridomestic environments, the need for flea control and confinement of pets, and the importance of avoiding contact with sick and dead animals. Other preventive measures include surveillance of rodent populations, use of insecticides and insect repellents, and rodent control measures by health authorities when surveillance indicates the occurrence of plague epizootics.

Vaccine. A recombinant fusion protein vaccine (rF1V) that provides protection from aerosolized plague is under development.

Pneumococcal Infections[1]

CLINICAL MANIFESTATIONS: Before routine use of heptavalent pneumococcal conjugate vaccine (PCV7), *Streptococcus pneumoniae* was the most common bacterial cause of invasive bacterial infections in children, including febrile bacteremia. Pneumococci also are a common cause of acute otitis media, sinusitis, community-acquired pneumonia, empyema, and conjunctivitis. Pneumococcus and meningococcus are the 2 most common causes of bacterial meningitis in infants and young children in the United States. Pneumococcus occasionally causes periorbital cellulitis, endocarditis, osteomyelitis, pericarditis, peritonitis, pyogenic arthritis, soft tissue infection, and neonatal septicemia. Pneumococcus also is associated with hemolytic-uremic syndrome, usually in the course of complicated invasive disease (eg, pneumonia with empyema).

ETIOLOGY: *S pneumoniae* organisms (pneumococci) are lancet-shaped, gram-positive catalase-negative diplococci. At least 90 pneumococcal serotypes have been identified on the basis of the polysaccharide capsule. Before implementation of routine immunization in infants with heptavalent pneumococcal conjugate vaccine (PCV7) in 2000, serotypes 4, 6B, 9V, 14, 18C, 19F, and 23F (Danish serotyping system) caused most invasive childhood pneumococcal infections in the United States; these 7 types are contained in PCV7. Serotypes 6A, 6B, 9V, 14, 19A, 19F, and 23F also were the most common serotypes associated with resistance to penicillin. Serotype 19A is the most common cause of invasive disease in PCV7-immunized children.

EPIDEMIOLOGY: Pneumococci are ubiquitous, with many people having transient colonization of their upper respiratory tract. In children, nasopharyngeal carriage rates range from 21% to 59%. Transmission is from person to person by respiratory droplet contact. The period of communicability is unknown and may be as long as the organism is present in respiratory tract secretions but probably is less than 24 hours after effective antimicrobial therapy is begun. Among young children who acquire a new pneumococcal serotype in the nasopharynx, illness (eg, otitis media) occurs in approximately 15%, usually within 1 month of acquisition. Viral upper respiratory tract infections, including influenza, can predispose to pneumococcal infections. Pneumococcal infections are most prevalent during winter months. Rates of infection are highest in infants, young children, elderly people, and black, Alaska Native, and some American Indian populations. The incidence and severity of infections are increased in people with congenital or acquired humoral immunodeficiency, human immunodeficiency virus (HIV) infection, absent or deficient splenic function (eg, sickle cell disease, congenital or surgical asplenia), or abnormal innate immune responses. Children with cochlear implants have high rates of pneumococcal

[1]American Academy of Pediatrics, Committee on Infectious Diseases. Recommendations for the prevention of pneumococcal infections, including the use of pneumococcal conjugate vaccine (Prevnar), pneumococcal polysaccharide vaccine, and antibiotic prophylaxis. *Pediatrics.* 2000;106(2 Pt 1):362–366

meningitis.[1] Other categories of children at presumed high risk or at moderate risk of developing invasive pneumococcal disease are outlined in Table 3.49 (p 526). Since introduction of the conjugate vaccine, racial disparities have diminished.

From 1998–1999 (before vaccine was introduced in 2000) to 2006, the incidence of vaccine-type invasive pneumococcal infections decreased by 99% and the incidence of invasive pneumococcal disease decreased by 77% in children younger than 5 years of age in the general US population. Disease also has decreased substantially in older children and adults, including the elderly. The reduction in cases in these latter groups indicates the significant indirect benefits of PCV7 immunization. Invasive disease caused by penicillin-nonsusceptible isolates also has decreased, especially among children younger than 2 years of age. Despite the success of PCV7 in preventing vaccine-type invasive pneumococcal infections, invasive disease caused by nonvaccine serotypes, especially 19A, has increased, with reduced overall rates of invasive pneumococcal disease leveling off after 2002. Overall rates of pneumococcal otitis media have not changed substantially since introduction of pneumococcal conjugate vaccine, although vaccine-type otitis media has been reduced.

The **incubation period** varies by type of infection and can be as short as 1 to 3 days.

DIAGNOSTIC TESTS: Material obtained from a suppurative focus should be Gram stained and cultured by appropriate microbiologic techniques. Blood cultures should be performed for all patients with suspected invasive pneumococcal disease; cultures of cerebrospinal fluid (CSF) and other specimens (eg, pleural fluid) also may be indicated. Recovery of pneumococci from an upper respiratory tract culture is not indicative of the etiologic diagnosis of pneumococcal disease in the middle ear, lower respiratory tract, or sinus. Rapid methods to detect pneumococcal capsular antigen in CSF, pleural and joint fluid, and concentrated urine as well as polymerase chain reaction (PCR) assay lack sufficient sensitivity or specificity to be of clinical value in children.

Susceptibility Testing. All *S pneumoniae* isolates from normally sterile body fluids (eg, CSF, blood, middle ear fluid, or pleural or joint fluid) should be tested for in vitro antimicrobial susceptibility to determine the minimum inhibitory concentration (MIC) of penicillin and cefotaxime or ceftriaxone. CSF isolates also should be tested for susceptibility to vancomycin and meropenem. *Nonsusceptible* is defined to include both *intermediate* and *resistant* isolates. Accordingly, current definitions by the Clinical and Laboratory Standards Institute (CLSI) of in vitro susceptibility and nonsusceptibility are provided in Table 3.50 for nonmeningeal and meningeal isolates.

For patients with meningitis whose organism is nonsusceptible to penicillin, susceptibility testing of rifampin also should be performed. If the patient has a nonmeningeal infection caused by an isolate that is nonsusceptible to penicillin, cefotaxime, and ceftriaxone, susceptibility testing to clindamycin, erythromycin, rifampin, trimethoprim-sulfamethoxazole, linezolid, meropenem, and vancomycin should be considered, depending on the patient's response to antimicrobial therapy.

Quantitative MIC testing using reliable methods, such as broth microdilution or antimicrobial gradient strips, should be performed on isolates from children with invasive infections. When quantitative testing methods are not available or for isolates from

---

[1]American Academy of Pediatrics, Committee on Infectious Diseases. Acute otitis media and meningitis in children with cochlear implants. *Pediatrics.* 2009; in press

Table 3.49. Children at High or Presumed High Risk of Invasive Pneumococcal Infection

High risk (incidence of invasive pneumococcal disease 150 or more cases/100 000 people per year in the absence of routine PCV7 immunization)

Children with:
- Sickle cell disease, congenital or acquired asplenia, or splenic dysfunction
- Human immunodeficiency virus infection
- Cochlear implants
- Children younger than 2 years of age who are Alaska Native and some American Indian populations

Presumed high risk (insufficient data to calculate rates)

Children with:
- Congenital immune deficiency; some B- (humoral) or T-lymphocyte deficiencies, complement deficiencies (particularly C1, C2, C3, and C4), or phagocytic disorders (excluding chronic granulomatous disease)
- Chronic cardiac disease (particularly cyanotic congenital heart disease and cardiac failure)
- Chronic pulmonary disease (including asthma if treated with high-dose oral corticosteroid therapy)
- Cerebrospinal fluid leaks from a congenital malformation, skull fracture, or neurologic procedure
- Chronic renal insufficiency, including nephrotic syndrome
- Diseases associated with immunosuppressive therapy or radiation therapy (including malignant neoplasms, leukemias, lymphomas, and Hodgkin disease) and solid organ transplantation
- Diabetes mellitus

PCV7 indicates heptavalent pneumococcal conjugate vaccine.

noninvasive infections, the qualitative screening test using a 1-μg oxacillin disk on an agar plate reliably identifies all penicillin-*susceptible* pneumococci on the basis of the criterion of a disk-zone diameter of 20 mm or greater. Organisms with an oxacillin disk-zone size of less than 20 mm potentially are nonsusceptible and require quantitative susceptibility testing. The oxacillin disk test is used as a screening test for resistance to beta-lactam drugs (ie, penicillins and cephalosporins).

TREATMENT: *S pneumoniae* strains that are nonsusceptible to penicillin G, cefotaxime, ceftriaxone, and other antimicrobial agents have been identified throughout the United States and worldwide. Among children in some geographic areas of the United States in the prevaccine era, more than 40% of isolates from sterile body sites were nonsusceptible to penicillin G, and as many as 50% of these isolates were resistant (MIC 2.0 μg/mL or greater). Approximately 50% of penicillin-nonsusceptible strains also were nonsusceptible to cefotaxime or ceftriaxone. Penicillin-nonsusceptible strains also have increased rates of resistance to trimethoprim-sulfamethoxazole, clindamycin, and especially, macrolides (eg, resistance greater than 50%). Rates of resistance to macrolides among penicillin-susceptible strains (eg, resistance greater than 10%), also have increased. However, the incidence of drug-resistant pneumococci has stabilized or decreased since 2000. Current national data on drug resistance are available from the Centers for Disease Control and Prevention (CDC) Web site (**www.cdc.gov/ncidod/dbmd/abcs**).

Table 3.50. Clinical and Laboratory Standards Institute Definitions of In Vitro Susceptibility and Nonsusceptibility Nonmeningeal and Meningeal Pneumococcal Isolates[a,b]

Drug and Isolate Location	Susceptible, µg/mL	Nonsusceptible, µg/mL	
		Intermediate	Resistant
Penicillin (oral)[c]	≤0.06	0.12–1.0	≥2.0
Penicillin (intravenous)[d]			
Nonmeningeal	≤2.0	4.0	≥8.0
Meningeal	≤0.06	None	≥0.12
Cefotaxime **OR** ceftriaxone			
Nonmeningeal	≤1.0	2.0	≥4.0
Meningeal	≤0.5	1.0	≥2.0

[a]Clinical and Laboratory Standards Institute. *Performance Standards for Antimicrobial Susceptibility Testing: 18th Informational Supplement.* CLSI Publication No. M100-S18. Wayne, PA: Clinical and Laboratory Standards Institute; 2008
[b]Centers for Disease Control and Prevention. Effects of new penicillin susceptibility breakpoints for *Streptococcus pneumoniae*—United States, 2006-2007. *MMWR Morb Mortal Wkly Rep.* 2008;57(50):1353–1355
[c]Without meningitis.
[d]Treated with intravenous penicillin.

Vancomycin resistance has not been reported in the United States. If a strain with an in vitro MIC greater than 1.0 µg/mL for vancomycin is isolated, the state health department should be notified promptly and arrangements should be made for confirmatory testing at the CDC.

Recommendations for treatment of pneumococcal infections are as follows.

Bacterial Meningitis Possibly or Proven to Be Caused by S pneumoniae. Combination therapy with vancomycin and cefotaxime or ceftriaxone should be administered initially to all children 1 month of age or older with definite or probable bacterial meningitis because of the increased prevalence of *S pneumoniae* resistant to penicillin, cefotaxime, and ceftriaxone.

For children with hypersensitivity to beta-lactam antimicrobial agents (ie, penicillins and cephalosporins), the combination of vancomycin and rifampin should be considered. Vancomycin should not be given alone, because bactericidal concentrations in CSF are difficult to sustain and clinical experience to support use of vancomycin as monotherapy is minimal. Rifampin also should not be given as monotherapy, because resistance may develop during therapy. Other possible antimicrobial agents for treatment of pneumococcal meningitis include meropenem or chloramphenicol (the latter of which only should be used for pneumococcal meningitis if the minimal bactericidal concentration is 4 µg/mL or less).

A lumbar puncture should be considered after 48 hours of therapy in the following circumstances: (1) the organism is penicillin nonsusceptible by oxacillin disk or quantitative (MIC) testing, and results from cefotaxime and ceftriaxone quantitative susceptibility testing are not yet available; (2) the patient's condition has not improved or has worsened; or (3) the child has received dexamethasone, which might interfere with the ability to interpret the clinical response, such as resolution of fever.

On the basis of available results of susceptibility testing of the pneumococcal isolate, therapy should be modified according to the guidelines in Table 3.51 (p 528). Vancomycin should be discontinued and penicillin, cefotaxime, or ceftriaxone should

Table 3.51. Antimicrobial Therapy for Infants and Children With Meningitis Caused by Streptococcus pneumoniae on the Basis of Susceptibility Test Results

Susceptibility Test Results	Antimicrobial Management[a]
• *Susceptible* to penicillin	**Discontinue vancomycin** **AND** Begin penicillin (and discontinue cephalosporin) **OR** Continue cefotaxime or ceftriaxone alone[b]
• *Nonsusceptible* to penicillin (*intermediate* or *resistant*) **AND** *Susceptible* to cefotaxime and ceftriaxone	**Discontinue vancomycin** **AND** Continue cefotaxime or ceftriaxone
• *Nonsusceptible* to penicillin (*intermediate* or *resistant*) **AND** *Nonsusceptible* to cefotaxime and ceftriaxone (*intermediate* or *resistant*) **AND** *Susceptible* to rifampin	Continue vancomycin and high-dose cefotaxime or ceftriaxone **AND** Rifampin may be added in selected circumstances (see text)

[a]See Table 3.52, p 529, for dosages. Some experts recommend the maximum dosages. Initial therapy of nonallergic children older than 1 month of age should be vancomycin and cefotaxime or ceftriaxone. See Bacterial Meningitis Possibly or Proven to Be Caused by *S pneumoniae*, p 527.
[b]Some physicians may choose this alternative for convenience and cost savings.

be continued if the organism is susceptible to penicillin, cefotaxime, or ceftriaxone. Vancomycin should be continued only if the organism is nonsusceptible to penicillin and to cefotaxime or ceftriaxone.

Addition of rifampin to vancomycin after 24 to 48 hours of therapy should be considered if the organism is susceptible to rifampin and (1) after 24 to 48 hours, despite therapy with vancomycin and cefotaxime or ceftriaxone, the clinical condition has worsened; (2) the subsequent culture of CSF indicates failure to eradicate or to decrease substantially the number of organisms; and/or (3) the organism has an unusually high cefotaxime or ceftriaxone MIC (4 µg/mL or greater). Consultation with an infectious disease specialist should be considered in such circumstances.

Dexamethasone. For infants and children 6 weeks of age and older, adjunctive therapy with dexamethasone may be considered after weighing the potential benefits and possible risks. Many experts recommend the use of corticosteroids in pneumococcal meningitis; but this issue is controversial and data are not sufficient to make a recommendation for children. If used, dexamethasone should be given before or concurrently with the first dose of the antimicrobial agent.

Nonmeningeal Invasive Pneumococcal Infections Requiring Hospitalization. For nonmeningeal invasive infections in previously well children who are not critically ill, antimicrobial agents currently in use to treat infections with *S pneumoniae* and other potential pathogens should be initiated at the usually recommended dosages (see Table 3.52, p 529).

Table 3.52. Dosages of Intravenous Antimicrobial Agents for Invasive Pneumococcal Infections in Infants and Children[a]

Antimicrobial Agent	Meningitis		Nonmeningeal Infections	
	Dose/kg per day	Dose Interval	Dose/kg per day	Dose Interval
Penicillin G	250 000–400 000 U[b]	4–6 h	250 000–400 000 U[b]	4–6 h
Cefotaxime	225–300 mg	8 h	75–100 mg	8 h
Ceftriaxone	100 mg	12–24 h	50–75 mg	12–24 h
Vancomycin	60 mg	6 h	40–45 mg	6–8 h
Rifampin[c]	20 mg	12 h	Not indicated	...
Chloramphenicol[d]	75–100 mg	6 h	75–100 mg	6 h
Clindamycin	Not indicated	...	25–40 mg	6–8 h
Meropenem[e]	120 mg	8 h	60 mg	8 h
Imipenem-cilastatin[f]	...	...	60 mg	6 h
Linezolid[g]	...	...	30 mg	8 h

[a]Doses are for children 1 month of age or older.
[b]Because 1 U = 0.6 μg/mL, this range is equal to 150 to 240 mg/kg per day.
[c]Indications for use are not defined completely.
[d]Drug should be considered only for patients with life-threatening allergic response after administration of beta-lactam antimicrobial agents.
[e]Drug is approved for pediatric patients 3 months of age and older.
[f]For dosing recommendations for infants 3 months of age of younger (weighing 1500 g or more), consult package insert. Drug is not recommended in patients with meningitis because of its potential epileptogenic properties.
[g]Use primarily is for children allergic to beta-lactam antimicrobial agents or children with multidrug-resistant isolates. Dose is for patients younger than 12 years of age. The dose for patients 12 years of age and older is 20 mg/kg per day in 2 doses (adult dose, 1200 mg/day in 2 doses).

For critically ill infants and children with invasive infections potentially attributable to *S pneumoniae*, vancomycin in addition to usual antimicrobial therapy (such as ampicillin, ampicillin-sulbactam, cefotaxime, or ceftriaxone) may be considered for strains that possibly are nonsusceptible to penicillin, cefotaxime, or ceftriaxone. Such patients include those with myopericarditis or severe multilobar pneumonia with hypoxia or hypotension. If vancomycin is administered, it should be discontinued as soon as antimicrobial susceptibility test results demonstrate effective alternative agents.

If the organism has in vitro resistance to penicillin, cefotaxime, and ceftriaxone by standards of the CLSI, therapy should be modified on the basis of clinical response, susceptibility to other antimicrobial agents, and results of follow-up cultures of blood and other body fluids. Consultation with an infectious disease specialist should be considered.

For children with severe hypersensitivity to beta-lactam antimicrobial agents (ie, penicillins and cephalosporins), initial management for a potential pneumococcal infection should include clindamycin or vancomycin in addition to antimicrobial agents for other potential pathogens as indicated. Vancomycin should not be continued if the organism is susceptible to other appropriate non–beta-lactam antimicrobial agents. Consultation with an infectious disease specialist should be considered.

Nonmeningeal Invasive Pneumococcal Infections in the Immunocompromised Host. The preceding recommendations for management of possible pneumococcal infections requiring hospitalization also apply to immunocompromised children, provided they are not critically ill. For critically ill patients, consideration should be given to initiating therapy with vancomycin and cefotaxime or ceftriaxone. Vancomycin should be discontinued as soon as antimicrobial susceptibility test results indicate that effective alternative antimicrobial agents are available.

Dosages. The recommended dosages of intravenous antimicrobial agents for treatment of invasive pneumococcal infections are given in Table 3.52 (p 529).

Acute Otitis Media.[1] According to clinical practice guidelines of the American Academy of Pediatrics (AAP) and the American Academy of Family Physicians (AAFP) on acute otitis media (AOM), amoxicillin (80–90 mg/kg/day) is recommended, except in select cases in which the option of observation without antimicrobial therapy is warranted. Optimal duration of therapy is uncertain. For younger children and children with severe disease at any age, a 10-day course is recommended; for children 6 years of age and older with mild or moderate disease, duration of 5 to 7 days is appropriate.

Patients who fail to respond to initial management should be reassessed at 48 to 72 hours to confirm the diagnosis of AOM and exclude other causes of illness. If AOM is confirmed in the patient managed initially with observation, amoxicillin should be given. If the patient has failed initial antibacterial therapy, a change in antibacterial agent is indicated. Suitable alternative agents should be active against penicillin-nonsusceptible pneumococci as well as beta-lactamase–producing *Haemophilus influenzae* and *Moraxella catarrhalis*. Such agents include high-dose oral amoxicillin-clavulanate; oral cefdinir, cefpodoxime, or cefuroxime; or intramuscular ceftriaxone in a 3-day course. Amoxicillin-clavulanate should be given at 80 to 90 mg/kg per day of the amoxicillin component in the 14:1 formulation to decrease the incidence of diarrhea. Patients who continue to fail therapy with one of the aforementioned oral agents should be treated with a 3-day course of parenteral ceftriaxone. Clarithromycin and azithromycin are appropriate alternatives for initial therapy in patients with type I (immediate, anaphylactic) reaction to a beta-lactam agent, although macrolide resistance among *S pneumoniae* is rising. For patients with a history of non-type I allergic reaction to penicillin, agents such as cefdinir, cefuroxime, or cefpodoxime may be used orally.

Myringotomy or tympanocentesis should be considered for children failing to respond to second-line therapy and for severe cases to obtain cultures to guide therapy. For multidrug-resistant strains of *S pneumoniae*, the use of clindamycin, rifampin, or other agents should be considered in consultation with an expert in infectious diseases.

For detailed information on the management of AOM, the clinical practice guideline of the AAP and AAFP should be consulted.[1]

Sinusitis. Antimicrobial agents effective for treatment of AOM also are likely to be effective for acute sinusitis and are recommended.

ISOLATION OF THE HOSPITALIZED PATIENT: Standard precautions are recommended, including for patients with infections caused by drug-resistant *S pneumoniae*.

---

[1] American Academy of Pediatrics, Clinical Practice Guideline. Subcommittee on Management of Acute Otitis Media. Diagnosis and management of acute otitis media. *Pediatrics.* 2004;113(5):1451–1465

CONTROL MEASURES:

Active Immunization. Two pneumococcal vaccines are available for use in children: PCV7 (Prevnar), which is recommended for all children from 2 through 59 months of age. This vaccine is composed of purified capsular polysaccharides of 7 serotypes (4, 6B, 9V, 14, 18C, 19F, and 23F) conjugated to a diphtheria protein (CRM[197]), and the 23-valent pneumococcal polysaccharide vaccine (PPSV23 [Pneumovax]) for children 2 years of age and older with certain underlying medical conditions. This vaccine is composed of the purified capsular polysaccharides of 23 serotypes. A 13-valent conjugated pneumococcal vaccine is under review by the FDA for licensure. Each available vaccine is recommended in a dose of 0.5 mL to be administered intramuscularly. PPSV23 induces antibody responses to the most common pneumococcal serotypes in the United States among children 2 years of age or older, although immune responses vary by serotype and the response to some serotypes (eg, 6A and 14) is decreased in children 2 through 5 years of age. Duration of protection after PPSV23 is unknown but likely is of relatively short duration. Immunization with PPSV23 does not include immunologic memory or boosting with subsequent doses, and no effect on nasopharyngeal carriage or indirect protection of unimmunized groups has been documented. By contrast, PCV7 elicits a protective antibody response in children as young as 2 months of age, induces immunologic memory, reduces carriage of vaccine-type isolates, and leads to herd protection of unimmunized people. At the time the first conjugate vaccine was licensed in 2000, the 7 serotypes of PCV7 accounted for approximately 88% of cases of bacteremia, 82% of cases of meningitis, and 70% of cases of pneumococcal otitis media in children younger than 6 years of age in the United States. Eighty percent of penicillin-nonsusceptible strains in the United States also were one of these 7 serotypes.

Routine Immunization With Pneumococcal Conjugate Vaccine. PCV7 is recommended for routine administration as a 4-dose series for infants at 2, 4, 6, and 12 through 15 months of age; catch-up immunization is recommended for all children 59 months of age or younger who are not completely immunized for age (Table 3.53, p 532). Each 0.5-mL dose of PCV7 should be administered intramuscularly. Infants should begin the PCV7 immunization series in conjunction with other recommended vaccines at the time of the first regularly scheduled health maintenance visit after 6 weeks of age. Infants of very low birth weight (1500 g or less) should be immunized when they attain a chronologic age of 6 to 8 weeks, regardless of their calculated gestational age. PCV7 may be administered concurrently with all other age-appropriate childhood immunizations using a separate syringe and a separate injection site. For children 23 months of age and younger who have not received the first PCV7 dose before 6 months of age, PCV7 doses should be administered according to the recommended catch-up schedule in Table 3.53 (p 532). For healthy children 24 through 59 months of age who have not completed any recommended schedule for PCV7, administer 1 dose of PCV7. Children who begin catch-up PCV7 immunization between 7 and 59 months of age should do so at the first opportunity. Dosing of PCV7 during vaccine shortages and catch-up regimens vary by degree and anticipated length of shortage and risk group (**www.cdc.gov/vaccines/vac-gen/ shortages/default.htm**).

Immunization of Children 24 Through 59 Months of Age at High Risk of Invasive Pneumococcal Disease. PCV7 is recommended for all children younger than 60 months of age, including children who are at high risk or presumed high risk of acquiring invasive pneumococcal infection, as defined in Table 3.49 (p 526). In addition, supplemental protection should

Table 3.53. Recommended Schedule for Doses of PCV7, Including Catch-up Immunizations in Previously Unimmunized and Partially Immunized Children

Age at Examination (mo)	Immunization History	Recommended Regimen[a]
2 through 6	0 doses	3 doses, 2 mo apart; fourth dose at 12 through 15 mo of age
	1 dose	2 doses, 2 mo apart; fourth dose at 12 through 15 mo of age
	2 doses	1 dose, 2 mo after the most recent dose; fourth dose at 12 through 15 mo of age
7 through 11	0 doses	2 doses, 2 mo apart; third dose at 12 mo of age
	1 or 2 doses before age 7 mo	1 dose at age 7 through 11 mo, with another dose at 12 through 15 mo of age ($\geq$2 mo later)
12 through 23	0 doses	2 doses, $\geq$2 mo apart
	1 dose at <12 mo	2 doses, $\geq$2 mo apart
	1 dose at $\geq$12 mo	1 dose, $\geq$2 mo after the most recent dose
	2 or 3 doses at <12 mo	1 dose, $\geq$2 mo after the most recent dose
24 through 59[b]		
Healthy children	Any incomplete schedule	1 dose, $\geq$2 mo after the most recent dose[c]
Children at high risk[d]	Any incomplete schedule of <3 doses	2 doses, one $\geq$2 mo after the most recent dose and another dose $\geq$2 mo later
	Any incomplete schedule of 3 doses	1 dose, $\geq$2 mo after the most recent dose

PCV7 indicates heptavalent pneumococcal conjugate vaccine.

[a]For children immunized at younger than 12 months of age, the minimum interval between doses is 4 weeks. Doses administered at 12 months of age or older should be at least 8 weeks apart.

[b]Centers for Disease Control and Prevention. Updated recommendation from the Advisory Committee on Immunization Practices (ACIP) for use of 7-valent pneumococcal conjugate vaccine (PCV7) in children aged 24–59 months who are not completely vaccinated. *MMWR Morb Mortal Wkly Rep.* 2008;57(13):33–344.

[c]Providers should administer a single dose to all healthy children 24 through 59 months of age with any incomplete schedule.

[d]Children with sickle cell disease, asplenia, chronic heart or lung disease, diabetes mellitus, cerebrospinal fluid leak, cochlear implant, human immunodeficiency virus infection, or another immunocompromising condition. PPV23 also is indicated. See Table 3.54, p 533.

be given with administration of PPSV23 vaccine at 24 months of age for children with certain underlying medical conditions or as soon as possible after the diagnosis for children 24 months of age or older with newly acquired or newly diagnosed chronic illness. Most children with underlying medical conditions will have received a series of 4 injections of PCV7 before 24 months of age; these children should be given 1 dose of PPSV23 at 24 months of age However, the clinical effectiveness of PPSV23 among children with underlying medical conditions who have received PCV7 is unknown. A second dose of PPSV23 at 5 years after the first dose is only recommended for children who are immuno-compromised or have sickle cell disease or functional asplenia. However, few studies have evaluated systematically the immunogenicity of multiple PPSV23 doses in children. The recommendations for children with underlying medical conditions who are 24 through 59 months of age and may have received previous doses of either PPSV23 or PCV7 are summarized in Table 3.54. All children 24 through 59 months of age with underlying medical conditions who previously received fewer than 3 doses of PCV7 should receive a series of 2 doses of PCV7 followed by 1 dose of PPSV23 given 8 weeks later. For chil-dren with underlying medical conditions 24 through 59 months of age who have received fewer than 3 doses, administer 2 doses of PCV7. Routine use of PPSV23 after PCV7 is not recommended for Alaska Native or American Indian children 24 through 59 months of age. However, in special situations, public health authorities may recommend use of PPSV23 after PVC7 for Alaska Native or American Indian children 24 through

Table 3.54. Recommendations for Pneumococcal Immunization With PCV7 or PPV23 Vaccine for Children at High Risk or Presumed High Risk of Pneumococcal Disease, as Defined in Table 3.49 (p 526)

Age	Previous Dose(s) of Any Pneumococcal Vaccine	Recommendations
23 mo or younger	None	PCV7, as in Table 3.53 (p 532)
24 through 59 mo	4 doses of PCV7	1 dose of PPSV23 vaccine at 24 mo of age, at least 8 wk after last dose of PCV7
		1 dose of PPSV23, 5 y after the first dose of PPV23
24 through 59 mo	1–3 previous doses of PCV7	1 dose of PCV7
		1 dose of PPSV23, 8 wk after the last dose of PCV7
		1 dose of PPSV23, 5 y after the first dose of PPSV23
24 through 59 mo	1 dose of PPSV23	2 doses of PCV7, 8 wk apart, beginning at 6–8 wk after last dose of PPSV23
		1 dose of PPSV23 vaccine, 5 y after the last dose of PPV23 and at least 8 wk after PCV7
24 through 59 mo	No previous dose of PPSV23 or PCV7	2 doses of PCV7, 8 wk apart
		1 dose of PPSV23 vaccine, 8 wk after the last dose of PCV7
		1 dose of PPSV23 vaccine, 5 y after the first dose of PPSV23 vaccine

PCV7 heptavalent pneumococcal conjugate vaccine; PPSV23, 23-valent pneumococcal polysaccharide vaccine. A second dose of PPSV23 5 years after the first dose is recommended only for children who are immunocompromised, have sickle cell -disease, or have functional or anatomic asplenia. All other children with underlying medical conditions should receive 1 dose of PPSV23.

59 months of age who are living in areas in which risk of invasive pneumococcal disease is increased.

Immunization of High-Risk Children 5 Years of Age and Older. Immunization using PCV7 at 5 years of age or older may be appropriate for certain unimmunized children who are at high risk because of chronic underlying disease. PCV7 is licensed by the Food and Drug Administration for children 9 years of age and younger. Limited safety and efficacy data are available for PCV7 or PPSV23 in children who are 60 months of age or older and are at high risk of pneumococcal disease. Studies of small numbers of children with sickle cell disease and HIV infection suggest that PCV7 is safe and immunogenic when administered to children up to 13 years of age. A multicenter study showed that a schedule of 2 doses of PCV7 followed by 1 dose of PPSV23 was safe and immunogenic in HAART-treated HIV-infected children and adolescents 2 through 19 years of age who had not received PCV7 in infancy. Therefore, administration of a single dose of PCV7 to children of any age who are at high risk of invasive pneumococcal disease, is not contraindicated. However, PPSV23 also may be effective and immunogenic in older children, and therefore, immunization with a single dose of PCV7 or PPSV23 is acceptable. If both vaccines are used, PCV7 should be administered first, and the administration of PPSV23 should follow at an interval of at least 8 weeks.

Immunization of Children With Severe or Recurrent Otitis Media. PPSV23 is not recommended for prevention of AOM.

Control of Transmission of Pneumococcal Infection and Invasive Disease Among Children Attending Out-of-Home Child Care. Before routine use of PCV7, children attending out-of-home child care were twofold to threefold more likely to acquire invasive pneumococcal infection than were healthy children of the same age not enrolled in out-of-home child care. PPSV23 has not been shown to decrease nasopharyngeal carriage of pneumococci. In contrast, PCV7 reduces carriage of vaccine serotype pneumococci, but nonvaccine serotype carriage increases at the same time, so overall colonization with pneumococci is not reduced. Available data are insufficient to recommend any antimicrobial regimen for preventing or interrupting the carriage or transmission of pneumococcal infection in out-of-home child care settings. Antimicrobial chemoprophylaxis is not recommended for contacts of children with invasive pneumococcal disease, regardless of their immunization status.

General Recommendations for Use of Pneumococcal Vaccines.
- Either PPSV23 or PCV7 may be given concurrently with other vaccines. Pneumococcal vaccine should be injected with a separate syringe in a separate injection site.
- When elective splenectomy is performed for any reason, immunization with PCV7 and/or PPSV23 should be completed at least 2 weeks before splenectomy. Immunization also should precede initiation of immune-compromising therapy or placement of a cochlear implant by at least 2 weeks.
- Generally, pneumococcal vaccines should be deferred during pregnancy, because whether pneumococcal vaccines can cause fetal harm when administered to a pregnant woman is not known. However, inactivated or killed vaccines, including other experimental and licensed polysaccharide vaccines, have been administered safely during pregnancy. The risk of severe pneumococcal disease in a pregnant woman who has underlying medical conditions that are vaccine indications should be considered when making decisions regarding the need for pneumococcal immunization.

- Children who have experienced invasive pneumococcal disease should receive all recommended doses of pneumococcal vaccines (PCV7 or PPSV23) appropriate for age and underlying condition. The full series of scheduled doses should be completed even if the series is interrupted by an episode of invasive pneumococcal disease.

Case Reporting. Cases of invasive pneumococcal disease in children younger than 5 years of age and drug-resistant infection in all ages should be reported according to state standards. Approximately 97% of invasive disease cases are caused by non-PCV7 serotypes. Therefore, the overwhelming majority of invasive pneumococcal disease cases occurring among unimmunized children do not represent vaccine failures. To differentiate a vaccine failure in an immunized child from disease caused by a serotype not included in PCV7, the isolate would need to be serotyped. A protocol for identifying pneumococcal serotypes included in PCV7 using polymerase chain reaction is available for state public health laboratories on the CDC Web site (**www.cdc.gov/ncidod/biotech/strep/ strepindex.htm**). If the isolate is a serotype included in the vaccine, an evaluation of the patient's HIV status and immunologic function should be considered.

Adverse Reactions to Pneumococcal Vaccines. Adverse reactions after administration of polysaccharide or conjugate vaccines generally are mild and limited to local reactions of redness or swelling. Fever may occur within the first 1 to 2 days after injections, particularly after use of conjugate vaccine.

Passive Immunization. Immune Globulin Intravenous administration is recommended for preventing pneumococcal infection in patients with congenital or acquired immunodeficiency diseases, including people with HIV infection who have recurrent pneumococcal infections (see Human Immunodeficiency Virus Infection, p 380).

Chemoprophylaxis. Daily antimicrobial prophylaxis is recommended for children with functional or anatomic asplenia, regardless of their immunization status, for prevention of pneumococcal disease on the basis of results of a large, multicenter study (see Children With Asplenia, p 84). Oral penicillin V (125 mg, twice a day, for children younger than 5 years of age; 250 mg, twice a day, for children 5 years of age and older) is recommended. The study, performed before the routine use of PCV7 in the United States, demonstrated that oral penicillin V given to infants and young children with sickle cell disease decreased the incidence of pneumococcal bacteremia by 84% compared with the placebo control group. Although overall incidence of invasive pneumococcal infection is decreased after penicillin prophylaxis, cases of penicillin-resistant invasive pneumococcal infections and nasopharyngeal carriage of penicillin-resistant strains in patients with sickle cell disease have increased in recent years. Parents should be informed that penicillin prophylaxis may not be effective in preventing all cases of invasive pneumococcal infections.

The age at which prophylaxis is discontinued often is an empiric decision. Most children with sickle cell disease who have received all recommended pneumococcal vaccines for age and who had received penicillin prophylaxis for prolonged periods, who are receiving regular medical attention, and who have not had a previous severe pneumococcal infection or a surgical splenectomy safely may discontinue prophylactic penicillin at 5 years of age. However, they must be counseled to seek medical attention for all febrile events. The duration of prophylaxis for children with asplenia attributable to other causes is unknown. Some experts continue prophylaxis throughout childhood.

Pneumocystis jirovecii Infections

CLINICAL MANIFESTATIONS: Infants and children develop a characteristic syndrome of subacute diffuse pneumonitis with dyspnea, tachypnea, oxygen desaturation, nonproductive cough, and fever. However, the intensity of these signs and symptoms can vary, and in some immunocompromised children and adults, onset can be acute and fulminant. Chest radiographs often show bilateral diffuse interstitial or alveolar disease; rarely, lobar, miliary, and nodular lesions or even no lesions are seen. The mortality rate in immunocompromised patients ranges from 5% to 40% if treated and approaches 100% if untreated.

ETIOLOGY: Nomenclature for *Pneumocystis* species is in evolution. *Pneumocystis jirovecii* has been proposed for human *Pneumocystis,* denoting the fact that *Pneumocystis carinii* only infects rats. At present, *Pneumocystis carinii* or *P carinii f sp hominis* continues to be used to refer to human *Pneumocystis. Pneumocystis jirovecii* is classified as a fungus on the basis of DNA sequence analysis. However, *P jirovecii* retains several morphologic and biologic similarities to protozoa, including susceptibility to a number of antiprotozoal agents but resistance to most antifungal agents. The 5- to 7-μm-diameter cysts contain up to 8 intracystic bodies.

EPIDEMIOLOGY: *Pneumocystis* species is ubiquitous in mammals worldwide, particularly rodents, and has a tropism for growth on respiratory tract epithelia. *Pneumocystis* isolates recovered from mice, rats, and ferrets are diverse genetically from each other and from human *Pneumocystis jirovecii;* isolates from one animal species do not cross-infect other animal species. Asymptomatic human infection occurs early in life, with more than 85% of healthy children acquiring antibody by 20 months of age. In resource-limited countries and in times of famine, *P jirovecii* pneumonia (PCP) has occurred in epidemics, primarily affecting malnourished infants and children. Epidemics also have occurred in preterm infants. In industrialized countries, PCP occurs almost entirely in immunocompromised people with deficient cell-mediated immunity, particularly people with human immunodeficiency virus (HIV) infection, recipients of immunosuppressive therapy after organ transplantation or treatment for malignant neoplasm, and children with congenital immunodeficiency syndromes. Although decreasing in frequency because of effective prophylaxis and antiretroviral therapy, PCP remains one of the most common serious opportunistic infections in infants and children with perinatally acquired HIV infection. Although onset of disease can occur at any age, including rare instances during the first month of life, PCP most commonly occurs in HIV-infected children in the first year of life. The mode of transmission is unknown. Animal studies have demonstrated animal-to-animal transmission by the airborne route, suggesting the possibility that person-to-person transmission may occur in humans. Primary infection probably accounts for disease during infancy. Although reactivation of latent infection with immunosuppression has been proposed as an explanation for disease after the first 2 years of life, animal models of PCP do not support the existence of latency. Studies of patients with acquired immunodeficiency syndrome (AIDS) with more than one episode of *P jirovecii* pneumonia suggest reinfection rather than relapse. In patients with cancer, the disease can occur during remission or relapse. The period of communicability is unknown.

The **incubation period** is unknown, but animal models suggest 4 to 8 weeks from exposure to clinically apparent infection.

DIAGNOSTIC TESTS: A definitive diagnosis of PCP is made by demonstration of organisms in lung tissue or respiratory tract secretion specimens. The most sensitive and specific diagnostic procedures are open lung biopsy and, in older children, transbronchial biopsy. However, bronchoscopy with bronchoalveolar lavage, induction of sputum in older children and adolescents, and intubation with deep endotracheal aspiration are less invasive, can be diagnostic, and are sensitive in patients with HIV infection who have a high number of organisms. Methenamine silver, toluidine blue O, calcofluor white, and fluorescein-conjugated monoclonal antibody are the most useful stains for identifying the thick-walled cysts of *P jirovecii*. Extracystic trophozoite forms are identified with Giemsa stain, modified Wright-Giemsa stain, and fluorescein-conjugated monoclonal antibody stain. Polymerase chain reaction assays for detecting *P jirovecii* infection are experimental and are not approved by the US Food and Drug Administration (FDA) for diagnosis.

TREATMENT[1]: The drug of choice is intravenous trimethoprim-sulfamethoxazole (see Drugs for Parasitic Infections, p 783). Oral therapy should be reserved for patients with mild disease who do not have malabsorption or diarrhea or for patients with a favorable clinical response to initial intravenous therapy. The rate of adverse reactions (rash, neutropenia, anemia, renal dysfunction, nausea, vomiting, and diarrhea) to trimethoprim-sulfamethoxazole is higher in HIV-infected children than in other patients. If the adverse reaction is not severe, continuation of therapy is recommended. Half of patients with adverse reactions can tolerate treatment with trimethoprim-sulfamethoxazole. Duration of therapy is 21 days.

Intravenously administered pentamidine is an alternative drug for children and adults who cannot tolerate trimethoprim-sulfamethoxazole or who have severe disease and have not responded to trimethoprim-sulfamethoxazole after 5 to 7 days of therapy. The therapeutic efficacy of parenteral pentamidine in adults with PCP is similar to that of trimethoprim-sulfamethoxazole. Pentamidine is associated with a high incidence of adverse reactions, including pancreatitis, renal dysfunction, hypoglycemia, hyperglycemia, hypotension, fever, and neutropenia. If a recipient of didanosine requires pentamidine, didanosine should be discontinued until 1 week after pentamidine therapy has been completed.

Atovaquone is approved for the oral treatment of mild to moderate PCP in adults who are intolerant of trimethoprim-sulfamethoxazole. Experience with the use of atovaquone in children is limited. Other potentially useful drugs in adults include clindamycin with primaquine, dapsone with trimethoprim, and trimetrexate with leucovorin. Experience with the use of these combinations in children is limited.

In patients with AIDS, prophylaxis should be initiated at the end of therapy for acute infection and should be continued until CD4+ T lymphocytes exceed the concentration no longer requiring prophylaxis (see Table 3.55, p 538) or lifelong if CD4+ T-lymphocyte cells do not respond to antiretroviral therapy. Children with PCP as a result of other conditions should be given lifelong prophylaxis as long as the patient continues to have immune compromise.

---

[1]Centers for Disease Control and Prevention. Guidelines for prevention and treatment of opportunistic infections among HIV-exposed and HIV-infected children. Recommendations from CDC, the National Institutes of Health, the HIV Medicine Association of the Infectious Diseases Society of America, the Pediatric Infectious Disease Society, and the American Academy of Pediatrics. *MMWR.* 2009; in press. Available at: **http://aidsinfo.nih.gov/contentfiles/Pediatric_OI.pdf**

Table 3.55. Recommendations for *Pneumocystis jirovecii* Pneumonia (PCP) Prophylaxis for Human Immunodeficiency Virus (HIV)-Exposed Infants and Children, by Age and HIV Infection Status[a]

Age and HIV Infection Status	PCP Prophylaxis[b]
Birth to 4 wk, HIV exposed	No prophylaxis
4 through 6 wk to 4 mo, HIV exposed	Prophylaxis
4 through 12 mo	
HIV infected or indeterminate	Prophylaxis
HIV infection excluded[c]	No prophylaxis
1 through 5 y, HIV-infected	Prophylaxis if:
	CD4+ T-lymphocyte count is less than 500 cells/μL or percentage is less than 15%[d,e]
6 y or older, HIV-infected	Prophylaxis if:
	CD4+ T-lymphocyte count is less than 200 cells/μL or percentage is less than 15%[e]

[a]Centers for Disease Control and Prevention. Guidelines for prevention and treatment of opportunistic infections in HIV-exposed and HIV-infected children. Recommendations from CDC, the National Institutes of Health, the HIV Medicine Association of the Infectious Diseases Society of America, the Pediatric Infectious Diseases Society, and the American Academy of Pediatrics. *MMWR*. 2009; in press. Available at: **http://aidsinfo.nih.gov/contentfiles/Pediatric_OI.pdf.**
[b]Children who have had PCP should receive lifelong PCP prophylaxis.
[c]HIV infection can be excluded reasonably among children who have had 2 or more negative results of HIV diagnostic tests, both of which are performed at 1 month of age or older and 1 of which is performed at 4 months of age or older; or 2 or more negative results of HIV immunoglobulin G antibody tests performed at 6 months of age or older among children who have no clinical evidence of HIV disease (see Human Immunodeficiency Virus Infection, p 380).
[d]Children 1 to 2 years of age who were receiving PCP prophylaxis and had a CD4+ T-lymphocyte count of less than 750/μL or percentage of less than 15% at younger than 12 months of age should continue prophylaxis.
[e]Prophylaxis should be considered on a case-by-case basis for children who might otherwise be at risk of PCP, such as children with rapidly declining CD4+ T-lymphocyte counts or percentages or children with category C status of HIV infection.

Corticosteroids appear to be beneficial in treatment of HIV-infected adults with moderate to severe PCP (as defined by an arterial oxygen pressure [PaO_2] of less than 70 mm Hg in room air or an arterial-alveolar gradient of more than 35 mm Hg). For adolescents older than 13 years of age and adults, 80 mg/day of oral prednisone in 2 divided doses for the first 5 days of therapy; 40 mg, once a day, on days 6 through 10; and 20 mg, once a day, on days 11 through 21 is recommended. Although no controlled studies of the use of corticosteroids in young children have been performed, most experts would include corticosteroids as part of therapy for children with moderate to severe PCP disease. The optimal dose and duration of corticosteroid therapy for children have not been determined, but small studies report improvement with methylprednisolone (1 mg/kg) or prednisone administered 2 to 4 times per day for 5 to 7 days, followed by a tapering dose during the next 7 to 12 days.

Chemoprophylaxis. Prophylaxis against a first episode of PCP is indicated for many patients with significant immunocompromise, including people with HIV infection (see Human Immunodeficiency Virus Infection, p 380) and people with primary or acquired immunodeficiency.

Because rapid changes in CD4+ T lymphocytes can occur in HIV-infected infants, prophylaxis for PCP is recommended for all infants born to HIV infected women beginning at 4 to 6 weeks of age unless the diagnosis has been excluded presumptively

(2 negative virologic test results, 1 performed at 2 weeks of age or older and 1 performed at 4 weeks of age or older; or 1 negative virologic test result, performed at 8 weeks of age or older) (see Table 3.55, p 538). Prophylaxis for PCP should be discontinued in children in whom HIV infection has been excluded definitively (2 negative virologic test results, 1 performed at 4 weeks of age or older and 1 performed at 24 months of age or older; or 2 negative HIV antibody test results from 2 separate specimens at 6 months of age or older). Children who are HIV infected or whose status is indeterminate should continue prophylaxis throughout the first year of life.

For older HIV-infected infants and children, PCP prophylaxis should be continued or administered in the following situations: (1) any CD4+ T-lymphocyte count that indicates severe immunosuppression for age (see Table 3.55, p 538); (2) a rapidly decreasing CD4+ T-lymphocyte count; or (3) severely symptomatic HIV disease (category C) (see Human Immunodeficiency Virus Infection, p 380, and Table 3.55, p 538). Criteria are the same for older children and adolescents, except for different age-specific definitions of low absolute CD4+ T-lymphocyte counts. For adolescents or adults, PCP prophylaxis has been recommended if the patient has a history of oropharyngeal candidiasis. On the basis of experience with discontinuing primary or secondary (after a case of PCP) prophylaxis for PCP in adolescents and adults after an adequate CD4+ T-lymphocyte response to antiretroviral therapy, cessation of prophylaxis also should be considered for children whose CD4+ T-lymphocyte counts are adequate, although only small numbers of children have been studied.

Children older than 1 year of age with HIV infection who are not receiving PCP prophylaxis (eg, children not previously identified or children whose PCP prophylaxis was discontinued) should begin prophylaxis if the CD4+ T-lymphocyte cell count indicates severe immunosuppression (see Table 3.55, p 538).

Prophylaxis for PCP is recommended[1] for children who have received hematopoietic stem cell transplants (HSCT) or organ transplants (except renal), children with lymphoproliferative malignancies (eg, leukemia or lymphoma) or severe cell-mediated immunodeficiency, or children who are immunosuppressed and have had a previous episode of PCP. Prophylaxis should be initiated at engraftment and administered for 6 months. Prophylaxis should be continued for more than 6 months in all children receiving immunosuppressive therapy (eg, prednisone or cyclosporin) or in those with chronic graft-versus-host disease.

The recommended drug regimen for PCP prophylaxis for all immunocompromised patients is trimethoprim-sulfamethoxazole (TMP-SMX) administered for 3 consecutive days each week (see Table 3.56 for dosage). Alternatively, TMP-SMX can be administered daily 7 days a week. For patients who cannot tolerate the drug, alternative choices would include oral atovaquone or dapsone. Atovaquone is effective and safe, but expensive. Dapsone is effective and inexpensive but associated with more serious adverse effects than atovaquone. Aerosolized pentamidine is recommended for children who cannot tolerate TMP-SMX, atovaquone, or dapsone and are old enough to use nebulization with a Respirgard II nebulizer. Intravenous pentamidine has been used but is more toxic than other prophylactic regimens.

---

[1]Centers for Disease Control and Prevention. Guidelines for preventing opportunistic infections among hematopoietic stem cell transplant recipients. Recommendations of the CDC, the Infectious Diseases Society of America, and the American Society of Blood and Barrow Transplantation. *MMWR Recomm Rep.* 2000;49(RR-10):1–128. Also see **www.hivatis.org.**

Table 3.56. Drug Regimens for *Pneumocystis jirovecii* Pneumonia Prophylaxis for Children 4 Weeks of Age or Older[a]

Recommended regimen:

Trimethoprim-sulfamethoxazole (trimethoprim, 150 mg/m^2 per day, with sulfamethoxazole, 750 mg/m^2 per day), orally, in divided doses twice a day, 3 times per week on consecutive days (eg, Monday-Tuesday-Wednesday).

Acceptable alternative trimethoprim-sulfamethoxazole dosage schedules:

- Trimethoprim (150 mg/m^2 per day) with sulfamethoxazole (750 mg/m^2 per day), orally, **as a single daily dose,** 3 times per week on consecutive days (eg, Monday-Tuesday-Wednesday).
- Trimethoprim (150 mg/m^2 per day) with sulfamethoxazole (750 mg/m^2 per day), orally, in divided doses, twice a day, and **administered 7 days per week.**
- Trimethoprim (150 mg/m^2 per day) with sulfamethoxazole (750 mg/m^2 per day), orally, in divided doses twice a day, and administered 3 times per week on alternate days (eg, Monday-Wednesday-Friday).

Alternative regimens if trimethoprim-sulfamethoxazole is not tolerated[b]:

- **Dapsone (children 1 mo of age or older)**
  2 mg/kg (maximum 100 mg), orally, once a day or 4 mg/kg (maximum 200 mg), orally, every week
- **Aerosolized pentamidine (children 5 y of age or older)**
  300 mg, inhaled monthly via Respirgard II nebulizer
- **Atovaquone (children 1–3 mo of age and older than 24 mo of age)**
  30 mg/kg, orally, once a day
- **(children 4–24 mo of age)**
  45 mg/kg, orally, once a day

[a]Centers for Disease Control and Prevention. Guidelines for prevention and treatment of opportunistic infections in HIV-exposed and HIV-infected children. Recommendations from CDC, the National Institutes of Health, the HIV Medicine Association of the Infectious Diseases Society of America, the Pediatric Infectious Diseases Society, and the American Academy of Pediatrics. *MMWR.* 2009; in press. Available at: **http://aidsinfo.nih.gov/contentfiles/Pediatric_OI.pdf**
[b]If dapsone, aerosolized pentamidine, and atovaquone are not tolerated, some clinicians use intravenous pentamidine (4 mg/kg) administered every 2 to 4 weeks.

Other drugs with potential for prophylaxis include pyrimethamine plus dapsone plus leucovorin or pyrimethamine-sulfadoxine. Experience with these drugs in adults and children is limited. These agents should be considered only in situations in which the recommended regimens are not tolerated or cannot be used.

ISOLATION OF THE HOSPITALIZED PATIENT: Standard precautions are recommended. Some experts recommend that patients with PCP not share a room with immunocompromised patients, although data are insufficient to support this recommendation as standard practice.

CONTROL MEASURES: Appropriate therapy for infected patients and prophylaxis in immunocompromised patients are the only available means of control. Detailed guidelines have been issued by the Centers for Disease Control and Prevention and the Infectious Diseases Society of America.

Poliovirus Infections

CLINICAL MANIFESTATIONS: Approximately 95% of poliovirus infections are asymptomatic. Nonspecific illness with low-grade fever and sore throat (minor illness) occurs in 4% to 8% of people who become infected. Aseptic meningitis, sometimes with paresthesias, occurs in 1% to 5% of patients a few days after the minor illness has resolved. Rapid onset of asymmetric acute flaccid paralysis with areflexia of the involved limb occurs in 0.1% to 2% of infections, and residual paralytic disease involving the motor neurons (paralytic poliomyelitis) occurs in approximately two thirds of people with acute motor neuron disease. Cranial nerve involvement and paralysis of respiratory tract muscles can occur. Findings in cerebrospinal fluid (CSF) are characteristic of viral meningitis with mild pleocytosis and lymphocytic predominance.

Adults who contracted paralytic poliomyelitis during childhood may develop the noninfectious postpolio syndrome 30 to 40 years later. Postpolio syndrome is characterized by slow and often significant onset of muscle pain and exacerbation of weakness.

ETIOLOGY: Polioviruses are enteroviruses and consist of serotypes 1, 2, and 3.

EPIDEMIOLOGY: Poliovirus infections occur only in humans. Spread is by the fecal-oral and respiratory routes. Infection is more common in infants and young children and occurs at an earlier age among children living in poor hygienic conditions. The risk of paralytic disease after infection increases with age. In temperate climates, poliovirus infections are most common during summer and autumn; in the tropics, the seasonal pattern is less pronounced.

The last reported case of poliomyelitis attributable to indigenously acquired, wild-type poliovirus in the United States occurred in 1979 and was caused by a wild type 1 poliovirus. In that outbreak, 10 paralytic cases and 4 other poliovirus infections occurred among unimmunized people. The only identified imported case of paralytic poliomyelitis since 1986 occurred in 1993 in a child transported to the United States for medical care. Since 1979, all other cases in the United States have been vaccine-associated paralytic poliomyelitis (VAPP) occurring in vaccine recipients or their contacts and attributable to oral poliovirus (OPV) vaccine. From 1980 to 1996, the average annual number of cases of VAPP reported in the United States was 8. Fewer VAPP cases were reported annually between 1997 and 1999, after a shift in United States immunization policy to a sequential inactivated poliovirus (IPV)-OPV immunization schedule. Implementation of an all-IPV vaccine schedule in 2000 ended the occurrence of new indigenously acquired VAPP cases. In 2005, however, a healthy, unimmunized young adult from the United States acquired VAPP abroad during a study program in Central America, most likely from an infant grandchild of the host family who recently had been immunized with OPV. Additionally, in 2005, a vaccine-derived poliovirus was identified in the stool of an unimmunized child in Minnesota, likely having been acquired from someone who received OPV in another country. Circulation of indigenous wild-type poliovirus strains ceased in the United States several decades ago, and the risk of contact with imported wild-type polioviruses is decreasing rapidly, in parallel with the success of the global eradication program of the World Health Organization (WHO) and WHO partners.

Communicability of poliovirus is greatest shortly before and after onset of clinical illness when the virus is present in the throat and excreted in high concentration in feces. The virus persists in the throat for approximately 1 week after onset of illness and is excreted in feces for several weeks. Patients potentially are contagious as long as fecal excretion persists. In recipients of OPV vaccine, the virus persists in the throat for 1 to 2 weeks and is excreted in feces for several weeks, although in rare cases, excretion for more than 2 months can occur. Immunocompromised patients have excreted virus for periods of more than 10 years.

The **incubation period** of asymptomatic or nonparalytic poliomyelitis is 3 to 6 days. For the onset of paralysis in paralytic poliomyelitis, the incubation period usually is 7 to 21 days.

DIAGNOSTIC TESTS: Poliovirus can be recovered from the pharynx, feces, urine, and rarely, cerebrospinal fluid by isolation in cell culture. Two or more stool and throat swab specimens for enterovirus isolation should be obtained at least 24 hours apart from patients with suspected paralytic poliomyelitis as early in the course of illness as possible, ideally within 14 days of onset of symptoms. Fecal material is most likely to yield virus.

Because OPV vaccine no longer is available in the United States, the chance of exposure to vaccine-type polioviruses has become remote. Therefore, if a poliovirus is isolated in the United States, the isolate should be reported promptly to the state health department and sent to the Centers for Disease Control and Prevention through the state health department for further testing. The diagnostic test of choice for confirming poliovirus disease is viral culture of stool specimens and throat swab specimens obtained as early in the course of illness as possible. Interpretation of acute and convalescent serologic test results can be difficult.

TREATMENT: Supportive.

ISOLATION OF THE HOSPITALIZED PATIENT: In addition to standard precautions, contact precautions are indicated for infants and young children for the duration of hospitalization.

CONTROL MEASURES:

Immunization of Infants and Children.

Vaccines. The 2 types of poliovirus vaccines are inactivated poliovirus (IPV) vaccine given parenterally (subcutaneously or intramuscularly) and live-virus vaccine given orally (OPV). IPV is the only poliovirus vaccine available in the United States. IPV vaccine contains the 3 types of poliovirus grown in Vero cells and inactivated with formaldehyde. Inactivated poliovirus vaccine also is available in several combined formulations (see Table 1.7, p 35). OPV vaccine contains attenuated poliovirus types 1, 2, and 3 produced in monkey kidney cells, human diploid cell cultures, or Vero cells.

Immunogenicity and Efficacy. Both IPV and OPV vaccines in their recommended schedules are highly immunogenic and effective in preventing poliomyelitis. Administration of IPV vaccine results in seroconversion in 95% or more of vaccine recipients to each of the 3 serotypes after 2 doses and in 99% to 100% of recipients after 3 doses. Immunity is prolonged, perhaps lifelong. During poliovirus infection, IPV-immunized children excrete polioviruses from stool but not from the oropharynx. Immunization with 3 or more doses of OPV vaccine induces excellent serum antibody responses and a high degree of intestinal immunity against poliovirus reinfection. A 3-dose series of OPV vaccine, as formerly used in the United States, results in sustained, probably lifelong immunity.

Administration With Other Vaccines. Either IPV or OPV vaccine may be given concurrently with other routinely recommended childhood vaccines (see Simultaneous Administration of Multiple Vaccines, p 33). For administration of combination vaccines containing IPV (see Table 1.7, p 35) with other vaccines and interchangeability of the combined vaccine with other vaccine products, see Pertussis (p 504), Hepatitis B (p 337), and *Haemophilus influenzae* infections (p 314).

Adverse Reactions. No serious adverse events have been associated with use of IPV vaccine. Because IPV vaccine may contain trace amounts of streptomycin, neomycin, and polymyxin B, allergic reactions are possible in recipients with hypersensitivity to one or more of these antimicrobial agents.

Oral poliovirus vaccine can cause VAPP. Before exclusive use of IPV vaccine in the United States, the overall risk of VAPP associated with OPV was approximately 1 case per 2.4 million doses of OPV vaccine distributed. The rate of VAPP after the first dose, including vaccine recipient and contact cases, was approximately 1 case per 750 000 doses.

Schedule. Four doses of IPV vaccine are recommended for routine immunization of all infants and children in the United States. The first 2 doses should be given at 2-month intervals beginning at 2 months of age (minimum age 6 weeks), and a third dose is recommended at 6 through 18 months of age. Doses may be given at 4-week intervals when accelerated protection is indicated. Administration of the third dose at 6 months of age has the potential advantage of enhancing the likelihood of completion of the primary series and does not compromise seroconversion. A supplemental dose of IPV vaccine should be given before the child enters school (ie, at 4 through 6 years of age). A fourth dose is not necessary if the third dose was given at 4 years of age or older.

Oral poliovirus vaccine remains the vaccine of choice for global eradication, although IPV may be adopted more widely to augment OPV in areas where poliomyelitis has been difficult to control.

OPV vaccine no longer is licensed or available in the United States.

Children Incompletely Immunized. Children who have not received the recommended doses of poliovirus vaccines on schedule should receive sufficient doses of IPV vaccine to complete the immunization series for their age (see Fig 1.3, p 28).

Vaccine Recommendations for Adults. Most adults residing in the United States are immune as a result of immunization received during childhood and have a small risk of exposure to wild-type poliovirus in the United States. Immunization is recommended only for certain adults who are at a greater risk of exposure to wild-type polioviruses than the general population, including the following:

• Travelers to areas or countries where poliomyelitis is or may be epidemic or endemic
• Members of communities or specific population groups with disease caused by wild-type polioviruses
• Laboratory workers handling specimens that may contain wild-type polioviruses
• Health care professionals in close contact with patients who may be excreting wild-type polioviruses

For unimmunized adults, primary immunization with IPV vaccine is recommended. Two doses of IPV vaccine should be given at intervals of 1 to 2 months (4–8 weeks); a third dose is given 6 to 12 months after the second unless the risk of exposure is increased, such as when traveling to areas where wild-type poliovirus is known to be circulating. If time does not allow 3 doses of IPV vaccine to be given according to the recommended schedule before protection is required, the following alternatives are recommended:

- If protection is not needed until 8 weeks or more, 3 doses of IPV vaccine should be given at least 4 weeks apart.
- If protection is not needed for 4 to 8 weeks, 2 doses of IPV vaccine should be given at least 4 weeks apart.
- If protection is needed in fewer than 4 weeks, a single dose of IPV vaccine should be given.

The remaining doses of vaccine to complete the primary immunization schedule should be given subsequently at the recommended intervals if the person remains at an increased risk.

Recommendations in other circumstances are as follows:

- **Incompletely immunized adults.** Adults who previously received less than a full primary course of OPV or IPV vaccine should be given the remaining required doses of IPV vaccine regardless of the interval since the last dose and the type of vaccine that was received previously.
- **Adults who are at an increased risk of exposure to wild-type poliovirus and who previously completed primary immunization with OPV or IPV vaccine.** These adults can receive a single dose of IPV vaccine.

Precautions and Contraindications to Immunization.

Immunocompromised Disorders. Immunocompromised patients, including HIV infection, combined immunodeficiency, abnormalities of immunoglobulin synthesis (ie, antibody deficiency syndromes), leukemia, lymphoma, or generalized malignant neoplasm, or people being given immunosuppressive therapy with pharmacologic agents (see Immunocompromised Children, p 72) or radiation therapy should receive IPV vaccine. A protective immune response to IPV vaccine in an immunocompromised patient cannot be ensured.

Household Contacts of Immunocompromised People or People With Altered Immune States, Immunosuppression Attributable to Therapy for Other Disease, or Known HIV Infection. IPV vaccine is recommended for these people, and OPV vaccine should not be used. If OPV vaccine inadvertently is introduced into a household of an immunocompromised or HIV-infected person, close contact between the patient and the OPV vaccine recipient should be minimized for approximately 4 to 6 weeks after immunization. Household members should be counseled on practices that will minimize exposure of the immunocompromised or HIV-infected person to excreted poliovirus vaccine. These practices include exercising hand hygiene after contact with the child by all and avoiding diaper changing by the immunosuppressed person.

Pregnancy. Immunization during pregnancy generally should be avoided for reasons of theoretical risk, although no convincing evidence indicates that the rates of adverse reactions to IPV vaccine are increased in pregnant women or in their developing fetuses. If immediate protection against poliomyelitis is needed, IPV is recommended.

Hypersensitivity or Anaphylactic Reactions to IPV Vaccine or Antimicrobial Agents Contained in IPV. The IPV vaccine is contraindicated for people who have experienced an anaphylactic reaction after a previous dose of IPV vaccine or to one of the following antimicrobial agents: streptomycin, neomycin, and polymyxin B.

Breastfeeding and mild diarrhea are not contraindications to IPV or OPV vaccine administration.

Reporting of Adverse Events After Immunization. All cases of VAPP and other serious adverse events associated temporally with poliomyelitis vaccine should be reported (see Reporting of Adverse Events, p 42).

Case Reporting and Investigation. A suspected case of poliomyelitis or isolation of a poliovirus should be reported promptly to the state health department and should result in an immediate epidemiologic investigation. Poliomyelitis should be considered in the differential diagnosis of all cases of acute flaccid paralysis, including Guillain-Barré syndrome and transverse myelitis. If the course is compatible clinically with poliomyelitis, specimens should be obtained for virologic studies (see Diagnostic Tests, p 542). If the evidence implicates wild-type or a genetically drifted vaccine-derived poliovirus infection, an intensive investigation will be conducted, and a public health decision will be made about the need for supplementary immunizations, choice of vaccine, and other action.

Polyomaviruses (BK Virus and JC Virus)

CLINICAL MANIFESTATIONS: BK virus (BKV) and James Canyon virus (JCV) infections in immunocompetent children usually are asymptomatic. Because of tropism for genitourinary tract epithelium, BKV may cause asymptomatic hematuria or cystitis in healthy children but is more likely to cause disease in immunocompromised people, in whom both lower tract renal disease (hemorrhagic cystitis in hematopoietic stem cell transplant recipients) and upper tract renal disease (interstitial nephritis and ureteral stenosis in renal transplant recipients) is possible. BKV-associated nephropathy occurs in 3% to 8% of renal transplant recipients and should be suspected in any renal transplant patient with allograft dysfunction. More than 50% of patients with BKV-associated nephropathy experience renal allograft loss. The primary symptom of BKV-associated hemorrhagic cystitis is painful hematuria. Passage of blood clots in the urine and secondary obstructive nephropathy can occur in patients with BKV-associated hemorrhagic cystitis.

JCV is the cause of progressive multifocal leukoencephalopathy (PML) that occurs in severely immune-compromised patients. PML, the only known disease caused by JCV, occurs in approximately 5% of untreated adults with acquired immunodeficiency syndrome (AIDS) but is less frequent in children with AIDS. PML is a rare demyelinating disease of the central nervous system. Symptoms of PML include cognitive disturbance, hemiparesis, ataxia, cranial nerve dysfunction, and aphasia. Cytocidal infection of oligodendrocytes with JCV produces the pathognomonic lesions of PML, which contain large numbers of JCV virions. In the absence of restored T-lymphocyte function, PML almost always is fatal. PML is an AIDS-defining illness in HIV-infected people.[1]

---

[1] Centers for Disease Control and Prevention. Guidelines for prevention and treatment of opportunistic infections among HIV-exposed and HIV-infected children. Recommendations from CDC, the National Institutes of Health, the HIV Medicine Association of the Infectious Diseases Society of America, the Pediatric Infectious Diseases Society, and the American Academy of Pediatrics. *MMWR.* 2009; in press. Available at **http://aidsinfo.nih.gov/contentfiles/Pediatric_OI.pdf**

Simian virus 40 (SV40) is a polyomavirus of Asian macaque monkeys and was a contaminant of some lots of Sabin and Salk poliovirus vaccines between 1955 and 1963. Two additional polyomaviruses, named KI and WU, have been detected in respiratory tract secretions and associated with respiratory tract infections in children and adults, respectively, but have not been associated with nephropathy. With the exception of SV40, the nomenclature for polyomaviruses reflects the initials of the patient from whom the virus initially was identified.

ETIOLOGY: BKV and JCV are members of the family Polyomaviridae.

EPIDEMIOLOGY: Humans are the only known natural hosts for BKV and JCV. The mode of transmission of BKV and JCV is uncertain. BKV and JCV are ubiquitous in the human population, with BKV infection occurring in early childhood and JCV infection occurring primarily in adolescence and adulthood. BKV persists in the kidney, gastrointestinal tract, and leukocytes of healthy subjects, with urinary excretion occurring in 3% to 5% of healthy adults. JCV persists in the kidney and brain of healthy people. The prevalence of urinary excretion of JCV increases with age.

DIAGNOSTIC TESTS: Detection of BKV T-antigen by immunohistochemical analysis of renal biopsy material is the gold standard for diagnosis of BK virus-associated nephropathy. Visualization of BKV particles in renal biopsy material by electron microscopy is a sensitive alternative to immunohistochemical analysis. Prospective monitoring of BK viral load in plasma commonly is used after renal transplantation. Detection of BKV nucleic acid in plasma by polymerase chain reaction (PCR) assay is associated with an increased risk of BKV-associated nephropathy, especially when BK viral loads exceed 10 000 genomes/mL. Detection of BKV in urine of renal transplant recipients is common and is not useful in evaluation of suspected BKV disease after renal transplantation.

The diagnosis of BKV-associated hemorrhagic cystitis is made clinically when other causes of urinary tract bleeding are excluded. Among hematopoietic stem cell transplant recipients, detection of BKV in urine is common (more than 50%), but BKV-associated hemorrhagic cystitis is much less common (10%–15%). Prolonged urinary shedding of BKV and detection of BKV in plasma after hematopoietic stem cell transplantation has been associated with increased risk of developing BKV-associated hemorrhagic cystitis. Urine cytologic testing may suggest urinary shedding of BKV on the basis of presence of decoy cells, which resemble renal carcinoma cells. However, decoy cells do not have high sensitivity or specificity for BKV infection.

A confirmed diagnosis of PML requires a compatible clinical syndrome and magnetic resonance imaging or computed tomographic findings showing lesions in the brain coupled with brain biopsy findings. JCV can be demonstrated by in situ hybridization or by electron microscopy for definitive diagnosis. Diagnosis of PML can be facilitated when JCV DNA is detected in cerebrospinal fluid by a nucleic acid amplification test, which may obviate the need for a brain biopsy. Early in the course of PML, false-negative PCR assay results have been reported, so repeat testing is warranted when the clinical suspicion of PML is high. Measurement of JCV DNA concentrations in cerebrospinal fluid samples may be a useful marker for managing PML in patients receiving highly active antiretroviral therapy (HAART).

TREATMENT: There have been no controlled clinical trials of antiviral agents active against BKV or JCV. In patients with biopsy-confirmed BKV-associated nephropathy, reduction of immune suppression may prevent allograft loss. Treatment of renal transplant recipients with BKV-associated nephropathy with cidofovir is being evaluated in a National Institutes of Health study being conducted by the Collaborative Antiviral Study Group; leflunomide also has been suggested as a possible therapeutic agent in this population. The role of Immune Globulin Intravenous in treatment of BKV-associated nephropathy is uncertain. In renal transplant patients with BKV plasma viral loads greater than 10 000 genomes/mL, judicious reduction of immune suppression has been shown to prevent development of BKV-associated nephropathy without increasing the risk of rejection.

Most patients with BKV-hemorrhagic cystitis after hematopoietic stem cell transplantation require only supportive care, because restoration of immune function by stem cell engraftment ultimately will control BKV replication. Cidofovir and leflunomide have been used in hematopoietic stem cell transplant recipients who have prolonged BKV hemorrhagic cystitis attributable to failure of engraftment. In severe cases, surgical intervention may be required to stop bladder hemorrhage.

Restoration of immune function (eg, HAART for patients with AIDS) is necessary for survival of patients with PML. Cidofovir sometimes is used but has not been shown to be effective in producing clinical improvement.

ISOLATION OF THE HOSPITALIZED PATIENT: Standard precautions are recommended.

CONTROL MEASURES: None.

PRION DISEASES

Transmissible Spongiform Encephalopathies[1]

CLINICAL MANIFESTATIONS: Transmissible spongiform encephalopathies (TSEs), or prion diseases, constitute a group of rare, rapidly progressive, universally fatal neurodegenerative syndromes of humans and animals that are characterized by neuronal degeneration, spongiform change, gliosis, and accumulation of an abnormal protease-resistant amyloid protein (protease-resistant prion protein [PrP^{res}], scrapie prion protein [PrP^{sc}], or as suggested by the World Health Organization [WHO], TSE-associated PrP [PrP^{TSE}]) distributed diffusely throughout the brain and sometimes also in discrete plaques.

Human TSEs include several diseases: Creutzfeldt-Jakob disease (CJD), Gerstmann-Sträussler-Scheinker disease, fatal familial and sporadic insomnia syndromes, kuru, and variant CJD (vCJD, or mad cow disease). Classic CJD can be sporadic (approximately 85% of cases), familial (approximately 15% of cases), or iatrogenic (fewer than 1% of cases). Sporadic CJD most commonly is a disease of the elderly (median age of death, 68 years in the United States) but also rarely has been described in adolescents older than 13 years of age and young adults. Iatrogenic CJD has been acquired through injection of cadaveric pituitary hormones (growth hormone and human gonadotropin), dura mater allografts, corneal transplantation, and instrumentation of the brain at neurosurgery or depth-electrode electroencephalographic recording. In 1996, an outbreak of vCJD linked to exposure to tissues from bovine spongiform encephalopathy (BSE)-infected cattle was reported in the United Kingdom. Since the end of 2003, 3

[1]American Academy of Pediatrics, Committee on Infectious Diseases. Transmissible spongiform encephalopathies: a review for pediatricians. *Pediatrics.* 2000;106(5):1160–1165

presumptive cases of transfusion-transmitted vCJD have been reported as well as 1 probable transfusion-transmitted preclinical vCJD infection. The best-known TSEs affecting animals are scrapie of sheep, BSE, and a chronic wasting disease of North American deer, elk, and moose. Except for vCJD, thought to have originated from BSE, no other human TSE has been attributed convincingly to infection with an agent of animal origin.

CJD manifests as a rapidly progressive, dementia-causing illness with defects in memory, personality, and other higher cortical functions. At presentation, approximately one third of patients have cerebellar dysfunction, including ataxia and dysarthria. Iatrogenic CJD may manifest as dementia or as cerebellar signs (as observed in virtually all people with inoculated disease). Myoclonus develops in at least 80% of affected patients at some point in the course of disease. Death usually occurs in weeks to months (median 4–5 months); approximately 10% to 15% of patients with sporadic CJD survive for more than 1 year.

vCJD is distinguished from classic CJD by younger age of onset, early "psychiatric" manifestations, and other features, such as painful sensory symptoms, delayed onset of overt neurologic signs, absence of diagnostic electroencephalographic changes, and a more prolonged duration of illness. In vCJD, the neuropathologic examination reveals numerous "florid" plaques and marked accumulation of protease-resistant prion protein (PrP^{res}). In addition, PrP^{res} readily is detectable in lymphoid tissues of patients with vCJD. In vCJD, but not in classic CJD, a high proportion of people exhibit high signal abnormalities on T2-weighted brain magnetic resonance imaging in the pulvinar region of the posterior thalamus (known as the "pulvinar sign").

ETIOLOGY: The infectious particle or prion responsible for human and animal prion diseases is thought to be the abnormal form of a normal ubiquitous glycoprotein, without a nucleic acid component. Proponents of the prion hypothesis postulate that sporadic CJD arises from a rare spontaneous structural change of the normal "cellular" protease-sensitive host-encoded glycoprotein (PrP^C or PrP^{sen}) that normally is found on the surface of neurons and many other cells in both humans and animals. Prion protein (PrP) conformational changes are postulated to be propagated by a "recruitment" reaction (the nature of which is unknown), in which abnormal PrP serves as a template or lattice for the conformational conversion of neighboring PrP^C molecules.

EPIDEMIOLOGY: Classic CJD is rare, occurring at a rate of approximately 1 case per million people annually. The onset of disease peaks in the 60- through 69-year age group. Familial CJD illnesses, which are associated with a variety of mutations of the PrP gene on chromosome 20, occurs at approximately one sixth the frequency of sporadic CJD, with onset of disease approximately 10 years earlier than sporadic CJD. Case-control studies of sporadic CJD have not identified any consistent environmental risk factor. As of December 2007, no statistically significant increased risk of sporadic CJD has been observed for treatment with blood, blood components, or plasma derivatives. The incidence of sporadic CJD is not increased in patients with several diseases associated with increased exposure to blood or blood products, specifically hemophilia A and B, thalassemia, and sickle cell disease, suggesting that the risk of transfusion transmission of classic CJD, if any, is very low and appropriately regarded as theoretical. CJD has not been reported in infants born to infected mothers.

As of September 2008 (**www.cjd.ed.ac.uk/vcjdworld.htm**), vCJD was reported in 164 patients in the United Kingdom, 23 in France, 4 in Ireland, 4 in Spain, 3 in the United States, 2 in the Netherlands, 2 in Portugal, and 1 each in Canada, Italy, Japan, and Saudi Arabia. Two of the 3 patients in the United States, 2 of the 3 in Ireland, and 1 each of the patients in France and Canada are believed to have acquired vCJD during prolonged residence in the United Kingdom. The CDC has concluded that the third vCJD patient in the United States probably was infected during prolonged residence in Saudi Arabia. Authorities suspect that the Japanese patient was infected during a short visit of 24 days to the United Kingdom, 12 years before the onset of vCJD. Most patients with vCJD were younger than 30 years of age, and several were adolescents. All but 2 patients with noniatrogenic vCJD died before 55 years of age (median age at death is 28 years). On the basis of animal inoculation studies, strain typing, and epidemiologic investigations, cases of vCJD are believed to have resulted from exposure to tissues from cattle infected with BSE. As noted, 4 patients are believed to have been infected with vCJD through blood transfusion.

The **incubation period** for iatrogenic CJD varies by route of exposure and ranges from 1.5 to more than 30 years.

DIAGNOSTIC TESTS: The diagnosis of human prion diseases can be made with certainty only by neuropathologic examination of affected brain tissue. In most patients with classic CJD, atypical 1-cycle to 2-cycles per second triphasic sharp-wave discharge on electroencephalographic tracing has been described. The likelihood of finding this abnormality is enhanced if serial electroencephalographic recordings are obtained. A protein assay that detects the 14-3-3 protein in cerebrospinal fluid has been reported to be reasonably sensitive, though not specific, as a marker for CJD. No validated blood test is available. A progressive neurologic syndrome in a person bearing a pathogenic mutation of the PrP gene (PRNP) is presumed to be prion disease. Failure to identify a unique prion nucleic acid component precludes detection of the infective particle by genome amplification. Performing a brain biopsy in patients with suspected or clinically diagnosed CJD is encouraged to confirm the diagnosis and detect other emerging forms of CJD, such as vCJD. Free state-of-the-art diagnostic testing, including 14-3-3 assays, PRNP gene sequencing, Western blot analysis to identify PrP^{TSE}, and histologic processing of biopsy and autopsy brain tissues with pathologic consultation are available at the National Prion Disease Pathology Surveillance Center (telephone, 216-368-0587; **www.cjdsurveillance.com**).

TREATMENT: No treatment has been shown in humans to slow or stop the progressive neurodegenerative syndromes of prion diseases. Experimental treatments are being studied. Supportive therapy is necessary to manage dementia, spasticity, rigidity, and seizures arising during the course of the illness. Psychological support may help families of affected people. Genetic counseling is indicated in familial disease, taking into account that penetrance has been variable in some kindred.

ISOLATION OF THE HOSPITALIZED PATIENT: Standard precautions are recommended. Available evidence indicates that even prolonged intimate contact with CJD-infected people has not resulted in transmission of disease. Tissues associated with high levels of infectivity (eg, brain, eyes, and spinal cord of affected people) and instruments in contact with those tissues are considered biohazards; incineration, prolonged autoclaving at high temperature and pressure after thorough cleaning, and especially exposure to a solution of sodium hydroxide of 1N or greater or a solution of sodium hypochlorite of 5.25% or greater (undiluted household chlorine bleach) for 1 hour has been reported to decrease infectivity of contaminated surgical instruments.[1] Detailed CJD infection-control recommendations, distribution of infectivity in various tissues, and specific decontamination protocols are available at **www.cdc.gov/ncidod/dvrd/cjd/qa_cjd_infection_ control.htm.** Person-to-person transmission of classic CJD by blood, milk, saliva, urine, or feces has not been reported. These body fluids should be handled using standard infection control procedures; universal blood precautions should be sufficient to prevent bloodborne transmission.

CONTROL MEASURES: Immunization against prion diseases is not available, and no protective immune response to infection has been demonstrated. Iatrogenic transmission of CJD through cadaveric pituitary hormones has been obviated by use of recombinant products. Recognition that CJD can be spread by transplantation of infected dura and corneas and that vCJD can be spread by blood transfusion has led to more stringent donor-selection criteria and improved collection protocols. Health care personnel should follow their state's prion disease reporting requirements, and any suspected or confirmed diagnosis of CJD for which a special public health response may be needed (eg, suspected iatrogenic disease or vCJD) should be reported promptly to the appropriate state or local health departments and to the Prion Diseases Surveillance Unit, Division of Viral and Rickettsial Diseases, Centers for Disease Control and Prevention, Atlanta, GA 30333; telephone, 404-639-3091. Current precautionary policies of the US Food and Drug Administration about risk of CJD and human blood or blood products are accessible on the Internet at **www.fda.gov/cber/whatsnew.htm.**

Q Fever

CLINICAL MANIFESTATIONS: Although up to 60% of initial infections are asymptomatic, disease attributable to Q fever occurs in 2 distinct forms: acute, which typically follows initial exposure; and chronic, which occurs months to years after acute infection. Acute Q fever usually is characterized by abrupt onset of fever, chills, weakness, headache, anorexia, and other nonspecific systemic symptoms. Weight loss and weakness can be pronounced. Cough and chest pain can accompany pneumonia and hepatitis, although jaundice is rare. Rash rarely is observed. The illness typically lasts 1 to 4 weeks and then resolves gradually. Life-threatening complications of acute infection, such as meningoencephalitis and myocarditis, occur rarely. Chronic Q fever occurs in approximately 1% of acutely ill patients and manifests as endocarditis in patients with underlying heart disease or prosthetic valves, vascular aneurysms, or vascular grafts. Hepatitis is another common manifestation. Pregnant and immunosuppressed people also are predisposed to chronic Q fever. Both acute and chronic Q fever may manifest as fever of undetermined origin. Although acute Q fever rarely is fatal, chronic Q fever often is fatal if untreated. With appropriate long-term antimicrobial therapy, mortality among patients with endocarditis is decreased to approximately 10%. Q fever during pregnancy is associated with abortion, preterm birth, and low birth weight.

---

[1] www.cdc.gov/ncidod/dvrd/prions

ETIOLOGY: *Coxiella burnetii*, the cause of Q fever, formerly was considered to be a *Rickettsia* organism, but it is an obligate intracellular bacterium that belongs to the order Legionellaceae. The infectious form of *C burnetii* is highly resistant to heat, desiccation, and disinfectant chemicals and can persist for long periods of time in the environment. *C burnetii* is classified in the gamma subgroup of Proteobacteria. *C burnetii* is a potential agent of bioterrorism.

EPIDEMIOLOGY: Q fever is a zoonotic infection that has been reported worldwide. In animals, *C burnetii* infection usually is asymptomatic. The most common reservoirs are domestic farm animals (especially sheep, goats, and cows), which most often are associated with human infection. Cats, dogs, rodents, marsupials, other mammalian species, and some wild and domestic bird species also may serve as reservoirs. Tick vectors may be important for maintaining animal and bird reservoirs but are not thought to be important in transmission to humans. Humans typically acquire infection by inhalation of *C burnetii* in fine-particle aerosols generated from birthing fluids during animal parturition or through inhalation of dust contaminated by these materials. Infection can occur by direct exposure to infected animals or tissues on farms and ranches or in research facilities or by exposure to contaminated materials, such as wool, straw, fertilizer, or laundry. Airborne particles containing infectious organisms can be carried downwind a half-mile or more, contributing to sporadic cases for which no apparent animal contact can be demonstrated. Unpasteurized dairy products can contain the organism. Seasonal trends occur in farming areas with predictable frequency, and the disease often coincides with the lambing season in early spring.

The **incubation period** usually is 14 to 22 days, with a range from 9 to 39 days, depending on the inoculum. Chronic Q fever can develop years to decades after initial infection.

DIAGNOSTIC TESTS: Isolation of *C burnetii* from blood usually is not attempted except in specialized laboratories because of the potential hazard to laboratory workers. Cell culture systems or the inoculation of animals or eggs can be used for isolating *C burnetii* from clinical samples. Confirmation of acute Q fever requires one of the following: (1) a four-fold change in immunoglobulin (Ig) G-specific antibody titer between acute and convalescent specimens taken 3 to 6 weeks apart by immunofluorescent antibody assay (IFA) or enzyme linked immunosorbent assay; (2) detection of *C burnetii* DNA in a clinical sample using polymerase chain reaction assay; (3) culture of *C burnetii* from a clinical specimen; or (4) positive immunohistochemical staining of *C burnetii* in a tissue sample. Confirmation of chronic Q fever is based on a single IgG titer of 800 or more by IFA.

TREATMENT: Acute Q fever generally is a self-limited illness, and many patients recover without antimicrobial therapy. Doxycycline is the drug of choice, and treatment can lessen the severity of illness and hasten recovery by several days. Fluoroquinolones or chloramphenicol are alternatives. Although tetracyclines generally should not be given to children younger than 8 years of age (see Antimicrobial Agents and Related Therapy, p 737), most experts consider the benefit of doxycycline in treating Q fever greater than the potential risk of dental staining. Fluoroquinolones also can be used but are not approved for this use in children younger than 18 years of age. Therapy should be initiated promptly and continued until the patient is afebrile and clinically improved, usually for 10 to 14 days. Chronic Q fever is much more difficult to treat, and relapses can occur despite appropriate therapy, necessitating repeated courses of therapy. The current recommended therapy for chronic Q fever endocarditis is a combination of doxycycline and hydroxy-chloroquine for a minimum of 18 months. Surgical replacement of the infected valve may be necessary in some patients.

ISOLATION OF THE HOSPITALIZED PATIENT: Standard precautions are recommended.

CONTROL MEASURES: Strict adherence to proper hygiene when handling parturient animals can help decrease the risk of infection in the farm setting. Improved prescreening of animal herds used by research facilities may decrease the risk of infection. Special safety practices are recommended for nonpropagative laboratory procedures involving *C burnetii* and for all propagative procedures, necropsies of infected animals, and manipulation of infected human and animal tissues. No specific management is recommended for people who have been exposed. Experimental vaccines for domestic animals and laboratory and other high-risk workers have been developed but are not licensed in the United States. Q fever is a nationally reportable disease, and all human cases should be reported to the state health department. For additional information about Q fever, see **www.cdc.gov/ncidod/dvrd/qfever/**.

Rabies[1]

CLINICAL MANIFESTATIONS: Infection with rabies virus characteristically produces an acute illness with rapidly progressive central nervous system manifestations, including anxiety, dysphagia, and seizures. Some patients may have paralysis. Illness almost invariably progresses to death. The differential diagnosis of acute encephalitic illnesses of unknown cause with atypical focal neurologic signs or with paralysis should include rabies.

ETIOLOGY: Rabies virus is an RNA virus classified in the Rhabdoviridae family, Lyssavirus genus.

EPIDEMIOLOGY: Understanding the epidemiology of rabies has been aided by viral variant identification using monoclonal antibodies and nucleotide sequencing. In the United States, human cases have decreased steadily since the 1950s, reflecting wide-spread immunization of dogs and the availability of effective prophylaxis after exposure to a rabid animal. Between 2000 and 2007, 20 of 25 cases of human rabies reported in the United States were acquired indigenously. Among the 20 indigenously acquired cases, 17 were associated with bat rabies virus variants, and 1 had a history of a bat bite, had rabies antibodies in serum and cerebrospinal fluid (CSF) samples, but rabies virus antigens were not detected. Despite the large focus of rabies in raccoons in the eastern United States, only 1 human death has been attributed to the raccoon rabies virus variant. Two cases of human rabies were attributable to probable aerosol exposure in laboratories, and 2 unusual cases have been attributed to possible airborne exposures in caves inhabited by millions of bats, although alternative infection routes cannot be discounted. Transmission also has occurred by transplantation of organs, corneas, and other tissues from patients dying of undiagnosed rabies. Person-to-person transmission by bite has not been documented in the United States, although the virus has been isolated from saliva of infected patients.

---

[1]For further information, see Centers for Disease Control and Prevention. Human rabies prevention: United States, 2008. Recommendations of the Advisory Committee on Immunization Practices. *MMWR Recomm Rep.* 2008;57(RR-3):1–28

Wildlife rabies persists throughout the United States except in Hawaii, which remains rabies free. Wildlife, including bats, raccoons, skunks, foxes, and coyotes, are the most important potential sources of infection for humans and domestic animals in the United States. Rabies in small rodents (squirrels, hamsters, guinea pigs, gerbils, chipmunks, rats, and mice) and lagomorphs (rabbits and hares) is rare. Rabies may occur in woodchucks or other large rodents in areas where raccoon rabies is common. The virus is present in saliva and is transmitted by bites or, rarely, by contamination of mucosa or skin lesions by saliva or other potentially infectious material (eg, neural tissue). Worldwide, most rabies cases in humans result from dog bites in areas where canine rabies is enzootic. Most rabid dogs, cats, and ferrets may shed virus for a few days before there are obvious signs of illness. No case of human rabies in the United States has been attributed to a dog, cat, or ferret that has remained healthy throughout the standard 10-day period of confinement.

The **incubation period** in humans averages 4 to 6 weeks but ranges from days to years. Incubation periods of up to 6 years have been confirmed by antigenic typing and nucleotide sequencing of rabies virus variants.

DIAGNOSTIC TESTS: Infection in animals can be diagnosed by demonstration of virus-specific fluorescent antigen in brain tissue. Suspected rabid animals should be euthanized in a manner that preserves brain tissue for appropriate laboratory diagnosis. Virus can be isolated in suckling mice or in tissue culture from saliva, brain, and other specimens and can be detected by identification of viral antigens or nucleotides in affected tissues. The diagnosis in suspected human cases can be made postmortem by either immunofluorescent or immunohistochemical examination of brain tissue. Antemortem diagnosis can be made by fluorescent microscopy of skin biopsy specimens from the nape of the neck, by isolation of the virus from saliva, by detection of antibody in the CSF or serum in unimmunized people, and by detection of viral antigens and nucleic acid in infected tissues. Laboratory personnel should be consulted before submission of specimens so that appropriate collection and transport of materials can be arranged.

TREATMENT: Once symptoms have developed, neither rabies vaccine nor Rabies Immune Globulin (RIG) improves the prognosis. There is no specific treatment. Very few patients with human rabies have survived, even with intensive supportive care. With 1 exception,[1] all other known survivors had received prophylaxis before clinical signs developed. In 2004, a 15-year-old female who had not received rabies postexposure prophylaxis survived rabies after receipt of a combination of drug-induced coma, antiviral administration, and intensive medical intervention. At least 2 other children have survived the disease using this strategy but later died of complications during rehabilitation. Details of the protocol used can be found at **www.mcw.edu/rabies.**

ISOLATION OF THE HOSPITALIZED PATIENT: Standard precautions are recommended for the duration of illness. If the patient has bitten another person or the patient's saliva has contaminated an open wound or mucous membrane, the involved area should be washed thoroughly and postexposure prophylaxis should be administered (see Care of Exposed People, p 556).

CONTROL MEASURES: Education of children to avoid contact with stray or wild animals is of primary importance. Children should be cautioned against provoking or attempting to capture stray or wild animals and against touching carcasses. Inadvertent contact of

---

[1]Willoughby RE Jr, Tieves KS, Hoffman GM, et al. Survival after treatment of rabies with induction of coma. *N Engl J Med*. 2005;352(24):2508–2514

family members and pets with potentially rabid animals, such as raccoons, foxes, coyotes, and skunks, may be decreased by securing garbage and refuse to decrease attraction of domestic and wild animals. Similarly, chimneys and other potential entrances for wildlife, including bats, should be identified and covered. Bats should be excluded from human living quarters. International travelers to areas with endemic canine rabies should be warned to avoid exposure to stray dogs, and if traveling to an area with enzootic infection where immediate access to medical care and biologicals is limited, preexposure prophylaxis is indicated.

Exposure Risk and Decisions to Give Prophylaxis. Exposure to rabies results from a break in the skin caused by the teeth of a rabid animal or by contamination of scratches, abrasions, or mucous membranes with saliva or other potentially infectious material, such as neural tissue, from a rabid animal. The decision to immunize a potentially exposed person should be made in consultation with the local health department, which can provide information on the risk of rabies in a particular area for each species of animal and in accordance with the guidelines in Table 3.57. In the United States, bats, raccoons, skunks, and foxes are more likely to be infected than other animals, but coyotes, cattle, dogs, cats, ferrets, and other species occasionally are infected. Bites of rodents (such as squirrels, mice, and rats) or lagomorphs (rabbits, hares, and pikas) rarely require prophylaxis. Additional factors must be considered when deciding whether immunoprophylaxis is indicated. An unprovoked attack may be more suggestive of a rabid animal than a bite that occurs during attempts to feed or handle an animal. Properly immunized dogs, cats,

Table 3.57. Rabies Postexposure Prophylaxis Guide

Animal Type	Evaluation and Disposition of Animal	Postexposure Prophylaxis Recommendations
Dogs, cats, and ferrets	Healthy and available for 10 days of observation	Prophylaxis only if animal develops signs of rabies[a]
	Rabid or suspected of being rabid[b]	Immediate immunization and RIG[c]
	Unknown (escaped)	Consult public health officials for advice
Bats, skunks, raccoons, foxes, and most other carnivores; woodchucks	Regarded as rabid unless geographic area is known to be free of rabies or until animal proven negative by laboratory tests[b]	Immediate immunization and RIG[c]
Livestock, rodents, and lagomorphs (rabbits, hares, and pikas)	Consider individually	Consult public health officials. Bites of squirrels, hamsters, guinea pigs, gerbils, chipmunks, rats, mice and other rodents, rabbits, hares, and pikas almost never require antirabies treatment.

RIG indicates Rabies Immune Globulin.
[a]During the 10-day observation period, at the first sign of rabies in the biting dog, cat, or ferret, treatment of the exposed person with RIG (human) and vaccine should be initiated. The animal should be euthanized immediately and tested.
[b]The animal should be euthanized and tested as soon as possible. Holding for observation is not recommended. Immunization is discontinued if immunofluorescent test result for the animal is negative.
[c]See text.

and ferrets have only a minimal chance of developing rabies. However, in rare instances, rabies has developed in properly vaccinated animals.

Postexposure prophylaxis for rabies is recommended for all people bitten by wild mammalian carnivores or bats or by domestic animals that may be infected. Rarely, exposures other than bites have resulted in infection. Postexposure prophylaxis is recommended for people who report an open wound, scratch, or mucous membrane that has been contaminated with saliva or other potentially infectious material (eg, brain tissue) from a rabid animal. Because the injury inflicted by a bat bite or scratch may be small and not readily evident or the circumstances of contact may preclude accurate recall (eg, a bat in a room of a sleeping person or previously unattended child), prophylaxis may be indicated for situations in which a bat physically is present if a bite or mucous membrane exposure cannot reliably be excluded, unless prompt testing of the bat has excluded rabies virus infection. Prophylaxis should be initiated as soon as possible after bites by known or suspected rabid animals.

Postexposure prophylaxis is recommended for people who report a possibly infectious exposure (eg, bite, scratch, or open wound or mucous membrane contaminated with saliva or other infectious material, such as cerebrospinal fluid or brain tissue) to a human with rabies. Rabies virus transmission after exposure to a human with rabies has not been documented in the United States, except after tissue or organ transplantation from donors who died of unsuspected rabies encephalitis. Casual contact with an infected person (eg, by touching a patient) or contact with noninfectious fluids or tissues (eg, blood or feces) alone does not constitute an exposure and is not an indication for prophylaxis (see Care of Hospital Contacts, below).

Handling of Animals Suspected of Having Rabies. A dog, cat, or ferret that is suspected of having rabies and has bitten a human should be captured, confined, and observed by a veterinarian for 10 days. Any illness in the animal should be reported immediately to the local health department. If signs of rabies develop, the animal should be euthanized in a manner to allow its head to be removed and shipped under refrigeration (not frozen) to a qualified laboratory for examination.

Other biting animals that may have exposed a person to rabies should be reported immediately to the local health department. Management of animals depends on the species, the circumstances of the bite, and the epidemiology of rabies in the area. Previous immunization of an animal may not preclude the necessity for euthanasia and testing. Because clinical manifestations of rabies in a wild animal cannot be interpreted reliably, a wild mammal suspected of having rabies should be euthanized at once, and its brain should be examined for evidence of rabies virus infection. The exposed person need not receive prophylaxis if the result of rapid examination of the brain by the direct fluorescent antibody test is negative for rabies virus infection.

Care of Hospital Contacts. Immunization of hospital contacts of a patient with rabies should be reserved for people who were bitten or whose mucous membranes or open wounds have come in contact with saliva, cerebrospinal fluid, or brain tissue of a patient with rabies (see Care of Exposed People). Other hospital contacts of a patient with rabies do not require prophylaxis.

Care of Exposed People.

Local Wound Care. The immediate objective of postexposure prophylaxis is to prevent virus from entering neural tissue. Prompt and thorough local treatment of all lesions is essential, because virus may remain localized to the area of the bite for a variable time. All wounds should be flushed thoroughly and cleaned with soap and water. Quaternary ammonium compounds (such as benzalkonium chloride) no longer are considered superior to soap. The need for tetanus prophylaxis and measures to control bacterial infection also should be considered. The wound, if possible, should not be sutured.

Prophylaxis (see Table 3.57, p 554). After wound care is completed, concurrent use of passive *and* active prophylaxis is optimal, with the exceptions of people who previously have received complete immunization regimens (preexposure or postexposure) with a cell culture vaccine and people who have been immunized with other types of rabies vaccines and previously have had a documented rabies virus-neutralizing antibody titer; these people should receive only vaccine. Prophylaxis should begin as soon as possible after exposure, ideally within 24 hours. However, a delay of several days or more may not compromise effectiveness, and prophylaxis should be initiated if indicated, regardless of the interval between exposure and initiation of therapy. In the United States, only the human product RIG is available for passive immunization. Licensed tissue culture rabies vaccine should be used for active immunization. Physicians can obtain expert counsel from their local or state health departments.

Active Immunization (Postexposure). Three rabies vaccines are licensed commercially for prophylaxis in the United States: human diploid cell vaccine (HDCV), rabies vaccine adsorbed (RVA), and purified chicken embryo cell vaccine (PCECV), but only HDCV and PCECV are available for use in the United States (see Table 3.58, p 557). A 1.0-mL dose of vaccine is given intramuscularly in the deltoid area or anterolateral aspect of the thigh on the first day of postexposure prophylaxis (day 0), and repeated doses are given on days 3, 7, 14, and 28 after the first dose, for a total of 5 doses. Ideally, an immunization series should be initiated and completed with 1 vaccine product unless serious allergic reactions occur. Clinical studies evaluating efficacy or frequency of adverse reactions when the series is completed with a second product have not been conducted. The volume of the dose is not decreased for children. Serologic testing to document seroconversion after administration of a rabies vaccine series is unnecessary but occasionally has been advised for recipients who may be immunocompromised but will not be useful if RIG also was administered, unless sufficient time has elapsed since RIG administration.

Care should be taken to ensure that the vaccine is administered intramuscularly. Intradermal vaccine is not advised for postexposure prophylaxis in the United States, although for reasons of cost and availability, intradermal regimens are used in some countries. Because antibody responses in adults who received vaccine in the gluteal area sometimes have been less than in those who were injected in the deltoid muscle, the deltoid site always should be used except in infants and young children, in whom the anterolateral thigh is the appropriate site.

• *Adverse reactions and precautions with HDCV and PCECV.* Reactions after immunization, primarily reported in adults, are less common than reactions after immunization with previously used rabies vaccines. Reactions are uncommon in children. In adults, local reactions, such as pain, erythema, and swelling or itching at the injection site, are reported in 15% to 25%, and mild systemic reactions, such as headache, nausea, abdominal pain, muscle aches, and dizziness, are reported in 10% to 20%

Table 3.58. US Food and Drug Administration-Licensed Rabies Vaccines[a] and Rabies Immune Globulin Products

Category	Product	Manufacturer	Dose and Route of Administration
Human rabies vaccine	Human diploid cell vaccine (HDCV) (Imovax)	sanofi pasteur	1 mL, IM
	Purified chicken embryo cell vaccine (PCECV) (RabAvert)	Novartis Vaccines and Diagnostics	1 mL, IM
Rabies Immune Globulin	Imogam Rabies-HT	sanofi pasteur	20 IU/kg, infiltrate around wound[b]
	HyperRab S/D	Talecris Biotherapeutics	20 IU/kg, infiltrate around wound[b]

IM indicates intramuscular.

[a]Rabies vaccine adsorbed (RVA) is licensed in the United States but no longer is distributed in the United States.

[b]Any remaining volume should be administered IM.

of recipients. Several cases of neurologic illness resembling Guillain-Barré syndrome that resolved without sequelae in 12 weeks and an acute, generalized, transient neurologic syndrome temporally associated with HDCV have been reported but are not thought to be related causally. A case of acute disseminated encephalomyelitis resulting in death has been reported after immunization with HDCV.

Immune complex-like reactions in people receiving booster doses of HDCV have been observed, possibly because of interaction between propiolactone contained in the vaccine and human albumin. The reaction, characterized by onset 2 to 21 days after inoculation, begins with generalized urticaria and can include arthralgia, arthritis, angioedema, nausea, vomiting, fever, and malaise. The reaction is not life threatening, occurs in as many as 6% of adults receiving booster doses as part of a preexposure immunization regimen, and is rare in people receiving primary immunization with HDCV. Similar allergic reactions with primary or booster doses have not been reported with PCECV.

If the patient has a serious allergic reaction to HDCV, PCECV may be given according to the same schedule as HDCV. All suspected serious, systemic, neuroparalytic, or anaphylactic reactions to the rabies vaccine should be reported immediately to the Vaccine Adverse Events Reporting System (see Reporting of Adverse Events, p 42).

Although safety of rabies vaccine during pregnancy has not been studied specifically in the United States, pregnancy should not be considered a contraindication to use of vaccine after exposure.

- **Nerve tissue vaccines.** Inactivated nerve tissue vaccines are not licensed in the United States but are available in many areas of the world. These preparations induce neuroparalytic reactions in 1:2000 to 1:8000 recipients. Immunization with nerve tissue vaccine should be discontinued if meningeal or neuroparalytic reactions develop. Corticosteroids can be used for treatment of complications but should be used only for life-threatening reactions, because they increase the risk of rabies in experimentally inoculated animals.

Passive Immunization. Human RIG should be used concomitantly with the first dose of vaccine for postexposure prophylaxis to bridge the time between possible infection and antibody production induced by the vaccine (see Table 3.58, p 557). If vaccine is not available immediately, RIG should be given alone and immunization should be started as soon as possible. If RIG is not available immediately, vaccine should be given and RIG given subsequently if obtained within 7 days after initiating immunization. If administration of both vaccine and RIG is delayed, both should be used regardless of the interval between exposure and treatment.

The recommended dose of RIG is 20 IU/kg. As much of the dose as possible should be used to infiltrate the wound(s), if present. The remainder is given intramuscularly. In cases of multiple severe wounds in which RIG is insufficient for infiltration, dilution in saline solution to an adequate volume (twofold or threefold) has been recommended to ensure that all wound areas receive infiltrate. For children with a small muscle mass, it may be necessary to administer RIG at multiple sites. Human RIG is supplied in 2-mL (300 IU) and 10-mL (1500 IU) vials. Passive antibody can inhibit the response to rabies vaccines; therefore, the recommended dose should not be exceeded. Vaccine never should be administered in the same parts of the body or with the same syringe used to give RIG. Hypersensitivity reactions to RIG occur rarely, if ever.

Purified equine RIG containing rabies antibodies may be available outside the United States and generally is accompanied by a low rate of serum sickness (less than 1%). Equine RIG is administered at a dose of 40 IU/kg, and desensitization may be required. Administration of RIG is not recommended for the following exposed people: (1) those who previously received postexposure prophylaxis with HDCV, RVA, or PCECV; (2) those who received a 3-dose, intramuscular, preexposure regimen of HDCV, RVA, or PCECV; (3) those who received a 3-dose, intradermal, preexposure regimen of HDCV with the product used in the United States; and (4) those who have a documented adequate rabies virus antibody titer after previous immunization with any other rabies vaccine. These people should receive two 1.0-mL booster doses of HDCV or PCECV; 1 dose is given on the day of exposure, and the second is given 3 days later.

Preexposure Control Measures, Including Immunization. The relatively low frequency of reactions to HDCV and PCECV has made provision of preexposure immunization practical for people in high-risk groups, including veterinarians, animal handlers, certain laboratory workers, and people moving to areas where canine rabies is common. Others, such as spelunkers, who have frequent exposures to bats and other wildlife, also should be considered for preexposure prophylaxis.

HDCV and PCECV are licensed for intramuscular administration. Previously, intradermal (0.1 mL) dosage formulations of HDCV were available for preexposure use. The preexposure immunization schedule is three 1-mL intramuscular injections each, given on days 0, 7, and 21 **or** 28. This series of immunizations has resulted in development of rabies virus-neutralizing antibodies in all people properly immunized. Therefore, routine serologic testing for antibody immediately after primary immunization is not indicated.

Serum antibodies usually persist for at least 2 years or more after the primary series given intramuscularly. Preexposure booster immunization with 1.0 mL of HDCV or PCEC intramuscularly will produce an effective anamnestic response. Rabies virus-neutralizing antibody titers should be determined at 6-month intervals for people at continuous risk of infection (rabies research laboratory workers, rabies biologicals production workers). Titers should be determined approximately every 2 years for people with risk of frequent exposure (rabies diagnostic laboratory workers, spelunkers, veterinarians and staff, animal-control and wildlife workers in rabies-enzootic areas, and all people who frequently handle bats). A single booster dose of vaccine should be administered only as appropriate to maintain adequate antibody concentrations. The Centers for Disease Control and Prevention currently specifies complete viral neutralization at a titer 1:5 or greater by the rapid fluorescent-focus inhibition test as acceptable; the World Health Organization specifies 0.5 IU/mL or greater as acceptable.

Public Health. A variety of approved public health measures, including immunization of dogs, cats, and ferrets and elimination of stray dogs and selected wildlife, are used to control rabies in animals.[1] In regions where oral immunization of wildlife with recombinant rabies vaccine is undertaken, the prevalence of rabies among foxes, coyotes, and raccoons may be decreased. Unimmunized dogs, cats, ferrets, or other pets bitten by a known rabid animal should be euthanized immediately. If the owner is unwilling to allow the animal to be euthanized, the animal should be placed in strict isolation for 6 months and immunized 1 month before release. If the exposed animal has been immunized within 1 to 3 years, depending on the vaccine administered and local regulations, the animal should be reimmunized and observed for 45 days.

Case Reporting. All suspected cases of rabies should be reported promptly to public health authorities.

Rat-Bite Fever

CLINICAL MANIFESTATIONS: Rat-bite fever is caused by *Streptobacillus moniliformis* or *Spirillum minus. S moniliformis* infection (streptobacillary fever or Haverhill fever) is characterized by fever, rash, and arthritis. There is an abrupt onset of fever, chills, muscle pain, vomiting, headache, and occasionally, adenopathy. A maculopapular or petechial rash develops, predominantly on the extremities including the palms and soles, typically within a few days of fever onset. The bite site usually heals promptly and exhibits no or minimal inflammation. Nonsuppurative migratory polyarthritis or arthralgia follows in approximately 50% of patients. Untreated infection usually has a relapsing course for a mean of 3 weeks. Complications include soft tissue and solid-organ abscesses, pneumonia, endocarditis, myocarditis, and meningitis. Disease can be severe or even fatal in infants younger than 3 months of age. The case-fatality rate is 7% to 10% in untreated patients. With *S minus* infection, a period of initial apparent healing at the site of the bite usually is followed by fever and ulceration at the site, regional lymphangitis and lymphadenopathy, and a distinctive rash of red or purple plaques. Arthritis is rare. Infection with *S minus* is rare in the United States.

ETIOLOGY: The causes of rat-bite fever are *Streptobacillus moniliformis,* a microaerophilic, gram-negative, pleomorphic bacillus, and *Spirillum minus,* a small, gram-negative, spiral organism with bipolar flagellar tufts.

EPIDEMIOLOGY: Rat-bite fever is a zoonotic illness. The natural habitat of *S moniliformis* and *S minus* is the upper respiratory tract of rodents. *S moniliformis* is transmitted by bites or scratches from or exposure to oral secretions of infected rats (eg, kissing the rodent); other rodents (eg, mice, gerbils, squirrels, weasels) and rodent-eating animals, including

---

[1]National Association of State Public Health Veterinarians Inc. Compendium of animal rabies prevention and control, 2008. *MMWR Recomm Rep.* 2008;57(RR-2):1–9

cats and dogs, also can transmit the infection. Haverhill fever refers to infection after ingestion of unpasteurized milk, water, or food contaminated with *S moniliformis*. *S minus* is transmitted by bites of rats and mice. *S moniliformis* infection accounts for most cases of rat-bite fever in the United States; *S minus* infections occur primarily in Asia.

The **incubation period** for *S moniliformis* usually is 3 to 10 days but can be as long as 3 weeks; for *S minus*, the incubation period is 7 to 21 days.

DIAGNOSTIC TESTS: *S moniliformis* is a fastidious, slow-growing organism isolated from specimens of blood, synovial fluid, aspirates from abscesses, or material from the bite lesion by inoculation into bacteriologic media enriched with blood, serum, or ascitic fluid. Cultures should be held up to 3 weeks if *S moniliformis* is suspected. Sodium polyanethol-sulfonate, present in most blood culture media, is inhibitory to *S moniliformis*. *S minus* has not been recovered on artificial media but can be visualized by darkfield microscopy in wet mounts of blood, exudate of a lesion, and lymph nodes. Blood specimens also should be viewed with Giemsa or Wright stain. *S minus* can be recovered from blood, lymph nodes, or local lesions by intraperitoneal inoculation of mice or guinea pigs.

TREATMENT: Penicillin G procaine intramuscularly or penicillin G intravenously should be administered for 7 to 10 days for rat-bite fever caused by either agent. Initial intravenous penicillin G therapy for 5 to 7 days followed by oral penicillin V for 7 days also has been successful. Limited experience exists for ampicillin, cefuroxime, and cefotaxime. Doxycycline or streptomycin can be substituted when a patient has a serious allergy to penicillin. Doxycycline should not be given to children younger than 8 years of age unless the benefits of therapy are greater than the risks of dental staining (see Antimicrobial Agents and Related Therapy, p 737). Patients with endocarditis should receive intravenous high-dose penicillin G for at least 4 weeks. The addition of streptomycin or another aminoglycoside for initial therapy may be useful.

ISOLATION OF THE HOSPITALIZED PATIENT: Standard precautions are recommended.

CONTROL MEASURES: Exposed people should be observed for symptoms. Because the occurrence of *S moniliformis* after a rat bite is approximately 10%, some experts recommend postexposure administration of penicillin. Rat control is important in the control of disease. People with frequent rodent exposure should wear gloves and avoid hand-to-mouth contact during animal handling. Regular hand hygiene should be practiced.

Respiratory Syncytial Virus

CLINICAL MANIFESTATIONS: Respiratory syncytial virus (RSV) causes acute upper respiratory tract infection in patients of all ages and is one of the most common diseases of childhood. Most infants are infected during the first year of life, with virtually all having been infected at least once by the second birthday. Most RSV-infected infants experience upper respiratory tract symptoms, and 20% to 30% develop lower respiratory tract disease with their first infection. During the first few weeks of life, particularly among preterm infants, infection with RSV may produce minimal respiratory tract signs. Lethargy, irritability, and poor feeding, sometimes accompanied by apneic episodes, may be the presenting manifestations in these infants. Most previously healthy infants who develop RSV bronchiolitis do not require hospitalization, and most who are hospitalized improve with supportive care and are discharged in fewer than 5 days. Characteristics that increase the risk of severe RSV lower respiratory tract illness are preterm birth; cyanotic or complicated congenital heart disease, especially conditions causing pulmonary hypertension; chronic lung disease of prematurity; and immunodeficiency disease or therapy causing immunosuppression at any age. The association between RSV bronchiolitis early in life and subsequent reactive airway disease remains poorly understood. RSV bronchiolitis may be associated with short-term or long-term complications that include recurrent wheezing, reactive airway disease, and abnormalities in pulmonary function. This association may reflect an underlying predisposition to reactive airway disease rather than a direct consequence of RSV infection.

Reinfection with RSV throughout life is common. RSV infection in older children and adults usually manifests as upper respiratory tract illness. More serious disease involving the lower respiratory tract may develop in older children and adults especially in immunocompromised patients, the elderly, and in people with cardiopulmonary disease.

ETIOLOGY: RSV is an enveloped, nonsegmented, negative strand RNA virus of the family *Paramyxoviridae*. The virus uses attachment (G) and fusion (F) surface glycoproteins that lack neuraminidase and hemagglutinin activities. Two major strains (groups A and B), each with numerous genotypes, have been identified, and strains of both groups often circulate concurrently. The clinical and epidemiologic significance of strain variation has not been determined, but evidence suggests that antigenic differences may affect susceptibility to infection and that some strains may be more virulent than others.

EPIDEMIOLOGY: Humans are the only source of infection. Transmission usually is by direct or close contact with contaminated secretions, which may occur from exposure to large-particle droplets at short distances (<3 feet) or fomites. RSV can persist on environmental surfaces for several hours and for a half-hour or more on hands. Infection among hospital personnel and others may occur by hand to eye or hand to nasal epithelium self-inoculation with contaminated secretions. Enforcement of infection-control policies is important to decrease the risk of health care-related transmission of RSV. Health care-related spread of RSV to bone marrow or solid organ transplant recipients or patients with cardiopulmonary abnormalities or immunocompromised conditions has been associated with severe and fatal disease in children and adults.

RSV usually occurs in annual epidemics during winter and early spring in temperate climates. Spread among household and child care contacts, including adults, is common. The period of viral shedding usually is 3 to 8 days, but shedding may last longer, especially in young infants and in immunosuppressed people, in whom shedding may continue for as long as 3 to 4 weeks.

The **incubation period** ranges from 2 to 8 days; 4 to 6 days is most common.

DIAGNOSTIC TESTS: Rapid diagnostic assays, including immunofluorescent and enzyme immunoassay techniques for detection of viral antigen in nasopharyngeal specimens, are available commercially and generally are reliable in infants and young children. In children, the sensitivity of these assays in comparison with culture varies between 53% and 96%, with most in the 80% to 90% range. The sensitivity may be lower in older children. As with all antigen detection assays, false-positive test results are more likely to occur when the incidence of disease is low. Therefore, antigen detection assays should not be the only basis on which the beginning and end of monthly prophylaxis is determined.

Viral isolation from nasopharyngeal secretions in cell culture requires 1 to 5 days (shell vial techniques can produce results within 24 to 48 hours), but results and sensitivity vary among laboratories. Experienced viral laboratory personnel should be consulted for optimal methods of collection and transport of specimens. Conventional serologic testing of acute and convalescent serum specimens cannot be relied on to confirm infection in young infants in whom sensitivity may be low. In some studies, polymerase chain reaction assays have increased RSV detection rates as much as twofold over viral isolation or antigen detection, but these assays are not widely available.

TREATMENT: Primary treatment is supportive and should include hydration, careful clinical assessment of respiratory status, including measurement of oxygen saturation, use of supplemental oxygen, suction of the upper airway, and if necessary, intubation and mechanical ventilation.[1] Ribavirin has in vitro antiviral activity against RSV, and aerosolized ribavirin therapy has been associated with a small but statistically significant increase in oxygen saturation during the acute infection in several small studies. However, a consistent decrease in need for mechanical ventilation, decrease in length of stay in the pediatric intensive care unit, or reduction in days of hospitalization among ribavirin recipients has not been demonstrated. The aerosol route of administration, concern about potential toxic effects among exposed health care professionals, and conflicting results of efficacy trials have led to decreasing use of this drug. Ribavirin is not recommended for routine use but may be considered for use in select patients with documented, potentially life-threatening RSV infection.

Beta-adrenergic Agents. Beta-adrenergic agents are not recommended for routine care of first-time wheezing associated with RSV bronchiolitis. Some physicians elect to use bronchodilator therapy because of concern that reactive airway disease may be misdiagnosed as bronchiolitis. Repeat doses of an inhaled bronchodilator may be continued in a minority of infants with well-documented improvement in respiratory function soon after the first dose, but its use is unlikely to alter the clinical course of RSV disease or to permit earlier hospital discharge.

Corticosteroid Therapy. In most randomized clinical trials of hospitalized infants as well as outpatients with RSV bronchiolitis, corticosteroid therapy has been found to have no effect on disease severity or length of stay and is not recommended.

Antimicrobial Therapy. Intravenous antimicrobial therapy is not indicated in infants hospitalized with RSV bronchiolitis or pneumonia unless there is evidence of secondary bacterial infection. Bacterial lung infections and bacteremia are uncommon in this setting. Otitis media occurs in infants with RSV bronchiolitis, but oral antimicrobial agents can be used if therapy for otitis media is necessary.

Prevention of RSV Infections. Respiratory Syncytial Virus Immune Globulin Intravenous (RSV-IGIV), a hyperimmune, polyclonal globulin prepared from donors selected for high serum titers of RSV neutralizing antibody, no longer is available. Palivizumab, a humanized mouse monoclonal antibody, is licensed for prevention of RSV lower respiratory tract disease in certain infants and children with chronic lung disease of prematurity (CLD [formerly called bronchopulmonary dysplasia]), or with a history of preterm birth (less than 35 weeks' gestation), or with congenital heart disease. Palivizumab is administered intramuscularly at a dose of 15 mg/kg once every 30 days. An attempt should be made to maintain compliance with monthly administration. In some reports, palivizumab administration in a home-based program has been shown to improve compliance and to reduce exposure to microbial pathogens compared with administration in office- or clinic-based settings. Additional doses of palivizumab should not be given to any patient with a

---

[1]American Academy of Pediatrics, Subcommittee on Diagnosis and Management of Bronchiolitis. Diagnosis and management of bronchiolitis. *Pediatrics.* 2006;118(4):1774–1793

history of a severe allergic reaction following a previous dose. Palivizumab is not effective in treatment of RSV disease and is not approved or recommended for this indication.

Cost Considerations. Immunoprophylaxis with 5 monthly doses of palivizumab is an effective, though costly, intervention that reduces hospitalization rates by 39% to 82% among high-risk infants. Optimal cost benefit from immunoprophylaxis is achieved during peak outbreak months when most RSV hospitalizations occur. If prophylaxis is initiated after widespread RSV circulation has begun, high-risk infants may not receive the full benefit of protection. Conversely, early initiation or continuation of monthly immuno-prophylaxis during months when RSV is not circulating widely is not cost-effective and provides little benefit to recipients.

The primary benefit of immunoprophylaxis is a decrease in the rate of RSV-associated hospitalization. No prospective, randomized clinical trial has demonstrated a significant decrease in the rate of mortality attributable to RSV or in the rate of recurrent wheezing following RSV infection among infants who receive prophylaxis. Economic analyses fail to demonstrate overall savings in health care dollars because of the high cost if all at risk infants receive prophylaxis.

Initiation and Termination of Immunoprophylaxis. In the temperate climates of North America, peak RSV activity typically occurs between November and March, whereas in equatorial countries, RSV seasonality patterns vary and may occur throughout the year. The inevitability of the RSV season is predictable, but the severity of the season, the time of onset, the peak of activity, and the end of the season cannot be predicted precisely. Substantial variation in timing of community outbreaks of RSV disease from year to year exists in the same community and between communities in the same year, even in the same region. These variations occur within the overall pattern of RSV outbreaks, usually beginning in November or December, peaking in January or February, and ending by the end of March or sometime in April. Communities in the southern United States, par-ticularly some communities in the state of Florida, tend to experience the earliest onset of RSV activity. In recent years, the national median duration of the RSV season has been 17 weeks or less. Results from clinical trials indicate that palivizumab trough serum concentrations more than 30 days after the fifth dose will be well above the protective concentration for most infants. Five monthly doses of palivizumab will provide more than 20 weeks of protective serum antibody concentration. In the continental United States, a total of 5 monthly doses for infants and young children with congenital heart disease or chronic lung disease of prematurity or preterm birth before 32 weeks' gestation (31 weeks, 6 days) will provide an optimal balance of benefit and cost, even with variation in season onset and end.

For infants who qualify for 5 doses, initiation of immunoprophylaxis in November and continuation for a total of 5 monthly doses will provide protection into April and is recommended for most areas of the United States. If prophylaxis is initiated in October, the fifth and final dose should be administered in February.

Data from the Centers for Disease Control and Prevention (CDC) have identified variations in the onset and offset of the RSV season in the state of Florida that should affect the timing of palivizumab administration. Northwest Florida has an onset in mid-November, which is consistent with other areas of the United States. In north central and southwest Florida, the onset of RSV season typically is late September to early October. The RSV season in southeast Florida (Miami-Dade County) typically has its onset in July. Despite varied onsets, the RSV season is of equal duration in the different regions of Florida. Children who qualify for palivizumab prophylaxis for the entire RSV season (infants and children with chronic lung disease of prematurity or congenital heart disease or preterm infants born before 32 weeks' gestation) should receive palivizumab only during the 5 months following the onset of RSV season in their region (maximum of 5 doses), which should provide coverage during the peak of the season, when prophylaxis is most effective (Table 3.59, p 565).

Specific groups of American Indian/Alaska Native children in certain geographic regions may experience more severe RSV disease and a longer RSV season. RSV hospitalizations for Navajo and White Mountain Apache infants and young children may be 2 to 3 times those of children of similar ages in the United States population. However, the timing and duration of the RSV season is similar to the remainder of the United States (November through March), so standard recommendations for children with congenital heart disease, chronic lung disease of prematurity, or preterm birth (before 32 weeks' gestation) still are appropriate. Alaska Native infants in the Yukon Kuskokwim (YK) Delta experience not only higher RSV hospitalization rates but also a longer RSV season. Pediatricians from the YK Delta may wish to use CDC-generated RSV hospitalization data from the YK Delta region to assist in determining the onset and offset of RSV season for the appropriate timing of palivizumab administration.

Infants and children with congenital heart disease or chronic lung disease or preterm infants less than 32 weeks' gestation who initiate palivizumab prophylaxis after start of the RSV season will not require all 5 doses (see Table 3.60, p 565).

ELIGIBILITY CRITERIA FOR PROPHYLAXIS OF HIGH-RISK INFANTS AND YOUNG CHILDREN.

- **Infants with CLD.** Palivizumab prophylaxis may be considered for infants and children younger than 24 months of age who receive medical therapy (supplemental oxygen, bronchodilator, diuretic or chronic corticosteroid therapy) for CLD within 6 months before the start of the RSV season. These infants and young children should receive a maximum of 5 doses. Patients with the most severe CLD who continue to require medical therapy may benefit from prophylaxis during a second RSV season. Data are limited regarding the effectiveness of palivizumab during the second year of life. Individual patients may benefit from decisions made in consultation with neonatologists, pediatric intensivists, pulmonologists, or infectious disease specialists. A maximum of 5 monthly doses is recommended for patients in this category.

- **Infants born before 32 weeks' gestation (31 weeks, 6 days or less). (See Table 3.61.)** Infants in this category may benefit from RSV prophylaxis, even if they do not have CLD. For these infants, major risk factors to consider include gestational age and chronologic age at the start of the RSV season. Infants born at 28 weeks of gestation or earlier may benefit from prophylaxis during the RSV season, whenever that occurs during the first 12 months of life. Infants born at 29 to 32 weeks of gestation may benefit most from prophylaxis if younger than 6 months of age at the start of the RSV season. In this setting, 32 weeks' gestation refers to an infant born before the 32nd week of gestation (31 weeks, 6 days or less). Once an infant qualifies for initiation of prophylaxis at the start of the RSV season, administration should continue throughout the season and not stop at the point an infant reaches either 6 months or 12 months of age. A maximum of 5 monthly doses is recommended for infants in this category.

Table 3.59. Palivizumab Prophylaxis for Infants and Young Children With Chronic Lung Disease of Prematurity or Congenital Heart Disease

Geographic Location	Earliest Date for Initiation of 5 Monthly Doses
Southeast Florida	July 1
North central and southwest Florida	September 15
Most other areas of United States	November 1

Table 3.60. Maximum Number of Monthly Doses of Palivizumab for Respiratory Syncytial Virus Prophylaxis

Infants Eligible for a Maximum of 5 Doses	Infants Eligible for a Maximum of 3 Doses
Infants younger than 24 months of age with chronic lung disease and requiring medical therapy	Preterm infants with gestational age of 32 weeks, 0 days to 34 weeks, 6 days with at least 1 risk factor and born 3 months before or during RSV season.
Infants younger than 24 months of age and requiring medical therapy for congenital heart disease	
Preterm infants born at 31 weeks, 6 days of gestation or less	
Certain infants with neuromuscular disease or congenital abnormalities of the airways	

- **Infants born at 32 to less than 35 weeks' gestation (defined as 32 weeks, 0 days through 34 weeks, 6 days). (See Table 3.61.)** Available data do not enable definition of a subgroup of infants at risk of prolonged hospitalization and admission to the intensive care unit. Therefore, current recommendations are intended to reduce the risk of RSV hospitalization during the period of greatest risk (the first 3 months of life) among infants with consistently identified risk factors for hospitalization. Palivizumab prophylaxis should be limited to infants in this group at greatest risk of hospitalization due to RSV, namely infants younger than 3 months of age at the start of the RSV season or who are born during the RSV season and who are likely to have an increased risk of exposure to RSV. Epidemiologic data suggest that RSV infection is more likely to occur and more likely to lead to hospitalization for infants in this gestational age group when at least one of the following two risk factors is present:
  - infant attends child care, defined as a home or facility where care is provided for any number of infants or young toddlers in the child care facility; or
  - infant has a sibling younger than 5 years of age.

    Prophylaxis may be considered for infants from 32 through less than 35 weeks' gestation (defined as 32 weeks, 0 days through 34 weeks, 6 days) who are born less than 3 months before the onset or during the RSV season and for whom at least 1

Table 3.61. Maximum Number of Palivizumab Doses for RSV Prophylaxis of Preterm Infants Without Chronic Lung Disease, on the Basis of Birth Date, Gestational Age, and Presence of Risk Factors (Shown for Geographic Areas Beginning Prophylaxis on November 1)[a]

Month of Birth	Maximum No. of Doses for Season Beginning November 1		
	≤28 Weeks, 6 Days of Gestation and <12 Months of Age at Start of Season	29 Weeks, 0 Days Through 31 Weeks, 6 Days of Gestation and <6 Months of Age at Start of Season	32 Weeks, 0 Days Through 34 Weeks, 6 Days of Gestation and With Risk Factor[b]
November 1– March 31 of previous RSV season	5[c]	0[d]	0[e]
April	5	0[d]	0[e]
May	5	0[d]	0[e]
June	5	5	0[e]
July	5	5	0[e]
August	5	5	1[f]
September	5	5	2[f]
October	5	5	3[f]
November	5	5	3[f]
December	4	4	3[f]
January	3	3	3[f]
February	2	2	2[f]
March	1	1	1[f]

[a]If infant is discharged from the hospital during RSV season, fewer doses may be required.
[b]For risk factors, see p 565–566.
[c]Some of these infants may have received 1 or more doses of palivizimab in the previous RSV season if discharged from the hospital during that season; if so, they still qualify for up to 5 doses during their second RSV season.
[d]Zero doses because infant will be older than 6 months of age at start of RSV season.
[e]Zero doses because infant will be older than 90 days of age at start of RSV season.
[f]On the basis of the age of patients at the time of discharge from the hospital, fewer doses may be required, because these infants will receive 1 dose every 30 days until the infant is 90 days of age.

of the 2 risk factors is present. Infants in this gestational age category should receive prophylaxis only until they reach 3 months of age and should receive a maximum of 3 monthly doses; many will receive only 1 or 2 doses until they reach 3 months of age. Once an infant has passed 3 months of age (90 days of age), the risk of hospitalization attributable to RSV lower respiratory tract disease is reduced. Administration of palivizumab is not recommended after 3 months of age.

Infants, especially high-risk infants, never should be exposed to tobacco smoke. In published studies, passive household exposure to tobacco smoke has not been associated with an increased risk of RSV hospitalization on a consistent basis. However, exposure to tobacco smoke is a known risk factor for many adverse health related outcomes. Exposure to tobacco smoke can be controlled by the family of an infant at increased risk of RSV disease, and preventive measures will be less costly than palivizumab prophylaxis.

In contrast to the well-documented beneficial effect of breastfeeding against many viral illnesses, existing data are conflicting regarding the specific protective effect of breastfeeding against RSV infection. Breastfeeding should be encouraged for all infants in accordance with recommendations of the American Academy of Pediatrics. High-risk infants should be kept away from crowds and from situations in which exposure to infected people cannot be controlled. Participation in group child care should be restricted during the RSV season for high-risk infants whenever feasible. Parents should be instructed on the importance of careful hand hygiene. In addition, all high-risk infants 6 months of age and older and their contacts should receive influenza vaccine as well as other recommended age-appropriate immunizations.

- **Infants with congenital abnormalities of the airway or neuromuscular disease.** Immunoprophylaxis may be considered for infants born before 35 weeks of gestation who have either congenital abnormalities of the airway or a neuromuscular condition that compromises handling of respiratory secretions. Infants and young children in this category should receive a maximum of 5 doses of palivizumab during the first year of life.

- **Infants and children with congenital heart disease.** Children who are 24 months of age or younger with hemodynamically significant cyanotic or acyanotic congenital heart disease may benefit from palivizumab prophylaxis. Decisions regarding prophylaxis with palivizumab in children with congenital heart disease should be made on the basis of the degree of physiologic cardiovascular compromise. Children younger than 24 months of age with congenital heart disease who are most likely to benefit from immunoprophylaxis include:
  - Infants who are receiving medication to control congestive heart failure
  - Infants with moderate to severe pulmonary hypertension
  - Infants with cyanotic heart disease

  Because a mean decrease in palivizumab serum concentration of 58% was observed after surgical procedures that use cardiopulmonary bypass, for children who still require prophylaxis, a postoperative dose of palivizumab (15 mg/kg) should be considered as soon as the patient is medically stable.

  The following groups of infants are **not** at increased risk of RSV and generally should not receive immunoprophylaxis:
  - Infants and children with hemodynamically insignificant heart disease (eg, secundum atrial septal defect, small ventricular septal defect, pulmonic stenosis, uncomplicated aortic stenosis, mild coarctation of the aorta, and patent ductus arteriosus)
  - Infants with lesions adequately corrected by surgery, unless they continue to require medication for congestive heart failure
  - Infants with mild cardiomyopathy who are not receiving medical therapy for the condition

  Dates for initiation and termination of prophylaxis should be based on the same considerations as for high-risk infants with CLD.

- **Immunocompromised children.** Palivizumab prophylaxis has not been evaluated in randomized trials in immunocompromised children. Although specific recommendations for immunocompromised patients cannot be made, infants and young children with severe immunodeficiencies (eg, severe combined immunodeficiency or advanced acquired immunodeficiency syndrome) may benefit from prophylaxis.

- **Patients with cystic fibrosis.** Limited studies suggest that some patients with cystic fibrosis may be at increased risk of RSV infection. Whether RSV infection exacerbates the chronic lung disease of cystic fibrosis is not known. In addition, insufficient data exist to determine the effectiveness of palivizumab use in this patient population. Therefore, a recommendation for routine prophylaxis in patients with cystic fibrosis cannot be made.
- **Other considerations.**
  - Hospitalized infants who qualify for prophylaxis during the RSV season should receive the first dose of palivizumab 48 to 72 hours before discharge or promptly after discharge.
  - If an infant or child who is receiving palivizumab immunoprophylaxis experiences a breakthrough RSV infection, monthly prophylaxis should continue until a maximum of 3 doses have been administered to infants in the 32 to less than 35 weeks' gestation group (defined as 32 weeks, 0 days through 34 weeks, 6 days) or until a maximum of 5 doses for infants with congenital heart disease, CLD, or preterm birth before 32 weeks' gestation. This recommendation is based on the observation that high-risk infants may be hospitalized more than once in the same season with RSV lower respiratory tract disease and the fact that more than one RSV strain often cocirculates in a community.
  - RSV is known to be transmitted in the hospital setting and to cause serious disease in high-risk infants. Among hospitalized infants, the major means to reduce RSV transmission is strict observance of infection control practices, including prompt initiation of precautions for RSV-infected infants. If an RSV outbreak occurs in a high-risk unit (eg, pediatric or neonatal intensive care unit or stem cell transplantation unit), primary emphasis should be placed on proper infection control practices, especially hand hygiene. No data exist to support palivizumab use in controlling outbreaks of health care-associated disease, and palivizumab use is not recommended for this purpose.
  - Palivizumab does not interfere with response to vaccines.

ISOLATION OF THE HOSPITALIZED PATIENT: In addition to standard precautions, contact precautions are recommended for the duration of RSV-associated illness among infants and young children, including patients treated with ribavirin. The effectiveness of these precautions depends on compliance and necessitates scrupulous adherence to appropriate hand hygiene practices. Patients with RSV infection should be cared for in single rooms or placed in a cohort.

CONTROL MEASURES: The control of health care-associated RSV transmission is complicated by the continuing chance of introduction through infected patients, staff, and visitors. Because the major source of spread is through direct contact, hand hygiene or, preferably, routine utilization of gloves during inpatient and outpatient contact appears to be the most effective means of preventing health care-associated spread. During the peak of the RSV season, many infants and children hospitalized with respiratory tract symptoms will be infected with RSV and should be cared for with contact precautions (see Isolation of the Hospitalized Patient, above). Early identification of RSV-infected patients (see Diagnostic Tests, p 561) is important so that appropriate precautions can be instituted promptly. During community outbreaks of RSV, a variety of measures have been demonstrated to reduce the risk of health care-associated transmission, including the following: (1) laboratory screening of symptomatic patients for RSV infection; (2) cohorting of infected patients and staff; (3) excluding visitors with current or recent respiratory tract infections; (4) excluding staff with respiratory tract illness or RSV infection from caring for susceptible infants; (5) using gowns and gloves and, possibly, goggles or masks for protection of health care workers' eyes; (6) emphasizing hand hygiene before and after direct contact with patients, after contact with inanimate objects in the direct vicinity of patients, and after glove removal; and (7) limiting young sibling visitation during the RSV season.

A critical aspect of RSV prevention among high-risk infants is education of parents and other caregivers about the importance of decreasing exposure to and transmission of RSV. Preventive measures include limiting, where feasible, exposure to contagious settings (eg, child care centers) and emphasis on hand hygiene in all settings, including the home, especially during periods when contacts of high-risk children have respiratory tract infections.

Rhinovirus Infections

CLINICAL MANIFESTATIONS: Rhinoviruses are the most frequent causes of the common cold or rhinosinusitis. Rhinoviruses also can be associated with pharyngitis and otitis media, less commonly with bronchiolitis and pneumonia, and with exacerbations of bronchitis and reactive airway disease. Nasal discharge usually is watery and clear at the onset but often becomes mucopurulent and viscous after a few days and may persist for 10 to 14 days. Malaise, headache, myalgia, and low-grade fever also may occur.

ETIOLOGY: Rhinoviruses are RNA viruses classified as picornaviruses. At least 100 antigenic serotypes have been identified by neutralizing antibodies. Infection with one type confers some type-specific immunity, but immunity is of variable degree and brief duration and offers little protection against other serotypes.

EPIDEMIOLOGY: Only humans, chimpanzees, and gibbons are infected with human rhinoviruses. Transmission occurs predominantly by person-to-person contact with self-inoculation by contaminated secretions on hands. Less commonly, transmission may occur by aerosol spread. Infections occur throughout the year, but peak activity occurs during autumn and spring. Several serotypes usually circulate simultaneously, but the prevalent serotypes circulating in a given population tend to change over time. By adulthood, antibodies to many serotypes have developed. Household spread is common. Viral shedding from nasopharyngeal secretions is most abundant during the first 2 to 3 days of infection and usually ceases by 7 to 10 days. However, shedding may continue for as long as 3 weeks.

The **incubation period** usually is 2 to 3 days but occasionally is up to 7 days.

DIAGNOSTIC TESTS: Inoculation of nasopharyngeal secretions in appropriate cell cultures for viral isolation has been the primary means to diagnose infection but is insensitive for many strains. Polymerase chain reaction (PCR) detection methods have become the best way to identify rhinoviruses infection. There are, however, no commercially available PCR assays for rhinoviruses. Diagnosis of rhinovirus infection is impractical because of the large number of antigenic types.

TREATMENT: In 2008, the US Food and Drug Administration (FDA) issued a safety warning that over-the-counter cold medications should be avoided in children younger than 4 years of age. Use of such medications also is discouraged for children younger than 6 years of age because of lack of efficacy and concerns regarding safety. Antimicrobial agents are not indicated for people with a common cold caused by a rhinovirus or other virus, because antimicrobial agents do not prevent secondary bacterial infection and their use may promote the emergence of resistant bacteria and complicate treatment for a bacterial infection (see Appropriate and Judicious Use of Antimicrobial Agents, p 740).

ISOLATION OF THE HOSPITALIZED PATIENT: In addition to standard precautions, droplet precautions are recommended for hospitalized infants and children for the duration of illness.

CONTROL MEASURES: Frequent hand hygiene, respiratory hygiene and general hygienic measures in schools, households, and other settings where transmission is common may help decrease the spread of rhinoviruses. Use of disinfectant sprays in the environment is of no proven benefit.

Rickettsial Diseases

Rickettsial diseases comprise infections caused by organisms of the genera *Rickettsia* (endemic and epidemic typhus and spotted fever group rickettsioses), *Orientia* (scrub typhus), *Ehrlichia* (ehrlichiosis), and *Anaplasma* (anaplasmosis).

CLINICAL MANIFESTATIONS: Rickettsial infections have many features in common, including the following:

- Fever, rash (especially in spotted fever and typhus group rickettsiae), headache, myalgia, and respiratory tract symptoms are prominent features.
- Local primary eschars occur with some rickettsial diseases, particularly spotted fever rickettsioses and scrub typhus.
- Systemic capillary and small vessel endothelial damage (ie, vasculitis) with increased microvascular permeability is the primary pathologic feature of spotted fever and typhus group rickettsial infections.
- Rickettsial diseases rapidly can become life threatening. Risk factors for severe disease include glucose-6-phosphate deficiency, male sex, and use of sulfonamides.

Immunity against reinfection by the same agent after natural infection usually is of long duration, except in the case of scrub typhus. Among the 4 groups of rickettsial diseases, some cross-immunity usually is conferred by infections within groups but not between groups. Reinfection with *Ehrlichia* and *Anaplasma* species has been described.

ETIOLOGY: The rickettsiae causing human disease include: *Rickettsia* species, *Orientia* tsutsugamushi, and *Ehrlichia* and *Anaplasma* species. Rickettsiae are small, coccobacillary gram-negative bacteria that are obligate intracellular pathogens and cannot be grown in cell-free media. They have a cell membrane characteristic of gram-negative microorganisms and divide by binary fission.

EPIDEMIOLOGY: Rickettsial diseases have arthropod vectors including ticks, fleas, mites, and lice. Humans are incidental hosts, except for epidemic (louseborne) typhus, for which humans are the principal reservoir and the human body louse is the vector. Rickettsia life cycles typically involve arthropod and mammalian reservoirs, and animal-to-human or vector-to-human transmission occurs as a result of environmental or occupational exposure. Thus, geographic and seasonal occurrence of rickettsial disease is related to arthropod vector life cycles, activity, and distribution.

The **incubation periods** vary according to organism (see specific chapters).

DIAGNOSIS: Group-specific antibodies are detectable in the serum of most people 7 to 14 days after onset of illness. Various serologic tests for detecting antirickettsial antibodies are available. The indirect immunofluorescent antibody assay is recommended in most circumstances because of its relative sensitivity and specificity; however, it cannot determine the causative agent to the species level. Treatment early in the course of illness can blunt or delay serologic responses. Polymerase chain reaction (PCR) assays can detect rickettsiae in whole blood or tissues collected during the acute stage of illness and before administration of antimicrobial agents, although availability of these tests is limited to reference and research laboratories. In laboratories with experienced personnel, immunohistochemical staining and PCR testing of skin biopsy specimens from patients with rash or eschar can help to diagnose rickettsial infections early in the course of disease. The Weil-Felix test is insensitive and nonspecific. Organism culture is not performed routinely.

TREATMENT: Prompt and specific therapy is important for optimal outcome. The drug of choice for rickettsioses is doxycycline. Although tetracyclines generally are not given to children younger than 8 years of age because of the risk of dental staining, most experts consider the risk of morbidity from rickettsial diseases greater than the minimal risk of dental staining from one course of doxycycline. Antimicrobial treatment is most effective when children are treated during the first week of illness. If the disease remains untreated during the second week, therapy is less effective in preventing complications of illness. Because confirmatory laboratory tests primarily are retrospective, treatment decisions should be made on the basis of clinical findings and epidemiologic data and should not be delayed until test results are known.

PREVENTION: Control measures primarily involve prevention of vector transmission of rickettsial agents to humans (see Prevention of Tickborne Infections, p 191).

Several rickettsial diseases, including Rocky Mountain spotted fever and ehrlichiosis, are nationally notifiable diseases and should be reported to state and local health departments.

For more details, the following chapters on rickettsial diseases should be consulted:
- *Ehrlichia* Infections (Human Ehrlichioses), p 284, or **www.cdc.gov/ticks/diseases/ehrlichiosis**
- Rickettsialpox, p 572
- Rocky Mountain Spotted Fever, p 573 or **www.cdc/ncidod/dvrd/qfever**
- Endemic Typhus (Murine Typhus), p 710
- Epidemic Typhus (Louseborne or Sylvatic Typhus), p 711

OTHER RICKETTSIAL SPOTTED FEVER INFECTIONS: A number of other epidemiologically distinct but clinically similar tickborne spotted fever infections caused by rickettsiae have been recognized. Many of them present with an eschar at the site of the tick bite. The causative agents of some of these infections share the same group antigen as *Rickettsia rickettsii*. These include:
- *Rickettsia africae,* the causative agent of African tick bite fever that is endemic to sub-Saharan Africa and some Caribbean Islands;

- *Rickettsia conorii,* the causative agent of boutonneuse fevers (Mediterranean spotted fever, India tick typhus, Marseilles fever, Israeli tick typhus, and Astrakhan spotted fever) that is endemic in southern Europe, Africa, the Middle East, and the Indian subcontinent;
- *Rickettsia parkeri,* the causative agent of maculatum infection in the Americas;
- *Rickettsia sibirica,* the causative agent of Siberian tick typhus, endemic in central Asia;
- *Rickettsia australis,* the causative agent of North Queensland tick typhus, endemic in eastern Australia;
- *Rickettsia japonica,* the causative agent of Japanese spotted fever, endemic in Japan;
- *Rickettsia honei,* the causative agent of Thai tick typhus and Flinders Island spotted fever;
- *Rickettsia slovaca,* the causative agent of tickborne lymphadenopathy, endemic in European countries;
- *Rickettsia felis,* the causative agent of cat flea rickettsiosis that occurs worldwide;
- *Rickettsia aeschlimannii,* reported from Africa;
- *Rickettsia heilongüangensis,* reported from the Russian Far East; and
- *Rickettsia helvetica, Rickettsia massiliae,* and *R sibirica* subspecies *mongolotimonae,* reported from European countries.

Each of these infections has some clinical and pathologic features similar to those of Rocky Mountain spotted fever. The specific diagnosis is confirmed using serologic assays. Demonstration of a fourfold or greater increase in specific antibodies (immunoglobulin G) in acute and convalescent serum samples taken 2 to 3 weeks apart is diagnostic of spotted fever rickettsioses; however, some PCR assays on DNA from acute whole blood or skin biopsy provide accurate identification of the etiologic agent. These diseases are of importance among people traveling to or returning from areas where these agents are endemic and people living in these areas.

Rickettsialpox

CLINICAL MANIFESTATIONS: Rickettsialpox is a febrile, eschar-associated illness that is characterized by generalized relatively sparse erythematous, papulovesicular eruptions on the trunk, face, and extremities (less often on palms and soles) or mucous membranes of the mouth. The rash develops 1 to 4 days after onset of fever and 3 to 10 days after appearance of an eschar at the site of the bite of a mouse mite. Regional lymph nodes in the area of the primary eschar typically become enlarged. Without specific antimicrobial therapy, systemic disease lasts approximately 7 to 10 days; manifestations include fever, headache, malaise, and myalgia. Less frequent manifestations include anorexia, vomiting, conjunctivitis, nuchal rigidity, and photophobia. The disease is mild compared with Rocky Mountain spotted fever, and no rickettsial-pox-associated deaths have been described; however, the disease occasionally is severe enough to warrant hospitalization.

ETIOLOGY: Rickettsialpox is caused by *Rickettsia akari,* which is classified with the spotted fever group rickettsiae and related antigenically to other members of that group.

EPIDEMIOLOGY: The natural host for *R akari* in the United States is *Mus musculus,* the common house mouse. The disease is transmitted by the house mouse mite *(Liponyssoides sanguineus).* Disease risk is heightened in areas infested with mice. The disease may be found wherever the hosts, pathogens, and humans coexist but is found mostly in large urban settings. In the United States, rickettsialpox has been described predominantly in northeastern metropolitan centers, especially in New York City. It also has been confirmed in many other countries, including Croatia, Ukraine, Turkey, Russia, and South Korea. All age groups can be affected. No seasonal pattern of disease occurs. The disease is not communicable and is reported rarely in the United States; however, it is likely that rickettsialpox is underdiagnosed.

The **incubation period** is 6 to 15 days.

DIAGNOSTIC TESTS: *R akari* can be isolated in cell culture from blood and eschar biopsy specimens during the acute stage of disease, but culture is not attempted routinely. Because antibodies to *R akari* have extensive cross-reactivity with antibodies against *R rickettsii* (the cause of Rocky Mountain spotted fever), an indirect immunofluorescent antibody assay for *R rickettsii* (the cause of Rocky Mountain spotted fever) can demonstrate a fourfold or greater change in antibody titers between acute and convalescent serum specimens taken 4 to 6 weeks apart. Direct fluorescent antibody or immunohistochemical testing of formalin-fixed paraffin-embedded eschars or papulovesicle biopsy specimens can detect rickettsiae in the samples and are useful diagnostic techniques.

TREATMENT: Doxycycline is the drug of choice and is effective when given for 3 to 5 days. Doxycycline will shorten the course of disease; symptoms resolve typically within 12 to 48 hours after initiation of therapy. Relapse is rare. Despite concerns regarding dental staining after use of tetracyclines in children younger than 8 years of age, a short course of doxycycline is not considered to cause dental staining (see Antimicrobial Agents and Related Therapy, p 737). Chloramphenicol and a fluoroquinolone are alternative drugs, although fluoroquinolones are not approved for this use in children younger than 18 years of age.

ISOLATION OF THE HOSPITALIZED PATIENT: Standard precautions are recommended.

CONTROL MEASURES: Disinfestation with residual acaricides can be used in heavily mite-infested environments to eliminate the vector locally. However, rodent-control measures particularly are important to limit or eliminate the spread of rickettsialpox. No specific management of exposed people is necessary.

Rocky Mountain Spotted Fever

CLINICAL MANIFESTATIONS: Rocky Mountain spotted fever (RMSF) is a systemic, small-vessel vasculitis with a characteristic rash that usually occurs before the sixth day of illness. Fever, myalgia, severe headache, nausea, vomiting, and anorexia are typical clinical features. Abdominal pain and diarrhea often are present and can obscure the diagnosis. The rash initially is erythematous and macular and later can become maculopapular and often petechial. Rash usually appears first on the wrists and ankles, often spreading within hours proximally to the trunk. The palms and soles typically are involved. The rash can be atypical. Although early development of a rash is a useful diagnostic sign, rash fails to develop in up to 20% of cases, and lack of rash is one reason why the diagnosis can be delayed. Thrombocytopenia of varying severity and hyponatremia develop in many cases. White blood cell count typically is normal, but leukopenia and anemia can occur. The illness can last as long as 3 weeks and can be severe, with prominent central nervous system, cardiac, pulmonary, gastrointestinal tract, and renal involvement; disseminated intravascular coagulation; and shock leading to death. Case-fatality rates of untreated RMSF approximate 25%. Significant long-term sequelae are common in patients with severe RMSF, including neurologic (paraparesis; hearing loss; peripheral neuropathy; bladder and bowel incontinence; and cerebellar, vestibular, and motor dysfunction) and nonneuro-logic (disability from limb amputation).

ETIOLOGY: *Rickettsia rickettsii*, an obligate intracellular pathogen and a member of the spotted fever group of rickettsiae, is the causative agent. The primary targets of infection in mammalian hosts are endothelial cells lining the small blood vessels of all major tissues and organs.

EPIDEMIOLOGY: The disease is transmitted to humans by the bite of an Ixodeae family tick. Many small wild animals and dogs have antibodies to *R rickettsii*, but their role as natural reservoirs is not clear. Ticks are both reservoirs and vectors of *R rickettsii*. In ticks, the agent is transmitted transovarially and between stages. People with occupational or recreational exposure to the tick vector (eg, pet owners, animal handlers, and people who spend time outdoors) are at increased risk of acquiring the organism. People of all ages can be infected. April through September are the months of highest incidence in the United States, although RMSF can occur year round in areas with endemic infection. Laboratory-acquired infection has resulted from accidental inoculation and aerosol contamination. Transmission has occurred on rare occasions by blood transfusion. Mortality is highest in males, people older than 50 years of age, children 5 to 9 years of age, and people with no recognized tick bite or attachment. Lack of confirmed recent tick bite does not exclude the diagnosis. Delay in disease recognition and initiation of antirickettsial therapy increase the risk of death. Factors contributing to delayed diagnosis include absence of rash, initial presentation before the fourth day of illness, and onset of illness during months other than May through August.

RMSF is widespread in the United States. Most cases are reported in the south Atlantic, southeastern, and south central states. The principal recognized vectors of *R rickettsii* are *Dermacentor variabilis* (the American dog tick) in the eastern and central United States and *Dermacentor andersoni* (the Rocky Mountain wood tick) in the western United States. Another common tick throughout the world that feeds on dogs, *Rhipicephalus sanguineus* (the brown dog tick), was implicated in 2005 as a vector of *R rickettsii* in a confined area of Arizona and Mexico. Transmission parallels the tick season in a given geographic area. Rocky Mountain spotted fever also occurs in Canada, Mexico, and Central and South America.

The **incubation period** is approximately 1 week (range, 2–14 days).

DIAGNOSTIC TESTS: The diagnosis can be established by one of the multiple rickettsial group-specific serologic tests.[1] A fourfold or greater change in immunoglobulin (Ig) G-specific antibody titer between acute and convalescent serum specimens obtained 2 to 3 weeks apart is diagnostic when determined by indirect immunofluorescent antibody (IFA) assay, enzyme immunoassay, complement fixation, latex agglutination, indirect hemagglutination, or microagglutination tests. The IFA assay is the most widely available confirmatory test. Antibodies generally are detected by IFA assay 7 to 10 days after onset of illness. Only a probable diagnosis can be established by a single serum IgG titer of 1:64 or greater by IFA assay. Commercially available enzyme immunoassays are not quantitative, cannot be used to evaluate changes in IgG titer, and should not be used.

---

[1]Centers for Disease Control and Prevention. Diagnosis and management of tickborne rickettsial diseases: Rocky Mountain spotted fever, ehrlichioses, and anaplasmosis. *MMWR Recomm Rep.* 2006;55(RR-4):1–27

Culture of *R rickettsii* should be conducted only by laboratories with adequate biohazard containment equipment. *R rickettsii* can be detected by immunohistochemical staining or polymerase chain reaction (PCR) of tissue specimens (biopsy or autopsy). Ideally, a specimen from the site of the rash should be obtained before antimicrobial therapy is initiated but no later than 24 hours after treatment is initiated, because sensitivity diminishes quickly afterward. Isolation or PCR assays for detection of *R rickettsii* in blood and biopsy specimens during the acute phase of illness confirm the diagnosis and are available at the Centers for Disease Control and Prevention reference laboratories.

TREATMENT: Doxycycline is the drug of choice; chloramphenicol or a fluoroquinolone are alternative drugs. Although tetracyclines generally are not given to children younger than 8 years of age because of the risk of dental staining (see Antimicrobial Agents and Related Therapy, p 737), most experts consider doxycycline to be the drug of choice for children of any age. Reasons for this preference include the following: (1) tetracycline staining of teeth is related to the total dose; (2) doxycycline is less likely than other tetracyclines to stain developing teeth; (3) doxycycline is effective against ehrlichiosis, which may mimic RMSF, but chloramphenicol may not be (see *Ehrlichia* Infections, p 284); and (4) use of chloramphenicol is problematic because of serious adverse effects, the need to monitor serum concentrations, and lack of an oral preparation in the United States. Also, retrospective studies indicate that chloramphenicol may be less effective than doxycycline for treatment of RMSF. Clinical data for fluoroquinolone treatment of RMSF are limited. Therapy is continued until the patient has been afebrile for at least 3 days and has demonstrated clinical improvement; the usual duration of therapy is 7 to 10 days. Treatment is initiated on the basis of clinical features and epidemiologic considerations. Treatment before day 5 of illness in children with compatible clinical manifestations affords the highest likelihood of good outcome.

ISOLATION OF THE HOSPITALIZED PATIENT: Standard precautions are recommended.

CONTROL MEASURES: Control of ticks in their natural habitat is difficult. Avoidance of tick-infested areas (ie, areas that border wooded regions) is the best preventive measure. If a tick-infested area is entered, people should wear protective clothing and apply tick or insect repellents to clothes and exposed body parts for added protection. Adults should be taught to inspect themselves, their children (bodies and clothing), and pets thoroughly for ticks after spending time outdoors during the tick season and to remove ticks promptly and properly (see Prevention of Tickborne Infections, p 191).

There is no role for prophylactic antimicrobial agents in preventing RMSF. No licensed *R rickettsii* vaccine is available in the United States. For additional information, see **www.cdc.gov/ticks/diseases/rocky_mountain_spotted_fever/.**

Rotavirus Infections

CLINICAL MANIFESTATIONS: Infection begins with acute onset of fever and vomiting followed 24 to 48 hours later by watery diarrhea. Symptoms generally persist for 3 to 8 days. In moderate to severe cases, dehydration, electrolyte abnormalities, and acidosis may occur. In immunocompromised children, including children with human immuno-deficiency virus infection, persistent infection and diarrhea can develop.

ETIOLOGY: Rotaviruses are segmented, double-stranded RNA viruses belonging to the family Reoviridae, with at least 7 distinct antigenic groups (A through G). Group A viruses are the major causes of rotavirus diarrhea worldwide. Serotyping is based on the 2 surface proteins, VP7 glycoprotein (G) and VP4 protease-cleaved hemagglutinin (P); G types 1 through 4 and 9 and P types 1A and 1B are most common in the United States.

EPIDEMIOLOGY: Most human infections result from direct or indirect contact with infected people. Rotavirus is present in high titer in stools of infected patients with diarrhea. Rotavirus can be detected in stool before onset of diarrhea and may persist for as long as 21 days after the onset of symptoms in immunocompetent hosts. Transmission is presumed to be by the fecal-oral route. Rotavirus can be found on toys and hard surfaces in child care centers, indicating that fomites may serve as a mechanism of transmission. Respiratory transmission likely plays a minor role in disease transmission. Spread within families and institutions is common. Rotavirus is the most common cause of health care-associated diarrhea in children and is an important cause of acute gastroenteritis in children attending child care. Rarely, common-source outbreaks from contaminated water or food have been reported.

Human rotavirus infections are ubiquitous. Virtually all children in the United States are infected by 5 years of age. Rotavirus gastroenteritis is the most common cause of severe diarrhea in children younger than 5 years of age. Severe rotavirus infections occur most commonly in infants and children between 3 and 24 months of age. Rotavirus-related hospitalizations can account for as many as 2.5% of all hospitalizations of children. Approximately 20% of adult household contacts of infected infants will develop symptomatic infection. Breastfeeding is associated with milder disease and should be encouraged. During the 2007–2008 rotavirus season in the United States, rotavirus activity was delayed substantially in onset and diminished in magnitude compared with previous years. These changes occurred coincident with increasing use of rotavirus vaccine among infants.[1]

In temperate climates, disease is most prevalent during the cooler months. In North America, the annual epidemic usually starts during the autumn in Mexico and the southwest United States and moves sequentially to reach the northeast United States and Canada by spring. The seasonal pattern of disease is less pronounced in tropical climates, where rotavirus infection is more common during the cooler, drier months.

The **incubation period** ranges from 1 to 3 days.

DIAGNOSTIC TESTS: It is not possible to diagnose rotavirus infection by clinical presentation or nonspecific laboratory tests. Enzyme immunoassay and latex agglutination assays for group A rotavirus antigen detection in stool are available commercially. Both assays have high specificity, but false-positive results and nonspecific reactions can occur

---

[1]Centers for Disease Control and Prevention. Delayed onset and diminished magnitude of rotavirus activity—United States, November 2007–May 2008. *MMWR Morb Mortal Wkly Rep.* 2008;57(25):697–700

in neonates and in people with underlying intestinal disease. Nonspecific reactions can be distinguished from true positive reactions by performance of confirmatory assays. Virus also can be identified in stool by electron microscopy and by specific nucleic acid amplification techniques.

TREATMENT: No specific antiviral therapy is available. Oral or parenteral fluids and electrolytes are given to prevent and correct dehydration. Orally administered Human Immune Globulin, administered as an investigational therapy in immunocompromised patients with prolonged infection, has decreased viral shedding and shortened the duration of diarrhea.

ISOLATION OF THE HOSPITALIZED PATIENT: In addition to standard precautions, contact precautions are indicated for diapered or incontinent children for the duration of illness.

CONTROL MEASURES:

Child Care. General measures for interrupting enteric transmission in child care centers are available (see Children in Out-of-Home Child Care, p 124). Surfaces should be washed with soap and water. A 70% ethanol solution or other disinfectants will inactivate rotavirus and may help prevent disease transmission resulting from contact with environmental surfaces.

Vaccines. In the United States, the rhesus rotavirus tetravalent vaccine (Rotashield) was licensed by the US Food and Drug Administration in August 1998 and incorporated into the 1999 recommended childhood immunization schedule. This product was withdrawn voluntarily from the market in October 1999 because of the association of this vaccine with intussusception. Children who received rotavirus vaccine during the period of approval are not at increased risk of developing intussusception in the future.

Two rotavirus vaccines are licensed for use among infants in the United States. In February 2006, a live, oral human-bovine reassortant pentavalent rotavirus (RotaTeq [RV5]) vaccine was licensed as a 3-dose series for use among infants in the United States. In April 2008, a live, oral human attenuated rotavirus (Rotarix [RV1]) vaccine was licensed as a 2-dose series for infants in the United States. The products differ in composition and schedule of administration. The American Academy of Pediatrics does not express a preference for either vaccine. As of May 2008, no association between RV5 vaccine and intussusception has been identified. Following are recommendations for use of these rotavirus vaccines,[1,2] (see Table 3.62, p 578):

• Infants in the United States routinely should be immunized with 3 doses of RV5 vaccine administered orally at 2, 4, and 6 months of age or 2 doses of RV1 vaccine administered orally at 2 and 4 months of age.

• The first dose of rotavirus vaccine should be administered from 6 weeks through 14 weeks, 6 days of age (the maximum age for the first dose is 14 weeks, 6 days). Immunization should not be initiated for infants 15 weeks, 0 days of age or older.

• The minimum interval between doses of rotavirus vaccine is 4 weeks.

• All doses of rotavirus vaccine should be administered by 8 months, 0 days of age.

---

[1] American Academy of Pediatrics, Committee on Infectious Diseases. Prevention of rotavirus disease: updated guidelines for use of rotavirus vaccine. *Pediatrics.* 2009; in press

[2] Centers for Disease Control and Prevention. Prevention of rotavirus gastroenteritis among infants and children. Recommendations of the Advisory Committee on Immunization Practices (ACIP). *MMWR Recomm Rep.* 2009;58(RR-2):1–25

Table 3.62. Recommended Schedule for Administration of Rotavirus Vaccine

Recommendation	RV5 (RotaTeq [Merck])	RV1 (Rotarix [GlaxoSmith Kline])
Number of doses in series	3	2
Recommended ages for doses	2, 4, and 6 months of age	2 and 4 months of age
Minimum age for first dose	6 weeks of age	6 weeks of age
Maximum age for first dose	14 weeks, 6 days of age	14 weeks, 6 days of age
Minimum interval between doses	4 weeks	4 weeks
Maximum age for last dose	8 months, 0 days of age	8 months, 0 days of age

- The rotavirus vaccine series should be completed with the same product whenever possible. However, immunization should not be deferred if the product used for previous doses is not available or is unknown. In this situation, the health care professional should continue or complete the series with the product available.
- If any dose in the series was RV5 vaccine or the product is unknown for any dose in the series, a total of 3 doses of rotavirus vaccine should be given.
- Rotavirus vaccine can be administered concurrently with other childhood vaccines.
- Infants with transient, mild illness with or without low-grade fever may receive rotavirus vaccine.
- Preterm infants may be immunized if the infant is at least 6 weeks of age and is clinically stable. Preterm infants should be immunized on the same schedule and with the same precautions as recommended for full-term infants. The first dose of vaccine should be given at the time of discharge or after the infant has been discharged from the nursery.
- Infants living in households with pregnant women or immunocompromised people can be immunized.
- Infants who regurgitate a dose of rotavirus vaccine should not be redosed.
- Rotavirus vaccine should not be administered to infants who have a history of a severe allergic reaction (eg, anaphylaxis) after a previous dose of rotavirus vaccine or to a vaccine component. Latex rubber is contained in the RV1 vaccine oral applicator, so infants with a severe (anaphylactic) allergy to latex should not receive human rotavirus vaccine. The RV5 vaccine dosing tube is latex free.
- Precautions for administration of rotavirus vaccine include altered immunocompetence; moderate to severe illness, including gastroenteritis; preexisting chronic intestinal tract disease; history of intussusception; and spina bifida or bladder exstrophy.
- Rotavirus vaccine may be administered at any time before, concurrent with, or after administration of any blood product, including antibody-containing blood products following the routinely recommended schedule for rotavirus vaccine among infants who are eligible for immunization.
- Breastfeeding infants should be immunized according to the same schedule as non-breastfed infants.
- Infants living in households with people who have or are suspected of having an immunodeficiency disorder, impaired immune status, or who are pregnant may be immunized.

- If an infant regurgitates, spits out, or vomits during or after vaccine administration, the vaccine dose should not be repeated.
- If a recently immunized infant is hospitalized for any reason, no precautions other than standard precautions need to be taken to prevent spread of vaccine virus in the hospital setting.
- Preterm infants may be immunized on the same schedule and with the same precautions as for full-term infants. The infant's postnatal age must meet the age requirements for rotavirus vaccine administration and the infant must be clinically stable. The infant may be immunized at the time of discharge from the neonatal intensive care unit or nursery.
- Infants who have had rotavirus gastroenteritis before receiving the full series of rotavirus immunization should begin or complete the schedule following the age and interval recommendations.

Rubella

CLINICAL MANIFESTATIONS:

Postnatal Rubella. Many cases of postnatal rubella are subclinical. Clinical disease usually is mild and characterized by a generalized erythematous maculopapular rash, lymphadenopathy, and slight fever. The rash starts on the face, becomes generalized in 24 hours, and lasts a median of 3 days. Lymphadenopathy, which may precede rash, often involves posterior auricular or suboccipital lymph nodes, can be generalized, and lasts between 5 and 8 days. Conjunctivitis and palatal enanthem have been noted. Transient polyarthralgia and polyarthritis rarely occur in children but are common in adolescents and adults, especially females. Encephalitis (1:5000 cases) and thrombocytopenia (1:3000 cases) are complications. Maternal rubella during pregnancy can result in miscarriage, fetal death, or a constellation of congenital anomalies (congenital rubella syndrome [CRS]).

Congenital Rubella Syndrome. The most commonly described anomalies/manifestations associated with CRS are ophthalmologic (cataracts, pigmentary retinopathy, microphthalmos, and congenital glaucoma), cardiac (patent ductus arteriosus, peripheral pulmonary artery stenosis), auditory (sensorineural hearing impairment), and neurologic (behavioral disorders, meningoencephalitis, and mental retardation). Neonatal manifestations of CRS include growth retardation, interstitial pneumonitis, radiolucent bone disease, hepatosplenomegaly, thrombocytopenia, and dermal erythropoiesis (so called "blueberry muffin" lesions). Mild forms of the disease can be associated with few or no obvious clinical manifestations at birth. The occurrence of congenital defects is up to 85% if maternal infection occurs during the first 12 weeks of gestation, 54% during the first 13 to 16 weeks of gestation, and 25% during the end of the second trimester.

ETIOLOGY: Rubella virus is an enveloped, positive-stranded RNA virus classified as a Rubivirus in the Togaviridae family.

EPIDEMIOLOGY: Humans are the only source of infection. Postnatal rubella is transmitted primarily through direct or droplet contact from nasopharyngeal secretions. The peak incidence of infection is during late winter and early spring. Approximately 25% to 50% of infections are asymptomatic. Immunity from wild-type or vaccine virus usually is prolonged, but reinfection on rare occasions has been demonstrated and rarely has resulted in CRS. The period of maximal communicability extends from a few days before to 7 days after onset of rash. Volunteer studies have demonstrated the presence of rubella virus in nasopharyngeal secretions from 7 days before to 14 days after onset of rash. A small number of infants with congenital rubella continue to shed virus in nasopharyngeal secretions and urine for 1 year or more and can transmit infection to susceptible contacts. Rubella virus has been recovered in high titer from lens aspirates in children with congenital cataracts for up to several years.

Before widespread use of rubella vaccine, rubella was an epidemic disease, occurring in 6- to 9-year cycles, with most cases occurring in children. In the vaccine era, most cases in the mid-1970s and 1980s occurred in young unimmunized adults in outbreaks on college campuses and in occupational settings. More recent outbreaks have occurred in foreign-born or underimmunized people. The risk of acquiring rubella has decreased in all age groups, and the incidence of rubella in the United States has decreased by more than 99% from the prevaccine era. Since 2003, fewer than 15 cases are reported in the United States annually. In 2004, an independent panel of internationally recognized experts reviewed available data and unanimously agreed that rubella no longer is endemic in the United States. Although the number of susceptible people has decreased since introduction and widespread use of rubella vaccine, recent serologic surveys indicate that approximately 10% of the US-born population older than 5 years of age is susceptible to rubella. In addition, epidemiologic studies of rubella and CRS have identified that susceptibility is higher among people born outside the United States or are from areas with poor vaccine coverage. The risk of CRS is highest in infants of women born outside the United States, because these women are more likely to be susceptible to rubella.

The **incubation period** for postnatally acquired rubella ranges from 14 to 23 days, usually 16 to 18 days.

DIAGNOSTIC TESTS: Detection of rubella-specific immunoglobulin (Ig) M antibody usually indicates recent postnatal infection or congenital infection in a newborn infant, but both false-negative and false-positive results occur. Most postnatal cases are IgM-positive by 5 days after symptom onset, and most congenital cases are IgM-positive at birth to 1 month of age. For diagnosis of postnatally acquired rubella, a fourfold or greater increase in antibody titer or seroconversion between acute and convalescent IgG serum titers also indicates infection. Congenital infection also can be confirmed by stable or increasing serum concentrations of rubella-specific IgG over several months. The hemagglutination-inhibition rubella antibody test, which previously was the most commonly used method of serologic screening for rubella infection, generally has been supplanted by a number of equally or more sensitive assays for determining rubella immunity, including enzyme immunoassays and latex agglutination tests. Diagnosis of congenital rubella infection in children older than 1 year of age is difficult; serologic testing usually is not diagnostic, and viral isolation, although confirmatory, is possible in only a small proportion of congenitally infected children of this age.

A false-positive IgM test result may be caused by rheumatoid factor, parvovirus IgM, and heterophile antibodies. The presence of high-avidity IgG or lack of increase in IgG titers can be useful in identifying false-positive rubella IgM results. Low-avidity IgG is associated with recent primary rubella infection, whereas high-avidity IgG is associated with past infection or reinfection. The avidity assay is not a routine test and should be performed in reference laboratories.

Rubella virus can be isolated most consistently from throat or nasal specimens by inoculation of appropriate cell culture. Detection of rubella virus RNA by reverse-transcriptase polymerase chain reaction from a throat swab or urine sample with subsequent genotyping of strains may be valuable for diagnosis and molecular epidemiology. Most postnatal cases are virus positive on the day of symptom onset, and most congenital cases are virus positive at birth. Laboratory personnel should be notified that rubella is suspected, because specialized testing is required to detect the virus. Blood, urine, and cataract specimens also can yield virus, particularly in infants with congenital infection. With the successful elimination of indigenous rubella and CRS in the United States, molecular typing of viral isolates is critical in defining a source in outbreak scenarios and for sporadic cases.

Every effort should be made to establish a laboratory diagnosis when rubella infection is suspected in pregnant women or newborn infants. Because laboratory tests are not completely specific, the risk of exposure to wild-type rubella virus (eg, travel to areas with endemic rubella infection) should be considered in the final evaluation of suspected cases of rubella in pregnant women.

TREATMENT: Supportive.

ISOLATION OF THE HOSPITALIZED PATIENT: In addition to standard precautions, for postnatal rubella, droplet precautions are recommended for 7 days after onset of the rash. Contact isolation is indicated for children with proven or suspected congenital rubella until they are at least 1 year of age, unless 2 nasopharyngeal and urine culture results after 3 months of age are negative consecutively for rubella virus.

CONTROL MEASURES:

School and Child Care. Children with postnatal rubella should be excluded from school or child care for 7 days after onset of the rash. Children with congenital rubella should be considered contagious until they are at least 1 year of age, unless nasopharyngeal and urine culture results are negative consecutively for rubella virus; infection control precautions should be considered in children up to 3 years of age who are hospitalized for congenital cataract extraction. Caregivers of these infants should be made aware of the potential hazard of the infants to susceptible pregnant contacts.

Care of Exposed People. When a pregnant woman is exposed to rubella, a blood specimen should be obtained as soon as possible and tested for rubella antibody (IgG and IgM). An aliquot of frozen serum should be stored for possible repeated testing at a later time. The presence of rubella-specific IgG antibody in a properly performed test at the time of exposure indicates that the person most likely is immune. If antibody is not detectable, a second blood specimen should be obtained 2 to 3 weeks later and tested concurrently with the first specimen. If the second test result is negative, another blood specimen should be obtained 6 weeks after the exposure and also tested concurrently with the first specimen; a negative test result in both specimens indicates that infection has not occurred, and a positive test result in the second or third specimen but not the first (seroconversion) indicates recent infection.

Immune Globulin. Limited data indicate that intramuscular Immune Globulin (IG) in a dose of 0.55 mL/kg may decrease clinically apparent infection, viral shedding, and rate of viremia significantly in exposed susceptible people. The reduction in virus multiplication theoretically may decrease the likelihood of fetal infection. IG can be considered for postexposure prophylaxis of rubella-susceptible women exposed to confirmed rubella early in pregnancy only if termination of pregnancy is declined. The absence of clinical signs in a woman who has received intramuscular IG does not guarantee that fetal infection has been prevented. Infants with congenital rubella have been born to mothers who were given IG shortly after exposure. Administration of IG eliminates the value of IgG antibody testing to detect maternal infection. IgM antibody can be used to detect maternal infection after exposure, even after receipt of IG.

Vaccine. Although live-virus rubella vaccine administered after exposure has not been demonstrated to prevent illness, vaccine theoretically could prevent illness if administered within 3 days of exposure. Immunization of exposed nonpregnant people may be indicated, because if the exposure did not result in infection, immunization will protect these people in the future. Immunization of a person who is incubating natural rubella or who already is immune is not associated with an increased risk of adverse effects.

Rubella Vaccine. The live-virus rubella vaccine distributed in the United States is the RA 27/3 strain grown in human diploid cell cultures. Vaccine is administered by subcutaneous injection as a combined vaccine containing measles-mumps-rubella (MMR) or measles-mumps-rubella-varicella (MMRV). Single-antigen rubella vaccine no longer is produced in the United States. Vaccine can be given simultaneously with other vaccines (see Simultaneous Administration of Multiple Vaccines, p 33). Serum antibody to rubella is induced in 95% or more of the recipients after a single dose at 12 months of age or older. Clinical efficacy and challenge studies have demonstrated that 1 dose confers long-term, probably lifelong, immunity against clinical and asymptomatic infection in more than 90% of immunized people. Asymptomatic reinfection has occurred.

Because of the 2-dose recommendations for measles vaccine (as MMR) and varicella vaccine (as MMRV), 2 doses of rubella vaccine now are given routinely. This provides an added safeguard against primary vaccine failures.

Vaccine Recommendations. At least 1 dose of live-attenuated rubella-containing vaccine is recommended for people 12 months of age or older. In the United States, rubella vaccine is recommended to be administered in combination with measles and mumps vaccines (MMR) or MMRV, which also contains varicella, when a child is 12 through 15 months of age, with a second dose of MMR or MMRV at school entry at 4 through 6 years of age, according to recommendations for routine measles and varicella immunization. People who have not received the dose at school entry should receive their second dose as soon as possible but optimally no later than 11 through 12 years of age (see Measles, p 444).

Special emphasis must continue to be placed on the immunization of at-risk postpubertal males and females, especially college students, military recruits, recent immigrants, health care professionals, teachers, and child care workers. People who were born in 1957 or after and have not received at least 1 dose of vaccine or who have no serologic evidence of immunity to rubella are considered susceptible and should be immunized with MMR vaccine. Clinical diagnosis of infection usually is unreliable and should not be accepted as evidence of immunity.

Specific recommendations are as follows:
- Postpubertal females without documentation of presumptive evidence of rubella immunity should be immunized unless they are known to be pregnant. Postpubertal females should be advised not to become pregnant for 28 days after receiving a rubella-containing vaccine (see Precautions and Contraindications, p 583, for further discussion).

- During annual health care examinations, premarital and family planning visits, and visits to sexually transmitted infection clinics, postpubertal females should be assessed for rubella susceptibility and, if deemed susceptible, should be immunized with MMR vaccine.
- Routine prenatal screening for rubella immunity should be undertaken. If a woman is found to be susceptible, rubella vaccine should be administered during the immediate postpartum period before discharge.
- Breastfeeding is not a contraindication to postpartum immunization of the mother (for additional information, see Human Milk, p 118).
- All susceptible health care professionals who may be exposed to patients with rubella or who take care of pregnant women, as well as people who work in educational institutions or provide child care, should be immunized for prevention or transmission of rubella to pregnant patients as well as for their own health.

Adverse Reactions.

- Of susceptible children who receive MMR or MMRV vaccines, fever develops in 5% to 15% from 6 to 12 days after immunization. Rash occurs in approximately 5% of immunized people. Mild lymphadenopathy occurs commonly. Febrile seizures occur more frequently among children 12 through 23 months of age after administration of MMRV vaccine compared with MMR and varicella given as separate injections during the same visit (see Measles, p 444).
- Joint pain, usually in small peripheral joints, has been reported in approximately 0.5% of young children. Arthralgia and transient arthritis tend to be more common in susceptible postpubertal females, occurring in approximately 25% and 10%, respectively, of vaccine recipients. Joint involvement usually begins 7 to 21 days after immunization and generally is transient.
- The incidence of joint manifestations after immunization is lower than that after natural infection at the corresponding age.
- Transient paresthesia and pain in the arms and legs also have been reported, although rarely.
- Central nervous system manifestations have been reported, but no causal relationship with rubella vaccine has been established.
- Other reactions that occur after immunization with MMR or MMRV are associated with the measles, mumps, and varicella components of the vaccine (see Measles, p 444, Mumps, p 468, and Varicella-Zoster Infections, p 714).

Precautions and Contraindications.

- ***Pregnancy.*** Rubella vaccine should not be given to pregnant women. If vaccine is given inadvertently or if pregnancy occurs within 28 days of immunization, the patient should be counseled on the theoretical risks to the fetus. A small percentage of offspring in such cases had signs of infection, but none had congenital defects. In view of these observations, receipt of rubella vaccine during pregnancy is not an indication for termination of pregnancy.
- ***Postpubertal women.*** Routine serologic testing of nonpregnant postpubertal women before immunization is unnecessary. Serologic testing is a potential impediment to protection against rubella, because it requires 2 visits.

- **Children of pregnant woman.** Immunizing susceptible children whose mothers or other household contacts are pregnant does not cause a risk. Most immunized people intermittently shed small amounts of virus from the pharynx 7 to 28 days after immunization, but no evidence of transmission of the vaccine virus from immunized children has been found.
- **Febrile illness.** Children with minor illnesses, such as upper respiratory tract infection, may be immunized (see Vaccine Safety and Contraindications, p 40). Fever is not a contraindication to immunization. However, if other manifestations suggest a more serious illness, the child should not be immunized until recovery has occurred.
- **Recent administration of IG.** IG preparations interfere with immune response to measles vaccine, and they theoretically may interfere with the serologic response to rubella vaccine (see p 37). Rubella vaccine may be given to women postpartum at the same time as anti-Rho (D) IG or after blood products are given, but these women should be tested 8 or more weeks later to determine whether they have developed an antibody response. Reimmunization may be necessary. Suggested intervals are the same as used between IG administration and measles immunization (see Table 3.34, p 448).
- **Altered immunity.** Immunocompromised patients with disorders associated with increased severity of viral infections should not receive live-virus rubella vaccine (see Immunocompromised Children, p 72). The exceptions are patients with human immunodeficiency virus infection who are not severely immunocompromised; these patients may be immunized against rubella with MMR or MMRV vaccine (see Human Immunodeficiency Virus Infection, p 380).
- **Household contacts of immunocompromised people.** The risk of rubella exposure for patients with altered immunity can be decreased by immunizing their close susceptible contacts.

  Precautions and contraindications appropriate for the measles, mumps, and varicella components of MMR or MMRV should be reviewed before administration (see Measles, p 444, Mumps, p 468, and Varicella-Zoster Infections, p 714).

Corticosteroids. For patients who have received high doses of corticosteroids (2 mg/kg or greater or more than 20 mg/day) for 14 days or more and who are not otherwise immunocompromised, the recommended interval before immunization is at least 1 month (see Immunocompromised Children, p 72) after steroids have been discontinued.

Surveillance for Congenital Infections. Accurate diagnosis and reporting of CRS are extremely important in assessing control of rubella. All birth defects in which rubella infection is suspected etiologically should be investigated thoroughly and reported to the Centers for Disease Control and Prevention through local or state health departments.

Salmonella Infections

CLINICAL MANIFESTATIONS: Nontyphoidal *Salmonella* organisms cause asymptomatic gastrointestinal tract carriage, gastroenteritis, bacteremia, and focal infections (such as meningitis and osteomyelitis). These disease categories are not mutually exclusive but represent a spectrum of illness. The most common illness associated with nontyphoidal *Salmonella* infection is gastroenteritis, in which diarrhea, abdominal cramps, and fever are common manifestations. The site of infection usually is the distal small intestine as well as the colon. Sustained or intermittent bacteremia can occur, and focal infections are recognized in as many as 10% of patients with *Salmonella* bacteremia.

Salmonella serotype Typhi and several other *Salmonella* serotypes can cause a protracted bacteremic illness often referred to as enteric or typhoid fever. The onset of illness typically is gradual, with manifestations such as fever, constitutional symptoms (eg, headache, malaise, anorexia, and lethargy), abdominal pain and tenderness, hepatomegaly, splenomegaly, rose spots, and change in mental status. Enteric fever can manifest as a mild, nondescript febrile illness in young children, in whom sustained or intermittent bacteremia can occur. Constipation can be an early feature. Diarrhea commonly occurs in children.

ETIOLOGY: *Salmonella* organisms are gram-negative bacilli that belong to the Enterobacteriaceae family. More than 2460 *Salmonella* serotypes exist; most serotypes causing human disease are divided among O-antigen groups A through E. *Salmonella* serotype Typhi is classified in serogroup D. In 2006, the most commonly reported human isolates in the United States were *Salmonella* serotype Typhimurium (greater than 20%), *Salmonella* serotype Enteritidis (approximately 39%), and *Salmonella* serotype Newport (approximately 9%); these 3 serotypes generally account for nearly half of all *Salmonella* infections. The *Salmonella* nomenclature is shown in Table 3.63.

EPIDEMIOLOGY: The principal reservoirs for nontyphoidal *Salmonella* organisms include poultry, livestock, reptiles, and pets. The major vehicle of transmission is food of animal origin, such as poultry, beef, eggs, and dairy products. Other food vehicles (eg, fruits, vegetables, peanut butter, frozen pot pies, powdered infant formula, cereal, and bakery products) have been implicated in outbreaks in which the food was contaminated by contact with an infected animal product or human. Other modes of transmission include ingestion of contaminated water; contact with infected reptiles or amphibians (eg, pet turtles, iguanas, lizards, snakes, frogs, toads, newts, salamanders) and possibly rodents; and exposure to contaminated medications, dyes, and medical instruments.

Unlike nontyphoidal *Salmonella* serotypes, *Salmonella* serotype Typhi is found only in humans, and infection implies direct contact with an infected person or with an item contaminated by a carrier. Although uncommon in the United States (approximately 400 cases/year), typhoid fever is endemic in many countries. Consequently, typhoid fever infections in people in the United States usually are acquired during international travel.

Age-specific attack rates for *Salmonella* infection are highest in people 1 to 4 years of age. Rates of invasive infections and mortality are higher in infants, elderly people, and people with immunosuppressive conditions, hemoglobinopathies (including sickle cell

Table 3.63. Nomenclature for *Salmonella* Organisms

Complete Name	CDC Designation	Commonly Used Name
S enterica[a] subspecies *enterica* serotype Typhi	*S* ser. Typhi	*S typhi*
S enterica subspecies *enterica* serotype Typhimurium	*S* ser. Typhimurium	*S typhimurium*
S enterica subspecies *enterica* serotype Newport	*S* ser. Newport	*S newport*
S enterica subspecies *enterica* serotype Choleraesuis	*S* ser. Choleraesuis	*S choleraesuis*
S enterica subspecies *enterica* serotype Enteritidis	*S* ser. Enteritidis	*S enteritidis*
S enterica subspecies *houtenae* serotype Marina	S ser. IV48:g,z$_{51}$:-	*S marina*

CDC indicates Centers for Disease Control and Prevention.
[a]Some also use *choleraesuis* and *enteritidis* as species names.

disease), malignant neoplasms, and human immunodeficiency virus (HIV) infection. Most reported cases are sporadic, but widespread outbreaks, including health care-associated and institutional outbreaks, have been reported. Every year, *Salmonella* organisms are one of the most common causes of laboratory-confirmed cases of enteric disease reported by the Foodborne Diseases Active Surveillance Network (FoodNet **[www.foodsafety.gov and www.cdc.gov/foodnet]**).

The risk of transmission exists for the duration of fecal excretion of organisms. Twelve weeks after infection, 45% of children younger than 5 years of age excrete *Salmonella* organisms, compared with 5% of older children and adults; antimicrobial therapy can prolong excretion. Approximately 1% of adults continue to excrete *Salmonella* organisms for more than 1 year (chronic carriers).

The **incubation period** for gastroenteritis usually is 12 to 36 hours (range, 6–72 hours). For enteric fever, the incubation period usually is 7 to 14 days (range, 3–60 days).

DIAGNOSTIC TESTS: Isolation of *Salmonella* organisms from cultures of stool, blood, urine, and material from foci of infection is diagnostic. Gastroenteritis is diagnosed by stool culture. Rapid tests using enzyme immunoassay, latex agglutination, DNA probes, and monoclonal antibodies have been developed and are in use in some laboratories. If enteric fever is suspected, blood or bone marrow culture is diagnostic since organisms often are absent from stool. The sensitivity of blood culture is approximately 60% and of bone marrow culture is approximately 90% in patients with enteric fever.

TREATMENT:
- Antimicrobial therapy usually is not indicated for patients with either asymptomatic infection or uncomplicated (noninvasive) gastroenteritis caused by nontyphoidal *Salmonella* species, because therapy does not shorten the duration of diarrheal disease and can prolong the duration of fecal excretion. Although of unproven benefit, antimicrobial therapy is recommended for gastroenteritis caused by *Salmonella* species in people at increased risk of invasive disease, including infants younger than 3 months of age and people with chronic gastrointestinal tract disease, malignant neoplasms, hemoglobinopathies, HIV infection, or other immunosuppressive illnesses or therapies.
- If antimicrobial therapy is initiated in people with gastroenteritis, ampicillin, amoxicillin, or trimethoprim-sulfamethoxazole is recommended for susceptible strains. Resistance to these antimicrobial agents is becoming more common, especially in resource-limited countries. In areas where ampicillin and trimethoprim-sulfamethoxazole resistance is common, ceftriaxone, cefotaxime, azithromycin, or fluoroquinolones usually are effective. However, fluoroquinolones are not approved for this indication in people younger than 18 years of age and are not recommended unless the benefits of therapy outweigh the potential risks with use of the drug (see Antimicrobial Agents and Related Therapy, p 737).
- For people with localized invasive disease (eg, osteomyelitis, abscess, meningitis, or bacteremia in people infected with HIV), empiric therapy with an expanded-spectrum cephalosporin (cefotaxime or ceftriaxone) is recommended. Once antimicrobial susceptibility test results are available, ampicillin, ceftriaxone, or cefotaxime for susceptible strains is recommended for at least 4 weeks (for meningitis 6 weeks) to prevent relapse.
- For invasive, nonfocal infections, such as bacteremia or enteric fever, caused by nontyphoidal *Salmonella* or *Salmonella* serotype Typhi, 10 to 14 days of therapy is recommended, although shorter courses (7–10 days) have been effective. Drugs of choice,

route of administration, and duration of therapy are based on susceptibility of the organism, site of infection, host, and clinical response. Multidrug-resistant isolates of *Salmonella* serotype Typhi are common, often requiring empirical treatment with an expanded-spectrum cephalosporin, azithromycin, or a fluoroquinolone. Relapse of enteric fever occurs in up to 15% of patients and requires retreatment. Treatment failures have occurred in people treated with cephalosporins, aminoglycosides, and furazolidone, despite in vitro testing indicating susceptibility.

- Chronic (1 year or more) *Salmonella* serotype Typhi carriage, which is unusual in children, may be eradicated by high-dose parenteral ampicillin or high-dose oral amoxicillin combined with probenecid (see Antimicrobial Agents and Related Therapy, p 737). Ciprofloxacin is the drug of choice for elimination of organisms from adult carriers of *Salmonella* serotype Typhi. Cholecystectomy can be indicated in some adults in whom gallstones contribute to chronic carrier states.

- Corticosteroids may be beneficial in patients with severe enteric fever, which is characterized by delirium, obtundation, stupor, coma, or shock. These drugs should be reserved for critically ill patients in whom relief of the manifestations of toxemia may be life saving. The usual regimen is high-dose dexamethasone given intravenously at an initial dose of 3 mg/kg, followed by 1 mg/kg, every 6 hours, for a total course of 48 hours.

ISOLATION OF THE HOSPITALIZED PATIENT: In addition to standard precautions, contact precautions should be used for diapered and incontinent children for the duration of illness. In children with typhoid fever, precautions should be continued until culture results for 3 consecutive stool specimens obtained at least 48 hours after cessation of antimicrobial therapy are negative.

CONTROL MEASURES: Important measures include proper sanitation methods for food preparation, sanitary water supplies, proper hand hygiene, sanitary sewage disposal, exclusion of infected people from handling food or providing health care, prohibiting the sale of pet turtles and restricting the sale of other reptiles for pets, limiting exposure of children younger than 5 years of age and immunocompromised children to reptiles and rodents (see Nontraditional Pets, p 198), reporting cases to appropriate health authorities, and investigating outbreaks. Eggs and other foods of animal origin should be cooked thoroughly. People should not eat raw eggs or foods containing raw eggs. There is evidence that breastfeeding and meticulous preparation of formula might prevent typhoid infection in areas with endemic infection. Notification of public health authorities and determination of serotype are of primary importance in detection and investigation of outbreaks.

Child Care. Outbreaks of *Salmonella* infection are rare but have occurred in child care centers. Specific strategies for controlling infection in out-of-home child care include adherence to hygiene practices, including meticulous hand hygiene and limiting exposure to reptiles and rodents (see Children in Out-of-Home Child Care, p 124).

When *Salmonella* serotype Typhi infection is identified in a symptomatic child care attendee or staff member, stool cultures should be collected from other attendees and staff members, and all infected people should be excluded. The recommended length of exclusion varies with the infected person's age; for children younger than 5 years of age, 3 negative stool specimens are recommended for return. For people 5 years of age and older, 24 hours without a diarrheal stool is recommended before return to a group setting.

When *Salmonella* serotypes other than Typhi are identified in a symptomatic child care attendee or staff member with enterocolitis, older children and staff members do not need to be excluded unless they are symptomatic. Stool cultures are not required for asymptomatic contacts. Antimicrobial therapy is not recommended for people with asymptomatic infection or uncomplicated diarrhea or for people who are contacts of an infected person.

Typhoid Vaccine. Resistance to infection with *Salmonella* serotype Typhi is enhanced by typhoid immunization, but the degree of protection with available vaccines is limited. Two typhoid vaccines are licensed for use in the United States (see Table 3.64).

The demonstrated efficacy of the 2 vaccines licensed by the US Food and Drug Administration ranges from 50% to 80%. Vaccine is selected on the basis of age of the child, need for booster doses, and possible contraindications (see Precautions and Contraindications, p 589) and reactions (see Adverse Events, p 589).

Indications. In the United States, immunization is recommended only for the following people:

- **Travelers to areas where risk of exposure to *Salmonella* serotype Typhi is recognized.** Risk is greatest for travelers to the Indian subcontinent, Latin America, Asia, the Middle East, and Africa who may have prolonged exposure to contaminated food and drink. Such travelers need to be cautioned that typhoid vaccine is not a substitute for careful selection of food and drink (see **www.cdc.gov/travel**).
- **People with intimate exposure to a documented typhoid fever carrier,** as occurs with continued household contact.
- **Laboratory workers with frequent contact with *Salmonella* serotype Typhi and people living in areas outside the United States with endemic typhoid infection.**

Dosages. For primary immunization, the following dosage is recommended for each vaccine:

- **Typhoid vaccine live oral Ty21a (Vivotif).** Children (6 years of age and older) and adults should take 1 enteric-coated capsule every other day for a total of 4 capsules. Each capsule should be taken with cool liquid, no warmer than 37°C (98°F), approximately 1 hour before a meal. The capsules must be kept refrigerated, and all 4 doses must be taken to achieve maximal efficacy. Immunization should be completed at least 1 week before possible exposure.

Table 3.64. Commercially Available Typhoid Vaccines in the United States

Typhoid Vaccine	Type	Route	Minimum Age of Receipt, y	No. of Doses[a]	Booster Frequency, y	Adverse Effects Incidence
Ty21a	Live-attenuated	Oral	6	4	5	Less than 5%
ViCPS	Polysaccharide	Intramusuclar	2	1	2	Less than 7%

ViCPS indicates Vi capsular polysaccharide vaccine.
[a]Primary immunization. For further information on dosage, schedules, and adverse events, see text.

- **Typhoid Vi polysaccharide vaccine (Typhim Vi).** Primary immunization of people 2 years of age and older with Vi capsular polysaccharide (ViCPS) vaccine consists of one 0.5-mL (25-µg) dose administered intramuscularly. Vaccine should be given at least 2 weeks before possible exposure.

  Booster Doses. In circumstances of continued or repeated exposure to *Salmonella* serotype Typhi, booster doses are recommended to maintain immunity after primary immunization. The optimal booster schedule for either vaccine has not been determined.

  Continued efficacy for 5 years after immunization with the oral Ty21a vaccine has been demonstrated; however, the manufacturer of oral Ty21a vaccine recommends reimmunization, completing the entire 4-dose series every 5 years if continued or renewed exposure to *Salmonella* serotype Typhi is expected.

  The manufacturer of ViCPS vaccine recommends a booster dose every 2 years after the primary dose if continued or renewed exposure is expected.

  No data have been reported concerning the use of one vaccine as a booster after primary immunization with the other.

  Adverse Events. The oral Ty21a vaccine produces mild adverse reactions that may include abdominal discomfort, nausea, vomiting, fever, headache, and rash or urticaria. Reported adverse reactions to ViCPS vaccine also are minimal and include fever, headache, and local reaction of erythema or induration of 1 cm or greater.

  Precautions and Contraindications. No data are available regarding the efficacy of typhoid vaccines in children younger than 2 years of age. A contraindication to administration of the parenteral ViCPS vaccine is a history of severe local or systemic reactions after a previous dose. No safety data have been reported for typhoid vaccines in pregnant women. The oral Ty21a vaccine is a live-attenuated vaccine and should not be administered to immunocompromised people, including people known to be infected with HIV; the parenteral ViCPS vaccine may be an alternative. The oral Ty21a vaccine requires replication in the gut for effectiveness; it should not be administered during gastrointestinal tract illness. Studies have demonstrated that simultaneous administration of either mefloquine or chloroquine with oral Ty21a results in an adequate immune response to the vaccine strain. However, if mefloquine is administered, immunization with Ty21a should be delayed for 24 hours. Also, the antimalarial agent proguanil should not be administered simultaneously with oral Ty21a vaccine but, rather, should be administered 10 or more days after the fourth dose of oral Ty21a vaccine. Atovaquone also can interfere with oral Ty21a immunogenicity. Antimicrobial agents should be avoided for 24 or more hours before the first dose of oral Ty21a vaccine and 7 days after the fourth dose of Ty21a vaccine.

Scabies

CLINICAL MANIFESTATIONS: Scabies is characterized by an intensely pruritic, erythematous, papular eruption caused by burrowing of adult female mites in upper layers of the epidermis, creating serpiginous burrows. Itching is most intense at night. In older children and adults, the sites of predilection are interdigital folds, flexor aspects of wrists, extensor surfaces of elbows, anterior axillary folds, waistline, thighs, navel, genitalia, areolae, abdomen, intergluteal cleft, and buttocks. In children younger than 2 years of age, the eruption generally is vesicular and often occurs in areas usually spared in older children and adults, such as the scalp, face, neck, palms, and soles. The eruption is caused by a hypersensitivity reaction to the proteins of the parasite.

Characteristic scabietic burrows appear as gray or white, tortuous, thread-like lines. Excoriations are common, and most burrows are obliterated by scratching before a patient is seen by a physician. Occasionally, 2- to 5-mm red-brown nodules are present, particularly on covered parts of the body, such as the genitalia, groin, and axilla. These scabies nodules are a granulomatous response to dead mite antigens and feces; the nodules can persist for weeks and even months after effective treatment. Cutaneous secondary bacterial infection can occur and usually is caused by *Streptococcus pyogenes* or *Staphylococcus aureus* (including methicillin-resistant *S aureus* [MRSA]). Studies have demonstrated a correlation between poststreptococcal glomerulonephritis and scabies.

Norwegian scabies is an uncommon clinical syndrome characterized by a large number of mites and widespread, crusted, hyperkeratotic lesions. Norwegian scabies usually occurs in debilitated, developmentally disabled, or immunologically compromised people but has occurred in otherwise healthy children after long-term use of topical corticosteroid therapy.

ETIOLOGY: The mite, *Sarcoptes scabiei* subspecies *hominis*, is the cause of scabies. The adult female mite lays eggs in burrows in the stratum corneum of the skin. Larvae emerge from the eggs in 2 to 4 days and molt to nymphs and then to adults, which mate and produce new eggs. The entire cycle takes approximately 10 to 17 days. *S scabiei* subspecies *canis*, acquired from dogs (with clinical mange), can cause a self-limited and mild infestation usually involving the area in direct contact with the infested animal that will resolve without specific treatment.

EPIDEMIOLOGY: Humans are the source of infestation. Transmission usually occurs through prolonged, close, personal contact. Because of the large number of mites in exfoliating scales, even minimal contact with a patient with crusted (Norwegian) scabies may result in transmission. Infestation acquired from dogs and other animals is uncommon, and these mites do not replicate in humans. Scabies of human origin can be transmitted as long as the patient remains infested and untreated, including the interval before symptoms develop. Scabies is endemic in many countries and occurs worldwide in cycles thought to be 15 to 30 years long. Scabies affects people from all socioeconomic levels without regard to age, sex, or standards of personal hygiene. Scabies in adults often is acquired sexually.

The **incubation period** in people without previous exposure usually is 4 to 6 weeks. People who previously were infested are sensitized and develop symptoms 1 to 4 days after repeated exposure to the mite; however, these reinfestations usually are milder than the original episode.

DIAGNOSTIC TESTS: Diagnosis is confirmed by identification of the mite or mite eggs or scybala (feces) from scrapings of papules or intact burrows, preferably from the terminal portion where the mite generally is found. Mineral oil, microscope immersion oil, or water applied to skin facilitates collection of scrapings. A broad-blade scalpel is used to scrape the burrow. Scrapings and oil can be placed on a slide under a glass coverslip and examined microscopically under low power. Adult female mites average 330 to 450 μm in length.

TREATMENT: Infested children and adults should apply lotion or cream containing a scabicide over their entire body below the head. Because scabies can affect the face, scalp, and neck in infants and young children, treatment of the entire head, neck, and body in this age group is required. Special attention should be given to trimming fingernails and ensuring application of medication to these areas. The drug of choice, particularly for infants, young children, and pregnant or nursing women, is 5% permethrin cream (not approved for children younger than 2 months of age), a synthetic pyrethroid. Permethrin cream should be removed by bathing after 8 to 14 hours. Alternative drugs are oral ivermectin or 10% crotamiton cream or lotion. Crotamiton is applied once followed by a second application 24 hours later. A cleansing bath should be taken 48 hours after the second application. Crotamiton is associated with frequent treatment failures and has not been approved for use in children. Ivermectin in a single dose administered orally is reported to be effective for treatment of severe or crusted (Norwegian) scabies and should be considered for patients whose infestation is refractory or who cannot tolerate topical therapy; at least 2 doses generally are necessary. Ivermectin is not approved for treatment of scabies by the US Food and Drug Administration. The safety of ivermectin in children weighing less than 15 kg (33 lbs) has not been determined (see Drugs for Parasitic Infections, p 783).

Because scabietic lesions are the result of a hypersensitivity reaction to the mite, itching may not subside for several weeks despite successful treatment. The use of oral antihistamines and topical corticosteroids can help relieve this itching. Topical or systemic antimicrobial therapy is indicated for secondary bacterial infections of the excoriated lesions.

Because of safety concerns and availability of other treatments, Lindane should not be used for the treatment of scabies.

ISOLATION OF THE HOSPITALIZED PATIENT: In addition to standard precautions, contact precautions are recommended until the patient has been treated with an appropriate scabicide.

CONTROL MEASURES:
- Prophylactic therapy is recommended for household members, particularly for household members who have had prolonged direct skin-to-skin contact. Manifestations of scabies infestation can appear as late as 2 months after exposure, during which time patients can transmit scabies. All household members should be treated at the same time to prevent reinfestation. Ivermectin is not recommended for women who are pregnant or who are lactating and intend to breastfeed. Bedding and clothing worn next to the skin during the 3 days before initiation of therapy should be laundered in a washer with hot water and dried using a hot cycle. Mites do not survive more than 3 days without skin contact. Clothing that cannot be laundered should be removed from the patient and stored for several days to a week to avoid reinfestation.
- Children should be allowed to return to child care or school after treatment has been completed.
- Epidemics and localized outbreaks may require stringent and consistent measures to treat contacts. Caregivers who have had prolonged skin-to-skin contact with infested patients may benefit from prophylactic treatment.
- Environmental disinfestation is unnecessary and unwarranted. Thorough vacuuming of environmental surfaces is recommended after use of a room by a patient with crusted (Norwegian) scabies.
- People with crusted (Norwegian) scabies and their close contacts must be treated promptly and aggressively to avoid outbreaks.

Schistosomiasis

CLINICAL MANIFESTATIONS: Initial entry of the infecting larvae (cercariae), which are shed by snails, is through skin and may be accompanied by a transient, pruritic, papular rash (cercarial dermatitis). After penetration, the organism enters the bloodstream and migrates through the lungs. Each of the 3 major human schistosome parasites lives in some part of the venous plexus that drains the intestines or the bladder. Four to 8 weeks after exposure, an acute illness can develop that manifests as fever, malaise, cough, rash, abdominal pain, hepatosplenomegaly, diarrhea, nausea, lymphadenopathy, and eosinophilia (Katayama fever). The severity of symptoms associated with chronic disease is related to the worm burden. People with low to moderate worm burdens may never develop overt clinical illness; people with significant worm burdens can have a range of symptoms caused primarily by inflammation and fibrosis triggered by eggs produced by adult worms. Heavy infection can result in mucoid bloody diarrhea accompanied by tender hepatomegaly. Portal hypertension can develop from intestinal forms of schistosomiasis and can cause hepatosplenomegaly, ascites, and esophageal varices and hematemesis. Long-term involvement of the colon produces abdominal pain and bloody diarrhea. In *Schistosoma haematobium* infections, the bladder can become inflamed and fibrotic. Symptoms and signs include dysuria, urgency, terminal microscopic and gross hematuria, secondary urinary tract infections, and nonspecific pelvic pain. An association between *S haematobium* and bladder cancer has been established. Other organ systems can be involved from embolized eggs, for example, to the lungs, causing pulmonary hypertension; or to the central nervous system, notably the spinal cord in *Schistosoma mansoni* or *S haematobium* infections and the brain in *Schistosoma japonicum* infection.

Cercarial dermatitis (swimmer's itch) is caused by the larvae of nonhuman schistosome species that penetrate human skin but are unable to complete their life cycle and do not cause systemic disease. Manifestations include pruritus at the penetration site a few hours after water exposure, followed in 5 to 14 days by an intermittent pruritic, sometimes papular, eruption. In previously sensitized people, more intense papular eruptions may occur for 7 to 10 days after exposure.

ETIOLOGY: The trematodes (flukes) *S mansoni*, *S japonicum*, *Schistosoma mekongi*, and *Schistosoma intercalatum* cause intestinal schistosomiasis, and *S haematobium* causes urinary tract disease. All species have similar life cycles. Swimmer's itch is caused by multiple avian and mammalian species of *Schistosoma*.

EPIDEMIOLOGY: Persistence of schistosomiasis depends on the presence of an appropriate snail as an intermediate host. Eggs excreted in stool (*S mansoni*, *S japonicum*, *S mekongi*, and *S intercalatum*) or urine *(S haematobium)* into fresh water hatch into motile miracidia, which infect snails. After development in snails, cercariae emerge and penetrate the skin of humans encountered in the water. Children commonly are infected after infancy when they begin to explore the environment. Children also are involved in transmission because of habits of uncontrolled defecation and urination and frequent wading in infected waters. Communicability lasts as long as live eggs are excreted in the urine and feces of humans and, in the case of *S japonicum*, in animals.

The distribution of schistosomiasis often is focal, limited by the presence of appropriate snail vectors, infected human reservoirs, and fresh water sources. *S mansoni* occurs throughout tropical Africa, in parts of several Caribbean islands, and in areas of Venezuela, Brazil, Suriname, and the Arabian Peninsula. *S japonicum* is found in

China, the Philippines, and Indonesia. *S haematobium* occurs in Africa and the eastern Mediterranean region. *S mekongi* is found in Cambodia, Laos, the Philippines, and Central Indonesia. *S intercalatum* is found in West and Central Africa. Adult worms of *S mansoni* can live as long as 30 years in the human host. Thus, schistosomiasis can be diagnosed in patients many years after they have left an area with endemic infection. Swimmer's itch can occur in all regions of the world after exposure to fresh water, brackish water, or salt water. Immunity is incomplete, and reinfection occurs commonly.

The **incubation period** is variable but is approximately 4 to 6 weeks for *S japonicum*, 6 to 8 weeks for *S mansoni*, and 10 to 12 weeks for *S haematobium*.

DIAGNOSTIC TESTS: Infection with *S mansoni* and other species (except *S haematobium*) is determined by microscopic examination of stool specimens to detect characteristic eggs. In light infections, several stool specimens examined by a concentration technique may be needed before eggs are found, or a biopsy of the rectal mucosa may be necessary. *S haematobium* is diagnosed by examining urine for eggs. Egg excretion in urine often peaks between noon and 3 pm. Biopsy of the bladder mucosa may be necessary. Serologic tests, available through the Centers for Disease Control and Prevention and some commercial laboratories, are 99%, 90%, and 50% sensitive for detecting infection attributable to *S mansoni*, *S haematobium*, and *S japonicum*, respectively. Specific serologic tests may be particularly helpful for detecting light infections or before eggs appear in the stool or urine. Results of these antibody-based tests remain positive for many years and are not useful in differentiating ongoing infection from past infection or reinfection.

Swimmer's itch can be difficult to differentiate from other causes of dermatitis. A skin biopsy may demonstrate larvae, but their absence does not exclude the diagnosis.

TREATMENT: The drug of choice for schistosomiasis caused by any species is praziquantel; the alternative drug for *S mansoni* is oxamniquine, although this drug is not available in the United States but is used in some areas of Brazil (see Drugs for Parasitic Infections, p 783). Praziquantel does not kill developing worms; therapy given within 4 to 8 weeks of exposure should be repeated 1 to 2 months later. Swimmer's itch is a self-limited disease that may require symptomatic treatment of the rash. More intense reactions may require a course of oral corticoids.

ISOLATION OF THE HOSPITALIZED PATIENT: Standard precautions are recommended.

CONTROL MEASURES: Elimination of the intermediate snail host is difficult to achieve in most areas. Thus, mass treatment of infected populations, sanitary disposal of human waste, and education about the source of infection are key elements of current control measures. Travelers to areas with endemic infection should be advised to avoid contact with freshwater streams and lakes.

Shigella Infections

CLINICAL MANIFESTATIONS: *Shigella* species primarily infect the large intestine, causing clinical manifestations that range from watery or loose stools with minimal or no constitutional symptoms to more severe symptoms, including high fever, abdominal cramps or tenderness, tenesmus, and mucoid stools with or without blood. Clinical presentations tend to vary with *Shigella* species; patients with *Shigella sonnei* infection usually exhibit watery diarrhea; people with *Shigella flexneri*, *Shigella boydii*, and *Shigella dysenteriae* infection more often have bloody diarrhea and severe systemic symptoms. Rare complications include bacteremia, Reiter syndrome (after *S flexneri* infection), hemolytic-uremic syndrome (after *S dysenteriae* type 1 infection), toxic megacolon and intestinal perforation, and toxic encephalopathy (ekiri syndrome).

ETIOLOGY: *Shigella* species are aerobic, gram-negative bacilli in the family Enterobacteriaceae. Four species (with more than 40 serotypes) have been identified. Among *Shigella* isolates reported in industrialized nations, including the United States, approximately 75% are *S sonnei*, 20% are *S flexneri*, 3% are *S boydii*, and less than 1% are *S dysenteriae*. In developing countries, especially in Africa and southeast Asia, *S flexneri* predominates, and *S dysenteriae* often causes outbreaks.

EPIDEMIOLOGY: Humans are the natural host for *Shigella*, although other primates may be infected. The primary mode of transmission is fecal-oral. Children 5 years of age or younger in child care settings, their caregivers, and other people living in crowded conditions are at increased risk of infection. Travel to resource-limited countries with inadequate sanitation can place the traveler at risk of infection. Ingestion of as few as 10 to 200 organisms is sufficient for infection to occur, depending on *Shigella* species. Predominant modes of transmission include person-to-person contact, contact with a contaminated inanimate object, ingestion of contaminated food or water, and sexual contact. Houseflies also may be vectors through physical transport of infected feces. *S flexneri, S boydii,* and *S dysenteriae* infections are more common in older children and adults, and these infections often are associated with sources outside the United States. Transmission can occur as long as the organism is present in feces. Even without antimicrobial therapy, the carrier state usually ceases within 1 week of the onset of illness; chronic carriage (1 year or longer) is rare.

The **incubation period** varies from 1 to 7 days but typically is 1 to 3 days.

DIAGNOSTIC TESTS: Isolation of *Shigella* organisms from feces or rectal swab specimens containing feces is diagnostic; sensitivity is improved by testing specimens as soon as they are received. The presence of fecal leukocytes on a methylene-blue stained stool smear is sensitive for the diagnosis of colitis but is not specific for *Shigella* species. An enzyme immunoassay for Shiga toxin may be useful for detection of *S dysenteriae* type 1 in stool. Although bacteremia is rare, blood should be cultured in severely ill, immunocompromised, or malnourished patients. Other testing modalities, including the fluorescent antibody test, polymerase chain reaction assay, and enzyme-linked DNA probes and microassays, are available in research laboratories.

TREATMENT:
- Correction of fluid and electrolyte losses, preferably by oral rehydration solutions, is the mainstay of treatment.
- Most clinical infections with *Shigella sonnei* are self-limited (48 to 72 hours) and do not require antimicrobial therapy. However, antimicrobial therapy is effective in shortening the duration of diarrhea and eradicating organisms from feces. Treatment is recommended for patients with severe disease, dysentery, or underlying immunosuppressive conditions; in these patients, empiric therapy should be given while awaiting culture and susceptibility results. In mild disease, the primary indication for treatment is to prevent spread of the organism.
- Antimicrobial susceptibility testing of clinical isolates is indicated, because resistance to antimicrobial agents is common and susceptibility data can guide appropriate therapy. Plasmid-mediated resistance has been identified in all *Shigella* species. In the United States, sentinel surveillance data indicate that approximately 80% of *Shigella* species

were resistant to ampicillin, 40% were resistant to trimethoprim-sulfamethoxazole, and less than 1% were resistant to ceftriaxone and ciprofloxacin (**www.cdc.gov/narms**).

- For cases in which treatment is required and susceptibility is unknown or an ampicillin and trimethoprim-sulfamethoxazole–resistant strain is isolated, parenteral ceftriaxone, a fluoroquinolone (such as ciprofloxacin), or azithromycin should be given. Oral cephalosporins are not useful for treatment. Fluoroquinolones are not approved by the FDA for use in people younger than 18 years of age with shigellosis, although fluoroquinolones have been shown to be beneficial (see Antimicrobial Agents and Related Therapy, p 737). For susceptible strains, ampicillin and trimethoprim-sulfamethoxazole are effective; amoxicillin is less effective because of its rapid absorption from the gastrointestinal tract. The oral route of therapy is recommended except for seriously ill patients.
- Antimicrobial therapy typically is administered for 5 days; a 2-day course of ceftriaxone may be used if there is a good clinical response and no extraintestinal infection.
- Antidiarrheal compounds that inhibit intestinal peristalsis are contraindicated, because they can prolong the clinical and bacteriologic course of disease and increase the rate of complications.
- Nutritional supplementation, including vitamin A (200 000 IU), can be given to hasten clinical resolution in geographic areas where children are at risk of malnutrition.

ISOLATION OF THE HOSPITALIZED PATIENT: In addition to standard precautions, contact precautions are indicated for the duration of illness.

CONTROL MEASURES:

Child Care Centers. General measures for interrupting enteric transmission in child care centers are recommended (see Children in Out-of-Home Child Care, p 124). Meticulous hand hygiene is the single most important measure to decrease transmission. Waterless hand sanitizers may be an effective option in circumstances where access to soap or clean water is limited and as an adjunct to washing hands with soap. Eliminating access to shared water-play areas and contaminated diapers also can decrease infection rates. Staff members who change diapers should not prepare food for child care attendees.

When *Shigella* infection is identified in a child care attendee or staff member, stool specimens from symptomatic attendees and staff members should be cultured. The local health department should be notified to evaluate and manage potential outbreaks. Ill children and staff should not be permitted to return to the child care facility until 24 or more hours after diarrhea has ceased and, depending on state regulations, until 2 stool cultures are negative for *Shigella* species.

Institutional Outbreaks. The most difficult outbreaks to control are those that involve young children (not yet toilet-trained), adults who are unable to care for themselves (mentally disabled people or skilled nursing facility residents), or an inadequate chlorinated water supply. A cohort system, combined with appropriate antimicrobial therapy, and a strong emphasis on hand hygiene, should be considered until stool cultures no longer yield *Shigella* species. In residential institutions, ill people and newly admitted patients should be housed in separate areas.

General Control Measures. Strict attention to hand hygiene is essential to limit spread. Other important control measures include improved sanitation, a safe water supply through chlorination, proper cooking and storage of food, the exclusion of infected people as food handlers, and measures to decrease contamination of food by houseflies. People should refrain from recreational water venues (eg, swimming pools, water parks) for 1 week after symptoms resolve. Breastfeeding provides some protection for infants. Case reporting to appropriate health authorities (eg, hospital infection control personnel and public health department) is essential.

Smallpox (Variola)

In 1979, the World Health Organization declared that smallpox (variola) had been eradicated successfully worldwide. The last naturally occurring case of smallpox occurred in Somalia in 1977, followed by 2 cases attributable to laboratory exposure in 1978. The United States discontinued routine childhood immunization against smallpox in 1972 and routine immunization of health care professionals in 1976. The US military continued to immunize military personnel until 1995. Two World Health Organization reference laboratories were authorized to maintain stocks of variola virus. There is concern that the virus and the expertise to use it as a weapon of bioterrorism may have been misappropriated. As a result, the United States resumed the military immunization program in 2002 and initiated a civilian preevent smallpox immunization program in 2003 to facilitate preparedness and response to a smallpox bioterrorism event.

CLINICAL MANIFESTATIONS: A person infected with variola major develops a severe prodromal illness characterized by high fever (102°F–104°F [38.9°C–40.0°C]) and constitutional symptoms, including malaise, severe headache, backache, abdominal pain, and prostration, lasting for 2 to 5 days. Infected children may suffer from vomiting and seizures during this prodromal period. Most patients with smallpox tend to be severely ill and bedridden during the febrile prodrome. The prodromal period is followed by development of lesions on mucosa of the mouth or pharynx, which may not be noticed by the patient. This stage occurs less than 24 hours before onset of rash, which usually is the first recognized manifestation of infectiousness. With onset of oral lesions, the patient becomes infectious and remains so until all skin crust lesions have separated. The rash typically begins on the face and rapidly progresses to involve the forearms, trunk, and legs, with the greatest concentration of lesions on the face and distal extremities. Many patients will have lesions on the palms and soles. With rash onset, fever decreases but does not resolve. Lesions begin as macules that progress to papules, followed by firm vesicles, and then deep-seated, hard pustules described as "pearls of pus," with each stage lasting 1 to 2 days. By the sixth or seventh day of rash, lesions may begin to umbilicate or become confluent. Lesions increase in size for approximately 8 to 10 days, after which they begin to crust. Once all the crusts have separated, 3 to 4 weeks after the onset of rash, the patient no longer is infectious. Variola minor is clinically indistinguishable except that it causes fewer systemic symptoms, less extensive rash, little persistent scarring, and fewer fatalities.

Varicella (chickenpox) is the condition most likely to be mistaken for smallpox. Generally, children with varicella do not have a febrile prodrome, while adults may have a brief, mild prodrome. Although the 2 diseases are confused easily in the first few days of the rash, smallpox lesions develop into pustules that are firm and deeply embedded in the dermis, whereas varicella lesions develop into superficial vesicles. Because varicella erupts in crops of lesions that evolve quickly, lesions on any one part of the body will be in different stages of evolution (papules, vesicles, and crusts), whereas all smallpox lesions on any one part of the body are in the same stage of development. The rash distribution of the 2 diseases differs; varicella most commonly affects the face and trunk with relative sparing of the extremities, and lesions on the palms or soles are rare.

Variola major in unimmunized people is associated with case-fatality rates of 30% during epidemics of smallpox. The mortality rate is highest in children younger than 1 year of age and adults older than 30 years of age. The potential for modern supportive therapy in improving outcome is not known.

In addition to the typical presentation of smallpox (90% of cases or greater), there are 2 uncommon forms of variola major: hemorrhagic (characterized by hemorrhage into skin lesions and disseminated intravascular coagulation) and malignant or flat type (in which the skin lesions do not progress to the pustular stage but remain flat and soft). Each variant occurs in approximately 5% of cases and is associated with a 95% to 100% mortality rate.

ETIOLOGY: Variola is a member of the Poxviridae family (genus *Orthopoxvirus*). Monkeypox, vaccinia, and cowpox are other members of the genus and can cause zoonotic infection of humans but usually do not spread from person to person. The Democratic Republic of Congo is experiencing an ongoing, isolated outbreak of monkeypox. In 2003, an outbreak of monkeypox linked to prairie dogs exposed to rodents imported from Ghana occurred in the United States. Humans are the only natural reservoir for variola virus (smallpox). Although the original vaccine used by Edward Jenner contained cowpox virus, the current vaccine contains vaccinia virus.

EPIDEMIOLOGY: Smallpox is spread most commonly in droplets from the oropharynx of infected people, although rare transmission from aerosol and direct contact with infected lesions, clothing, or bedding has been reported. Because most patients with smallpox are extremely ill and bedridden, spread generally is limited to household contacts, hospital workers, and other health care professionals. Secondary household attack rates for smallpox were considerably lower than for measles and similar to or lower than the rates for varicella.

The **incubation period** is 7 to 17 days (mean, 12 days).

DIAGNOSTIC TESTS: Variola virus can be detected in vesicular or pustular fluid by culture or by polymerase chain reaction assay. Screening is available through state health departments, and laboratory confirmation is available only at the Centers for Disease Control and Prevention (CDC). Diagnostic work-up includes the exclusion of varicella-zoster virus as the cause of the rash illness.

TREATMENT: There is no known effective antiviral therapy available to treat smallpox. Infected patients should receive supportive care. Cidofovir has been suggested as having a role in smallpox therapy, but data to support its use in smallpox are not available. Vaccinia Immune Globulin (VIG) is reserved for certain complications of immunization (see Control Measures, p 598) and has no role in treatment of smallpox.

ISOLATION OF THE HOSPITALIZED PATIENT: On admission, a patient suspected of having smallpox should be placed in a private, airborne infection isolation room equipped with negative-pressure ventilation with high-efficiency particulate air filtration. Standard, contact, and airborne precautions should be implemented immediately, and hospital infection control personnel and the state (and/or local) health department should be alerted at once. After evaluation by the state or local health department, if smallpox laboratory diagnostics are considered necessary, the CDC Rash Illness Evaluation Team should be consulted at 770-488-7100.

CONTROL MEASURES:

Care of Exposed People. Cases of febrile rash illness for which smallpox is considered in the differential diagnosis should be reported immediately to local or state health departments.

Use of vaccine. Postexposure immunization (within 3–4 days of exposure) provides some protection against disease and significant protection against a fatal outcome. Any person with a significant exposure to a patient with proven smallpox during the infectious stage of illness requires immunization as soon after exposure as possible, but within 4 days of first exposure ("ring vaccination"). Because infected people are not contagious until the rash (and/or oral lesions) appears, people exposed only during the prodromal period are not at risk.

Preexposure Immunization of Adults.

Smallpox vaccine. The only smallpox vaccine licensed in the United States is ACAM2000, a live vaccinia virus smallpox vaccine.[1] The vaccines do not contain variola virus but contain a related virus called vaccinia virus, distinct from the cowpox virus initially used for immunization by Jenner. Vaccinia vaccines are highly effective in preventing smallpox, with protection waning after 5 to 10 years after 1 dose; protection after reimmunization has lasted longer. However, substantial protection against death from smallpox persisted in the past for more than 30 years after immunization during infancy on the basis of experience at a time of worldwide smallpox virus circulation and routine smallpox immunization practices. Smallpox revaccination recommendations can be found at **http://emergency.cdc.gov/agent/smallpox/revaxmemo.asp.** Information about vaccine administration and adverse events[2] can be found in the vaccine package insert or at **www.bt.cdc.gov/agent/smallpox/index.asp.**

Sporotrichosis

CLINICAL MANIFESTATIONS: Sporotrichosis manifests as either cutaneous or extracutaneous disease. The lymphocutaneous manifestation is the most common **cutaneous** form. Inoculation occurs at a site of minor trauma, causing a painless papule that enlarges slowly to become a nodular lesion that can develop a violaceous hue or can ulcerate. Secondary lesions follow the same evolution and develop along the lymphatic distribution proximal to the initial lesion. A localized cutaneous form of sporotrichosis, also called fixed cutaneous form, common in children, presents as a solitary crusted papule or papuloulcerative or nodular lesion in which lymphatic spread is not observed. The extremities and face are the most common sites of infection. A disseminated cutaneous form with multiple lesions is rare, usually occurring in immunocompromised children.

Extracutaneous sporotrichosis most commonly is limited to bones and joints, particularly those of the hands, elbows, ankles, or knees. Osteoarticular structures are involved after local inoculation or hematogenous spread. Pulmonary sporotrichosis clinically resembles tuberculosis and occurs after inhalation or aspiration of aerosolized spores. Disseminated disease generally occurs after hematogenous spread from primary skin or lung infection. Disseminated sporotrichosis can involve multiple foci (eg, eyes, genitourinary tract, central nervous system) and occurs predominantly in

---

[1] Centers for Disease Control and Prevention. Notice to readers: newly licensed smallpox vaccine to replace old smallpox vaccine. *MMWR Morb Mortal Wkly Rep.* 2008;57(8):207–208

[2] Centers for Disease Control and Prevention. Surveillance guidelines for smallpox vaccine (vaccinia) adverse reactions. *MMWR Recomm Rep.* 2006;55(RR-1):1–16

immunocompromised patients. Pulmonary and disseminated forms of sporotrichosis are uncommon in children.

ETIOLOGY: *Sporothrix schenckii* is a thermally dimorphic fungus that grows as a mold or mycelial form at room temperature and as a yeast at 37°C (98°F) and in host tissues.

EPIDEMIOLOGY: *S schenckii* is a ubiquitous organism that has worldwide distribution but is most common in tropical and subtropical regions of Central and South America and parts of North America. The fungus is isolated from soil and plants, including hay, straw, thorny plants (especially roses), sphagnum moss, and decaying vegetation. Cutaneous disease occurs from inoculation of debris containing the organism. People engaging in gardening or farming are at risk of infection. Inhalation of spores can lead to pulmonary disease. Transmission from infected cats has led to cutaneous disease.

The **incubation period** is 7 to 30 days after cutaneous inoculation but can be as long as 3 months.

DIAGNOSTIC TESTS: Culture of *S schenckii* from a tissue, wound drainage, or sputum specimen is diagnostic. Culture of *S schenckii* from a blood specimen suggests the disseminated form of infection associated with immunodeficiency. Histopathologic examination of tissue may not be helpful, because the organism seldom is abundant. Special fungal stains to visualize the oval or cigar-shaped organism are required. A latex agglutination assay for detection of *Sporothrix* antibody in serum or cerebrospinal fluid is available commercially. Serologic testing and polymerase chain reaction assay show promise for accurate and specific diagnosis but are available only in research laboratories.

TREATMENT: Sporotrichosis usually does not resolve without treatment. Itraconazole is the drug of choice for lymphocutaneous and localized cutaneous disease. The duration of therapy is 3 to 6 months. Oral fluconazole is less effective. The time-honored treatment for sporotrichosis, a saturated solution of potassium iodide, is much less costly and still is recommended as an alternative treatment for cutaneous and lymphocutaneous disease. Saturated solution of potassium iodide (1 drop 3 times daily, increasing as tolerated to a maximum of 1 drop/kg of body weight or 40 to 50 drops 3 times daily, whichever is lowest) is given orally until several weeks after all lesions are healed, is much less costly, and still is recommended as an alternative treatment for cutaneous and extracutaneous disease.

For extracutaneous disease, amphotericin B or itraconazole are the drugs of choice (see Recommended Doses of Parenteral and Oral Antifungal Drugs, p 768). Itraconazole is the treatment of choice for osteoarticular infection, because this form of sporotrichosis rarely is accompanied by systemic illness; therapy should be continued for at least 12 months. Amphotericin B and itraconazole are treatment options for pulmonary infections, depending on severity. Amphotericin B is the drug of choice for disseminated sporotrichosis, including meningeal sporotrichosis, and for infection in children with immunodeficiency, including human immunodeficiency virus infection. Itraconazole may be required for lifelong maintenance therapy after initial treatment with amphotericin B in children with HIV infection. Pulmonary and disseminated infections respond less well than cutaneous infection, despite prolonged therapy. Surgical débridement or excision may be necessary to achieve resolution of cavitary pulmonary disease.

ISOLATION OF THE HOSPITALIZED PATIENT: Standard precautions are indicated.

CONTROL MEASURES: Use of protective gloves and clothing in occupational and avocational activities associated with infection can decrease risk of disease.

Staphylococcal Food Poisoning

CLINICAL MANIFESTATIONS: Staphylococcal foodborne illness is characterized by the abrupt and sometimes violent onset of severe nausea, abdominal cramps, vomiting, and prostration, often accompanied by diarrhea. Low-grade fever or mild hypothermia can occur. The duration of illness typically is 1 to 2 days, but the intensity of symptoms may require hospitalization. The short incubation period, brevity of illness, and usual lack of fever help distinguish staphylococcal from other types of food poisoning except that caused by *Bacillus cereus*. Chemical food poisoning usually has an even shorter incubation period. *Clostridium perfringens* food poisoning usually has a longer incubation period and commonly is not accompanied by vomiting. Patients with foodborne *Salmonella* or *Shigella* infection usually have fever and a longer incubation period (see Appendix IX, Clinical Syndromes Associated With Foodborne Diseases, p 860).

ETIOLOGY: Enterotoxins produced by strains of *Staphylococcus aureus* and, rarely, *Staphylococcus epidermidis* elicit the symptoms of staphylococcal food poisoning. Of the 8 immunologically distinct heat-stable enterotoxins (A, B, C1–3, D, E, and F), enterotoxin A is the most commonly identified cause of staphylococcal food poisoning outbreaks in the United States.

EPIDEMIOLOGY: Illness is caused by ingestion of food containing staphylococcal enterotoxins. Foods usually implicated are those that come in contact with hands of food handlers without food subsequently being cooked or foods that are heated or refrigerated inadequately, such as pastries, custards, salad dressings, sandwiches, poultry, sliced meats, and meat products. When these foods remain at room temperature for several hours before being eaten, toxin-producing staphylococci multiply and produce heat-stable toxin. The organisms can be of human origin from purulent discharges of an infected finger or eye, abscesses, acneiform facial eruptions, nasopharyngeal secretions, or apparently normal skin or, less commonly, can be of bovine origin, such as contaminated milk or milk products, especially cheese.

The **incubation period** ranges from 30 minutes to 8 hours after ingestion, usually 2 to 4 hours.

DIAGNOSTIC TESTS: Recovery of large numbers of staphylococci or of enterotoxin from stool or vomitus supports the diagnosis. In an outbreak setting, demonstration of either enterotoxin or a large number of staphylococci (greater than 10^5 colony-forming units/g of specimen) in an epidemiologically implicated food confirms the diagnosis. Identification (by pulsed-field gel electrophoresis or phage typing) of the same type of *S aureus* from stool or vomitus of 2 or more ill people, from stool or vomitus of an ill person and an implicated food, or stool or vomitus of an ill person and a person who handled the food also confirms the diagnosis. Local health authorities should be notified to help determine the source of the outbreak.

TREATMENT: Treatment is supportive. Antimicrobial agents are not indicated.

ISOLATION OF THE HOSPITALIZED PATIENT: Standard precautions are recommended.

CONTROL MEASURES: Prompt consumption or immediate cooling or refrigeration of cooked or baked foods will help to prevent the illness. Cooked foods should be refrigerated at temperatures less than 5°C (41°F). People with boils, abscesses, and other purulent lesions of the hands, face, or nose should be excluded temporarily from food preparation and handling. Strict hand hygiene before food handling should be enforced.

Staphylococcal Infections

CLINICAL MANIFESTATIONS: *Staphylococcus aureus* causes a variety of localized and invasive suppurative infections and 3 toxin-mediated syndromes: toxic shock syndrome, scalded skin syndrome, and food poisoning (see Staphylococcal Food Poisoning, p 600). Localized infections include hordeola, furuncles, carbuncles, impetigo (bullous and nonbullous), paronychia, ecthyma, cellulitis, omphalitis, parotitis, lymphadenitis, and wound infections. *S aureus* also causes infections associated with foreign bodies, including intravascular catheters or grafts, pacemakers, peritoneal catheters, cerebrospinal fluid shunts, and prosthetic joints, which can be associated with bacteremia. Bacteremia can be complicated by septicemia; endocarditis; pericarditis; pneumonia; pleural empyema; soft tissue, muscle, or visceral abscesses; arthritis; osteomyelitis; septic thrombophlebitis of large vessels; and other foci of infection. Primary *S aureus* pneumonia also can occur after aspiration of organisms from the upper respiratory tract and typically is associated with mechanical ventilation or viral infections in the community (eg, influenza). Meningitis is rare unless accompanied by an intradermal foreign body (eg, ventriculoperitoneal shunt) or a congenital or acquired defect in the dura. *S aureus* infections can be fulminant and commonly are associated with metastatic foci and abscess formation, often requiring prolonged antimicrobial therapy, drainage, and foreign body removal to achieve cure. Risk factors for severe *S aureus* infections include chronic diseases, such as diabetes mellitus and cirrhosis, immunodeficiency, nutritional disorders, surgery, and transplantation.

Staphylococcal toxic shock syndrome (TSS), a toxin-mediated disease, usually is caused by strains producing TSS toxin-1 or possibly other related staphylococcal enterotoxins. This toxin acts as a superantigen that stimulates production of tumor necrosis factor and other mediators that cause capillary leak, leading to hypotension and multiorgan failure. Staphylococcal TSS is characterized by acute onset of fever, generalized erythroderma, rapid-onset hypotension, and signs of multisystem organ involvement, including profuse watery diarrhea, vomiting, conjunctival injection, and severe myalgia (see Table 3.65, p 602). Although approximately 50% of reported cases of staphylococcal TSS occur in menstruating females using tampons, nonmenstrual TSS cases occur after childbirth or abortion, after surgical procedures, and in association with cutaneous lesions. TSS also can occur in males and females without a readily identifiable focus of infection. Prevailing clones of community-associated methicillin-resistant *S aureus* (MRSA) rarely produce TSS toxin. People with TSS, especially menses-associated illness, are at risk of a recurrent episode.

Staphylococcal scalded skin syndrome (SSSS) is a toxin-mediated disease caused by circulation of exfoliative toxins A and B. The manifestations of SSSS are age related and include Ritter disease (generalized exfoliation) in the neonate, a tender scarlatiniform eruption and localized bullous impetigo in older children, and a combination of these with thick white/brown flaky desquamation of the entire skin, especially on the face and neck, in older infants and toddlers. The hallmark of SSSS is the toxin-mediated

Table 3.65. *Staphylococcus aureus* Toxic Shock Syndrome: Clinical Case Definition[a]

Clinical Findings

- Fever: temperature 38.9°C (102.0°F) or greater
- Rash: diffuse macular erythroderma
- Desquamation: 1–2 wk after onset, particularly on palms, soles, fingers, and toes
- Hypotension: systolic pressure 90 mm Hg or less for adults; lower than fifth percentile for age for children younger than 16 years of age; orthostatic drop in diastolic pressure of 15 mm Hg or greater from lying to sitting; orthostatic syncope or orthostatic dizziness
- Multisystem organ involvement: 3 or more of the following:
  - Gastrointestinal: vomiting or diarrhea at onset of illness
  - Muscular: severe myalgia or creatinine phosphokinase concentration greater than twice the upper limit of normal
  - Mucous membrane: vaginal, oropharyngeal, or conjunctival hyperemia
  - Renal: serum urea nitrogen or serum creatinine concentration greater than twice the upper limit of normal or urinary sediment with 5 white blood cells/high-power field or greater in the absence of urinary tract infection
  - Hepatic: total bilirubin, aspartate transaminase, or alanine transaminase concentration greater than twice the upper limit of normal
  - Hematologic: platelet count 100 000/mm³ or less
  - Central nervous system: disorientation or alterations in consciousness without focal neurologic signs when fever and hypotension are absent

Laboratory Criteria

- *Negative* results on the following tests, if obtained:
  - Blood, throat, or cerebrospinal fluid cultures; blood culture may be positive for *S aureus*
  - Serologic tests for Rocky Mountain spotted fever, leptospirosis, or measles

Case Classification

- ***Probable:*** a case that meets the laboratory criteria and in which 4 of 5 clinical findings are present
- ***Confirmed:*** a case that meets laboratory criteria and all 5 of the clinical findings, including desquamation, unless the patient dies before desquamation occurs.

[a]Adapted from Wharton M, Chorba TL, Vogt RL, Morse DL, Buehler JW. Case definitions for public health surveillance. *MMWR Recomm Rep.* 1990;39(RR-13):1–43

cleavage of the stratum granulosum layer of the epidermis (ie, Nikolsky sign). Healing occurs without scarring. Bacteremia is rare, but dehydration and superinfection can occur with extensive exfoliation.

Coagulase-Negative Staphylococci. Most coagulase-negative staphylococci (CoNS) isolates from patient specimens typically represent contamination of culture material (see Diagnostic Tests, p 606). Of the isolates that do not represent contamination, most come from infections that are associated with health care, in patients who have obvious disruptions of host defenses caused by surgery, medical device insertion, immunosuppression, or developmental maturity (eg, infants with very low birth weight). CoNS are the most common cause of late-onset bacteremia and septicemia among preterm infants, especially infants weighing less than 1500 g at birth, and of episodes of health care-associated bacteremia in all age groups. CoNS are responsible for bacteremia in children with intravascular catheters, cerebrospinal fluid shunts, peritoneal catheters, vascular grafts or intracardiac patches, prosthetic cardiac valves, pacemaker wires, or prosthetic joints. Mediastinitis after open-heart surgery, endophthalmitis after intraocular trauma, and omphalitis and scalp abscesses in neonates have been described. CoNS also can enter the bloodstream from the respiratory tract of mechanically ventilated preterm infants or from the gastrointestinal tract of infants with necrotizing enterocolitis. Some species of CoNS are associated with urinary tract infection, including *Staphylococcus saprophyticus* in adolescent females and young adult women, often after sexual intercourse, and *Staphylococcus epidermidis* and *Staphylococcus haemolyticus* in hospitalized patients with urinary tract catheters. In general, CoNS infections have an indolent clinical course in children with intact immune function and even in children who are immunocompromised.

ETIOLOGY: Staphylococci are catalase-positive, gram-positive cocci that appear microscopically as grape-like clusters. There are 32 species that are related closely on the basis of DNA base composition, but only 17 species are indigenous to humans. *S aureus* is the only species that produces coagulase. Of the 16 CoNS species, *S epidermidis, S haemolyticus, S saprophyticus, Staphylococcus schleiferi*, and *Staphylococcus lugdunensis* most often are associated with human infections. Staphylococci are ubiquitous and can survive extreme conditions of drying, heat, and low-oxygen and high-salt environments. *S aureus* has many surface proteins, including the microbial surface components recognizing adhesive matrix molecule (MSCRAMM) receptors that allow the organism to bind to tissues and foreign bodies coated with fibronectin, fibrinogen, and collagen. This permits a low inoculum of organisms to adhere to sutures, catheters, prosthetic valves, and other devices. Many CoNS produce an exopolysaccharide slime biofilm that makes these organisms, as they bind to medical devices (eg, catheters), relatively inaccessible to host defenses and antimicrobial agents.

EPIDEMIOLOGY:

Staphylococcus aureus. *S aureus,* which is second only to CoNS as a cause of health care-associated bacteremia, is equal to *Pseudomonas aeruginosa* as the most common cause of health care-associated pneumonia in adults and is responsible for most health care-associated surgical site infections. *S aureus* colonizes the skin and mucous membranes of 30% to 50% of healthy adults and children. The anterior nares, throat, axilla, perineum, vagina, or rectum are usual sites of colonization. Rates of carriage of more than 50% occur in children with desquamating skin disorders or burns and in people with frequent needle use (eg, diabetes mellitus, hemodialysis, illicit drug use, allergy shots).

    S aureus-mediated TSS was recognized in 1978, and many early cases were associated with tampon use. Although changes in tampon composition and use have resulted in a decreased proportion of cases associated with menses, menstrual and nonmenstrual cases of TSS continue to occur and are reported with similar frequency. Risk factors for TSS include absence of antibody to TSS toxin-1 and focal *S aureus* infection with a TSS toxin-1-producing strain. TSS toxin-1 producing strains can be part of normal flora of anterior nares or vagina, and colonization at these sites is believed to result in protective antibody in more than 90% of adults. Health care-associated TSS can occur and most often follows surgical procedures. In postoperative cases, the organism generally originates from the patient's own flora.

    ***Transmission of* S aureus.** *S aureus* is transmitted most often by direct contact in community settings and indirectly from patient to patient via transiently colonized hands of health care professionals. Health care professionals and family members who are colonized with *S aureus* in the nares or on the skin also can serve as a reservoir for transmission.

Contaminated environmental surfaces and objects also can play a role in transmission of *S aureus*, although their contribution to spread is probably minor. Although not transmitted by the droplet route routinely, *S aureus* can be dispersed into the air over short distances. Dissemination of *S aureus* from people, including infants, with nasal carriage is related to density of colonization, and increased dissemination occurs during viral upper respiratory tract infections. Additional risk factors for health care-associated acquisition of *S aureus* include illness requiring care in neonatal or pediatric intensive care or burn units; surgical procedures; prolonged hospitalization; local epidemic of *S aureus* infection; and the presence of indwelling catheters or prosthetic devices.

Staphylococcus aureus *Colonization and Disease.* Nasal, skin, vaginal, and rectal carriage are the primary reservoirs for *S aureus*. Although domestic animals can be colonized, data suggest that colonization is acquired from humans. Adults who carry MRSA in the nose preoperatively are more likely to develop surgical site infections after general, cardiac, orthopedic, or solid organ transplant surgery than are patients who are not carriers. Heavy cutaneous colonization at an insertion site is the single most important predictor of intravenous catheter-related infections for short-term percutaneously inserted catheters. For hemodialysis patients with *S aureus* skin colonization, the incidence of vascular access-related bacteremia is sixfold higher than for patients without skin colonization. After head trauma, adults who are nasal carriers of *S aureus* are more likely to develop *S aureus* pneumonia than are noncolonized patients.

Health Care-Associated MRSA. MRSA has been endemic in most US hospitals since the 1980s, recently accounting for more than 60% of health care-associated *S aureus* infections in intensive care units reporting to the Centers for Disease Control and Prevention (CDC). Health care-associated MRSA strains are resistant to all beta-lactamase resistant (BLR) beta-lactam and cephalosporin antimicrobial agents as well as to antimicrobial agents of several other classes (multi-drug resistance). Methicillin-susceptible *S aureus* (MSSA) strains can be heterogeneous for methicillin resistance (see Diagnostic Tests, p 606).

Risk factors for nasal carriage of health care-associated MRSA include hospitalization within the previous year, recent (within the previous 60 days) antimicrobial use, prolonged hospital stay, frequent contact with a health care environment, presence of an intravascular or peritoneal catheter or tracheal tube, increased number of surgical procedures, or frequent contact with a person with one or more of the preceding risk factors. A discharged patient known to have had colonization with MRSA should be assumed to have continued colonization when rehospitalized, because carriage can persist for years.

MRSA, both health care- and community-associated strains, and methicillin-resistant CoNS are responsible for a large portion of infections acquired in health care settings. Health care-associated MRSA strains are difficult to treat, because they usually are multidrug resistant and predictably susceptible only to vancomycin, linezolid, and agents not approved for use in children.

Community-Associated MRSA. Unique clones of MRSA increasingly are responsible for community-associated infections in healthy children and adults without typical risk factors for health care-associated MRSA infections. The most frequent manifestation of community-associated MRSA infections is skin and soft tissue infection, but invasive disease also occurs. Antimicrobial susceptibility patterns of these strains differ from those of health care-associated MRSA strains. Although community-associated MRSA are resistant to all beta-lactam antimicrobial agents, they typically are susceptible to multiple other antimicrobial agents, including trimethoprim-sulfamethoxazole, gentamicin, and doxycycline; clindamycin susceptibility is variable. Community-associated MRSA infections have occurred in settings where there is crowding; frequent skin-to-skin contact; sharing of personal items, such as towels and clothing; and poor personal hygiene, such as occurs among athletic teams, in correctional facilities, and in military training facilities. However, most community-associated MRSA infections occur in people without direct links to those settings. Transmission of community-associated MRSA colonization from an infected classmate has been described in child care centers and among sports teams. Although community-associated MRSA arose from the community, in many health care settings, these clones are overtaking health care-associated MRSA strains as a cause of health care-associated MRSA infections, making the usefulness of the epidemiologic terms "health care-associated" and "community-associated" of less value.

Vancomycin-Intermediately Susceptible S aureus. Strains of MRSA with intermediate susceptibility to vancomycin (minimum inhibitory concentration [MIC], 4–8 µg/mL) have been isolated from people (historically, dialysis patients) who had received multiple courses of vancomycin for a MRSA infection. Strains of MRSA can be heterogeneous for vancomycin resistance (see Diagnostic Tests, p 606). Extensive vancomycin use allows vancomycin-intermediately susceptible *S aureus* (VISA) strains to grow. These strains may emerge during therapy. Recommended control measures from the Centers for Disease Control and Prevention (CDC) have included using proper methods to detect VISA, using appropriate infection control measures, and adopting measures to ensure appropriate vancomycin use. Although rare, outbreaks of VISA and heteroresistant VISA have been reported in France, Spain, and Japan. Communicability persists as long as lesions or the carrier state are present.

Vancomycin-Resistant S aureus. In 2002, 2 isolates of vancomycin-resistant *S aureus* (VRSA [MIC 16 µg/mL or greater]) were identified in adults from 2 different states. As of November 2007, VRSA had been isolated from 8 adults in the United States. Each of the adults with VRSA infections had underlying medical conditions, a history of MRSA infections and prolonged exposure to vancomycin. No spread of VRSA beyond case patients has been documented. A concern is that most automated antimicrobial susceptibility testing methods commonly used in the United States were unable to detect vancomycin resistance in these isolates.

Coagulase-Negative Staphylococci. CoNS are common inhabitants of the skin and mucous membranes. Virtually all infants have colonization at multiple sites by 2 to 4 days of age. The most frequently isolated CoNS organism is *S epidermidis*. Different species colonize specific areas of the body. *S haemolyticus* is found on areas of skin with numerous apocrine glands. The frequency of health care-associated CoNS infections increased steadily during the past 3 decades and appears to have plateaued. Infants and children in intensive care units, including neonatal intensive care units, have the highest incidence of CoNS bloodstream infections. Coagulase-negative staphylococci can be introduced at the time of medical device placement, through mucous membrane or skin breaks, through loss of bowel wall integrity (eg, necrotizing enterocolitis in very preterm neonates), or during catheter manipulation. Less often, health care personnel with environmental CoNS colonization on the hands transmit the organism. The roles of the environment or fomites in CoNS transmission are not known.

Methicillin-Resistant CoNS. Methicillin-resistant CoNS account for most health care-associated CoNS infections. Methicillin-resistant strains are resistant to all beta-lactam drugs, including cephalosporins, and usually several other drug classes. Once these strains become endemic in a hospital, eradication is difficult, even when strict infection-control practices are followed.

The **incubation period** is variable for staphylococcal disease. A long delay can occur between acquisition of the organism and onset of disease. For toxin-mediated SSSS, the **incubation period** usually is 1 to 10 days; for postoperative TSS it can be as short as 12 hours. Menses-related cases can develop at any time during menses.

DIAGNOSTIC TESTS: Gram-stained smears of material from skin lesions or pyogenic foci can provide presumptive evidence of infection. Isolation of organisms from culture of otherwise sterile body fluid is definitive. *S aureus* almost never is a contaminant when isolated from a blood culture. CoNS isolated from a blood culture commonly are dismissed as "contaminants." In a very preterm neonate, an immunocompromised person, or a patient with an indwelling catheter or prosthetic device, repeated isolation of the same phenotypic strain of CoNS (on the basis of antimicrobial susceptibility testing) from blood cultures or another normally sterile body fluid suggests true infection, but genotyping more strongly supports the diagnosis by confirming the same strain. For catheter-related bacteremia, quantitative blood cultures from the catheter will have 5 to 10 times more organisms than cultures from a peripheral blood vessel. Criteria that suggest CoNS as pathogens rather than contaminants include the following: (1) 2 or more positive blood cultures from different collection sites; (2) a positive culture from blood or a usually sterile site (eg, cerebrospinal fluid, joint) with identical or nearly identical antimicrobial susceptibility patterns for all isolates; (3) growth in a continuously monitored blood culture system within 15 hours of incubation; (4) clinical findings of infection; (5) an intravascular catheter that has been in place for 3 days or more; and (6) similar or identical genotypes among all isolates.

S aureus-mediated TSS is a clinical diagnosis (Table 3.65, p 602). Blood cultures grow *S aureus* in fewer than 5% of patients. Specimens for culture should be obtained from an identified site of infection, because these sites usually will yield the organism. Because approximately one third of isolates of *S aureus* from nonmenstrual cases produce toxins other than TSS toxin-1, and TSS toxin-1-producing organisms can be present as normal flora, TSS-1 production by an isolate is not useful diagnostically.

Quantitative antimicrobial susceptibility testing should be performed for all staphylococci, including CoNS, isolated from normally sterile sites. Health care-associated MRSA heterogeneous or heterotypic strains appear susceptible by disk testing. However, when a parent strain is cultured on methicillin-containing media, resistant subpopulations are apparent. When these resistant subpopulations are cultured on methicillin-free media, they can continue as stable resistant mutants or revert to susceptible strains (heterogeneous resistance). Cells expressing heteroresistance grow more slowly than the oxacillin-susceptible cells and can be missed at growth conditions above 35°C (95°F).

An increasing proportion of community-associated *S aureus* strains are methicillin resistant, and more than 90% of health care-associated *S aureus* as well as CoNS strains are methicillin and multidrug resistant. Because of the high rates of community-associated MRSA infections in the United States, clindamycin has become an often-used drug for treatment of nonlife-threatening presumed *S aureus* infections. Routine antimicrobial susceptibility testing of *S aureus* strains historically did not include a method to detect strains susceptible to clindamycin that rapidly become clindamycin-resistant when exposed to this agent. This clindamycin-inducible resistance can be detected by the D zone test. When a MRSA isolate is determined to be erythromycin resistant and clindamycin susceptible by routine methods, the D zone test is performed. Patients with MRSA isolates that demonstrate clindamycin-inducible resistance should not receive clindamycin routinely. All *S aureus* strains with an MIC to vancomycin of 4 µg/mL or greater should be confirmed and further characterized. Early detection of VISA is critical to trigger aggressive infection-control measures (see Table 3.66).

Table 3.66. Recommendations for Detecting and Preventing Spread of *Staphylococcus aureus* With Decreased Susceptibility to Vancomycin[a]

Definitions:
- **Vancomycin-susceptible *S aureus***
  MIC 2 µg/mL or less
- **Vancomycin-intermediately susceptible *S aureus* (VISA)**
  MIC 4 through 8 µg/mL
  Not transferable to susceptible strains
- **Vancomycin-resistant *S aureus* (VRSA)**
  MIC 16 µg/mL or greater
  Potentially transferable to susceptible strains
- **Confirmation of VISA and VRSA**
  Possible VISA and VRSA isolates should be retested using vancomycin screen plates or a validated MIC method.
  VISA and VRSA isolates should be reported to the local health department or CDC.

Infection control[b]:
- Isolate patient in a private room.
- Minimize numbers of people caring for VISA/VRSA patients.
- Implement appropriate infection-control precautions:
  - Use contact precautions (gown and gloves).
  - Wear mask/eye protection or face shield if performing procedures (eg, wound manipulations, suctioning) likely to generate splash or splatter of VISA/VRSA-contaminated materials (eg, blood, body fluids, secretions).
  - Perform hand hygiene using appropriate agent (eg, hand washing with soap and water or alcohol-based hand sanitizer).
  - Dedicate nondisposable items for patient use.
  - Monitor and strictly enforce compliance with contact precautions and other measures.
- Educate and inform health care professionals about the need for contact isolation.
- Consult with state health department and CDC before discharging and/or transferring the patient, and notify receiving institution or unit of presence of VISA and of appropriate precautions.

MIC indicates minimum inhibitory concentration; MRSA, methicillin-resistant *S aureus;* VISA, vancomycin-intermediately susceptible *S aureus;* CDC, Centers for Disease Control and Prevention.
[a]Hageman JC, Patel JB, Carey RC, Tenover FC, McDonald LC. *Investigation and Control of Vancomycin-Intermediate and –Resistant Staphylococcus aureus (VISA/VRSA): A Guide for Health Departments and Infection Control Personnel.* Atlanta, GA: Centers for Disease Control and Prevention; 2006. Available at: **www.cdc.gov/ncidod/dhqp/pdf/ar/visa_vrsa_guide.pdf**
[b]For information regarding control of spread of VISA and vancomycin-resistant *S aureus,* e-mail SEARCH@cdc.gov or visit **www.cdc.gov/ncidod/dhqp.**

Guidelines for laboratory detection of VISA and VRSA are available at **http://www.cdc.gov/ncidod/dhqp/ar_visavrsa_lab.html.** *S aureus* and CoNS strain genotyping has become a necessary adjunct for determining whether several isolates from one patient or from different patients are the same. Typing, in conjunction with epidemiologic information, can facilitate identification of the source, extent, and mechanism of transmission of an outbreak. Antimicrobial susceptibility testing is the most readily available method for typing by a phenotypic characteristic. A number of molecular typing methods are available for *S aureus*. Choice of method should consider purpose of typing and available resources. The primary method currently used by the CDC is pulsed-field gel electrophoresis.

TREATMENT: The most frequent manifestation of community-associated MRSA infection is skin and soft tissue infection. Fig 3.3 shows the initial management of skin and soft tissue infections caused by community-associated MRSA.

Serious MSSA infections require intravenous therapy with a beta lactamase-resistant (BLR) beta-lactam antimicrobial agent, such as nafcillin or oxacillin, because most *S aureus* strains produce beta-lactamase enzymes and are resistant to penicillin and ampicillin (see Table 3.67, p 610). First- or second-generation cephalosporins (eg, cefazolin or cefuroxime) or vancomycin are effective but less so than nafcillin or oxacillin, especially for some sites of infection (eg, endocarditis, meningitis). Furthermore, nafcillin or oxacillin, rather than vancomycin (or clindamycin if the *S aureus* strain is susceptible to this agent), is recommended for treatment of serious MSSA infections to minimize emergence of vancomycin- or clindamycin-resistant strains. The addition of gentamicin or rifampin to the regimen should be considered for certain MSSA or MRSA infections, such as endocarditis, persistent bacteremia, meningitis, or ventriculitis, and in consultation with an infectious diseases specialist. A patient who is allergic to penicillin can be treated with a first- or second-generation cephalosporin, if the patient is not also allergic to cephalosporins; with vancomycin; or with clindamycin, if endocarditis or central nervous system infection is not a consideration and the *S aureus* strain is susceptible.

Intravenous vancomycin is recommended for treatment of serious infections caused by staphylococcal strains resistant to BLR beta-lactam antimicrobial agents (eg, MRSA and all CoNS). For empiric therapy of life-threatening *S aureus* infections, initial therapy should include vancomycin and a BLR beta-lactam antimicrobial agent (eg, nafcillin, oxacillin). For hospital-acquired CoNS infections, vancomycin is the drug of choice. Subsequent therapy should be determined by antimicrobial susceptibility results.

VISA infection is rare in children. For seriously ill patients with a history of recurrent MRSA infections or for patients failing vancomycin therapy for whom VISA strains are a consideration, initial therapy could include linezolid or trimethoprim-sulfamethoxazole, with or without gentamicin. If antimicrobial susceptibility results document multidrug resistance, alternative agents, such as quinupristin-dalfopristin, daptomycin, or tigecycline, could be considered, but quinupristin-dalfopristin is not approved for use in children younger than 16 years of age, and daptomycin and tigecycline are not approved for use in people younger than 18 years of age.

Duration of therapy for serious MSSA or MRSA infections depends on the site and severity of infection but usually is 4 weeks or more for endocarditis, osteomyelitis, necrotizing pneumonia, or disseminated infection. After initial parenteral therapy and documented clinical improvement, completion of the course with an oral drug can be considered in older children if adherence can be ensured and endocarditis or CNS

Fig 3.3. Algorithm for Initial Management of Skin and Soft Tissue Infections Caused by Community-Acquired *Staphylococcus aureus*

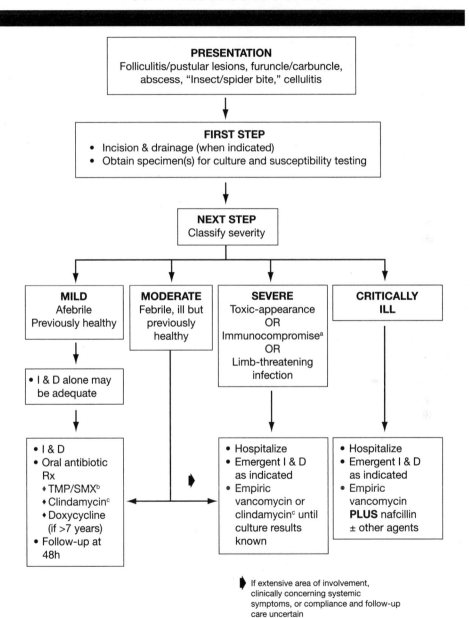

PRESENTATION
Folliculitis/pustular lesions, furuncle/carbuncle, abscess, "Insect/spider bite," cellulitis

FIRST STEP
- Incision & drainage (when indicated)
- Obtain specimen(s) for culture and susceptibility testing

NEXT STEP
Classify severity

MILD
Afebrile
Previously healthy

MODERATE
Febrile, ill but previously healthy

SEVERE
Toxic-appearance
OR
Immunocompromise[a]
OR
Limb-threatening infection

CRITICALLY ILL

- I & D alone may be adequate

- I & D
- Oral antibiotic Rx
  - TMP/SMX[b]
  - Clindamycin[c]
  - Doxycycline (if >7 years)
- Follow-up at 48h

- Hospitalize
- Emergent I & D as indicated
- Empiric vancomycin or clindamycin[c] until culture results known

- Hospitalize
- Emergent I & D as indicated
- Empiric vancomycin **PLUS** nafcillin ± other agents

If extensive area of involvement, clinically concerning systemic symptoms, or compliance and follow-up care uncertain

[a]Immunocompromise: any chronic illness except asthma or eczema.
[b]TMP/SMX = trimethoprim/sulfamethoxazole if group A *Streptococcus* unlikely.
[c]Consider prevalence of clindamycin-susceptible MSSA and "D" test-negative community-associated MRSA strains in the community.

Table 3.67. Parenteral Antimicrobial Agent(s) for Treatment of Bacteremia and Other Serious *Staphylococcus aureus* Infections

Susceptibility	Antimicrobial Agents	Comments
I. Initial empiric therapy (organism of unknown susceptibility)		
Drugs of choice:	Vancomycin + nafcillin or oxacillin + gentamicin	For life-threatening infections (ie, septicemia, endocarditis, CNS infection); linezolid could be substituted for vancomycin if the patient has received several recent courses of vancomycin
	Nafcillin or oxacillin[a]	For nonlife-threatening infection without signs of sepsis (eg, skin infection, cellulitis, osteomyelitis, pyarthrosis) when rates of MRSA colonization and infection in the community are low
	Clindamycin	For nonlife-threatening infection without signs of sepsis when rates of MRSA colonization and infection in the community are substantial and prevalence of clindamycin resistance is low
	Vancomycin	For nonlife-threatening infections without signs of sepsis when rates of MRSA colonization and infection in the community are substantial and when prevalence of clindamycin resistant strains in the community is substantial
II. Methicillin-susceptible, penicillin-resistant *S aureus* (MSSA)		
Drugs of choice:	Nafcillin or oxacillin[a,b]	
Alternatives:	Cefazolin[a]	
	Clindamycin	Only for patients with a serious penicillin allergy and clindamycin-susceptible strain
	Vancomycin	Only for patients with a serious penicillin and cephalosporin allergy
	Ampicillin + sulbactam	
III. MRSA (oxacillin MIC, 4 µg/mL or greater)		
A. Health care–associated (multidrug resistant)		
Drugs of choice:	Vancomycin ± gentamicin or ± rifampin[b]	

Table 3.67. Parenteral Antimicrobial Agent(s) for Treatment of Bacteremia and Other Serious *Staphylococcus aureus* Infections, continued

Susceptibility	Antimicrobial Agents	Comments
Alternatives: susceptibility testing results available before alternative drugs are used	Trimethoprim-sulfamethoxazole	
	Linezolid[c]	
	Quinupristin-dalfopristin[c]	
	Fluoroquinolones	Not recommended for people younger than 18 years of age or as monotherapy
B. Community-associated (not multidrug resistant)		
Drugs of choice:	Vancomycin ± gentamicin (or ± rifampin[b])	For life-threatening infections
	Clindamycin (if strain susceptible)	For pneumonia, septic arthritis, osteomyelitis, skin or soft tissue infections
	Trimethoprim-sulfamethoxazole	For skin or soft tissue infections
Alternative:	Vancomycin[b]	
IV. Vancomycin-intermediately susceptible *S aureus* (MIC, 4 to 16 μg/mL)[b]		
Drugs of choice:	Optimal therapy is not known	Dependent on in vitro susceptibility test results
	Linezolid[c]	
	Daptomycin[d]	
	Quinupristin-dalfopristin[c]	
	Tigecycline[c]	
Alternatives:	Vancomycin + linezolid ± gentamicin	
	Vancomycin + trimethoprim-sulfamethoxazole[b]	

CNS indicates central nervous system; MRSA, methicillin-resistant *S aureus*; MIC, minimum inhibitory concentration.

[a]Penicillin and cephalosporin-allergic patients should receive vancomycin as initial therapy for serious infections.

[b]One of the adjunctive agents, gentamicin or rifampin, should be added to the therapeutic regimen for life-threatening infections such as endocarditis or CNS infection or infections with a vancomycin-intermediate *S aureus* strain. Consultation with an infectious diseases specialist should be considered to determine which agent to use and duration of use.

[c]Linezolid, quinupristin-dalfopristin, and tigecycline are agents with activity in vitro and efficacy in adults with multidrug-resistant, gram-positive organisms, including *S aureus*. Because experience with these agents in children is limited, consultation with an infectious diseases specialist should be considered before use.

[d]Daptomycin is active in vitro against multidrug-resistant, gram-positive organisms, including *S aureus*, but has not been evaluated in children. Daptomycin is approved by the US Food and Drug Administration only for treatment of complicated skin and skin structure infections and for *S aureus* bloodstream infections. It is not indicated for treatment of pneumonia in patients 18 years of age and older.

infection is not a consideration. For endocarditis and CNS infection, parenteral therapy is recommended for the entire treatment. Drainage of abscesses and removal of foreign bodies is desirable and almost always is required for treatment to be effective.

As summarized in Table 3.68, the first priority in management of S aureus TSS is aggressive fluid management as well as management of respiratory or cardiac failure, if present. Initial antimicrobial therapy should include a parentally administered beta-lactam antistaphylococcal antimicrobial agent and a protein synthesis-inhibiting drug, such as clindamycin, at maximum dosages. Vancomycin should be substituted for BLR penicillins or cephalosporins in regions where community-associated MRSA infections are common (see Table 3.67, p 610). Once the organism is identified and susceptibility is known, therapy for S aureus should be modified, but an active antimicrobial agent should be continued for 10 to 14 days. Administration of antimicrobial agents can be changed to the oral route once the patient is tolerating oral alimentation. The total duration of therapy is based on the usual duration of established foci of infection (eg, pneumonia, osteomyelitis). Aggressive drainage and irrigation of accessible sites of purulent infection should be performed as soon as possible. All foreign bodies, including those recently inserted during surgery, should be removed if possible. Immune Globulin Intravenous (IGIV) can be considered in patients with severe staphylococcal TSS unresponsive to all other therapeutic measures, because IGIV may neutralize circulating toxin. The optimal IGIV regimen is unknown, but 150 to 400 mg/kg per day for 5 days or a single dose of 1 to 2 g/kg has been used. Animal studies have suggested that parentally administered corticosteroids may be useful in refractory cases of TSS.

SSSS in infants should be treated with a parenteral BLR beta-lactam antimicrobial agent or, if MRSA is a consideration, vancomycin. In older children, depending on severity, oral agents can be considered. Skin and soft tissue infections, such as impetigo or cellulitis attributable to S aureus, can be treated with oral penicillinase-resistant beta-lactam drugs, such as cloxacillin, dicloxacillin, or a first- or second-generation cephalosporin unless the prevalence of community-associated MRSA in the region is substantial. In the latter circumstance or for the penicillin-allergic patient, trimethoprim-sulfamethoxazole, doxycycline in children 8 years of age and older, or clindamycin can be used.

The duration of therapy for central venous catheter infections is controversial and depends on consideration of a number of factors, including the organism (S aureus vs CoNS), the type and location of the catheter, the site of infection (exit site vs tunnel vs

Table 3.68. Management of Staphylococcal Toxic Shock Syndrome

- Fluid management to maintain adequate venous return and cardiac filling pressures to prevent end-organ damage
- Anticipatory management of multisystem organ failure
- Parenteral antimicrobial therapy at maximum doses
  - Kill organism with bactericidal cell wall inhibitor (eg, beta-lactamase–resistant antistaphylococcal antimicrobial agent)
  - Stop enzyme, toxin, or cytokine production with protein synthesis inhibitor (eg, clindamycin)
- Immune Globulin Intravenous may be considered for infection refractory to several hours of aggressive therapy, or in the presence of an undrainable focus, or persistent oliguria with pulmonary edema

bacteremia), the feasibility of using an alternative vessel at a later date, and the presence or absence of a catheter-related thrombus. Infections are more difficult to treat when associated with a thrombus, thrombophlebitis, or intra-atrial thrombus. If a catheter can be removed, there is no demonstrable thrombus, and bacteremia resolves promptly, a 3- to 5-day course of therapy seems appropriate for CoNS infections in the immunocompetent host. A longer course (eg, 7 to 10 days) is suggested if the patient is immunocompromised or the organism is *S aureus;* experts differ on recommended duration. If the patient needs a new catheter, waiting 48 to 72 hours after bacteremia apparently has resolved before insertion is optimal. If a tunneled catheter is needed for ongoing care, in situ treatment of the infection can be attempted. If the patient responds to antimicrobial therapy with immediate resolution of the *S aureus* bacteremia, treatment should be continued for 10 to 14 days parenterally. Antimicrobial lock therapy of tunneled catheters may result in a higher rate of catheter salvage in adults with CoNS infections, but experience with this approach is limited in children. If blood cultures remain positive for staphylococci for more than 3 to 5 days or if the clinical illness fails to improve, the catheter should be removed, parenteral therapy should be continued, and the patient should be evaluated for metastatic foci of infection. Vegetations or a thrombus in the heart or great vessels always should be considered when an intravascular catheter becomes infected. Transesophageal echocardiography, if feasible, is the most sensitive technique for identifying vegetations.

ISOLATION OF THE HOSPITALIZED PATIENT: Standard precautions are recommended for many patients infected or colonized with MSSA, including patients with TSS. However, contact precautions should be used for patients with abscesses or draining wounds that cannot be covered, regardless of staphylococcal strain, and should be maintained until draining ceases or can be contained by a dressing. Patients infected or colonized with MRSA should be managed with contact precautions for the duration of hospitalization and subsequent hospitalizations, because MRSA carriage can persist for years. For MSSA or MRSA pneumonia, droplet precautions are recommended for the first 24 hours of antimicrobial therapy. Droplet precautions should be maintained throughout the illness for MSSA or MRSA tracheitis with a tracheostomy tube in place.

To prevent transmission of VISA and VRSA, the CDC has issued specific infection-control recommendations that should be followed (see Table 3.66, p 607). For CoNS, standard precautions are recommended. For known epidemic MRSA strains, contact precautions should be used.

CONTROL MEASURES:
Coagulase-Negative Staphylococci. Prevention and control of CoNS infections have focused on prevention of intraoperative contamination by skin flora and sterile insertion of intra-vascular and intraperitoneal catheters and other prosthetic devices. Prophylactic admin-istration of an antimicrobial agent intraoperatively lowers the incidence of infection after cardiac surgery and implantation of synthetic vascular grafts and prosthetic devices and often has been used at the time of cerebrospinal fluid shunt placement.

Staphylococcus aureus. Measures to prevent and control *S aureus* infections can be con-sidered separately for people and for health care facilities.

Individual Patient. Community-associated *S aureus* infections in immunocompetent hosts usually cannot be prevented, because the organism is ubiquitous and there is no vaccine. However, strategies focusing on hand hygiene and wound care have been effective at lim-iting transmission of *S aureus* and preventing spread of infections in community settings.

Specific strategies include appropriate wound care, minimizing skin trauma and keeping abrasions and cuts covered, optimizing hand hygiene and personal hygiene practices (eg, shower after activities involving skin-to-skin contact), avoiding sharing of personal items (eg, towels, razors, clothing), cleaning shared equipment between uses, and regular cleaning of frequently touched environmental surfaces. For patients who experience recurrent *S aureus* infections or who are predisposed to *S aureus* infections because of disorders of neutrophil function, chronic skin conditions, or obesity, a variety of techniques have been used to prevent infection, including scrupulous attention to skin hygiene and to use of clothing and bed linens that minimize sweating, but none have been shown to be effective in preventing recurrent infections with community-associated MRSA.

Measures to prevent health care-associated *S aureus* infections in individual patients include strict adherence to recommended infection-control precautions, appropriate intraoperative antimicrobial prophylaxis, and in some circumstances, use of antimicrobial regimens to eradicate nasal carriage.

Child Care or School Settings. Children with *S aureus* colonization or infection should not be excluded routinely from child care or school settings. Children with draining or open abrasions or wounds should have these covered with a clean, dry dressing. Routine hand hygiene should be emphasized for personnel and children in these facilities.

General Measures. Published recommendations of the CDC Healthcare Infection Control Practices Advisory Committee (HICPAC)[1] for prevention of health care-associated pneumonia should be effective for decreasing the incidence of *S aureus* pneumonia. Careful preparation of the skin before surgery, including cleansing of skin before placement of intravascular catheters using barrier methods, will decrease the incidence of *S aureus* wound and catheter infections. Meticulous surgical technique with minimal trauma to tissues, maintenance of good oxygenation, and minimal hematoma and dead space formation will minimize risk of surgical site infection. Appropriate hand hygiene, including before and after use of gloves, by health care professionals and strict adherence to contact precautions are of paramount importance.

Intraoperative Antimicrobial Prophylaxis. The efficacy of prophylaxis for clean surgery is established. The antimicrobial agent is administered 30 minutes before the operation, and a total duration of therapy of less than 24 hours is recommended. Staphylococci are the most common pathogens causing surgical site infections, and cefazolin is the most commonly recommended drug.

Eradication of Nasal Carriage. Detection and eradication of nasal carriage using mupirocin twice a day for 5 to 7 days before surgery can decrease the incidence of *S aureus* infections in some colonized adult patients after cardiothoracic, general, or neurosurgical procedures. The use of intermittent or continuous intranasal mupirocin for eradication of nasal carriage also has been shown to decrease the incidence of invasive *S aureus* infections in adult patients undergoing long-term hemodialysis or ambulatory peritoneal dialysis. However, eradication of nasal carriage of *S aureus* is difficult, and mupirocin-resistant strains can emerge with repeated or widespread use; therefore, this treatment is not recommended for routine use.

---

[1] Centers for Disease Control and Prevention. Guidelines for preventing health-care–associated pneumonia, 2003: recommendations of CDC and the Healthcare Infection Control Practices Advisory Committee. *MMWR Recomm Rep.* 2004;53(RR-3):1–36

Institutions. Measures to control spread of *S aureus* within health care facilities involve use and careful monitoring of HICPAC guidelines.[1,2] Strategies for controlling spread of MRSA also are found in recommendations for controlling spread of multidrug-resistant organisms (**www.cdc.gov/drugresistance/clinical.htm**). These include general recommendations for all settings and focus on administrative issues; engagement, education, and training of personnel; judicious use of antimicrobial agents; monitoring of prevalence trends over time; use of standard precautions for all patients; and use of contact precautions when appropriate. When endemic rates are not decreasing despite implementation of and adherence to the aforementioned measures, additional interventions, such as use of active surveillance cultures to identify colonized patients and to place them in contact precautions, are warranted. When a patient or health care professional is found to be a carrier of *S aureus*, attempts to eradicate carriage with topical nasal mupirocin therapy may be useful. Both low level (MIC 8–256 µg/mL) and high level (MIC greater than 512 µg/mL) resistance to mupirocin have been identified in *S aureus*, with high-level resistance associated with failure of decolonization therapy. Other topical preparations for intranasal application to be considered if mupirocin fails are ointments containing bacitracin and polymyxin B or a povidone-iodine cream. These preparations have not been studied in children. Minimizing prolonged use of vancomycin will decrease the emergence of VISA. Recommendations for investigation and control of VISA and VRSA have been published by the CDC (Table 3.66, p 607). Ongoing review and restriction of vancomycin use is critical in attempts to control the emergence of VISA and VRSA (see Appropriate and Judicious Use of Antimicrobial Agents, p 740). To date, the use of catheters impregnated with various antimicrobial agents or metals to prevent health care-associated infections has not been evaluated adequately in children.

Nurseries. Outbreaks of *S aureus* infections in newborn nurseries require unique measures of control. Hand hygiene should be emphasized to all personnel and visitors. Application of triple dye, iodophor ointment, or 1% chlorhexidine powder to the umbilical stump has been used to delay or prevent colonization. Other measures recommended during outbreaks include reinforcement of hand hygiene, alleviating overcrowding and understaffing, colonization surveillance cultures of newborn infants at admission and periodically thereafter, use of contact precautions for colonized or infected infants, and cohorting of colonized or infected infants and their caregivers. For hand hygiene, soaps containing chlorhexidine or alcohol-based hand rubs are preferred during an outbreak. Colonized health care personnel epidemiologically implicated in transmission should receive decolonization therapy, but eradication of colonization may not occur.

---

[1] Hageman JC, Patel JB, Carey RC, Tenover FC, McDonald LC. *Investigation and Control of Vancomycin-Intermediate and –Resistant Staphylococcus aureus (VISA/VRSA): A Guide for Health Departments and Infection Control Personnel.* Atlanta, GA: Centers for Disease Control and Prevention; 2006. Available at: **www.cdc.gov/ncidod/dhqp/pdf/ar/visa_vrsa_guide.pdf**

[2] Siegel JD, Rhinehart E, Jackson M, Chianello L, and the Healthcare Infection Control Practices Advisory Committee. *Guideline for Isolation Precautions: Preventing Transmission of Infectious Agents in Healthcare Settings. Recommendations of the Healthcare Infection Control Practices Advisory Committee.* Atlanta, GA: Centers for Disease Control and Prevention; 2007. Available at: **www.cdc.gov/ncidod/dhqp/gl_isolation.html**

Group A Streptococcal Infections

CLINICAL MANIFESTATIONS: The most common group A streptococcal (GAS) infection is acute pharyngotonsillitis. Purulent complications, including otitis media, sinusitis, peritonsillar and retropharyngeal abscesses, and suppurative cervical adenitis develop in some patients, usually people who are untreated. The value of antimicrobial therapy for GAS upper respiratory tract disease is to reduce acute morbidity and to decrease nonsuppurative sequelae (acute rheumatic fever and acute glomerulonephritis).

Scarlet fever occurs most often in association with pharyngitis and, rarely, with pyoderma or an infected wound. Scarlet fever has a characteristic confluent erythematous sandpaper-like rash that is caused by one or more of several erythrogenic exotoxins produced by GAS strains. Severe scarlet fever occurs rarely. Other than the occurrence of rash, the epidemiologic features, symptoms, signs, sequelae, and treatment of scarlet fever are the same as those of streptococcal pharyngitis.

Toddlers (1 through 3 years of age) with GAS respiratory tract infection initially can have serous rhinitis and then develop a protracted illness with moderate fever, irritability, and anorexia (streptococcal fever). The classic presentation of streptococcal upper respiratory tract infection as acute pharyngitis is uncommon in children younger than 3 years of age. Rheumatic fever also is rare in children younger than 3 years of age.

The second most common site of GAS infection is skin. Streptococcal skin infections (ie, pyoderma or impetigo) can result in acute glomerulonephritis, which occasionally occurs in epidemics. Acute rheumatic fever is not a sequela of streptococcal skin infection.

Other GAS infections include erysipelas, perianal cellulitis, vaginitis, bacteremia, pneumonia, endocarditis, pericarditis, septic arthritis, cellulitis, necrotizing fasciitis, osteomyelitis, myositis, puerperal sepsis, surgical wound infection, acute otitis media, sinusitis, mastoiditis, and neonatal omphalitis. Invasive GAS infections can be severe, with or without an identified focus of local infection, and can be associated with streptococcal toxic shock syndrome or necrotizing fasciitis. Infection can follow minor or unrecognized trauma. An association between GAS infection and sudden onset of obsessive-compulsive and/or tic disorders—pediatric autoimmune neuropsychiatric disorders associated with streptococcal infections (PANDAS)—has been proposed but is unproven.

Streptococcal toxic shock syndrome (TSS) is caused by toxin-producing GAS strains and typically manifests as an acute illness characterized by fever, generalized erythroderma, rapid-onset hypotension, and signs of multiorgan involvement including rapidly accelerated renal failure (see Table 3.69, p 617). Evidence of local soft tissue infection (eg, cellulitis, myositis, or necrotizing fasciitis) associated with severe increasing pain is common, but streptococcal TSS can occur without an identifiable focus of infection. Streptococcal TSS also can be associated with invasive infections, such as bacteremia, pneumonia, osteomyelitis, pyarthrosis, or endocarditis.

ETIOLOGY: More than 120 distinct serotypes or genotypes of group A beta-hemolytic streptococci *(Streptococcus pyogenes)* have been identified based on M-protein serotype or M-protein gene sequence *(emm* types). Because of a variety of factors, including M nontypability and *emm* sequence variation within given M types, *emm* typing generally is more discriminating than M typing. Epidemiologic studies suggest an association between certain serotypes (eg, types 1, 3, 5, 6, 18, 19, and 24) and rheumatic fever, but a specific rheumatogenic factor has not been identified. Several serotypes (eg, types 49, 55, 57, and 59) are associated with pyoderma and acute glomerulonephritis. Other serotypes

Table 3.69. Streptococcal Toxic Shock Syndrome: Clinical Case Definition[a]

I. Isolation of group A streptococcus *(Streptococcus pyogenes)*
- A. From a normally sterile site (eg, blood, cerebrospinal fluid, peritoneal fluid, or tissue biopsy specimen)
- B. From a nonsterile site (eg, throat, sputum, vagina, open surgical wound, or superficial skin lesion)

II. Clinical signs of severity
- A. Hypotension: systolic pressure 90 mm Hg or less in adults or lower than the fifth percentile for age in children

AND

- B. Two or more of the following signs:
  - Renal impairment: creatinine concentration 177 μmol/L (2 mg/dL) or greater for adults or 2 times or more the upper limit of normal for age
  - Coagulopathy: platelet count 100 000/mm³ or less or disseminated intravascular coagulation
  - Hepatic involvement: elevated alanine transaminase, aspartate transaminase, or total bilirubin concentrations 2 times or more the upper limit of normal for age
  - Adult respiratory distress syndrome
  - A generalized erythematous macular rash that may desquamate
  - Soft tissue necrosis, including necrotizing fasciitis or myositis, or gangrene

Adapted from The Working Group on Severe Streptococcal Infections. Defining the group A streptococcal toxic shock syndrome: rationale and consensus definition. *JAMA.* 1993;269(3):390–39

[a]An illness fulfilling criteria IA and IIA and IIB can be defined as a *definite* case. An illness fulfilling criteria IB and IIA and IIB can be defined as a *probable* case if no other cause for the illness is identified.

(eg, types 1, 6, and 12) are associated with pharyngitis and acute glomerulonephritis. Most cases of streptococcal TSS are caused by strains producing at least 1 of several different pyrogenic exotoxins. These toxins act as superantigens that stimulate production of tumor necrosis factor and other mediators that cause capillary leak, leading to hypotension and organ damage.

EPIDEMIOLOGY: Pharyngitis usually results from contact with a person who has GAS pharyngitis. Fomites and household pets, such as dogs, are not vectors of GAS infection. Transmission of GAS infection, including in school outbreaks of pharyngitis, almost always follows contact with respiratory tract secretions. Pharyngitis and impetigo (and their nonsuppurative complications) can be associated with crowding, which often is present in socioeconomically disadvantaged populations. The close contact that occurs in schools, child care centers, and military installations facilitates transmission. Foodborne outbreaks of pharyngitis have occurred and are a consequence of human contamination of food in conjunction with improper food preparation or improper refrigeration procedures.

Streptococcal pharyngitis occurs at all ages but is most common among school-aged children and adolescents. GAS pharyngitis and pyoderma are less common in adults than in children.

Geographically, GAS pharyngitis and pyoderma are ubiquitous. Pyoderma is more common in tropical climates and warm seasons, presumably because of antecedent insect bites and other minor skin trauma. Streptococcal pharyngitis is more common during late autumn, winter, and spring in temperate climates, presumably because of close person-to-person contact in schools. Communicability of patients with streptococcal pharyngitis is highest during acute infection and, in untreated people, gradually diminishes over a period of weeks. Patients no longer are contagious within 24 hours after initiation of appropriate antimicrobial therapy.

Throat culture surveys of healthy asymptomatic children during school outbreaks of pharyngitis have yielded GAS prevalence rates as high as 15%. These surveys include children who were pharyngeal carriers with no subsequent immune response to GAS cellular or extracellular antigens. Carriage of GAS can persist for months, but the risk of transmission to others is minimal.

The incidence of acute rheumatic fever in the United States has decreased sharply over several decades, but focal outbreaks of rheumatic fever in school-aged children occurred throughout the 1990s. Although the reason(s) for these focal outbreaks is not clear, their occurrence reemphasizes the importance of diagnosing GAS pharyngitis and of adherence to recommended antimicrobial regimens.

In streptococcal impetigo, the organism usually is acquired from another person with impetigo by direct contact. GAS colonization of healthy skin usually precedes development of skin infection, but GAS does not penetrate intact skin. Impetiginous lesions occur at the site of breaks in skin (eg, insect bites, burns, traumatic wounds). After development of impetiginous lesions, the upper respiratory tract often becomes colonized with GAS. Infection of surgical wounds and postpartum (puerperal) sepsis usually result from contact transmission. Anal or vaginal carriers and people with skin infection, such as pyoderma or local suppurative infections, can transmit GAS to surgical and obstetrical patients, resulting in health care-associated outbreaks. Infections in neonates can result from intrapartum or contact transmission; in the latter situation, infection can begin as omphalitis, cellulitis, or necrotizing fasciitis.

The incidence of invasive GAS infections is highest in infants and older people. Before use of varicella vaccine, varicella was the most commonly identified risk factor in children. Other risk factors for invasive disease include exposure to other children and household crowding. The portal of entry is unknown in almost 50% of invasive GAS infections; in most cases, the entry site is believed to be skin or mucous membranes. Such infections rarely follow GAS pharyngitis. Although case reports have described a temporal association between use of nonsteroidal anti-inflammatory drugs and invasive GAS infections in children with varicella, a causal relationship has not been established.

The incidence of GAS-mediated TSS is highest among young children and the elderly, although TSS can occur in people of any age. Of all cases of severe invasive streptococcal infections in children, fewer than 10% are associated with TSS. Among children, TSS has been reported with focal lesions (eg, varicella, cellulitis, trauma, osteomyelitis), pneumonia, and bacteremia without a defined focus. Mortality rates are lower for children than for adults with GAS-mediated TSS.

The **incubation period** for streptococcal pharyngitis is 2 to 5 days. For impetigo, a 7- to 10-day period between acquisition of GAS on healthy skin and development of lesions has been demonstrated. For TSS, the incubation period is not defined clearly. The incubation period has been as short as 14 hours in cases associated with subcutaneous inoculation of organisms (eg, childbirth, penetrating trauma).

DIAGNOSTIC TESTS: Laboratory confirmation of GAS pharyngitis is recommended for children, because accurate clinical differentiation of viral and GAS pharyngitis is not possible. A specimen should be obtained by vigorous swabbing of both tonsils and the posterior pharynx. Culture on sheep blood agar can confirm GAS infection, and latex agglutination, fluorescent antibody assay, coagglutination, or precipitation techniques performed on colonies growing on an agar plate can differentiate GAS from other beta-hemolytic streptococci. Appropriate use of bacitracin susceptibility disks (containing 0.04 units of bacitracin) allows presumptive identification of GAS but is a less accurate method of diagnosis. False-negative culture results occur in fewer than 10% of symptomatic patients when an adequate throat swab specimen is obtained and cultured properly by trained personnel. Recovery of GAS from the pharynx does not distinguish patients with true streptococcal infection (defined by a serologic antibody response) from streptococcal carriers who have an intercurrent viral pharyngitis. The number of colonies of GAS on an agar culture plate also does not differentiate true infection from carriage. Cultures that are negative for GAS after 24 hours should be incubated for a second day to optimize recovery of GAS.

Several rapid diagnostic tests for GAS pharyngitis are available. Most are based on nitrous acid extraction of group A carbohydrate antigen from organisms obtained by throat swab. The specificities of these tests generally are high, but the reported sensitivities vary considerably. As with throat cultures, the sensitivity of these tests is highly dependent on the quality of the throat swab specimen, the experience of the person performing the test, and the rigor of the culture method used for comparison. Therefore, when a child or adolescent suspected of having GAS pharyngitis has a negative rapid streptococcal test result, a throat culture should be obtained to ensure that the patient does not have GAS infection. Because of the high specificity of these rapid tests, a positive test result does not require throat culture confirmation. Rapid diagnostic tests using techniques such as optical immunoassay and chemiluminescent DNA probes have been developed. These tests may be as sensitive as standard throat cultures on sheep blood agar. The diagnosis of acute rheumatic fever is based on the Jones criteria (Table 3.70, p 620).

Indications for GAS Testing. Factors to be considered in the decision to obtain a throat swab specimen for testing in children with pharyngitis are the patient's age; clinical signs and symptoms; the season; and family and community epidemiology, including contact with a case of GAS infection or presence in the family of a person with a history of acute rheumatic fever or with poststreptococcal glomerulonephritis. GAS pharyngitis is uncommon in children younger than 3 years of age, but outbreaks of GAS pharyngitis have been reported in young children in child care settings. The risk of acute rheumatic fever is so remote in young children in industrialized countries that diagnostic studies for GAS pharyngitis are indicated considerably less often for children younger than 3 years of age than for older children. Children with manifestations highly suggestive of viral infection, such as coryza, conjunctivitis, hoarseness, cough, anterior stomatitis, discrete ulcerative lesions, or diarrhea, are unlikely to have GAS infection as the cause of their pharyngitis and generally should not be tested for GAS infection. Children with acute onset of sore throat and clinical signs and symptoms such as pharyngeal exudate, pain on swallowing, fever, and enlarged tender anterior cervical lymph nodes or exposure to a person with GAS pharyngitis are more likely to have GAS infection as the cause of their pharyngitis and should have a rapid antigen test and/or throat culture performed.

Table 3.70. Jones Criteria for Diagnosis of Acute Rheumatic Fever

Diagnosis: requires 2 major criteria or 1 major and 2 minor criteria with supporting evidence of antecedent group A streptococcal infection

Major Criteria	Minor Criteria	Supporting Evidence
Carditis	Clinical findings:	Positive throat culture or rapid test
Polyarthritis	Fever, arthralgia	OR
Chorea	Laboratory findings:	Elevated or rising streptococcal
Erythema marginatum	Elevated acute phase reac-	antibody test
Subcutaneous nodules	tants; prolonged PR interval	

Testing Contacts for GAS Infection. Indications for testing contacts for GAS infection vary according to circumstances. Testing asymptomatic household contacts for GAS is not recommended except when contacts are at increased risk of developing sequelae of GAS infection. Throat swab specimens should be obtained from all household contacts of a child who has acute rheumatic fever or acute glomerulonephritis, and if test results are positive, contacts should be treated.

In schools, child care centers, or other environments in which a large number of people are in close contact, the prevalence of GAS pharyngeal carriage in healthy children can be as high as 15% in the absence of an outbreak of streptococcal disease. Therefore, classroom or more widespread culture surveys are not indicated.

Follow-up Throat Cultures. Post-treatment throat swab cultures are indicated only for patients at particularly high risk of acute rheumatic fever or who have symptoms compatible with GAS pharyngitis. Repeated courses of antimicrobial therapy are not indicated for asymptomatic patients with GAS-positive cultures; the exceptions are people who have had or whose family members have had acute rheumatic fever or other uncommon epidemiologic circumstances, such as outbreaks of rheumatic fever or acute poststreptococcal glomerulonephritis.

Patients in whom repeat episodes of pharyngitis occur at short intervals and GAS infection is documented by culture or antigen detection test present a special problem. Often, these people are chronic GAS carriers who are experiencing frequent viral illnesses. In assessing such patients, inadequate adherence to oral treatment also should be considered. Although uncommon, in some areas, erythromycin resistance among GAS strains occurs, resulting in erythromycin treatment failures. Such strains also are resistant to clarithromycin and azithromycin. Testing asymptomatic household contacts usually is not helpful. However, if multiple household members have pharyngitis or other GAS infections, such as pyoderma, simultaneous cultures of all household members and treatment of all people with positive cultures or rapid antigen test results may be of value.

Testing for GAS in Nonpharyngitis Infections. Cultures of impetiginous lesions are not indicated routinely, because lesions often yield both streptococci and staphylococci, and determination of the primary pathogen is not possible.

In suspected invasive GAS infections, cultures of blood and focal sites of possible infection are indicated. In necrotizing fasciitis, imaging studies often delay, rather than facilitate, the diagnosis. Clinical suspicion of necrotizing fasciitis should prompt surgical inspection of the deep tissues with Gram stain and culture of surgical specimens.

Streptococcal TSS is diagnosed on the basis of clinical findings and isolation of GAS (see Table 3.69, p 617). Blood culture results are positive for *S pyogenes* in more than 50% of patients with streptococcal TSS. Culture results from a focal site of infections also usually are positive and can remain so for several days after appropriate antimicrobial agents have been initiated. *S pyogenes* uniformly is susceptible to beta-lactam antimicrobial agents, and susceptibility testing is needed only for nonbeta-lactam agents, such as erythromycin or clindamycin, to which *S pyogenes* can be resistant. A significant increase in antibody titers to streptolysin O, deoxyribonuclease B, or other streptococcal extracellular enzymes 4 to 6 weeks after infection may help to confirm the diagnosis if culture results are negative.

TREATMENT:

Pharyngitis.

- Although penicillin V is the drug of choice for treatment of GAS pharyngitis, ampicillin or amoxicillin equally are effective. A clinical isolate of GAS resistant to penicillin never has been documented. Prompt administration of penicillin therapy shortens the clinical course, decreases the risk of suppurative sequelae and transmission, and prevents acute rheumatic fever even when given up to 9 days after illness onset. For all patients with acute rheumatic fever, a complete course of penicillin or other appropriate antimicrobial agents for GAS pharyngitis should be given to eradicate GAS organisms from the throat, even though GAS organisms may not be recovered in the initial throat culture.

  The dose of orally administered penicillin V is 400 000 U (250 mg), 2 to 3 times per day, for 10 days for children weighing less than 27 kg (60 lb) and 800 000 U (500 mg), 2 to 3 times per day, for heavier children, adolescents, and adults. To prevent acute rheumatic fever, oral treatment with penicillin should be given for the full 10 days, regardless of the promptness of clinical recovery. Although different preparations of oral penicillin vary in absorption, their clinical efficacy is similar. Treatment failures may occur more often with oral penicillin than with intramuscularly administered penicillin G benzathine as a result of inadequate adherence to oral therapy. In addition, short-course treatment for GAS pharyngitis, particularly with penicillin V, is associated with inferior bacteriologic eradication rates.

- Orally administered amoxicillin given as a single daily dose (50 mg/kg, maximum 1000 mg) for 10 days is as effective as orally administered penicillin V or amoxicillin given multiple times per day for 10 days. This approach is an acceptable treatment option if strict adherence to once-daily dosing can be ensured.

- Intramuscular penicillin G benzathine is appropriate therapy. It ensures adequate blood concentrations and avoids the problem of adherence, but administration is painful. For children who weigh less than 27 kg, penicillin G benzathine is given in a single dose of 600 000 U (375 mg); for heavier children and adults, the dose is 1.2 million U (750 mg). Discomfort is less if the preparation of penicillin G benzathine is brought to room temperature before intramuscular injection. Mixtures containing shorter-acting penicillins (eg, penicillin G procaine) in addition to penicillin G benzathine have not been demonstrated to be more effective than penicillin G benzathine alone but are less painful when administered. Although supporting data are limited, the combination of 900 000 U (562.5 mg) of penicillin G benzathine and 300 000 U (187.5 mg) of penicillin G procaine is satisfactory therapy for most children; however, the efficacy of this combination for heavier patients, such as adolescents and adults, has not been demonstrated.

- For some patients who are allergic to penicillin, a 10-day course of a narrow-spectrum (first-generation) oral cephalosporin is indicated. However, as many as 5% of penicillin-allergic people also are allergic to cephalosporins. Patients with immediate or type I hypersensitivity to penicillin should not be treated with a cephalosporin. Oral clindamycin (20 mg/kg per day in 3 divided doses, maximum 1.8 g/day) is an acceptable alternative to penicillin in people with intermediate or type 1 hypersensitivity to penicillin.
- An oral macrolide or azalide like erythromycin, clarithromycin, or azithromycin is acceptable for patients allergic to penicillins. Therapy for 10 days is indicated except for azithromycin, which is given for 5 days. Erythromycin is associated with substantially higher rates of gastrointestinal tract adverse effects than are the other agents. Strains of GAS resistant to these agents have been highly prevalent in some areas of the world and have resulted in treatment failures. In recent years, macrolide resistance rates in most areas of the United States have been 5% to 8%, but resistance rates need continued monitoring.
- Tetracyclines; sulfonamides, including trimethoprim-sulfamethoxazole; and fluoroquinolones should not be used for treating GAS pharyngitis.

Children who have a recurrence of GAS pharyngitis shortly after completing a 10-day course of a recommended oral antimicrobial agent can be retreated with the same antimicrobial agent, given an alternative oral drug, or given an intramuscular dose of penicillin G benzathine, especially if inadequate adherence to oral therapy is likely. Alternative drugs include a narrow-spectrum cephalosporin, amoxicillin-clavulanate, clindamycin, a macrolide, or azalide. Expert opinions differ about the most appropriate therapy in this circumstance.

Management of a patient who has repeated and frequent episodes of acute pharyngitis associated with a positive laboratory test for GAS infection is problematic. To determine whether the patient is a long-term streptococcal pharyngeal carrier who is experiencing repeated episodes of intercurrent viral pharyngitis (which is the situation in most cases), the following should be determined: (1) whether the clinical findings are more suggestive of a GAS or a viral cause; (2) whether epidemiologic factors in the community are more suggestive of a GAS or a viral cause; (3) the nature of the clinical response to the antimicrobial therapy (in true GAS pharyngitis, response to therapy usually is rapid); (4) whether laboratory test results are positive for GAS infection between episodes of acute pharyngitis; and (5) whether a serologic response to GAS extracellular antigens (eg, antistreptolysin O) has occurred. Serotyping of GAS isolates generally is available only in research laboratories, but if performed, repeated isolation of the same serotype suggests carriage, and isolation of differing serotypes indicates repeated infections.

Pharyngeal Carriers. Antimicrobial therapy is not indicated for most GAS pharyngeal carriers. Exceptions (ie, specific situations in which eradication of carriage may be indicated) include the following: (1) an outbreak of acute rheumatic fever or poststreptococcal glomerulonephritis occurs; (2) an outbreak of GAS pharyngitis in a closed or semiclosed community occurs; (3) a family history of acute rheumatic fever exists; or (4) multiple episodes of documented symptomatic GAS pharyngitis continue to occur within a family during a period of many weeks despite appropriate therapy.

Streptococcal carriage can be difficult to eradicate with conventional antimicrobial therapy. A number of antimicrobial agents, including clindamycin, cephalosporins, amoxicillin-clavulanate, azithromycin, and a combination of rifampin for the last 4 days of treatment with either penicillin V or penicillin G benzathine have been demonstrated to be more effective than penicillin in eliminating chronic streptococcal carriage. Of these drugs, oral clindamycin, given as 20 mg/kg per day in 3 doses (maximum, 1.8 g/day) for 10 days, has been reported to be the most effective. Documented eradication of the carrier state is helpful in the evaluation of subsequent episodes of acute pharyngitis; however, long-term carriage may recur after reacquisition of GAS infection.

Nonbullous Impetigo. Local mupirocin or retapamulin ointment may be useful for limiting person-to-person spread of nonbullous impetigo and for eradicating localized disease. With multiple lesions or with nonbullous impetigo in multiple family members, child care groups, or athletic teams, impetigo should be treated with antimicrobial regimens administered systemically. Because episodes of nonbullous impetigo may be caused by *Staphylococcus aureus* or *S pyogenes*, children with nonbullous impetigo usually should be treated with an antimicrobial agent active against both GAS and *S aureus* infections.

Toxic Shock Syndrome. As outlined in Tables 3.71 and 3.72 (p 624), most aspects of management are the same for TSS caused by *S pyogenes* or *S aureus*. Paramount are immediate aggressive fluid replacement and management of respiratory and cardiac failure, if present, and aggressive surgical débridement of any deep-seated GAS infection. Because *S pyogenes* and *S aureus* TSS cannot be distinguished clinically, initial antimicrobial therapy should include an antistaphylococcal agent and a protein synthesis-inhibiting antimicrobial agent, such as clindamycin. The addition of clindamycin is more effective than penicillin alone for treating well-established *S pyogenes* infections, because the antimicrobial activity of clindamycin is not affected by inoculum size, has a long postantimicrobial effect, and acts on bacteria by inhibiting protein synthesis. Inhibition of protein synthesis results in suppression of synthesis of the *S pyogenes* antiphagocytic M-protein and bacterial toxins. Clindamycin should not be used alone as initial antimicrobial therapy, because in the United States, 1% to 2% of *S pyogenes* strains are resistant to clindamycin.

Once GAS has been identified, antimicrobial therapy can be changed to penicillin and clindamycin. Intravenous therapy should be continued until the patient is afebrile and stable hemodynamically and blood culture results are negative. The total duration of therapy is based on duration established for the primary infection.

Aggressive drainage and irrigation of accessible sites of infection should be performed as soon as possible. If necrotizing fasciitis is suspected, immediate surgical exploration or biopsy is crucial to identify deep soft tissue infection that should be débrided immediately.

Table 3.71. Management of Streptococcal Toxic Shock Syndrome Without Necrotizing Fasciitis

- Fluid management to maintain adequate venous return and cardiac filling pressures to prevent end-organ damage
- Anticipatory management of multisystem organ failure
- Parenteral antimicrobial therapy at maximum doses
  - Kill organism with bactericidal cell wall inhibitor (eg, beta-lactamase–resistant antistaphylococcal antimicrobial agent)
  - Stop enzyme, toxin, or cytokine production with protein synthesis inhibitor (eg, clindamycin)
- Immune Globulin Intravenous may be considered for infection refractory to several hours of aggressive therapy or in the presence of an undrainable focus or persistent oliguria with pulmonary edema

Table 3.72. Management of Streptococcal Toxic Shock Syndrome With Necrotizing Fasciitis

- Principles outlined in Table 3.71 (p 623)
- Immediate surgical evaluation
  - Exploration or incisional biopsy for diagnosis and culture
  - Resection of all necrotic tissue
- Repeated resection of tissue may be needed if infection persists or progresses

The use of Immune Globulin Intravenous (IGIV) can be considered as adjunctive therapy of GAS-associated TSS or necrotizing fascitis if the patient is severely ill. Various regimens of IGIV, including 150 to 400 mg/kg per day for 5 days or a single dose of 1 to 2 g/kg, have been used, but the optimal regimen is unknown.

Other Infections. Parenteral antimicrobial therapy is required for severe infections, such as endocarditis, pneumonia, septicemia, meningitis, arthritis, osteomyelitis, erysipelas, necrotizing fasciitis, neonatal omphalitis, and streptococcal toxic shock syndrome. Treatment often is prolonged (2–6 weeks).

Prevention of Sequelae. Acute rheumatic fever and acute glomerulonephritis are serious nonsuppurative sequelae of GAS infections. During epidemics of GAS infections on military bases in the 1950s, rheumatic fever developed in 3% of untreated patients with acute GAS pharyngitis. The current incidence after endemic infections is not known but is believed to be less than 1%. The risk of acute rheumatic fever virtually can be eliminated by adequate treatment of the antecedent GAS infection; however, rare cases have occurred even after apparently appropriate therapy. The effectiveness of antimicrobial therapy for preventing acute poststreptococcal glomerulonephritis after pyoderma has not been established. Suppurative sequelae, such as peritonsillar abscesses and cervical adenitis, usually are prevented by treatment of the primary infection.

ISOLATION OF THE HOSPITALIZED PATIENT: In addition to standard precautions, droplet precautions are recommended for children with GAS pharyngitis or pneumonia until 24 hours after initiation of appropriate antimicrobial therapy. For burns with secondary GAS infection and extensive or draining cutaneous infections that cannot be covered or contained adequately by dressings, contact precautions should be used for at least 24 hours after the start of appropriate therapy.

CONTROL MEASURES: The most important means of controlling GAS disease and its sequelae is prompt identification and treatment of infections.

School and Child Care. Children with streptococcal pharyngitis or skin infections should not return to school or child care until at least 24 hours after beginning appropriate antimicrobial therapy. Close contact with other children during this time should be avoided.

Care of Exposed People. People who are contacts of documented cases of GAS infection and who have recent or current clinical evidence of a GAS infection should undergo appropriate laboratory tests and should be treated if test results are positive. Rates of GAS carriage are higher among sibling contacts of children with GAS pharyngitis than among parent contacts in nonepidemic settings; rates as high as 50% for sibling contacts and 20% for parent contacts have been reported during epidemics. More than half of contacts who acquire GAS organisms will become ill. Asymptomatic acquisition of GAS infection may pose some risk of nonsuppurative complications; studies indicate that as many as one third of patients with acute rheumatic fever had no history of recent streptococcal infection and another third had minor respiratory tract symptoms that were not brought to medical attention. However, routine laboratory evaluation of asymptomatic household contacts usually is not indicated except during outbreaks or when the contacts are at increased risk of developing sequelae of infection (see Indications for GAS Testing, p 619). Short courses (less than 10 days) of an antimicrobial agent for healthy contacts are inappropriate. In rare circumstances, such as a large family with documented, repeated, intrafamilial transmission resulting in frequent episodes of GAS pharyngitis during a prolonged period, physicians may elect to treat all family members identified by laboratory tests as harboring GAS organisms.

Household contacts of patients with severe invasive GAS disease, including toxic shock syndrome, are at increased risk of developing severe invasive GAS disease compared with the general population, but the risk is not sufficiently high to warrant routine testing for GAS colonization or routine chemoprophylaxis of all household contacts of people with invasive GAS disease. However, because of increased risk of sporadic, invasive GAS disease among certain populations and because of increased risk of death in people 65 years of age and older who develop invasive GAS disease, health care professionals may choose to offer targeted chemoprophylaxis to household contacts who are 65 years of age and older or who are members of other high-risk populations (eg, people with human immunodeficiency virus infection, varicella, or diabetes mellitus). Because of the rarity of subsequent cases and the low risk of invasive GAS infections in children in general, chemoprophylaxis is not recommended in schools or child care facilities.

Secondary Prophylaxis for Rheumatic Fever. Patients who have a well-documented history of acute rheumatic fever (including cases manifested solely as Sydenham chorea) and patients who have documented evidence of rheumatic heart disease should be given continuous antimicrobial prophylaxis to prevent recurrent attacks (secondary prophylaxis), because asymptomatic and symptomatic GAS infections can result in a recurrence of rheumatic fever. Continuous prophylaxis should be initiated as soon as the diagnosis of acute rheumatic fever or rheumatic heart disease is made.

Duration. Secondary prophylaxis should be long-term, perhaps for life, for patients with rheumatic heart disease (even after prosthetic valve replacement), because these patients remain at risk of recurrence of rheumatic fever. The risk of recurrence decreases as the interval from the most recent episode increases, and patients without rheumatic heart disease are at a lower risk of recurrence than are patients with residual cardiac involvement. These considerations, as well as the estimate of exposure to people with streptococcal infections, influence the duration of secondary prophylaxis in adults but should not alter the practice of secondary prophylaxis for children and adolescents. Secondary prophylaxis for all patients who have had rheumatic fever should be continued for at least 5 years or until the person is 21 years of age, whichever is longer (see Table 3.73, p 626). Prophylaxis also should be continued if the risk of contact with people with GAS infection is high, such as for parents with school-aged children and for teachers.

The drug regimens in Table 3.74 (p 627) are effective for secondary prophylaxis. The intramuscular regimen has been shown to be the most reliable, because the success of oral prophylaxis depends primarily on patient adherence; however, inconvenience and pain of injection may cause some patients to discontinue intramuscular prophylaxis. In populations in which the risk of rheumatic fever is high, administration of penicillin G benzathine given every 3 weeks is justified and recommended, because drug concentrations in

Table 3.73. Duration of Prophylaxis for People Who Have Had Acute Rheumatic Fever (ARF): Recommendations of the American Heart Association[a]

Category	Duration
Rheumatic fever without carditis	5 y since last episode of ARF or until 21 y of age, whichever is longer
Rheumatic fever with carditis but without residual heart disease (no valvular disease[b])	10 y since last episode of ARF or until age 21 y, whichever is longer
Rheumatic fever with carditis and residual heart disease (persistent valvular disease[b])	10 y since last episode of ARF or until 40 y of age, whichever is longer; consider lifelong prophylaxis for people with severe valvular disease or ongoing exposure to group A streptococcal infection

[a]Modified from Gerber M, Baltimore R, Eaton C, et al. Prevention of rheumatic fever and diagnosis and treatment of acute streptococcal pharyngitis. A scientific statement from the American Heart Association, Rheumatic Fever, Endocarditis, and Kawasaki Disease Committee, Council on Cardiovascular Disease in the Young, and the Quality of Care and Outcomes Research Interdisciplinary Working Group. *Circulation*. 2009; in press
[b]Clinical or echocardiographic evidence.

serum may decrease below a protective level before the fourth week after administration of this dose of penicillin. In the United States, administration every 4 weeks seems adequate except for people who have recurrent acute rheumatic fever despite adherence to an every-4-week regimen. Oral sulfadiazine is as effective as oral penicillin for secondary prophylaxis but may not be available readily in the United States. By extrapolating from data demonstrating effectiveness of sulfadiazine, sulfisoxazole has been deemed an appropriate alternative drug.

Allergic reactions to oral penicillin are similar to reactions with intramuscular penicillin, but usually these are less severe and occur less commonly. These reactions also occur less commonly in children than in adults. Anaphylaxis is rare in patients receiving oral penicillin. Severe allergic reactions in patients receiving continuous penicillin G benzathine prophylaxis also are rare. The rare reports of anaphylaxis and death generally have involved patients older than 12 years of age with severe rheumatic heart disease. Most severe reactions seem to represent vasovagal responses rather than anaphylaxis. Reactions also can include a serum sickness-like reaction characterized by fever and joint pains, which can be mistaken for recurrence of acute rheumatic fever.

Reactions to continuous sulfadiazine or sulfisoxazole prophylaxis are rare and usually minor; evaluation of blood cell counts may be advisable after 2 weeks of prophylaxis, because leukopenia has been reported. Prophylaxis with a sulfonamide during late pregnancy is contraindicated because of interference with fetal bilirubin metabolism. Febrile mucocutaneous syndromes (erythema multiforme, Stevens-Johnson syndrome, or toxic epidermal necrolysis) have been associated with penicillin and with sulfonamides. When an adverse event occurs with any of these therapeutic regimens, the drug should be stopped immediately and an alternative drug should be selected. For the rare patient allergic to both penicillins and sulfonamides, erythromycin is recommended. Other macrolides, such as azithromycin or clarithromycin, also should be acceptable; they have less risk of gastrointestinal tract intolerance but increased costs.

Table 3.74. Chemoprophylaxis for Recurrences of Acute Rheumatic Fever[a]

Drug	Dose	Route
Penicillin G benzathine	1.2 million U, every 4 wk[b]; 600 000 U, every 4 wk for patients weighing less than 27.3 kg (60 lb)	Intramuscular
OR		
Penicillin V	250 mg, twice a day	Oral
OR		
Sulfadiazine or sulfisoxazole	0.5 g, once a day for patients weighing 27 kg (60 lb) or less	Oral
	1.0 g, once a day for patients weighing greater than 27 kg (60 lb)	
For people who are allergic to penicillin and sulfonamide drugs		
Macrolide or azalide	Variable (see text)	Oral

[a]Gerber M, Baltimore R, Eaton C, Gewitz M, Rowley A, Shulman S, Taubert K. Prevention of rheumatic fever and diagnosis and treatment of acute streptococcal pharyngitis. A scientific statement from the American Heart Association, Rheumatic Fever, Endocarditis, and Kawasaki Disease Committee, Council on Cardiovascular Disease in the Young, and the Quality of Care and Outcomes Research Interdisciplinary Working Group. *Circulation*. 2009; in press
[b]In high-risk situations, administration every 3 weeks is recommended.

Poststreptococcal Reactive Arthritis. After an episode of acute GAS pharyngitis, reactive arthritis may develop in the absence of sufficient clinical manifestations and laboratory findings to fulfill the Jones criteria for the diagnosis of acute rheumatic fever. This syndrome has been termed poststreptococcal reactive arthritis (PSRA). The precise relationship of PSRA to acute rheumatic fever is unclear. In contrast with the arthritis of acute rheumatic fever, PSRA does not respond dramatically to nonsteroidal anti-inflammatory agents. Because a small proportion of patients with PSRA have been reported to later develop valvular heart disease, these patients should be observed carefully for several months for carditis. Some experts recommend secondary prophylaxis for these patients for several months to a year if carditis does not develop. If carditis occurs, the patient should be considered to have had acute rheumatic fever, and secondary prophylaxis should be continued (see Secondary Prophylaxis for Rheumatic Fever, p 625).

Bacterial Endocarditis Prophylaxis.[1] The American Heart Association (AHA) has published updated recommendations regarding use of antimicrobial agents to prevent infective endocarditis (see prevention of Bacterial Endocarditis, p 826). The AHA no longer recommends prophylaxis for patients with rheumatic heart disease. However, use of oral antiseptic solutions and maintenance of assiduous oral health care remain important components of an overall health care program. For the relatively few patients with rheumatic heart disease in whom infective endocarditis prophylaxis still is recommended (eg, people with prosthetic valves), the current AHA recommendations should

---

[1]Wilson W, Taubert KA, Gewitz M, et al. Prevention of infective endocarditis. Recommendations by the American Heart Association. A guideline from the American Heart Association Rheumatic Fever, Endocarditis, and Kawasaki Disease Committee, Council on Cardiovascular Disease in the Young, and the Council on Clinical Cardiology, Council on Cardiovascular Surgery and Anesthesia, and the Quality of Care and Outcomes Research Interdisciplinary Working Group. *Circulation*. 2007;116(15):1736–1754

be followed, recognizing that the agent selected should be one other than a penicillin, because penicillin-resistant alpha-hemolytic streptococci may be present when penicillin is used for secondary prevention of rheumatic fever.

Group B Streptococcal Infections

CLINICAL MANIFESTATIONS: Group B streptococci are a major cause of perinatal bacterial infections, including bacteremia, endometritis, chorioamnionitis, and urinary tract infections in pregnant women and systemic and focal infections in infants from birth until 3 months of age or, rarely, older. Invasive disease in young infants is categorized on the basis of chronologic age at onset. Early-onset disease usually occurs within the first 24 hours of life (range, 0–6 days) and is characterized by signs of systemic infection, respiratory distress, apnea, shock, pneumonia, and less often, meningitis (5%–10% of cases). Late-onset disease, which typically occurs at 3 to 4 weeks of age (range, 7–89 days), commonly manifests as occult bacteremia or meningitis; other focal infections, such as osteomyelitis, septic arthritis, pneumonia, adenitis, and cellulitis, can occur. Late, late-onset disease occurs beyond 89 days of age in very preterm infants requiring prolonged hospitalization. Group B streptococci also cause systemic infections in nonpregnant adults with underlying medical conditions, such as diabetes mellitus, chronic liver or renal disease, malignancy, or other immunocompromising conditions and in adults 65 years of age and older.

ETIOLOGY: Group B streptococci *(Streptococcus agalactiae)* are gram-positive, aerobic diplococci that typically produce a narrow zone of beta hemolysis on 5% sheep blood agar. These organisms are divided into 9 serotypes on the basis of capsular polysaccharides (Ia, Ib, II, and III through VIII). Serotypes Ia, Ib, II, III, and V account for approximately 95% of cases in infants in the United States. Serotype III is the predominant cause of early-onset meningitis and most late-onset infections in infants. Pilus-like structures are important virulence factors and potential vaccine candidates.

EPIDEMIOLOGY: Group B streptococci are common inhabitants of the human gastrointestinal and genitourinary tracts. Less commonly, they colonize the pharynx. The colonization rate in pregnant women ranges from 15% to 40%. Colonization during pregnancy can be constant or intermittent. Before recommendations for prevention of early-onset group B streptococcal (GBS) disease by maternal intrapartum antimicrobial prophylaxis (see Control Measures, p 630) were made, the incidence was 1 to 4 cases per 1000 live births; early-onset disease accounted for approximately 75% of cases in infants and occurred in approximately 1 infant per 100 colonized women. Associated with widespread maternal intrapartum antimicrobial prophylaxis, the incidence of early-onset disease has decreased by approximately 80% to approximately 0.35 cases per 1000 live births in 2005 and now equals that of late-onset disease. Case-fatality rates in term infants range from 3% to 5% but are higher in preterm neonates. Transmission from mother-to-infant occurs shortly before or during delivery. After delivery, person-to-person transmission can occur. Although uncommon, GBS infection can be acquired in the nursery from hospital personnel (probably via hand contamination) or more commonly in the community from healthy colonized people. The risk of early-onset disease is increased in preterm infants born at less than 37 weeks of gestation, in infants born after the amniotic membranes have been ruptured 18 hours or more, and in infants born to women with high genital GBS inoculum, intrapartum fever (temperature 38°C [100.4°F] or greater), chorioamnionitis, GBS bacteriuria during the pregnancy, or a previous infant with invasive GBS disease. A low or an absent concentration of serotype-specific serum antibody also is a predisposing factor. Other risk factors are intrauterine fetal monitoring, maternal age younger than 20 years, and black ethnicity. Rates of early-onset disease increased from 2003 to 2005 among black infants (0.52–0.89 cases per 1000 live births) and decreased among white infants (0.26–0.22 cases per 1000 live births). The period of communicability is unknown but may extend throughout the duration of colonization or of disease. Infants can remain colonized for several months after birth and after treatment for systemic infection. Recurrent GBS disease affects an estimated 1% to 3% of appropriately treated infants.

The **incubation period** of early-onset disease is fewer than 7 days. In late-onset and late, late-onset disease, the incubation period from GBS acquisition to disease is unknown. The incidence of GBS disease declines dramatically after 89 days of age, but up to 10% of pediatric cases occur beyond early infancy, and many, but not all, of these are in infants who were born preterm.

DIAGNOSTIC TESTS: Gram-positive cocci in Gram stain of body fluids that typically are sterile (eg, cerebrospinal [CSF], pleural, or joint fluid) provide presumptive evidence of infection. Cultures of blood, other typically sterile body fluids, or a suppurative focus are necessary to establish the diagnosis. Serotype identification is available in reference laboratories. Rapid tests that identify group B streptococcal antigen in body fluids other than CSF are not recommended because of poor specificity. Commercially available real-time polymerase chain reaction tests for group B streptococci in vaginal swab specimens have high sensitivity and specificity, but data are limited regarding their usefulness for women with unknown colonization status at admission for delivery.

TREATMENT:
- Ampicillin plus an aminoglycoside is the initial treatment of choice for a newborn infant with presumptive invasive GBS infection.
- Penicillin G alone can be given when group B streptococci have been identified as the cause of the infection and when clinical and microbiologic responses have been documented.
- For infants with meningitis attributable to group B streptococci, the recommended dosage of penicillin G for infants 7 days of age or younger is 250 000 to 450 000 U/kg per day, intravenously, in 3 divided doses; for infants older than 7 days of age, 450 000 to 500 000 U/kg per day, intravenously, in 4 divided doses is recommended. For ampicillin, the recommended dosage for infants with meningitis 7 days of age or younger is 200 to 300 mg/kg per day, intravenously, in 3 divided doses; for infants older than 7 days of age, 300 mg/kg per day, intravenously, in 4 divided doses is recommended.
- For meningitis, some experts believe that a second lumbar puncture approximately 24 to 48 hours after initiation of therapy assists in management and prognosis. If CSF sterility is not achieved, a complicated course (eg, cerebral infarcts) can be expected; also, an increasing protein concentration suggests an intracranial complication (eg, infarction, ventricular obstruction). Additional lumbar punctures and diagnostic imaging studies are indicated if response to therapy is in doubt, neurologic abnormalities persist, or focal neurologic deficits occur. Consultation with a specialist in pediatric infectious diseases often is useful.

- For infants with bacteremia without a defined focus, treatment should be continued for 10 days. For infants with uncomplicated meningitis, 14 days of treatment is satisfactory, but longer periods of treatment may be necessary for infants with prolonged or complicated courses. Septic arthritis or osteomyelitis requires treatment for 3 to 4 weeks; endocarditis or ventriculitis requires treatment for at least 4 weeks.
- Because of the reported increased risk of infection, the sibling of a multiple birth index case with early- or late-onset disease should be observed carefully and evaluated and treated empirically for suspected systemic infection if any signs of illness occur.

ISOLATION OF THE HOSPITALIZED PATIENT: Standard precautions are recommended, except during a nursery outbreak of disease attributable to group B streptococci (see Control Measures, Nursery Outbreak, p 634).

CONTROL MEASURES:

Chemoprophylaxis. Recommendations for prevention of early-onset neonatal GBS infection are based on data comparing a maternal culture screening method to a risk-based method to identify women who should receive intrapartum antimicrobial prophylaxis that demonstrated significantly better efficacy for culture screening than with a risk-based method. Recommendations from the Centers for Disease Control and Prevention (CDC)[1] include the following:

- All pregnant women should be screened at 35 to 37 weeks' gestation for vaginal and rectal GBS colonization (see Fig 3.4, p 631). The only exceptions to this recommendation for universal culture screening are women with GBS bacteriuria during the current pregnancy or women who have had a previous infant with invasive GBS disease; these women always should receive intrapartum chemoprophylaxis. At the onset of labor or rupture of membranes, intrapartum chemoprophylaxis should be given to all pregnant women identified as carriers of group B streptococci. Colonization during a previous pregnancy is *not* an indication for intrapartum chemoprophylaxis unless screening results are positive in the current pregnancy.
- Women with group B streptococci isolated from urine in any concentration during their current pregnancy should receive intrapartum chemoprophylaxis, because these women usually are heavily colonized with group B streptococci and are at increased risk of delivering an infant with early-onset GBS disease; culture screening at 35 to 37 weeks' gestation is not necessary.
- Women who previously have given birth to an infant with invasive GBS disease should receive intrapartum chemoprophylaxis; culture screening is not necessary.
- If GBS status is not known at onset of labor or rupture of membranes, intrapartum chemoprophylaxis should be administered to women with any of the following risk factors: gestation less than 37 weeks, duration of membrane rupture 18 hours or longer, or intrapartum temperature of 38.0°C (100.4°F) or greater.
- Culture techniques that maximize the likelihood of recovery of group B streptococci are required for prenatal screening. The optimal method for GBS screening cultures is collection of 1 or 2 swabs of the lower vagina and rectum; placement of swabs in a nonnutrient transport medium; removal of swabs and inoculation into selective broth medium, such as Trans-Vag Broth supplemented with 5% defibrinated sheep blood or Lim broth; overnight incubation; and subculture onto solid blood agar medium.

[1]Centers for Disease Control and Prevention. Prevention of perinatal group B streptococcal disease. Revised guidelines from CDC. *MMWR Recomm Rep.* 2002;52(RR–11):1–22

Fig 3.4. Indications for Intrapartum Antimicrobial Prophylaxis (IAP) to Prevent Early-Onset Group B Streptococcal (GBS) Disease Using a Universal Prenatal Culture Screening Strategy at 35 to 37 Weeks' Gestation for All Women.

Vaginal and Rectal GBS Cultures at 35–37 Weeks' Gestation for ALL Pregnant Women[a]

IAP INDICATED	IAP *NOT* INDICATED
• Previous infant with invasive GBS disease	• Previous pregnancy with a positive GBS screening culture (unless a culture also was positive during the current pregnancy or previous infant with invasive GBS disease)
• GBS bacteriurua during *current* pregnancy	
• Positive GBS screening culture during current pregnancy (*unless* a planned cesarean delivery is performed in the absence of labor or membrane rupture)	• Planned cesarean delivery performed in the absence of labor or membrane rupture (regardless of GBS culture status)
• Unknown GBS status AND any of the following:	• Negative vaginal and rectal GBS screening culture in late gestation, regardless of intrapartum risk factors
♦ Delivery at <37 weeks' gestation	
♦ Membranes ruptured for ≥18 hours	
♦ Intrapartum fever (temperature ≥38.0°C [≥100.4°F])[b]	

[a]Exceptions: women with GBS bacteriuria during the current pregnancy or women with a previous infant with invasive GBS disease.
[b]If chorioamnionitis is suspected, broad-spectrum antimicrobial therapy that includes an agent known to be active against group B streptococci should replace GBS IAP.

- Oral antimicrobial agents should *not* be used to treat women who are found to have GBS colonization during culture screening unless there is a GBS urinary tract infection warranting treatment according to obstetric standards of care. Such treatment is *not* effective in eliminating carriage of group B streptococci or preventing neonatal disease.
- Women who have GBS colonization and have a planned cesarean delivery performed before rupture of membranes and onset of labor should *not* receive intrapartum chemoprophylaxis routinely.

- For intrapartum chemoprophylaxis, intravenous penicillin G (5 million U initially, then 2.5 million U every 4 hours until delivery) is the preferred agent because of its efficacy and narrow spectrum of antimicrobial activity. An alternative regimen is intravenous ampicillin (2 g initially, then 1 g every 4 hours until delivery).
- Because of increasing prevalence of GBS resistance to both erythromycin and clindamycin (20%–40%), cefazolin (2 g initially, then 1 g every 8 hours) is recommended for women who are allergic to penicillin but at low risk of anaphylaxis. Cefazolin is recommended because of its narrow spectrum of activity and ability to achieve high amniotic fluid concentrations. Women whose GBS isolates are tested and found to be clindamycin susceptible and who are at high risk of anaphylaxis with penicillin can receive this drug at a dose of 900 mg every 8 hours. Vancomycin should be reserved for penicillin-allergic women who are at high risk of anaphylaxis (ie, type I hypersensitivity) and for whom GBS isolate susceptibility testing has not been performed; vancomycin should be administered intravenously, 1 g every 12 hours until delivery. The efficacy of clindamycin or vancomycin is not established.
- Routine use of antimicrobial agents as chemoprophylaxis for neonates born to mothers who have received adequate intrapartum chemoprophylaxis for GBS disease is *not* recommended. However, therapeutic use of these agents is appropriate for infants with clinically suspected systemic infection.

An approach for empiric management of newborn infants born to women who receive intrapartum chemoprophylaxis to prevent early-onset GBS disease or to treat suspected chorioamnionitis is provided in Fig 3.5, p 633. These guidelines are based on published information as well as expert opinion and are as follows:

- If a woman receives intrapartum antimicrobial agents for treatment of suspected chorioamnionitis, her newborn infant should have a full diagnostic evaluation and empiric antimicrobial therapy pending culture results, regardless of clinical condition at birth, duration of maternal therapy before delivery, or weeks of gestation at delivery. Empiric therapy for the infant should include antimicrobial agents active against group B streptococci as well as other organisms that might cause early-onset neonatal sepsis (eg, ampicillin and gentamicin).
- If clinical signs in the infant suggest sepsis, a full diagnostic evaluation should include a lumbar puncture, if feasible. Blood cultures can be sterile in as many as 15% to 38% of newborn infants with GBS meningitis, and the clinical management of an infant with abnormal CSF differs from that of an infant with normal CSF. If a lumbar puncture has been deferred for a neonate receiving empiric antimicrobial therapy and therapy is continued beyond 48 hours because of ongoing clinical findings suggesting infection, CSF should be obtained for measurement of white blood cell count and differential, glucose, and protein and for culture.
- Initiation of intrapartum antimicrobial prophylaxis for the woman with nontype I allergy to penicillin with cefazolin if administered at least 4 hours before delivery can be considered adequate. The effectiveness of other agents (eg, clindamycin or vancomycin) in preventing early-onset GBS disease has not been studied, and no data are available to suggest the duration before delivery of these regimens that can be considered adequate.
- On the basis of the demonstrated effectiveness of intrapartum antimicrobial prophylaxis in preventing early-onset GBS disease and data indicating that clinical onset occurs within the first 24 hours of life in more than 90% of infants, hospital discharge

FIG 3.5. EMPIRIC MANAGEMENT OF A NEONATE WHOSE MOTHER RECEIVED INTRAPARTUM ANTIMICROBIAL PROPHYLAXIS (IAP) FOR PREVENTION OF EARLY-ONSET GROUP B STREPTOCOCCAL (GBS) DISEASE[a] OR SUSPECTED CHORIOAMNIONITIS.

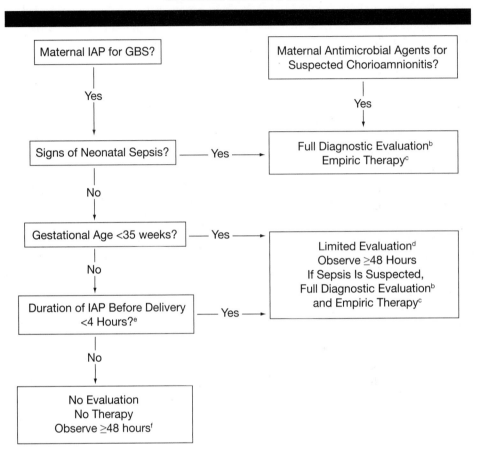

[a] If no maternal IAP for GBS infection was administered despite an indication being present, data are insufficient on which to recommend a single management strategy.

[b] Includes complete blood cell (CBC) count with differential, blood culture, and chest radiograph if respiratory abnormalities are present. When signs of sepsis are present, a lumbar puncture, if feasible, should be performed.

[c] Duration of therapy varies depending on results of blood culture, cerebrospinal fluid findings (if obtained), and the clinical course of the infant. If laboratory results and clinical course do not indicate bacterial infection, duration may be as short as 48 hours.

[d] CBC including white blood cell count with differential and blood culture.

[e] Applies only to penicillin, ampicillin, or cefazolin and assumes recommended dosing regimens.

[f] A healthy-appearing infant who was 38 weeks' gestation or more at delivery and whose mother received 4 hours or more of IAP before delivery may be discharged home after 24 hours if other discharge criteria have been met and a person able to comply fully with instructions for home observation will be present. If any one of these conditions is not met, the infant should be observed in the hospital for at least 48 hours and until criteria for discharge are achieved.

This algorithm is not an exclusive course of management. Variations that incorporate individual circumstances or institutional preferences may be appropriate.

at 24 hours after birth may be reasonable under certain circumstances. Specifically, a healthy-appearing infant who is at least 38 weeks' gestation at delivery and whose mother received 4 or more hours of intrapartum penicillin, ampicillin, or cefazolin before delivery may be discharged home as early as 24 hours after delivery if other discharge criteria have been met and a person able to comply fully with instructions for home observation will be present. A key component of following instructions is the ability of the person observing the infant to communicate with health care professionals by telephone and to transport the infant promptly to an appropriate health care facility if clinical signs of systemic infection develop. If these conditions are not met, the infant should remain in the hospital for at least 48 hours of observation.

Neonatal Infection Control. Routine cultures to determine whether infants are colonized with group B streptococci are not recommended. Epidemiologic evaluation of late-onset or late, late-onset cases in a special care nursery may be required to exclude a health care-associated source.

Nursery Outbreak. Cohorting of ill and colonized infants and use of contact precautions during an outbreak are recommended. Other methods of control (eg, treatment of asymptomatic carriers with penicillin) are ineffective. Routine hand hygiene by health care professionals caring for infants colonized or infected with GBS is the best way to prevent spread to other infants.

Non-Group A or B Streptococcal and Enterococcal Infections

CLINICAL MANIFESTATIONS: Streptococci of Lancefield groups other than A or B can be associated with invasive disease in infants, children, adolescents, and adults. The principal clinical syndromes of groups C, F, and G streptococci are septicemia, upper and lower respiratory tract infections, skin and soft tissue infections, septic arthritis, meningitis with a parameningeal focus, brain abscess, and endocarditis. Viridans streptococci are associated with endocarditis in patients with congenital or valvular heart disease and bacteremia in neutropenic patients with cancer. Among the viridans streptococci, organisms from the anginosus group often are isolated from patients with brain abscess or abscesses in other sites, including lymph nodes, liver, and lung. Enterococci are associated with bacteremia in neonates and bacteremia, device-associated infections, intra-abdominal abscesses, and urinary tract infections in older children and adults.

ETIOLOGY: Changes in taxonomy and nomenclature of the *Streptococcus* genus have evolved with advances in molecular technology. Among gram-positive organisms that are catalase negative and that display chains by Gram stain, the 2 genera associated most often with human disease are *Streptococcus* and *Enterococcus*. The *Streptococcus* genus contains organisms that are (1) beta-hemolytic on blood agar plates (*Streptococcus pyogenes* [see Group A Streptococcal Infections, p 616], *Streptococcus agalactiae* [see Group B Streptococcal Infections, p 628], and groups C, F, and G streptococci); (2) non-beta–hemolytic (alpha-hemolytic or non-hemolytic) on blood agar plates (*Streptococcus pneumoniae* [see Pneumococcal Infections, p 524], *Streptococcus bovis group*, *Streptococcus milleri* group and more than 20 species of viridans streptococci commonly isolated from humans, which are divided into 6 groups by phenotypic characteristics; (3) nutritionally variant streptococci (now referred to as *Abiotrophia* and *Granulicatella*); and (4) unusual streptococcal species that do not fit into any of the other *Streptococcus* species groups. *S milleri* group organisms (*Streptococcus anginosus*, *Streptococcus constellatus*, and *Streptococcus intermedins*) may have variable hemolysis, and approximately one third possess group A, C, F, or G antigens.

The genus *Enterococcus* (previously included with Lancefield group D streptococci) contains at least 12 species, with *Enterococcus faecalis* and *Enterococcus faecium* accounting for most human enterococcal infections.

EPIDEMIOLOGY: The habitats that non-group A and B streptococci and enterococci occupy in humans include skin (groups C, F, and G streptococci), oropharynx (groups C, F, and G streptococci and the mutans group streptococci), gastrointestinal tract (groups C, F, and G and the bovis group streptococci and *Enterococcus* species), and vagina (groups C, D, F, and G streptococci and *Enterococcus* species). Typical human habitats of different species of viridans streptococci are the oropharynx, epithelial surfaces of the oral cavity, teeth, skin, and gastrointestinal and genitourinary tracts. Intrapartum transmission probably is responsible for most cases of early-onset neonatal infection caused by non-group A and B streptococci and enterococci. Environmental contamination or transmission via hands of health care professionals can lead to colonization of patients. Groups C and G streptococci have been known to cause foodborne outbreaks of pharyngitis.

The **incubation period** and the period of communicability are unknown.

DIAGNOSTIC TESTS: Diagnosis is established by culture of sterile body fluids and serogrouping of the isolate, using group-specific antisera. Antimicrobial susceptibility testing of enterococci isolated from sterile sites is important to determine ampicillin and vancomycin susceptibility as well as lack of high-level gentamicin resistance to assess potential for synergy when used in combination with a cell wall active agent (ampicillin or vancomycin). Some susceptibility testing methods may not detect vancomycin resistance reliably; the addition of testing on vancomycin screening agar can increase reliability.

TREATMENT: For many streptococcal infections, treatment with penicillin G alone is adequate. However, for penicillin-resistant isolates, options include penicillin with gentamicin, other beta-lactam agents, vancomycin, and vancomycin with rifampin. Enterococci and some streptococcal strains (especially viridans streptococci and nutritionally variant streptococci requiring growth media additives) are resistant to penicillin. Enterococci uniformly are resistant to cephalosporins and can be resistant to ampicillin and vancomycin as well, making treatment challenging. Invasive enterococcal infections, such as endocarditis, should be treated with ampicillin or vancomycin in combination with an aminoglycoside (usually gentamicin). However, the aminoglycoside should be discontinued if in vitro susceptibility testing demonstrates high-level gentamicin resistance, in which case synergy cannot be achieved. Linezolid is approved for use in children, including neonates, for treatment of vancomycin-resistant enterococcal infections, including *E faecium* and *E faecalis.* Daptomycin has been approved for use in adults for treatment of infections attributable to vancomycin-susceptible *E faecalis.* Most vancomycin-resistant isolates of *E faecalis* and *E faecium* demonstrate susceptibility to daptomycin, but the efficacy of daptomycin in treating infections attributed to these isolates has not been established. Quinupristin-dalfopristin has been approved for use in adults for treatment of infections attributable to vancomycin-resistant *E faecium.* Quinupristin-dalfopristin is not effective against *E faecalis.*

Endocarditis. Guidelines for antimicrobial therapy in adults have been formulated by the American Heart Association and should be consulted for regimens that may be appropriate for children and adolescents.

ISOLATION OF THE HOSPITALIZED PATIENT: Standard precautions are recommended. For patients with infection or colonization attributable to vancomycin-resistant entero-cocci (VRE), contact as well as standard precautions are indicated. Common practice is to maintain precautions until the patient no longer harbors the organism or is discharged from the health care facility. Criteria of negative culture results from body fluid or tissue specimens from multiple sites (may include stool or rectal swab, perineal area, axilla or umbilicus, wound, and indwelling urinary catheter or colostomy sites, if present) on at least 3 separate occasions obtained after cessation of antimicrobial therapy and more than 1 week apart have been used to define resolution of VRE colonization.

CONTROL MEASURES: Patients with a prosthetic valve, previous infective endocarditis, or congenital heart disease associated with the highest risk of adverse outcome from endocarditis should receive antimicrobial prophylaxis to prevent endocarditis at the time of dental and other selected surgical procedures (see Prevention of Bacterial Endocarditis, p 826). Use of vancomycin and treatment with broad-spectrum antimicrobial agents are risk factors for colonization and infection with VRE. Hospitals should develop institution-specific guidelines for the proper use of vancomycin.[1] Early instruction in proper diet; oral health, including use of dental sealants and adequate fluoride intake; and prevention or cessation of smoking will aid in the prevention of dental caries.[2]

Strongyloidiasis
(Strongyloides stercoralis)

CLINICAL MANIFESTATIONS: Because most infections with *Strongyloides stercoralis* are asymptomatic, strongyloidiasis should be considered in any patient with unexplained eosinophilia and potential risk of exposure. When symptoms occur, they are most often related to larval skin invasion, tissue migration, and/or the presence of adult worms in the intestine. Infective (filariform) larvae are acquired from skin contact with contaminated soil, producing transient pruritic papules at the site of penetration. Larvae migrate to the lungs and can cause a transient pneumonitis or Loeffler-like syndrome. After ascending the tracheobronchial tree, larvae are swallowed and mature into adults within the gastrointestinal tract. Symptoms of intestinal infection include vague abdominal pain, malabsorption, vomiting, and diarrhea. Larval migration from defecated stool can result in pruritic skin lesions in the perianal area, buttocks, and upper thighs, which may present as serpiginous, erythematous tracks called larva currens. Immunocompromised people, usually people receiving glucocorticoids for underlying malignancy or autoimmune disease and people with human T-lymphotropic virus (HTLV-1), are at risk of *Strongyloides* hyperinfection, which results from dissemination of larvae via the systemic circulation to a variety of tissues with subsequent abdominal pain, diffuse pulmonary infiltrates, and septicemia or meningitis from enteric gram-negative bacilli.

ETIOLOGY: *S stercoralis* is a nematode (roundworm).

---

[1]Hageman JC, Patel JB, Carey RC, Tenover FC, McDonald LC. *Investigation and Control of Vancomycin-Intermediate and −Resistant Staphylococcus aureus (VISA/VRSA): A Guide for Health Departments and Infection Control Personnel.* Atlanta, GA: Centers for Disease Control and Prevention; 2006. Available at: **www.cdc.gov/ncidod/dhqp/pdf/ar/visa_vrsa_guide.pdf**

[2]Centers for Disease Control and Prevention. Surveillance for dental caries, dental sealants, tooth retention, edentulism, and enamel fluorosis—United States, 1988–1994 and 1999–2002. *MMWR Surveill Summ.* 2005;54(SS-3):1–43

EPIDEMIOLOGY: Strongyloidiasis is endemic in the tropics and subtropics, including the southeastern United States, wherever suitable moist soil and improper disposal of human waste coexist. Humans are the principal hosts, but dogs, cats, and other animals can serve as reservoirs. Transmission involves penetration of skin by infective (filariform) larvae from contact with infected soil. Infections rarely can be acquired from intimate skin contact or from inadvertent coprophagy, such as from ingestion of contaminated food or within institutional settings. Adult females release eggs in the small intestine, where they hatch as first-stage (rhabditiform) larvae that are excreted in feces. A small percentage of larvae molt to the infective (filariform) stage during intestinal transit, at which point they can penetrate the bowel mucosa or perianal skin, thus maintaining the life cycle within a single person (autoinfection). Because of this capacity for autoinfection, people can remain infected for decades after leaving a geographic area with endemic infection.

The **incubation period** in humans is unknown.

DIAGNOSTIC TESTS: Strongyloidiasis can be difficult to diagnose in immunocompetent people, because the total worm burden generally is low and excretion of larvae is variable. Eosinophilia (blood eosinophil count greater than $500/\mu L$) is common. At least 3 consecutive stool specimens should be examined microscopically for characteristic larvae (not eggs), but stool concentration techniques may be required to establish the diagnosis. The use of agar plate culture methods may have greater sensitivity than fecal microscopy, and examination of duodenal contents obtained using the string test (Entero-Test) or a direct aspirate through a flexible endoscope may also demonstrate larvae. Serodiagnosis using immunoassay is helpful and should be considered in all people with unexplained eosinophilia. Although sensitive, cross-reaction with other helminths limits the specificity of serodiagnosis. The serologic test typically yields negative results approximately 6 to 12 months after successful therapy.

In disseminated strongyloidiasis, filariform larvae may be isolated from sputum or bronchoalveolar lavage fluid as well as spinal fluid. Gram-negative bacillary meningitis is a common associated finding in disseminated disease and carries a high mortality rate.

TREATMENT: Ivermectin is the treatment of choice for both chronic (asymptomatic) and disseminated disease with hyperinfection. Alternative agents include albendazole and thiabendazole, although both drugs are associated with slightly lower cure rates (see Drugs for Parasitic Infections, p 873). Prolonged or repeated treatment may be necessary in people with hyperinfection and disseminated strongyloidiasis, and relapse can occur.

ISOLATION OF THE HOSPITALIZED PATIENT: Standard precautions are recommended.

CONTROL MEASURES: Sanitary disposal measures for human waste should be followed, and education about risk of infection through bare skin is important.

Examination of stool and serologic specimens for *S stercoralis* should be considered for all people with unexplained eosinophilia, especially for people who are immunosuppressed or for whom administration of glucocorticoids is planned. If a patient's condition requires initiation of immunosuppressive therapy before results of diagnostic tests can be obtained, risks of empiric antiparasitic therapy for strongyloidiasis must be weighed against risks of possible dissemination.

Syphilis

CLINICAL MANIFESTATIONS:

Congenital Syphilis. Intrauterine infection with *Treponema pallidum* can result in stillbirth, hydrops fetalis, or preterm birth or may be asymptomatic at birth. Infected infants can have hepatosplenomegaly, snuffles, lymphadenopathy, mucocutaneous lesions, pneumonia, osteochondritis and pseudoparalysis, edema, rash, hemolytic anemia, or thrombocytopenia at birth or within the first 4 to 8 weeks of age. Skin lesions or moist nasal secretions of congenital syphilis are highly infectious. However, organisms rarely are found in lesions more than 24 hours after treatment has begun. Untreated infants, regardless of whether they have manifestations in early infancy, may develop late manifestations, which usually appear after 2 years of age and involve the central nervous system (CNS), bones and joints, teeth, eyes, and skin. Some consequences of intrauterine infection may not become apparent until many years after birth, such as interstitial keratitis (5–20 years of age), eighth cranial nerve deafness (10–40 years of age), Hutchinson teeth (peg-shaped, notched central incisors), anterior bowing of the shins, frontal bossing, mulberry molars, saddle nose, rhagades, and Clutton joints (symmetric, painless swelling of the knees). The first 3 manifestations are referred to as the Hutchinson triad. Late manifestations can be prevented by treatment of early infection.

Acquired Syphilis. Infection with *T pallidum* in childhood or adulthood can be divided into 3 stages. The **primary stage** appears as one or more painless indurated ulcers (chancres) of the skin or mucous membranes at the site of inoculation, but chancres may not be recognized. These lesions most commonly appear on the genitalia but may appear elsewhere, depending on the sexual contact responsible for transmission (ie, oral). These lesions appear, on average, 3 weeks after exposure (10–90 days) and heal spontaneously in a few weeks. The **secondary stage,** beginning 1 to 2 months later, is characterized by rash, mucocutaneous lesions, and lymphadenopathy. The polymorphic maculopapular rash is generalized and typically includes the palms and soles. In moist areas around the vulva or anus, hypertrophic papular lesions (condylomata lata) can occur and can be confused with condyloma acuminata secondary to human papillomavirus (HPV) infection. Generalized lymphadenopathy, fever, malaise, splenomegaly, sore throat, headache, and arthralgia can be present. This stage also resolves spontaneously without treatment in approximately 3 to 12 weeks, leaving the infected person completely asymptomatic. A variable latent period follows but sometimes is interrupted during the first few years by recurrences of symptoms of secondary syphilis. **Latent syphilis** is defined as the period after infection when patients are seroreactive but demonstrate no clinical manifestations of disease. Latent syphilis acquired within the preceding year is referred to as **early latent syphilis**; all other cases of latent syphilis are **late latent syphilis** (greater than one year's duration) or **syphilis of unknown duration**. The tertiary stage of infection refers to gumma formation and cardiovascular involvement but not neurosyphilis. The **tertiary stage,** occurring 15 to 30 years after the initial infection, can be marked by aortitis or gummatous changes of the skin, bone, or viscera. Neurosyphilis is defined as infection of the central nervous system with *T pallidum*. Manifestations of neurosyphilis can occur at any stage of infection, especially in people infected with human immunodeficiency virus (HIV).

ETIOLOGY: *T pallidum* is a thin, motile spirochete that is extremely fastidious, surviving only briefly outside the host. The organism has not been cultivated successfully on artificial media.

EPIDEMIOLOGY: Syphilis, which is rare in much of the industrialized world, persists in the United States and in developing countries. The incidence of acquired and congenital syphilis increased dramatically in the United States during the late 1980s and early 1990s but subsequently decreased, and in 2000, the incidence was the lowest since reporting began in 1941. Since 2001, however, the rate of primary and secondary syphilis has increased, primarily among men who have sex with men. Among women, the rate of primary and secondary syphilis has increased since 2005, with a concomitant increase in cases of congenital syphilis. Rates of infection remain disproportionately high in large urban areas and in the southern United States. In adults, syphilis is more common among people with HIV infection.

Congenital syphilis is contracted from an infected mother via transplacental transmission of *T pallidum* at any time during pregnancy or possibly at birth from contact with maternal lesions. Among women with untreated early syphilis, as many as 40% of pregnancies result in spontaneous abortion, stillbirth, or perinatal death. Infection can be transmitted to the fetus at any stage of maternal disease. The rate of transmission is 60% to 100% during primary and secondary syphilis and slowly decreases with later stages of maternal infection (approximately 40% with early latent infection and 8% with late latent infection). The World Health Organization estimates that 1 million pregnancies are affected by syphilis worldwide. Of these, 460 000 will result in stillbirth, hydrops fetalis, abortion, or perinatal death; 270 000 will result in an infant born preterm or with low birth weight; and 270 000 will result in an infant with stigmata of congenital syphilis.

Acquired syphilis almost always is contracted through direct sexual contact with ulcerative lesions of the skin or mucous membranes of infected people. Sexual abuse must be suspected in any young child with acquired syphilis. Open, moist lesions of the primary or secondary stages are highly infectious. Relapses of secondary syphilis with infectious mucocutaneous lesions can occur up to 4 years after primary infection.

The **incubation period** for acquired primary syphilis typically is 3 weeks but ranges from 10 to 90 days.

DIAGNOSTIC TESTS: Definitive diagnosis is made when spirochetes are identified by microscopic darkfield examination or direct fluorescent antibody tests of lesion exudate, nasal discharge, or tissue, such as placenta, umbilical cord, or autopsy specimens. Specimens should be scraped from moist mucocutaneous lesions or aspirated from a regional lymph node. Specimens from mouth lesions are best examined by direct fluorescent antibody techniques to distinguish *T pallidum* from nonpathogenic treponemes that may be seen on darkfield microscopy. Although such testing can provide definitive diagnosis, in most instances, serologic testing is necessary. Polymerase chain reaction tests and immunoglobulin (Ig) M immunoblotting have been developed but are not yet available commercially.

Presumptive diagnosis is possible using nontreponemal and treponemal serologic tests. The use of only one type of test is insufficient for diagnosis, because false-positive nontreponemal test results occur with various medical conditions, and treponemal test results remain positive long after syphilis has been treated adequately and can be falsely positive with other spirochetal diseases.

The standard nontreponemal tests for syphilis include the Venereal Disease Research Laboratory (VDRL) slide test and the rapid plasma reagin (RPR) test. These tests measure antibody directed against lipoidal antigen from *T pallidum,* antibody interaction with host tissues, or both. These tests are inexpensive and performed rapidly and provide quantitative results. Quantitative results help define disease activity and monitor response to therapy. Nontreponemal test results may be falsely negative (ie, nonreactive) with early primary syphilis, latent acquired syphilis of long duration, and late congenital syphilis. Occasionally, a nontreponemal test performed on serum samples containing high concentrations of antibody against *T pallidum* will be weakly reactive or falsely negative, a reaction termed the *prozone* phenomenon. Diluting the serum results in a positive test. When nontreponemal tests are used to monitor treatment response, the same specific test (eg, VDRL or RPR) must be used throughout the follow-up period, preferably by the same laboratory, to ensure comparability of results.

A reactive nontreponemal test result from a patient with typical lesions indicates the need for treatment. However, any reactive nontreponemal test result must be confirmed by one of the specific treponemal tests to exclude a false-positive test result. False-positive results can be caused by certain viral infections (eg, Epstein Barr virus infection, hepatitis, varicella, and measles), lymphoma, tuberculosis, malaria, endocarditis, connective tissue disease, pregnancy, abuse of injection drugs, laboratory or technical error, or Wharton jelly contamination when umbilical cord blood specimens are used. Treatment should not be delayed while awaiting the results of the treponemal test results if the patient is symptomatic or at high risk of infection. A sustained fourfold decrease in titer, equivalent to a change of 2 dilutions (eg, from 1:32 to 1:8), of the nontreponemal test result after treatment usually demonstrates adequate therapy, whereas a fourfold increase in titer after treatment suggests reinfection or relapse. The quantitative nontreponemal test titer usually decreases fourfold within 6 to 12 months after therapy for primary or secondary syphilis, and usually becomes nonreactive within 1 year after successful therapy if the infection (primary or secondary syphilis) was treated early. The patient usually becomes seronegative within 2 years even if the initial titer was high or the infection was congenital. Some people will continue to have low stable nontreponemal antibody titers despite effective therapy. This serofast state is more common in patients treated for latent or tertiary syphilis.

Treponemal tests in use are fluorescent treponemal antibody absorption (FTA-ABS) and *T pallidum* particle agglutination (TP-PA) tests. Some clinical laboratories and blood banks have begun to screen samples using treponemal enzyme immunoassay (EIA) tests. People who have reactive treponemal test results usually remain reactive for life, even after successful therapy. However, 15% to 25% of patients treated during the primary stage revert to being serologically nonreactive after 2 to 3 years. Treponemal test antibody titers correlate poorly with disease activity and should not be used to assess response to therapy.

Treponemal tests also are not 100% specific for syphilis; positive reactions variably occur in patients with other spirochetal diseases, such as yaws, pinta, leptospirosis, rat-bite fever, relapsing fever, and Lyme disease. Nontreponemal tests can be used to differentiate Lyme disease from syphilis, because the VDRL test is nonreactive in Lyme disease.

Usually, a serum nontreponemal test is obtained initially, and if it is reactive, a treponemal test is then performed. The probability of syphilis is high in a sexually active person whose serum is reactive on both nontreponemal and treponemal tests.

Differentiating syphilis treated in the past from reinfection often is difficult unless the nontreponemal titer is increasing.

In summary, nontreponemal antibody tests (VDRL and RPR) are used for screening, and treponemal tests (FTA-ABS and TP-PA) are used to establish a presumptive diagnosis. Quantitative nontreponemal antibody tests are useful in assessing the adequacy of therapy and in detecting reinfection. All patients who have syphilis should be tested for HIV infection.

Cerebrospinal Fluid Tests. For evaluation of possible neurosyphilis, the VDRL test should be performed on cerebrospinal fluid (CSF). The CSF VDRL is highly specific, but it is insensitive. In addition, evaluation of CSF protein and white blood cell count is used to assess the likelihood of CNS involvement. The CSF leukocyte count usually is elevated in neurosyphilis (greater than 5 white blood cells [WBCs]/mm^3). Although the FTA-ABS test of CSF is less specific than the VDRL test, some experts recommend using the FTA-ABS test, believing it to be more sensitive than the VDRL test. Results from the VDRL test should be interpreted cautiously, because a negative result on a VDRL test of CSF does not exclude a diagnosis of neurosyphilis. Alternatively, a reactive VDRL test in the CSF of neonates can be the result of nontreponemal IgG antibodies that cross the blood-brain barrier. Fewer data exist for the TP-PA test for CSF, and none exist for the RPR test; these tests should not be used for CSF evaluation.

Testing During Pregnancy. All women should be screened serologically for syphilis early in pregnancy with a nontreponemal test (eg, RPR or VDRL) and preferably again at delivery. In areas of high prevalence of syphilis and in patients considered at high risk of syphilis, a nontreponemal serum test at the beginning of the third trimester (28 weeks of gestation) and at delivery is indicated. For women treated during pregnancy, follow-up serologic testing is necessary to assess the efficacy of therapy. Low-titer false-positive nontreponemal antibody test results occasionally occur in pregnancy. The result of a positive nontreponemal antibody test should be confirmed with a treponemal antibody test (eg, FTA-ABS or TP-PA). When a pregnant woman has a reactive nontreponemal test result and a persistently negative treponemal test result, a false-positive test result is confirmed. As noted above, some laboratories are screening pregnant women using an EIA treponemal test, but this is not recommended during pregnancy. Pregnant women with reactive treponemal screening tests should have confirmatory testing with a nontreponemal test with titers. Any woman who delivers a stillborn infant after 20 weeks' gestation should be tested for syphilis.

Evaluation of Infants for Congenital Infection During the First Month of Age. No newborn infant should be discharged from the hospital without determination of the mother's serologic status for syphilis at least once during pregnancy and also at delivery in communities and populations in which the risk for congenital syphilis is high. Testing of umbilical cord blood or an infant serum sample is inadequate for screening, because these can be nonreactive if the mother's serologic test result is of low titer or she was infected late in pregnancy. All infants born to seropositive mothers require a careful examination and a quantitative nontreponemal syphilis test. The test performed on the infant should be the same as that performed on the mother to enable comparison of titer results. A negative maternal RPR or VDRL test result at delivery does not rule out completely the possibility of the infant having congenital syphilis, although such a situation is rare. The diagnostic and therapeutic approach to infants being evaluated for congenital syphilis is summarized in Fig 3.6 (p 642).

FIG 3.6. ALGORITHM FOR EVALUATION AND TREATMENT OF INFANTS BORN TO MOTHERS WITH REACTIVE SEROLOGIC TESTS FOR SYPHILIS.

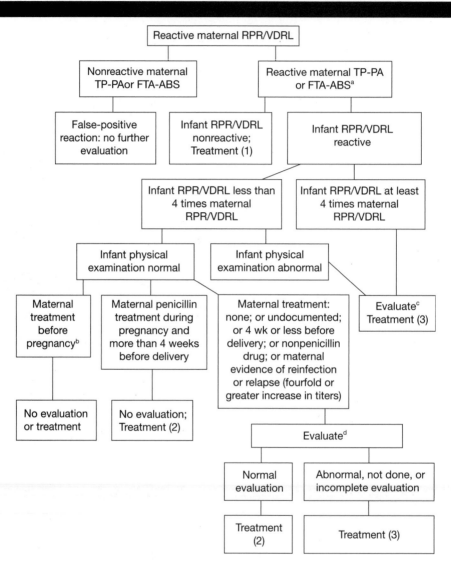

RPR indicates rapid plasma reagin (test); VDRL, Venereal Disease Research Laboratory (test); TP-PA, *Treponema pallidum* particle agglutination (test); FTA-ABS, fluorescent treponema antibody absorption (test).

[a] Test for human immunodeficiency virus (HIV) antibody. Infants of HIV-infected mothers do not require different evaluation or treatment.

[b] Women who maintain a VDRL titer 1:2 or less (RPR 1:4 or less) beyond 1 year after successful treatment are considered serofast.

[c] Evaluation consists of complete blood cell (CBC) and platelet count; cerebrospinal fluid (CSF) examination for cell count, protein, and quantitative VDRL. Other tests as clinically indicated: long-bone and chest radiographs, neuroimaging, auditory brainstem response, eye examination, liver function tests.

[d] CBC, platelet count; CSF examination for cell count, protein, and quantitative VDRL; long-bone radiography.

TREATMENT:
(1) If the mother has had no treatment, undocumented treatment, treatment 4 weeks or less before delivery or evidence of reinfection or relapse (fourfold or greater increase in titers) AND the infant's physical examination is normal, THEN treat infant with a single intramuscular (IM) injection of benzathine penicillin (50 000 U/kg). If these criteria are not met, no treatment is required. In both scenarios, no additional evaluation is needed.
(2) Benzathine penicillin G, 50 000 U/kg, IM, x 1 dose.
(3) Aqueous penicillin G, 50 000 U/kg, IV, every 12 hours (1 week of age or younger), every 8 hours (older than 1 week), or procaine penicillin G, 50 000 U/kg, IM, single daily dose, x 10 days.

Further management of an infant depends on the maternal treatment history as well as results of the infant's nontreponemal serologic test, physical examination, long bone radiography, and laboratory tests. Infants born to mothers who are coinfected with syphilis and HIV do not require different evaluation, therapy, or follow-up for syphilis than is recommended for all infants.

Evaluation and Treatment of Older Infants and Children. Children who are identified as having reactive serologic tests for syphilis after the neonatal period (ie, older than 1 month of age) should have maternal serologic test results and records reviewed to assess whether they have congenital or acquired syphilis. The recommended evaluation includes: 1) CSF analysis for VDRL testing, cell count, and protein concentration; 2) complete blood cell, differential, and platelet count; and 3) other tests as indicated clinically (eg, long-bone or chest radiography, liver function tests, abdominal ultrasonography, ophthalmologic examination, auditory brain stem response testing, and neuroimaging studies).

Cerebrospinal Fluid Testing. Guidance for examination of CSF in the evaluation for possible congenital syphilis is provided under Evaluation of Newborn Infants for Congenital Infection (p 641). CSF test results obtained during the neonatal period can be difficult to interpret; normal values differ by gestational age and are higher in preterm infants. Values as high as 25 WBCs/mm^3 and/or protein up to 150 mg/dL might occur among normal term neonates; some specialists, however, recommend that lower values (ie, 5 WBCs/mm^3 and protein of 40 mg/dL) be considered the upper limits of normal when assessing a term infant for congenital syphilis. Other causes of elevated values should be considered when an infant is being evaluated for congenital syphilis.

CSF should be examined in all patients with neurologic or ophthalmic signs or symptoms, evidence of active tertiary syphilis (eg, aortitis and gumma), treatment failure, or HIV infection with late latent syphilis or syphilis of unknown duration. Abnormalities in CSF in patients with neurosyphilis include increased protein concentration, increased white blood cell count, and/or a reactive VDRL test result. Some experts also recommend performing the FTA-ABS test on CSF, believing it to be more sensitive but less specific than VDRL testing of CSF for neurosyphilis.

TREATMENT[1]**:** Parenteral penicillin G remains the preferred drug for treatment of syphilis at any stage. Recommendations for penicillin G use and duration of therapy vary, depending on the stage of disease and clinical manifestations. Parenteral penicillin G is the only documented effective therapy for patients who have neurosyphilis, congenital syphilis, or syphilis during pregnancy and is recommended for HIV-infected patients. Such patients always should be treated with penicillin, even if desensitization for penicillin allergy is necessary. If shortages of aqueous penicillin G exist, alternate treatment recommendations can be found online (**www.cdc.gov/nchstp/dstd/penicillinG.htm**). Neither combinations of benzathine penicillin and procaine penicillin nor oral penicillin preparations are considered adequate for the treatment of syphilis of any stage.

Penicillin Allergy. Skin testing for penicillin hypersensitivity with the major and minor determinants reliably can identify people at high risk of reacting to penicillin, although only the major determinant (benzylpenicilloyl poly-L-lysine [Pre-Pen]) and penicillin G skin tests have been available commercially. Skin testing without the minor determinant

[1]Centers for Disease Control and Prevention. Sexually transmitted infection treatment guidelines—United States, 2006. *MMWR Recomm Rep.* 2006;55(RR-11):1–94

misses 3% to 10% of allergic patients who are at risk of serious or fatal reactions. Thus, a cautious approach to penicillin therapy is advised when a patient cannot be tested with all of the penicillin skin test reagents. If the major determinant is not available for skin testing, all patients with IgE-mediated reactions to penicillin should be desensitized in a hospital setting. In patients with non-IgE–mediated reactions, outpatient oral desensitization or monitored test doses may be considered. An oral or intravenous desensitization protocol for patients with a positive skin test result is available and should be performed in a hospital setting.[1] Oral desensitization is regarded as safer and easier to perform. Desensitization usually can be completed in approximately 4 hours, after which the first dose of penicillin can be given.

Congenital Syphilis: Infants in the First Month of Age (see Table 3.75, p 645). Infants should be treated for congenital syphilis if they have proven or probable disease demonstrated by one or more of the following: (1) physical, laboratory, or radiographic evidence of active disease; (2) positive placenta or umbilical cord test results for treponemes using direct fluorescent antibody-*T pallidum* staining or darkfield test; (3) a reactive result on VDRL testing of CSF; or (4) a serum quantitative nontreponemal titer that is at least fourfold higher than the mother's titer using the same test and preferably the same laboratory. If the infant's titer is less than 4 times higher than that of the mother, congenital syphilis still can be present. In infants with proven or highly probable disease, aqueous crystalline penicillin G is preferred. The dosage should be based on chronologic age rather than gestational age (see Table 3.75, p 645). Alternatively, some experts recommend penicillin G procaine for treatment of congenital syphilis, because no treatment failures have occurred with its use despite low CSF concentrations. If more than 1 day of therapy is missed, the entire course should be restarted. Data supporting the use of other antimicrobial agents (eg, ampicillin) for treatment of congenital syphilis are not available. When possible, a full 10-day course of penicillin is preferred, even if ampicillin initially was provided for possible sepsis. The use of agents other than penicillin requires close serologic follow-up to assess adequacy of therapy.

In all other situations, maternal history of infection with *T pallidum* and treatment for syphilis must be considered in deciding whether to treat the infant. For an infant with a normal physical examination and a serum quantitative nontreponemal serologic titer that is the same or less than fourfold the maternal titer and whose mother was not treated, inadequately treated, or has no documentation of having received treatment; whose mother was treated with erythromycin or other nonpenicillin regimen; or whose mother received treatment less than 4 weeks before delivery, 3 treatment options are available: (1) aqueous crystalline penicillin G; (2) aqueous penicillin G procaine; or (3) penicillin G benzathine in a single dose.

Some experts would treat all such infants, especially infants born to mothers with untreated early syphilis, with aqueous crystalline penicillin G (or aqueous penicillin G procaine) for 10 days, because physical examination and laboratory test results cannot exclude the diagnosis reliably in all cases. However, if the infant's physical examination, CSF findings, radiographs of long bones, and complete blood cell and platelet counts all are normal, some experts would treat these infants with a single dose of penicillin G benzathine (50 000 U/kg intramuscularly). If the evaluation of these infants is incomplete (ie, a lumbar puncture cannot be performed), then 10 days of treatment is recommended.

[1]Centers for Disease Control and Prevention. Sexually transmitted infection treatment guidelines—United States, 2006. *MMWR Recomm Rep.* 2006;55(RR-11):1–94

Table 3.75. Recommended Management of Neonates (1 Month of Age or Younger) Born to Mothers With Reactive Serologic Tests for Syphilis

Clinical Status	Evaluation (in Addition to Physical Examination and Quantitative Non-treponemal Testing)	Antimicrobial Therapy[a]
Proven or highly probable disease[b]	CSF analysis for VDRL, cell count, and protein CBC and platelet count Other tests as clinically indicated (eg, long-bone radiography, liver function tests, ophthalmologic examination)	Aqueous crystalline penicillin G, 100 000–150 000 U/kg/day, administered as 50 000 U/kg/dose, IV, every 12 h during the first 7 days of age and every 8 h thereafter for a total of 10 days **OR** Penicillin G procaine,[c] 50 000 U/kg/day, IM, in a single dose for 10 days
Normal physical examination and serum quantitative nontreponemal titer the same or less than fourfold the maternal titer:		
(a) (i) Mother was not treated or inadequately treated or has no documented treatment; (ii) mother was treated with erythromycin or other nonpenicillin regimen; (iii) mother received treatment 4 wk or less before delivery; (iv) maternal evidence of reinfection or relapse (less than fourfold decrease in titers)	CSF analysis for VDRL, cell count, and protein[d] CBC and platelet count[d] Long-bone radiography[d]	Aqueous crystalline penicillin G, IV, for 10 days[d] **OR** Penicillin G procaine,[c] 50 000 U/kg, IM, in a single dose for 10 days[d] **OR** Penicillin G benzathine,[c] 50 000 U/kg, IM, in a single dose[d]
(b) (i) Adequate maternal therapy given more than 4 wk before delivery; (ii) mother has no evidence of reinfection or relapse	None	Clinical, serologic follow-up, and penicillin G benzathine, 50 000 U/kg, IM, in a single dose[e]
(c) Adequate therapy before pregnancy and mother's nontreponemal serologic titer remained low and stable during pregnancy and at delivery	None	None[f]

Table 3.75. Recommended Management of Neonates (1 Month of Age or Younger) Born to Mothers With Reactive Serologic Tests for Syphilis, continued

CSF indicates cerebrospinal fluid; VDRL, Venereal Disease Research Laboratory; CBC, complete blood cell; IV, intravenously; IM, intramuscularly.

[a]If more than 1 day of therapy is missed, the entire course should be restarted.

[b]Abnormal physical examination, serum quantitative nontreponemal titer that is fourfold greater than the mother's titer, or positive result of darkfield or fluorescent antibody test of body fluid(s).

[c]Penicillin G benzathine and penicillin G procaine are approved for IM administration only.

[d]A complete evaluation (CSF analysis, bone radiography, CBC) is not necessary if 10 days of parenteral therapy is administered but may be useful to support a diagnosis of congenital syphilis. If a single dose of penicillin G benzathine is used, then the infant must be evaluated fully, results of the full evaluation must be normal, and follow-up must be certain. If any part of the infant's evaluation is abnormal or not performed or if the CSF analysis is uninterpretable, the 10-day course of penicillin is required.

[e]Some experts would not treat the infant but would provide close serologic follow-up.

[f]Some experts would treat with penicillin G benzathine, 50 000 U/kg, as a single IM injection, if follow-up is uncertain.

Infants who have a normal physical examination and a serum quantitative non-treponemal serologic titer the same or less than fourfold the maternal titer are at minimal risk of syphilis if (1) they are born to mothers who completed appropriate penicillin treatment for syphilis more than 4 weeks before delivery, and (2) the mother had no evidence of reinfection or relapse. Although a full evaluation may be unnecessary, these infants should be treated with a single injection of penicillin G benzathine, because fetal treatment failure can occur despite adequate maternal treatment during pregnancy. Alternatively, these infants may be examined carefully, preferably monthly, until their nontreponemal serologic test results are negative.

Infants who have a normal physical examination and a serum quantitative non-treponemal serologic titer the same or less than fourfold the maternal titer and (1) whose mother's treatment was adequate before pregnancy, and (2) whose mother's nontrepone-mal serologic titer remained low and stable before and during pregnancy and at delivery (VDRL less than 1:2; RPR less than 1:4) require no evaluation. Some specialists, however, would treat with penicillin G benzathine as a single intramuscular injection if follow-up is uncertain.

Congenital Syphilis: Older Infants and Children. Because establishing the diagnosis of neurosyphilis is difficult, infants older than 1 month of age who possibly have con-genital syphilis or who have neurologic involvement should be treated with aqueous crystalline penicillin for 10 days (see Table 3.76, p 647). This regimen also should be used to treat children older than 2 years of age who have late and previously untreated congenital syphilis. Some experts suggest giving such patients a single dose of penicil-lin G benzathine, 50 000 U/kg, intramuscularly after the 10-day course of intravenous aqueous crystalline penicillin. If the patient has no clinical manifestations of disease, the CSF examination is normal, and the result of the VDRL test of CSF is negative, some experts would treat with 3 weekly doses of penicillin G benzathine (50 000 U/kg, intramuscularly).

Syphilis in Pregnancy. Regardless of the stage of pregnancy, patients should be treated with penicillin according to the dosage schedules appropriate for the stage of syphilis as recommended for nonpregnant patients (see Table 3.76, p 647). For penicillin-allergic patients, no proven alternative therapy has been established. A pregnant woman with

Table 3.76. Recommended Treatment for Syphilis in People Older Than 1 Month of Age

Status	Children	Adults
Congenital syphilis	Aqueous crystalline penicillin G, 200 000–300 000 U/kg/day, IV, administered as 50 000 U/kg every 4–6 h for 10 days[a]	
Primary, secondary, and early latent syphilis[b]	Penicillin G benzathine,[c] 50 000 U/kg, IM, up to the adult dose of 2.4 million U in a single dose	Penicillin G benzathine, 2.4 million U, IM, in a single dose **OR** _If allergic to penicillin and not pregnant,_ Doxycycline, 100 mg, orally, twice a day for 14 days **OR** Tetracycline, 500 mg, orally, 4 times/day for 14 days
Late latent syphilis[d] **or latent syphilis of unknown duration**	Penicillin G benzathine, 50 000 U/kg, IM, up to the adult dose of 2.4 million U, administered as 3 single doses at 1-wk intervals (total 150 000 U/kg, up to the adult dose of 7.2 million U)	Penicillin G benzathine, 7.2 million U total, administered as 3 doses of 2.4 million U, IM, each at 1-wk intervals **OR** _If allergic to penicillin and not pregnant,_ Doxycycline, 100 mg, orally, twice a day for 4 wk **OR** Tetracycline, 500 mg, orally, 4 times/day for 4 wk
Tertiary	…	Penicillin G benzathine 7.2 million U total, administered as 3 doses of 2.4 million U, IM, at 1-wk intervals _If allergic to penicillin and not pregnant, same as for late latent syphilis_
Neurosyphilis[e]	Aqueous crystalline penicillin G, 200 000–300 000 U/kg/day, given every 4–6 h for 10–14 days in doses not to exceed the adult dose	Aqueous crystalline penicillin G, 18–24 million U per day, administered as 3–4 million U, IV, every 4 h for 10–14 days[f] **OR** Penicillin G procaine,[c] 2.4 million U, IM, once daily **PLUS** probenecid, 500 mg, orally, 4 times/day, both for 10–14 days[f]

IV indicates intravenously; IM, intramuscularly.

[a] If the patient has no clinical manifestations of disease, the CSF examination is normal, and the CSF VDRL result is negative, some experts would treat with up to 3 weekly doses of penicillin G benzathine, 50 000 U/kg, IM. Some experts also suggest giving these patients a single dose of penicillin G benzathine, 50 000 U/kg, IM, after the 10-day course of IV aqueous penicillin.

[b] Early latent syphilis is defined as being acquired within the preceding year.

[c] Penicillin G benzathine and penicillin G procaine are approved for IM administration only.

[d] Late latent syphilis is defined as syphilis beyond 1 year's duration.

[e] Patients who are allergic to penicillin should be desensitized.

[f] Some experts administer penicillin G benzathine, 2.4 million U, IM, once per week for up to 3 weeks after completion of these neurosyphilis treatment regimens.

a history of penicillin allergy should be treated with penicillin after desensitization. Desensitization should be performed in consultation with a specialist and only in facilities in which emergency assistance is available (see Penicillin Allergy, p 643).

Erythromycin, azithromycin, or any other nonpenicillin treatment of syphilis during pregnancy cannot be considered reliable to cure infection in the fetus. Tetracycline is not recommended for pregnant women because of potential adverse effects on the fetus.

Early Acquired Syphilis (Primary, Secondary, Early Latent Syphilis). A single intramuscular dose of penicillin G benzathine is the preferred treatment for children and adults (see Table 3.76, p 647). All children should have a CSF examination before treatment to exclude a diagnosis of neurosyphilis. Evaluation of CSF in adolescents and adults is necessary only if clinical signs or symptoms of neurologic or ophthalmic involvement are present. Neurosyphilis should be considered in the differential diagnosis of neurologic disease in HIV-infected people.

For nonpregnant patients who are allergic to penicillin, doxycycline or tetracycline should be given for 14 days. Children younger than 8 years of age should not be given tetracycline or doxycycline unless the benefits of therapy are greater than the risks of dental staining (see Antimicrobial Agents and Related Therapy, p 737). Clinical studies, along with biologic and pharmacologic considerations, suggest ceftriaxone should be effective for early-acquired syphilis. The recommended dose and duration of ceftriaxone therapy are 1 g once daily via either the intramuscular or intravenous route for 8 to 10 days (for adolescents and adults). Because efficacy of ceftriaxone is not well documented, close follow-up is essential. Single-dose therapy with ceftriaxone is not effective. Preliminary data suggest that azithromycin might be effective as a single oral dose of 2 g. However, several cases of azithromycin treatment failures have been reported, and resistance to azithromycin has been documented in several geographic areas. When follow-up cannot be ensured, especially for children younger than 8 years of age, consideration must be given to hospitalization and desensitization followed by administration of penicillin G (see Penicillin Allergy, p 643).

Syphilis of More Than 1 Year's Duration (Late Latent Syphilis, Except Neurosyphilis) or of Unknown Duration. Penicillin G benzathine should be given intramuscularly weekly for 3 successive weeks (see Table 3.76, p 647). In patients who are allergic to penicillin, doxycycline or tetracycline for 4 weeks should be given only with close serologic and clinical follow-up. Limited clinical studies suggest that ceftriaxone might be effective, but the optimal dose and duration have not been defined. Patients who have syphilis and who demonstrate any of the following criteria should have a prompt CSF examination:

1. Neurologic or ophthalmic signs or symptoms;
2. Evidence of active tertiary syphilis (eg, aortitis, gumma, iritis, uveitis);
3. Treatment failure; or
4. HIV infection with late latent syphilis or syphilis of unknown duration.

If dictated by circumstances and patient or parent preferences, a CSF examination may be performed for patients who do not meet these criteria. Some experts recommend performing a CSF examination on all patients who have latent syphilis and a nontreponemal serologic test result of 1:32 or greater or if the patient is HIV infected and has a serum CD4+ T-lymphocyte count 350 or less. The risk of neurosyphilis in this circumstance is unknown. If a CSF examination is performed and the results indicate abnormalities consistent with neurosyphilis, the patient should be treated for neurosyphilis (see Neurosyphilis). Children younger than 8 years of age should not be given tetracycline or doxycycline unless the benefits of therapy are greater than the risks of dental staining (see Antimicrobial Agents and Related Therapy, p 737).

Neurosyphilis. The recommended regimen for adults is aqueous crystalline penicillin G, intravenously, for 10 to 14 days (see Table 3.76, p 647). If adherence to therapy can be ensured, patients may be treated with an alternative regimen of daily intramuscular penicillin G procaine plus oral probenecid for 10 to 14 days. Some experts recommend following both of these regimens with penicillin G benzathine, 2.4 million U, intramuscularly, weekly for 1 to 3 doses. For children, aqueous crystalline penicillin G for 10 to 14 days is recommended, and some experts recommend additional therapy with penicillin G benzathine, 50 000 U/kg per dose (not to exceed 2.4 million U) for up to 3 single weekly doses.

If the patient has a history of allergy to penicillin, consideration should be given to desensitization, and the patient should be managed in consultation with an allergy specialist (see Penicillin Allergy, p 643).

Other Considerations.

- Mothers of infants with congenital syphilis should be tested for other sexually transmitted infections (STIs), including *Neisseria gonorrhoeae, Chlamydia trachomatis,* HIV, hepatitis B, and human papillomavirus infections. If injection drug use is suspected, the mother also may be at risk of hepatitis C virus infection.
- All recent sexual contacts of people with acquired syphilis should be evaluated for other STIs as well as syphilis (see Control Measures, p 651). Partners who were exposed within 90 days preceding the diagnosis of primary, secondary, or early latent syphilis in the index patient should be treated presumptively for syphilis, even if they are seronegative.
- All patients with syphilis should be tested for other STIs, including HIV, hepatitis B, and human papillomavirus infection. Patients who have primary syphilis should be retested for HIV after 3 months if the first HIV test result is negative.
- For HIV-infected patients with syphilis, careful follow-up is essential. Patients infected with HIV who have early syphilis may be at increased risk of neurologic complications and higher rates of treatment failure with currently recommended regimens.
- Children with acquired primary, secondary, or latent syphilis should be evaluated for possible sexual assault or abuse.

Follow-up and Management.

Congenital syphilis. All infants who have reactive serologic tests for syphilis or were born to mothers who were seroreactive at delivery should receive careful follow-up evaluations during regularly scheduled well-child care visits at 2, 4, 6, and 12 months of age. Serologic nontreponemal tests should be performed every 2 to 3 months until the nontreponemal test becomes nonreactive or the titer has decreased fourfold. Nontreponemal antibody titers should decrease by 3 months of age and should be nonreactive by 6 months of age if the infant was infected and adequately treated or was not infected and initially seropositive because of transplacentally acquired maternal antibody. The serologic response after therapy may be slower for infants treated after the neonatal period. Patients with increasing titers or with persistent stable titers 6 to 12 months after initial treatment should be reevaluated, including a CSF examination, and treated with a 10-day course of parenteral penicillin G, even if they were treated previously.

Treponemal tests should not be used to evaluate treatment response, because results for an infected child can remain positive despite effective therapy. Passively transferred maternal treponemal antibodies can persist in an infant until 15 months of age. A reactive treponemal test after 18 months of age is diagnostic of congenital syphilis. If the nontreponemal test is nonreactive at this time, no further evaluation or treatment is necessary. If the nontreponemal test is reactive at 18 months of age, the infant should be fully evaluated (or reevaluated) and treated for congenital syphilis.

Treated infants with congenital neurosyphilis and initially positive results of VDRL tests of CSF or abnormal CSF cell counts and/or protein concentrations should undergo repeated clinical evaluation and CSF examination at 6-month intervals until their CSF examination is normal. A reactive result of VDRL testing of CSF at the 6-month interval is an indication for retreatment. Abnormal CSF indices that cannot be attributed to other ongoing illness also require retreatment. Neuroimaging studies, such as magnetic resonance imaging, should be considered in these children.

Acquired syphilis. Treated pregnant women with syphilis should have quantitative nontreponemal serologic tests repeated at 28 to 32 weeks of gestation, at delivery, and following the recommendations for the stage of disease. Serologic titers may be repeated monthly in women at high risk of reinfection or in geographic areas where the prevalence of syphilis is high. The clinical and antibody response should be appropriate for stage of disease. Most women will deliver before their serologic response to treatment can be assessed definitively. Therapy should be judged inadequate if the maternal antibody titer has not decreased fourfold by delivery. Inadequate maternal treatment is likely if clinical signs of infection are present at delivery or if maternal antibody titer is fourfold higher than the pretreatment titer. Fetal treatment is considered inadequate if delivery occurs within 28 days of maternal therapy.

Indications for Retreatment.

Primary/secondary syphilis:
- If clinical signs or symptoms persist or recur or if a fourfold increase in titer of a nontreponemal test occurs, evaluate CSF and HIV status and repeat therapy.
- If the nontreponemal titer fails to decrease fourfold within 6 months after therapy, evaluate for HIV; repeat therapy unless follow-up for continued clinical and serologic assessment can be ensured. Some experts recommend CSF evaluation.

Latent syphilis: In the following situations, CSF examination should be performed and retreatment should be provided:
- Titers increase fourfold;
- An initially high titer (greater than 1:32) fails to decrease at least fourfold within 12 to 24 months; or
- Signs or symptoms attributable to syphilis develop.

In all these instances, retreatment, when indicated, should be performed with 3 weekly injections of penicillin G benzathine, 2.4 million U, intramuscularly, unless CSF examination indicates that neurosyphilis is present, at which time treatment for neurosyphilis should be initiated. Retreated patients should be treated with the schedules recommended for patients with syphilis for more than 1 year. In general, only 1 retreatment course is indicated. The possibility of reinfection or concurrent HIV infection always should be considered when retreating patients with early syphilis.

Patients with neurosyphilis must have periodic serologic testing, clinical evaluation at 6-month intervals, and repeat CSF examinations. If the CSF cell count has not decreased after 6 months or CSF is not entirely normal after 2 years, retreatment should be considered. CSF abnormalities may persist for extended periods of time in HIV-infected people with neurosyphilis. Close follow-up is warranted.

ISOLATION OF THE HOSPITALIZED PATIENT: Standard precautions are recommended for all patients, including infants with suspected or proven congenital syphilis. Because moist open lesions, secretions, and possibly blood are contagious in all patients with syphilis, gloves should be worn when caring for patients with congenital, primary, and secondary syphilis with skin and mucous membrane lesions until 24 hours of treatment has been completed.

Control Measures:

- All women should be screened for syphilis early in pregnancy. For communities and populations in which the prevalence of syphilis is high or for patients at high risk, serologic testing should be performed at 28 to 32 weeks of gestation and at delivery. No newborn infant should leave the hospital without the maternal serologic status having been determined at least once during the pregnancy.
- Education of patients and populations about STIs, treatment of sexual contacts, reporting of each case to local public health authorities for contact investigation and appropriate follow-up, and serologic screening of high-risk populations are indicated.
- All recent sexual contacts of a person with acquired syphilis should be identified, examined, serologically tested, and treated appropriately. Sexual contacts of people with primary, secondary, or early latent syphilis who were exposed within the preceding 3 months may be infected even if seronegative and should be treated for early-acquired syphilis. People exposed more than 3 months previously should be treated presumptively if serologic test results are not available immediately and follow-up is uncertain. For identification of at-risk sexual partners, the periods before treatment are (1) 3 months plus duration of symptoms for primary syphilis; (2) 6 months plus duration of symptoms for secondary syphilis; and (3) 1 year for early latent syphilis. Recommendations for partner service programs provided to partners of people with syphilis are available.[1]
- All people, including hospital personnel, who have had close unprotected contact with a patient with early congenital syphilis before identification of the disease or during the first 24 hours of therapy should be examined clinically for the presence of lesions 2 to 3 weeks after contact. Serologic testing should be performed and repeated 3 months after contact or sooner if symptoms occur. If the degree of exposure is considered substantial, immediate treatment should be considered.

---

[1]Centers for Disease Control and Prevention. Recommendations for partner service programs for HIV infection, syphilis, gonorrhea, and chlamydial infection. *MMWR Recomm Rep.* 2008;57(RR-9):1–83

Tapeworm Diseases
(Taeniasis and Cysticercosis)

CLINICAL MANIFESTATIONS:

Taeniasis. Infection often is asymptomatic; however, mild gastrointestinal tract symptoms, such as nausea, diarrhea, and pain, can occur. Tapeworm segments can be seen migrating from the anus or in feces.

Cysticercosis. Manifestations depend on the location and number of pork tapeworm cysts (cysticerci) and the host response. Cysts may be found anywhere in the body. The most common and serious manifestations are caused by cysts in the central nervous system. Cysts of *Taenia solium* in the brain (neurocysticercosis) can cause seizures, behavioral disturbances, obstructive hydrocephalus, and other neurologic signs and symptoms. In some countries, neurocysticercosis is a leading cause of epilepsy. The host reaction to degenerating cysts can produce signs and symptoms of meningitis. Cysts in the spinal column can cause gait disturbance, pain, or transverse myelitis. Subcutaneous cysts produce palpable nodules, and ocular involvement can cause visual impairment.

ETIOLOGY: Taeniasis is caused by intestinal infection by the adult tapeworm, *Taenia saginata* (beef tapeworm) or *T solium* (pork tapeworm). *Taenia asiatica* causes taeniasis in Asia. Human cysticercosis is caused only by the larvae of *T solium (Cysticercus cellulosae)*.

EPIDEMIOLOGY: These tapeworm diseases have worldwide distribution. Prevalence is high in areas with poor sanitation and human fecal contamination in areas where cattle graze or swine are fed. Most cases of *T solium* infection in the United States are imported from Latin America or Asia. High rates of *T saginata* infection occur in Mexico, parts of South America, East Africa, and central Europe. *T asiatica* is common in China, Taiwan, and Southeast Asia. Taeniasis is acquired by eating undercooked beef *(T saginata)* or pork *(T solium)*. *T asiatica* is acquired by eating viscera of infected pigs that contain encysted larvae. Infection often is asymptomatic.

Cysticercosis in humans is acquired by ingesting eggs of the pork tapeworm *(T solium)*, through fecal-oral contact with a person harboring the adult tapeworm, or by autoinfection. Eggs are found only in human feces, because humans are the obligate definitive host. Eggs liberate oncospheres in the intestine that migrate through the blood and lymphatics to tissues throughout the body, including the central nervous system, where cysts form. Although most cases of cysticercosis in the United States have been imported, cysticercosis can be acquired in the United States from tapeworm carriers who emigrated from an area with endemic infection and still have *T solium* intestinal stage infection.

The **incubation period** for taeniasis—the time from ingestion of the larvae until segments are passed in the feces—is 2 to 3 months. For cysticercosis, the time between infection and onset of symptoms may be several years.

DIAGNOSIS: Diagnosis of taeniasis (adult tapeworm infection) is based on demonstration of the proglottids or ova in feces or the perianal region. However, these techniques are insensitive. Species identification of the parasite is based on the different structures of the terminal gravid segments. Diagnosis of neurocysticercosis is made primarily on the basis of computed tomography (CT) scanning or magnetic resonance imaging (MRI) of the brain or spinal cord. Antibody assays that detect specific antibody to larval *T solium* in serum and cerebrospinal fluid (CSF) are the confirmatory tests of choice. In the United

States, this test is available through the Centers for Disease Control and Prevention and several commercial laboratories. The test is more sensitive with serum specimens than with CSF specimens. Serum antibody assay results often are negative in children with solitary parenchymal lesions but usually are positive in patients with multiple lesions.

TREATMENT:

Taeniasis. Praziquantel is highly effective for eradicating infection with the adult tapeworm, and niclosamide is an alternative (see Drugs for Parasitic Infections, p 783). Praziquantel is not approved for this indication, but dosing is provided for children older than 4 years of age for some other indications. Niclosamide is not approved for *T solium* but is approved for *T saginata.*

Cysticercosis. Neurocysticercosis treatment should be individualized on the basis of the number and viability of cysticerci as assessed by neuroimaging studies (MRI or CT scan) and where they are located. For patients with only nonviable cysts (eg, only calcifications on CT scan), management should be aimed at symptoms and should include anticonvulsants for patients with seizures and insertion of shunts for patients with hydrocephalus. Two antiparasitic drugs—albendazole and praziquantel—are available. Praziquantel is not approved for this indication, but dosing is provided for children older than 4 years of age for some other indications. Although both drugs are cysticercidal and hasten radiologic resolution of cysts, most symptoms result from the host inflammatory response and may be exacerbated by treatment. In some clinical trials, patients treated with albendazole had better radiologic and clinical responses than patients treated with low doses of praziquantel. Several studies have indicated that patients with single inflamed cysts within the brain parenchyma do well without antiparasitic therapy. Most experts recommend therapy with albendazole or praziquantel for patients with nonenhancing or multiple cysticerci. Albendazole is preferred over praziquantel, because it has fewer drug-drug interactions with anticonvulsants. Coadministration of corticosteroids for the first 2 to 3 days of therapy may decrease adverse effects if more extensive viable central nervous system cysts are suspected. Arachnoiditis, vasculitis, or diffuse cerebral edema (cysticercal encephalitis) is treated with corticosteroid therapy until cerebral edema is controlled and albendazole or praziquantel therapy is completed.

Seizures may recur for months or years. Anticonvulsant therapy is recommended until there is neuroradiologic evidence of resolution and seizures have not occurred for 1 to 2 years. Calcification of cysts may require prolonged or indefinite use of anticonvulsants. Intraventricular cysts and hydrocephalus usually require surgical therapy. Intraventricular cysts often can be removed by endoscopic surgery, which is the treatment of choice. If cysts cannot be removed easily, hydrocephalus should be corrected with placement of intraventricular shunts. Adjunctive chemotherapy with antiparasitic agents and corticosteroids may decrease the rate of subsequent shunt failure. Ocular cysticercosis is treated by surgical excision of the cysts. Ocular and spinal cysts generally are not treated with anthelmintic drugs, which can exacerbate inflammation. An ophthalmic examination should be performed before treatment to rule out intraocular cysts.

ISOLATION OF THE HOSPITALIZED PATIENT: Standard precautions are recommended.

CONTROL MEASURES: Eating raw or undercooked beef or pork should be avoided. People known to harbor the adult tapeworm of *T solium* should be treated immediately. Careful attention to hand hygiene and appropriate disposal of fecal material is important.

Examination of stool specimens obtained from food handlers who recently have emigrated from countries with endemic infection for detection of eggs and proglottids is advisable. To prevent fecal-oral transmission of *T solium* eggs, people traveling to developing countries with high endemic rates of cysticercosis should avoid eating uncooked vegetables and fruits that cannot be peeled.

Other Tapeworm Infections
(Including Hydatid Disease)

Most infections are asymptomatic, but nausea, abdominal pain, and diarrhea have been observed in people who are heavily infected.

ETIOLOGIES

Hymenolepis nana. This tapeworm, also called dwarf tapeworm because it is the smallest of the adult tapeworms, has its entire cycle within humans. New infection is acquired by ingestion of eggs passed in feces of infected people. More problematic is autoinfection, which tends to perpetuate infection in the host, because eggs can hatch within the intestine and reinitiate the cycle, leading to development of new worms and a large worm burden. If infection persists after treatment, retreatment with praziquantel is indicated. Nitazoxanide is an alternative drug. Praziquantel and nitazoxanide are not approved for this indication, but dosing is provided for children 4 years of age and older (praziquantel) and 1 year of age and older (nitazoxanide) for other indications.

Dipylidium caninum. This tapeworm is the most common and widespread adult tapeworm of dogs and cats. *Dipylidium caninum* infects children when they inadvertently swallow a dog or cat flea, which serves as the intermediate host. Diagnosis is made by finding the characteristic eggs or motile proglottids in stool. Proglottids resemble rice kernels. Therapy with praziquantel is effective. Niclosamide is an alternative therapeutic option. Praziquantel and niclosamide are not approved for this indication, but dosing is provided for children 4 years of age and older (praziquantel) and 2 years of age and older (niclosamide) for other indications.

Diphyllobothrium latum **(and related species).** The *Diphyllobothrium latum* tapeworm, also called fish tapeworm, has fish as one of its intermediate hosts. Consumption of infected, raw freshwater fish (including salmon) leads to infection. Three to 5 weeks are needed for the adult tapeworm to mature and begin to lay eggs. The worm sometimes causes mechanical obstruction of the bowel or diarrhea, abdominal pain, or rarely, megaloblastic anemia secondary to vitamin B12 deficiency. Diagnosis is made by recognition of the characteristic eggs or proglottids passed in stool. Therapy with praziquantel is effective; niclosamide is an alternative. Praziquantel is not approved for this indication, but dosing is provided for children 4 years of age and older for other indications.

Echinococcus granulosus **and** *Echinococcus multilocularis.* The larval forms of these tapeworms are the causes of hydatid disease. The distribution of *Echinococcus granulosus* is related to sheep or cattle herding. Areas of high prevalence include parts of South America, East Africa, Eastern Europe, the Middle East, the Mediterranean region, China, and Central Asia. Disease also is endemic in Australia and New Zealand. In the United States, small foci of endemic infection exist in Arizona, California, New Mexico, and Utah, and a strain adapted to wolves, moose, and caribou occurs in Alaska and Canada. Dogs, coyotes, wolves, dingoes, and jackals can become infected by swallowing protoscolices of the parasite within hydatid cysts in the organs of sheep or other intermediate hosts. Dogs pass embryonated eggs in their stools, and sheep become infected by swallowing the eggs. If humans swallow *Echinococcus* eggs, they can become inadvertent intermediate hosts, and cysts can develop in various organs, such as the liver, lungs, kidney, and spleen. These cysts usually grow slowly (1 cm in diameter per year) and eventually can contain several liters of fluid. If a cyst ruptures, anaphylaxis and multiple secondary cysts from seeding of protoscolices can result. Clinical diagnosis often is difficult. A history of contact with dogs in an area with endemic infection is helpful. Cystic lesions can be demonstrated by radiography, ultrasonography, or computed tomography of various organs. Serologic tests, available at the Centers for Disease Control and Prevention, are helpful, but false-negative results occur. In uncomplicated cases, treatment of choice is **p**ercutaneous **a**spiration, **i**nfusion of scolicidal agents, and **r**easpiration (PAIR). PAIR should be performed at least a few days after initiation of albendazole chemotherapy. Contraindications to PAIR include communication of the cyst with the biliary tract (eg, bile staining after initial aspiration), superficial cysts, and heavily septated cysts. Surgical therapy is indicated for complicated cases and requires meticulous care to prevent spillage. Surgical drapes should be soaked in hypertonic saline. In general, the cyst should be removed intact, because leakage of contents is associated with a higher rate of complications. Treatment with albendazole generally should be initiated days to weeks before surgery and continued for several months afterwards.

Echinococcus multilocularis, a species whose life cycle involves foxes, dogs, and rodents, causes the alveolar form of hydatid disease, which is characterized by invasive growth of the larvae in the liver with occasional metastatic spread. The alveolar form of hydatid disease is limited to the northern hemisphere and usually is diagnosed in people 50 years of age or older. The preferred treatment is surgical removal of the entire larval mass. In nonresectable cases, continuous treatment with albendazole has been associated with clinical improvement. Efficacy of albendazole in the therapy of alveolar hydatid disease caused by *E multilocularis* has not been clearly demonstrated in clinical studies.

ISOLATION OF THE HOSPITALIZED PATIENT: Standard precautions are recommended.

CONTROL MEASURES: Preventive measures for *H nana* include educating the public about personal hygiene and sanitary disposal of feces.

Infection with *D caninum* is prevented by keeping dogs and cats free of fleas and worms.

Thorough cooking (56°C [133°F] for 5 minutes), freezing (−18°C [0°F] for 24 hours), or irradiation of freshwater fish ensures protection against *D latum.*

Control measures for prevention of *E granulosus* and *E multilocularis* include educating the public about hand hygiene and avoiding exposure to dog feces. Prevention and control of infection in dogs decreases the risk.

Tetanus
(Lockjaw)

CLINICAL MANIFESTATIONS: Generalized tetanus (lockjaw) is a neurologic disease manifesting as trismus and severe muscular spasms. Tetanus is caused by neurotoxin produced by the anaerobic bacterium *Clostridium tetani* in a contaminated wound. Onset is gradual, occurring over 1 to 7 days, and symptoms progress to severe generalized muscle spasms, which often are aggravated by any external stimulus. Severe spasms persist for 1 week or more and subside over several weeks in people who recover.

Neonatal tetanus is a form of generalized tetanus occurring in newborn infants lacking protective passive immunity because their mothers are not immune. Localized tetanus manifests as local muscle spasms in areas contiguous to a wound. Cephalic tetanus is a dysfunction of cranial nerves associated with infected wounds on the head and neck. Both of the latter conditions may precede generalized tetanus.

ETIOLOGY: *C tetani* is a spore-forming, anaerobic, gram-positive bacillus. This organism is a wound contaminant that causes neither tissue destruction nor an inflammatory response. The vegetative form of *C tetani* produces a potent plasmid-encoded exotoxin (tetanospasmin), which binds to gangliosides at the myoneural junction of skeletal muscle and on neuronal membranes in the spinal cord, blocking inhibitory impulses to motor neurons. The action of tetanus toxin on the brain and sympathetic nervous system is less well documented.

EPIDEMIOLOGY: Tetanus occurs worldwide and is more common in warmer climates and during warmer months, in part because of the higher frequency of contaminated wounds associated with those locations and seasons. The organism, a normal inhabitant of soil and animal and human intestines, is ubiquitous in the environment, especially where contamination by excreta is common. Organisms multiply in wounds, recognized or unrecognized, and elaborate toxins in the presence of anaerobic conditions. Contaminated wounds, especially wounds with devitalized tissue and deep-puncture trauma, are at greatest risk. Neonatal tetanus is common in many developing countries where women are not immunized appropriately against tetanus and nonsterile umbilical cord-care practices are followed. Widespread active immunization against tetanus has modified the epidemiology of disease in the United States, where 40 or fewer cases have been reported annually since 1999. Tetanus is not transmissible from person to person.

The **incubation period** ranges from 3 to 21 days, with most cases occurring within 8 days. Shorter incubation periods have been associated with more heavily contaminated wounds, more severe disease, and a worse prognosis. In neonatal tetanus, symptoms usually appear from 4 to 14 days after birth, averaging 7 days.

DIAGNOSTIC TESTS: The diagnosis of tetanus is made clinically by excluding other causes of tetanic spasms, such as hypocalcemic tetany, phenothiazine reaction, strychnine poisoning, and hysteria. Attempts to culture *C tetani* are associated with poor yield, and a negative culture does not rule out disease. A protective serum antitoxin concentration should not be used to exclude the diagnosis of tetanus.

TREATMENT:
- Human Tetanus Immune Globulin (TIG), 3000 to 6000 U, given in a single dose, is recommended for treatment; however, the optimal therapeutic dose has not been established. Some experts recommend 500 U, which appears to be as effective as higher doses and causes less discomfort. Available preparations must be given intramuscularly. Infiltration of part of the dose locally around the wound is recommended, although the efficacy of this approach has not been proven. Results of studies on the benefit from intrathecal administration of TIG are conflicting. The TIG preparation in use in the United States is not licensed or formulated for intrathecal or intravenous use.
- In countries where TIG is not available, equine tetanus antitoxin may be available. This product no longer is available in the United States. Equine antitoxin is administered after appropriate testing for sensitivity and desensitization if necessary (see Sensitivity Tests for Reactions to Animal Sera, p 62, and Desensitization to Animal Sera, p 63).

- Immune Globulin Intravenous (IGIV) contains antibodies to tetanus and can be considered for treatment in a dose of 200 to 400 mg/kg if TIG is not available. The US Food and Drug Administration has not licensed IGIV for this use.
- All wounds should be cleaned and débrided properly, especially if extensive necrosis is present. In neonatal tetanus, wide excision of the umbilical stump is not indicated.
- Supportive care and pharmacotherapy to control tetanic spasms are of major importance.
- Oral (or intravenous) metronidazole (30 mg/kg per day, given at 6-hour intervals; maximum, 4 g/day) is effective in decreasing the number of vegetative forms of *C tetani* and is the antimicrobial agent of choice. Parenteral penicillin G (100 000 U/kg per day, given at 4- to 6-hour intervals; maximum 12 million U/day) is an alternative treatment. Therapy for 10 to 14 days is recommended.

ISOLATION OF THE HOSPITALIZED PATIENT: Standard precautions are recommended.

CONTROL MEASURES:

Care of Exposed People (see Table 3.77). After primary immunization with tetanus toxoid, antitoxin persists at protective concentrations in most people for at least 10 years and for a longer time after a booster immunization.

- The use of tetanus toxoid with or without TIG in management of wounds depends on the nature of the wound and the history of immunization with tetanus toxoid, as described in Table 3.77.
- For infants younger than 6 months of age who have not received a full 3-dose primary series of tetanus toxoid-containing vaccine, decisions on the need for TIG with wound care should be based on the mother's tetanus toxoid immunization history at the time of delivery, applying the guidelines in Table 3.77.
- Although any open wound is a potential source of tetanus, wounds contaminated with dirt, feces, soil, or saliva are at increased risk. Punctures and wounds containing devitalized tissue, including necrotic or gangrenous wounds, frostbite, crush and avulsion injuries, and burns particularly are conducive to *C tetani* infection.

Table 3.77. Guide to Tetanus Prophylaxis in Routine Wound Management in Children 7 Years of Age and Older and Adolescents

History of Absorbed Tetanus Toxoid (Doses)	Clean, Minor Wounds		All Other Wounds[a]	
	Td or Tdap[b]	TIG[c]	Td or Tdap[b]	TIG[c]
Less than 3 or unknown	Yes	No	Yes	Yes
3 or more[d]	No[e]	No	No[f]	No

Td indicates adult-type diphtheria and tetanus toxoids vaccine; Tdap, booster tetanus toxoid, reduced diphtheria toxoid, and acellular pertussis; TIG, Tetanus Immune Globulin (human).

[a] Such as, but not limited to, wounds contaminated with dirt, feces, soil, and saliva; puncture wounds; avulsions; and wounds resulting from missiles, crushing, burns, and frostbite.

[b] Tdap is preferred to Td vaccine for adolescents who never have received Tdap vaccine. Td is preferred to tetanus toxoid (TT) vaccine for adolescents who received Tdap vaccine previously or when Tdap vaccine is not available.

[c] Immune Globulin Intravenous should be used when TIG is not available.

[d] If only 3 doses of fluid toxoid have been received, a fourth dose of toxoid, preferably an adsorbed toxoid, should be given. Although licensed, fluid tetanus toxoid rarely is used.

[e] Yes, if 10 years or longer since last tetanus-containing vaccine dose.

[f] Yes, if 5 years or longer since last tetanus-containing vaccine dose. More frequent boosters are not needed and can accentuate adverse effects.

- If tetanus immunization is incomplete at the time of wound treatment, a dose of vaccine should be given, and the immunization series should be completed according to the age-appropriate primary immunization schedule. TIG should be administered for tetanus-prone wounds in patients infected with human immunodeficiency virus, regardless of the history of tetanus immunizations.
- Diphtheria and tetanus toxoids and acellular pertussis (DTaP) is the recommended and preferred vaccine for children 6 weeks through 6 years of age and for catch-up immunization for children 4 months through 6 years of age (see Fig 1.3, p 28). When a booster injection is indicated for wound prophylaxis in a child younger than 7 years of age, DTaP should be used unless pertussis vaccine is contraindicated (see Pertussis, p 504), in which case immunization with diphtheria and tetanus toxoids (DT) vaccine is recommended.
- When tetanus toxoid is required for wound prophylaxis in a child 7 through 10 years of age, use of adult-type diphtheria and tetanus toxoids (Td) vaccine instead of tetanus toxoid alone is advisable so that diphtheria immunity also is maintained.
- Adolescents 10 through 18 years of age who require a tetanus toxoid-containing vaccine as part of wound management should receive a single dose of tetanus toxoid, reduced diphtheria toxoid, and acellular pertussis (Tdap) instead of Td if they have not received Tdap previously. If Tdap is not available or was administered previously, adolescents who need a tetanus toxoid-containing vaccine should receive Td (see Pertussis, p 504). People 19 through 64 years of age who require a tetanus toxoid-containing vaccine as part of wound management should receive Tdap instead of Td if they previously have not received Tdap.
- When TIG is required for wound prophylaxis, it is given intramuscularly in a dose of 250 U (regardless of age or weight). IGIV or equine tetanus antitoxin is recommended if TIG is unavailable. Equine antitoxin should be given after appropriate testing of the patient for sensitivity (see Sensitivity Tests for Reactions to Animal Sera, p 62). Equine antitoxin is not available in the United States. If tetanus toxoid and TIG, IGIV, or equine tetanus antitoxin are given concurrently, separate syringes and sites should be used. Administration of TIG, IGIV, or equine tetanus antitoxin does not preclude initiation of active immunization with adsorbed tetanus toxoid. Efforts should be made to initiate immunization and arrange for its completion. Administration of tetanus toxoid simultaneously or at an interval after receipt of Immune Globulin does not impair development of protective antibody substantially.
- Regardless of immunization status, wounds should be cleaned and débrided properly if dirt or necrotic tissue is present. Wounds should receive prompt surgical treatment to remove all devitalized tissue and foreign material as an essential part of tetanus prophylaxis. It is not necessary or appropriate to débride puncture wounds extensively.

Immunization. Active immunization with tetanus toxoid is recommended for all people. For all appropriate indications, tetanus immunization is administered with diphtheria toxoid-containing vaccines or with diphtheria toxoid- and acellular pertussis-containing vaccines. Vaccine is given intramuscularly and may be given concurrently with other vaccines (see Simultaneous Administration of Multiple Vaccines, p 33). *Haemophilus influenzae* type b conjugate vaccines containing tetanus toxoid (PRP-T) are not substitutes for tetanus toxoid immunization. Recommendations for use of tetanus toxoid-containing vaccines (summarized in Fig 1.1–1.3 [p 24–28]) are as follows:

- Immunization for children from 2 months of age to the seventh birthday (see Fig 1.1, p 24–25, and Fig 1.3, p 28) should consist of 5 doses of tetanus and diphtheria toxoid-containing vaccine. The initial 3 doses are given as DTaP administered at 2-month intervals beginning at approximately 2 months of age. A fourth dose is recommended 6 to 12 months after the third dose, usually at 15 through 18 months of age (see Pertussis, p 504). The final dose of DTaP is recommended before school entry (kindergarten or elementary school) at 4 through 6 years of age, unless the fourth dose was given after the fourth birthday. DTaP can be given concurrently with other vaccines (see Simultaneous Administration of Multiple Vaccines, p 33).
- For children younger than 7 years of age who have received fewer than the recommended number of doses of pertussis vaccine but who have received the recommended number of DT doses for their age (ie, children in whom immunization was started with DT and who then were given DTaP [or DTP]), dose(s) of DTaP should be given to complete the recommended pertussis immunization schedule (see Pertussis, p 504). However, the total number of doses of diphtheria and tetanus toxoids (as DT, DTaP, or DTP) should not exceed 6 before the seventh birthday.
- Immunization against tetanus and diphtheria for children younger than 7 years of age in whom pertussis immunization is contraindicated (see Pertussis, p 504) should be accomplished with DT instead of DTaP, as follows:
  - For children younger than 1 year of age, 3 doses of DT are given at 2-month intervals; a fourth dose should be given 6 to 12 months after the third dose, and the fifth dose should be given before school entry at 4 through 6 years of age.
  - For children 1 through 6 years of age who have not received previous doses of DT, DTaP, or diphtheria and tetanus toxoids and whole-cell pertussis vaccine (DTP), 2 doses of DT approximately 2 months apart should be given, followed by a third dose 6 to 12 months later to complete the initial series. DT can be given concurrently with other vaccines. An additional dose is recommended before school entry at 4 through 6 years of age unless the preceding dose was given after the fourth birthday.
  - For children 1 through 6 years of age who have received 1 or 2 doses of DTaP, DTP, or DT during the first year of life and for whom further pertussis immunization is contraindicated, additional doses of DT should be given until a total of 5 doses of diphtheria and tetanus toxoids are received by the time of school entry. The fourth dose is administered 6 to 12 months after the third dose. The preschool (fifth) dose is omitted if the fourth dose was given after the fourth birthday.

Other recommendations for tetanus immunization, including recommendations for older children, are as follows:

- For children 7 through 10 years of age (see Fig 1.3, p 28), tetanus immunization should be accomplished with Td (ie, adult-type diphtheria and tetanus toxoids). Because of the lower dose of diphtheria toxoid, Td is less likely than DTaP or DT to produce adverse reactions in older children and adults. Two doses are given 1 to 2 months apart; a third dose should be given 6 to 12 months after the second.
- Adolescents 11 through 18 years of age should receive a single dose of Tdap instead of Td for booster immunization against tetanus, diphtheria, and pertussis if they have completed the recommended childhood DTP/DTaP immunization series and have not received Td or Tdap. The preferred age for Tdap immunization is 11 through 12 years; routinely administering Tdap to young adolescents will reduce the morbidity associated with pertussis in adolescents.

- Adolescents 11 through 18 years of age who received Td but not Tdap are encouraged to receive a single dose of Tdap to provide protection against pertussis if they have completed the recommended childhood DTP/DTaP immunization series. An interval of 5 years from the last Td dose is encouraged when Tdap is used as a booster dose, but a shorter interval may be used. The benefits of protection from pertussis generally outweigh the risk of local or systemic reactions in settings with increased risk of pertussis (eg, pertussis outbreaks and close contact with an infant younger than 6 months of age).
- If more than 5 years have elapsed since the last dose, a booster of a tetanus-containing vaccine should be considered for people at risk of occupational or avocational exposure where tetanus boosters may not be available readily. Tdap is preferred to Td if the person has not received Tdap previously.
- Prevention of neonatal tetanus can be accomplished by prenatal immunization of the previously unimmunized mother. Pregnant women who have not completed their primary series should do so before delivery if time permits. If there is insufficient time, 2 doses of Td should be administered at least 4 weeks apart, and the second dose should be given at least 2 weeks before delivery. Immunization with tetanus toxoid Td or Tdap is not contraindicated during pregnancy (see Pertussis, p 504).
- Active immunization against tetanus always should be undertaken during convalescence from tetanus, because this exotoxin-mediated disease usually does not confer immunity.

Adverse Events, Precautions, and Contraindications. Severe anaphylactic reactions, Guillain-Barré syndrome (GBS), and brachial neuritis attributable to tetanus toxoid have been reported but are rare. No increased risk of GBS has been observed with use of DTaP in children, and therefore, no special precautions are recommended when immunizing children with a history of GBS.

An immediate anaphylactic reaction to tetanus and diphtheria toxoid-containing vaccines (ie, DTaP, Tdap, DT, or Td) is a contraindication to further doses unless the patient can be desensitized to these toxoids (see Pertussis, p 504). Because of uncertainty about which vaccine component (ie, diphtheria, tetanus, or pertussis) might be responsible and the importance of tetanus immunization, people who experience anaphylactic reactions may be referred to an allergist for evaluation and possible desensitization to tetanus toxoid.

Other Control Measures. Sterilization of hospital supplies will prevent the rare instances of tetanus that may occur in a hospital from contaminated sutures, instruments, or plaster casts.

For prevention of neonatal tetanus, preventive measures (in addition to maternal immunization) include community immunization programs for adolescent girls and women of childbearing age and appropriate training of midwives in recommendations for immunization and sterile technique.

Tinea Capitis
(Ringworm of the Scalp)

CLINICAL MANIFESTATIONS: Fungal infection of the scalp may manifest as one of the following distinct clinical syndromes:
- Patchy areas of dandruff-like scaling, with subtle or extensive hair loss, which easily is confused with dandruff, seborrheic dermatitis, or atopic dermatitis;
- Discrete areas of hair loss studded by stubs of broken hairs, which is referred to as *black-dot ringworm;*
- Numerous discrete pustules or excoriations with little hair loss or scaling; or
- Kerion, a boggy inflammatory mass surrounded by follicular pustules, which is a hypersensitivity reaction to the fungal infection (may be accompanied by fever and local lymphadenopathy and commonly is misdiagnosed as impetigo, cellulitis, or an abscess of the scalp).

A pruritic, fine, papulovesicular eruption (dermatophytid or id reaction) involving the trunk, hands, or face caused by a hypersensitivity response to the infecting fungus, may accompany scalp lesions.

Tinea capitis may be confused with many other diseases, including seborrheic dermatitis, atopic dermatitis, psoriasis, alopecia areata, trichotillomania, folliculitis, impetigo, and lupus erythematosus.

ETIOLOGY: *Trichophyton tonsurans* is the cause of tinea capitis in more than 90% of cases in North and Central America. *Microsporum canis, Microsporum audouinii,* and *Trichophyton mentagrophytes* are less common. Causative agents may vary in different geographic areas.

EPIDEMIOLOGY: Infection of the scalp with *T tonsurans* results from person-to-person transmission. Although the organism remains viable on combs, hairbrushes, and other fomites for long periods of time, the role of fomites in transmission has not been defined. Occasionally, *T tonsurans* is cultured from the scalp of asymptomatic children or family members of an index case. Asymptomatic carriers are thought to have a significant role as reservoirs for infection and reinfection within families, schools, and communities. Tinea capitis attributable to *T tonsurans* occurs most commonly in children between 3 and 9 years of age and appears to be more common in black children.

M canis infection results from animal-to-human transmission. Infection often is the result of contact with household pets.

The **incubation period** is unknown.

DIAGNOSTIC TESTS: Potassium hydroxide wet mount, cultures, and/or Wood light examination may be used to confirm the diagnosis before treatment. Hairs obtained by gentle scraping of a moistened area of the scalp with a blunt scalpel, toothbrush, tweezers, or a moistened cotton swab are used for potassium hydroxide wet mount examination and culture. In black-dot ringworm, broken hairs should be obtained for diagnosis. In cases of *T tonsurans* infection, microscopic examination of a potassium hydroxide wet mount preparation will disclose numerous arthroconidia within the hair shaft. In *Microsporum* infection, spores surround the hair shaft. Use of dermatophyte test medium also is a reliable, simple, and inexpensive method of diagnosing tinea capitis. Skin scrapings, brushings, or hairs from lesions are inoculated directly onto culture medium and incubated at room temperature. After 1 to 2 weeks, a phenol red indicator in the agar will turn from yellow to red in the area surrounding a dermatophyte colony. When necessary, the diagnosis also may be confirmed by culture on Sabouraud dextrose agar by direct plating technique or by moistened cotton-tipped applicators or by Culturettes transported to reference laboratories.

Examination of hair of patients with *Microsporum* infection using Wood light results in brilliant green fluorescence. However, because *T tonsurans* does not fluoresce under Wood light, this diagnostic test is not helpful for most patients with tinea capitis.

TREATMENT: Because topical antifungal medications are not effective for treatment of tinea capitis, systemic antifungal therapy is required. Microsize griseofulvin, 10 to 20 mg/kg per day (maximum, 1 g), or ultramicrosize griseofulvin, 5 to 15 mg/kg per day (maximum, 750 mg), is given orally once daily. Optimally, griseofulvin is given after a meal containing fat (eg, peanut butter or ice cream). Treatment for 4 to 6 weeks typically is necessary and should be continued 2 weeks beyond clinical resolution. Some children may require higher doses to achieve clinical cure. Griseofulvin is approved for children older than 2 years of age. Children who have no history or clinical evidence of liver disease are not required to have serum hepatic enzyme values tested either before or during a standard course of therapy lasting up to 8 weeks. Prolonged therapy may be associated with a greater risk of hepatotoxicity, and enzyme testing every 8 weeks during treatment should be considered. A 6-week course of terbinafine in the form of oral granules has been shown to be as effective as a 6-week course of griseofulvin for treatment of *Tinea capitis* in children 4 years of age and older. Terbinafine dosage is based on body weight (67.5 mg/day for patients weighing less than 20 kg; 125 mg/day for patients weighing 20-40 kg; and 250 mg for patients weighing more than 40 kg). Baseline serum transaminase (alanine transaminase and aspartate transaminase) testing is advised. Treatment with oral itraconazole or fluconazole may be effective for tinea capitis; itraconazole is not approved for use in children. Selenium sulfide shampoo, either 1% or 2.5%, used twice a week, decreases fungal shedding and may help curb the spread of infection.

Kerion is treated with griseofulvin. Corticosteroid therapy consisting of prednisone or prednisolone given orally in dosages of 1.5 to 2 mg/kg per day (maximum, 20 mg/day) may be used in addition. Treatment with corticosteroids should be continued for approximately 2 weeks, with tapering doses toward the end of therapy. Antibacterial agents generally are not needed, except if there is suspected secondary infection. Surgery is not indicated.

ISOLATION OF THE HOSPITALIZED PATIENT: Standard precautions are recommended.

CONTROL MEASURES: Early treatment of infected people is indicated, as is examination of siblings and other household contacts for evidence of tinea capitis. Sharing of ribbons, combs, and hairbrushes should be discouraged.

Children receiving treatment for tinea capitis may attend school once they start therapy with griseofulvin or other effective systemic agent, with or without the addition of selenium sulfide shampoo. Haircuts, shaving of the head, or wearing a cap during treatment are unnecessary.

Tinea Corporis
(Ringworm of the Body)

CLINICAL MANIFESTATIONS: Superficial tinea infections of the nonhairy (glabrous) skin may involve the face, trunk, or limbs but not the scalp, beard, groin, hands, or feet. The lesion generally is circular (hence, the term "ringworm"), slightly erythematous, and well demarcated with a scaly, vesicular, or pustular border. Pruritus is common. Lesions often are mistaken for atopic, seborrheic, or contact dermatitis. A frequent source of confusion is an alteration in the appearance of lesions as a result of application of a topical corticosteroid preparation, termed *tinea incognito*. In patients with diminished T-lymphocyte function (eg, human immunodeficiency virus infection), the rash may appear as grouped papules or pustules unaccompanied by scaling or erythema.

A pruritic, fine, papulovesicular eruption (dermatophytic or id reaction) involving the trunk, hands, or face, caused by a hypersensitivity response to infecting fungus, may accompany the rash.

ETIOLOGY: The prime causes of the disease are fungi of the genus *Trichophyton*, especially *Trichophyton rubrum*, *Trichophyton mentagrophytes*, and *Trichophyton tonsurans;* the genus *Microsporum*, especially *Microsporum canis;* and *Epidermophyton floccosum.*

EPIDEMIOLOGY: These causative fungi occur worldwide and are transmissible by direct contact with infected humans, animals, or fomites. Fungi in lesions are communicable.

The **incubation period** is unknown.

DIAGNOSIS: The fungi responsible for tinea corporis can be detected by microscopic examination of a potassium hydroxide wet mount of skin scrapings. Use of dermatophyte test medium also is a reliable, simple, and inexpensive method of diagnosis. Skin scrapings from lesions are inoculated directly onto culture medium and incubated at room temperature. After 1 to 2 weeks, a phenol red indicator in the agar will turn from yellow to red in the area surrounding a dermatophyte colony. When necessary, the diagnosis also can be confirmed by culture on Sabouraud dextrose agar.

TREATMENT: Topical application of a miconazole, clotrimazole, terbinafine (12 years of age and older), tolnaftate, naftifine, or ciclopirox (10 years of age and older) preparation twice a day or of a ketoconazole, econazole, oxiconazole, butenafine (12 years of age and older), or sulconazole preparation once a day is recommended (see Topical Drugs for Superficial Fungal Infections, p 773). Topical econazole, ketoconazole, naftifine, and sulconazole are not approved by the US Food and Drug Administration for use as antifungal agents in children. Although clinical resolution may be evident within 2 weeks of therapy, a minimum duration of 4 to 6 weeks generally is indicated. Topical preparations of antifungal medication mixed with high-potency corticosteroids should not be used because of the potential for local and systemic adverse events.

If lesions are extensive or unresponsive to topical therapy, griseofulvin is administered orally for 4 weeks (see Tinea Capitis, p 661). Oral itraconazole and terbinafine are more effective therapies for tinea corporis in adults.

ISOLATION OF THE HOSPITALIZED PATIENT: Standard precautions are recommended.

CONTROL MEASURES: Direct contact with known or suspected sources of infection should be avoided. Periodic inspections of contacts for early lesions and prompt therapy are recommended.

Tinea Cruris
(Jock Itch)

CLINICAL MANIFESTATIONS: Tinea cruris is a common superficial fungal disorder of the groin and upper thighs. The eruption is marginated sharply and usually is bilaterally symmetric. Involved skin is erythematous and scaly and varies from red to brown; occasionally, the eruption is accompanied by central clearing and a vesiculopapular border. In chronic infections, the margin may be subtle, and lichenification may be present. Tinea cruris skin lesions may be extremely pruritic. These lesions should be differentiated from intertrigo, seborrheic dermatitis, psoriasis, primary irritant dermatitis, allergic contact dermatitis (generally caused by the therapeutic agents applied to the area), or erythrasma, which is a superficial bacterial infection of the skin caused by *Corynebacterium minutissimum*.

ETIOLOGY: The fungi *Epidermophyton floccosum, Trichophyton rubrum,* and *Trichophyton mentagrophytes* are the most common causes.

EPIDEMIOLOGY: Tinea cruris occurs predominantly in adolescent and adult males, mainly via indirect contact from desquamated epithelium or hair. Moisture, close-fitting garments, friction, and obesity are predisposing factors. Direct or indirect person-to-person transmission may occur. This infection commonly occurs in association with tinea pedis.

The **incubation period** is unknown.

DIAGNOSTIC TESTS: The fungi responsible for tinea cruris may be detected by microscopic examination of a potassium hydroxide wet mount of scales. Use of dermatophyte test medium also is a reliable, simple, and inexpensive method of diagnosing tinea cruris. Skin scrapings from lesions are inoculated directly onto culture medium and incubated at room temperature. After 1 to 2 weeks, a phenol red indicator in the agar will turn from yellow to red in the area surrounding a dermatophyte colony. When necessary, the diagnosis also can be confirmed by culture on Sabouraud dextrose agar. A characteristic coral-red fluorescence under Wood light can identify the presence of erythrasma and, thus, exclude tinea cruris.

TREATMENT: Twice-daily topical application for 4 to 6 weeks of a clotrimazole, miconazole, terbinafine (12 years of age and older), tolnaftate, or ciclopirox (10 years of age and older) preparation rubbed or sprayed onto the affected areas and surrounding skin is effective. Once-daily therapy with topical econazole, ketoconazole, naftifine, oxiconazole, butenafine (12 years of age and older), or sulconazole preparation also is effective (see Topical Drugs for Superficial Fungal Infections, p 773). Topical econazole, ketoconazole, naftifine, and sulconazole are not approved by the US Food and Drug Administration for use as antifungal agents in children. Tinea pedis, if present, should be treated concurrently (see Tinea Pedis, p 665).

Topical preparations of antifungal medication mixed with high-potency corticosteroids should be avoided because of the potential for local and systemic adverse events. Corticosteroids may cause local and/or systemic effects or predispose to recurrence. Loose-fitting, washed cotton underclothes to decrease chafing as well as the use of an absorbent powder can be helpful adjuvants to therapy. Griseofulvin, given orally for 2 to 6 weeks, may be effective in unresponsive cases (see Tinea Capitis, p 661). Oral itraconazole and terbinafine are more effective therapies in adults. Because many conditions mimic tinea cruris, a differential diagnosis should be considered if primary treatments fail.

ISOLATION OF THE HOSPITALIZED PATIENT: Standard precautions are recommended.

CONTROL MEASURES: Infections should be treated promptly. Potentially involved areas should be kept dry, and loose undergarments should be worn. Patients should be advised to dry the groin area before drying their feet to avoid inoculating dermatophytes of tinea pedis into the groin area.

Tinea Pedis and Tinea Unguium
(Athlete's Foot, Ringworm of the Feet)

CLINICAL MANIFESTATIONS: Tinea pedis manifests as fine vesiculopustular or scaly lesions that commonly are pruritic. The lesions can involve all areas of the foot, but usually lesions are patchy in distribution, with a predisposition to fissures and scaling between toes, particularly in the third and fourth interdigital spaces. Toenails may be infected and can be dystrophic (tinea unguium). Tinea pedis must be differentiated from dyshidrotic eczema, atopic dermatitis, contact dermatitis, juvenile plantar dermatosis, and erythrasma (a superficial bacterial infection caused by *Corynebacterium minutissimum*). Tinea pedis commonly occurs in association with tinea cruris and onychomycosis (tinea unguium) a nail infection by any fungus. Dermatophyte infections commonly affect otherwise healthy people, but immunocompromised people have increased susceptibility.

Tinea pedis and many other fungal infections can be accompanied by a hypersensitivity reaction to the fungi (the dermatophytid or id reaction), with resulting vesicular eruptions on the palms and the sides of fingers and, occasionally, by an erythematous vesicular eruption on the extremities and trunk.

ETIOLOGY: The fungi *Trichophyton rubrum*, *Trichophyton mentagrophytes*, and *Epidermophyton floccosum* are the most common causes.

EPIDEMIOLOGY: Tinea pedis is a common infection worldwide in adolescents and adults but is relatively uncommon in young children. The fungi are acquired by contact with skin scales containing fungi or with fungi in damp areas, such as swimming pools, locker rooms, and shower rooms. Tinea pedis can spread throughout the household among family members and is communicable for as long as infection is present.

The **incubation period** is unknown.

DIAGNOSIS: Tinea pedis usually is diagnosed by clinical manifestations and may be confirmed by microscopic examination of a potassium hydroxide wet mount of the cutaneous scrapings. Use of dermatophyte test medium is a reliable, simple, and inexpensive method of diagnosis in complicated or unresponsive cases. Skin scrapings are inoculated directly onto the culture medium and incubated at room temperature. After 1 to 2 weeks, a phenol red indicator in the agar will turn from yellow to red in the area surrounding a dermatophyte colony. When necessary, the diagnosis also can be confirmed by culture on Sabouraud dextrose agar. Infection of the nail can be verified by direct microscopic examination and fungal culture of desquamated subungual material.

TREATMENT: Topical application of terbinafine, twice daily, or an azole agent (clotrimazole, miconazole, econazole, oxiconazole, sertaconazole), once or twice daily, usually is adequate for milder cases. Acute vesicular lesions may be treated with intermittent use of open wet compresses (eg, with Burrow solution, 1:80). Tinea cruris, if present, should be treated concurrently (see Tinea Cruris, p 664).

Tinea pedis that is severe, chronic or refractory to topical treatment may be treated with oral griseofulvin, administered orally for 6 to 8 weeks. Fluconazole administered orally once per week for 1 to 4 weeks may be an effective alternative therapy. Oral itraconazole or terbinafine may also be effective alternative therapies for tinea pedis unresponsive to topical therapy. Id (hypersensitivity response) reactions are treated by wet compresses, topical corticosteroids, occasionally systemic corticosteroids, and eradication of the primary source of infection.

Recurrence is prevented by proper foot hygiene, which includes keeping the feet dry and cool, gentle cleaning, drying between the toes, use of absorbent antifungal foot powder, frequent airing of affected areas, and avoidance of occlusive footwear and nylon socks or other fabrics that interfere with dissipation of moisture.

In people with onychomycosis (tinea unguium), topical therapy should be used only when the infection is confined to the distal ends of the nail; this approach frequently is not effective, and therapy must be continued for 6 to 12 months. Topical ciclopirox (8%) may be applied to affected toenail(s) once daily (best evaluated in people 12 years of age and older). Studies in adults have demonstrated a modest cure rate after therapy with oral itraconazole or terbinafine. In adults, pulse therapy with terbinafine (1 week each month for 3 to 6 months) is preferred treatment. Recurrences are common. Removal of the nail plate followed by use of oral therapy during the period of regrowth can help to effect a cure in resistant cases.

ISOLATION OF THE HOSPITALIZED PATIENT: Standard precautions are recommended.

CONTROL MEASURES: Treatment of patients with active infections should decrease transmission. Public areas conducive to transmission (eg, swimming pools) should not be used by people with active infection. Chemical foot baths are of no value and can facilitate spread of infection. Because recurrence after treatment is common, proper foot hygiene is important (as described in Treatment). People should be advised to dry the groin area before drying their feet to avoid inoculating tinea pedis dermatophytes into the groin area.

Toxocariasis
(Visceral Larva Migrans, Ocular Larva Migrans)

CLINICAL MANIFESTATIONS: The severity of symptoms depends on the number of larvae ingested and the degree of allergic response. Most people who are infected lightly are asymptomatic. Visceral larva migrans typically occurs in children 1 to 4 years of age with a history of pica but can occur in older children and adults. Characteristic manifestations include fever, leukocytosis, eosinophilia, hypergammaglobulinemia, and hepatomegaly. Other manifestations include malaise, anemia, cough, and in rare instances, pneumonia, myocarditis, and encephalitis. When ocular invasion (endophthalmitis or retinal granulomas) occurs (usually in older children or adolescents), other evidence of infection usually is lacking, suggesting that the visceral and ocular manifestations are distinct syndromes. Atypical manifestations include hemorrhagic rash and seizures. In some cases, so-called covert toxocariasis may manifest only as asymptomatic eosinophilia or pulmonary wheezing.

ETIOLOGY: Toxocariasis is caused by *Toxocara* species, which are common roundworms of dogs and cats (especially puppies or kittens), specifically *Toxocara canis* and *Toxocara cati* in the United States; most cases are caused by *T canis.* Other nematodes of animals also can cause this syndrome, although rarely.

EPIDEMIOLOGY: Humans are infected by ingestion of soil containing infective eggs of the parasite. A history of pica, particularly eating soil, is common. Direct contact with dogs is of secondary importance, because eggs are not infective immediately when shed in the feces. Most reported cases involve children. Toxocariasis is endemic wherever dogs are present. Infection risk is highest in hot, humid regions where eggs persist in soil. The infection is endemic in many underserved urban areas in the United States. Eggs may be found wherever dogs and cats defecate.

The **incubation period** is unknown.

DIAGNOSTIC TESTS: Hypereosinophilia and hypergammaglobulinemia associated with increased titers of isohemagglutinin to the A and B blood group antigens are presumptive evidence of infection. Microscopic identification of larvae in a liver biopsy specimen is diagnostic, but this finding is rare. A liver biopsy negative for larvae, therefore, does not exclude the diagnosis. An enzyme immunoassay for *Toxocara* antibodies in serum, available at the Centers for Disease Control and Prevention and some commercial laboratories, can provide confirmatory evidence of toxocariasis. This assay is specific and sensitive for diagnosis of visceral larva migrans but is less sensitive for diagnosis of ocular larva migrans.

TREATMENT: Albendazole is the recommended drug for treatment of toxocariasis (see Drugs for Parasitic Infections, p 783). The drug has been approved by the US Food and Drug Administration, but not for this indication. In severe cases with myocarditis or involvement of the central nervous system, corticosteroid therapy is indicated. Correcting the underlying causes of pica helps prevent reinfection.

Recommended treatment of ocular larva migrans may not be effective. Inflammation may be decreased by injection of corticosteroids, and secondary damage may be aided by surgery.

ISOLATION OF THE HOSPITALIZED PATIENT: Standard precautions are recommended.

CONTROL MEASURES: Proper disposal of cat and dog feces is essential. Treatment of puppies and kittens with anthelmintics at 2, 4, 6, and 8 weeks of age prevents excretion of eggs by worms acquired transplacentally or through mother's milk. Covering sandboxes when not in use is helpful. No specific management of exposed people is recommended.

Toxoplasma gondii Infections
(Toxoplasmosis)

CLINICAL MANIFESTATIONS: Infants with congenital infection are asymptomatic at birth in 70% to 90% of cases, although visual impairment, learning disabilities, or mental retardation will become apparent in a large proportion of children several months to years later. Signs of congenital toxoplasmosis at birth can include a maculopapular rash, generalized lymphadenopathy, hepatomegaly, splenomegaly, jaundice, and thrombocytopenia. As a consequence of intrauterine infection, meningoencephalitis, cerebrospinal fluid (CSF) abnormalities, hydrocephalus, microcephaly, chorioretinitis, seizures, and deafness can develop. Some severely affected infants die in utero or within a few days of birth. Cerebral calcifications may be demonstrated by radiography, ultrasonography, or computed tomography of the head.

Toxoplasma gondii infection acquired after birth may be asymptomatic, except in immunocompromised people. When symptoms develop, they are nonspecific and include malaise, fever, sore throat, and myalgia. Lymphadenopathy, frequently cervical, is the most common sign. Occasionally, patients may have a mononucleosis-like illness associated with a macular rash and hepatosplenomegaly. The clinical course usually is benign and self-limited. Myocarditis, pericarditis, and pneumonitis are rare complications.

Isolated ocular toxoplasmosis commonly results from reactivation of untreated congenital infection but also occurs in a small percentage of people with acquired infection. However, because many people become infected with *T gondii* after birth, even this small percentage results in a large proportion of all toxoplasmic ocular disease being attributable to infection after birth. Characteristic retinal lesions (chorioretinitis) develop in up to 85% of young adults after untreated congenital infection. Acute ocular involvement manifests as blurred vision. Ocular disease can become reactivated years after the initial infection in healthy and immunocompromised people.

In chronically infected immunodeficient patients, including people with human immunodeficiency virus (HIV) infection, reactivated infection can result in encephalitis, pneumonitis, or less commonly, systemic toxoplasmosis. Rarely, infants who are born to HIV-infected mothers or mothers who are immunocompromised for other reasons and who have chronic infection with *T gondii* may have acquired congenital toxoplasmosis in utero as a result of reactivated maternal parasitemia.

ETIOLOGY: *T gondii*, a protozoan parasite, is the only known species of *Toxoplasma*.

EPIDEMIOLOGY: *T gondii* is worldwide in distribution and infects most species of warm-blooded animals. Members of the feline family are definitive hosts. Cats generally acquire the infection by feeding on infected animals, such as mice or uncooked household meats. The parasite replicates sexually in the feline small intestine. Cats may begin to excrete oocysts in their stools 3 to 30 days after primary infection and may shed oocysts for 7 to 14 days. After excretion, oocysts require a maturation phase (sporulation) of 24 to 48 hours in temperate climates before they are infective by the oral route. Intermediate hosts (including sheep, pigs, and cattle) can have tissue cysts in the brain, myocardium, skeletal muscle, and other organs. These cysts remain viable for the lifetime of the host. Humans usually become infected by consumption of raw or undercooked meat that contains cysts or by accidental ingestion of sporulated oocysts from soil or in contaminated food or water. A large outbreak linked epidemiologically to contamination of a municipal water supply also has been reported. Transmission of *T gondii* has been documented to result from blood or blood product transfusion and organ (eg, heart) or stem cell transplantation from a seropositive donor with latent infection. Rarely, infection has occurred as a result of a laboratory accident. In most cases, congenital transmission occurs as a result of primary maternal infection during gestation. The incidence of congenital toxoplasmosis in the United States has been estimated to be 1 in 1000 to 1 in 10 000 live births.

The **incubation period** of acquired infection, on the basis of a well-studied outbreak, is estimated to be approximately 7 days, with a range of 4 to 21 days.

DIAGNOSTIC TESTS: Serologic tests are the primary means of diagnosis, but results must be interpreted carefully. Laboratories with special expertise in *Toxoplasma* serologic assays and their interpretation, such as the Remington lab (**www.pamf.org/serology**), are useful to the practitioner. Immunoglobulin (Ig) G-specific antibodies achieve a peak concentration 1 to 2 months after infection and remain positive indefinitely. To determine the approximate time of infection in IgG-positive adults, specific IgM antibody determinations should be performed. The lack of *T gondii*-specific IgM antibodies in a person with IgG antibodies indicates infection more than 6 months ago. The presence of *T gondii*-specific IgM antibodies can indicate recent infection or can result from a false-positive reaction. Enzyme immunoassays are the more sensitive tests for IgM, and indirect fluorescent antibody tests are the least sensitive tests for detecting IgM. IgM-specific antibodies can be detected 2 weeks after infection, achieve peak concentrations in 1 month, decrease thereafter, and usually become undetectable within 6 to 9 months. In adults, when determining the timing of infection is important clinically (eg, in a pregnant woman), a positive IgM test should be followed by an IgG avidity test. The presence of high-avidity IgG antibodies indicates that infection occurred at least 12 to 16 weeks previously. However, the presence of low-avidity antibodies is not a reliable indication of recent infection and treatment may affect the maturation of IgG avidity and prolong the presence of low-avidity antibodies. Tests to detect IgA and IgE antibodies, which decrease to undetectable concentrations sooner than do IgM antibodies, are useful for diagnosis of congenital infections and infections in other patients, such as pregnant women, for whom more precise information about the duration of infection is needed. *T gondii*-specific IgA and IgE antibody tests are available in *Toxoplasma* reference laboratories but not generally in other laboratories. Diagnosis of *Toxoplasma* infection during pregnancy should be made on the basis of results of serologic assays performed in a reference laboratory.

Special Situations.

Prenatal. A definitive diagnosis of congenital toxoplasmosis can be made prenatally by detecting parasite DNA in amniotic fluid or fetal blood or by isolating the parasite by mouse or tissue culture inoculation. Serial fetal ultrasonographic examinations can be performed in cases of suspected congenital infection to detect any increase in size of the lateral ventricles of the central nervous system or other signs of fetal infection.

Postnatal. Infants who are born to women who have evidence of primary *T gondii* infection during gestation or women who are infected with HIV and have serologic evidence of past infection with *T gondii* should be assessed for congenital toxoplasmosis.

If the diagnosis for an infant is unclear at the time of delivery, *Toxoplasma*-specific laboratory tests for IgG, IgM, IgA, and IgE on newborn and maternal serum samples should be performed. Peripheral blood white blood cells, CSF, and amniotic fluid specimens should be assayed for *T gondii* by polymerase chain reaction assay in a reference laboratory. Evaluation of the infant should include ophthalmologic, auditory, and neurologic examinations; lumbar puncture; and computed tomography of the head. An attempt may be made to isolate *T gondii* from the placenta, umbilical cord, or blood specimen from the infant by mouse inoculation.

Congenital infection is confirmed serologically by persistently positive IgG titers beyond the first 12 months of life. Before 12 months of age, a persistently positive or increasing IgG antibody concentration in the infant compared with the mother, and/or a positive *Toxoplasma*-specific IgM or IgA assay indicate congenital infection. Although placental leak occasionally can lead to false-positive IgM or IgA reactions in the newborn infant, repeat testing in approximately 10 days can help resolve the diagnosis, because the half-life of these immunoglobulins is short and the titers in an infant who is not infected should decrease rapidly. The sensitivity of *T gondii*-specific IgM by the double-sandwich enzyme immunoassay or an immunosorbent assay is 75% to 80%. IgA antibodies are found more frequently than IgM antibodies; some infants may have only IgA or only IgM antibodies. The indirect fluorescent assay for IgM should not be relied on to diagnose congenital infection. In an uninfected infant, a continuous decrease in IgG titer without detection of IgM or IgA antibodies will occur. Transplacentally transmitted IgG antibody usually will become undetectable by 6 to 12 months of age.

HIV Infection. Patients with HIV infection who are infected latently with *T gondii* have variable titers of IgG antibody to *T gondii* but rarely have IgM antibody. Although seroconversion and fourfold increases in IgG antibody titers may occur, the ability to diagnose active disease in patients with acquired immunodeficiency syndrome commonly is impaired by immunosuppression. In HIV-infected patients who are seropositive for *T gondii* IgG, *T gondii* encephalitis is diagnosed presumptively on the basis of the presence of characteristic clinical and radiographic findings. If the infection does not respond to an empiric trial of anti-*T gondii* therapy, demonstration of *T gondii* organisms, antigen, or DNA in sites such as blood, CSF, or bronchoalveolar fluid, where the organism would not be expected to reside in the chronic cyst form, may be necessary to confirm the diagnosis.

Infants born to women who are infected simultaneously with HIV and *T gondii* should be evaluated for congenital toxoplasmosis because of an increased likelihood of maternal reactivation and congenital transmission in this setting.

Ocular toxoplasmosis usually is diagnosed on the basis of observation of characteristic retinal lesions in conjunction with serum *T gondii*-specific IgG or IgM antibodies.

TREATMENT: Most cases of acquired infection in an immunocompetent host do not require specific antimicrobial therapy unless infection occurs during pregnancy. When indicated (eg, chorioretinitis or significant organ damage), the combination of pyrimethamine and sulfadiazine,[1] with supplemental leucovorin (folinic acid) to minimize pyrimethamine-associated hematologic toxicity, is the regimen most widely accepted for children and adults with acute symptomatic disease (see Drugs for Parasitic Infections, p 783). Alternatively, pyrimethamine can be used in combination with clindamycin if the patient does not tolerate sulfadiazine. Corticosteroids appear to be useful in the management of ocular complications and central nervous system disease in certain patients.

Patients infected with HIV who have had toxoplasmic encephalitis should receive lifelong suppressive therapy to prevent recurrence. Regimens for primary treatment also are effective for suppressive therapy.

For HIV-infected adults, primary chemoprophylaxis with trimethoprim-sulfamethoxazole (TMP-SMX) against toxoplasmosis has been recommended as the preferred regimen by the Centers for Disease Control and Prevention, the National Institutes of Health, and the HIV Medicine Association of the Infectious Diseases Society of America[2] for people who are *T gondii*-seropositive and have CD4+ T-lymphocyte counts less than

---

[1]Available from Eon Labs, Laurelton, NY (800-526-0225)

[2]Centers for Disease Control and Prevention. Guidelines for prevention and treatment of opportunistic infections in HIV-infected adults and adolescents. Recommendations from CDC, the National Institutes of Health, and the HIV Medicine Association of the Infectious Diseases Society of America. *MMWR Early Release.* 2009;58(March 24, 2009):1–207. Available at: **http://www.cdc.gov/mmwr/pdf/rr/rr58e324.pdf.**

100 x 10^6/L (100/μL). Alternative regimens and discontinuation of prophylaxis after CD4+ T-lymphocyte count increases in association with highly active antiretroviral therapy are discussed in the guidelines.[1]

Prophylaxis to prevent the first episode of toxoplasmosis generally is recommended for HIV-infected children (see Table 3.78, p 672).[1] Trimethoprim-sulfamethoxazole, when administered for *Pneumocystis jirovecii* pneumonia (PCP) prophylaxis, also provides prophylaxis against toxoplasmosis. Atovaquone also may provide protection. Children older than 12 months of age who qualify for PCP prophylaxis and who are receiving an agent other than TMP-SMX or atovaquone should have serologic testing for *Toxoplasma* antibodies, because alternative drugs for PCP prophylaxis might not be effective against *Toxoplasma* species. Severely immunosuppressed children who are not receiving TMP-SMX or atovaquone who are found to be seropositive for *Toxoplasma* infection should receive prophylaxis for both PCP and toxoplasmosis (ie, dapsone plus pyrimethamine). HIV-infected children with a history of toxoplasmosis should receive lifelong prophylaxis to prevent recurrence (see Table 3.78, p 672). The safety of discontinuing primary or secondary prophylaxis in HIV-infected children receiving highly active antiretroviral therapy has not been studied extensively.

For symptomatic and asymptomatic congenital infections, pyrimethamine combined with sulfadiazine (supplemented with folinic acid) is recommended as initial therapy. Duration of therapy is prolonged and often is 1 year. However, the optimal dosage and duration are not established definitively and should be determined in consultation with appropriate specialists.

Treatment of primary *T gondii* infection in pregnant women, including women with HIV infection, is recommended. Appropriate specialists should be consulted for management. Spiramycin treatment of primary infection during gestation is used in an attempt to decrease transmission of *T gondii* from the mother to the fetus. Spiramycin treatment in pregnant women may reduce congenital transmission but does not treat the fetus in utero if infection has spread to the placenta. Maternal therapy may decrease the severity of sequelae in the fetus once congenital toxoplasmosis has occurred. Spiramycin is available only as an investigational drug in the United States. Spiramycin may be obtained from the manufacturer with authorization from the US Food and Drug Administration.[2] If fetal infection is confirmed after 17 weeks of gestation or if the mother acquires infection during the third trimester, consideration should be given to starting therapy with pyrimethamine and sulfadiazine.

ISOLATION OF THE HOSPITALIZED PATIENT: Standard precautions are recommended.

CONTROL MEASURES: Pregnant women whose serostatus for *T gondii* is negative or unknown should avoid activities that potentially expose them to cat feces (such as changing litter boxes, gardening, and landscaping), or they should wear gloves and wash their hands if such activities are unavoidable. Daily changing of cat litter will decrease the chance of infection, because oocysts are not infective during the first 1 to 2 days after passage. Domestic cats can be protected from infection by feeding them commercially

---

[1]Centers for Disease Control and Prevention. Guidelines for prevention and treatment of opportunistic infections in HIV-infected adults and adolescents. Recommendations from CDC, the National Institutes of Health, and the HIV Medicine Association of the Infectious Diseases Society of America. *MMWR Early Release.* 2009; 58(March 24, 2009):1–207. Available at: **http://www.cdc.gov/mmwr/pdf/rr/rr58e324.pdf.**

[2]US Food and Drug Administration, Division of Special Pathogens and Transplant Drug Products. Telephone, 301-796-1600; fax, 301-796-9882.

Table 3.78. Prophylaxis to Prevent First Episode and Recurrence of Toxoplasmosis in Children

Prevention of	Indication	First Choice	Alternatives
First episode of toxoplasmosis[a]	Severe immuno-suppression and presence of immuno-globulin G antibody to *Toxoplasma*	Trimethoprim-sulfamethoxazole, 150–750 mg/m²/day in 2 divided doses, orally, every day	Dapsone (children 1 mo of age or older), 2 mg/kg or 15 mg/m² (max 25 mg), orally, every day; **PLUS** pyrimethamine, 1 mg/kg, orally every day; **PLUS** leucovorin, 5 mg, orally, every 3 days Atovaquone, children 1 through 3 mo or older than 24 mo of age; 30 mg/kg, orally, every day; children 14–24 mo of age: 45 mg/kg, orally, every day
Recurrence of toxoplasmosis[b]	Prior to toxoplasmic encephalitis	Sulfadiazine, 85–120 mg/kg/day in 2–4 divided doses, orally, every day, **PLUS** pyrimethamine, 1 mg/kg or 15 mg/m² (maximum, 25 mg), orally, every day; **PLUS** leucovorin, 5 mg, orally, every 3 days	Clindamycin, 20–30 mg/kg/day in 3 divided doses, orally, every day, **PLUS** pyrimethamine 1 mg/kg, orally, every day; **PLUS** leucovorin, 5 mg, orally, every 3 days

[a]Protection against toxoplasmosis is provided by the preferred antipneumocystis regimens and possibly by atovaquone. Atovaquone may be used with or without pyrimethamine. Pyrimethamine alone probably provides little, if any, protection (for information about severe immunosuppression, see Table 3.55, p 538).
[b]Only pyrimethamine plus sulfadiazine confers protection against *Pneumocystis jirovecii* pneumonia as well as toxoplasmosis. Although the clindamycin plus pyrimethamine regimen is recommended in adults, this regimen has not been tested in children. However, these drugs are safe and are used for other infections.

prepared cat food and preventing them from eating undercooked kitchen meat scraps and hunting wild rodents and birds.

Oral ingestion of *T gondii* can be avoided by the following measures: (1) avoiding eating raw or undercooked meat and cooking meat—particularly pork, lamb, beef, and venison—to an internal temperature of 65.5°C to 76.6°C (150°F–170°F [no longer pink]) before consumption (smoked meat and meat cured in brine are considered safe); (2) washing fruits and vegetables; (3) washing hands and cleaning kitchen surfaces after handling fruits, vegetables, and raw meat; (4) washing hands after gardening or other contact with soil; (5) preventing contamination of food with raw or undercooked meat or soil; and (6) avoiding ingestion of untreated water, particularly in developing countries. All HIV-infected people and pregnant women should be counseled about the various sources of toxoplasmic infection.

Trichinellosis
(Trichinella spiralis)

CLINICAL MANIFESTATIONS: The clinical spectrum of infection ranges from inapparent to fulminant and fatal illness, but most infections are inapparent. The severity of the disease is proportional to the infective dose. During the first week after ingesting infected meat, a person may be asymptomatic or experience abdominal discomfort, nausea, vomiting, and/or diarrhea. Two to 8 weeks later, as larvae migrate into tissues, fever, myalgia, periorbital edema, urticarial rash, and conjunctival and subungual hemorrhages may develop. Larvae may remain viable in tissues for years; calcification of some larvae in skeletal muscle usually occurs within 6 to 24 months and may be detected on radiographs. In severe infections, myocarditis, neurologic involvement, and pneumonitis can follow in 1 or 2 months.

ETIOLOGY: Infection is caused by nematodes (roundworms) of the genus *Trichinella*. At least 5 species capable of infecting only warm-blooded animals have been identified. Worldwide, *Trichinella spiralis* is the most common cause of human infection.

EPIDEMIOLOGY: The infection is enzootic worldwide in many carnivores, especially scavengers. Infection occurs as a result of ingestion of raw or insufficiently cooked meat containing encysted larvae of *T spiralis*. The usual source of human infections is pork, but horse meat and wild carnivorous game, such as bear, seal, and walrus meat in North America, can be sources. *Trichinella nativa* is the causative organism in most of these arctic sources. Feeding pigs uncooked garbage perpetuates the cycle of infection. In the United States, the incidence of infection in humans has decreased considerably as pork production standards have improved, but infection occurs sporadically, often in people who have ingested undercooked bear meat. The disease is not transmitted from person to person.

The **incubation period** usually is 1 to 2 weeks.

DIAGNOSTIC TESTS: Eosinophilia approaching 70%, in conjunction with compatible symptoms and dietary history, suggests the diagnosis. Increases in concentrations of muscle enzymes, such as creatinine phosphokinase and lactic dehydrogenase, also occur. Encapsulated larvae in a skeletal muscle biopsy specimen (particularly deltoid and gastrocnemius) can be visualized microscopically beginning 2 weeks after infection. Fresh tissue, compressed between 2 microscope slides, should be examined. Digestion of muscle tissue in artificial gastric juice followed by examination of the sediment for larvae is more sensitive. Identification of larvae in suspect meat can be the most rapid source of diagnostic information. Serologic tests are available through some private and state laboratories and the Centers for Disease Control and Prevention. Serum antibody titers rarely become positive before the second week of illness. Testing paired acute and convalescent serum specimens usually is diagnostic.

TREATMENT: Albendazole and mebendazole have comparable efficacy for treatment of trichinosis (see Drugs for Parasitic Infections, p 783). Neither albendazole nor mebendazole is effective for *Trichinella* larvae already in the muscles, and neither drug is approved by the US Food and Drug Administration for trichinellosis. Coadministration of corticosteroids with mebendazole or albendazole often is recommended when symptoms are severe. Corticosteroids alleviate symptoms of the inflammatory reaction and can be life-saving when the central nervous system or heart is involved.

ISOLATION OF THE HOSPITALIZED PATIENT: Standard precautions are recommended.

CONTROL MEASURES: Transmission to pigs can be prevented by not feeding pigs garbage, by preventing cannibalism, and by effective rat control. The public should be educated about the necessity of cooking pork and meat of wild animals thoroughly (until the meat no longer is pink). Freezing pork at −23°C (−10°F) for 10 days kills larvae. However, *Trichinella* organisms in wild animals, such as bears and raccoons, can survive this procedure. People known to have ingested contaminated meat recently should be treated with albendazole (or mebendazole).

Trichomonas vaginalis Infections
(Trichomoniasis)

CLINICAL MANIFESTATIONS: Infection with *Trichomonas vaginalis* is asymptomatic in up to 90% of men and 50% of women infected with this organism. Clinical manifestations in symptomatic postpubertal female patients consist of a diffuse vaginal discharge and vulvovaginal pruritus and irritation. Dysuria and, less often, lower abdominal pain can occur. Vaginal discharge usually is yellow-green in color and may have a musty odor. Symptom exacerbation can occur after menstruation. The vulva and vaginal mucosa can be erythematous and edematous, and the cervix can be friable and inflamed, sometimes covered with numerous punctate cervical hemorrhages with ulceration (colpitis macularis), commonly known as "strawberry cervix." Urethritis and, more rarely, epididymitis or prostatitis can develop in infected males, but most males are asymptomatic. Reinfection is common. *T vaginalis* infection can increase both the acquisition and transmission of human immunodeficiency virus (HIV).

ETIOLOGY: *T vaginalis* is a flagellated protozoan that is the size of a leukocyte. It requires adherence to host cells for survival. The genome of *T vaginalis* has been sequenced.

EPIDEMIOLOGY: *T vaginalis* infection is the second most common sexually transmitted infection in the United States and commonly coexists with other conditions, particularly with *Neisseria gonorrhoeae* and *Chlamydia trachomatis* infections and with bacterial vaginosis. The presence of *T vaginalis* in a prepubertal child should raise suspicion of sexual abuse. *T vaginalis* acquired during birth by female newborn infants can cause vaginal discharge during the first weeks of life but usually resolves as maternal hormones are metabolized.

The **incubation period** averages 1 week but ranges from 5 to 28 days.

DIAGNOSTIC TESTS: Diagnosis usually is established by examination of a wet-mount preparation of vaginal discharge. Lashing of the flagella and jerky motility of the organism are distinctive. Microscopy has 60% to 70% sensitivity for diagnosis of *T vaginalis* in vaginal secretions. Positive identification of the organism is more common in women who have symptoms and is related directly to the number of organisms. Culture of the organism is the most sensitive and specific method of diagnosis. Two point-of-care tests are available: an immunochromatographic capillary flow dipstick and a nucleic acid probe test. These tests are more sensitive than microscopy, but they may result in more false-positive results in populations with a low prevalence of disease. They have not been approved for use in men. Culture is required for the diagnosis of *T vaginalis* in men.

TREATMENT: Treatment of adults with metronidazole (2 g, orally, in a single dose) results in cure rates of approximately 90% to 95%, and treatment with tinidazole (2 g, orally, in a single dose) results in cure rates of approximately 86% to 100%; both drugs are approved for this indication in adults but not in children and adolescents (see Drugs for

Parasitic Infections, p 783). Topical preparations should not be used, because they do not achieve therapeutic concentrations in the urethra or perivaginal glands. Sexual partners should be treated concurrently, even if asymptomatic, because reinfection is a major factor in treatment failures. Patients should abstain from alcohol during treatment and for 24 hours after completing metronidazole or 72 hours after completing tinidazole because of the disulfiram-like effects of these drugs. *T vaginalis* strains with decreased susceptibility to metronidazole have been reported. If treatment failure occurs with metronidazole and reinfection is excluded, either metronidazole (500 mg, orally, twice daily for 7 days) or tinidazole (2 g, orally, in a single dose) can be used. If treatment failure occurs with either of these regimens, then either metronidazole (2 g daily for 5 days) or tinidazole (2 g daily for 5 days) can be used. In the event of continued treatment failure, consultation with an expert is advised. Consultation is available from the Centers for Disease Control and Prevention at **www.cdc.gov/std** or 770-488-4115. Pregnant women can be treated with metronidazole (2 g in a single dose). Metronidazole is a pregnancy category B drug (animal studies have revealed no evidence of harm to the fetus, but no adequate and well-controlled studies in pregnant women have been conducted). Tinidazole is a pregnancy category C drug (animal studies have demonstrated an adverse effect, and no adequate and well-controlled studies in pregnant women have been conducted), and its safety in pregnant women has not been well evaluated. Some specialists would defer therapy in asymptomatic pregnant women until after 37 weeks' gestation. In lactating women to whom metronidazole is administered, withholding breastfeeding during treatment and for 12 to 24 hours after the last dose will reduce the exposure of metronidazole to the infant. While using tinidazole, interruption of breastfeeding is recommended during treatment and for 3 days after the last dose.

People infected with *T vaginalis* should be evaluated for other sexually transmitted infections, including syphilis, gonorrhea, chlamydia, hepatitis B, and HIV infection. Newborn infection is self-limited and treatment generally is not recommended.

ISOLATION OF THE HOSPITALIZED PATIENT: Standard precautions are recommended.

CONTROL MEASURES: Measures to prevent sexually transmitted infections, particularly the consistent and correct use of condoms, are indicated. Patients should be instructed to avoid sexual activity until they and their sexual partners are treated and asymptomatic.

Trichuriasis
(Whipworm Infection)

CLINICAL MANIFESTATIONS: Most infected children harbor only small numbers of the organism and are asymptomatic. Children with heavy infestations can develop a *Trichuris trichiura* dysentery syndrome consisting of abdominal pain, tenesmus, and bloody diarrhea with mucus or a chronic *T trichiura* colitis. *T trichiura* colitis can mimic other forms of inflammatory bowel disease and lead to physical growth retardation. Even otherwise asymptomatic infections may have adverse effects on nutritional status. Chronic illness associated with heavy infestation also can be associated with rectal prolapse.

ETIOLOGY: *T trichiura*, the whipworm, is the causative agent. Adult worms are 30 to 50 mm long with a large, thread-like anterior end that is embedded in the mucosa of the large intestine.

EPIDEMIOLOGY: The parasite has a worldwide distribution but is more common in the tropics and in areas of poor sanitation. In some areas of Asia, the prevalence of infection is 50%. In the United States, trichuriasis no longer is a public health problem, although migrants from tropical areas may be infected. Eggs require a minimum of 10 days of incubation in the soil before they are infectious. The disease is not communicable from person to person.

The **incubation period** is unknown. However, the time required for mature worms to begin laying eggs that are passed in feces is approximately 90 days after ingestion of eggs.

DIAGNOSTIC TESTS: Eggs may be found on direct examination of stool or by using concentration techniques.

TREATMENT: Mebendazole, albendazole, or ivermectin given for 3 days usually is effective in eradicating most of the worms, with mebendazole being the treatment of choice. In mass treatment efforts involving entire communities, a single dose of either mebendazole (500 mg) or albendazole (400 mg) will reduce worm burdens (see Drugs for Parasitic Infections, p 783). In 1-year-old children, the World Health Organization recommends reducing the albendazole dose to half of that given to older children and adults for single-dose and 3-day treatment. Reexamination of stool specimens 2 weeks after therapy to determine whether the worms have been eliminated is helpful for assessing therapy but is not essential.

ISOLATION OF THE HOSPITALIZED PATIENT: Only standard precautions are recommended, because there is no direct person-to-person transmission.

CONTROL MEASURES: Proper disposal of fecal material is indicated. Mass treatment of infected school-aged populations can reduce whipworm transmission in communities with endemic infection.

African Trypanosomiasis
(African Sleeping Sickness)

CLINICAL MANIFESTATIONS: The rapidity and severity of clinical manifestations vary with the infecting subspecies. With *Trypanosoma brucei gambiense* (West African) infection, a cutaneous nodule or chancre may appear at the site of parasite inoculation within a few days of a bite by an infected tsetse fly. Systemic illness is chronic, occurring months to years later, and is characterized by intermittent fever, posterior cervical lymphadenopathy (Winterbottom sign), and multiple nonspecific complaints, including malaise, weight loss, arthralgia, rash, pruritus, and edema. If the central nervous system (CNS) is involved, chronic meningoencephalitis with behavioral changes, cachexia, headache, hallucinations, delusions, and somnolence can occur. In contrast, *Trypanosoma brucei rhodesiense* (East African) infection is an acute, generalized illness that develops days to weeks after parasite inoculation, with manifestations including high fever, cutaneous chancre, myocarditis, hepatitis, anemia, thrombocytopenia, and laboratory evidence of disseminated intravascular coagulopathy. Clinical meningoencephalitis can develop as early as 3 weeks after onset of the untreated systemic illness. Both forms of African trypanosomiasis have high fatality rates; without treatment, infected patients usually die within weeks to months after clinical onset of disease caused by *T brucei rhodesiense* and within a few years from disease caused by *T brucei gambiense*.

ETIOLOGY: The West African (Gambian) form of sleeping sickness is caused by *T brucei gambiense*, whereas the East African (Rhodesian) form is caused by *T brucei rhodesiense*. Both are extracellular protozoan hemoflagellates that live in blood and tissue of the human host. The genome of *T brucei* has been sequenced.

EPIDEMIOLOGY: Approximately 15 000 human cases are reported annually worldwide, although only a few cases, which are acquired in Africa, are reported every year in the United States. Transmission is confined to an area in Africa between the latitudes of 15° north and 20° south, corresponding precisely with the distribution of the tsetse fly vector (*Glossina* species). In East Africa, wild animals, such as antelope, bushbuck, and hartebeest, constitute the major reservoirs for sporadic infections with *T brucei rhodesiense*, although cattle serve as reservoir hosts in local outbreaks. Domestic pigs and dogs have been found as incidental reservoirs of *T brucei gambiense;* however, humans are the only important reservoir in West and Central Africa.

The **incubation period** for *T brucei rhodesiense* infection is 3 to 21 days and usually is 5 to 14 days; for *T brucei gambiense* infection, the incubation period usually is longer and variable, ranging from several months to years.

DIAGNOSTIC TESTS: Diagnosis is made by identification of trypomastigotes in specimens of blood, cerebrospinal fluid (CSF), or fluid aspirated from a chancre or lymph node or by inoculation of susceptible laboratory animals (mice) with heparinized blood. Examination of the CSF is critical to management and should be performed using the double-centrifugation technique. Concentration and Giemsa staining of the buffy coat layer of peripheral blood also can be helpful. *T brucei gambiense* is more likely to be found in lymph node aspirates. Although an increased concentration of immunoglobulin M in serum or CSF is considered characteristic of African trypanosomiasis, polyclonal hyperglobulinemia is common.

TREATMENT: When no evidence of CNS involvement is present (including absence of trypanosomes and CSF pleocytosis), the drug of choice for the acute hemolymphatic stage of infection is pentamidine for *T brucei gambiense* infection and suramin for *T brucei rhodesiense* infection. For treatment of hemolymphatic and CNS disease, see Drugs for Parasitic Infections (p 783). Eflornithine kills trypanosomes by inhibiting ornithine decarboxylase, but its expense limits its use in Africa. Because of the risk of relapse, patients who have had CNS involvement should undergo repeated CSF examinations every 6 months for 2 years.

ISOLATION OF THE HOSPITALIZED PATIENT: Standard precautions are recommended.

CONTROL MEASURES: Travelers to areas with endemic infection should avoid known foci of sleeping sickness and tsetse fly infestation and minimize fly bites by the use of protective clothing and insect repellents. Infected patients should not breastfeed or donate blood. Refer to the chapter on preventing insect bites (see Prevention of Mosquitoborne Infections, p 193).

American Trypanosomiasis
(Chagas Disease)

CLINICAL MANIFESTATIONS: Patients can have acute or chronic disease. The early phase of this disease commonly is asymptomatic. However, children are more likely to exhibit symptoms than are adults. In some patients, a red nodule known as a *chagoma* develops at the site of the original inoculation, usually on the face or arms. The surrounding skin becomes indurated and, later, hypopigmented. Unilateral firm edema of the eyelids, known as Romaña sign, is the earliest indication of the infection when the portal of entry is the conjunctiva; it is not always present. The edematous skin is violaceous and associated with conjunctivitis and enlargement of the ipsilateral preauricular lymph node. A few days after appearance of Romaña sign, fever, generalized lymphadenopathy, and malaise can develop. In rare instances, acute myocarditis, hepatosplenomegaly, edema, and meningoencephalitis can follow. In nearly all cases, acute Chagas disease resolves after 1 to 3 months, and an asymptomatic or indeterminate period follows. In 20% to 30% of cases, serious sequelae, consisting of cardiomyopathy, megaesophagus, and/or megacolon, develop many years after the initial infection (chronic phase). Cardiomyopathy causes conduction system abnormalities, arrhythmias, and eventually congestive heart failure. Patients with Chagas cardiomyopathy may die suddenly from ventricular arrhythmias or complete heart block or may die from intractable congestive heart failure or embolic phenomena. Congenital disease may be characterized by low birth weight, hepatosplenomegaly, and/or meningoencephalitis with seizures and tremors, but most infants infected in utero have no signs or symptoms of disease. Reactivation may occur, especially in immunocompromised people, including people infected with human immunodeficiency virus and those who are immunosuppressed after transplantation.

ETIOLOGY: *Trypanosoma cruzi*, a protozoan hemoflagellate, is the cause.

EPIDEMIOLOGY: Parasites are transmitted through feces of infected triatomine insects (cone-nose or kissing bugs). These insects defecate during or after taking blood. The bitten person is inoculated by inadvertently rubbing the insect feces containing the parasite into the site of the bite or mucous membranes of the eye or the mouth. The parasite also can be transmitted congenitally, during organ transplantation, through blood transfusion, and by consumption of the vector or the vector's excretion. Accidental laboratory infections can result from handling blood from infected people or laboratory animals, usually through needlestick injuries. Vectorborne transmission of the disease is limited to the Western hemisphere, predominantly Mexico and Central and South America. Although some small mammals in the southern and southwestern United States harbor *T cruzi*, documented vectorborne transmission to humans is rare in the United States. Several transfusion- and transplantation-associated cases have been documented in the United States. Infection is more common in immigrants from Central and South America. The disease is an important cause of death in South America, where an estimated 8 to 10 million people are infected.

The **incubation period** for the acute phase of disease is 1 to 2 weeks or longer. Chronic manifestations do not appear for years to decades.

DIAGNOSTIC TESTS: During the acute phase of disease, the parasite is demonstrable in blood specimens by Giemsa staining after a concentration technique or by direct wet-mount or buffy coat preparation. During the indeterminate and chronic phases, which are characterized by low-level parasitemia, recovery of the parasite requires culture on special media (available at the Centers for Disease Control and Prevention [CDC]), but the result of culture often is negative because of a low parasite burden. Xenodiagnosis (isolation of trypanosomes from the intestine of a triatomine bug that has fed on patient blood) is available in Central and South America. Serologic tests include indirect immunofluorescent and enzyme immunosorbent assays, which are the primary diagnostic modality in chronic disease. Serologic testing is available at the CDC. The diagnosis of congenital Chagas disease can be made during the first 3 months of life by identification of motile trypomastigotes on direct microscopy of fresh anticoagulated blood specimens. However, the sensitivity of this technique is not high, and all infants of seropositive mothers should be screened using conventional serologic testing after 9 months of age, when immunoglobulin G measurements reflect infant response.

TREATMENT: Antitrypanosomal treatment is recommended for all cases of acute and congenital Chagas disease, reactivated infection, and chronic *T cruzi*-infection in children younger than 18 years old. The only drugs with proven efficacy are benznidazole and nifurtimox (see Drugs for Parasitic Infections, p 783).

ISOLATION OF THE HOSPITALIZED PATIENT: Standard precautions should be followed.

CONTROL MEASURES: Travelers to areas with endemic infection should avoid contact with triatomine bugs by avoiding habitation in buildings that do not have control measures for these insects, particularly buildings constructed of mud, palm thatch, or adobe brick and especially those with cracks in the walls or roof. The use of insecticide-impregnated bed nets also may be beneficial. Camping or sleeping outdoors in areas with highly endemic infection is not recommended. Blood and serologic testing should be performed on members of households with an infected patient if they have had exposure to the vector similar to that of the patient. All children of infected mothers should be tested.

Education about the mode of spread and the methods of prevention is warranted in areas with endemic infection. Homes should be examined for the presence of the vectors, and if found, measures to eliminate the vector should be taken.

In December 2006, the US Food and Drug Administration (FDA) approved a test to detect antibodies to *T cruzi*. The American Red Cross tested almost 150 000 samples from areas of the United States where some blood donors were expected to have undiagnosed Chagas disease and found that 61 donors repeatedly were reactive for antibodies to *T cruzi*.[1] The AABB (formerly known as the American Association of Blood Banks) offered recommendations to member facilities regarding appropriate use of the test. The American Red Cross and Blood Systems Inc voluntarily began screening all blood donations in January 2008. As of November 2007, the FDA has concluded that the test offers an important new safety measure and is expected to issue specific guidance for appropriate use of the test for all blood donations (see Blood Safety, p 106).

---

[1] Centers for Disease Control and Prevention. Blood donor screening for Chagas disease—United States, 2006–2007. *MMWR Morb Mortal Wkly Rep.* 2007;56(7):141–143

Tuberculosis

CLINICAL MANIFESTATIONS: Tuberculosis disease is caused by infection with organisms of the *Mycobacterium tuberculosis* complex, which includes *M tuberculosis, Mycobacterium bovis,* and *Mycobacterium africanum. M africanum* is rare in the United States, and clinical laboratories do not distinguish it routinely. *M bovis* can be distinguished routinely, and although the spectrum of illness that is caused by *M bovis* is similar to that of *M tuberculosis,* the epidemiology, treatment, and prevention are distinct. Most infections caused by *M tuberculosis* complex in children and adolescents are asymptomatic. When tuberculosis disease does occur, clinical manifestations most often appear 1 to 6 months after infection and include fever, weight loss, or poor weight gain and possibly growth delay, cough, night sweats, and chills. Chest radiographic findings after infection range from normal to diverse abnormalities, such as lymphadenopathy of the hilar, subcarinal, paratracheal, or mediastinal nodes; atelectasis or infiltrate of a segment or lobe; pleural effusion; cavitary lesions; or miliary disease. Extrapulmonary manifestations include meningitis and granulomatous inflammation of the lymph nodes, bones, joints, skin, and middle ear and mastoid. Renal tuberculosis and progression to disease from latent tuberculosis infection ("adult-type pulmonary tuberculosis") are unusual in younger children but can occur in adolescents. In addition, chronic abdominal pain with intermittent partial intestinal obstruction can be present in disease caused by *M bovis.* Clinical findings in patients with drug-resistant tuberculosis disease are indistinguishable from manifestations in patients with drug-susceptible disease.

ETIOLOGY: The agent is *M tuberculosis* complex, a group of closely related acid-fast bacilli (AFB): *M tuberculosis, M bovis,* and *M africanum.*

DEFINITIONS:

- **Positive tuberculin skin test (TST) result.** A positive TST result (see Table 3.79, p 681) indicates possible infection with *M tuberculosis* complex. Tuberculin reactivity appears 2 to 10 weeks after initial infection; the median interval is 3 to 4 weeks (see Tuberculin Testing, p 683).
- **Positive interferon-gamma release assay (IGRA).** A positive IGRA result indicates possible infection with *M tuberculosis* complex.
- **Exposed person** refers to a person who has had recent contact with another person with suspected or confirmed contagious pulmonary tuberculosis disease and who has a negative TST or IGRA result, normal physical examination findings, and chest radiographic findings that are not compatible with tuberculosis. Some exposed people become infected (and subsequently, most have a positive TST or IGRA result) and some people do not become infected after exposure; the 2 groups cannot be distinguished initially.
- **Source case** is defined as the person who has transmitted infection with *M tuberculosis* complex to another person who subsequently has either latent tuberculosis infection or tuberculosis disease.
- **Latent tuberculosis infection (LTBI)** is defined as *M tuberculosis* complex infection in a person who has a positive TST or IGRA result, no physical findings of disease, and chest radiograph findings that are normal or reveal evidence of healed infection (eg, calcification in the lung, hilar lymph nodes, or both).

Table 3.79. Definitions of Positive Tuberculin Skin Test (TST) Results in Infants, Children, and Adolescents[a]

Induration 5 mm or greater

Children in close contact with known or suspected contagious people with tuberculosis disease

Children suspected to have tuberculosis disease:
- Findings on chest radiograph consistent with active or previous tuberculosis disease
- Clinical evidence of tuberculosis disease[b]

Children receiving immunosuppressive therapy[c] or with immunosuppressive conditions, including human immunodeficiency (HIV) infection

Induration 10 mm or greater

Children at increased risk of disseminated tuberculosis disease:
- Children younger than 4 years of age
- Children with other medical conditions, including Hodgkin disease, lymphoma, diabetes mellitus, chronic renal failure, or malnutrition (see Table 3.80, p 684)

Children with likelihood of increased exposure to tuberculosis disease:
- Children born in high-prevalence regions of the world
- Children frequently exposed to adults who are HIV infected, homeless, users of illicit drugs, residents of nursing homes, incarcerated or institutionalized, or migrant farm workers
- Children who travel to high-prevalence regions of the world

Induration 15 mm or greater

Children 4 years of age or older without any risk factors

[a]These definitions apply regardless of previous bacille Calmette-Guérin (BCG) immunization (see also Interpretation of TST Results in Previous Recipients of BCG Vaccine, p 685); erythema alone at TST site does not indicate a positive test result. Tests should be read at 48 to 72 hours after placement.
[b]Evidence by physical examination or laboratory assessment that would include tuberculosis in the working differential diagnosis (eg, meningitis).
[c]Including immunosuppressive doses of corticosteroids (see Corticosteroids, p 694).

- **Tuberculosis disease** is defined as disease in a person with infection in whom symptoms, signs, or radiographic manifestations caused by *M tuberculosis* complex are apparent; disease may be pulmonary, extrapulmonary, or both. Infectious tuberculosis refers to tuberculosis disease of the lungs or larynx in a person who has the potential to transmit the infection to other people.
- **Directly observed therapy (DOT)** is defined as an intervention by which medication is administered directly to the patient by a health care professional or trained third party (not a relative or friend), who observes and documents that the patient ingests each dose of medication.
- **Multiply drug-resistant (MDR) tuberculosis** is defined as tuberculosis infection or disease caused by a strain of *M tuberculosis* complex that is resistant to at least isoniazid and rifampin, the 2 first-line drugs with greatest efficacy.
- **Extensively drug-resistant (XDR) tuberculosis** is a subset of MDR tuberculosis. It is defined as infection or disease caused by a strain of *M tuberculosis* complex that is resistant to isoniazid and rifampin, at least 1 fluoroquinolone, and at least 1 of the following parenteral drugs: amikacin, kanamycin, or capreomycin.

- **Bacille Calmette-Guérin (BCG)** is an attenuated vaccine strain of *M bovis*. BCG rarely is administered to children in the United States but is probably the most widely used vaccine in the world. An isolate of BCG can be distinguished from wild-type *M bovis* only in a reference laboratory.

EPIDEMIOLOGY: Case rates of tuberculosis for all ages are higher in urban, low-income areas and in nonwhite racial and ethnic groups; two thirds of reported cases in the United States occur in nonwhite people. In recent years, foreign-born children have accounted for more than one quarter of newly diagnosed cases in children 14 years of age or younger. Specific groups with greater LTBI and disease rates include immigrants, international adoptees, and refugees from or travelers to high-prevalence regions (eg, Asia, Africa, Latin America, and countries of the former Soviet Union); homeless people; and residents of correctional facilities.

Infants and postpubertal adolescents are at increased risk of progression of LTBI to tuberculosis disease. Other predictive factors for development of disease include recent infection (within the past 2 years); immunodeficiency, especially from human immunodeficiency virus (HIV) infection; use of immunosuppressive drugs, such as prolonged or high-dose corticosteroid therapy or chemotherapy; intravenous drug use; and certain diseases or medical conditions, including Hodgkin disease, lymphoma, diabetes mellitus, chronic renal failure, and malnutrition. There have been reports of tuberculosis disease in adolescents and adults being treated for arthritis, inflammatory bowel disease, and other conditions with tumor necrosis factor alpha (TNF-alpha) antagonists, such as infliximab and etanercept. Before use of TNF-alpha antagonists, patients should be screened for risk factors for *M tuberculosis* complex infection and have a TST or IGRA performed.

A diagnosis of LTBI or tuberculosis disease in a young child is a public health sentinel event usually representing recent transmission. Transmission of *M tuberculosis* complex is airborne, with inhalation of droplet nuclei usually produced by an adult or adolescent with contagious pulmonary or laryngeal tuberculosis disease. *M bovis* is transmitted most often by unpasteurized dairy products. The duration of contagiousness of an adult receiving effective treatment depends on drug susceptibilities of the organism, the number of organisms in sputum, and frequency of cough. Although contagiousness usually lasts only a few days to weeks after initiation of effective drug therapy, it can last longer, especially when the adult patient has cavitary disease, does not adhere to medical therapy, or is infected with a drug-resistant strain. If the sputum smear is negative for AFB organisms on 3 separate days and the patient has improved clinically, the treated person can be considered at low risk of disease transmission. Children younger than 10 years of age with pulmonary tuberculosis rarely are contagious, because their pulmonary lesions are small (paucibacillary disease), cough is not productive, and few or no bacilli are expulsed. Unusual cases of adult-form pulmonary disease in young children can be highly contagious.

The **incubation period** from infection to development of a positive TST or IGRA result is 2 to 10 weeks. The risk of developing tuberculosis disease is highest during the 6 months after infection and remains high for 2 years; however, many years can elapse between initial tuberculosis infection and tuberculosis disease.

DIAGNOSTIC TESTS: Isolation of *M tuberculosis* complex by culture from specimens of gastric aspirates, sputum, bronchial washings, pleural fluid, cerebrospinal fluid (CSF), urine, or other body fluids or a biopsy specimen establishes the diagnosis. Children older than 5 years of age and adolescents frequently can produce sputum by induction with aerosolized hypertonic saline. Studies have demonstrated successful collections of induced sputum from infants with pulmonary tuberculosis, but this requires special expertise. The best specimen for diagnosis of pulmonary tuberculosis in any child or adolescent in whom the cough is nonproductive or absent and sputum cannot be induced is an early morning gastric aspirate. Gastric aspirate specimens should be obtained with a nasogastric tube on awakening the child and before ambulation or feeding.[1] Aspirates collected on 3 separate days should be submitted for testing. Results of AFB smears of gastric aspirates usually are negative, and false-positive smear results caused by the presence of nontuberculous mycobacteria can occur. Gastric aspirates have the highest culture yield in young children on the first day of collection. Fluorescent staining methods for gastric aspirate smears are more sensitive and, if available, are preferred. The overall diagnostic yield of gastric aspirates is less than 50%. Histologic examination for and demonstration of AFB and granulomas in biopsy specimens from lymph node, pleura, mesentery, liver, bone marrow, or other tissues can be useful, but *M tuberculosis* complex organisms cannot be distinguished reliably from other mycobacteria in stained specimens. Regardless of results of the AFB smears, each specimen should be cultured.

Because *M tuberculosis* complex organisms are slow growing, detection of these organisms may take as long as 10 weeks using solid media; use of liquid media allows detection within 1 to 6 weeks and usually within 3 weeks. Even with optimal culture techniques, *M tuberculosis* complex organisms are isolated from fewer than 50% of children and 75% of infants with pulmonary tuberculosis diagnosed by other clinical criteria. Species identification of isolates from culture can be more rapid if a DNA probe or high pressure liquid chromatography is used. The differentiation between *M tuberculosis* and *M bovis* usually is based on pyrazinamide resistance, which is characteristic of almost all *M bovis* isolates.

One nucleic acid amplification test for rapid diagnosis is licensed by the Food and Drug Administration (FDA) for acid-fast stain positive respiratory tract specimens only, and another one is approved for any respiratory tract specimens, but these tests have decreased sensitivity for gastric aspirate, CSF, and tissue specimens, with false-negative and false-positive results reported.

Identification of the culture-positive source case supports the child's presumptive diagnosis and provides the likely drug susceptibility of the child's organism. Culture material should be collected from children with evidence of tuberculosis disease, especially when (1) an isolate from a source case is not available; (2) the presumed source case has drug-resistant tuberculosis; (3) the child is immunocompromised (eg, HIV infection); or (4) the child has extrapulmonary disease. Drug resistance cannot be confirmed without a bacterial isolate.

Tuberculin Testing. The TST is the most common method for diagnosing LTBI in asymptomatic people. The Mantoux method consists of 5 tuberculin units of purified protein derivative (0.1 mL) injected intradermally using a 27-gauge needle and a 1.0-mL syringe into the volar aspect of the forearm. Creation of a palpable induration 6 to 10 mm in diameter is crucial to accurate testing. Multiple puncture tests are not recommended, because they lack adequate sensitivity and specificity.

---

[1]**www.nationaltbcenter.edu/catalogue/epub/index.cfm?tableName=GAP**

A TST should be administered to children who are at increased risk of acquiring LTBI and tuberculosis disease (see Table 3.80). Routine TST administration, including programs based at schools, child care centers, and camps that include populations at low risk, is discouraged, because it results in either a low yield of positive results or a large proportion of false-positive results, leading to an inefficient use of health care resources. Simple questionnaires can identify children with risk factors for LTBI who then should be tested with a TST (see Table 3.81, p 685). Risk assessment for tuberculosis should be performed at first contact with a child and every 6 months thereafter for the first 2 years of life (eg, 2 weeks and 6, 12, 18, and 24 months of age). If at any time, tuberculosis disease is suspected, a TST should be performed, although a negative result should be considered as especially unreliable in infants younger than 3 months of age. After 2 years of age, risk assessment for tuberculosis should be performed annually, if possible.

Recommendations for use of the TST are independent of those for immunization. Tuberculin testing at any age is not required before administration of live-virus vaccines. A TST can be applied at the same visit during which these vaccines are administered. Measles vaccine temporarily can suppress tuberculin reactivity for at least 4 to 6 weeks. The effect of live-virus varicella, yellow fever, and live-attenuated influenza vaccines on TST reactivity and IGRA results is not known. In the absence of

Table 3.80. Tuberculin Skin Test (TST) Recommendations for Infants, Children, and Adolescents[a]

Children for whom immediate TST or IGRA is indicated[b]:
- Contacts of people with confirmed or suspected contagious tuberculosis (contact investigation)
- Children with radiographic or clinical findings suggesting tuberculosis disease
- Children immigrating from countries with endemic infection (eg, Asia, Middle East, Africa, Latin America, countries of the former Soviet Union), including international adoptees
- Children with travel histories to countries with endemic infection and substantial contact with indigenous people from such countries[c]

Children who should have annual TST or IGRA:
- Children infected with HIV infection (TST only)
- Incarcerated adolescents

Children at increased risk of progression of LTBI to tuberculosis disease: Children with other medical conditions, including diabetes mellitus, chronic renal failure, malnutrition, and congenital or acquired immunodeficiencies deserve special consideration. Without recent exposure, these people are not at increased risk of acquiring tuberculosis infection. Underlying immune deficiencies associated with these conditions theoretically would enhance the possibility for progression to severe disease. Initial histories of potential exposure to tuberculosis should be included for all of these patients. If these histories or local epidemiologic factors suggest a possibility of exposure, immediate and periodic TST or IGRA should be considered. **An initial TST or IGRA should be performed before initiation of immunosuppressive therapy, including prolonged steroid administration, use of tumor necrosis factor-alpha antagonists, or other immunosuppressive therapy in any child requiring these treatments.**

IGRA indicates interferon-gamma release assay; HIV, human immunodeficiency virus; LTBI, latent tuberculosis infection.
[a]Bacille Calmette-Guérin immunization is not a contraindication to a TST.
[b]Beginning as early as 3 months of age.
[c]If the child is well, the TST or IGRA should be delayed for up to 10 weeks after return.

Table 3.81. Validated Questions for Determining Risk of LTBI in Children in the United States

- Has a family member or contact had tuberculosis disease?
- Has a family member had a positive tuberculin skin test result?
- Was your child born in a high-risk country (countries other than the United States, Canada, Australia, New Zealand, or Western European countries)?
- Has your child traveled (had contact with resident populations) to a high-risk country for more than 1 week?

LTBI indicates latent tuberculosis infection.

data, the same TST spacing recommendation should be applied to these vaccines as described for MMR. There is no evidence that inactivated vaccines, polysaccharide vaccines, or recombinant or subunit vaccines or toxoids interfere with immune response to TST.

Administration of TSTs and interpretation of results should be performed by experienced health care professionals who have been trained in the proper methods, because administration and interpretation by unskilled people and family members are unreliable. The recommended time for assessing the TST result is 48 to 72 hours after administration. However, induration that develops at the site of administration more than 72 hours later should be measured, and some experts advise that this should be considered the result. The diameter of induration in millimeters is measured transversely to the long axis of the forearm. Positive test results, as defined in Table 3.79 (p 681), can persist for several weeks.

A negative TST result does not exclude LTBI or tuberculosis disease. Approximately 10% to 40% of immunocompetent children with culture-documented tuberculosis disease do not react initially to a TST. Host factors, such as young age, poor nutrition, immunosuppression, other viral infections (especially measles, varicella, and influenza), recent tuberculosis infection, and disseminated tuberculosis disease can decrease TST reactivity. Many children and adults coinfected with HIV and *M tuberculosis* complex do not react to a TST. Control skin tests to assess cutaneous anergy are not recommended routinely.

Interpretation of TST Results (see Table 3.79, p 681). Classification of TST results is based on epidemiologic and clinical factors. The size of induration (mm) for a positive result varies with the person's risk of LTBI and progression to tuberculosis disease.

Current guidelines from the Centers for Disease Control and Prevention (CDC), American Thoracic Society, and American Academy of Pediatrics accept 15 mm or greater of induration as a positive TST result for any person. Interpretation of 5 mm or more or 10 mm or more induration is summarized in Table 3.79 (p 681). Interpretation is aided by knowledge of the child's risk factors for LTBI and tuberculosis disease. Prompt clinical and radiographic evaluation of all children and adolescents with a positive TST reaction is recommended.

Interpretation of TST Results in Previous Recipients of BCG Vaccine. Generally, interpretation of TST results in BCG recipients is the same as for people who have not received BCG vaccine. After BCG immunization, distinguishing between a positive TST result caused by pathogenic *M tuberculosis* complex infection and that caused by BCG can be impossible. Reactivity of the TST after receipt of BCG vaccine does not occur in some patients. The size of the TST reaction (ie, mm of induration) attributable to BCG immunization depends on many factors, including age at BCG immunization, quality and strain of BCG vaccine used, number of doses of BCG vaccine received, nutritional and immunologic status of the vaccine recipient, frequency of TST administration, and time lapse between immunization and TST.

Tuberculosis disease should be suspected strongly in any symptomatic person regardless of a TST result and history of BCG immunization. When evaluating an asymptomatic child who has a positive TST result and who possibly received BCG vaccine, certain factors, such as documented receipt of multiple BCG immunizations (as evidenced by BCG scars), decrease the likelihood that the positive TST result is attributable to LTBI. Evidence that increases the probability that a positive TST result is attributable to LTBI includes known contact with a person with contagious tuberculosis, a family history of tuberculosis disease, a long interval (more than 5 years) since neonatal BCG immunization, and a TST reaction 15 mm or greater.

Prompt clinical and radiographic evaluation of all children with a positive TST reaction is recommended. Chest radiographic findings of a granuloma, calcification, or adenopathy can be caused by infection with *M tuberculosis* complex but not by BCG immunization. BCG can cause suppurative lymphadenitis in the regional lymph node drainage of the infectious site of a healthy child and can cause disseminated disease in children with some forms of immunodeficiency.

Recommendations for TST Use. The most reliable strategies for preventing LTBI and tuberculosis disease in children are based on thorough and expedient contact investigations rather than nonselective skin testing of large populations. Contact investigations are public-health interventions that should be coordinated through the local public health department. Specific recommendations for TST use are given in Table 3.80 (p 684). All children need routine health care evaluations that include an assessment of their risk of exposure to tuberculosis. Only children deemed to have increased risk of contact with people with contagious tuberculosis or children with suspected tuberculosis disease should be considered for a TST. Household investigation is indicated whenever a TST result of a household member converts from negative to positive (indicating recent infection).

Immunologic-Based Testing.[1] QuantiFERON-TB Gold and Gold In-Tube and T-SPOT. TB are IGRAs. These FDA-approved tests measure ex vivo interferon-gamma production from T lymphocytes in response to stimulation with antigens that are fairly specific to *M tuberculosis* complex. As with TSTs, IGRAs cannot distinguish between latent infection and disease, and a negative result from these tests cannot exclude the possibility of tuberculosis infection or disease in a patient with findings that raise suspicion for these conditions. The sensitivity of these blood tests is similar to that of TSTs for detecting infection in adults and children who have untreated culture-confirmed tuberculosis. The specificity of IGRAs is higher than that for TSTs, because the antigens used are not found in BCG or most pathogenic nontuberculous mycobacteria (eg, are not found in *M avium* complex but are found in *M kansasii*, *M fortuitum*, and *M marinum*). IGRAs are recommended by the Centers for Disease Control and Prevention, and some experts prefer IGRAs for use in adults in all circumstances in which a TST is used. The published experience with testing children with IGRAs is less extensive than for adults, but a number of studies have demonstrated that IGRAs perform well in most children 4 years of age and older. Some children who received BCG vaccine may have a false-positive TST result, and LTBI

---

[1]Centers for Disease Control and Prevention. Guidelines for using the QuantiFERON-TB Gold test for detecting *Mycobacterium tuberculosis* infection, United States. *MMWR Recomm Rep.* 2005;54(RR-15):49–55

is overestimated by use of the TST, even in these circumstances. However, the correct interpretation of a negative IGRA test result in a child with a positive TST result remains challenging because of the current absence of longitudinal studies to determine the negative predictive value of the IGRAs (when the TST result is positive and the IGRA result is negative).

At this time, neither an IGRA nor the TST can be considered a "gold standard" for diagnosis of LTBI. Current recommendations for use of IGRAs in children are as follows:

- For immune-competent children 5 years of age and older, IGRAs can be used in place of a TST to confirm cases of tuberculosis or cases of LTBI and likely will yield fewer false-positive test results.
- Children with a positive result from an IGRA should be considered infected with *M tuberculosis* complex. A negative IGRA result cannot universally be interpreted as absence of infection.
- Because of their higher specificity and lack of cross-reaction with BCG, IGRAs may be useful in children who have received BCG vaccine. IGRAs may be useful to determine whether a BCG-immunized child with a reactive TST more likely has LTBI or has a false-positive TST reaction caused by the BCG.
- IGRAs cannot be recommended routinely for use in children younger than 5 years of age or for immune-compromised children of any age because of a lack of published data about their utility with these groups.
- Indeterminate IGRA results do not exclude tuberculosis infection and should not be used to make clinical decisions.

Serologic tests for tuberculosis disease that are used in some Asian and African countries have unsatisfactory sensitivity and specificity, and none of them have been approved for use in the United States.

HIV Infection. Children with HIV infection are considered at high risk of tuberculosis, and an annual TST beginning at 3 through 12 months of age is recommended. Children who have tuberculosis disease should be tested for HIV infection.

TREATMENT (SEE TABLE 3.82, P 688):

Specific Drugs. Antituberculosis drugs kill *M tuberculosis* complex organisms or inhibit multiplication of the organism, thereby arresting progression of LTBI and preventing most complications of early tuberculosis disease. Chemotherapy does not cause rapid disappearance of already caseous or granulomatous lesions (eg, mediastinal lymphadenitis). Dosage recommendations and the more commonly reported adverse reactions of major antituberculosis drugs are summarized in Tables 3.82 (p 688) and 3.83 (p 689). For treatment of tuberculosis disease, these drugs always must be used in recommended combination to minimize emergence of drug-resistant strains. Use of nonstandard regimens for any reason (eg, drug allergy or drug resistance) should be undertaken only in consultation with an expert in treating tuberculosis.

Isoniazid is bactericidal, rapidly absorbed, and well tolerated and penetrates into body fluids, including cerebrospinal fluid (CSF). Isoniazid is metabolized in the liver and excreted primarily through the kidneys. Hepatotoxic effects are rare in children but can be life threatening. In children and adolescents given recommended doses, peripheral neuritis or seizures caused by inhibition of pyridoxine metabolism are rare, and most do not need pyridoxine supplements. Pyridoxine supplementation is recommended for exclusively breastfed infants and for children and adolescents on meat- and milk-deficient diets; children with nutritional deficiencies, including all symptomatic HIV-infected children;

Table 3.82. Recommended Treatment Regimens for Drug-Susceptible Tuberculosis in Infants, Children, and Adolescents

Infection or Disease Category	Regimen	Remarks
Latent tuberculosis infection (positive TST or IGRA result, no disease)		
• Isoniazid susceptible	9 mo of isoniazid, once a day	If daily therapy is not possible, DOT twice a week can be used for 9 mo.
• Isoniazid resistant	6 mo of rifampin, once a day	If daily therapy is not possible, DOT twice a week can be used for 6 mo.
• Isoniazid-rifampin resistant[a]	Consult a tuberculosis specialist	
Pulmonary and extrapulmonary (except meningitis)	2 mo of isoniazid, rifampin, pyrazinamide, and ethambutol daily, followed by 4 mo of isoniazid and rifampin[b] by DOT[c] for drug-susceptible *Mycobacterium tuberculosis* 9 to 12 mo of isoniazid and rifampin for drug-susceptible *Mycobacterium bovis*	If possible drug resistance is a concern (see text), another drug (ethambutol or an aminoglycoside) is added to the initial 3-drug therapy until drug susceptibilities are determined. DOT is highly desirable. If hilar adenopathy only, a 6-mo course of isoniazid and rifampin is sufficient. Drugs can be given 2 or 3 times/wk under DOT in the initial phase if nonadherence is likely.
Meningitis	2 mo of isoniazid, rifampin, pyrazinamide, and an aminoglycoside or ethambutol or ethionamide, once a day, followed by 7–10 mo of isoniazid and rifampin, once a day or twice a week (9–12 mo total) for drug-susceptible *M tuberculosis* At least 12 mo of therapy without pyrazinamide for drug-susceptible *M bovis*	A fourth drug, such as an aminoglycoside, is given with initial therapy until drug susceptibility is known. For patients who may have acquired tuberculosis in geographic areas where resistance to streptomycin is common, kanamycin, amikacin, or capreomycin can be used instead of streptomycin.

TST indicates tuberculin skin test; IGRA, interferon-gamma release assay; DOT, directly observed therapy.

[a]Duration of therapy is longer for human immunodeficiency virus (HIV)-infected people, and additional drugs may be indicated (see Tuberculosis Disease and HIV Infection, p 694).

[b]Medications should be administered daily for the first 2 weeks to 2 months of treatment and then can be administered 2 to 3 times per week by DOT.

[c]If initial chest radiograph shows cavitary lesions and sputum after 2 months of therapy remains positive, duration of therapy is extended to 9 months.

Table 3.83. Commonly Used Drugs for Treatment of Tuberculosis in Infants, Children, and Adolescents

Drugs	Dosage Forms	Daily Dosage, mg/kg	Twice a Week Dosage, mg/kg per Dose	Maximum Dose	Adverse Reactions
Ethambutol	Tablets 100 mg 400 mg	20–25	50	2.5 g	Optic neuritis (usually reversible), decreased red-green color discrimination, gastrointestinal tract disturbances, hypersensitivity
Isoniazid[a]	Scored tablets 100 mg 300 mg Syrup 10 mg/mL	10–15[b]	20–30	Daily, 300 mg Twice a week, 900 mg	Mild hepatic enzyme elevation, hepatitis,[b] peripheral neuritis, hypersensitivity
Pyrazinamide[a]	Scored tablets 500 mg	30–40	50	2 g	Diarrhea and gastric irritation caused by vehicle in the syrup Hepatotoxic effects, hyperuricemia, arthralgia, gastrointestinal tract upset
Rifampin[a]	Capsules 150 mg 300 mg Syrup formulated capsules	10–20	10–20	600 mg	Orange discoloration of secretions or urine, staining of contact lenses, vomiting, hepatitis, influenza-like reaction, thrombocytopenia, pruritus; oral contraceptives may be ineffective

[a]Rifamate is a capsule containing 150 mg of isoniazid and 300 mg of rifampin. Two capsules provide the usual adult (greater than 50 kg) daily doses of each drug. Rifater is a capsule containing 50 mg of isoniazid, 120 mg of rifampin, and 300 mg of pyrazinamide. Isoniazid and rifampin also are available for parenteral administration.

[b]When isoniazid in a dosage exceeding 10 mg/kg/day is used in combination with rifampin, the incidence of hepatotoxic effects may be increased.

and pregnant adolescents and women. For infants and young children, isoniazid tablets can be pulverized.

Rifampin is a bactericidal agent in the rifamycin class of drugs that is absorbed rapidly and penetrates into body fluids, including CSF. Other drugs in this class approved for treating tuberculosis are rifabutin and rifapentine. Rifampin is metabolized by the liver and can alter the pharmacokinetics and serum concentrations of many other drugs. Rare adverse effects include hepatotoxicity, influenza-like symptoms, and pruritus. Rifampin is excreted in bile and urine and can cause orange urine, sweat, and tears and discoloration of soft contact lenses. Rifampin can make oral contraceptives ineffective, so other birth control methods should be adopted when rifampin is administered to sexually active female adolescents and adults. For infants and young children, the contents of the capsules can be suspended in wild cherry-flavored syrup or sprinkled on semisoft foods (eg, applesauce). *M tuberculosis* complex isolates that are resistant to rifampin are uncommon in the United States. Rifabutin is a suitable alternative to rifampin in children with HIV infection receiving highly active antiretroviral therapy that proscribes the use of rifampin; however, experience in children is limited. Major toxicities of rifabutin include leukopenia, gastrointestinal tract upset, polyarthralgia, rash, increased transaminase concentrations, and skin and secretion discoloration (pseudojaundice). Anterior uveitis has been reported among children receiving rifabutin as prophylaxis or as part of a combination regimen for treatment, usually when administered at high doses. Rifabutin also increases hepatic metabolism of many drugs but is a less potent inducer of cytochrome P450 enzymes than rifampin and has fewer problematic drug interactions than rifampin. However, adjustments in dose of rifabutin and the coadministered antiretroviral drugs may be necessary for certain combinations. Rifapentine is a long-acting rifamycin that permits weekly dosing in select adults, but it has not been evaluated in pediatric patients.

Pyrazinamide attains therapeutic CSF concentrations, is detectable in macrophages, is administered orally, and is metabolized by the liver. Administration of pyrazinamide with isoniazid and rifampin allows for 6-month regimens in patients with drug-susceptible tuberculosis. Almost all isolates of *M bovis* are resistant to pyrazinamide, precluding 6-month therapy for this pathogen. In daily doses of 40 mg/kg per day or less, pyrazinamide seldom has hepatotoxic effects and is well tolerated by children. Some adolescents and many adults develop arthralgia and hyperuricemia because of inhibition of uric acid excretion. Pyrazinamide must be used with caution in people with underlying liver disease. Pyrazinamide, when administered with rifampin, is associated with high rates of hepatotoxicity.

Ethambutol is well absorbed after oral administration, diffuses well into tissues, and is excreted in urine. However, concentrations in the CSF are low. At 20 mg/kg per day, ethambutol is bacteriostatic, and its primary therapeutic role is to prevent emergence of drug resistance. Ethambutol can cause reversible or irreversible optic neuritis, but reports in children with normal renal function are rare. Children who are receiving ethambutol should be monitored monthly for visual acuity and red-green color discrimination if they are old enough to cooperate. Use of ethambutol in young children whose visual acuity cannot be monitored requires consideration of risks and benefits.

Streptomycin is regarded as a "second-line" drug and is available only on a limited basis. It is administered intramuscularly. When streptomycin is not available, kanamycin, amikacin, or capreomycin are alternatives that can be prescribed for the initial 4 to 8 weeks of therapy. Patients who receive any of these drugs should be monitored for otic, vestibular, and renal toxicity.

The less commonly used (eg, "second-line") antituberculosis drugs, their doses, and adverse effects are listed in Table 3.84 (p 692). These drugs have limited usefulness because of decreased effectiveness and greater toxicity and should be used only in consultation with a specialist familiar with childhood tuberculosis. Ethionamide is an orally administered antituberculosis drug that is well tolerated by children, achieves therapeutic CSF concentrations, and may be useful for treatment of people with meningitis or drug-resistant tuberculosis. Fluoroquinolones have antituberculosis activity and can be used in special circumstances. Because some fluoroquinolones are approved by the FDA for use only in people 18 years of age and older, their use in younger patients necessitates careful assessment of the potential risks and benefits (see Antimicrobial Agents and Related Therapy, p 737).

Occasionally, a patient cannot tolerate oral medications. Isoniazid, rifampin, streptomycin and related drugs, and fluoroquinolones can be administered parenterally.

Therapy for LTBI. Isoniazid given to adults who have LTBI (ie, no clinical or radiographic abnormalities suggesting tuberculosis disease) provides substantial protection (54%–88%) against development of tuberculosis disease for at least 20 years. Among children, efficacy approaches 100% with appropriate adherence to therapy. All infants, children, and adolescents who have a positive TST result but no evidence of tuberculosis disease and who never have received antituberculosis therapy should be considered for isoniazid unless resistance to isoniazid is suspected (ie, known exposure to a person with isoniazid-resistant tuberculosis) or a specific contraindication exists. Isoniazid, in this circumstance, is therapeutic and prevents development of disease. A physical examination and chest radiograph should be obtained at the time isoniazid therapy is initiated to exclude tuberculosis disease; if the radiograph is normal, the child remains asymptomatic, and treatment is completed, radiography need not be repeated.

Duration of Therapy for LTBI. For infants, children, and adolescents, the recommended duration of isoniazid therapy is 9 months. Isoniazid is given daily in a single dose. Clinicians who treat LTBI should educate patients and their families about the adverse effects of isoniazid and should prescribe it in monthly allocations, with clinic visits scheduled for monthly face-to-face monitoring. Successful completion of therapy is based on total number of doses taken. When adherence with daily therapy with isoniazid cannot be ensured, twice-a-week DOT can be considered. The twice-weekly regimen should not be prescribed unless each dose is by DOT. Routine determination of serum transaminase values during the 9 months of therapy for LTBI is not indicated.

Therapy for Contacts of Patients With Isoniazid-Resistant M tuberculosis. The incidence of isoniazid resistance among *M tuberculosis* complex isolates from US patients is approximately 9%. Risk factors for drug resistance are listed in Table 3.85, p 693. However, most experts recommend that isoniazid be used to treat LTBI in children unless the child has had contact with a person known to have isoniazid-resistant tuberculosis. If the source case is found to have isoniazid-resistant, rifampin-susceptible organisms, isoniazid should be discontinued and rifampin should be given for a total course of 6 months. A 2-month course of rifampin and pyrazinamide for treatment of LTBI that once was recommended only for adults no longer is recommended for any age group because of unacceptable hepatotoxicity. Optimal therapy for children with LTBI caused by organisms with resistance to isoniazid and rifampin (ie, MDR) is not known. In these circumstances,

Table 3.84. Less Commonly Used Drugs for Treatment of Drug-Resistant Tuberculosis in Infants, Children, and Adolescents[a]

Drugs	Dosage, Forms	Daily Dosage, mg/kg	Maximum Dose	Adverse Reactions
Amikacin[b]	Vials, 500 mg and 1 g	15–30 (intravenous or intramuscular administration)	1 g	Auditory and vestibular toxic effects, nephrotoxic effects
Capreomycin[b]	Vials, 1 g	15–30 (intramuscular administration)	1 g	Auditory and vestibular toxicity and nephrotoxic effects
Cycloserine	Capsules, 250 mg	10–20, given in 2 divided doses	1 g	Psychosis, personality changes, seizures, rash
Ethionamide	Tablets, 250 mg	15–20, given in 2–3 divided doses	1 g	Gastrointestinal tract disturbances, hepatotoxic effects, hypersensitivity reactions, hypothyroid
Kanamycin	Vials 75 mg/2 mL 500 mg/2 mL 1 g/3 mL	15–30 (intramuscular or intravenous administration)	1 g	Auditory and vestibular toxic effects, nephrotoxic effects
Levofloxacin[c]	Tablets 250 mg 500 mg Vials 25 mg/mL	Adults 500–1000 mg (once daily) Children: not recommended	1 g	Theoretical effect on growing cartilage, gastrointestinal tract disturbances, rash, headache, restlessness, confusion
Para-aminosalicylic acid (PAS)	Packets, 3 g	200–300 (2–4 times a day)	10 g	Gastrointestinal tract disturbances, hypersensitivity, hepatotoxic effects
Streptomycin[b]	Vials 1 g 4 g	20–40 (intramuscular administration)	1 g	Auditory and vestibular toxic effects, nephrotoxic effects, rash

[a]These drugs should be used in consultation with a specialist in tuberculosis.
[b]Dose adjustment in renal insufficiency.
[c]Levofloxacin is not approved for use in children younger than 18 years of age; its use in younger children necessitates assessment of the potential risks and benefits (see Antimicrobial Agents and Related Therapy, p 737).

Table 3.85. People at Increased Risk of Drug-Resistant Tuberculosis Infection or Disease

- People with a history of treatment for tuberculosis disease (or whose source case for the contact received such treatment)
- Contacts of a patient with drug-resistant contagious tuberculosis disease
- People born in countries with high prevalence of drug-resistant tuberculosis
- Infected people whose source case has positive smears for acid-fast bacilli or cultures after 2 months of appropriate antituberculosis therapy and patients who do not respond to a standard treatment regimen.
- Residence in geographic area with a high percentage of drug-resistant isolates.

multidrug regimens have been used. Drugs to consider include pyrazinamide, a fluoro-quinolone, and ethambutol, depending on susceptibility of the isolate. Consultation with a tuberculosis specialist is indicated.

Treatment of Tuberculosis Disease. The goal of treatment is to achieve sterilization of the tuberculous lesion in the shortest possible time. Achievement of this goal minimizes the possibility of development of resistant organisms. The major problem limiting successful treatment is poor adherence to prescribed treatment regimens. The use of DOT decreases the rates of relapse, treatment failures, and drug resistance; therefore, DOT is recommended strongly for treatment of children and adolescents with tuberculosis disease in the United States.

For tuberculosis disease, a 6-month 4-drug regimen consisting of isoniazid, rifampin, pyrazinamide, and ethambutol for the first 2 months and isoniazid and rifampin for the remaining 4 months is recommended for treatment of pulmonary disease, pulmonary disease with hilar adenopathy, and hilar adenopathy disease in infants, children, and adolescents when an MDR case is not suspected as the source of infection or when drug-susceptibility results are available. Some experts would administer 3 drugs (isoniazid, rifampin, and pyrazinamide) as the initial regimen if a source case has been identified with known pansusceptible *M tuberculosis*, if the presumed source case has no risk factors for drug-resistant *M tuberculosis*, or if the source case is unknown but the child resides in an area with low rates of isoniazid resistance. If the chest radiograph shows one or more cavitary lesions and sputum culture remains positive after 2 months of therapy, the duration of therapy should be extended to 9 months. For children with hilar adenopathy in whom drug resistance is not a consideration, a 6-month regimen of only isoniazid and rifampin is considered adequate by some experts.

In the 6-month regimen with 4-drug therapy, isoniazid, rifampin, pyrazinamide, and ethambutol are given once a day for the first 2 weeks by DOT. Between 2 weeks and 2 months of treatment, these drugs can be given daily or twice or 3 times a week by DOT. After the initial 2-month period, a DOT regimen of isoniazid and rifampin given 2 or 3 times a week is acceptable (see Table 3.82, p 688, for doses). Several alternative regimens with differing durations of daily therapy and total therapy have been used successfully in adults and children. These alternative regimens should be prescribed and managed by a specialist in tuberculosis.

When **drug resistance** is possible (see Table 3.85, above), initial therapy should be adjusted to match the presumed drug susceptibility pattern until drug susceptibility results are available. If an isolate from the pediatric case under treatment is not available, drug susceptibilities can be inferred by the drug susceptibility pattern of isolates from the adult source case. Data for guiding drug selection may not be available for foreign-born children or in circumstances of international travel. If this information is not available, a 4-drug initial regimen is recommended with close monitoring for clinical response.

Therapy for Drug-Resistant Tuberculosis Disease. Drug resistance is most common in the following: (1) people born in areas such as Russia and the former Soviet Union, Asia, Africa, and Latin America; (2) people previously treated for tuberculosis disease; and (3) contacts, especially children, with tuberculosis disease whose source case is a person from one of these groups (see also Table 3.85, p 693). Most cases of pulmonary tuberculosis in children that are caused by an isoniazid-resistant but rifampin- and pyrazinamide-susceptible strain of *M tuberculosis* complex can be treated with a 6-month regimen of rifampin, pyrazinamide, and ethambutol. For cases of MDR tuberculosis disease, the treatment regimen should include at least 4 antituberculosis drugs to which the organism is susceptible. In cases of tuberculosis with isoniazid- and rifampin-resistant strains, 6-month drug regimens are not recommended. A regimen lasting 12 to 24 months of therapy usually is necessary for cure. Regimens in which drugs are administered 2 or 3 times per week also are not recommended for drug-resistant disease; daily DOT is critical to cure children with drug-resistant tuberculosis disease and to prevent emergence of further resistance.

Extrapulmonary M tuberculosis Tuberculosis Disease. In general, extrapulmonary tuberculosis—with the exception of meningitis—can be treated with the same regimens as used for pulmonary tuberculosis. For suspected drug-susceptible tuberculous meningitis, daily treatment with isoniazid, rifampin, pyrazinamide, and ethambutol or ethionamide, if possible, or an aminoglycoside should be initiated. When susceptibility to all drugs is established, the ethambutol, ethionamide, or aminoglycoside can be discontinued. Pyrazinamide is given for a total of 2 months and isoniazid and rifampin are given for a total of 9 to 12 months. Isoniazid and rifampin can be given daily or 2 or 3 times per week after the first 2 months of treatment.

Corticosteroids. The evidence supporting adjuvant treatment with corticosteroids for children with tuberculosis disease is incomplete. Corticosteroids are indicated for children with tuberculous meningitis, because corticosteroids decrease rates of mortality and long-term neurologic impairment. Corticosteroids can be considered for children with pleural and pericardial effusions (to hasten reabsorption of fluid), severe miliary disease (to mitigate alveolocapillary block), endobronchial disease (to relieve obstruction and atelectasis), and abdominal tuberculosis (to decrease the risk of strictures). Corticosteroids should be given only when accompanied by appropriate antituberculosis therapy. Most experts consider 2 mg/kg per day of prednisone (maximum, 60 mg/day) or its equivalent for 4 to 6 weeks followed by tapering to be appropriate.

Tuberculosis Disease and HIV Infection.[1] Adults and children with HIV infection have an increased incidence of tuberculosis disease. Hence, *HIV testing is indicated for all patients with tuberculosis disease.* The clinical manifestations and radiographic appearance of tuberculosis disease in children with HIV infection tend to be similar to those in immunocompetent children, but manifestations in these children can be more severe and unusual and

[1] Centers for Disease Control and Prevention. Guidelines for prevention and treatment of opportunistic infections in HIV-infected adults and adolescents. Recommendations from CDC, the National Institutes of Health, and the HIV Medicine Association of the Infectious Diseases Society of America. *MMWR Early Release.* 2009;58(March 24, 2009):1–207. Available at: **http://www.cdc.gov/mmwr/pdf/rr/rr58e324.pdf.**

can include extrapulmonary involvement of multiple organs. In HIV-infected patients, a TST result of 5-mm induration or more is considered positive (see Table 3.79, p 681); however, a negative TST result attributable to HIV-related immunosuppression also can occur. Specimens for culture should be obtained from all HIV-infected children with suspected tuberculosis.

Most HIV-infected adults with drug-susceptible tuberculosis respond well to antituberculosis drugs when appropriate therapy is given early. However, optimal therapy for tuberculosis in children with HIV infection has not been established. Treating tuberculosis in an HIV-infected child is complicated by antiretroviral drug interactions with the rifamycins and overlapping toxicities caused by antiretroviral drugs and medications used to treat tuberculosis. Therapy always should include at least 4 drugs initially and be continued for at least 9 months. Isoniazid, rifampin, and pyrazinamide, usually with ethambutol or an aminoglycoside, should be given for at least the first 2 months. A 3-drug regimen can be used once drug-resistant tuberculosis disease is excluded. Rifampin may be contraindicated in people who are receiving highly active antiretroviral therapy. Rifabutin can be substituted for rifampin in some circumstances. Consultation with a specialist who has experience in managing HIV-infected patients with tuberculosis is advised strongly.

Evaluation and Monitoring of Therapy in Children and Adolescents. Careful monthly monitoring of the clinical and bacteriologic responses to therapy is important. With DOT, clinical evaluation is an integral component of each visit for drug administration. For patients with pulmonary tuberculosis, chest radiographs should be obtained after 2 months of therapy to evaluate response. Even with successful 6-month regimens, hilar adenopathy can persist for 2 to 3 years; normal radiographic findings are not necessary to discontinue therapy. Follow-up chest radiography beyond termination of successful therapy usually is not necessary unless clinical deterioration occurs.

If therapy has been interrupted, the date of completion should be extended. Although guidelines cannot be provided for every situation, factors to consider when establishing the date of completion include the following: (1) length of interruption of therapy; (2) time during therapy (early or late) when interruption occurred; and (3) the patient's clinical, radiographic, and bacteriologic status before, during, and after interruption of therapy. The total doses administered by DOT should be calculated to guide the duration of therapy. Consultation with a specialist in tuberculosis is advised.

Untoward effects of isoniazid therapy, including severe hepatitis in otherwise healthy infants, children, and adolescents, are rare. Routine determination of serum transaminase concentrations is not recommended. However, for children with severe tuberculosis disease, especially children with meningitis or disseminated disease, transaminase concentrations should be monitored approximately monthly during the first several months of treatment. Other indications for testing include the following: (1) having concurrent or recent liver or biliary disease; (2) being pregnant or in the first 6 weeks postpartum; (3) having clinical evidence of hepatotoxic effects; or (4) concurrently using other hepatotoxic drugs (eg, anticonvulsant or HIV agents). In most other circumstances, monthly clinical evaluations to observe for signs or symptoms of hepatitis and other adverse effects of drug therapy without routine monitoring of transaminase concentrations is appropriate follow-up. In all cases, regular physician-patient contact to assess drug adherence, efficacy, and adverse effects is an important aspect of management. Patients should be advised to call a physician immediately if signs of adverse effects, in particular hepatotoxicity (eg, vomiting, abdominal pain, jaundice), develop.

Immunizations. Patients who are receiving treatment for tuberculosis can be given measles and other age-appropriate attenuated live-virus vaccines unless they are receiving high-dose corticosteroids, are severely ill, or have other specific contraindications to immunization.

Tuberculosis During Pregnancy and Breastfeeding. Tuberculosis treatment during pregnancy varies because of the complexity of management decisions. During pregnancy, if tuberculosis disease is diagnosed, a regimen of isoniazid, rifampin, and ethambutol is recommended. Pyrazinamide commonly is used in a 3- or 4-drug regimen, but safety during pregnancy has not been established. At least 6 months of therapy is indicated for drug-susceptible tuberculosis disease if pyrazinamide is used; at least 9 months of therapy is indicated if pyrazinamide is not used. Prompt initiation of therapy is mandatory to protect mother and fetus.

Asymptomatic pregnant women with a positive TST or IGRA result, normal chest radiographic findings, and recent contact with a contagious person should be considered for isoniazid therapy. The recommended duration of therapy is 9 months. Therapy in these circumstances should begin after the first trimester. Pyridoxine supplementation is indicated for all pregnant and breastfeeding women receiving isoniazid.

Isoniazid, ethambutol, and rifampin are relatively safe for the fetus. The benefit of ethambutol and rifampin for therapy of tuberculosis disease in the mother outweighs the risk to the infant. Because streptomycin can cause ototoxic effects in the fetus, it should not be used unless administration is essential for effective treatment. The effects of other second-line drugs on the fetus are unknown.

Although isoniazid is secreted in human milk, no adverse effects of isoniazid on nursing infants have been demonstrated (see Human Milk, p 118). Breastfed infants do not require pyridoxine supplementation unless they are receiving isoniazid.

Congenital Tuberculosis. Women who have only pulmonary tuberculosis are not likely to infect the fetus but can infect their infant after delivery. Congenital tuberculosis is rare, but in utero infections can occur after maternal bacillemia.

If a newborn infant is suspected of having congenital tuberculosis, a TST, chest radiography, lumbar puncture, and appropriate cultures should be performed promptly. The TST result usually is negative in newborn infants with congenital or perinatally acquired infection. Only case reports of results of IGRAs in selected newborn infants have been published, and IGRAs should not be substituted for the TST in newborn infants. Hence, regardless of the TST results, treatment of the infant should be initiated promptly with isoniazid, rifampin, pyrazinamide, and an aminoglycoside (eg, amikacin). The placenta should be examined histologically for granulomata and AFB, and a specimen should be cultured for *M tuberculosis* complex. The mother should be evaluated for presence of pulmonary or extrapulmonary disease, including uterine tuberculosis disease. If the maternal physical examination and chest radiographic findings support the diagnosis of tuberculosis disease, the newborn infant should be treated with regimens recommended for tuberculosis disease. If meningitis is confirmed, corticosteroids should be added (see Corticosteroids, p 694). Drug susceptibility testing of the organism recovered from the mother or household contact, infant, or both should be performed.

Management of the Newborn Infant Whose Mother (or Other Household Contact) Has LTBI or Tuberculosis Disease. Management of the newborn infant is based on categorization of the maternal (or household contact) infection. Although protection of the infant from exposure and infection is of paramount importance, contact between infant and mother should be allowed when possible. Differing circumstances and resulting recommendations are as follows:

- **Mother (or household contact) has a positive TST or IGRA result and normal chest radiographic findings.** If the mother (or household contact) is asymptomatic, no separation is required. The mother usually is a candidate for treatment of LTBI after the initial postpartum period. The newborn infant needs no special evaluation or therapy. Because the positive TST or IGRA result could be a marker of an unrecognized case of contagious tuberculosis within the household, other household members should have a TST or IGRA and further evaluation, but this should not delay the infant's discharge from the hospital. These mothers can breastfeed their infants.

- **Mother (or household contact) has clinical signs and symptoms or abnormal findings on chest radiograph consistent with tuberculosis disease.** Cases of suspected or proven tuberculosis disease in mothers (or household contacts) should be reported immediately to the local health department, and investigation of all household members should start within 7 days. If the mother has tuberculosis disease, the infant should be evaluated for congenital tuberculosis (see Congenital Tuberculosis), and the mother should be tested for HIV infection. The mother (or household contact) and the infant should be separated until the mother (or household contact) has been evaluated and, if tuberculosis disease is suspected, until the mother (or household contact) and infant are receiving appropriate antituberculosis therapy, the mother wears a mask, and the mother understands and is willing to adhere to infection-control measures. Once the infant is receiving isoniazid, separation is not necessary unless the mother (or household contact) has possible MDR tuberculosis disease or has poor adherence to treatment and DOT is not possible. In this circumstance, the infant should be separated from the mother (or household contact), and BCG immunization should be considered for the infant. If the mother is suspected of having MDR tuberculosis disease, an expert in tuberculosis disease treatment should be consulted. Women with tuberculosis disease who have been treated appropriately for 2 or more weeks and who are not considered contagious can breastfeed.

  If congenital tuberculosis is excluded, isoniazid is given until the infant is 3 or 4 months of age, when a TST should be performed. If the TST result is positive, the infant should be reassessed for tuberculosis disease. If tuberculosis disease is excluded, isoniazid should be continued for a total of 9 months. The infant should be evaluated at monthly intervals during treatment. If the TST result is negative at 3 to 4 months of age and the mother (or household contact) has good adherence and response to treatment and no longer is contagious, isoniazid is discontinued.

- **Mother (or household contact) has abnormal findings on chest radiography but no evidence of tuberculosis disease.** If the chest radiograph of the mother (or household contact) appears abnormal but is not characteristic of tuberculosis disease and the history, physical examination, and sputum smear indicate no evidence of tuberculosis disease, the infant can be assumed to be at low risk of tuberculosis infection and need not be separated from the mother (or household contact). The mother and her infant should receive follow-up care and the mother should be treated for LTBI. Other household members should have a TST or IGRA and further evaluation.

ISOLATION OF THE HOSPITALIZED PATIENT: Most children with tuberculosis disease, especially children younger than 10 years, are not contagious. Exceptions are the following: (1) children with cavitary pulmonary tuberculosis; (2) children with positive sputum AFB smears; (3) children with laryngeal involvement; (4) children with extensive pulmonary infection; or (5) children with congenital tuberculosis undergoing procedures that involve the oropharyngeal airway (eg, endotracheal intubation). In these instances, isolation for tuberculosis or AFB are indicated until effective therapy has been initiated, sputum smears demonstrate a diminishing number of organisms, and cough is abating. Children with no cough and negative sputum AFB smears can be hospitalized in an open ward. Infection-control measures for hospital personnel exposed to contagious patients should include the use of personally "fitted" and "sealed" particulate respirators for all patient contacts (see Infection Control for Hospitalized Children, p 148). The contagious patient should be placed in an airborne infection isolation room in the hospital.

The major concern in infection control relates to adult household members and contacts who can be the source of infection. Visitation should be limited to people who have been evaluated medically. Household members and contacts should be managed with tuberculosis precautions when visiting until they are demonstrated not to have contagious tuberculosis. Nonadherent household contacts should be excluded from hospital visitation until evaluation is complete and tuberculosis disease is excluded or treatment has rendered source cases noncontagious.

TUBERCULOSIS CAUSED BY *M BOVIS*: Infections with *M bovis* account for approximately 1% to 2% of tuberculosis cases in the United States. Children who come from countries where *M bovis* is prevalent in cattle or whose parents come from those countries are more likely to be infected. Most infections in humans are transmitted from cattle by unpasteurized milk and its products, such as fresh cheese, although human-to-human transmission by the airborne route has been documented. In children, *M bovis* more commonly causes cervical lymphadenitis, intestinal tuberculosis disease, and meningitis. In adults, latent *M bovis* infection can progress to advanced pulmonary disease, with a risk of transmission to others.

The diagnosis of tuberculosis caused by *M bovis* infection requires a culture isolate. The commonly used methods for identifying *M tuberculosis* complex do not distinguish *M bovis* from *M tuberculosis*, *M africanum*, and BCG; *M bovis* is identified in clinical laboratories routinely by its resistance to pyrazinamide. However, this approach can be unreliable, and species confirmation at a reference laboratory should be requested when *M bovis* is suspected. Resistance to first-line drugs in addition to pyrazinamide has been reported. BCG rarely is isolated from pediatric clinical specimens; however, it should be suspected from the characteristic lesions or localized BCG suppuration or draining lymphadenitis in children who have received BCG vaccine. Only a reference laboratory can distinguish an isolate of BCG from an isolate of *M bovis*.

Therapy for* M bovis *Disease. Controlled clinical trials for treatment of *M bovis* disease have not been conducted, and treatment recommendations for *M bovis* disease in adults and children are based on results from treatment trials for *M tuberculosis* disease. Although most strains of *M bovis* are pyrazinamide-resistant and resistance to other first-line drugs has been reported, MDR strains are rare. Initial therapy should include 3 or 4 drugs besides pyrazinamide that would be used to treat disease from *M tuberculosis* infection. For isoniazid- and rifampin-susceptible strains, a total treatment course of at least 9 to 12 months is recommended.

Parents should be counseled about the many infectious diseases transmitted by unpasteurized milk and its products, and parents who might import traditional dairy products from countries where *M bovis* infection is prevalent in cattle should be advised against giving those products to their children. When people are exposed to an adult who has pulmonary disease caused by *M bovis* infection, they should be evaluated by the same methods as other contacts to contagious tuberculosis.

CONTROL MEASURES[1]: Control of tuberculosis disease in the United States requires collaboration between health care professionals and health department personnel, obtaining a thorough history of exposure(s) to people with infectious tuberculosis, timely and effective contact investigations, proper interpretation of TST or IGRA results, and appropriate antituberculosis therapy, including DOT services. A plan to control and prevent extensively drug-resistant tuberculosis has been published.[2] Eliminating ingestion of unpasteurized dairy products will prevent most *M bovis* infection.

Management of Contacts, Including Epidemiologic Investigation.[3] Children with a positive TST or IGRA result or tuberculosis disease should be the starting point for epidemiologic investigation by the local health department. Close contacts of a TST- or IGRA-positive child should have a TST or IGRA, and people with a positive TST or IGRA result or symptoms consistent with tuberculosis disease should be investigated further. Because children with tuberculosis usually are not contagious unless they have an adult-type multibacillary form of pulmonary or laryngeal disease, their contacts are not likely to be infected unless they also have been in contact with the same adult source case. After the presumptive adult source of the child's tuberculosis is identified, other contacts of that adult should be evaluated.

Therapy for Contacts. Children and adolescents exposed to a contagious case of tuberculosis disease should have a TST or IGRA and an evaluation for tuberculosis disease (chest radiography and physical examination). For exposed contacts with impaired immunity (eg, HIV infection) and all contacts younger than 4 years of age, isoniazid therapy should be initiated, even if the TST result is negative, once tuberculosis disease is excluded (see Therapy for LTBI, p 691). Infected people can have a negative TST or IGRA result because a cellular immune response has not yet developed or because of cutaneous anergy. People with a negative TST or IGRA result should be retested 8 to 10 weeks after the last exposure to a source of infection. If the TST or IGRA result still is negative in an immunocompetent person, isoniazid is discontinued. If the contact is immunocompromised and LTBI cannot be excluded, treatment should be continued for 9 months. If a TST or IGRA result of a contact becomes positive, isoniazid should be continued for 9 months.

Child Care and Schools. Children with tuberculosis disease can attend school or child care if they are receiving therapy (see Children in Out-of-Home Child Care, p 124). They can return to regular activities as soon as effective therapy has been instituted, adherence to therapy has been documented, and clinical symptoms have diminished. Children with LTBI can participate in all activities whether they are receiving treatment or not.

---

[1]American Thoracic Society, Centers for Disease Control and Prevention, and Infectious Diseases Society of America. Controlling tuberculosis in the United States. Recommendations from the American Thoracic Society, CDC, and the Infectious Diseases Society of America. *MMWR Recomm Rep.* 2005;54(RR-12):1–81

[2]Centers for Disease Control and Prevention. Plan to combat extensively drug-resistant tuberculosis: recommendations of the Federal Tuberculosis Task Froce. *MMWR Recomm Rep.* 2009;58(RR-3):1–43

[3]National Tuberculosis Controllers Association and Centers for Disease Control and Prevention. Guidelines for the investigation of contacts of persons with infectious tuberculosis. Recommendations from the National Tuberculosis Controllers Association and CDC. *MMWR Recomm Rep.* 2005;54(RR-15):1–47

BCG Vaccines. The bacille Calmette-Guérin (BCG) vaccine is a live vaccine originally prepared from attenuated strains of *M bovis*. Use of BCG vaccine is recommended by the Expanded Programme on Immunization of the World Health Organization for administration at birth (see Table 1.3, p 10) and is used in more than 100 countries. BCG vaccine is used to reduce the incidence of disseminated and other life-threatening manifestations of tuberculosis in infants and young children. Although BCG immunization appears to decrease the risk of serious complications of tuberculosis disease in children, the various BCG vaccines used throughout the world differ in composition and efficacy.

Two meta-analyses of published clinical trials and case-control studies concerning the efficacy of BCG vaccines concluded that BCG vaccine has relatively high protective efficacy (approximately 80%) against meningeal and miliary tuberculosis in children. The protective efficacy against pulmonary tuberculosis differed significantly among the studies, precluding a specific conclusion. Protection afforded by BCG vaccine in one meta-analysis was estimated to be 50%. Two BCG vaccines, one manufactured by Organon Teknika Corporation and the other by sanofi pasteur, are licensed in the United States. Comparative evaluations of these and other BCG vaccines have not been performed.

Indications. In the United States, administration of BCG vaccine should be considered only in limited and select circumstances, such as unavoidable risk of exposure to tuberculosis and failure or unfeasibility of other control methods. Recommendations for use of BCG vaccine for control of tuberculosis among children and health care professionals have been published by the Advisory Committee on Immunization Practices of the CDC and the Advisory Council for the Elimination of Tuberculosis.[1] For infants and children, BCG immunization should be considered only for people with a negative TST result who are not infected with HIV in the following circumstances:

- The child is exposed continually to a person or people with contagious pulmonary tuberculosis resistant to isoniazid and rifampin, and the child cannot be removed from this exposure.
- The child is exposed continually to a person or people with untreated or ineffectively treated contagious pulmonary tuberculosis, and the child cannot be removed from such exposure or given antituberculosis therapy.

Careful assessment of the potential risks and benefits of BCG vaccine and consultation with personnel in local tuberculosis control programs are recommended strongly before use of BCG vaccine.

Healthy infants from birth to 2 months of age may be given BCG vaccine without a TST unless congenital infection is suspected; thereafter, BCG vaccine should be given only to children with a negative TST result.

Adverse Reactions. Uncommonly (1%–2% of immunizations), BCG vaccine can result in local adverse reactions, such as subcutaneous abscess and regional lymphadenopathy, which generally are not serious. One rare complication, osteitis affecting the epiphysis of long bones, can occur as long as several years after BCG immunization. Disseminated fatal infection occurs rarely (approximately 2 per 1 million people), primarily in people who are immunocompromised severely. Antituberculosis therapy is recommended to treat osteitis and disseminated disease caused by BCG vaccine. Pyrazinamide is not believed to be effective against BCG and should not be included in treatment regimens. Most experts

---

[1]Centers for Disease Control and Prevention. The role of BCG vaccine in the prevention and control of tuberculosis in the United States: a joint statement by the Advisory Committee for the Elimination of Tuberculosis and the Advisory Committee on Immunization Practices. *MMWR Recomm Rep.* 1996;45(RR-4):1–18

do not recommend treatment of draining skin lesions or chronic suppurative lymph-adenitis caused by BCG vaccine, because spontaneous resolution occurs in most cases. Large-needle aspiration of suppurative lymph nodes can hasten resolution. People with complications caused by BCG vaccine should be referred for management, if possible, to a tuberculosis expert.

Contraindications. People with burns, skin infections, and primary or secondary immu-nodeficiencies, including HIV infection, should not receive BCG vaccine. Because an increasing number of cases of localized and disseminated BCG have been described in infants and children with HIV infection, the World Health Organization no longer rec-ommends BCG in healthy, HIV-infected children. Use of BCG vaccine is contraindicated for people receiving immunosuppressive medications, including high-dose corticosteroids (see Corticosteroids, p 694). Although no untoward effects of BCG vaccine on the fetus have been observed, immunization during pregnancy is not recommended.

Reporting of Cases. Reporting of suspected and confirmed cases of tuberculosis disease is mandated by law in all states. A diagnosis of LTBI or tuberculosis disease in a child is a sentinel event representing recent transmission of *M tuberculosis* in the community. Physicians should assist local health department personnel in the search for a source case and others infected by the source case. Members of the household, such as relatives, babysitters, au pairs, boarders, domestic workers, and frequent visitors or other adults, such as child care providers and teachers with whom the child has frequent contact, potentially are source cases.

Diseases Caused by Nontuberculous Mycobacteria
(Atypical Mycobacteria, Mycobacteria Other Than *Mycobacterium tuberculosis*)

CLINICAL MANIFESTATIONS: Several syndromes are caused by nontuberculous mycobac-teria (NTM). In children, the most common of these syndromes is cervical lymphadenitis. Less common infections include soft tissue infection, osteomyelitis, otitis media, central vascular catheter-associated infections, and pulmonary infection, especially in adolescents with cystic fibrosis. NTM, especially *Mycobacterium avium* complex (MAC [including *M avium* and *Mycobacterium intracellulare*]) and *Mycobacterium abscessus,* can be recovered from sputum in 10% to 20% of adolescents and young adults with cystic fibrosis and can be associated with fever and declining clinical status. Disseminated infections almost always are associated with impaired cell-mediated immunity, as found in congenital immune defects or advanced human immunodeficiency virus (HIV) infection. Disseminated MAC is rare in HIV-infected children during the first year of life. Its frequency increases with increasing age and declining CD4+ T-lymphocyte counts, typically less than 50 cells/μL) in children older than 6 years of age. Manifestations of disseminated NTM infections depend on the species and route of infection but include fever, night sweats, weight loss, abdominal pain, fatigue, diarrhea, and anemia. In HIV-infected patients developing immune restoration with initiation of highly active antiretroviral therapy (HAART), local MAC symptoms can worsen. This immune reconstitution syndrome usually occurs 2 to 4 weeks after initiation of HAART. Symptoms can include worsening fever, swollen lymph nodes, local pain, and laboratory abnormalities.

ETIOLOGY: Of the more than 130 species of NTM that have been identified, only a few account for most human infections. The species most commonly infecting children in the United States are MAC, *Mycobacterium fortuitum, M abscessus,* and *Mycobacterium marinum* (see Table 3.86, p 703). Several new species that can be detected by nucleic acid amplification testing but cannot be grown by routine culture methods have been identified in lymph nodes of children with cervical adenitis. NTM disease in patients with HIV infection usually is caused by MAC. *M fortuitum, Mycobacterium chelonae,* and *M abscessus* commonly are referred to as "rapidly growing" mycobacteria, because sufficient growth and identification can be achieved in the laboratory within 3 to 7 days, whereas other NTM and *Mycobacterium tuberculosis* usually require several weeks before sufficient growth occurs for identification. Rapidly growing mycobacteria have been implicated in wound, soft tissue, bone, pulmonary, central venous catheter, and middle-ear infections. Other mycobacterial species that usually are not pathogenic have caused infections in immunocompromised hosts or have been associated with the presence of a foreign body.

EPIDEMIOLOGY: Many NTM species are ubiquitous in nature and are found in soil, food, water, and animals. The major reservoir for *Mycobacterium kansasii, Mycobacterium lenteflavum, Mycobacterium xenopi, Mycobacterium simiae,* and health care-associated infections attributable to the rapidly growing mycobacteria is tap water. For *M marinum,* water in a fish tank or aquarium or an injury in a salt-water environment is the major source of infections. The environmental reservoir for *M abscessus* and MAC causing pulmonary infection is unknown. Although many people are exposed to NTM, only a few exposures result in chronic infection or disease. The usual portals of entry for NTM infection are believed to be abrasions in the skin (eg, cutaneous lesions caused by *M marinum*), surgical sites (especially for central vascular catheters), oropharyngeal mucosa (the presumed portal of entry for cervical lymphadenitis), gastrointestinal or respiratory tract for disseminated MAC, and respiratory tract (including tympanostomy tubes for otitis media). Pulmonary disease and rare cases of mediastinal adenitis and endobronchial disease occur. Most infections remain localized at the portal of entry or in regional lymph nodes. Dissemination to distal sites primarily occurs in immunocompromised hosts. No definitive evidence of person-to-person transmission of NTM exists. Outbreaks of otitis media caused by *M abscessus* have been associated with polyethylene ear tubes and use of contaminated equipment or water. A waterborne route of transmission has been implicated for MAC infection in some immunodeficient hosts. Buruli ulcer disease is a skin and bone infection caused by *Mycobacterium ulcerans,* an emerging disease causing significant morbidity and disability in tropical areas, such as Africa, Asia, South America, Australia, and the western Pacific.

The **incubation periods** are variable.

DIAGNOSTIC TESTS: Definitive diagnosis of NTM disease requires isolation of the organism. Consultation with the laboratory should be obtained to ensure that culture specimens are handled correctly. Because these organisms commonly are found in the environment, contamination of cultures or transient colonization can occur. Caution must be exercised in interpretation of cultures obtained from nonsterile sites, such as gastric washing specimens, endoscopy material, a single expectorated sputum specimen, or a urine specimen and if the species cultured usually is nonpathogenic (eg, *Mycobacterium terrae* complex or *Mycobacterium gordonae*). An acid-fast bacilli smear-positive sample or repeated isolation of a single species on culture media is more likely to indicate disease than culture contamination or transient colonization. Diagnostic criteria for NTM lung disease in adults include 2 or more separate sputum samples that grow NTM or 1 from a bronchial alveolar lavage

Table 3.86. Diseases Caused by Nontuberculous *Mycobacterium* Species

Clinical Disease	Common Species	Less Common Species in the United States
Cutaneous infection	*M chelonae, M fortuitum, M abscessus, M marinum*	*M ulcerans*[a]
Lymphadenitis	MAC; *M haemophilus*; *M lenteflavum*	*M kansasii, M fortuitum, M malmoense*[b]
Otologic infection	*M abscessus*	*M fortuitum*
Pulmonary infection	MAC, *M kansasii, M abscessus*	*M xenopi, M malmoense*,[b] *M szulgai, M fortuitum, M simiae*
Catheter-associated infection	*M chelonae, M fortuitum*	*M abscessus*
Skeletal infection	MAC, *M kansasii, M fortuitum*	*M chelonae, M marinum, M abscessus, M ulcerans*[a]
Disseminated	MAC	*M kansasii, M genavense, M haemophilum, M chelonae*

MAC indicates *Mycobacterium avium* complex.
[a]Not endemic in the United States.
[b]Found primarily in Northern Europe.

specimen.[1] These criteria have not been validated in children and apply best to MAC, *M kansasii*, and *M abscessus*. Unlike other bacteria, NTM isolates from draining sinus tracts or wounds almost always are significant clinically. Recovery of NTM from sites that usually are sterile, such as cerebrospinal fluid, pleural fluid, bone marrow, blood, lymph node aspirates, middle ear or mastoid aspirates, or surgically excised tissue, is the most reliable diagnostic test. With radiometric or nonradiometric broth techniques, blood cultures are highly sensitive in recovery of disseminated MAC and other bloodborne NTM species. Disseminated MAC disease should prompt a search for underlying immunodeficiency.

Patients with NTM infection, such as *M marinum* or MAC cervical lymphadenitis, can have a positive tuberculin skin test (TST) result, because the purified protein derivative preparation, derived from *M tuberculosis*, shares a number of antigens with NTM species. These TST reactions usually measure less than 10 mm of induration but can measure more than 15 mm (see Tuberculosis, p 680).

TREATMENT: Many NTM relatively are resistant in vitro to antituberculosis drugs. In vitro resistance to these agents, however, does not necessarily correlate with clinical response, especially with MAC infections. Only limited controlled trials of antituberculous drugs have been performed in patients with NTM infections. The approach to therapy should be dictated by the following: (1) the species causing the infection; (2) the results of drug-susceptibility testing; (3) the site(s) of infection; (4) the patient's immune status; and (5) the need to treat a patient presumptively for tuberculosis while awaiting culture reports that subsequently reveal NTM.

---

[1]American Thoracic Society and Infectious Disease Society of America. An official ATS/IDSA statement: diagnosis, treatment, and prevention of nontuberculous mycobacterial diseases. *Am J Respir Crit Care Med.* 2007;175(4):367–416

For NTM lymphadenitis in otherwise healthy children, especially when the disease is caused by MAC, complete surgical excision is curative. Antimicrobial therapy has been shown in a randomized, controlled trial to provide no additional benefit. Therapy with clarithromycin or azithromycin combined with ethambutol or rifampin or rifabutin may be beneficial for children in whom surgical excision is incomplete or for children with recurrent disease (see Table 3.87, p 705).

Isolates of rapidly growing mycobacteria (*M fortuitum, M abscessus,* and *M chelonae*) should be tested in vitro against drugs to which they commonly are susceptible and that have been used with some therapeutic success (eg, amikacin, imipenem, sulfamethoxazole or trimethoprim-sulfamethoxazole, cefoxitin, ciprofloxacin, clarithromycin, linezolid, and doxycycline).[1] Clarithromycin and at least one other agent is the treatment of choice for cutaneous (disseminated) infections attributable to *M chelonae* or *M abscessus.* Indwelling foreign bodies should be removed, and surgical débridement for serious localized disease is optimal. The choice of drugs, dosages, and duration should be reviewed with a consultant experienced in the management of NTM infections.

In patients with acquired immunodeficiency syndrome (AIDS) and in other immuno-compromised people with disseminated MAC infection, multidrug therapy is recommended. Clinical isolates of MAC usually are resistant to many of the approved antituberculosis drugs, including isoniazid, but are susceptible to clarithromycin and azithromycin and often are susceptible to combinations of ethambutol, rifabutin or rifampin, and amikacin or streptomycin. Susceptibility testing to these agents has not been standardized and, thus, is not recommended routinely. The optimal regimen is yet to be determined. Treatment of disseminated MAC infection should be undertaken in consultation with an expert. In addition, the following treatment guidelines should be considered:

- Susceptibility testing to drugs other than the macrolides is not predictive of in vivo response and should not be used to guide therapy.
- Unless there is clinical or laboratory evidence of macrolide resistance, treatment regimens should contain clarithromycin (preferred) or azithromycin, combined with ethambutol. This 2-drug regimen is the foundation for any MAC treatment.
- Many clinicians have added a third agent (rifampin or rifabutin), especially for pulmonary disease and, in some situations, a fourth agent (amikacin or streptomycin).
- Drug-drug interactions can occur between medications used to treat disseminated MAC and HIV infections. Protease inhibitors (PIs) can increase and efavirenz can decrease clarithromycin concentrations. Available data are not adequate to make recommendations for clarithromycin dose adjustments in these circumstances. Azithromycin is not metabolized by the cytochrome P450 (CYP 450) system, and drug-drug interactions with PIs and efavirenz is not a concern. Rifampin and rifabutin increase CYP 450 activity and lead to more rapid clearance of PIs and efavirenz and increase toxicity. Rifampin and rifabutin should be avoided in HIV-infected children receiving PIs or efavirenz.[2]

---

[1]American Thoracic Society and Infectious Disease Society of America. An official ATS/IDSA statement: diagnosis, treatment, and prevention of nontuberculous mycobacterial diseases. *Am J Respir Crit Care Med.* 2007;175(4):367–416

[2]Centers for Disease Control and Prevention. Guidelines for prevention and treatment of opportunistic infections among HIV-exposed and HIV-infected children. Recommendations from CDC, the National Institutes of Health, the HIV Medicine Association of the Infectious Diseases Society of America, the Pediatric Infectious Diseases Society, and the American Academy of Pediatrics. *MMWR.* 2009; in press. Available at: **http://aidsinfo.nih.gov/contentfiles/Pediatric_OI.pdf.**

Table 3.87. Treatment of Nontuberculous Mycobacteria Infections in Children

Organism	Disease	Treatment
Slowly Growing Species		
Mycobacterium avium complex (MAC); *Mycobacterium haemophilus*; *Mycobacterium lentiflavum*	Lymphadenitis	Complete excision of lymph nodes; if excision incomplete or disease recurs, clarithromycin or azithromycin plus ethambutol or rifampin (or rifabutin).
	Pulmonary infection	Clarithromycin or azithromycin plus ethambutol with rifampin or rifabutin (pulmonary resection in some patients who fail to respond to drug therapy). For severe disease, an initial course of amikacin or streptomycin often is included. Clinical data in adults support that 3-times-weekly therapy is as effective as daily therapy, with less toxicity.
	Disseminated	See text.
Mycobacterium kansasii	Pulmonary infection	Rifampin plus ethambutol with isoniazid.
	Osteomyelitis	Surgical débridement and prolonged antimicrobial therapy using rifampin plus ethambutol with isoniazid.
Mycobacterium marinum	Cutaneous infection	None, if minor; rifampin, trimethoprim-sulfamethoxazole, clarithromycin, or doxycycline[a] for moderate disease; extensive lesions may require surgical débridement. Susceptibility testing not required.
Mycobacterium ulcerans	Cutaneous and bone infections	Excision of tissue; rifampicin plus streptomycin under investigation.
Rapidly Growing Species		
Mycobacterium fortuitum group	Cutaneous infection	Initial therapy for serious disease is amikacin plus meropenem, IV, followed by clarithromycin, doxycycline,[a] or trimethoprim-sulfamethoxazole or ciprofloxacin, orally, on the basis of in vitro susceptibility testing; may require surgical excision.
	Catheter infection	Catheter removal and amikacin plus meropenem, IV; clarithromycin, trimethoprim-sulfamethoxazole, or ciprofloxacin, orally, on the basis of in vitro susceptibility testing.

Table 3.87. Treatment of Nontuberculous Mycobacteria Infections in Children, continued

Organism	Disease	Treatment
Mycobacterium abscessus	Otitis media	Clarithromycin plus initial course of amikacin plus cefoxitin; may require surgical débridement on the basis of in vitro susceptibility testing (50% are amikacin resistant).
	Pulmonary infection (in cystic fibrosis)	Serious disease, clarithromycin, amikacin, and cefoxitin on the basis of susceptibility testing; may require surgical resection.
Mycobacterium chelonae	Catheter infection	Catheter removal and tobramycin (initially) plus clarithromycin.
	Disseminated cutaneous infection	Tobramycin and meropenem or linezolid (initially) plus clarithromycin.

IV indicates intravenously.

[a]Doxycycline should not be given to children younger than 8 years of age unless the benefits of therapy are greater than the risks of dental staining (see Antimicrobial Agents and Related Therapy, p 737). Only 50% of isolates of *M marinum* are susceptible to doxycycline.

- The optimal time to initiate HAART in a child in whom HIV and disseminated MAC are diagnosed newly is not established. Many experts would provide treatment of disseminated MAC for 2 weeks before initiating HAART in an attempt to minimize occurrence of the immune reconstitution syndrome and minimize confusion relating to the cause of drug-associated toxicity.
- Clofazimine is ineffective for treatment of MAC infection and should not be used.
- Patients receiving therapy should be monitored. Considerations are as follows:
  - Most patients who respond ultimately show substantial clinical improvement in the first 4 to 6 weeks of therapy. Elimination of the organisms from blood cultures can take longer, often up to 12 weeks.
  - Patients receiving clarithromycin plus rifabutin or high-dose rifabutin (with another drug) should be observed for the rifabutin-related development of leukopenia, uveitis, polyarthralgias, and pseudojaundice.

The duration of therapy for NTM infections will depend on host status, site(s) of involvement, and severity. Most experts recommend a minimum of 3 to 6 months or longer.

Chemoprophylaxis. The most effective way to prevent disseminated MAC in HIV-infected children is to preserve their immune function. According to the 2007 American Thoracic Society/Infectious Diseases Society of America guidelines[1] for preventing the first MAC episode in HIV infected children with advanced immunosuppression, prophylaxis with azithromycin or clarithromycin is recommended. Age-related advanced immunosuppression is defined as follows: (1) 6 years of age or older: CD4+ T-lymphocyte count

---

[1]American Thoracic Society and Infectious Disease Society of America. An official ATS/IDSA statement: diagnosis, treatment, and prevention of nontuberculous mycobacterial diseases. *Am J Respir Crit Care Med.* 2007;175(4):367–416

less than 50 cells/µL; (2) 3 through 5 years of age: CD4+ T-lymphocyte count less than 75 cells/µL; 1 through 2 years of age: CD4+ T-lymphocyte count less than 500 cells/ µL; and younger than 1 year of age: CD4+ T-lymphocyte count of less than 750 cells/ µL. Rifabutin is a less effective alternative agent but should not be used until tuberculosis disease has been excluded. Disseminated MAC should be excluded by a negative blood culture result before prophylaxis is initiated.

Oral suspensions of clarithromycin and azithromycin are available in the United States. Appropriate doses would be: clarithromycin, 7.5 mg/kg (maximum, 500 mg), orally, twice daily; azithromycin, 20 mg/kg (maximum, 1200 mg), orally, weekly; or azithromycin, 5 mg/kg (maximum, 250 mg), orally, daily. No pediatric formulation of rifabutin is available, but a dosage of 5 mg/kg per day (maximum, 300 mg) seems appropriate. Rifabutin should be used only for children older than 6 years of age. Prophylaxis can be discontinued in some HIV-infected children after immune reconstitution (see Table 3.88).

Table 3.88. Criteria for Discontinuing and Restarting MAC Prophylaxis in HIV-Infected Children

Age	Criteria for Discontinuing Primary Prophylaxis	Criteria for Restarting Primary Prophylaxis	Criteria for Discontinuing Secondary Prophylaxis	Criteria for Restarting Secondary Prophylaxis
Younger than 2 y	Do not discontinue	...	Do not discontinue	...
2 through 5 y	HAART 6 mo or more CD4+ T-lymphocyte count greater than 200 cells/mm³ for more than 3 consecutive mo	CD4+ T-lymphocyte count less than 200/mm³	HAART 6 mo or more More than 12 mo MAC therapy Asymptomatic CD4+ T-lymphocyte count greater than 200/mm³ for 6 mo or more	CD4+ T-lymphocyte count less than 200/mm³
6 y or older	HAART 6 mo or longer CD4+ T-lymphocyte count greater than 200 cells/mm³ for more than 3 consecutive mo	CD4+ T-lymphocyte count less than 100/mm³	HAART 6 mo or more More than 12 mo MAC therapy Asymptomatic CD4+ T-lymphocyte count less than 100/mm³ for 6 mo or more	CD4+ T-lymphocyte count less than 100/mm³

HIV indicates human immunodeficiency virus; MAC, *Mycobacterium avian* complex; HAART, highly active antiretroviral therapy.

ISOLATION OF THE HOSPITALIZED PATIENT: Standard precautions are recommended.

CONTROL MEASURES: Control measures include chemoprophylaxis for high-risk patients with HIV infection (see Treatment, p 703), avoidance of tap water contamination of central venous catheters, and use of sterile equipment for middle-ear instrumentation, including otoscopic equipment, for prevention of *M abscessus* otitis media. Because MAC and *M abscessus* are common in environmental sources, current information does not support specific recommendations about avoidance of exposure for HIV-infected people (MAC) or adolescents with cystic fibrosis (MAC or *M abscessus*).

Tularemia

CLINICAL MANIFESTATIONS: Most patients with tularemia experience an abrupt onset of fever, chills, myalgia, and headache. Illness usually conforms to one of several tularemic syndromes. Most common is the ulceroglandular syndrome, characterized by a maculopapular lesion at the entry site, with subsequent ulceration and slow healing associated with painful, acutely inflamed regional lymph nodes, which can drain spontaneously. The glandular syndrome (regional lymphadenopathy with no ulcer) also is common. Less common disease syndromes are: oculoglandular (severe conjunctivitis and preauricular lymphadenopathy), oropharyngeal (severe exudative stomatitis, pharyngitis, or tonsillitis and cervical lymphadenopathy), vesicular skin lesions that can be mistaken for herpes simplex virus or varicella zoster virus, typhoidal (high fever, hepatomegaly, and splenomegaly), intestinal (intestinal pain, vomiting, and diarrhea), and pneumonic. Pneumonic tularemia, characterized by fever, dry cough, chest pain, and hilar adenopathy, would be the typical syndrome after intentional aerosol release of organisms.

ETIOLOGY: *Francisella tularensis,* the causative agent, is a gram-negative pleomorphic coccobacillus.

EPIDEMIOLOGY: Sources of the organism include approximately 100 species of wild mammals (eg, rabbits, hares, prairie dogs, skunks, raccoons, and muskrats, rats, voles, and other rodents), at least 9 species of domestic animals (eg, sheep, cattle, and cats), blood-sucking arthropods that bite these animals (eg, ticks and deerflies), and water and soil contaminated by infected animals. In the United States, ticks and rabbits are major sources of human infection. Infected animals and arthropods, especially ticks, are infective for prolonged periods; frozen rabbits can remain infective for more than 3 years. People at risk are people with occupational or recreational exposure to infected animals or their habitats, such as rabbit hunters and trappers, people exposed to certain ticks or biting insects, and laboratory technicians working with *F tularensis,* which is highly infectious and aerosolized easily when grown in culture. In the United States, most cases occur during June to October. Approximately two thirds of cases occur in males and one quarter of cases occur in children 1 to 14 years of age. Since 2000, when tularemia was redesignated a nationally notifiable disease, there have been 90 to 154 cases reported per year. Ticks are the most important arthropod vectors. Infection also may be acquired by direct contact with infected animals, ingestion of contaminated water or inadequately cooked meat, or inhalation of aerosolized organisms or contaminated particles related to lawn mowing, brush cutting, piling contaminated hay, or bioterrorism. Person-to-person transmission does not occur. Organisms can be present in blood during the first 2 weeks of disease and in cutaneous lesions for as long as 1 month if untreated.

The **incubation period** usually is 3 to 5 days, with a range of 1 to 21 days.

DIAGNOSTIC TESTS: Diagnosis is established most often by serologic testing. A single serum antibody titer of 1:128 or greater determined by microagglutination (MA) or of 1:160 or greater determined by tube agglutination (TA) is consistent with recent or past infection and constitutes a presumptive diagnosis. Confirmation by serologic testing requires a fourfold or greater titer change between 2 serum samples obtained at least 2 weeks apart, with one of the specimens having a minimum titer of 1:128 or greater by MA or 1:160 or greater by TA. Nonspecific cross-reactions can occur with specimens containing heterophil antibodies or antibodies to *Brucella* species, *Legionella* species, or other gram-negative bacteria. However, cross-reactions rarely result in MA or TA titers that are diagnostic. Some clinical laboratories can identify presumptively *F tularensis* in ulcer exudate or aspirate material by direct fluorescent antibody or polymerase chain reaction assays. Suspect growth on culture may be identified presumptively by direct fluorescent antibody or polymerase chain reaction. Isolation of *F tularensis* from specimens of blood, skin, ulcers, lymph node drainage, gastric washings, or respiratory tract secretions is best achieved by inoculation of cysteine-enriched media. Immunohistochemical staining is specific for detection of *F tularensis* in fixed tissues; however, this method is not available in most clinical laboratories. Because of its propensity for causing laboratory-acquired infections, laboratory personnel should be alerted to the suspicion of *F tularensis.*

TREATMENT: Streptomycin, gentamicin, or amikacin are recommended for treatment of tularemia. Duration of therapy usually is 10 days. A longer course is required for more severe illness. Alternative drugs for less severe disease include ciprofloxacin (which is approved only for specific indications in patients younger than 18 years of age), doxycycline (which should not be given to children younger than 8 years of age unless the benefits of therapy are greater than the risks of dental staining [see Antimicrobial Agents and Related Therapy, p 737]), or chloramphenicol. These drugs are associated with prompt clinical response, but relapses have been reported after treatment with tetracyclines. *F tularensis* generally is resistant to beta-lactams, including penicillin and cephalosporins, and carbapenems.

ISOLATION OF THE HOSPITALIZED PATIENT: Standard precautions are recommended.

CONTROL MEASURES:

- People should protect themselves against arthropod bites by wearing protective clothing, by frequent inspection for and removal of ticks from the skin and scalp, and by using insect repellents (see Prevention of Tickborne Infections, p 191).
- Children should be instructed not to handle sick or dead animals.
- Rubber gloves should be worn by hunters, trappers, and food preparers when handling the carcasses of wild rabbits and other potentially infected animals.
- Game meats should be cooked thoroughly.
- Face masks and rubber gloves should be worn by people working with cultures or infective material in the laboratory, and the work should be performed in a biologic safety cabinet.
- Standard precautions should be used for handling clinical materials.
- A 14-day course of doxycycline (which should not be given to children younger than 8 years of age unless the benefits are greater than the risks of dental staining) or ciprofloxacin (which is only approved for specific indications in patients younger than 18 years of age) is recommended for children and adults after exposure to an intentional release of tularemia.

- A live-attenuated vaccine derived from the avirulent live vaccine biovar (Type B) strain has been used to protect people routinely working with *F tularensis* in the laboratory. This vaccine currently is under review by the US Food and Drug Administration.

Endemic Typhus
(Murine Typhus)

CLINICAL MANIFESTATIONS: Endemic typhus resembles epidemic (louseborne) typhus but usually has a less abrupt onset with less severe systemic symptoms. In young children, the disease can be mild. Fever, present in almost all patients, can be accompanied by persistent headache, which usually is severe, and myalgia. Nausea and vomiting also develop in approximately half of patients. A rash typically appears on day 4 to 7 of illness, is macular or maculopapular, lasts 4 to 8 days, and tends to remain discrete, with sparse lesions and no hemorrhage. Rash is present in approximately 50% of patients. Illness seldom lasts longer than 2 weeks; visceral involvement is uncommon, but untreated severe disease can be fatal.

ETIOLOGY: Endemic typhus is caused by *Rickettsia typhi*.

EPIDEMIOLOGY: Rats, in which infection is inapparent, are the natural reservoirs. Opossums and domestic cats and dogs also can be infected and can serve as hosts. The primary vector for transmission among rats and to humans is a rat flea (usually *Xenopsylla cheopis*), although other fleas and mites have been implicated. Infected flea feces are rubbed into broken skin or mucous membranes or inhaled. The disease is worldwide in distribution and tends to occur most commonly in adults, in males, and during the months of April to October; in children, males and females are affected equally. Endemic typhus is rare in the United States, with most cases occurring in southern California, southern Texas, the southeastern Gulf Coast, and Hawaii. Since 2002, an increased number of cases have been reported from Hawaii. Exposure to rats and their fleas is the major risk factor for infection, although a history of such exposure often is absent. In some regions, peridomestic cycles involving cats, dogs, opossums, and their fleas may exist.

The **incubation period** is 6 to 14 days.

DIAGNOSTIC TESTS: Antibody titers determined by an indirect fluorescent antibody test, enzyme immunoassay, or latex agglutination test peak around 4 weeks after infection. A fourfold titer change between acute and convalescent serum specimens taken 2 to 3 weeks apart is diagnostic, and immunoassays demonstrating rises in specific immunoglobulin M antibody can aid in confirmation of clinical diagnoses. However, serologic tests may not differentiate reliably murine typhus from epidemic (louseborne) typhus without antibody cross-absorption tests, which are not available routinely. Isolation of the organism in culture potentially is hazardous and requires use of specialized laboratories, such as the Centers for Disease Control and Prevention (CDC). Molecular diagnostic assays on infected whole blood and skin biopsies can distinguish endemic and epidemic typhus reliably and are performed at the CDC. Immunohistochemical procedures on formalin-fixed skin biopsy tissues can be performed at the CDC.

TREATMENT: Doxycycline, administered intravenously or orally, is the treatment of choice. Treatment should be continued for at least 3 days after defervescence and evidence of clinical improvement is documented, usually for 5 to 10 days. Despite concerns regarding dental staining after the use of tetracyclines in young children (see Antimicrobial Agents and Related Therapy, p 737), doxycycline provides superior therapy for this potentially severe or life-threatening disease. Fluoroquinolones or chloramphenicol are alternative drugs for therapy.

ISOLATION OF THE HOSPITALIZED PATIENT: Standard precautions are recommended.

CONTROL MEASURES: Fleas should be controlled by appropriate insecticides before use of rodenticides, because fleas will seek alternative hosts, including humans. Suspected animal populations should be controlled by animal-appropriate means. No prophylaxis is recommended for exposed people. The disease should be reported to local or state public health departments.

Epidemic Typhus
(Louseborne or Sylvatic Typhus)

CLINICAL MANIFESTATIONS: Epidemic louseborne typhus is characterized by the abrupt onset of high fever, chills, and myalgia accompanied by severe headache and malaise. A rash appears 4 to 7 days after illness onset, beginning on the trunk and spreading to the limbs. A concentrated eruption can be present in the axillae. The rash typically is maculopapular, becomes petechial or hemorrhagic, and then develops into brownish pigmented areas. The face, palms, and soles usually are not affected. There is no eschar, as often is present in many other rickettsial diseases. Changes in mental status are common, and delirium or coma can occur. Myocardial and renal failure can occur when the disease is severe. The fatality rate in untreated people is as high as 30%. Mortality is less common in children, and the rate increases with advancing age. Untreated patients who recover typically have an illness lasting 2 weeks. Brill-Zinsser disease is a relapse of epidemic louseborne typhus that can occur years after the initial episode. Factors that reactivate the rickettsiae are unknown, but relapse often is more mild and of shorter duration.

ETIOLOGY: Epidemic typhus is caused by *Rickettsia prowazekii.*

EPIDEMIOLOGY: Humans are the primary reservoir of the organism, which is transmitted from person to person by the human body louse, *Pediculus humanus.* Infected louse feces are rubbed into broken skin or mucous membranes or inhaled. All ages are affected. Poverty, crowding, poor sanitary conditions, and poor personal hygiene contribute to the spread of lice and, hence, the disease. Currently, cases of epidemic louseborne typhus are rare in the United States but have occurred throughout the world, including Asia, Africa, some parts of Europe, and Central and South America. Typhus is most common during winter, when conditions favor person-to-person transmission of the vector, the body louse. Rickettsiae are present in the blood and tissues of patients during the early febrile phase but are not found in secretions. Direct person-to-person spread of the disease does not occur in the absence of the louse vector. In the United States, sporadic human cases associated with close contact with infected flying squirrels, their nests, or their ectoparasites occasionally are reported in the eastern United States. Flying squirrel-associated disease, called sylvatic typhus, typically presents as a milder illness than body louse transmitted infection.

The **incubation period** is 1 to 2 weeks.

DIAGNOSTIC TESTS: *R prowazekii* can be isolated from acute blood specimens by animal passage or through tissue culture but can be hazardous. Definitive diagnosis requires immunohistochemical visualization of rickettsiae in tissues, isolation of the organism, detection of the DNA of rickettsiae by polymerase chain reaction assay, or antibody detection in paired serum specimens obtained during the acute and convalescent phases of disease. The indirect fluorescent antibody test is the preferred serologic assay, but enzyme immunoassay, dot immunoassay, and latex agglutination tests also are available. A fourfold change in antibody titer between acute and convalescent serum specimens taken 2 to 3 weeks apart is diagnostic. Specific molecular assays, isolation, and an immunohistochemical assay for typhus group rickettsiae in formalin-fixed tissue specimens are available at the Centers for Disease Control and Prevention.

TREATMENT: Doxycycline, administered intravenously or orally, is the treatment of choice for epidemic louseborne typhus. Children weighing 45 kg or more would receive a standard adult dose of doxycycline. Therapy should be administered until the patient is afebrile for at least 3 days and clinical improvement is documented; the usual duration of therapy is 7 to 10 days. Severe disease can require a longer course of treatment. Despite concerns regarding dental staining after use of a tetracycline-class antimicrobial agent in children 8 years of age or younger (see Antimicrobial Agents and Related Therapy, p 737), doxycycline provides superior therapy for this potentially life-threatening disease. Fluoroquinolones or chloramphenicol are alternative drugs for therapy. To halt the spread of disease to other people, louse-infested patients should be treated with cream or gel pediculicides containing pyrethrins or permethrin; malathion is prescribed most often when pyrethroids fail. In epidemic situations in which antimicrobial agents may be limited (eg, refugee camps), a single dose of doxycycline may provide effective treatment (4.4 mg/kg for children weighing less than 45 kg, or 200 mg for heavier children).

ISOLATION OF THE HOSPITALIZED PATIENT: Standard precautions are recommended. Precautions should be taken to delouse hospitalized patients with louse infestations.

CONTROL MEASURES: Thorough delousing in epidemic situations, particularly among exposed contacts of cases, is recommended. Several applications of pediculicides may be needed, because lice eggs are resistant to most insecticides. Washing clothes in hot water kills lice and eggs. During epidemics, insecticides dusted onto clothes of louse-infested populations are effective. Prevention and control of flying squirrel-associated typhus requires precautions to prevent contact with these animals and their ectoparasites and to exclude them from human dwellings. No prophylaxis is recommended for people exposed to flying squirrels. Cases should be reported to local or state public health departments.

Ureaplasma urealyticum Infections

CLINICAL MANIFESTATIONS: The most common syndrome associated with *Ureaplasma urealyticum* infections is nongonococcal urethritis (NGU). Although 15% to 55% of cases of NGU are caused by *Chlamydia trachomatis*, *U urealyticum* has been implicated as an etiologic agent in many of the remaining cases. Without treatment, the disease usually resolves within 1 to 6 months, although asymptomatic infection may persist thereafter. Prostatitis and epididymitis also have been associated with *U urealyticum* infection in men. In women, salpingitis, endometritis, and chorioamnionitis can occur. There is an association between infection and infectivity and recurrent pregnancy loss. Recently, association of *U urealyticum* as a cofactor with HPV in the development of cervical cancer has been described.

U urealyticum has been isolated from the lower respiratory tract and from lung biopsy specimens of preterm infants and contributes to intrauterine pneumonia and chronic lung disease of prematurity. Although the organism also has been recovered from respiratory tract secretions of infants 3 months of age or younger with pneumonia, its role in development of lower respiratory tract disease in otherwise healthy young infants is controversial. *U urealyticum* has been isolated from cerebrospinal fluid of newborn infants with meningitis, intraventricular hemorrhage, and hydrocephalus. The contribution of *U urealyticum* to the outcome of these newborn infants is unclear given the confounding effects of preterm birth and intraventricular hemorrhage.

Isolated cases of *U urealyticum* arthritis, osteomyelitis, pneumonia, pericarditis, meningitis, and progressive sinopulmonary disease in immunocompromised patients have been reported.

ETIOLOGY: *Ureaplasma* and *Mycoplasma* are genera in the Mycoplasmataceae family. *Ureaplasma* organisms are small pleomorphic bacteria that lack a cell wall. The genus *Ureaplasma* contains 2 species capable of causing human infection, *U urealyticum* and *Ureaplasma parvum*. At least 14 serotypes have been described.

EPIDEMIOLOGY: The principal reservoir of human *U urealyticum* is the genital tract of sexually active adults. Colonization occurs in approximately half of sexually active women; the incidence in sexually active men is lower. Colonization is uncommon in prepubertal children and adolescents who are not sexually active, but a positive genital tract culture is not in itself an indication of sexual abuse. Transmission during delivery is likely from an asymptomatic colonized mother to her newborn infant. *U urealyticum* may colonize the throat, eyes, umbilicus, and perineum of newborn infants and may persist for several months after birth.

Because *U urealyticum* commonly is isolated from the female lower genital tract and neonatal respiratory tract in the absence of disease, a positive culture does not establish its causative role in acute infection. However, recovery from an upper genital tract or lower respiratory tract specimen is much more indicative of infection.

The **incubation period** for NGU after sexual transmission is 10 to 20 days.

DIAGNOSTIC TESTS: Specimens for culture require specific *Ureaplasma* transport media with refrigeration at 4°C (39°F). Dacron or calcium alginate swabs should be used; cotton swabs should be avoided. Several rapid, sensitive polymerase chain reaction assays for detection of *U urealyticum* have been developed and have greater sensitivity than culture but are not available routinely. *U urealyticum* can be cultured in urea-containing broth in 1 to 2 days. Serologic testing for *U urealyticum* antibodies is of limited value and should not be used for routine diagnosis.

TREATMENT: A positive culture does not indicate need for therapy if the patient is asymptomatic. Mycoplasmas generally are susceptible to tetracyclines (eg, minocycline, doxycycline) and quinolones, but because they lack a cell wall, mycoplasmas are not susceptible to penicillins or cephalosporins. For symptomatic older children, adolescents, and adults, doxycycline is the drug of choice. Recurrences are common. Azithromycin is the preferred antimicrobial agent for children younger than 8 years of age, people who are allergic to tetracycline, and people with infections caused by tetracycline-resistant strains. Studies in adult men with NGU indicate that single-dose azithromycin (1 g orally) is effective. Antimicrobial treatment with erythromycin has failed both in small randomized trials and in reports of cohort studies in pregnant women to prevent preterm delivery and in preterm infants to prevent pulmonary disease. Although better in vitro efficacy is observed with clarithromycin and newer quinolones, adequate efficacy trials that control for confounding attributable to concurrent infections or concomitant medications, such as anti-inflammatory agents, have not yet been completed. Neither clarithromycin nor ciprofloxacin are approved by the US Food and Drug Administration for the treatment of *Ureaplasma*, although both are approved for other indications in pediatric patients. Clarithromycin and ciprofloxacin cannot be recommended for *Ureaplasma* infection in preterm infants. Similarly, definitive evidence of efficacy of antimicrobial agents in treatment of central nervous system infections in infants and children is lacking.

ISOLATION OF THE HOSPITALIZED PATIENT: Standard precautions are recommended.

CONTROL MEASURES: Partners of patients with NGU attributable to *U urealyticum* should be offered treatment.

Varicella-Zoster Infections

CLINICAL MANIFESTATIONS: Primary infection results in varicella (chickenpox), manifesting as a generalized, pruritic, vesicular rash typically consisting of 250 to 500 lesions in varying stages of development and resolution (crusting), mild fever, and other systemic symptoms. Complications include bacterial superinfection of skin lesions, pneumonia, central nervous system involvement (acute cerebellar ataxia, encephalitis), thrombocytopenia, and other rare complications, such as glomerulonephritis, arthritis, and hepatitis. Varicella tends to be more severe in adolescents and adults than in young children. Breakthrough chickenpox cases usually are mild and can occur in immunized children, as described later in Active Immunization (p 721). Reye syndrome can follow cases of chickenpox, although today Reye syndrome is very rare because of decreased use of salicylates during varicella. In immunocompromised children, progressive, severe varicella characterized by continuing eruption of lesions and high fever persisting into the second week of illness as well as encephalitis, hepatitis, and pneumonia can develop. Hemorrhagic varicella is much more common among immunocompromised patients than among immunocompetent hosts. Pneumonia is relatively less common among immunocompetent children but is the most common complication in adults. In children with human immunodeficiency virus (HIV) infection, recurrent varicella or disseminated herpes zoster can develop. Severe and even fatal varicella has been reported in otherwise healthy children receiving intermittent courses of high-dose corticosteroids (greater than 2 mg/kg of prednisone or equivalent) for treatment of asthma and other illnesses. The risk especially is high when corticosteroids are given during the incubation period for chickenpox.

Varicella-zoster virus (VZV) establishes latency in the dorsal root ganglia during primary infection. Reactivation results in herpes zoster ("shingles"), characterized by grouped vesicular lesions in the distribution of 1 to 3 sensory dermatomes, sometimes accompanied by pain localized to the area. *Postherpetic neuralgia*, which may last for weeks to months, is defined as pain that persists after resolution of the zoster rash. Zoster occasionally can become disseminated in immunocompromised patients, with lesions appearing outside the primary dermatomes and with visceral complications.

Fetal infection after maternal varicella during the first or early second trimester of pregnancy occasionally results in fetal death or varicella embryopathy, characterized by limb hypoplasia, cutaneous scarring, eye abnormalities, and damage to the central nervous system (the congenital varicella syndrome). The incidence of congenital varicella syndrome among infants born to mothers with varicella is approximately 1% to 2% when infection occurs before 20 weeks of gestation. Children exposed to VZV in utero during the second 20 weeks of pregnancy can develop inapparent varicella and subsequent zoster early in life without having had extrauterine varicella. Two cases of congenital varicella syndrome have been reported after 20 weeks of pregnancy, the latest occurring at 28 weeks. Varicella infection can be fatal for an infant if the mother develops varicella from 5 days before to 2 days after delivery. When varicella develops in a mother more than 5 days before delivery and gestational age is 28 weeks or more, the severity of disease in the newborn infant is modified by transplacental transfer of VZV-specific maternal immunoglobulin (Ig) G antibody.

ETIOLOGY: VZV is a member of the herpesvirus family.

EPIDEMIOLOGY: Humans are the only source of infection for this highly contagious virus. Humans are infected when the virus comes in contact with the mucosa of the upper respiratory tract or the conjunctiva. Person-to-person transmission occurs from patients with varicella by direct contact, airborne droplets, or infected respiratory tract secretions, and from contact with vesicular zoster lesions. In utero infection also can occur as a result of transplacental passage of virus during maternal varicella infection. VZV infection in a household member usually results in infection of almost all susceptible people in that household. Children who acquire their infection at home (secondary family cases) often have more skin lesions than the index case. Health care-associated transmission is well documented in pediatric units, but transmission is rare in newborn nurseries.

In temperate climates in the prevaccine era, varicella was a childhood disease with a marked seasonal distribution with peak incidence during late winter and early spring. In tropical climates, the epidemiology of varicella is different; acquisition of disease occurs at later ages, resulting in a higher proportion of adults being susceptible to varicella compared with adults in temperate climates. In the prevaccine era, most cases of varicella in the United States occurred in children younger than 10 years of age. Following implementation of universal immunization in 1995, varicella disease has declined in all age groups with evidence of herd protection. The age of peak varicella incidence is shifting from children younger than 10 years of age to children 10 through 14 years of age, although the incidence in this and all age groups is lower than in the prevaccine era. Immunity generally is lifelong. Cellular immunity is more important than humoral immunity for limiting the extent of primary infection with VZV and for preventing reactivation of virus with herpes zoster. Symptomatic reinfection is uncommon in immunocompetent people; asymptomatic reinfection is more frequent. Asymptomatic primary infection is unusual, but because some cases are mild, they may not be recognized.

In 2007, 90% of 19- through 35-month-old children in the United States had received 1 dose of varicella vaccine. As vaccine coverage increases and the incidence of wild-type varicella decreases, a greater number of varicella cases are occurring in immunized people as breakthrough disease. This should not be confused as an increasing rate of breakthrough disease or as evidence of increasing vaccine failure. In the surveillance areas with high vaccine coverage, the rate of varicella disease decreased by approximately 85% from 1995 to 2004 with use of varicella vaccine.

Immunocompromised people with primary (varicella) or recurrent (zoster) infection are at increased risk of severe disease. Severe varicella and disseminated zoster are more likely to develop in children with congenital T-lymphocyte defects or acquired immuno-deficiency syndrome than in people with B-lymphocyte abnormalities. Other groups of pediatric patients who may experience more severe or complicated disease include infants, adolescents, patients with chronic cutaneous or pulmonary disorders, and patients receiving systemic corticosteroids or long-term salicylate therapy.

Patients are contagious from 1 to 2 days before the rash to crusting of all lesions.

The **incubation period** usually is 14 to 16 days and occasionally is as short as 10 or as long as 21 days after contact. The incubation period may be prolonged for as long as 28 days after receipt of Varicella-Zoster Immune Globulin (VariZIG) or Immune Globulin Intravenous (IGIV) and shortened in immunocompromised patients. Varicella can develop between 1 and 16 days of life in infants born to mothers with active varicella around the time of delivery; the usual interval from onset of rash in a mother to onset in her neonate is 9 to 15 days.

DIAGNOSTIC TESTS: Diagnostic tests for VZV are summarized in Table 3.89, p 717. Vesicular fluid or a scab can be used to identify VZV using a polymerase chain reaction (PCR) test. VZV also can be isolated from scrapings of a vesicle base during the first 3 to 4 days of the eruption, sometimes from saliva or buccal swabs, but rarely from other sites (except with severe, disseminated disease), including respiratory tract secretions. Isolation of virus or rapid diagnostic tests (PCR, direct fluorescent antibody) are the methods of choice. Viral culture is less sensitive than PCR testing. Strain identification (genotyping) can distinguish wild-type VZV from the vaccine strain; however, testing is only available at highly specialized reference laboratories (eg, the Centers for Disease Control and Prevention [CDC]). A significant increase in serum varicella IgG antibody from acute and convalescent samples by any standard serologic assay can confirm a diagnosis retrospectively. These antibody tests are fairly reliable for diagnosing natural infection in healthy hosts but may not be reliable in immunocompromised people (see Care of Exposed People, p 718). Commercially available tests are not sufficiently sensitive to demonstrate reliably a vaccine-induced antibody response. IgM tests are not reliable for routine confirmation or ruling out of acute infection, but positive results suggest current or recent VZV infection or reactivation.

TREATMENT: The decision to use antiviral therapy and the route and duration of therapy should be determined by specific host factors, extent of infection, and initial response to therapy. Antiviral drugs have a limited window of opportunity to affect the outcome of VZV infection. In immunocompetent hosts, most virus replication has stopped by 72 hours after onset of rash; the duration of replication may be extended in immuno-compromised hosts. Oral acyclovir is not recommended for routine use in otherwise healthy children with varicella. Administration within 24 hours of onset of rash results in only a modest decrease in symptoms. Oral acyclovir should be considered for otherwise healthy people at increased risk of moderate to severe varicella, such as people older than 12 years of age, people with chronic cutaneous or pulmonary disorders, people receiving long-term salicylate therapy, and people receiving short, intermittent, or aerosolized courses of corticosteroids. Some experts also recommend use of oral acyclovir for secondary household cases in which the disease usually is more severe than in the primary case. For recommendations on dosage and duration of therapy, see Antiviral Drugs (p 777).

Table 3.89. Diagnostic Tests for Varicella-Zoster Virus (VZV) Infection

Test	Specimen	Comments
Tissue culture	Vesicular fluid, CSF, biopsy tissue	Distinguish VZV from HSV. Cost, limited availability, requires up to a week for result.
PCR	Vesicular swabs or scrapings, scabs from crusted lesions, biopsy tissue, CSF	Very sensitive method. Specific for VZV. Real-time methods (not widely available) have been designed that distinguish vaccine strain from wild-type (rapid, within 3 hours). Requires special equipment.
DFA	Vesicle scraping, swab of lesion base (must include cells)	Specific for VZV. More rapid and more sensitive than culture, less sensitive than PCR.
Tzanck smear	Vesicle scraping, swab of lesion base (must include cells)	Observe multinucleated giant cells with inclusions. Not specific for VZV. Less sensitive and accurate than DFA.
Serology (IgG)	Acute and convalescent serum specimens for IgG	Specific for VZV. May not be sensitive enough to identify vaccine-induced immunity.
Capture IgM	Acute serum specimens for IgM	Specific for VZV. IgM inconsistently detected. Not reliable method for routine confirmation but positive result indicates current/recent VZV activity. Requires special equipment.

CSF indicates cerebrospinal fluid; HSV, herpes simplex virus; PCR, polymerase chain reaction; DFA, direct fluorescent antibody; IgG, immunoglobulin G; IgM, immunoglobulin M.

Acyclovir is a category B drug based on US Food and Drug Administration (FDA) Drug Risk Classification in pregnancy. Some experts recommend oral acyclovir for pregnant women with varicella, especially during the second and third trimesters. Intravenous acyclovir is recommended for the pregnant patient with serious complications of varicella. VariZIG or IGIV can be used during pregnancy for susceptible women who are exposed to VZV.

Intravenous antiviral therapy is recommended for immunocompromised patients, including patients being treated with chronic corticosteroids. Therapy initiated early in the course of the illness, especially within 24 hours of rash onset, maximizes efficacy. Oral acyclovir should not be used to treat immunocompromised children with varicella because of poor oral bioavailability. Some experts have used high-dose oral acyclovir, valacyclovir, or famciclovir in selected immunocompromised patients perceived to be at lower risk of developing severe varicella, such as HIV-infected patients with relatively normal concentrations of CD4+ T-lymphocytes and children with leukemia in whom careful follow-up is ensured. Although VariZIG or, if not available, IGIV given shortly after exposure can prevent or modify the course of disease, Immune Globulin preparations are not effective once disease is established (see Care of Exposed People, p 718).

Famciclovir and valacyclovir have been licensed for treatment of zoster in adults. Famciclovir is converted to penciclovir, which has an extended half-life in infected cells. Valacyclovir is converted to acyclovir and produces fourfold greater serum concentrations than those produced by oral acyclovir. No pediatric formulation is available for either medication, and insufficient data exist on the use or dose of these drugs in children to support therapeutic recommendations. Infections caused by acyclovir-resistant VZV strains, which generally are limited to immunocompromised hosts, should be treated with parenteral foscarnet.

Children with varicella should not receive salicylates or salicylate-containing products, because administration of salicylates to such children increases the risk of Reye syndrome. Salicylate therapy should be stopped in a child who is exposed to varicella.

ISOLATION OF THE HOSPITALIZED PATIENT: In addition to standard precautions, airborne and contact precautions are recommended for patients with varicella for a minimum of 5 days after onset of rash and until all lesions are crusted, which in immunocompromised patients can be a week or longer. For immunized patients with breakthrough varicella with only maculopapular lesions, isolation is recommended until no new lesions occur or the lesions have faded; lesions do not have to be completely resolved. For exposed patients without evidence of immunity (see Evidence of Immunity to Varicella, p 724), airborne and contact precautions from 8 until 21 days after exposure to the index patient also are indicated; these precautions should be maintained until 28 days after exposure for those who received VariZIG or IGIV.

Airborne and contact precautions are recommended for neonates born to mothers with varicella and, if still hospitalized, should be continued until 21 or 28 days of age if they received VariZIG or IGIV. Infants with varicella embryopathy do not require isolation if they do not have active lesions.

Immunocompromised patients who have zoster (localized or disseminated) and immunocompetent patients with disseminated zoster require airborne and contact precautions for the duration of illness. For immunocompetent patients with localized zoster, contact precautions are indicated until all lesions are crusted.

CONTROL MEASURES:

Child Care and School. Children with uncomplicated chickenpox who have been excluded from school or child care may return when the rash has crusted, or in immunized people without crusts, until lesions are resolving.

Exclusion of children with zoster whose lesions cannot be covered is based on similar criteria. Children who are excluded may return after the lesions have crusted. Lesions that are covered pose little risk to susceptible people. Older children and staff members with zoster should be instructed to wash their hands if they touch potentially infectious lesions.

CARE OF EXPOSED PEOPLE: Potential interventions for people without evidence of immunity exposed to a person with varicella include either varicella vaccine administered ideally within 3 days but up to 5 days after exposure or, when indicated, VariZIG (1 dose up to 96 hours after exposure). If VariZIG is not available, IGIV (1 dose up to 96 hours after exposure) can be used (see Unavailability of VariZIG, p 721).[1] Prophylactic administration of oral acyclovir beginning 7 days after exposure also may prevent or attenuate varicella disease.

Hospital Exposure. If an inadvertent exposure in the hospital to an infected patient, health care professional, or visitor occurs, the following control measures are recommended:

---

[1] Centers for Disease Control and Prevention. A new product (VariZIG) for postexposure prophylaxis of varicella available under an investigational new drug application expanded access protocol. *MMWR Morb Mortal Wkly Rep.* 2006;55(8):209–210

- Health care professionals and patients who have been exposed (see Table 3.90, p 720) and who lack evidence of immunity to varicella should be identified.
- Varicella immunization is recommended for people without evidence of immunity, provided there are no contraindications to vaccine use.
- VariZIG should be administered to appropriate candidates (see Table 3.91, p 721). If VariZIG is not available, IGIV is recommended.
- All exposed patients without evidence of immunity should be discharged as soon as possible.
- All exposed susceptible patients who cannot be discharged should be placed in isolation from day 8 to day 21 after exposure to the index patient. For people who received VariZIG or IGIV, isolation should continue until day 28.
- All exposed health care professionals without evidence of immunity should be furloughed or excused from patient contact from day 8 to day 21 after exposure to an infectious patient or to day 28 for people who have received VariZIG or IGIV.
- Serologic testing for immunity is not necessary for health care professionals who have been immunized, because most adults are immune after the second vaccine dose and because most serologic assays will not reliably detect immunity resulting from vaccines. For more information, see the recommendations of the Advisory Committee on Immunization Practices (ACIP) of the CDC.[1]
- Immunized health care professionals who develop breakthrough infection should be considered infectious.

Postexposure Immunization. Administration of varicella vaccine to people without evidence of immunity 12 months of age or older, including adults, as soon as possible within 72 hours and possibly up to 120 hours after varicella exposure may prevent or modify disease and should be considered in these circumstances if there are no contraindications to vaccine use. Physicians should advise parents and their children that the vaccine may not protect against disease in all cases, because some children may have been exposed at the same time as the index case. However, if exposure to varicella does not cause infection, postexposure immunization with varicella vaccine will result in protection against subsequent exposure. There is no evidence that administration of varicella vaccine during the presymptomatic or prodromal stage of illness increases the risk of vaccine-associated adverse events or more severe natural disease.

Passive Immunoprophylaxis. The decision to administer VariZIG depends on 3 factors: (1) the likelihood that the exposed person has no evidence of immunity to varicella; (2) the probability that a given exposure to varicella or zoster will result in infection; and (3) the likelihood that complications of varicella will develop if the person is infected.

Data are unavailable regarding the sensitivity and specificity of serologic tests in immunocompromised patients. However, no test is 100% sensitive or specific and, consequently, false-positive results can occur. Therefore, regardless of serologic test results, careful questioning of children's parents about potential past exposure to disease or clinical description of disease can be helpful in determining immunity. Administration of VariZIG or IGIV as soon as possible within 96 hours to exposed immunocompromised children with no history of varicella and unknown or negative serologic test results usually is advised. The degree and type of immunosuppression should be considered in making this decision. VariZIG is given intramuscularly at the recommended dose of

---

[1]Centers for Disease Control and Prevention. Prevention of varicella: recommendations of the Advisory Committee on Immunization Practices (ACIP). *MMWR Recomm Rep.* 2007;56(RR-4):1–40

Table 3.90. Types of Exposure to Varicella or Zoster for Which VariZIG Is Indicated for People Without Evidence of Immunity[a]

- Household: residing in the same household
- Playmate: face-to-face[b] indoor play
- Hospital:

  Varicella: In same 2- to 4-bed room or adjacent beds in a large ward, face-to-face[b] contact with an infectious staff member or patient, or visit by a person deemed contagious

  Zoster: Intimate contact (eg, touching or hugging) with a person deemed contagious.

  Newborn infant: onset of varicella in the mother 5 days or less before delivery or within 48 h after delivery; VariZIG or IGIV is not indicated if the mother has zoster

VariZIG indicates Varicella-Zoster Immune Globulin; IGIV, Immune Globulin Intravenous.

[a]Patients should meet criteria of both significant exposure and candidacy for receiving VariZIG, as given in Table 3.91, p 721. VariZIG should be administered as soon as possible and no later than 96 hours after exposure.

[b]Experts differ in opinion about the duration of face-to-face contact that warrants administration of VariZIG. However, the contact should be nontransient. Some experts suggest a contact of 5 or more minutes as constituting significant exposure for this purpose; others define close contact as more than 1 hour.

125 units/10 kg body weight, up to a maximum of 625 units (ie, 5 vials). IGIV is given intravenously at the dose of 400 mg/kg.

Patients receiving monthly high-dose IGIV (400 mg/kg or greater) at regular intervals are likely to be protected if the last dose of IGIV was given 3 weeks or less before exposure.

Where to Obtain VariZIG. VariZIG is available under an investigational new drug (IND) protocol and can be requested by calling the 24-hour telephone number of FFF Enterprises (800-843-7477).

Indications for VariZIG. Tables 3.90 (above) and 3.91 (p 721) indicate people without evidence of immunity who should receive VariZIG if exposed, including immunocompromised people, pregnant women, and certain newborn infants.

For healthy term infants exposed postnatally to varicella, including infants whose mother's rash developed more than 48 hours after delivery, VariZIG is not indicated. However, some experts advise use of VariZIG for any exposed newborn who has severe skin disease and whose mother does not have evidence of immunity.

- **Subsequent exposures and follow-up of VariZIG recipients.** Because administration of VariZIG can cause varicella infection to be asymptomatic, testing of recipients 2 months or later after administration of VariZIG to ascertain their immune status may be helpful in the event of subsequent exposure. Some experts, however, would advise VariZIG administration after subsequent exposures regardless of serologic results because of the unreliability of serologic test results in immunocompromised people and the uncertainty about whether asymptomatic infection after VariZIG administration confers lasting protection.

Any patient to whom VariZIG is administered to prevent varicella subsequently should receive age-appropriate varicella vaccine, provided the vaccine is not contraindicated. Varicella immunization should be delayed until 5 months after VariZIG administration. Varicella vaccine is not needed if the patient develops varicella after administration of VariZIG.

Table 3.91. Candidates for VariZIG or Acyclovir, Provided Significant Exposure Has Occurred[a]

- Immunocompromised children[b] without history of varicella or varicella immunization[c]
- Pregnant women without evidence of immunity[d]
- Newborn infant whose mother had onset of chickenpox within 5 days before delivery or within 48 h after delivery
- Hospitalized preterm infant (28 wk or more of gestation) whose mother lacks a reliable history of chickenpox or serologic evidence of protection against varicella
- Hospitalized preterm infants (less than 28 wk of gestation or birth weight 1000 g or less), regardless of maternal history of varicella or varicella-zoster virus serostatus

VariZIG indicates Varicella-Zoster Immune Globulin.
[a]See text and Table 3.90, p 720 for additional discussion.
[b]Including children who are infected with human immunodeficiency virus.
[c]Immunocompromised adolescents and adults without evidence of immunity should receive VariZIG.
[d]If VariZIG is not available, clinicians may choose to administer Immune Globulin Intravenous or closely monitor the pregnant woman for signs and symptoms of varicella and institute treatment with acyclovir if disease develops.

Unavailability of VariZIG. If VariZIG is not available, IGIV can be used. The recommendation for use of IGIV is based on "best judgment of experts" and is supported by reports comparing VZV IgG antibody titers measured in both IGIV and VariZIG preparations and patients given IGIV and VariZIG. Although licensed IGIV preparations contain antivaricella antibodies, the titer of any specific lot of IGIV is uncertain, because IGIV is not tested routinely for antivaricella antibodies. No clinical data demonstrating effectiveness of IGIV for postexposure prophylaxis of varicella are available. The recommended IGIV dose for postexposure prophylaxis of varicella is 400 mg/kg, intravenously administered once.

Chemoprophylaxis. If VariZIG is not available or more than 96 hours have passed since exposure, some experts recommend prophylaxis with acyclovir (80 mg/kg per day, administered 4 times/day for 7 days; maximum dose, 800 mg, 4 times/day) beginning 7 to 10 days after exposure for immunocompromised patients without evidence of immunity who have been exposed to varicella. A 7-day course of acyclovir also may be given to adults without evidence of immunity if vaccine is contraindicated. Limited data on acyclovir as postexposure prophylaxis are available for healthy children; no studies were performed for adults. However, limited data support use of acyclovir as postexposure prophylaxis, and clinicians may choose this option if active or passive immunization is not possible. Most adults with no history or an uncertain history of chickenpox are immune if they were raised in the continental United States or Canada.

Active Immunization.[1,2]

Vaccine. Varicella vaccine is a live-attenuated preparation of the serially propagated and attenuated wild Oka strain. The product contains trace amounts of neomycin and gelatin. The monovalent vaccine was licensed in March 1995 by the FDA for use in

[1]Centers for Disease Control and Prevention. Prevention of varicella: recommendations of the Advisory Committee on Immunization Practices (ACIP). *MMWR Recomm Rep.* 2007;56(RR-4):1–40
[2]American Academy of Pediatrics, Committee on Infectious Diseases. Prevention of varicella: recommendations for use of varicella vaccines in children, including a recommendation for a routine 2-dose varicella immunization schedule. *Pediatrics.* 2007;120(1):221–231

healthy people 12 months of age or older who have not had varicella illness. Quadrivalent measles-mumps-rubella-varicella (MMRV) vaccine was licensed in September 2005 by the FDA for use in healthy children 12 months through 12 years of age.

Dose and Administration. The recommended dose of the vaccine is 0.5 mL administered subcutaneously.

Immunogenicity. Approximately 85% of immunized healthy children older than 12 months of age develop humoral and cell-mediated immune response to VZV at levels associated with protection after a single dose of varicella vaccine. Seroprotection rates are significantly higher (approaching 100%) after 2 doses.

Effectiveness. The efficacy of 1 dose of varicella vaccine ranges from 70% to 90% against infection and 95% against severe disease. In general, postlicensure effectiveness studies have reported a similar range for prevention against infection, with a few studies yielding lower or higher values. The vaccine is highly effective (97% or greater) in preventing severe varicella in postlicensure evaluations.

Recipients of 2 doses of varicella vaccine are 3.3-fold less likely to have breakthrough varicella as compared with recipients of 1 dose (2.2% vs 7.3% [P <0.001]) during the first 10 years after immunization. Breakthrough cases developed in 0.0% to 0.8% in recipients of 2 doses of vaccine per year, compared with 0.2% to 2.3% of recipients of 1 dose of vaccine.

Varicella in vaccine recipients is milder than that occurring in unimmunized children, usually with a median of fewer than 50 vesicles, lower rate of fever (10% with temperature 39°C [102°F] or higher), and faster recovery. At times, the disease is so mild that it is not easily recognizable as varicella, because skin lesions may resemble insect bites. In contrast, the median number of lesions in unimmunized children with varicella is more than 250. However, varicella transmission from vaccine recipients with mild breakthrough disease may occur; in household settings, the risk of transmission is approximately one third that of unimmunized cases.

Duration of Immunity. Although there has been concern about waning immunity, follow-up evaluations of children immunized during prelicensure clinical trials in the United States indicate persistence of antibodies for at least 8 years. Studies in Japan indicate persistence of antibodies for at least 20 years; however, these studies were conducted during a period when a substantial amount of wild-type VZV was present in the community, with many opportunities for boosting of immunity by subclinical infection. Available data are inconclusive regarding waning of immunity after one dose of varicella vaccine. For measles prevention, the primary reason for the second dose of measles vaccine is to induce protection in children without an adequate response to the first dose, not because of waning immunity. Similarly, a 2-dose schedule for varicella vaccine for all children was recommended by the American Academy of Pediatrics and CDC in 2006–2007. Postlicensure surveillance studies are being performed to determine the persistence of antibodies and the effectiveness of the 2-dose varicella vaccine strategy.

Simultaneous Administration With Other Vaccines or Antiviral Agents. Varicella-containing vaccines may be given simultaneously with other recommended childhood immunizations recommended for children 12 through 15 months of age and 4 through 6 years of age (see Fig 1.1, p 24–25). If not administered at the same visit or as MMRV vaccine, the interval between administration of a varicella-containing vaccine and measles-mumps-rubella (MMR) vaccine should be at least 28 days. Because of susceptibility of vaccine virus to acyclovir, valacyclovir, or famciclovir, these antiviral agents should be avoided from 1 day before to 21 days after receipt of a varicella-containing vaccine.

Adverse Events. Varicella vaccine is safe; reactions generally are mild and occur with an overall frequency of approximately 5% to 35%. Approximately 20% of immunized people will experience minor injection site reactions (eg, pain, redness, swelling). In approximately 3% to 5% of immunized children, a localized rash develops, and in an additional 3% to 5%, a generalized varicella-like rash develops. However, all observed postimmunization rashes cannot be attributed to vaccine. These rashes typically consist of 2 to 5 lesions and may be maculopapular rather than vesicular; lesions usually appear 5 to 26 days after immunization. Many generalized varicelliform rashes that occur within the first 2 weeks after varicella immunization are attributable to wild-type VZV infection and are not an adverse effect of the vaccine. In a 2-dose regimen of monovalent vaccine separated by 3 months, injection site complaints were slightly higher after the second dose. After 1 dose, recipients of MMRV are more likely than are recipients of monovalent varicella vaccine and MMR given at separate injection sites to have fever (21.5% vs 14.9%, respectively) and a measles-like rash (3% vs 2.1%, respectively). Both fever and measles-like rash usually occurred within 5 to 12 days of immunization, were of short duration, and resolved without long-term sequelae. A 2.3 times higher relative risk for confirmed febrile seizures was found in children 12 through 23 months of age during the period of 5 through 12 days after MMRV immunization when compared with same-aged children immunized with MMR vaccine and varicella vaccine given separately at the same visit.[1] After the second dose, there were no differences in incidence of fever or rash among recipients of MMRV compared with recipients of simultaneous MMR and varicella vaccines. Serious adverse events, such as anaphylaxis, encephalitis, ataxia, erythema multiforme, Stevens-Johnson syndrome, pneumonia, thrombocytopenia, seizures, neuropathy, Guillain-Barré syndrome, secondary bacterial infections, and death have been reported rarely in temporal association with varicella vaccine. In rare instances, a causal relationship between the varicella vaccine and some of these serious adverse events has been established, most often in children with immunocompromising conditions, although the frequency of serious adverse events is much lower than after natural infection. In most cases, data are insufficient to determine a causal association.

Herpes Zoster After Immunization. Varicella vaccine virus has been associated with development of herpes zoster in immunocompetent and immunocompromised people. However, data from postlicensure surveillance indicate that the clinical severity seems to be milder and the age-specific risk of herpes zoster seems to be lower among immunocompetent children immunized with varicella vaccine than among children who have had natural varicella infection. Wild-type VZV has been identified in vesicles in people with herpes zoster after immunization, indicating that herpes zoster in immunized people also may result from natural varicella infection that occurred before or after immunization. Therefore, it is important that physicians obtain event-appropriate clinical specimens for strain identification when a vaccine adverse event (eg, herpes zoster, meningitis, encephalitis) is suspected. A zoster vaccine for older adults has been licensed by the FDA in the United States and is recommended by the CDC for healthy people 60 years of

---

[1]Centers for Disease Control and Prevention. Update: recommendations from the Advisory Committee on Immunization Practices (ACIP) regarding administration of combination MMRV vaccine. *MMWR Morb Mortal Wkly Rep.* 2008;57(10):258–260

age and older for the prevention of herpes zoster.[1] Among zoster vaccinees who develop zoster, postherpetic neuralgia is reduced by two thirds in vaccine recipients, compared with placebo recipients.

Transmission of Vaccine-Associated Virus. Vaccine-associated virus transmission to contacts is rare (only 5 instances, resulting in 6 secondary cases), and the risk of transmission exists only if a rash develops on the immunized person.

Postexposure prophylaxis with VariZIG, IGIV, acyclovir, or varicella vaccine in high-risk people exposed to immunized people with lesions has not been studied. However, some experts believe that immunocompromised people in whom skin lesions develop, possibly related to vaccine virus, should receive acyclovir treatment. Attempts to identify VZV by laboratory means should be made in these patients.

Storage. The lyophilized vaccine should be stored in a frost-free freezer at an average temperature of −15°C (+5°F) or colder. The diluent used for reconstitution should be stored separately in a refrigerator or at room temperature. Once the vaccine has been reconstituted, it should be injected as soon as possible and discarded if not used within 30 minutes.

Evidence of Immunity to Varicella. Evidence of immunity to VZV in the pediatric population includes any of the following:

1. Documentation of 2 appropriately timed doses of varicella vaccine.
2. Laboratory evidence of immunity or laboratory confirmation of disease.
3. Varicella diagnosed by a health care professional or verification of history of varicella disease.
    *   For people reporting or presenting with typical disease, verification can be performed by any health care professional (eg, school or occupational clinic nurse, nurse practitioner, physician assistant, physician)
    *   For people reporting or presenting with atypical and/or mild cases, assessment by a physician or physician's designee is recommended, and one of the following should be sought: (i) an epidemiologic link to a typical varicella case or to a laboratory-confirmed case; or (ii) evidence of laboratory confirmation, if it was performed at the time of acute disease. When such documentation is lacking, people should not be considered as having a valid history of disease, because other diseases may mimic mild atypical varicella.
4. History of herpes zoster diagnosed by a health care professional.

Recommendations for Immunization.

Children 12 Months Through 12 Years of Age. Both monovalent varicella vaccine and MMRV have been licensed for use for healthy children 12 months through 12 years of age. Children in this age group should receive two 0.5-mL doses of varicella vaccine administered subcutaneously, separated by at least 3 months. The recommendation for at least a 3-month interval between doses is based on the design of the studies evaluating 2 doses in this age group; if the second dose inadvertently is administered between 28 days and 3 months after the first dose, the second dose does not need to be repeated.

All children routinely should receive the first dose of varicella-containing vaccine at 12 through 15 months of age. Because of the potential for increased febrile seizures after the first dose of MMRV vaccine in children 12 through 15 months of age, the American

---

[1]Centers for Disease Control and Prevention. Prevention of herpes zoster: recommendations of the Advisory Committee on Immunization Practices (ACIP). *MMWR Recomm Rep.* 2008;57(RR-5):1–30

Academy of Pediatrics and the ACIP do not express a preference for use of MMRV vaccine over separate injections of equivalent component vaccines (MMR and varicella vaccines).[1] Information about changes in recommendations for use of MMRV vaccine can be found at **www.cdc.gov/vaccines** and **www.aapredbook.aappublications. org.** The varicella vaccine should be administered to all children in this age range unless there is evidence of immunity to VZV or a contraindication to administration of the vaccine. The second dose of varicella-containing vaccine is recommended routinely when children are 4 through 6 years of age (ie, before a child enters kindergarten or first grade) but can be administered at an earlier age. A routine health maintenance visit at 11 through 12 years of age is recommended for all adolescents to evaluate immunization status and administer necessary vaccines, including the varicella vaccine.

People 13 Years of Age or Older. People 13 years of age or older without evidence of immunity should receive two 0.5-mL doses of varicella vaccine separated by at least 28 days. The recommendation for at least a 28-day interval between doses is based on the design of the studies evaluating 2 doses in this age group. For people who previously received only 1 dose of varicella vaccine, a second dose is necessary to provide evidence of immunity. Monovalent varicella vaccine, but not MMRV vaccine, is licensed for use in this age group.

Contraindications and Precautions.

Intercurrent Illness. As with other vaccines, varicella vaccine should not be administered to people who have moderate or severe illnesses, with or without fever (see Vaccine Safety and Contraindications, p 40).

Immunization of Immunocompromised Patients.

General recommendations. Varicella vaccine should not be administered routinely to children who have congenital or acquired T-lymphocyte immunodeficiency, including people with leukemia, lymphoma, and other malignant neoplasms affecting the bone marrow or lymphatic systems, as well as children receiving long-term immunosuppressive therapy. An exception includes certain children infected with HIV, as discussed later. Children with impaired humoral immunity may be immunized.

Immunodeficiency should be excluded before immunization in children with a family history of hereditary immunodeficiency. The presence of an immunodeficient or HIV-seropositive family member does not contraindicate vaccine use in other family members.

When immunizing people with altered immunity against chickenpox, only monovalent varicella vaccine should be used. The Oka vaccine strain remains susceptible to acyclovir, and if a high-risk patient develops vaccine-related varicella, then acyclovir should be used as treatment.

Acute lymphocytic leukemia. Before routine immunization of healthy children against varicella was instituted in the United States in 1995, many young children with leukemia were susceptible to chickenpox. To protect them against serious and fatal varicella, a research protocol for immunization against chickenpox was in place, but the protocol has been terminated. Considering the variability of chemotherapy regimens and the current decreasing incidence of varicella in the United States, however, these high-risk children should not be immunized routinely. Immunization of leukemic children without evidence

---

[1] Centers for Disease Control and Prevention. Update: recommendations from the Advisory Committee on Immunization Practices (ACIP) regarding administration of combination MMRV vaccine. *MMWR Morb Mortal Wkly Rep.* 2008;57(10):258–260

of immunity in remission should be undertaken only with expert guidance and with availability of antiviral therapy should complications occur.

Live-virus vaccines usually are withheld for an interval of at least 3 months after immunosuppressive cancer chemotherapy has been discontinued. The interval until immune reconstruction varies with the intensity and type of immunosuppressive therapy, radiation therapy, underlying disease, and other factors. Therefore, it often is not possible to make a definitive recommendation for an interval after cessation of immunosuppressive therapy when live-virus vaccines can be administered safely and effectively.

HIV infection.[1] Screening for HIV infection is not indicated before routine VZV immunization. After weighing potential risks and benefits, varicella vaccine should be considered for HIV-infected children with a CD4+ T-lymphocyte percentage of 15% or greater. Eligible children should receive 2 doses of monovalent varicella vaccine with a 3-month interval between doses and return for evaluation if they experience a postimmunization varicella-like rash. With increased use of varicella vaccine and the resulting decrease in incidence of varicella in the community, exposure of immunocompromised hosts to VZV will decrease. As the risk of exposure decreases and more data are generated on the use of varicella vaccine in high-risk populations, the risk versus benefit of VZV immunization in HIV-infected children will need to be reassessed.

Children receiving corticosteroids. Varicella vaccine should not be administered to people who are receiving high doses of systemic corticosteroids (2 mg/kg per day or more of prednisone or its equivalent or 20 mg/day of prednisone or its equivalent) for 14 days or more. The recommended interval between discontinuation of corticosteroid therapy and immunization with varicella vaccine is at least 1 month. Varicella vaccine may be administered to people on inhaled, nasal, and topical steroids.

Children with nephrotic syndrome. The results of one small study indicate that 2 doses of the varicella vaccine in 29 children between 12 months and 18 years of age generally were well tolerated and immunogenic, including children receiving low-dose, alternate-day prednisone.

Households with potential contact with immunocompromised people. Transmission of vaccine-strain VZV from healthy people has been documented in 5 instances, resulting in 6 secondary cases. Even in families with immunocompromised people, including people with HIV infection, no precautions are needed after immunization of healthy children in whom a rash does not develop. Immunized people in whom a rash develops should avoid direct contact with immunocompromised hosts without evidence of immunity for the duration of the rash.

Pregnancy and Lactation. Varicella vaccine should not be administered to pregnant women, because the possible effects on fetal development are unknown, although no pattern of malformation has been identified after inadvertent immunization of pregnant women. When postpubertal females are immunized, pregnancy should be avoided for at least 1 month after immunization. A pregnant mother or other household member is not a contraindication for immunization of a child in the household. Reporting of instances of inadvertent immunization with a varicella-zoster–containing vaccine during preg-

---

[1] Centers for Disease Control and Prevention. Guidelines for prevention and treatment of opportunistic infections in HIV-infected adults and adolescents. Recommendations from CDC, the National Institutes of Health, and the HIV Medicine Association of the Infectious Diseases Society of America. *MMWR Early Release.* 2009; 58(March 24, 2009):1–207. Available at: **http://www.cdc.gov/mmwr/pdf/rr/rr58e324.pdf**

nancy by telephone is encouraged (1-800-986-8999). (See Pregnancy, p 70–71, and **www.merckpregnancyregistries.com/varivax.html**).

A study of nursing mothers and their infants showed no evidence of excretion of vaccine strain in human milk or of transmission to infants who are breastfeeding. Varicella vaccine should be administered to nursing mothers who lack evidence of immunity.

Immune Globulin. Whether Immune Globulin (IG) can interfere with varicella vaccine-induced immunity is unknown, although IG can interfere with immunity induction by measles vaccine. Pending additional data, varicella vaccine should be withheld for the same intervals after receipt of any form of IG or other blood product as measles vaccine (see Measles, p 444). Conversely, IG should be withheld for at least 2 weeks after receipt of varicella vaccine. Transplacental antibodies to VZV do not interfere with the immunogenicity of varicella vaccine administered at 12 months of age or older.

Salicylates. Whether Reye syndrome results from administration of salicylates after immunization for varicella in children is unknown. No cases have been reported. However, because of the association among Reye syndrome, natural varicella infection, and salicylates, the vaccine manufacturer recommends that salicylates be avoided for 6 weeks after administration of varicella vaccine. Physicians need to weigh the theoretical risks associated with varicella vaccine against the known risks of wild-type virus in children receiving long-term salicylate therapy.

Allergy to Vaccine Components. Varicella vaccine should not be administered to people who have had an anaphylactic-type reaction to any component of the vaccine, including gelatin and neomycin. Most people with allergy to neomycin have resulting contact dermatitis, a reaction that is not a contraindication to immunization. Monovalent varicella vaccine does not contain preservatives or egg protein, and although the measles and mumps vaccines included in MMRV vaccine are produced in chick embryo culture, the amounts of egg cross-reacting proteins are not significant. Therefore, children with egg allergy routinely may be given MMRV without previous skin testing.

VIBRIO INFECTIONS

Cholera
(Vibrio cholerae)

CLINICAL MANIFESTATIONS: Cholera is characterized by painless voluminous watery diarrhea without abdominal cramps or fever. Dehydration, hypokalemia, metabolic acidosis, and occasionally, hypovolemic shock can occur in 4 to 12 hours if fluid losses are not replaced. Coma, seizures, hypoglycemia, and death also can occur, particularly in children. Stools are colorless, with small flecks of mucus ("rice-water"), and contain high concentrations of sodium, potassium, chloride, and bicarbonate. Most infected people with toxigenic *Vibrio cholerae* O1 have no symptoms, and some have only mild to moderate diarrhea lasting 3 to 7 days; fewer than 5% have severe watery diarrhea, vomiting, and dehydration (cholera gravis).

ETIOLOGY: *V cholerae* is a gram-negative, curved, motile bacillus with many serogroups. Only serogroups O1 and O139 cause epidemic clinical cholera associated with enterotoxin. There are 3 serotypes of *V cholerae* O1: Inaba, Ogawa, and Hikojima. The 2 biotypes of *V cholerae* are classical and El Tor. El Tor is more commonly observed. Since 1992, toxigenic *V cholerae* serogroup O139 has been recognized as a cause of cholera in Asia. Nontoxigenic strains of *V cholerae* O1 and some toxigenic non-O1 serogroups (eg, 0141) can cause sporadic diarrheal illness, but they have not caused epidemics.

EPIDEMIOLOGY: During the last 5 decades, *V cholerae* O1 biotype El Tor has spread from India and Southeast Asia to Africa, the Middle East, Southern Europe, and the Western Pacific Islands (Oceania). In 1991, epidemic cholera caused by toxigenic *V cholerae* O1, serotype Inaba, biotype El Tor, appeared in Peru and spread to most countries in South, Central and North America. In the United States, cases resulting from travel to or ingestion of contaminated food transported from Latin America or Asia have been reported. In addition, the Gulf Coast of Louisiana and Texas has an endemic focus of a unique strain of toxigenic *V cholerae* O1. Most cases of disease from this strain have resulted from consumption of raw or undercooked shellfish.

Humans are the only documented natural host, but free-living *V cholerae* organisms can exist in the aquatic environment. The usual mode of infection is ingestion of large numbers of organisms from contaminated water or food (particularly raw or undercooked shellfish, raw or partially dried fish, or moist grains or vegetables held at ambient temperature). Direct person-to-person spread has not been documented. People with low gastric acidity and with blood group O are at increased risk of cholera infection.

The **incubation period** usually is 1 to 3 days, with a range of a few hours to 5 days.

DIAGNOSTIC TESTS: *V cholerae* can be cultured from fecal specimens or vomitus plated on thiosulfate citrate bile salts sucrose agar. Because most laboratories in the United States do not culture routinely for *V cholerae* or other *Vibrio* organisms, clinicians should request appropriate cultures for clinically suspected cases. Isolates of *V cholerae* should be sent to a state health department laboratory for serogrouping; isolates of serogroup O1 or O139 then are sent to the Centers for Disease Control and Prevention (CDC) for testing for production of enterotoxin. A fourfold increase in vibriocidal antibody titers between acute and convalescent serum specimens or a fourfold decrease in vibriocidal titers available through CDC laboratories between early and late convalescent (more than a 2-month interval) serum specimens can confirm the diagnosis.

TREATMENT: Oral or parenteral rehydration therapy to correct dehydration and electrolyte abnormalities is the most important modality of therapy and should be initiated as soon as the diagnosis is suspected.[1] Oral rehydration is preferred unless the patient is in shock, is obtunded, or has intestinal ileus. The World Health Organization's Oral Rehydration Solution (ORS) has been the standard, but data suggest that rice-based ORS or amylase-resistant starch ORS is more effective.

Antimicrobial therapy results in prompt eradication of vibrios, decreases the duration of diarrhea, and decreases fluid losses. Antimicrobial therapy should be considered for people who are moderately to severely ill. Oral doxycycline as a single dose or tetracycline for 3 days are the drugs of choice for cholera. Although tetracyclines generally are not recommended for children younger than 8 years of age, in cases of severe cholera, the benefits may outweigh the small risk of staining of developing teeth (see Antimicrobial Agents and Related Therapy, p 737). If strains are resistant to tetracyclines,

---

[1]Centers for Disease Control and Prevention. Managing acute gastroenteritis among children: oral rehydration, maintenance, and nutritional therapy. *MMWR Recomm Rep.* 2003;52(RR-16):1–16

then ciprofloxin, ofloxacin, or trimethoprim-sulfamethoxazole can be used. Antimicrobial susceptibility testing of newly isolated organisms should be determined.

ISOLATION OF THE HOSPITALIZED PATIENT: In addition to standard precautions, contact precautions are indicated for diapered or incontinent children for the duration of illness.

CONTROL MEASURES:

Hygiene. Disinfection or boiling of water prevents transmission. Thoroughly cooking crabs, oysters, and other shellfish from the Gulf Coast before eating is recommended to decrease the likelihood of transmission. Foods such as fish, rice, or grain gruels should be refrigerated promptly after meals and thoroughly reheated before eating. Appropriate hand hygiene after defecating and before preparing or eating food is important for preventing transmission.

Treatment of Contacts. The administration of doxycycline, tetracycline, ciprofloxacin, ofloxacin, or trimethoprim-sulfamethoxazole within 24 hours of identification of the index case may prevent coprimary cases of cholera among household contacts. However, because secondary transmission of cholera is rare, chemoprophylaxis of contacts is not recommended by the World Health Organization, except in special circumstances in which the probability of fecal exposure is high and the medication can be delivered rapidly.

Vaccine. No cholera vaccines are available in the United States. An oral vaccine is available in other countries (Dukoral from SBL vaccines in Sweden). Cholera immunization is not required for travelers entering the United States from cholera-affected areas, and the World Health Organization no longer recommends immunization for travel to or from areas with cholera infection. No country requires cholera vaccine for entry.

Reporting. Confirmed cases of cholera must be reported to health authorities in any country in which they occur or were contracted. Local and state health departments should be notified immediately of presumed or known cases of cholera attributable to *V cholerae* O1 or O139.

Other *Vibrio* Infections

CLINICAL MANIFESTATIONS: Several noncholera *Vibrio* species can cause a variety of clinical syndromes, including gastroenteritis, wound infection, and bacteremia. Gastroenteritis is the most common syndrome and is characterized by acute onset of watery stools and crampy abdominal pain. Approximately half of those afflicted will have low-grade fever, headache, and chills; approximately 30% will have vomiting. Spontaneous recovery follows in 2 to 5 days. Wound infection especially is severe in people with liver disease or who are immunocompromised. These people can develop septicemia or hemorrhagic bullous or necrotic skin lesions or die after wound infections, especially those caused by *Vibrio vulnificus.* Primary septicemia is uncommon but can develop in immunocompromised people with preceding gastroenteritis or wound infection.

ETIOLOGY: *Vibrio* organisms are facultatively anaerobic, motile, gram-negative bacilli that are tolerant of salt. The most commonly reported noncholera *Vibrio* species associated with diarrhea are *Vibrio parahaemolyticus, Vibrio cholerae* non-O1, *Vibrio mimicus, Vibrio hollisae,* and *Vibrio fluvialis. V vulnificus* causes primary septicemia and severe wound infections. *Vibrio alginolyticus, Vibrio parahaemolyticus, Vibrio fluvialis,* and others also are associated with wound infections.

EPIDEMIOLOGY: Noncholera *Vibrio* species are natural inhabitants of marine and estuarine environments. Most infections occur during summer and fall months, when *Vibrio* populations in seawater are highest. Enteritis usually follows ingestion of undercooked seafood, especially oysters, crabs, and shrimp. Wound infections can result from exposure of a preexisting wound to contaminated seawater or from punctures resulting from handling of contaminated shellfish. Exposure to contaminated water during natural disasters such as hurricanes has resulted in wound infections attributable to *V vulnificus*. Enteritis, caused by vibrio infection or toxins, is not communicable person-to-person. People with liver disease, low gastric acidity, and immunodeficiency have increased susceptibility to infection with *Vibrio* species.

The **incubation period** for enteritis is 23 hours, with a range of 5 to 92 hours.

DIAGNOSTIC TESTS: *Vibrio* organisms can be isolated from stool or vomitus of patients with gastroenteritis, from blood specimens, and from wound exudates. Because identification of the organism in stool requires special techniques, laboratory personnel should be notified when infection with *Vibrio* species is suspected.

TREATMENT: Most episodes of diarrhea are mild and self-limited and do not require treatment other than oral rehydration. Antimicrobial therapy can benefit people with severe diarrhea, wound infection, or septicemia. Septicemia with or without hemorrhagic bullae should be treated with a third generation cephalosporin plus a tetracycline.

ISOLATION OF THE HOSPITALIZED PATIENT: In addition to standard precautions, contact precautions are recommended for diapered or incontinent children.

CONTROL MEASURES: Seafood should be cooked adequately and, if not ingested immediately, should be refrigerated. Uncooked mollusks and crustaceans should be handled with care. Abrasions suffered by ocean bathers should be rinsed with clean fresh water. All children, immunocompromised people, and people with chronic liver disease should avoid eating raw oysters or clams and should be advised of risks associated with seawater exposure if a wound is present or likely to occur. Vibriosis is a nationally notifiable disease, and cases should be reported to local or state health departments.

West Nile Virus

CLINICAL MANIFESTATIONS: Most infections attributable to West Nile virus (WNV) are asymptomatic. Approximately 20% of infected people will develop a systemic febrile illness called West Nile fever (WNF), and less than 1% will develop neuroinvasive disease, such as aseptic meningitis, encephalitis, or flaccid paralysis. The risk of neuroinvasive disease increases with age and is highest among adults older than 60 years of age. Patients with WNF typically have an abrupt onset of fever, headache, myalgia, weakness, and often, abdominal pain, nausea, vomiting, or diarrhea. Some patients have a transient maculopapular rash. The acute phase of illness usually resolves within several days, but fatigue, malaise, and weakness can linger for weeks. Patients with neuroinvasive disease may present with neck stiffness and headache typical of aseptic meningitis, mental status changes indicating encephalitis, focal neurologic deficits, movement disorders, such as tremor or Parkinsonism, seizures, or acute flaccid paralysis with or without meningitis or encephalitis. Isolated limb paralysis can occur without fever or apparent viral prodrome. Flaccid paralysis caused by WNV infection is identical clinically and pathologically to poliomyelitis caused by poliovirus, with damage of anterior horn cells, and may progress to respiratory muscle paralysis requiring mechanical ventilation. Guillain-Barré syndrome also has been reported after WNV infection and can be distinguished from anterior horn cell damage by clinical manifestations and electrophysiologic testing. Cardiac dysrhythmias, myocarditis, rhabdomyolysis, optic neuritis, uveitis, chorioretinitis, orchitis, pancreatitis, and hepatitis have been described rarely after WNV infection.

Most patients who develop WNF or aseptic meningitis recover completely. Patients with encephalitis may have residual neurologic deficits, and patients with flaccid paralysis may not recover full neuromuscular function. The case-fatality rate after neuroinvasive WNV disease is approximately 9% among adult patients and less than 1% in children.

Most women known to have been infected with WNV during pregnancy have delivered infants without evidence of infection or clinical abnormalities. In the single known instance of confirmed congenital WNV infection, the mother developed WNV encephalitis during the 27th week of gestation, and the infant was born with cystic destruction of cerebral tissue and chorioretinitis.

ETIOLOGY: WNV is an RNA flavivirus that is related antigenically to St Louis and Japanese encephalitis viruses.

EPIDEMIOLOGY: WNV is transmitted to humans primarily through the bite of infected mosquitoes. The predominant vectors worldwide are *Culex* mosquitoes, which tend to feed most avidly from dusk to dawn and breed mostly in either peridomestic standing water with high organic content or pools created by irrigation or rainfall. Mosquitoes acquire the virus by feeding on infected birds and then transmit the virus to humans and other mammals during subsequent feeding. Viremia usually lasts fewer than 7 days in immunocompetent people, and viral concentrations in human blood are too low to effectively infect mosquitoes. However, WNV can be transmitted through transfusion of infected blood and through organ transplantation. Both intrauterine transmission and probable transmission through human milk have been described but appear to be uncommon. Percutaneous and aerosol infection has occurred in laboratory workers, and an outbreak of WNV infection among turkey handlers also raised the possibility of aerosol transmission.

The risk of severe WNV disease increases with age and may be slightly higher among males. Organ-transplant recipients also are at higher risk of severe illness. Risk of infection is higher during warmer months, when mosquitoes are more abundant. WNV transmission has been described in Europe and the Middle East, Africa, India, parts of Asia, and Australia (in the form of Kunjin virus, a subtype of WNV). WNV first was detected in North America in 1999 and has spread across the continent, north into Canada, and south into Mexico, Central America, and the Caribbean. In the United States, WNV transmission has been reported in all states except Alaska and Hawaii. From 1999 to 2006, 9906 cases of West Nile neuroinvasive disease were reported in the United States, including 393 (4%) cases among children younger than 18 years of age.

The **incubation period** usually is 2 to 6 days but ranges from 2 to 14 days and can be up to 21 days in immunocompromised people.

DIAGNOSTIC TESTS: WNV infection should be considered in the differential diagnosis of any child with a febrile or acute neurologic illness who has had recent exposure to mosquitoes, blood transfusion, or organ transplantation or was born to a mother infected during pregnancy or while breastfeeding. Serum and, if indicated, cerebrospinal fluid, should be tested for WNV-specific immunoglobulin (Ig) M antibody. Enzyme immunoassays or immunofluorescent assays for WNV-specific IgM are available commercially or through state public health laboratories. Positive test results for WNV-specific IgM provide good evidence of recent WNV infection but may indicate cross-reaction with antibody to other flaviviruses. Because WNV IgM can persist in some patients for more than 1 year, a positive WNV IgM test result occasionally may reflect past rather than recent WNV infection. Serum collected within 8 days of illness onset may not have detectable IgM, and the test may need to be repeated on a later sample. Acute infection may be documented with a fourfold change in WNV-specific antibody titer between acute and convalescent serum samples collected 2 to 3 weeks apart. Other arboviruses also should be considered in the differential etiology of suspected WNV illness. Plaque-reduction neutralization tests performed in reference laboratories, including some state public health laboratories and the Centers for Disease Control and Prevention (CDC), can help determine the infecting flavivirus (see Arboviruses, p 214).

Viral culture and nucleic acid amplification (NAA) tests for WNV RNA can be performed on serum, cerebrospinal fluid, and tissue specimens that are collected early in the course of illness, and if results are positive, can confirm WNV infection. However, results of viral culture and NAA tests are not positive routinely during the acute illness; they may be more likely to be positive with samples from the elderly or immunocompromised hosts. Immunohistochemical staining (IHC) can detect WNV antigen in formalin-fixed tissue. Negative results of these tests do not rule out WNV infection. Viral culture, NAA testing, and IHC can be requested through state public health laboratories or the CDC.

If WNV disease is diagnosed during pregnancy, detailed examination of the fetus and of the newborn infant should be performed. Interim guidelines for the evaluation of the fetus and infant born to mothers infected with West Nile virus during pregnancy have been published by the CDC.[1]

TREATMENT: Management of WNV disease is supportive. Although various therapies have been evaluated or used for West Nile disease, none has shown specific benefit thus far. Information regarding ongoing clinical trials for treating West Nile disease can be found at **www.cdc.gov/ncidod/dvbid/westnile/clinicalTrials.htm.**

ISOLATION OF THE HOSPITALIZED PATIENT: Standard precautions are recommended.

CONTROL MEASURES: WNV infection can be prevented by avoiding exposure to infected mosquitoes and screening blood and organ donors. Coordinated mosquito-control programs in areas with endemic infection can reduce the abundance of mosquito vectors. People who live in areas with WNV-infected mosquitoes should apply insect repellent to skin and clothes and avoid being outdoors during peak mosquito-feeding times (usually dusk to dawn). The most effective repellents for use on the skin are diethyltoluamide (DEET), picaridin, and oil of lemon eucalyptus (see Prevention of Mosquitoborne Infections, p 193). Products containing DEET or permethrin also can be applied to clothing. The American Academy of Pediatrics recommends using formulations of no more than 30% DEET on infants and children and not using DEET on infants younger than 2 months of age. Screening of the blood supply in the United States has been implemented since 2003, but health care professionals should remain vigilant for the possible

---

[1] Centers for Disease Control and Prevention. Interim guidelines for the evaluation of infants born to mothers infected with West Nile virus during pregnancy. *MMWR Morb Mortal Wkly Rep.* 2004;53(7):154–157. Available at: **www.cdc.gov/mmwr/preview/mmwrhtml/mm5307a4.htm**

transmission of WNV through blood transfusion or organ transplantation. Any suspected WNV infections temporally associated with blood transfusion or organ transplantation should be reported promptly to the appropriate state health department.

Pregnant women should take the aforementioned precautions to avoid mosquito bites. Products containing DEET can be used in pregnancy without adverse effects. Pregnant women who develop meningitis, encephalitis, flaccid paralysis, or unexplained fever in areas of ongoing WNV transmission should be tested for WNV infection. Confirmed WNV infections during pregnancy should be reported to the local or state health department, and the women should be followed to determine the outcomes of their pregnancies. Although WNV probably has been transmitted through human milk, such transmission appears rare and no adverse effects on infants have been described. Because the benefits of breastfeeding seem to outweigh the risk of any WNV illness in breastfeeding infants, mothers should be encouraged to breastfeed even in areas of ongoing WNV transmission.

Four vaccines against WNV are licensed for use in horses, but human vaccines are not yet available. Several candidate WNV vaccines are being evaluated in preclinical or clinical trials.

Yersinia enterocolitica and *Yersinia pseudotuberculosis* Infections
(Enteritis and Other Illnesses)

CLINICAL MANIFESTATIONS: *Yersinia enterocolitica* causes several age-specific syndromes and a variety of other less common presentations. Infection with *Y enterocolitica* typically manifests as fever and diarrhea in young children; stool often contains leukocytes, blood, and mucus. Relapsing disease and, rarely, necrotizing enterocolitis also have been described. In older children and adults, a pseudoappendicitis syndrome (fever, abdominal pain, tenderness in the right lower quadrant of the abdomen, and leukocytosis) predominates. Bacteremia with *Y enterocolitica* most often occurs in children younger than 1 year of age and in older children with predisposing conditions, such as excessive iron storage (eg, desferrioxamine use, sickle cell disease, beta-thalassemia) and immunosuppressive states. Focal manifestations of *Y enterocolitica* are uncommon and include pharyngitis, meningitis, osteomyelitis, pyomyositis, conjunctivitis, pneumonia, empyema, endocarditis, acute peritonitis, abscesses of the liver and spleen, and primary cutaneous infection. Postinfectious sequelae with *Y enterocolitica* infection include erythema nodosum, proliferative glomerulonephritis, and reactive arthritis; these sequelae occur most often in older children and adults, particularly people with HLA-B27 antigen.

The major manifestations of *Yersinia pseudotuberculosis* infection are fever, scarlatiniform rash, and abdominal symptoms. Acute pseudoappendiceal abdominal pain is common, resulting from ileocecal mesenteric adenitis, or terminal ileitis. Other findings include diarrhea, erythema nodosum, septicemia, and sterile pleural and joint effusions. Clinical features can mimic those of Kawasaki disease; in Hiroshima, Japan nearly 10% of children with a diagnosis of Kawasaki disease have serologic or culture evidence of *Y pseudotuberculosis* infection.

ETIOLOGY: The genus *Yersinia* consists of 11 species of gram-negative bacilli. *Y enterocolitica*, *Y pseudotuberculosis*, and *Yersinia pestis* are the 3 pathogens most commonly encountered. Fifteen pathogenic O groups of *Y enterocolitica* are recognized. Differences in virulence exist among various O groups of *Y enterocolitica;* serotype O:3 now predominates as the most common type in the United States.

EPIDEMIOLOGY: *Y enterocolitica* infections are uncommon in the United States. According to the Foodborne Disease Active Surveillance Network (FoodNet), the mean annual incidence is 0.4 per 100 000 people, the incidence for infants is 9.4 per 100 000, and the incidence for other age groups is 0.2 per 100 000. *Y pseudotuberculosis* accounts for less than 1% of reported cases. The principal reservoir of *Y enterocolitica* is swine; feral *Y pseudotuberculosis* has been isolated from ungulates (deer, elk, goats, sheep, cattle), rodents (rats, squirrels, beaver), rabbits, and many bird species. Infection with *Y enterocolitica* is believed to be transmitted by ingestion of contaminated food (raw or incompletely cooked pork products, tofu, and unpasteurized or inadequately pasteurized milk), by contaminated surface or well water, by direct or indirect contact with animals, by transfusion with contaminated packed red blood cells, and rarely by person-to-person transmission. Cross-contamination can lead to infection in infants if their caregivers handle raw pork intestines (chitterlings) and do not cleanse their hands adequately before handling the infant or the infant's toys, bottles, or pacifiers. *Y enterocolitica* and *Y pseudotuberculosis* are isolated most often during the cool months of temperate climates. Recent outbreaks of *Y pseudotuberculosis* infection in Finland have been associated with eating fresh produce, presumably contaminated by wild animals carrying the organism.

The **incubation period** typically is 4 to 6 days, with a range of 1 to 14 days. Organisms are excreted for a mean of 2 to 3 weeks, and prolonged asymptomatic carriage is possible.

DIAGNOSTIC TESTS: *Y enterocolitica* and *Yersinia pseudotuberculosis* can be recovered from stool, throat swabs, mesenteric lymph nodes, peritoneal fluid, and blood. *Y enterocolitica* also has been isolated from synovial fluid, bile, urine, cerebrospinal fluid, sputum, and wounds. Stool cultures generally are positive during the first 2 weeks of illness, regardless of the nature of gastrointestinal tract manifestations. Because of the relatively low incidence of *Yersinia* infection in the United States, *Yersinia* is not sought routinely in stool specimens by most laboratories. Consequently, laboratory personnel should be notified when *Yersinia* infection is suspected so that stool can be cultured on suitable media (eg, CIN agar). Biotyping and serotyping for further identification of pathogenic strains are available through public health reference laboratories. Infection can be confirmed by demonstrating increases in serum antibody titer after infection, but these tests generally are available only in reference or research laboratories. Cross-reactions of these antibodies with *Brucella, Vibrio, Salmonella,* and *Rickettsia* organisms and *Escherichia coli* lead to false-positive *Y enterocolitica* and *Y pseudotuberculosis* titers. In patients with thyroid disease, persistently increased *Y enterocolitica* antibody titers can result from antigenic similarity of the organism with antigens of the thyroid epithelial cell membrane. Characteristic ultrasonographic features demonstrating edema of the wall of the terminal ileum and cecum help to distinguish pseudoappendicitis from appendicitis and can help avoid exploratory surgery.

TREATMENT: Patients with septicemia or sites of infection other than the gastrointestinal tract and immunocompromised hosts with enterocolitis should receive antimicrobial therapy. Other than decreasing the duration of fecal excretion of *Y enterocolitica* and *Y pseudotuberculosis,* a clinical benefit of antimicrobial therapy for immunocompetent patients with enterocolitis, pseudoappendicitis syndrome, or mesenteric adenitis has not been established. *Y enterocolitica* and *Y pseudotuberculosis* usually are susceptible to trimethoprim-sulfamethoxazole, aminoglycosides, cefotaxime, fluoroquinolones (for patients 18 years of age and older), tetracycline or doxycycline (for children 8 years of age and older), and chloramphenicol. *Y enterocolitica* isolates usually are resistant to first-generation cephalosporins and most penicillins.

ISOLATION OF THE HOSPITALIZED PATIENT: In addition to standard precautions, contact precautions are indicated for diapered or incontinent children for the duration of diarrheal illness.

CONTROL MEASURES: Ingestion of uncooked meat, unpasteurized milk, or contaminated water should be avoided. People who handle raw pork intestines should not care for young children at the same time and should wash their hands thoroughly after they have finished.

Antimicrobial Agents and Related Therapy

....
INTRODUCTION

In some instances, antimicrobial agents are recommended for specific indications other than indications in the product label (package insert) approved by the US Food and Drug Administration (FDA). The FDA maintains a general Web site (**www.fda.gov/cder/orange/default.htm**) of approved drug products with therapeutic equivalence evaluations. Another site (**www.fda.gov/cder/ob/default.htm**) enables searches by active ingredient and proprietary name. An FDA-approved indication means that adequate and well-controlled studies were conducted and then reviewed by the FDA. However, accepted medical practice often includes drug use that is not reflected in approved drug labeling. Lack of approval for an indication does not necessarily mean lack of effectiveness but indicates that the appropriate studies have not been performed or data have not been submitted to the FDA for approval for that indication. Unapproved use does not imply improper use, provided that reasonable medical evidence justifies such use and that use of the drug is deemed in the best interest of the patient. The decision to prescribe a drug resides with the physician, who must weigh risks and benefits of using the drug, regardless of whether the drug has received FDA approval for the specific indication and age of the patient. In addition, occasional drug shortages occur, which require alternative therapy (**www.fda.gov/cder/drug/shortages/default.htm**).

Some antimicrobial agents with proven therapeutic benefit in humans are not approved by the FDA for use in pediatric patients or are considered contraindicated in children because of possible toxicity. Some of these drugs, however, such as fluoroquinolones (in people younger than 18 years of age), tetracyclines (in children younger than 8 years of age), and other agents approved for use in adults may be used in special circumstances after careful assessment of risks and benefits. Obtaining informed consent before use is prudent. The following information delineates general principles for use of fluoroquinolones, tetracyclines, and other agents that generally are approved for adults with serious bacterial infections.

Fluoroquinolones

Use of fluoroquinolones (eg, ciprofloxacin, levofloxacin, lomefloxacin, gatifloxacin, gemifloxacin, moxifloxacin, ofloxacin) generally is contraindicated, according to FDA-approved product labeling, in children and adolescents younger than 18 years of age, because fluoroquinolones have been shown to cause cartilage damage in every juvenile animal model tested at doses that approximate those needed to be therapeutic. The mechanism for this damage is unknown. Pefloxacin, a fluoroquinolone that had been used extensively in France, causes adverse musculoskeletal effects in children and adults and is not available in the United States.

Ciprofloxacin and levofloxacin are the fluoroquinolones that have been used most extensively in children and adolescents. On the basis of past experience, these drugs appear to be well tolerated, do not appear to cause arthropathy, and are effective as oral agents for treating a number of diseases in children that otherwise would require parenteral therapy. Fluoroquinolones are associated with an increased risk of tendonitis and tendon rupture, especially in people older than 60 years of age and in recipients of renal, heart, and lung transplants and with concomitant use of steroid therapy (**www.fda. gov/cder/drug/InfoSheets/HCP/fluoroquinolonesHCP.htm**). In special circumstances after careful assessment of risks and benefits for the individual patient, use of a fluoroquinolone can be justified. Circumstances in which fluoroquinolones may be useful include those in which (1) parenteral therapy is not feasible and no other effective oral agent is available; and (2) infection is caused by multidrug-resistant pathogens, such as certain *Pseudomonas* and *Mycobacterium* strains, for which there is no other effective oral agent available. The only indications for which a fluoroquinolone is approved by the FDA for use in patients younger than 18 years of age are complicated urinary tract infection, pyelonephritis, and postexposure treatment for inhalation anthrax. Possible uses, accordingly, include the following[1]:

- Exposure to aerosolized *Bacillus anthracis* to decrease the incidence or progression of disease (FDA approved)
- Urinary tract infections caused by *Pseudomonas aeruginosa* or other multidrug-resistant, gram-negative bacteria (FDA approved for complicated *Escherichia coli* urinary tract infections and pyelonephritis attributable to *E coli* in patients 1 through 17 years of age)
- Chronic suppurative otitis media or malignant otitis externa caused by *P aeruginosa*
- Chronic or acute osteomyelitis or osteochondritis caused by *P aeruginosa* but not for prophylaxis of nail puncture wounds to the foot
- Exacerbation of pulmonary disease in patients with cystic fibrosis who are colonized with *P aeruginosa* and who can be treated in an ambulatory setting
- Mycobacterial infections caused by isolates known to be susceptible to fluoroquinolones
- Gram-negative bacterial infections in immunocompromised hosts in which oral therapy is desired or resistance to alternative agents is present
- Gastrointestinal tract infection caused by multidrug-resistant *Shigella* species, *Salmonella* species, *Vibrio cholerae,* or *Campylobacter jejuni*
- Documented bacterial septicemia or meningitis attributable to organisms with in vitro resistance to approved agents or in immunocompromised infants and children who have failed to respond to parenteral therapy with other appropriate antimicrobial agents
- Serious infections attributable to fluoroquinolone-susceptible pathogen(s) in children with life-threatening allergy to alternative agents

If use of a fluoroquinolone is recommended for a patient younger than 18 years of age, the risks and benefits should be explained to the patients and parents. Inappropriate use of fluoroquinolones in children and adults is likely to be associated with increasing resistance to these agents.

---

[1]American Academy of Pediatrics, Committee on Infectious Diseases. The use of systemic fluoroquinolones. *Pediatrics.* 2006;118(3):1287–1292

Tetracyclines

Use of tetracyclines in pediatric patients has been limited, because these drugs can cause permanent dental discoloration in children younger than 8 years of age. Studies have documented that tetracyclines and their colored degradation products that are bound to teeth are observed in the dentin and incorporated diffusely in the enamel. The period of odontogenesis to completion of formation of enamel in permanent teeth appears to be the critical time for the effects of these drugs and virtually is complete by 8 years of age, at which time the drug can be given without concern for dental staining. The degree of staining appears to depend on dosage and duration of therapy, with the total dosage received being the most important factor. In addition to dental discoloration, tetracyclines also may cause enamel hypoplasia and reversible delay in rate of bone growth.

These possible adverse events have resulted in use of alternative, equally effective antimicrobial agents in most circumstances in young children in which tetracyclines are likely to be effective. However, in some cases, the benefits of therapy with a tetracycline can exceed the risks, particularly if alternative drugs are associated with significant adverse effects or may be less effective. In these cases, the use of tetracyclines in young children is justified. Examples include life-threatening rickettsial infections such as Rocky Mountain spotted fever (see p 573), ehrlichiosis (see p 284), cholera (see p 727), and anthrax (see p 211). Doxycycline usually is the agent of choice in children with these infections, because the risk of dental staining is less with this product than with other tetracyclines. In addition, the drug is given only twice a day, in contrast to the more frequent dosing regimens of other tetracyclines.

Other Agents

Other antimicrobial agents in a variety of classes have been studied and approved by the FDA for use in adults with certain serious infectious diseases. These agents include but are not limited to dalfopristin-quinupristin, daptomycin, doripenem, tigecycline, and telithromycin. Evaluations of the pharmacokinetics, efficacy, and safety of these antimicrobial agents for various clinical indications generally have not been performed in pediatric age groups, specifically neonates. These drugs should be used in children only when no other safe and effective agents that are FDA approved for use in children are available and should be used in consultation with an expert in pediatric infectious diseases.

··

APPROPRIATE AND JUDICIOUS USE OF ANTIMICROBIAL AGENTS[1]

The increasing prevalence of antimicrobial resistance is an issue of major concern to patients as well as health care professionals. This issue has been reviewed by the Infectious Diseases Society of America.[1] Rarely, highly resistant gram-negative (*Pseudomonas aeruginosa, Acinetobacter* species, *Klebsiella pneumoniae,* and *Burkholderia cepacia*) and gram-positive (*Staphylococcus aureus* and *Enterococcus faecium*) pathogens are susceptible only to one available agent. More commonly, the presence of resistant pathogens complicates therapy, increases expense, and makes treatment failure more likely. Resistant community-associated pathogens, such as drug-resistant *Streptococcus pneumoniae* and methicillin-resistant *S aureus* (MRSA) as well as hospital-associated pathogens, such as vancomycin-resistant enterocacci, have unique epidemiologic features and require comprehensive infection control measures. Overuse, inappropriate selection, and unnecessarily prolonged administration of antimicrobial agents are likely to place increased and unnecessary antimicrobial pressure on bacteria, leading to an increase in development and spread of resistant pathogens or susceptibility to opportunistic pathogens, such as *Clostridium difficile,* or both. The principles for appropriate use of antimicrobial agents, combined with infection-control programs, have become a central focus of measures to combat development and spread of resistant organisms.[2] Health care organizations caring for both inpatients and outpatients are encouraged to embrace antimicrobial stewardship programs that are designed to optimize clinical outcomes while minimizing inappropriate antimicrobial exposures and toxicities, unnecessary costs, and selection of antimicrobial-resistant pathogens. Application of principles of appropriate use of antimicrobial agents for respiratory tract infections in children has led to a decrease in number of prescriptions written for antimicrobial agents. Additional information on judicious use of antimicrobial agents and antimicrobial resistance is available at **www.cdc.gov/drugresistance**.

Principles of Appropriate Use for Upper Respiratory Tract Infections

Approximately three quarters of all outpatient prescriptions of antimicrobial agents for children are given for 5 conditions: otitis media, sinusitis, cough illness/bronchitis, pharyngitis, and nonspecific upper respiratory tract infection (the common cold). Antimicrobial agents are prescribed, even though many of these illnesses are caused by viruses and are unresponsive to antimicrobial therapy. Physicians report that many patients and parents try to persuade them to dispense unnecessary antimicrobial agents. Children treated with an antimicrobial agent are at increased risk of becoming carriers of resistant bacteria, including *S pneumoniae* and *Haemophilus influenzae.* Carriers of a resistant strain who develop illness from that strain are more likely to have failure of antimicrobial therapy. In some conditions, such as otitis media with effusion (OME), observation without antimicrobial therapy is recommended, and in other conditions, such as the common cold or cough, antimicrobial therapy is not indicated. The following

---

[1]Boucher HW, Talbot GH, Bradley JS, et al. Bad bugs, no drugs: no ESKAPE! An update from the Infectious Diseases Society of America. *Clin Infect Dis.* 2009;48(1):1–12

[2]Dellit TH, Owens RC, McGowan JE Jr, et al. Infectious Diseases Society of America and the Society for Healthcare Epidemiology of America guidelines for developing an institutional program to enhance antimicrobial stewardship. *Clin Infect Dis.* 2007;44(2):159–177

principles, with detailed supporting evidence, were published by the American Academy of Pediatrics, American Academy of Family Physicians, and Centers for Disease Control and Prevention (CDC) to identify clinical conditions for which antimicrobial therapy could be curtailed without compromising patient care (**www.aafp.org/online/en/ home/clinical/clinicalrecs/aom.htm**).

OTITIS MEDIA

- Antimicrobial agents are indicated for treatment of acute otitis media (AOM) but not for OME. Diagnosis of AOM requires a history of acute onset, evidence of middle ear effusion, and signs or symptoms of inflammation of the middle ear.
- Observation without use of an antimicrobial agent in a child with uncomplicated AOM is an option for selected children on the basis of diagnostic certainty, age, illness severity, and assurance of follow-up.[1]
- When antimicrobial agents are used for AOM, a narrow-spectrum antimicrobial agent (eg, amoxicillin, 80–90 mg/kg per day) in 2 divided doses for 5 to 7 days should be used for episodes in most children 6 years of age or older.
- Younger children and children with underlying medical conditions, craniofacial abnormalities, chronic or recurrent otitis media, or perforation of the tympanic membrane should be treated with a 10-day course of an antimicrobial agent.[2]
- Persistent middle ear effusion (OME) for 2 to 3 months after therapy for AOM is expected and does not require routine retreatment; treatment for 10 to 14 days may be considered an option if effusions persist for 3 months, especially if hearing is impaired. Repetitive or prolonged courses of antimicrobial agents are not recommended.

ACUTE SINUSITIS

- Clinical diagnosis of acute bacterial sinusitis requires the presence of nasal or postnasal discharge (of any quality) without improvement for 10 to 14 days, with or without daytime cough (cough may be worse at night); or temperature of 39°C (102°F) or higher and purulent nasal discharge present concurrently for at least 3 consecutive days in a child who seems ill.
- Findings on plain radiographs of sinuses correlate poorly with disease and should not be used. Computed tomography of sinuses may be indicated when symptoms of sinusitis are persistent or recurrent or when complications are suspected.
- Initial antimicrobial treatment of acute sinusitis should be with a narrow-spectrum agent (eg, amoxicillin, 80–90 mg/kg per day in 2 divided doses) for most children, with the same considerations for antimicrobial resistance following amoxicillin treatment failure as outlined previously.

---

[1] American Academy of Pediatrics, Subcommittee on Management of Acute Otitis Media; American Academy of Family Physicians. Clinical practice guideline: diagnosis and management of acute otitis media. *Pediatrics.* 2004;113(5):1451–1465

[2] American Academy of Family Physicians; American Academy of Otolaryngology-Head and Neck Surgery; and American Academy of Pediatrics, Subcommittee on Otitis Media With Effusion. Clinical practice guideline: otitis media with effusion. *Pediatrics.* 2004;113(5):1412–1429

COUGH ILLNESS/BRONCHITIS

- Nonspecific cough illness/bronchitis in children, regardless of duration, does not warrant antimicrobial treatment.
- Prolonged cough (10–14 days or more) may be caused by *Bordetella pertussis, Bordetella parapertussis, Mycoplasma pneumoniae,* and *Chlamydophila pneumoniae.* When infection caused by these organisms is suspected clinically or is confirmed, appropriate antimicrobial therapy is indicated (see Pertussis, p 504, *Mycoplasma pneumoniae* Infections, p 473, and Chlamydial Infections, p 252).

PHARYNGITIS

(See Group A Streptococcal Infections, p 616)
- Diagnosis of group A streptococcal pharyngitis should be made on the basis of results of appropriate laboratory tests in conjunction with clinical and epidemiologic findings.
- Most cases of pharyngitis are viral in origin. Antimicrobial therapy should not be given to a child with pharyngitis in the absence of identified group A streptococci. Rarely, other bacteria may cause pharyngitis (eg, *Corynebacterium diphtheriae, Francisella tularensis,* groups G and C hemolytic streptococci, *Neisseria gonorrhoeae, Arcanobacterium haemolyticum*), and treatment should be provided according to recommendations in disease-specific chapters in Section 3.
- Penicillin remains the drug of choice for treating group A streptococcal pharyngitis. Amoxicillin and other oral antimicrobial agents may have improved efficacy of microbiologic eradication of group A streptococci from the pharynx, but this potential advantage must be considered against the disadvantage of increased antimicrobial pressure from use of more broad-spectrum antimicrobial agents.

THE COMMON COLD

- Antimicrobial agents should not be given for the common cold.
- Mucopurulent rhinitis (thick, opaque, or discolored nasal discharge) commonly accompanies the common cold and is not an indication for antimicrobial treatment unless it persists without signs of improvement for 10 to 14 days, suggesting possible acute bacterial sinusitis.

Principles of Appropriate Use of Vancomycin[1]

Increased use of vancomycin is responsible for the frequent occurrence of vancomycin-resistant enterococcal colonizations and infections as well as the infrequent emergence of vancomycin-intermediately susceptible and vancomycin-resistant strains of *S aureus.* Risk occurs particularly among patients receiving hematology-oncology, nephrology, neonatology, cardiac surgery, and neurosurgery services. Prevention of further emergence of vancomycin resistance will depend on more limited use of vancomycin for treatment and prophylaxis.

---

[1]Centers for Disease Control and Prevention. Recommendations for preventing the spread of vancomycin resistance: recommendations of the Hospital Infection Control Practices Advisory Committee. *MMWR Recomm Rep.* 1995;44(RR-12):1–13

SITUATIONS IN WHICH USE OF VANCOMYCIN IS APPROPRIATE INCLUDE THE FOLLOWING:

- Treatment of serious infections attributable to beta-lactam–resistant gram-positive organisms.
- Treatment of infections attributable to gram-positive microorganisms in patients with serious allergy to beta-lactam agents.
- Antimicrobial-associated colitis that fails to respond to metronidazole therapy or colitis that is severe and potentially life threatening (see *Clostridium difficile*, p 263).
- Prophylaxis, as recommended by the 2007 American Heart Association guidelines (**http://circ.ahajournals.org/cgi/content/full/116/15/1736**), for endocarditis after certain procedures in patients at high risk of endocarditis caused by MRSA, or in people intolerant of beta-lactam agents (see Prevention of Bacterial Endocarditis, p 826).
- Prophylaxis for major surgical procedures involving implantation of prosthetic materials or devices at institutions with a high rate of infections attributable to MRSA or methicillin-resistant coagulase-negative staphylococci.

SITUATIONS IN WHICH USE OF VANCOMYCIN IS DISCOURAGED INCLUDE THE FOLLOWING:

- Routine prophylaxis for the following:
  - Surgical patients other than patients with a life-threatening allergy to beta-lactam antimicrobial agents or in a setting delineated previously;
  - Infants with very low birth weight;
  - Patients receiving continuous ambulatory peritoneal dialysis or hemodialysis; or
  - Preventing infection or colonization of indwelling central or peripheral intravascular catheters (either systemic or antimicrobial lock).
- Empiric antimicrobial therapy for a patient with neutropenia and fever, unless strong evidence indicates an infection attributable to gram-positive microorganisms and the prevalence of infections attributable to MRSA in the hospital is substantial.
- Treatment in response to a single positive result of a blood culture for coagulase-negative staphylococcus, if other blood culture results obtained in the same period are negative.
- Continued empiric use for presumed infections in patients whose culture results are negative for beta-lactam–resistant, gram-positive microorganisms.
- Selective decontamination of the digestive tract.
- Attempted eradication of MRSA colonization.
- Primary treatment of nonlife-threatening antimicrobial-associated colitis (see *Clostridium difficile*, p 263).
- Treatment of infections attributable to beta-lactam–susceptible gram-positive micro-organisms, including vancomycin given for dosing convenience in patients with renal failure.
- Topical application or irrigation.
- When vancomycin is started for empiric therapy its use should be discontinued when cultures reveal that alternate antimicrobial agents are available (eg, nafcillin to treat MSSA) or if cultures fail to provide evidence that vancomycin is needed (eg, lack of beta-lactamase resistant gram-positive organisms).

DRUG INTERACTIONS

The use of multiple drugs for therapy of seriously ill patients increases the probability of drug-drug interactions. Drug-drug interactions can be considered as producing either changes in drug concentrations (pharmacokinetics) or changes in the drug effect/toxicity profile (pharmacodynamics). Pharmacokinetic interactions result from alterations in the absorption, distribution, metabolism, or elimination of a drug and thereby result in a change in concentration in the body. Pharmacodynamic drug-drug interactions may produce synergistic, additive, or antagonistic drug effects or toxicities. Many of the serious adverse interactions between drugs are attributable to inhibition (some macrolides, quinolones, and azole agents) or induction (rifabutin, rifampin) of hepatic intestinal cytochrome P450 (CYP) isoenzymes, especially CYP3A, which is thought to be involved in metabolism of more than 50% of prescribed drugs.

For information on drug interactions, see **www.fda.gov/cder/drug/ drugInteractions/default.htm.**

Tables of Antibacterial Drug Dosages

Recommended dosages for antibacterial agents commonly used for newborn infants (see Table 4.1, p 745) and for older infants and children (see Table 4.2, p 747) are given separately because of the physiologic immaturity of the newborn infant and resulting different pharmacokinetics. The table for newborn infants is divided by postnatal age and birth weight because of age-related differences in pharmacokinetics.

Recommended dosages are not absolute and are intended only as a guide. Clinical judgment about the disease, alterations in renal or hepatic function, coadministration of other drugs, and other factors affecting pharmacokinetics, patient response, and laboratory results may dictate modifications of these recommendations in an individual patient. In some cases, monitoring of serum drug concentrations is recommended to avoid toxicity and to ensure therapeutic efficacy.

Product label information should be consulted for details, such as the diluent for reconstitution of injectable preparations, measures to be taken to avoid incompatibilities, drug interactions, and other precautions.

Table 4.1 Antibacterial Drugs for Newborn Infants: Dose[a] (mg/kg or U/kg) and Frequency of Administration

Drug	Route	Infants 0–4 wk of Age BW <1200 g	Infants <1 wk of Age BW 1200–2000 g	Infants <1 wk of Age BW >2000 g	Infants ≥1 wk of Age BW 1200–2000 g	Infants ≥1 wk of Age BW >2000 g
Aminoglycosides[b,c]						
Amikacin	IV, IM	7.5 every 18–24 h	7.5 every 12 h	7.5–10 every 12 h	7.5–10 every 8 or 12 h	10 every 8 h
Gentamicin	IV, IM	2.5 every 18–24 h	2.5 every 12 h	2.5 every 12 h	2.5 every 8 or 12 h	2.5 every 8 h
Neomycin	PO only	...	25 every 6 h	25 every 6 h	25 every 6 h	25 every 6 h
Tobramycin	IV, IM	2.5 every 18–24 h	2.5 every 12 h	2.5 every 12 h	2.5 every 8 or 12 h	2.5 every 8 h
Antistaphylococcal penicillins[d]						
Methicillin	IV, IM	25 every 12 h	25–50 every 12 h	25–50 every 8 h	25–50 every 8 h	25–50 every 6 h
Nafcillin	IV, IM	25 every 12 h	25 every 12 h	25 every 8 h	25 every 8 h	25–35 every 6 h
Oxacillin	IV, IM	25 every 12 h	25–50 every 12 h	25–50 every 8 h	25–50 every 8 h	25–50 every 6 h
Monobactam						
Aztreonam	IV, IM	30 every 12 h	30 every 12 h	30 every 8 h	30 every 8 h	30 every 6 h
Carbapenems[e]						
Imipenem/cilastatin	IV	25 every 12 h	25 every 12 h	25 every 12 h	25 every 8 h	25 every 8 h
Cephalosporins						
Cefotaxime	IV, IM	50 every 12 h	50 every 12 h	50 every 8 or 12 h	50 every 8 h	50 every 6 or 8 h
Ceftazidime	IV, IM	50 every 12 h	50 every 12 h	50 every 8 or 12 h	50 every 8 h	50 every 8 h
Ceftriaxone[f]	IV, IM	50 every 24 h	50 every 24 h	50 every 24 h	50 every 24 h	50–75 every 24 h

Table 4.1 Antibacterial Drugs for Newborn Infants: Dose[a] (mg/kg or U/kg) and Frequency of Administration, continued

Drug	Route	Infants 0–4 wk of Age BW <1200 g	Infants <1 wk of Age BW 1200–2000 g	Infants <1 wk of Age BW >2000 g	Infants ≥1 wk of Age BW 1200–2000 g	Infants ≥1 wk of Age BW >2000 g
Clindamycin	IV, IM, PO	5 every 12 h	5 every 12 h	5 every 8 h	5 every 8 h	5–7.5 every 6 h
Erythromycin	PO	10 every 12 h	10 every 12 h	10 every 12 h	10 every 8 h	10 every 8 h
Metronidazole[e]	IV, PO	7.5 every 24–48 h	7.5 every 24 h	7.5 every 12 h	7.5 every 12 h	15 every 12 h
Oxazolidinone						
Linezolid	IV	10 every 8–12 h[g]	10 every 8–12 h[g]	10 every 8–12 h	10 every 8 h	10 every 8 h
Penicillins						
Ampicillin[e]	IV, IM	25–50 every 12 h	25–50 every 12 h	25–50 every 8 h	25–50 every 8 h	25–50 every 6 h
Penicillin G,[d] aqueous	IV, IM	25 000–50 000 U every 12 h	25 000–50 000 U every 12 h	25 000–50 000 U every 8 h	25 000–50 000 U every 8 h	25 000–50 000 U every 6 h
Penicillin G procaine	IM	…	50 000 U every 24 h	50 000 U every 24 h	50 000 U every 24 h	50 000 U every 24 h
Ticarcillin[h]	IV, IM	75 every 12 h	75 every 12 h	75 every 8 h	75 every 8 h	100 every 8 h
Vancomycin[b]	IV	15 every 24 h	10–15 every 12–18 h	10–15 every 8–12 h	10–15 every 8–12 h	10–15 every 6–8 h

BW indicates birth weight; IV, intravenous; IM, intramuscular; PO, oral.

[a] Unless otherwise listed, dosages are given as mg/kg.

[b] Optimal dosage should be based on determination of serum concentrations, especially in low birth weight infants (less than 1500 g) infants. In very low birth weight infants (less than 1200 g) infants, dosing every 18 to 24 hours may be appropriate in the first week of life.

[c] Dosages for aminoglycosides may differ from dosages recommended by the manufacturer in the package insert.

[d] For meningitis, the larger dosage is recommended. Some experts recommend even larger dosages for group B streptococcal meningitis.

[e] Safety in infants and children has not been established. Meropenem is preferred if a carbapenem is to be used in newborn infants.

[f] Drug should not be administered to neonates with hyperbilirubinemia, especially infants born preterm. Neonates should not receive ceftriaxone intravenously while receiving calcium in any form (including hyperalimentation).

[g] Dosing every 12 hours is recommended for infants less than 34 weeks' gestation and less than 1 week of age.

[h] Same dosage for ticarcillin and clavulanate potassium.

Table 4.2. Antibacterial Drugs for Pediatric Patients Beyond the Newborn Period

Drug Generic (Trade Name)	Route	Dosage per kg per Day		Comments
		Mild to Moderate Infections	Severe Infections	
Aminoglycosides[a]				
Amikacin (Amikin)	IV, IM	Inappropriate	15–22.5 mg in 3 doses (daily adult dose, 15 mg/kg; maximum, 1.5 g)	30 mg in 3 doses is recommended by some consultants.
Gentamicin	IV, IM	Inappropriate	3–7.5 mg in 3 doses (daily adult dose is the same)	Once-daily dosing (5–6 mg/kg every 24 h) is investigational in children.
Kanamycin	IV, IM	Inappropriate	15–22.5 mg in 3 doses (daily adult dose, 1–1.5 g)	30 mg in 3 doses is recommended by some consultants.
Neomycin (numerous types)	PO only	100 mg in 4 doses	100 mg in 4 doses	For some enteric infections.
Tobramycin (Nebcin)	IV, IM	Inappropriate	3–7.5 mg in 3 doses (daily adult dose, 3–5 mg in 3 doses)	Once daily dosing (5–6 mg/kg every 24 h) is investigational in children.
Carbapenems				
Doripenem (Doribax)	IV	…	500 mg every 8 h	Not approved for use in children.
Imipenem/cilastatin[b] (Primaxin)	IV, IM	See package insert	See package insert	Approved for use in pediatric patients, neonates to 16 years of age. Caution in use for treatment of meningitis because of possible seizures.
Meropenem[b] (Merrem)	IV	See package insert	See package insert	Approved for use in children 3 mo of age and older. Daily dose varies by indication with higher dosage used for treatment of meningitis.
Ertapenem (Invanz)	IV	See package insert	See package insert	Approved for children 3 mo to 12 y of age. Less active against *Pseudomonas* species, *Acinetobacter* species, and gram-positive cocci.

Table 4.2. Antibacterial Drugs for Pediatric Patients Beyond the Newborn Period, continued

Drug Generic (Trade Name)	Route	Dosage per kg per Day		Comments
		Mild to Moderate Infections	Severe Infections	
Cephalosporins[b]				
Cefaclor (Ceclor)	PO	20–40 mg in 2 or 3 doses (daily adult dose, 750 mg–1.5 g)	Inappropriate	A twice-daily regimen has been demonstrated to be effective for treatment of acute otitis media (AOM).
Cefadroxil (Duricef)	PO	30 mg in 2 doses (maximum daily adult dose, 2 g)	Inappropriate	First-generation activity.
Cefazolin (Ancef, Kefzol)	IV, IM	100 mg in 3 doses (maximum 4–6 g/day)	100 mg in 3 doses (maximum 4–6 g/day)	First-generation activity.
Cefdinir (Omnicef)	PO	14 mg in 1 or 2 doses (maximum 600 mg/day)	Inappropriate	Inadequate activity against resistant pneumococci.
Cefditoren (Spectracef)	PO	800 mg total dose divided (maximum 800 mg/day) in 2 doses	No data available	Not approved for children younger than 12 y of age.
Cefepime (Maxipime)	IV, IM	≥2 mo of age: 100–150 mg in 3 doses (daily adult dose, 1–2 g)	≥2 mo of age: 150 mg in 3 doses (daily adult dose, 2–4 g)	Not approved for treatment of meningitis. Considered fourth generation.
Cefixime (Suprax)	PO	8 mg in 1 or 2 doses (maximum adult dose, 400 mg)	Inappropriate	Single-dose treatment for gonorrhea (400 mg × 1).
Cefoperazone (Cefobid)	IV, IM	100–150 mg in 2 or 3 doses (maximum daily adult dose, 4 g)	No data available	Not approved for use in children.
Cefotaxime (Claforan)	IV, IM	75–100 mg in 3 or 4 doses (daily adult dose, 4–6 g)	150–200 mg in 3 or 4 doses (daily adult dose, 8–10 g)	A regimen of 300 mg in 3 or 4 doses can be used for treatment of meningitis.

Table 4.2. Antibacterial Drugs for Pediatric Patients Beyond the Newborn Period, continued

| Drug Generic (Trade Name) | Route | Dosage per kg per Day | | Comments |
		Mild to Moderate Infections	Severe Infections	
Cefotetan (Cefotan)	IV, IM	Inappropriate	40–80 mg in 2 doses (maximum daily adult dose, 6 g)	Not licensed for use in children.
Cefoxitin (Mefoxin)	IV, IM	80–100 mg in 3–4 doses (daily adult dose, 3–4 g)	80–160 mg in 4–6 doses (daily adult dose, 6–12 g)	Improved activity against *Bacteroides fragilis*.
Cefpodoxime (Vantin)	PO	10 mg in 2 doses (maximum daily adult dose, 800 mg)	Inappropriate	Similar to cefixime with greater activity against methicillin-susceptible staphylococci.
Cefprozil (Cefzil)	PO	15–30 mg in 2 doses (maximum daily adult dose, 1 g)	Inappropriate	30 mg dosage recommended for treatment of acute otitis media.
Ceftazidime (Ceptaz, Fortaz, Tazidime)	IV, IM	75–100 mg in 3 doses (daily adult dose, 3 g)	125–150 mg in 3 doses (daily adult dose, 6 g)	Anti-*Pseudomonas* activity; has been approved for use in children.
Ceftibuten (Cedax)	PO	9 mg in 1 dose (maximum adult dose: 400 mg/day)	Inappropriate	Approved for people ≥6 mo of age. Inadequate activity against intermediate and resistant pneumococci.
Ceftizoxime (Cefizox)	IV, IM	100–150 mg in 3 doses (daily adult dose, 3–4 g)	150–200 mg in 3 or 4 doses (daily adult dose, 4–6 g)	Third-generation activity.
Ceftriaxone (Rocephin)	IV, IM	50–75 mg in 1 or 2 doses (daily adult dose, 2 g)	80–100 mg in 1 or 2 doses (daily adult dose, 4 g)	Larger dosage appropriate for penicillin-resistant pneumococcal meningitis.
Cefuroxime (Zinacef)	IV, IM	75–100 mg in 3 doses (daily adult dose, 2–4 g)	100–150 mg in 3 doses (daily adult dose, 4–6 g)	Second-generation activity, less active than third-generation cephalosporins against penicillin-resistant *Streptococcus pneumoniae*.
Cefuroxime axetil (Ceftin)	PO	20–30 mg in 2 doses (daily adult dose, 1–2 g)	Inappropriate	The higher dosage recommended for treatment of otitis media. Limited activity against penicillin-resistant *S pneumoniae*.

Table 4.2. Antibacterial Drugs for Pediatric Patients Beyond the Newborn Period, continued

Drug Generic (Trade Name)	Route	Dosage per kg per Day		Comments
		Mild to Moderate Infections	Severe Infections	
Cephalexin (Keflex)	PO	25–50 mg in 3–4 doses (daily adult dose, 1–4 g)	Inappropriate	First-generation activity.
Cephalothin (Keflin)	IV, IM	80–100 mg in 4 doses (daily adult dose, 2–4 g)	100–150 mg in 4–6 doses (daily adult dose, 8–12 g)	First-generation activity.
Cephradine (Velosef)	PO	25–50 mg in 2–4 doses (daily adult dose, 1–4 g)	Inappropriate	First-generation activity.
Chloramphenicol (Chloromycetin)				
Chloramphenicol	IV	Inappropriate	50–100 mg in 4 doses (daily adult dose, 2–4 g)	Optimal dosage is determined by measurement of serum concentrations with resulting modifications to achieve therapeutic concentrations. Use only for serious infections because of the rare occurrence of aplastic anemia after administration. Oral formulation (palmitate) not available in the United States.
Clindamycin (Cleocin)	IM, IV	15–25 mg in 3–4 doses (daily adult dose, 600 mg–3.6 g)	25–40 mg in 3–4 doses (daily adult dose, 1.2–2.7 g)	Active against anaerobes, especially *Bacteroides* species. Active against many multidrug-resistant pneumococci.
	PO	10–20 mg in 3–4 doses (daily adult dose, 600 mg–1.8 g)	Inappropriate	Effective for otitis media caused by many multidrug-resistant pneumococci.
Fluoroquinolones[d]				
Ciprofloxacin (Cipro)	PO	20–30 mg in 2 doses (daily adult dose, 0.5–1.5 g)	30 mg in 2 doses (daily adult dose, 1.0–1.5 g)	Only licensed for children younger than 18 y of age for specific indications[d] (see p 737).

Table 4.2. Antibacterial Drugs for Pediatric Patients Beyond the Newborn Period, continued

Drug Generic (Trade Name)	Route	Dosage per kg per Day		Comments
		Mild to Moderate Infections	Severe Infections	
Ciprofloxacin (Cipro), continued	IV	Inappropriate	18–30 mg in 2 or 3 doses (daily adult dose, 400–800 mg in 2 doses)	...
Ketolides				
Telithromycin	PO	800 mg total dose, once daily (maximum adult dose 800 mg/day)		Not approved for people younger than 18 y of age. Used for treatment of community-acquired pneumonia.
Macrolides/ streptogramins				
Azithromycin (Zithromax)	PO	5–12 mg once daily (maximum daily adult dose, 600 mg)	Inappropriate	Pharyngitis, 6 mo of age or older: 12 mg/kg per day for 5 days.
Clarithromycin (Biaxin)	PO	15 mg in 2 doses (maximum daily adult dose, 1 g)	Inappropriate	Similar to erythromycin; more activity against *Mycobacterium avium* and *Helicobacter pylori* and preventing *Mycobacterium tuberculosis*.
Erythromycins (numerous types)	PO	30–50 mg in 2–4 doses (daily adult dose, 1–2 g)	Inappropriate	Available in base, stearate, ethylsuccinate, and estolate preparations.
	IV	Inappropriate	15–50 mg in 4 doses (daily adult dose, 1–4 g)	Administer in a continuous drip or by slow infusion over 60 min or longer. May cause cardiac arrhythmia.
Metronidazole (Flagyl)	PO	15–50 mg in 3 doses (maximum daily adult dose, 1–2.25 g)	Inappropriate	Safety in infants and children has not been established, except for intestinal amebiasis.

Table 4.2. Antibacterial Drugs for Pediatric Patients Beyond the Newborn Period, continued

| Drug Generic (Trade Name) | Route | Dosage per kg per Day | | Comments |
		Mild to Moderate Infections	Severe Infections	
Miscellaneous				
Daptomycin	IV	Inappropriate	4 mg, once daily	Not approved for people <18 y of age. Effective for complicated skin and soft tissue infections caused by staphylococci, streptococci, and enterococci.
Monobactam				
Aztreonam[b] (Azactam)	IV, IM	90 mg in 3 doses (daily adult dose, 3 g)	90–120 mg in 3 or 4 doses (maximum daily adult dose, 8 g)	...
Loracarbef (Lorabid)	PO	6 mo–12 y of age: 15 mg/kg per day, every 12 h ≥13 y of age: 400 mg/day, in 2 doses	6 mo–12 y of age: 30 mg/kg per day, every 12 h ≥13 y of age: 800 mg/day, in 2 doses	Pharyngitis, tonsillitis, sinusitis, and skin and soft tissue infections (use higher dose for sinusitis).
Nitrofurantoin (Furadantin)	PO	5–7 mg in 4 doses (daily adult dose, 200–400 mg)	Inappropriate	Should not be used for young infants; prophylactic dose is 1–2 mg/kg per day in 1 dose.
Oxazolidinones				
Linezolid (Zyvox)	PO, IV	30 mg in 3 doses (children <12 y of age) 20 mg in 2 doses (adolescents and adults up to 1200 mg maximum)	30 mg in 3 doses (children <12 y of age) 20 mg in 2 doses (adolescents and adults up to 1200 mg maximum)	Myelosuppression may occur. Active against Enterococcus faecium, E faecalis, oxacillin-resistant S aureus, and penicillin-resistant S pneumoniae.

Table 4.2. Antibacterial Drugs for Pediatric Patients Beyond the Newborn Period, continued

Drug Generic (Trade Name)	Route	Dosage per kg per Day		Comments
		Mild to Moderate Infections	Severe Infections	
PENICILLINS[b]				
Broad-spectrum penicillins				
Ampicillin (numerous types)	IV, IM	100–150 mg in 4 doses (daily adult dose, 2–4 g)	200–400 mg in 4 doses (daily adult dose, 6–12 g)	Larger dosage recommended for treatment of meningitis.
	PO	50–100 mg in 4 doses (daily adult dose, 2–4 g)	Inappropriate	Diarrhea occurs in approximately 20% of recipients.
Ampicillin-sulbactam (Unasyn)	IV	100–150 mg of ampicillin in 4 doses	200–400 mg of ampicillin in 4 doses (daily adult dose, 6–12 g)	Licensed for use in children 1 y of age and older.
Amoxicillin (numerous types)	PO	25–50 mg in 3 doses (daily adult dose, 750 mg–1.5 g); 90 mg/kg in 2 doses for AOM	Inappropriate	90 mg/kg dose recommended for initial therapy of AOM.[c]
Amoxicillin-clavulanic acid				
(Augmentin ES-600; 14:1 ratio)	PO	90 mg of amoxicillin in 2 doses	Inappropriate	Preferred for recurrent AOM and treatment failures.
(Augmentin XR)	PO	4 g total, in 2 doses (total 4000 mg)	Inappropriate	Oral extended-release formulation licensed for adults.
Piperacillin[f]	IV, IM	100–150 mg in 4 doses (daily adult dose, 6–8 g)	200–300 mg in 4–6 doses (daily adult dose, 12–18 g)	…

Table 4.2. Antibacterial Drugs for Pediatric Patients Beyond the Newborn Period, continued

Drug Generic (Trade Name)	Route	Dosage per kg per Day		Comments
		Mild to Moderate Infections	Severe Infections	
Piperacillin-tazobactam[f] (Zosyn)	IV	Inappropriate	300 mg of piperacillin in 3 doses (children >9 months of age) 240 mg of piperacillin in 3 doses (children 2–9 months of age) (daily adult dose 12–18 g)	Approved for use in children 2 mo of age and older with appendicitis and/or peritonitis.
Ticarcillin (Ticar)	IV, IM	100–200 mg in 4 doses (daily adult dose, 4–6 g)	200–300 mg in 4 doses (daily adult dose, 12–24 g)	Contains 5.2 mEq of sodium/g.
Ticarcillin-clavulanate (Timentin)	IV, IM	100–200 mg of ticarcillin in 4 doses (daily adult dose, 4–6 g)	200–300 mg of ticarcillin in 4 doses (daily adult dose, 12–24 g)	…
Penicillin G and V[a,f]				
Penicillin G, crystalline potassium or sodium (numerous types)	IV, IM	25 000–50 000 U in 4 doses	250 000–400 000 U in 4–6 doses. Maximum adult dose 24 million U/24 h.	Larger dosage appropriate for central nervous system infections.
Penicillin G procaine (numerous types)	IM	25 000–50 000 U in 1–2 doses. Maximum adult dose 4.8 million U/24 h.	Inappropriate	Contraindicated for procaine allergy.
Penicillin G benzathine (Bicillin LA, Permapen)	IM	<27.3 kg (60 lb) in body weight: 600 000 U once ≥27.3 kg (60 lb): 1.2 million U once	Inappropriate	Major use is prevention of rheumatic fever by treatment and prophylaxis of streptococcal infections.

Table 4.2. Antibacterial Drugs for Pediatric Patients Beyond the Newborn Period, continued

Drug Generic (Trade Name)	Route	Dosage per kg per Day		Comments
		Mild to Moderate Infections	Severe Infections	
Penicillin V (numerous types)	PO	25–50 mg in 3 or 4 doses. Maximum adult dose 500 mg/dose, every 6–8 h. (2 g/24 h).	Inappropriate	Optimal to administer on an empty stomach.
Penicillinase-resistant penicillins[b]				Methicillin (oxacillin)-resistant staphylococci usually are resistant to all other semisynthetic antistaphylococcal penicillins and cephalosporins.
Penicillinase-resistant penicillins[b]				Methicillin (oxacillin)-resistant staphylococci usually are resistant to all other semisynthetic antistaphylococcal cephalosporins.
Oxacillin	IV, IM	100–150 mg in 4 doses (daily adult dose, 2–4 g)	150–200 mg in 4–6 doses (daily adult dose, 4–12 g)	…
Nafcillin	IV, IM, PO	50–100 mg in 4 doses (daily adult dose, 2–4 g)	100–150 mg in 4 doses (daily adult dose, 4–12 g)	Oral formulation not used because of poor absorption.
Cloxacillin (Tegopen, Cloxapen)	PO	50–100 mg in 4 doses (daily adult dose, 2–4 g)	Inappropriate	…
Dicloxacillin	PO	25–50 mg in 4 doses (daily adult dose, 1–2 g)	Inappropriate	Excellent serum concentrations after oral administration.
Rifampin (numerous types)	PO	10–20 mg in 1–2 doses (daily adult dose, 600 mg)	20 mg in 2 doses. Maximum adult dose 600 mg/24 h.	Should not be used as monotherapy except when given for prophylaxis.
	IV	10–20 mg in 1–2 doses (daily adult dose, 600 mg)	20 mg in 2 doses. Maximum adult dose 600 mg/24 h.	…
Rifaximin (Xifaxan)	PO	≥12 y of age: 600 mg/day, given 3 times/day	Inappropriate	Treatment of travelers' diarrhea caused by noninvasive *Escherichia coli*. Nonabsorbable.

Table 4.2. Antibacterial Drugs for Pediatric Patients Beyond the Newborn Period, continued

Drug Generic (Trade Name)	Route	Dosage per kg per Day		Comments
		Mild to Moderate Infections	Severe Infections	
Streptogramin				
Quinupristin/dalfo-pristin (Synercid)	IV	15 mg in 2 doses (daily adult dose, same)	22.5 mg in 3 doses (daily adult dose, same)	Modestly effective for vancomycin-resistant *E faecium* (but not *Enterococcus faecalis*) as well as *Staphylococcus aureus*. Limited use in children.
Sulfonamides				
Sulfadiazine	PO	100–150 mg in 4 doses (daily adult dose 4–6 g)	120–150 mg in 4–6 doses (daily adult dose 4–6 g)	…
Sulfisoxazole (Gantrisin)	PO	120–150 mg in 4–6 doses (daily adult dose 2–4 g)	120-150 mg in 4–6 doses (daily adult dose 2–4 g)	…
Triple sulfonamides (numerous types)	PO	120–150 mg in 4 doses	120–150 mg in 4 doses	…
Trimethoprim-sulfamethoxazole (Bactrim, Septra)	PO	8–12 mg of trimethoprim, 40–60 mg of sulfamethoxazole in 2 doses (daily adult dose, 320 mg of trimethoprim, 1.6 g of sulfamethoxazole)	20 mg of trimethoprim, 100 mg of sulfamethoxazole in 4 doses (for use only in *Pneumocystis jiroveci* pneumonia)	For prophylaxis in immunocompromised patients, recommended dose is 5 mg of trimethoprim, 25 mg of sulfamethoxazole per kg per day in 2 doses.
	IV	Inappropriate	8–12 mg of trimethoprim, 40–60 mg of sulfamethoxazole in 4 doses **OR** 20 mg of trimethoprim, 100 mg of sulfamethoxazole in 4 doses	Use intravenous formulation when PO formulation cannot be administered. Treatment of *Pneumocystis* infection.

Table 4.2. Antibacterial Drugs for Pediatric Patients Beyond the Newborn Period, continued

Drug Generic (Trade Name)	Route	Dosage per kg per Day		Comments
		Mild to Moderate Infections	Severe Infections	
Tetracyclines (numerous types)	IV	Inappropriate	10–25 mg in 2–4 doses (daily adult dose, 1–2 g)	Responsible for staining of developing teeth; use only in children 8 y of age or older except in circumstances in which the benefits of therapy exceed the risks and alternative drugs are less effective or more toxic (see p 739).
Doxycycline (numerous types)	PO	20–50 mg in 4 doses (daily adult dose, 1–2 g)	Inappropriate	Responsible for staining of developing teeth; use only in children 8 y of age or older except in circumstances in which the benefits of therapy exceed the risks and alternative drugs are less effective or more toxic (see p 739).
	PO, IV	2–4 mg in 1–2 doses (daily adult dose, 100–200 mg)	Inappropriate	Adverse effects similar to those of other tetracycline products except that risk of dental staining in children younger than 8 y of age is less.
Vancomycin (Vancocin, Vancoled, Vancor)	IV	40 mg in 3–4 doses (daily adult dose,[g] 1–2 g)	40–60 mg in 4 doses (daily adult dose,[g] 2–4 g)	In meningitis, 60 mg/kg dose should be given over a period of at least 60 min; routine monitoring of serum concentrations is unnecessary.

IV, indicates intravenous; IM, intramuscular; PO, oral; AOM, acute otitis media.

[a] Dosages for aminoglycosides may differ from those recommended by the manufacturers (see package insert).

[b] In patients with history of allergy to penicillin or one of its many congeners, alternative drugs are recommended. In some circumstances, a cephalosporin or other beta-lactam–class drug may be acceptable. However, these drugs should not be used in patients with an immediate hypersensitivity (anaphylaxis) to penicillin, because approximately 5% to 15% of penicillin-allergic patients also will be allergic to cephalosporins.

[c] Not licensed for use in patients younger than 12 years of age.

[d] Only licensed for use in patients younger than 18 years of age for complicated urinary tract infections and postexposure inhalation anthrax. Some fluoroquinolones are being studied in selected children and adolescents (see Fluoroquinolones, p 737).

[e] American Academy of Pediatrics, Subcommittee on Management of Acute Otitis Media. Diagnosis and management of acute otitis media. *Pediatrics.* 2004;113(5):1451–1465

[f] Patients with a history of allergy to penicillin G or penicillin V should be considered for subsequent skin testing. Many such patients can be treated safely with penicillin, because only 10% of children with such history are proven allergic when skin tested.

[g] In adults, daily dose is given in 2 to 4 divided doses.

For more information on individual drugs, see *Physician's Desk Reference* or **www.pdr.net** (for registered users only).

SEXUALLY TRANSMITTED INFECTIONS

Table 4.3. Guidelines for Treatment of Sexually Transmitted Infections in Children and Adolescents According to Syndrome

Preferred regimens are listed. For further information concerning other acceptable regimens and diseases not included, see recommendations in disease-specific chapters in Section 3. In addition, revised recommendations on treatment of sexually transmitted infections have been issued by the Centers for Disease Control and Prevention in 2006[a]; updates are posted at **www.cdc.gov/std/treatment.**

Syndrome	Organisms/ Diagnoses	Treatment of Adolescent	Treatment of Infant/Child
Urethritis and cervicitis Urethritis: Inflammation of urethra with mucoid, mucopurulent, or purulent discharge Cervicitis: Inflammation of cervix with mucopurulent or purulent cervical discharge. Cervicitis occurs rarely in prepubertal girls (see Prepubertal vaginitis)	*Neisseria gonorrhoeae, Chlamydia trachomatis* Other causes of urethritis and cervicitis include *Ureaplasma urealyticum,* possibly *Mycoplasma genitalium,* and sometimes *Trichomonas vaginalis* and herpes simplex virus (HSV)	Cefixime, 400 mg, orally, in a single dose[b] **OR** Ceftriaxone, 125 mg, IM, in a single dose[b] **PLUS (if chlamydial infection not ruled out) EITHER** Azithromycin, 1 g, orally, in a single dose **OR** Doxycycline, 100 mg, orally, twice a day for 7 days	*Children <45 kg:* Ceftriaxone, 125 mg, IM, in a single dose **OR** Cefixime, 8 mg/kg (maximum 400 mg, orally, in a single dose) **OR** Spectinomycin, 40 mg/kg (maximum 2 g), IM, in a single dose **PLUS (if chlamydial infection not ruled out) EITHER** Erythromycin base or ethylsuccinate, 50 mg/kg per day, orally, in 4 divided doses (maximum 2 g/day) for 14 days *Children ≥45 kg but younger than 8 y of age:* Azithromycin, 1 g, orally, in a single dose *Children 8 y of age or older:* Azithromycin, 1 g, orally, in a single dose **OR** Doxycycline, 100 mg, orally, twice a day for 7 days

Table 4.3. Guidelines for Treatment of Sexually Transmitted Infections in Children and Adolescents According to Syndrome, continued

Syndrome	Organisms/ Diagnoses	Treatment of Adolescent	Treatment of Infant/Child
Prepubertal vaginitis (STI related):	*N gonorrhoeae*[a]	...	***Children <45 kg:*** Ceftriaxone, 125 mg, in a single dose
	C trachomatis[a]	...	***Children <45 kg:*** Erythromycin base or ethylsuccinate, 50 mg/kg per day, orally, in 4 divided doses (maximum 2 g/day) for 14 days ***Children ≥45 kg but younger than 8 y of age:*** Azithromycin, 1 g, orally, in a single dose ***Children 8 y of age or older:*** Azithromycin, 1 g, orally, in a single dose **OR** Doxycycline, 100 mg, orally, twice a day for 7 days
	T vaginalis	...	***Children <45 kg:*** Metronidazole, 15 mg/kg per day, orally, in 3 divided doses (maximum 2 g/day) for 7 days

Table 4.3. Guidelines for Treatment of Sexually Transmitted Infections in Children and Adolescents According to Syndrome, continued

Syndrome	Organisms/ Diagnoses	Treatment of Adolescent	Treatment of Infant/Child
	Bacterial vaginosis	…	**Children <45 kg:** Metronidazole, 15 mg/kg per day, orally, in 2 divided doses (maximum 1 g/day) for 7 days
	HSV—primary infection	Acyclovir, 400 mg, orally, 3 times/day for 7–10 days **OR** Acyclovir, 200 mg, orally, 5 times/day for 7–10 days **OR** Famciclovir (250 mg, orally, 3 times/day) for 7–10 days **OR** Valacyclovir (1 g, orally, twice daily) for 7–10 days	**Children <45 kg:** Acyclovir, 80 mg/kg per day, orally, in 3–4 divided doses (maximum 1.2 g/day) for 7–10 days
Adolescent vulvovaginitis	*T vaginalis*	Metronidazole, 2 g, orally, in a single dose **OR** Tinidazole, 2 g, orally, in a single dose	…
	Bacterial vaginosis	Metronidazole, 500 mg, orally, twice daily for 7 days **OR** Metronidazole gel 0.75%, 1 full applicator (5 g), intravaginally, once a day for 5 days **OR** Clindamycin cream 2%, 1 full applicator (5 g), intravaginally at bedtime, for 7 days	…
	Candida species	See Table 4.4, Recommended Regimens for Vulvovaginal Candidiasis (p 764)	…

Table 4.3. Guidelines for Treatment of Sexually Transmitted Infections in Children and Adolescents According to Syndrome, continued

Syndrome	Organisms/Diagnoses	Treatment of Adolescent	Treatment of Infant/Child
	HSV—primary infection	Acyclovir, 400 mg, orally, 3 times/day for 7–10 days **OR** Famcyclovir, 250 mg, orally, 3 times/day for 7–10 days **OR** Valcyclovir, 1 g, orally twice/day for 7–10 days	…
Pelvic inflammatory disease (PID)	*N gonorrhoeae, C trachomatis,* anaerobes, coliform bacteria, and *Streptococcus* species	See Pelvic Inflammatory Disease (Table 3.43, p 503)	PID occurs rarely, if at all, in prepubertal girls
Syphilis	*Treponema pallidum*	See Syphilis, p 638	*Children <45 kg:* Same as for congenital syphilis (see p 644 and Table 3.75, p 645)
Genital ulcer disease	*T pallidum*	Same as for syphilis	*Children <45 kg:* Same as for congenital syphilis (see p 644 and Table 3.75, p 645)
	HSV—primary infection	See prepubertal vaginitis	*Children <45 kg:* See prepubertal vaginitis
	Haemophilus ducreyi (chancroid)	Azithromycin, 1 g, orally, in a single dose **OR** Ceftriaxone, 250 mg, IM, in a single dose **OR** Ciprofloxacin, 500 mg, orally, twice daily for 3 days[c] **OR** Erythromycin base, 500 mg, orally, 3 times/day for 7 days	*Children <45 kg:* Ceftriaxone, 50 mg/kg, IM, in a single dose **OR** *Children <45 kg:* Azithromycin, 20 mg/kg, orally, in a single dose (maximum 1 g)

Table 4.3. Guidelines for Treatment of Sexually Transmitted Infections in Children and Adolescents According to Syndrome, continued

Syndrome	Organisms/ Diagnoses	Treatment of Adolescent	Treatment of Infant/Child
	Klebsiella granulomatis (granuloma inguinale [Donovanosis])	Doxycycline, 100 mg, orally, twice a day for at least 3 wk and until all lesions have healed completely **OR** Azithromycin, 1 g, orally, once/wk for at least 3 wk and until all lesions have healed completely **OR** Ciprofloxacin, 750 mg, orally, twice a day for at least 3 wk and until all lesions have healed completely **OR** Erythromycin base, 500 mg, orally, 4 times/day for at least 3 wk and until all lesions have healed completely **OR** Trimethoprim-sulfamethoxazole, 1 double-strength (160 gm/800 mg) tablet, orally, twice a day for at least 3 wk and until all lesions have healed completely	
Sexually acquired epididymitis	*C trachomatis, N gonorrhoeae*	Ceftriaxone, 250 mg, IM, in a single dose **PLUS** Doxycycline, 100 mg, orally, twice daily for 10 days	...
	Enteric organisms (for patients allergic to cephalosporins and/or tetracycline or for patients >35 y of age)	Ofloxacin, 300 mg, orally, twice a day for 10 days **OR** Levofloxacin, 500 mg, orally, once daily for 10 days	...

Table 4.3. Guidelines for Treatment of Sexually Transmitted Infections in Children and Adolescents According to Syndrome, continued

Syndrome	Organisms/ Diagnoses	Treatment of Adolescent	Treatment of Infant/Child
Gonococcal infections of the pharynx	*N gonorrhoeae*	Ceftriaxone, 125 mg, IM, in a single dose	⋯
Anogenital warts	Human papillomavirus	*Patient-applied:* Podofilox 0.5% solution or gel[c] **OR** Imiquimod 5% cream *Provider-administered:* Cryotherapy **OR** Podophyllin resin 10%–25%[c] **OR** Trichloroacetic acid **OR** Bichloroacetic acid **OR** Surgical removal	*Children <45 kg:* Same as for adolescents

IM indicates intramuscularly; STI, sexually transmitted infection.

[a]For additional information and recommendations, see Centers for Disease Control and Prevention. Sexually transmitted infection treatment guidelines—2006. *MMWR Recomm Rep.* 2006;55(RR11):1–94, and for updates, see **www.cdc.gov/std/treatment**. Some regimens are not indicated for pregnant adolescents.

[b]Flouroquinolones no longer are recommended for treatment of gonococcal infections because of increasing prevalence of resistant organisms (Centers for Disease Control and Prevention. Update to CDC's sexually transmitted diseases treatment guidelines, 2006: fluoroquinolones no longer recommended for treatment of gonococcal infections. *MMWR Morb Mortal Wkly Rep.* 2007;56[14]:332–336).

[c]Not tested for safety in children and contraindicated in pregnancy.

Table 4.4. Recommended Regimens for Vulvovaginal Candidiasis

Intravaginal agents:

Butoconazole, 2% cream, 5 g, intravaginally, for 3 days[a,b]

OR

Butoconazole, 2% cream (sustained release), 5 g, single intravaginal application

OR

Clotrimazole, 1% cream, 5 g, intravaginally, for 7–14 days[a,b]

OR

Clotrimazole, 100-mg vaginal tablet for 7 days[a]

OR

Clotrimazole, 100-mg vaginal tablet, 2 tablets for 3 days[a]

OR

Miconazole, 2% cream, 5 g, intravaginally, for 7 days[a,b]

OR

Miconazole, 200-mg vaginal suppository, 1 suppository for 3 days[a,b]

OR

Miconazole, 100-mg vaginal suppository, 1 suppository for 7 days[a,b]

OR

Miconazole, 1200 mg vaginal suppository, one suppository for one day

OR

Nystatin, 100 000-U vaginal tablet, 1 tablet for 14 days

OR

Tioconazole, 6.5% ointment, 5 g, intravaginally, in a single application[a,b]

OR

Terconazole, 0.4% cream, 5 g, intravaginally, for 7 days[a]

OR

Terconazole, 0.8% cream, 5 g, intravaginally, for 3 days[a]

OR

Terconazole, 80-mg vaginal suppository, 1 suppository for 3 days[a]

Oral agent:

Fluconazole, 150-mg oral tablet, 1 tablet in single dose

[a] These creams and suppositories are oil-based and might weaken latex condoms and diaphragms. Refer to condom or diaphragm product labeling for additional information.
[b] Over-the-counter preparations.

ANTIFUNGAL DRUGS FOR SYSTEMIC FUNGAL INFECTIONS

Polyenes

Amphotericin B is the drug of choice for many disseminated, potentially life-threatening fungal infections. Amphotericin B is a fungicidal agent that is effective against a broad array of fungal species. Amphotericin B, especially the deoxycholate formulation, can cause adverse reactions, particularly renal toxicity, that limit its use in certain patients. Lipid-associated formulations of amphotericin B, especially liposomal amphotericin B, limit renal toxicity but also can cause adverse effects.

Amphotericin B deoxycholate is the preferred formulation for treatment of neonates and young infants, because it is able to penetrate into the central nervous system, urinary tract, and eye, which often are involved in *Candida* species infections; lipid-associated formulations do not penetrate well into these body sites. Amphotericin B deoxycholate is given intravenously in a single daily dose of 0.5 to 1.5 mg/kg (maximum, 1.5 mg/kg/day). Amphotericin B is administered in 5% dextrose in water at a concentration of 0.1 mg/mL and delivered through a central or peripheral venous catheter (see Table 4.5, p 768). Infusion times of 1 to 2 hours have been shown to be well tolerated in adults and older children and theoretically increase the blood-to-tissue gradient, thereby improving drug delivery. After completing 1 week of daily therapy, adequate serum concentrations of the drug usually can be maintained by administering double the daily dose (maximum, 1.5 mg/kg) on alternate days. The duration of therapy depends on the type and extent of the specific fungal infection.

Amphotericin B deoxycholate is eliminated by a renal mechanism for approximately 2 weeks after therapy is discontinued. No adjustment in dose is required for neonates or for children with impaired renal function, because serum concentrations are not significantly increased in these patients. If renal toxicity occurs, alternate-day dosing is preferred to a decrease in daily dose. Neither hemodialysis nor peritoneal dialysis significantly decreases serum concentrations of the drug.

Infusion-related reactions to amphotericin B deoxycholate include fever, chills, and sometimes nausea, vomiting, headache, generalized malaise, hypotension, and arrhythmias. Onset usually is within 1 to 3 hours after starting the infusion; duration typically is less than an hour. Hypotension and arrhythmias are idiosyncratic reactions that are unlikely to occur if not observed after the initial dose but also can occur in association with very rapid infusion. Multiple regimens have been used to prevent infusion-related reactions, but few have been studied in controlled clinical trials. Pretreatment with acetaminophen, alone or combined with diphenhydramine, may alleviate febrile reactions; these reactions appear to be less common in children than in adults. Hydrocortisone (25–50 mg in adults and older children) also can be added to the infusion to decrease febrile and other systemic reactions. Tolerance to febrile reactions develops with time, allowing tapering and eventual discontinuation of the hydrocortisone and often diphenhydramine and antipyretic agents.

Meperidine and ibuprofen have been effective in preventing or treating fever and chills in some patients who are refractory to the conventional premedication regimen. Toxicity from amphotericin B deoxycholate can include nephrotoxicity, hepatotoxicity, thrombophlebitis, anemia, or neurotoxicity. Nephrotoxicity is caused by decreased renal blood flow and can be prevented or ameliorated by hydration, saline solution loading (0.9% saline solution over 30 minutes) before infusion of amphotericin B, and avoiding diuretic drugs. Hypokalemia is common and can be exacerbated by sodium loading. Renal tubular acidosis can occur but usually is mild. Permanent nephrotoxicity is related to cumulative dose. Nephrotoxicity can be enhanced by concomitant administration of amphotericin B and aminoglycosides, cyclosporine, tacrolimus, cisplatin, nitrogen mustard compounds, and acetazolamide. Anemia is secondary to inhibition of erythropoietin production. Neurotoxicity occurs rarely and can manifest as confusion, delirium, obtundation, psychotic behavior, seizures, blurred vision, or hearing loss.

Lipid-associated formulations of amphotericin B have a role in some children who are intolerant of or refractory to amphotericin B deoxycholate or can be considered in children who have renal insufficiency or at risk of significant renal toxicity from concomitant medications (see Table 4.5, p 768). In adults, none of the lipid-associated formulations have been demonstrated to be more efficacious than has conventional amphotericin B deoxycholate. Amphotericin B lipid formulations approved by the US Food and Drug Administration (FDA) for treatment of invasive fungal infections in children and adults who are refractory to or intolerant of amphotericin B deoxycholate therapy are amphotericin B lipid complex (ABLC, Abelcet), and liposomal amphotericin B (L-AmB, AmBisome). Compared with amphotericin B deoxycholate, acute infusion-related reactions occur with both formulations but are less frequent with AmBisome. Nephrotoxicity is less common with lipid-associated products than with amphotericin B deoxycholate. Liver toxicity, which generally is not associated with amphotericin B deoxycholate, has been reported with the lipid formulations.

Pyrimidines

Among pyrimidine antifungal agents, only flucytosine (5-fluorocytosine) is approved by the FDA for use in children. Flucytosine has a limited spectrum of activity against fungi and potential for toxicity (see Table 4.5, p 768), and when flucytosine is used as a single agent, resistance often emerges. Flucytosine is used in combination with amphotericin B for cryptococcal meningitis and some life-threatening *Candida* infections, such as meningitis. It is critical to monitor serum concentrations of flucytosine to avoid bone marrow toxicity.

Azoles

Five oral azoles are available in the United States and include ketoconazole, fluconazole, itraconazole, voriconazole, and posaconazole. All have relatively broad activity against common fungi but differ in their activity, bioavailability, adverse effects, and potential for drug interactions (see Table 4.5, p 768). Limited data are available regarding the safety and efficacy of azoles in pediatric patients, and trials comparing these agents to amphotericin B have been limited. Azoles are easy to administer and have little toxicity, but their use can be limited by the frequency of their interactions with coadministered drugs. These drug interactions can result in decreased serum concentrations of the azole (ie, poor therapeutic activity) or unexpected toxicity from the coadministered drug (ie, increased serum concentrations of the coadministered drug). When considering use of azoles, the patient's concurrent medications should be reviewed to avoid potential adverse clinical outcomes. Another potential limitation of azoles is emergence of resistant fungi, especially *Candida* species resistant to fluconazole. *Candida krusei* are intrinsically resistant to fluconazole and strains of *Candida glabrata* are showing increasing resistance to fluconazole and voriconazole. Itraconazole is approved by the FDA for treatment of blastomycosis, histoplasmosis (nonmeningeal), and aspergillosis in patients who are intolerant to amphotericin B and for empiric therapy of febrile neutropenic patients with suspected fungal infection. Itraconazole does not cross the blood-brain barrier and should not be used for infections of the central nervous system. Voriconazole has been approved by the FDA for primary treatment of invasive *Aspergillus* species, for esophageal candidiasis, and for refractory infection with *Scedosporium apiospermum* (the asexual form of *Pseudallescheria boydii*) and *Fusarium* species. Limited data are available regarding use of voriconazole in children. Posaconazole is approved for use in adults for prophylaxis against fungal infections and as salvage therapy for invasive aspergillosis. Ketoconazole seldom is used, because other azoles have fewer adverse effects and generally are preferred.

Echinocandins

Caspofungin, micafungin, and anidulafungin are the only echinocandins approved by the FDA. Caspofungin is approved for treatment of esophageal candidiasis, invasive candidiasis, and aspergillosis in adults who are refractory to or intolerant of other antifungal drugs. Clinical trials assessing safety or efficacy in pediatric patients are being conducted. Table 4.6 (p 772) provides recommendations for treatment of serious fungal infections with amphotericin B, flucytosine, azoles, echinocandins, and other antifungal agents. Micafungin is approved by the FDA for intravenous treatment of esophageal candidiasis and prophylaxis of invasive *Candida* infections in patients undergoing hematopoietic stem cell transplantation. Anidulafungin is approved by the FDA for intravenous treatment of candidemia, *Candida* infections, and esophageal candidiasis.

RECOMMENDED DOSES OF PARENTERAL AND ORAL ANTIFUNGAL DRUGS

Table 4.5. Recommended Doses of Parenteral and Oral Antifungal Drugs

Drug	Route	Dose (per day)	Adverse Reactions[a,b]
Amphotericin B deoxycholate (see Antifungal Drugs for Systemic Fungal Infections, p 765, for detailed information)	IV	1.0–1.5 mg/kg; infuse as single dose over 2 h	Fever, chills, gastrointestinal tract symptoms, headache, hypotension, renal dysfunction, hypokalemia, anemia, cardiac arrhythmias, neurotoxicity, anaphylaxis
	IT	0.025 mg, increase to 0.5 mg, twice a week	Headache, gastrointestinal tract symptoms, arachnoiditis/radiculitis
Amphotericin B lipid complex (Abelcet)[c,d]	IV	5 mg/kg, infused over 2 h	Fever, chills, other reactions associated with amphotericin B deoxycholate, but less nephrotoxicity; hepatotoxicity has been reported with lipid complex
Anidulafungin[c,d]	IV	Adults: 100–200 mg loading dose, then 50–100 mg once daily (higher dose for candidemia) Children: load with 1.5 to 3 mg/kg once, then 0.75–1.5 mg/kg per day	Fever, headache, nausea, vomiting, diarrhea, leukopenia, hepatic enzyme elevations, and phlebitis
Liposomal amphotericin B (AmBisome)[c,d]	IV	3–5 mg/kg, infused over 1–2 h	Fever, chills, other reactions associated with amphotericin B, but less nephrotoxicity; hepatotoxicity has been reported
Caspofungin[c,d]	IV	Adults: 70 mg loading dose, then 50 mg once daily Children: 70 mg/m² loading dose, then 50 mg/m² once daily	Fever, rash, pruritus, phlebitis, headache, gastrointestinal tract symptoms, anemia. Concomitant use with cyclosporine is not recommended unless potential benefits outweigh potential risks.

Table 4.5. Recommended Doses of Parenteral and Oral Antifungal Drugs, continued

Drug	Route	Dose (per day)	Adverse Reactions[a,b]
Clotrimazole	PO	10-mg tablet 5 times per day (dissolved slowly in mouth)	Gastrointestinal tract symptoms, hepatotoxicity
Fluconazole[b,d]	IV	Children: 3–6 mg/kg per day, single dose (up to 12 mg/kg per day for serious infections)	Rash, gastrointestinal tract symptoms, hepatotoxicity, Stevens-Johnson syndrome, anaphylaxis
	PO	Children: 6 mg/kg once, then 3 mg/kg per day for oropharyngeal or esophageal candidiasis; 6–12 mg/kg per day for invasive fungal infections; 6 mg/kg per day for suppressive therapy in HIV-infected children with cryptococcal meningitis	
		Adults: 200 mg once, followed by 100 mg/day for oropharyngeal or esophageal candidiasis; 400–800 mg/day for other invasive fungal infections; 200 mg/day for suppressive therapy in HIV-infected patients with cryptococcal meningitis	
Flucytosine	PO	50–150 mg/kg per day in 4 doses at 6-h intervals (adjust dose if renal dysfunction); follow trough levels closely	Bone marrow suppression, renal dysfunction, gastrointestinal tract symptoms, rash, neuropathy, hepatotoxicity, confusion, hallucinations
Griseofulvin	PO	Ultramicrosize: 5–15 mg/kg, single dose; maximum dose, 750 mg Microsize: 10–20 mg/kg per day divided in 2 doses; maximum dose, 1000 mg	Rash, paresthesias, leukopenia, gastrointestinal tract symptoms, proteinuria, hepatotoxicity, mental confusion, headache

Table 4.5. Recommended Doses of Parenteral and Oral Antifungal Drugs, continued

Drug	Route	Dose (per day)	Adverse Reactions[a,b]
Itraconazole[b,d]	IV, PO	Children: 5–10 mg/kg per day divided into 2 doses Adults: 200–400 mg/day once or twice a day; 200 mg once a day for suppressive therapy in HIV-infected patients with histoplasmosis	Gastrointestinal tract symptoms, rash, edema, headache, hypokalemia, hepatotoxicity; thrombocytopenia, leukopenia; cardiac toxicity is possible in patients also taking terfenadine or astemizole
Ketoconazole[b,d]	PO	Children[c]: 3.3–6.6 mg/kg per day, single dose Adults: 200 mg, twice a day for 4 doses, then 200 mg, once a day	Hepatotoxicity, gastrointestinal tract symptoms, rash, anaphylaxis, thrombocytopenia, hemolytic anemia, gynecomastia, adrenal insufficiency; cardiac toxicity is possible in patients also taking terfenadine or astemizole
Micafungin[c,d]	IV	Adults: 50–150 mg once daily Children: 4–12 mg/kg per day once daily (higher dose needed for patients <8 y of age)	Fever, headache, nausea, vomiting, diarrhea, leukopenia, hepatic enzyme elevations, and phlebitis
Nystatin	PO	Infants: 200 000 U, 4 times a day; after meals Children and adults: 400 000–600 000 U, 3 times a day; after meals	Gastrointestinal tract symptoms, rash
Posaconazole[c,d]	PO	Adults: 400 mg 2 times a day with meals (or liquid nutritional supplement) for treatment, 200 mg 3 times a day (prophylaxis) Children: Not known	Gastrointestinal tract symptoms, rash, edema, headache, anemia, neutropenia, thrombocytopenia, fatigue, arthralgia, myalgia, fever
Terbinafine[c]	PO	Adults: 250 mg, once a day Children: <20 kg: 67.5 mg/day; 20–40 kg: 125 mg/day; >40 kg: 250 mg/day	Gastrointestinal tract symptoms, rash, taste abnormalities, cholestatic hepatitis

Table 4.5. Recommended Doses of Parenteral and Oral Antifungal Drugs, continued

Drug	Route	Dose (per day)	Adverse Reactions[a,b]
Voriconazole[d]	IV	Children: 7 mg/kg every 12 h for one day, then 7 mg/kg every 12 h Adults: 6 mg/kg every 12 h for one day (loading dose), then 4 mg/kg every 12 h	Visual disturbance, photosensitive rash, increased liver function tests
	PO	Children: 10 mg/kg every 12 h for one day, then 7 mg/kg every 12 h Adults: <40 kg: 200 mg every 12 h for one day, then 100 mg every 12 h; >40 kg: 400 mg every 12 h for one day, then 200 mg every 12 h	

IV indicates intravenous; IT, intrathecal; PO, oral; HIV, human immunodeficiency virus.

[a]See package insert or listing in current edition of the *Physicians' Desk Reference* or **www.pdr.net** (for registered users only).

[b]Interactions with other drugs are common. Consult **www.fda.gov/cder/drug/drugInteractions/default**.htm and the *Physicians' Desk Reference* (a drug interaction reference or database) or a pharmacist before prescribing these medications.

[c]Experience with drug in children is limited.

[d]Limited or no information about use in newborn infants is available.

[e]For children 2 years of age and younger, the daily dose has not been established.

DRUGS FOR INVASIVE AND OTHER SERIOUS FUNGAL INFECTIONS IN CHILDREN

Table 4.6. Drugs for Invasive and Other Serious Fungal Infections

| Disease | Intravenous | | Oral | Intravenous or Oral | | |
	Amphotericin B	Caspofungin,[a] Micafungin,[a,b] or Anidulafungin[a,b]	Flucytosine	Itraconazole[a]	Fluconazole[a]	Voriconazole[a]
Aspergillosis	A	A	…	M	…	P
Blastomycosis	P	…	…	M	M	…
Candidiasis:						
Chronic, mucocutaneous	A	A	…	A	P	A
Oropharyngeal, esophageal	P	P	…	A	P	A
	(severe cases)					
Systemic	P[d]	P	S	…	P, M	A
Coccidioidomycosis	P	…	…	P, M	P, M	…
Cryptococcosis	P, S	…	S	…	A, M	…
Fusariosis	P	…	…	…	…	P
Histoplasmosis	P	…	…	P, A	A, M	…
Mucormycosis (zygomycosis)	P	…	…	…	…	…
Paracoccidioidomycosis	P[c]	…	…	P, M	…	…
Pseudallescheriasis	…	…	…	M	…	P
Sporotrichosis	P	…	…	M	…	…

P indicates preferred treatment in most cases; A, efficacy less well established or alternative drug; M, for mild and moderately severe cases; S, combination recommended if infection is severe or central nervous system is involved.

[a] Approved by the Food and Drug Administration for adults.

[b] Efficacy has not been established for children.

[c] Usually in combination with itraconazole or a sulfonamide.

[d] Preferred treatment in neonates; alternate treatment for children and adults.

TOPICAL DRUGS FOR SUPERFICIAL FUNGAL INFECTIONS

Table 4.7. Topical Drugs for Superficial Fungal Infections

Drug	Strength	Formulation	Trade Name Examples	Application(s) per Day	Adverse Reactions/Notes
Amorolfine (OTC)	5%	NL	Loceryl	1–2 weekly (mild onychomycosis)	Well-tolerated; minor local
Basic fuchsin, phenol, resorcinol, and acetone (Rx)		S	Castellani Paint Modified	1	Excellent for intertriginous areas. Stains everything. Also available as a colorless solution with alcohol and without basic fuchsin. This is an alternative if the patient cannot tolerate other topical antifungals.
Butenafine (Rx)	1%	C	Mentax	1	Safety and efficacy in patients younger than 12 y of age have not been established. Do not occlude. Sensitivity to allylamines.
Ciclopirox olamine (Rx)	1%; 8%	C, L, S, P, Gel	Loprox; Penlac nail lacquer	2	Irritant dermatitis, hair discoloration; shake lotion vigorously before application; safety and efficacy in children younger than 10 y of age have not been established. Precautions: diabetes mellitus; immune compromise; seizures.
Clotrimazole (Rx and OTC)	1%	C, L, S, P, Com, SpP, SpL; check with pharmacist[a]	Topical solution (more than 10 preparations); Lotrimin, Mycelex, Desenex	1 (Rx) 2 (OTC)	Irritant dermatitis. Avoid topical steroid combinations.[b]

Table 4.7. Topical Drugs for Superficial Fungal Infections, continued

Drug	Strength	Formulation	Trade Name Examples[c]	Application(s) per Day	Adverse Reactions/Notes
Clotrimazole and betamethasone dipropionate (Rx)		C, L	Lotrisone[c]	2[b]	Irritant dermatitis: safety and efficacy in children have been established. Beware of topical steroid combinations,[b] especially when applied to the diaper area, because high systemic steroid exposure can occur. Contraindications: varicella or vaccinia.
Econazole (Rx)	1%	C, L, P, S (foaming)	Spectazole, Pevaryl-Ecreme	1 (dermatophyte) 2 (candidiasis)	Irritant dermatitis; safety and efficacy in children have not been established.
Ketoconazole (Rx and OTC)	1, 2%	C, Sh	Nizoral, Nizoral AD, Sebizol, Xolegel	1 (tinea dermatophyte) 2 (candidiasis)	Potential sulfite reaction with anaphylactic or asthmatic reaction; shampoo can cause dry or oily hair and increase hair loss; irritant dermatitis. May interfere with permanent waving or changes in hair texture.
Miconazole (Rx and OTC)	2%	O, C, P, S, SpP, SpL; check with pharmacist[a]	More than 10 preparations; Monistat-Derm, Zeasorb AF, Micatin, Daktarin tincture, Vusion	2 (seborrhea), apply 2–3 times/day for several months 2 (C, L) 2 (P, L)	Irritant and allergic contact dermatitis.
Naftifine HC (Rx)	1%	C, Gel	Naftin	1 (C) 2 (Gel)	Burning/stinging, irritant dermatitis, safety and efficacy in children have not been established.
Nystatin (Rx and OTC)	100 000 U/mL or 100 000 U/g	C, P, O, Com	Nystatin, Nystop powder, Pedi-Dri powder, Mycostatin	2 (C) 2–3 (P)	Nontoxic except with topical steroid combinations.[d]

Table 4.7. Topical Drugs for Superficial Fungal Infections, continued

Drug	Strength	Formulation	Trade Name Examples	Application(s) per Day	Adverse Reactions/Notes
Nystatin and triamcinolone acetonide (Rx)		C, O	Mytrex cream, Mytrex ointment, Mycolog-II	2^3	Contraindications: varicella or vaccinia. Do not occlude. Use lowest effective dose.
Oxiconazole (Rx)	1%	C, L	Oxistat	1–2 (tinea dermatophyte)	Pruritus, burning, irritant dermatitis.
Sulconazole (Rx)	1%	C, S	Exelderm	1–2 (tinea vesicular)	Irritant dermatitis; safety and efficacy in children have not been established.
Terbinafine (Rx and OTC)	1%	C, Gel, Sp	Lamisil, Lamisil AT	1–2	Irritant dermatitis; avoid use of occlusive clothing or dressings. Do not apply spray to faces. Safety and efficacy in children have not been established.
Tolnaftate (OTC)	1%	C, P, S, Gel, SpP, SpL Check with pharmacist[a]	>10 preparations; Tinactin, Zeasorb AF, Fungicure	2	Irritant and allergic contact dermatitis. Not recommended if younger than 2 y of age.
Triacetin (Rx)	% varies	S, C, Sp	Fungoid tincture, Fungoid cream only-clean nail	3 (C, S)	Irritant dermatitis; active ingredient is miconazole 2%.
Undecylenic acid and derivatives (OTC)	8%–25%	C, O, S, F, SpP, P, soap	See pharmacist for formulations and applications[a]	2 (tincture); spray 1–2 sec	Irritant dermatitis.
Undecylenic acid and chloroxylenol	25% 3%	S	Gordochom solution	2 for 4 wk	Local hypersensitivity.

Table 4.7. Topical Drugs for Superficial Fungal Infections, continued

Drug	Strength	Formulation	Trade Name Examples	Application(s) per Day	Adverse Reactions/Notes
Other Remedies					
Gentian violet (OTC)	2%	S	…	2	Staining.
Selenium sulfide (OTC)	2.5%	Sh	Selsun 2.5%	Use twice weekly for 2 wk	Irritant dermatitis and ulceration. For tinea capitis, to decrease spore formation and to decrease the potential spread of the dermatophyte.
	1%	Sh	Head & Shoulders, Selsun Blue	Use twice weekly for 2 wk	For tinea capitis, to decrease spore formation and to decrease the potential spread of the dermatophyte.
Sertaconazole nitrate	2%	C	Ertaczo	2	Contact dermatitis, local hypersensitivity; safety and efficacy in children have not been established.

OTC indicates over the counter; NL, nail lacquer; Rx, prescription; S, solution; C, cream; L, lotion; P, powder; Com, combinations; SpP, spray powder; SpL, spray lotion; Sh, shampoo; O, ointment; F, foam.

[a]Pharmacists are the best resource to check formulations that are available and new (they use *Facts and Comparisons* reference products).

[b]Topical steroids must be used with caution in young children and in areas of thin skin (eg, diaper area). In these circumstances, high systemic exposure may occur, resulting in endogenous synthesis suppression with the potential for serious adverse effects. Potential adverse effects include irritant dermatitis, folliculitis, hypertrichosis, acneiform eruptions, hypopigmentation, perioral dermatitis, allergic contact dermatitis, maceration, secondary infection, skin atrophy, striae, and miliaria.

[c]Lotrisone cream no longer is available; lotion is available. Also available are Lotrim and Fungizid spray.

[d]Any topical preparation has the potential to irritate the skin and cause itching, burning, stinging, erythema, edema, vesicles, and blister formation.

For more information on individual drugs, see *Physician's Desk Reference* or **www.pdr.net** (for registered users only).

ANTIVIRAL DRUGS[1]

Table 4.8. Antiviral Drugs

Generic (Trade Name)	Indication	Route	Age	Usually Recommended Dosage
Acyclovir[a,b,c] (Zovirax)	Neonatal herpes simplex virus (HSV) infection	IV	Birth to 3 mo	60 mg/kg per day in 3 divided doses for 14–21 days.
	HSV encephalitis	IV	≥3 mo to 12 y	60 mg/kg per day in 3 divided doses for 14–21 days; some experts recommend a dosing of 45 mg/kg per day in 3 divided doses for 14–21 days.[d]
		IV	≥12 y	30 mg/kg per day in 3 divided doses for 14–21 days.
	Varicella in immunocompetent host[e]	Oral	≥2 y	80 mg/kg per day in 4 divided doses for 5 days; maximum dose, 3200 mg/day.
	Varicella in immunocompetent host	IV	≥2 y	30 mg/kg per day for 7–10 days or 1500 mg/m² per day in 3 doses for 7–10 days
	Varicella in immunocompromised host	IV	<1 y	30 mg/kg per day in 3 divided doses for 7–10 days.
	Varicella in immunocompromised host	IV	≥1 y	1500 mg/m² per day in 3 doses for 7–10 days; some experts recommend the 30 mg/kg per day dose.
	Zoster in immunocompetent host	IV	All ages	Same as for varicella in immunocompromised host.
		Oral	≥12 y	4000 mg/day in 5 divided doses for 5–7 days.
	Zoster in immunocompromised host	IV	<12 y	30 mg/kg per day in 3 divided doses, for 7–10 days.
		IV	≥12 y	30 mg/kg per day in 3 divided doses, for 7–10 days.
	HSV infection in immunocompromised host (localized, progressive, or disseminated)	IV	<12 y	30 mg/kg per day in 3 divided doses for 7–14 days.
		IV	≥12 y	15 mg/kg per day in 3 divided doses for 7–14 days.
		Oral	≥2 y	1000 mg/day in 3–5 divided doses for 7–14 days.
	Prophylaxis of HSV in immunocompromised host	Oral	≥2 y	600–1000 mg/day in 3–5 divided doses during period of risk.

[1] Drugs for human immunodeficiency virus infection are not included.

Table 4.8. Antiviral Drugs, continued

Generic (Trade Name)	Indication	Route	Age	Usually Recommended Dosage
Acyclovir[a,b,c] (Zovirax), continued	HSV-seropositive patients	IV	All ages	15 mg/kg in 3 divided doses during period of risk.
	Genital HSV infection: first episode	Oral	≥12 y	1000–1200 mg/day in 3–5 divided doses for 7–10 days. Oral pediatric dose: 40–80 mg/kg per day divided in 3–4 doses for 5–10 days (maximum 1.0 g/day).
		IV	≥12 y	15 mg/kg per day in 3 divided doses for 5–7 days.
	Genital HSV infection: recurrence	Oral	≥12 y	1000 mg in 5 divided doses for 5 days, or 1600 mg in 2 divided doses for 5 days, or 2400 mg in 3 divided doses for 2 days.
	Chronic suppressive therapy for recurrent genital and cutaneous (ocular) HSV episodes	Oral	≥12 y	800 mg/day in 2 divided doses for as long as 12 continuous mo.
Adefovir (Hepsera)	Chronic hepatitis B	Oral	≥18 y	10 mg once daily for 1–3 y; optimal duration of therapy unknown.
Amantadine (Symmetrel)[f]	Influenza A: treatment and prophylaxis (see Influenza, p 400)[f]	Oral	1–9 y	Treatment or prophylaxis: 5 mg/kg per day, maximum 150 mg/day, in 2 divided doses.
		Oral	≥10 y	Treatment or prophylaxis: <40 kg: 5 mg/kg per day, in 2 divided doses; ≥40 kg: 200 mg/day in 2 divided doses.
		Oral	Dose by weight, not age	Alternative prophylactic dose for children >20 kg and adults: 100 mg/day.
Cidofovir (Vistide)	Cytomegalovirus (CMV) retinitis	IV	Adult dose[g]	Induction: 5 mg/kg once weekly × 2 doses with probenecid and hydration. Maintenance: 5 mg/kg once every 2 weeks with probenecid and hydration.

Table 4.8. Antiviral Drugs, continued

Generic (Trade Name)	Indication	Route	Age	Usually Recommended Dosage
Entecavir (Baraclude)	Chronic hepatitis B	Oral	≥16 y[g]	0.5 mg once daily; optimum duration of therapy unknown.
Famciclovir (Famvir)	Genital HSV infection, first episode	Oral	Adult dose[g]	750 mg/day in 3 divided doses for 7–10 days.
	Episodic recurrent genital HSV infection	Oral	Adult dose[g]	Immunocompetent: 250 mg/day in 2 divided doses for 5 days, or 2000 mg in 2 divided doses for 1 day. Immunocompromised: 1500 mg/day in 3 divided doses for 7 days.
	Daily suppressive therapy	Oral	Adult dose[g]	500 mg/day in 2 divided doses for 1 y; then reassess for recurrence of HSV infection.
	Recurrent herpes labialis	Oral	Adult dose[g]	Immunocompetent: 1500 mg as a single dose. Immunocompromised: 1500 mg/day in 3 divided doses for 7 days.
	Herpes zoster	Oral	Adult dose[g]	1500 mg/day in 3 divided doses for 7 days.
Foscarnet[a] (Foscavir)	CMV retinitis in patients with acquired immunodeficiency syndrome	IV	Adult dose[g]	180 mg/kg per day in 2–3 divided doses for 14–21 days, then 90–120 mg/kg once a day as maintenance dose.
	HSV infection resistant to acyclovir in immunocompromised host	IV	Adult dose[g]	80–120 mg/kg per day in 2–3 divided doses until infection resolves.

Table 4.8. Antiviral Drugs, continued

Generic (Trade Name)	Indication	Route	Age	Usually Recommended Dosage
Ganciclovir[a] (Cytovene)	Acquired CMV retinitis in immunocompromised host[h]	IV	Adult dose[g]	Treatment: 10 mg/kg per day in 2 divided doses for 14–21 days; Long-term suppression; 5 mg/kg per day for 7 days/wk or 6 mg/kg per day for 5 days/wk.
	Prophylaxis of CMV in high-risk host	IV	Adult dose[g]	10 mg/kg per day in 2 divided doses for 1–2 wk, then 5 mg/kg per day in 1 dose for 100 days or 6 mg/kg per day for 5 days/wk.
Interferon alfa	Chronic hepatitis B	SC	1–18 y	6 million IU/m^2 3 times/wk; optimum duration of therapy unknown.
			>18 y	5 million IU/day; or 10 million IU 3 times/wk.
	Chronic hepatitis C	SC; IM	>18 y[g]	3 million IU, 3 times/wk, for 24–48 wk.
Lamivudine (Epivir-HBV)	Treatment of chronic hepatitis B	Oral	≥2 y	3 mg/kg once a day (maximum 100 mg/day) (children coinfected with HIV and hepatitis B should use the approved dose for HIV).
Oseltamivir[i] (Tamiflu)	Influenza A and B: treatment (see Influenza, p 400)	Oral[i]	1–12 y	≤15 kg: 30 mg, twice daily; 16–23 kg: 45 mg, twice daily; 24–40 kg: 60 mg, twice daily; >40 kg: 75 mg, twice daily.
		Oral	≥13 y	75 mg, twice daily for treatment.
	Influenza A and B: prophylaxis	Oral	1–12 y	Same as treatment for patients 1–12 y of age, except dose given once daily.
		Oral	≥13 y	75 mg once daily.
Pegylated interferon	Chronic hepatitis B or C	SC	>18 y[g]	180 µg or 1.5 µg/kg once weekly, for 24–48 wk.

Table 4.8. Antiviral Drugs, continued

Generic (Trade Name)	Indication	Route	Age	Usually Recommended Dosage
Ribavirin (Rebetol)	Treatment of hepatitis C in combination with interferon	Oral/capsule	Dose by weight	Fixed dose by weight is suggested: 25–36 kg: 200 mg AM and PM; >36–49 kg: 200 mg AM and 400 mg PM; >49–61 kg: 400 mg AM and PM; >61–75 kg: 400 mg AM and 600 mg PM; >75 kg: 600 mg AM and PM.
		Oral/solution	≥3 y (<25 kg)	15 mg/kg per day in 2 divided doses.
Rimantadine (Flumadine)[f]	Influenza A: treatment[h]	Oral	≥13 y	200 mg/day in 2 divided doses.
	Influenza A: prophylaxis (see Influenza, p 400)[f]	Oral	≥1 y	1–9 y of age: 5 mg/kg per day, maximum 150 mg/day, once daily; ≥10 y of age, <40 kg: 5 mg/kg per day, in 2 divided doses; ≥40 kg: 200 mg/day in 2 divided doses.
Telbivudine (Tyzeka)	Chronic hepatitis B	Oral	Adult dose[g]	600 mg once daily.
Valacyclovir (Valtrex)	Genital HSV infection, first episode	Oral	Adult dose[g]	2 g/day in 2 divided doses for 7–10 days.
	Episodic recurrent genital HSV infection	Oral	Adult dose[g]	1 g/day in 2 divided doses for 3 days or 1000 mg once a day for 5 days.
	Daily suppressive therapy for HSV infection	Oral	Adult dose[g]	500–1000 mg, once daily for 1 year, then reassess for recurrences.
	Recurrent herpes labialis	Oral	Adult dose[g]	4 g/day in 2 divided doses for 1 day.
	Herpes zoster	Oral	Adult dose[g]	3 g/day in 3 divided doses for 7 days.
Valganciclovir	Acquired CMV retinitis in immunocompromised host	Oral	Adult dose[g]	Treatment: 900 mg twice daily for 3 weeks Long-term suppression: 900 mg once daily.

Table 4.8. Antiviral Drugs, continued

Generic (Trade Name)	Indication	Route	Age	Usually Recommended Dosage
Zanamivir (Relenza)	Influenza A and B: treatment (see Influenza, p 400)	Inhalation	≥7 y (treatment)	10 mg, twice daily for 5 days.
	Influenza A and B: prophylaxis	Inhalation	≥5 y (prophylaxis)	10 mg, once daily for 28 days (community outbreaks) or 10 days (household setting).

IV indicates intravenous; IO, intraocular; IM, Intramuscular; SC, subcutaneous; IU, international units.

[a]Dose should be decreased in patients with impaired renal function.

[b]Oral dosage of acyclovir in children should not exceed 80 mg/kg per day.

[c]Acyclovir doses listed in this table are based on clinical trials and clinical experience and may not be identical to doses approved by the US Food and Drug Administration.

[d]Monitor for nephrotoxicity and neurologic irritation.

[e]Selective indications; see Varicella-Zoster Infections (p 714).

[f]Since 2005-2006, most influenza A (H3N2) strains tested have been resistant to adamantanes. See Influenza (p 400) for specific recommendations.

[g]There are not sufficient clinical data to identify the appropriate dose for use in children.

[h]Some experts use ganciclovir in immunocompromised hosts with CMV gastrointestinal tract disease and CMV pneumonitis (with or without CMV Immune Globulin Intravenous).

[i]In 2008-2009, most influenza A (H1N1) strains tested were resistant to oseltamivir. See Influenza (p 400) for specific recommendations.

For more information on individual drugs, see *Physician's Desk Reference* or **www.pdr.net** (for registered users only).

DRUGS FOR PARASITIC INFECTIONS

The following tables (4.9, 4.10, and 4.11) are reproduced from *The Medical Letter*.[1] These tables provide recommendations that are likely to be consistent in many cases with those of the American Academy of Pediatrics (AAP) Committee on Infectious Diseases, as given in the disease-specific chapters in Section 3. However, because *The Medical Letter* recommendations are developed independently, these recommendations occasionally may differ from recommendations of the AAP. Accordingly, both should be consulted. The AAP appreciates the consideration of *The Medical Letter* in allowing this information to be reprinted.

In Table 4.9 (p 784), first-choice and alternative drugs with recommended adult and pediatric dosages for most parasitic infections are given. In each case, the need for treatment must be weighed against the toxic effects of the drug. A decision to withhold therapy often may be correct, particularly when the drugs can cause severe adverse effects. When the first-choice drug initially is ineffective and the alternative is more hazardous, a second course of treatment with the first drug before giving the alternative may be prudent.

Several drugs recommended in Table 4.9 (p 784) have not been approved by the US Food and Drug Administration and, thus, are investigational (see footnotes). When prescribing an unlicensed drug, the physician should inform the patient of the investigational status and adverse effects of the drug.

These recommendations periodically (usually every other year) are updated by *The Medical Letter* (**www.medicalletter.com**) and, thus, likely are to be superseded by new ones before the next edition of the *Red Book* is published.

---

[1]Reprinted with permission from Drugs for parasitic infections. *Treatment Guidelines from the Medical Letter.* 2007;5(Suppl):e1–e15

Table 4.9. Drugs for Parasitic Infections

With increasing travel, immigration, use of immunosuppressive drugs and the spread of AIDS, physicians anywhere may see infections caused by parasites. The table below lists first-choice and alternative drugs for most parasitic infections. The table on page 811 summarizes the known prenatal risks of antiparasitic drugs. The brand names and manufacturers of the drugs are listed on page 814.

Infection	Drug	Adult dosage	Pediatric dosage
***ACANTHAMOEBA* keratitis**			
Drug of choice:	See footnote 1		
AMEBIASIS (*Entamoeba histolytica*)			
asymptomatic			
Drug of choice:	Iodoquinol[2]	650 mg PO tid × 20d	30-40 mg/kg/d (max. 2g) PO in 3 doses × 20d
OR	Paromomycin[3]	25–35 mg/kg/d PO in 3 doses × 7d	25–35 mg/kg/d PO in 3 doses × 7d
OR	Diloxanide furoate[4*]	500 mg PO tid × 10d	20 mg/kg/d PO in 3 doses × 10d
mild to moderate intestinal disease			
Drug of choice:[5]	Metronidazole	500–750 mg PO tid × 7–10d	35–50 mg/kg/d PO in 3 doses × 7–10d
OR	Tinidazole[6]	2 g once PO daily × 3d	>3yrs: 50 mg/kg/d (max. 2g) PO in 1 dose × 3d
	either followed by		
OR	Iodoquinol[2]	650 mg PO tid × 20d	30-40 mg/kg/d (max. 2g) PO in 3 doses × 20d
	Paromomycin[3]	25–35 mg/kg/d PO in 3 doses × 7d	25–35 mg/kg/d PO in 3 doses × 7d

* Availability problems. See table on page 814.

1. Topical 0.02% chlorhexidine and polyhexamethylene biguanide (PHMB, 0.02%), either alone or in combination, have been used successfully in a large number of patients. Treatment with either chlorhexidine or PHMB is often combined with propamidine isethionate (*Brolene*) or hexamidine (*Desmodine*). None of these drugs is commercially available or approved for use in the US, but they can be obtained from compounding pharmacies (see footnote 2). Leiter's Park Avenue Pharmacy, San Jose, CA (800-292-6773; **www.leiterrx.com**) is a compounding pharmacy that specializes in ophthalmic drugs. Propamidine is available over the counter in the UK and Australia. Hexamidine is available in France. The combination of chlorhexidine, natamycin (pimaricin) and debridement also has been successful (K Kitagawa et al,Jpn J Ophthalmol 2003; 47:616). Debridement is most useful during the stage of corneal epithelial infection. Most cysts are resistant to neomycin; its use is no longer recommended. Azole antifungal drugs (ketoconazole, itraconazole) have been used as oral or topical adjuncts (FL Shuster and GS Visvesvara, Drug Resist Update 2004; 7:41). Use of corticosteroids is controversial (K Hammersmith, Curr Opinions Ophthal 2006; 17:327; ST Awwad et al, Eye Contact Lens 2007; 33:1).

2. Iodoquinol should be taken after meals.

3. Paromomycin should be taken with a meal.

4. Not available commercially. It may be obtained through compounding pharmacies such as Panorama Compounding Pharmacy, 6744 Balboa Blvd, Van Nuys, CA 91406 (800-247-9767) or Medical Center Pharmacy, New Haven, CT (203-688-6816). Other compounding pharmacies may be found through the National Association of Compounding Pharmacies (800-687-7850) or the Professional Compounding Centers of America (800-331-2498, **www.pccarx.com**).

5. Nitazoxanide may be effective against a variety of protozoan and helminth infections (DA Bobak, Curr Infect Dis Rep 2006; 8:91; E Diaz et al, Am J Trop Med Hyg 2003; 68:384). It was effective against mild to moderate amebiasis, 500 mg bid × 3d, in a recent study (JF Rossignol et al, Trans R Soc Trop Med Hyg 2007 Oct; 101:1025 E pub 2007 July 20). It is FDA-approved only for treatment of diarrhea caused by *Giardia* or *Cryptosporidium* (Med Lett Drugs Ther 2003; 45:29). Nitazoxanide is available in 500-mg tablets and an oral suspension; it should be taken with food.

6. A nitroimidazole similar to metronidazole, tinidazole appears to be as effective as metronidazole and better tolerated (Med Lett Drugs Ther 2004; 46:70). It should be taken with food to minimize GI adverse effects. For children and patients unable to take tablets, a pharmacist can crush the tablets and mix them with cherry syrup (*Humco*, and others). The syrup suspension is good for 7 days at room temperature and must be shaken before use (HB Fung and TL Doan et al, Clin Ther 2005; 27:1859). Ornidazole, a similar drug, is also available outside the US.

Table 4.9. Drugs for Parasitic Infections, continued

Infection	Drug	Adult dosage	Pediatric dosage
AMEBIASIS (*Entamoeba histolytica*), continued			
severe intestinal and extraintestinal disease			
Drug of choice:	Metronidazole	750 mg PO tid × 7-10d	35-50 mg/kg/d PO in 3 doses × 7-10d
OR	Tinidazole[6]	2 g once PO daily × 5d	>3yrs: 50 mg/kg/d (max. 2g) PO in 1 dose × 3d
either followed by			
	Iodoquinol[2]	650 mg PO tid × 20d	30-40 mg/kg/d (max. 2g) PO in 3 doses × 20d
OR	Paromomycin[3]	25-35 mg/kg/d PO in 3 doses × 7d	25-35 mg/kg/d PO in 3 doses × 7d
AMEBIC MENINGOENCEPHALITIS, primary and granulomatous			
Naegleria			
Drug of choice:	Amphotericin B[7,8]	1.5 mg/kg/d IV in 2 doses × 3d, then 1 mg/kg/d × 6d plus 1.5 mg/d intrathecally × 2d, then 1 mg/d every other day × 8d	1.5 mg/kg/d IV in 2 doses × 3d, then 1 mg/kg/d × 6d plus 1.5 mg/d intrathecally × 2d, then 1 mg/d every other day × 8d
Acanthamoeba			
Drug of choice:	See footnote 9		

*Availability problems. See table on page 814.

7. Not FDA-approved for this indication.

8. Although A.*Naegleria fowleri* infection was treated successfully in a 9-year old girl with combination of amphotericin B and miconazole both intravenous and intrathecal, plus oral rifampin (JS Seidel et al NEJM 1982;306:346). Amphotericin B and miconazole appear to have a synergistic effect, but Medical Letter consultants believe the rifampin probably had no additional effect (GS Visvesvara et al, FEMS Immunol Med Microbiol 2007; 50:1). Parenteral miconazole is no longer available in the US. Azithromycin is more active than clarithromycin against *Naegleria*, so may be a better choice combined with amphotericin B for treatment of *Naegleria* (TR Deetz et al, Clin Infect Dis 2003; 37:1304; FL Schuster and GS Visvesvara, Drug Resistance Updates 2004; 7:41). Combinations of amphotericin B, ornidazole and rifampin (R Jain et al, Neurol Indian 2002; 50:470) and amphotericin B fluconazole and rifampin have also been used (J Vargas-Zepeda et al, Arch Med Research 2005;36:83). Case reports of other successful therapy have been published (FL Schuster and GS Visvesvara, Int J Parasitol 2004; 34:1001).

9. Several patients with granulomatous amebic encephalitis (GAE) have been successfully treated with combinations of pentamidine, sulfadiazine, flucytosine, and either fluconazole or itraconazole (GS Visvesvara et al, FEMS Immunol Med Microbiol 2007; 50:1, epub Apr 11). GAE in an AIDS patient was treated successfully with sulfadiazine, primethamine and fluconazole combined with surgical resection of the CNS lesion (M Seijo Martinez, et al, J Clin Microbiol 2000; 38:3892). Chronic *Acanthamoeba* meningitis was successfully treated in 2 children with a combination of oral trimethoprim/sulfamethoxazole, rifampin and ketoconazole (T Singhal et al, Pediatr Infect Dis J 2001; 20:623). Disseminated cutaneous infection in an immunocompromised patient was treated successfully with IV pentamidine, topical chlorhexidine and 2% ketoconazole cream, followed by oral itraconazole (CA Slater et al, N Engl J Med 1994; 331:85) and with voriconazole and amphotericin B lipid complex (R Walia et al, Transplant Infect Dis 2007; 9:51). Other reports of successful therapy have been described (FL Schuster and GS Visvesvara, Drug Resistance Updates 2004; 7:41). Susceptibility testing of *Acanthamoeba* isolates has shown differences in drug sensitivity between species and even among strains of a single species; antimicrobial susceptibility testing is advisable (FL Schuster and GS Visvesvara, Int J Parasitol 2004; 34:1001).

Table 4.9. Drugs for Parasitic Infections, continued

Infection	Drug	Adult dosage	Pediatric dosage
AMEBIC MENINGOENCEPHALITIS, primary and granulomatous, continued			
Balamuthia mandrillaris			
Drug of choice:	See footnote 10		
Sappinia diploidea			
Drug of choice:	See footnote 11		
ANCYLOSTOMA caninum (Eosinophilic enterocolitis)			
Drug of choice:	Albendazole[7,12]	400 mg PO once	400 mg PO once
OR	Mebendazole	100 mg PO bid × 3d	100 mg PO bid × 3d
OR	Pyrantel pamoate[7,13]*	11 mg/kg (max. 1g) PO × 3d	11 mg/kg (max. 1g) PO × 3d
OR	Endoscopic removal		
Ancylostoma duodenale, see HOOKWORM			
ANGIOSTRONGYLIASIS (*Angiostrongylus cantonensis, Angiostrongylus costaricensis*)			
Drug of choice:	See footnote 14		
ANISAKIASIS (*Anisakis* spp.)			
Treatment of choice:[15]	Surgical or endoscopic removal		

*Availability problems. See table on page 814.

10. *B. mandrillaris* is a free-living ameba that causes subacute to fatal granulomatous amebic encephalitis (GAE) and cutaneous disease. Two cases of *Balamuthia* encephalitis have been successfully treated with flucytosine, pentamidine, fluconazole and sulfadiazine plus either azithromycin or clarithromycin (phenothiazines were also used) combined with surgical resection of the CNS lesion (TR Deetz et al, Clin Infect Dis 2003; 37:1304). Another case was successfully treated following open biopsy with pentamidine, fluconazole, sulfadiazine and clarithromycin (S Jung et al, Arch Pathol Lab Med 2004; 128:466).

11. A free-living ameba once thought not to be pathogenic to humans. *S. diploidea* has been successfully treated with azithromycin, pentamidine, itraconazole and flucytosine combined with surgical resection of the CNS lesion (BB Gelman et al, J Neuropathol Exp Neurol 2003; 62:990). 12. Albendazole must be taken with food; a fatty meal increases oral bioavailability.

13. Pyrantel pamoate suspension can be mixed with milk or fruit juice.

14. *A. cantonensis* causes predominantly neurotropic disease. *A. costaricensis* causes gastrointestinal disease. Most patients infected with either species have a self-limited course and recover completely. Analgesics, corticosteroids and careful removal of CSF at frequent intervals can relieve symptoms from increased intracranial pressure (V Lo Re III and SJ Gluckman, Am J Med 2003; 114:217). Treatment of *A. cantonensis* is controversial and varies across endemic areas. No antihelminthic drug is proven to be effective and some patients have worsened with therapy (TJ Slom et al, N Engl J Med 2002; 346:668). Mebendazole and a corticosteroid, however, appear to shorten the course of infection (H-C Tsai et al, Am J Med 2001; 111:109; V Chotmongkol et al, Am J Trop Med Hyg 2006; 74:1122). Albendazole has also relieved symptoms of angiostrongyliasis (XG Chen et al, Emerg Infect Dis 2005; 11:1645).

Table 4.9. Drugs for Parasitic Infections, continued

Infection	Drug	Adult dosage	Pediatric dosage
ASCARIASIS (*Ascaris lumbricoides*, roundworm)			
Drug of choice:[5]	Albendazole[7,12]	400 mg PO once	400 mg PO once
OR	Mebendazole	100 mg bid PO × 3d or 500 mg once	100 mg PO bid × 3d or 500 mg once
OR	Ivermectin[7,16]	150–200 mcg/kg PO once	150–200 mcg/kg PO once
BABESIOSIS (*Babesia microti*)			
Drug of choice:[17]	Clindamycin[7,18]	1.2 g bid IV or 600 mg tid PO × 7–10d	20–40 mg/kg/d PO in 3 doses × 7–10d
	plus quinine[7,19]	650 mg PO tid × 7–10d	30 mg/kg/d PO in 3 doses × 7–10d
OR	Atovaquone[7,20]	750 mg PO bid × 7–10d	40 mg/kg/d PO in 2 doses × 7–10d
	plus azithromycin[7]	600 mg PO daily × 7–10d	12 mg/kg/d PO × 7–10d
Balamuthia mandrillaris, see AMEBIC MENINGOENCEPHALITIS, PRIMARY			
BALANTIDIASIS (*Balantidium coli*)			
Drug of choice:	Tetracycline[7,21]	500 mg PO qid × 10d	40 mg/kg/d (max. 2 g) PO in 4 doses × 10d
Alternative:	Metronidazole[7]	750 mg PO tid × 5d	35–50 mg/kg/d PO in 3 doses × 5d
OR	Iodoquinol[2,7]	650 mg PO tid × 20d	30–40 mg/kg/d (max 2 g) PO in 3 doses × 20d

*Availability problems. See table on page 814.

15. A Repiso Ortega et al, Gastroenterol Hepatol 2003; 26:341. Successful treatment of *Anisakiasis* with albendazole 400 mg PO bid × 3–5d has been reported, but the diagnosis was presumptive (DA Moore et al, Lancet 2002; 360:54; E Pacios et al, Clin Infect Dis 2005; 41:1825).

16. Safety of ivermectin in young children (<15 kg) and pregnant women remains to be established. Ivermectin should be taken on an empty stomach with water.

17. Exchange transfusion has been used in severely ill patients and those with high (>10%) parasitemia (VI Powell and K Grima, Transfus Med Rev 2002; 16:239). In patients who were not severely ill, combination therapy with atovaquone and azithromycin was as effective as clindamycin and quinine and may have been better tolerated (PJ Krause et al, N Engl J Med 2000; 343:1454). Longer treatment courses may be needed in immunosuppressed patients and those with asplenia. Patients are commonly co-infected with Lyme disease (Med Lett Drugs Ther 2007; 49:49; AC Steere et al, Clin Infect Dis 2003; 36:1078).

18. Oral clindamycin should be taken with a full glass of water to minimize esophageal ulceration.

19. Quinine should be taken with or after a meal to decrease gastrointestinal adverse effects.

20. Atovaquone is available in an oral suspension that should be taken with a meal to increase absorption.

21. Use of tetracyclines is contraindicated in pregnancy and in children <8 years old. Tetracycline should be taken 1 hour before or 2 hours after meals and/or dairy products.

Table 4.9. Drugs for Parasitic Infections, continued

Infection	Drug	Adult dosage	Pediatric dosage
BAYLISASCARIASIS (*Baylisascaris procyonis*)			
Drug of choice:	See footnote 22		
BLASTOCYSTIS hominis infection			
Drug of choice:	See footnote 23		
CAPILLARIASIS (*Capillaria philippinensis*)			
Drug of choice:	Mebendazole[7]	200 mg PO bid × 20d	200 mg PO bid × 20d
Alternative:	Albendazole[7,12]	400 mg PO daily × 10d	400 mg PO daily × 10d
Chagas' disease, see TRYPANOSOMIASIS			
Clonorchis sinensis, see FLUKE infection			
CRYPTOSPORIDIOSIS (*Cryptosporidium*) **Non-HIV infected**			
Drug of choice:	Nitazoxanide[5]	500 mg PO bid × 3d	1–3yrs: 100 mg PO bid × 3d
			4–11yrs: 200 mg PO bid × 3d
			>12yrs: 500 mg PO q12h × 3d
HIV infected			
Drug of choice:	See footnote 24		

*Availability problems. See table on page 814.

22. No drug has been demonstrated to be effective. Albendazole 25 mg/kg/d PO × 20d started as soon as possible (up to 3d after possible infection) might prevent clinical disease and is recommended for children with known exposure (ingestion of raccoon stool or contaminated soil) (WJ Murray and KR Kazacos, Clin Infect Dis 2004; 39:1484). Mebendazole, levamisole or ivermectin could be tried if albendazole is not available. Steroid therapy may be helpful, especially in eye and CNS infections (PJ Gavin et al, Clin Microbiol Rev 2005; 18:703). Ocular baylisascariasis has been treated successfully using laser photocoagulation therapy to destroy the intraretinal larvae (CA Garcia et al, Eye 2004; 18:624).

23. Clinical significance of these organisms is controversial; metronidazole 750 mg PO tid × 10d, iodoquinol 650 mg PO tid × 20d or trimethoprim/sulfamethoxazole 1 DS tab PO bid × 7d have been reported to be effective (DJ Stenzel and PFL Borenam, Clin Microbiol Rev 1996; 9:563; UZ Ok et al, Am J Gastroenterol 1999; 94:3245). Metronidazole resistance may be common in some areas (K Haresh et al, Trop Med Int Health 1999; 4:274). Nitazoxanide has been effective in clearing organism and improving symptoms (E Diaz et al, Am J Trop Med Hyg 2003; 68:384; JF Rossignol, Clin Gastroenterol Hepatol 2005; 18:703).

24. No drug has proven efficacy against cryptosporidiosis in advanced AIDS (I Abubakar et al, Cochrane Database Syst Rev 2007; 1:CD004932). Treatment with HAART is the mainstay of therapy. Nitazoxanide (JF Rossignol, Aliment Pharmacol Ther 2006; 24:807), paromomycin (P Maggi et al, Clin Infect Dis 2000; 33:1609), or a combination of paromomycin and azithromycin (NH Smith et al, J Infect Dis 1998; 178:900) may be tried to decrease diarrhea and recalcitrant malabsorption of antimicrobial drugs, which can occur with chronic cryptosporidiosis.

Table 4.9. Drugs for Parasitic Infections, continued

Infection	Drug	Adult dosage	Pediatric dosage
CUTANEOUS LARVA MIGRANS (creeping eruption, dog and cat hookworm)			
Drug of choice:[25]	Albendazole[7,12]	400 mg PO daily × 3d	400 mg PO daily × 3d
OR	Ivermectin[7,16]	200 mcg/kg PO daily × 1–2d	200 mcg/kg PO daily × 1–2d
CYCLOSPORIASIS (*Cyclospora cayetanensis*)			
Drug of choice:[26]	Trimethoprim/ sulfamethoxazole[7]	TMP 160 mg/SMX 800 mg (1 DS tab) PO bid × 7–10d	TMP 5 mg/kg/SMX 25 mg/kg/d PO in 2 doses × 7–10d
CYSTICERCOSIS, see TAPEWORM infection			
DIENTAMOEBA fragilis infection[27]			
Drug of choice:	Iodoquinol[2,7]	650 mg PO tid × 20d	30–40 mg/kg/d (max. 2g) PO in 3 doses × 20d
OR	Paromomycin[3,7]	25–35 mg/kg/d PO in 3 doses × 7d	25–35 mg/kg/d PO in 3 doses × 7d
OR	Tetracycline[7,21]	500 mg PO qid × 10d	40 mg/kg/d (max. 2g) PO in 4 doses × 10d
OR	Metronidazole[7]	500–750 mg PO tid × 10d	35–50 mg/kg/d PO in 3 doses × 10d
Diphyllobothrium latum, see TAPEWORM infection			
DRACUNCULUS medinensis (guinea worm) infection			
Drug of choice:	See footnote 28		
Echinococcus, see TAPEWORM infection			
Entamoeba histolytica, see AMEBIASIS			

*Availability problems. See table on page 814.

25. G Albanese et al, Int J Dermatol 2001; 40:67; D Malvy et al, J Travel Med 2006; 13:244.

26. HIV-infected patients may need higher dosage and long-term maintenance. Successful use of nitazoxanide (see also footnote 5) has been reported in one patient with sulfa allergy (SM Zimmer et al, Clin Infect Dis 2007; 44:466).

27. A Norberg et al, Clin Microbiol Infect 2003; 9:65; O Vandenberg et al, Int J Infect Dis 2006; 10:255.

28. No drug is curative against *Dracunculus*. A program for monitoring local sources of drinking water to eliminate transmission has dramatically decreased the number of cases worldwide (M Barry, N Engl J Med 2007; 356:25). The treatment of choice is slow extraction of worm combined with wound care and pain management (C Greenaway; CMAJ 2004; 170:495).

Table 4.9. Drugs for Parasitic Infections, continued

Infection	Drug	Adult dosage	Pediatric dosage
ENTEROBIUS *vermicularis* (pinworm) infection			
Drug of choice:[29]	Mebendazole	100 mg PO once; repeat in 2wks	100 mg PO once; repeat in 2wks
OR	Pyrantel pamoate[13]*	11 mg/kg base PO once (max. 1 g); repeat in 2wks	11 mg/kg base PO once (max. 1 g); repeat in 2wks
OR	Albendazole7,[12]	400 mg PO once; repeat in 2wks	400 mg PO once; repeat in 2wks
Fasciola hepatica, see FLUKE infection			
FILARIASIS[30]			
Wuchereria bancrofti, Brugia malayi, Brugia timori			
Drug of choice:[31]	Diethylcarbamazine*	6 mg/kg/d PO in 3 doses × 12d[32,33]	6 mg/kg/d PO in 3 doses × 12d[32,33]
Loa loa			
Drug of choice:[34]	Diethylcarbamazine*	6 mg/kg/d PO in 3 doses × 12d[32,33]	6 mg/kg/d PO in 3 doses × 12d[32,33]

* Availability problems. See table on page 814.

29. Since family members are usually infected, treatment of the entire household is recommended.

30. Antihistamines or corticosteroids may be required to decrease allergic reactions to components of disintegrating microfilariae that result from treatment, especially in infection caused by *Loa loa*. Endosymbiotic *Wolbachia* bacteria may have a role in filarial development and host response, and may represent a potential target for therapy. Addition of doxycycline 100 or 200 mg/d PO × 6–8wks in lymphatic filariasis and onchocerciasis has resulted in substantial loss of *Wolbachia* and decrease in both micro- and macrofilariae (MJ Taylor et al, Lancet 2005; 365:2116; AY Debrah et al, Plos Pathog 2006; e92:0829); but use of tetracyclines is contraindicated in pregnancy and in children <8 yrs old.

31. Most symptoms are caused by adult worm. A single-dose combination of albendazole (400 mg PO) with either ivermectin (200 mcg/kg PO) or diethylcarbamazine (6 mg/kg PO) is effective for reduction or suppression of *W. bancrofti* microfilaria, but the albendazole/ivermectin combination does not kill all the adult worms (D Addiss et al, Cochrane Database Syst Rev 2004; CD003753).

32. For patients with microfilaria in the blood, Medical Letter consultants start with a lower dosage and scale up: d1: 50 mg; d2: 50 mg tid; d3: 100 mg tid; d4–14: 6 mg/kg in 3 doses (for *Loa Loa* d4–14: 9 mg/kg in 3 doses). Multi-dose regimens have been shown to provide more rapid reduction in microfilaria than single-dose diethylcarbamazine, but microfilaria levels are similar 6–12 months after treatment (LD Andrade et al, Trans R Soc Trop Med Hyg 1995; 89:319; PE Simonsen et al, Am J Trop Med Hyg 1995; 53:267). A single dose of 6 mg/kg is used in endemic areas for mass treatment (J Figueredo-Silva et al, Trans R Soc Trop Med Hyg 1996; 90:192; J Noroes et al, Trans R Soc Trop Med Hyg 1997; 91:78).

33. Diethylcarbamazine should not be used for treatment of *Onchocerca volvulus* due to the risk of increased ocular side effects including blindness associated with rapid killing of the worms. It should be used cautiously in geographic regions where *O. volvulus* coexists with other filariae. Diethylcarbamazine is contraindicated during pregnancy. See also footnote 38.

34. In heavy infections with *Loa loa*, rapid killing of microfilariae can provoke encephalopathy. Apheresis has been reported to be effective in lowering microfilarial counts in patients heavily infected with *Loa loa* (EA Ottesen, Infect Dis Clin North Am 1993; 7:619). Albendazole may be useful for treatment of loiasis when diethylcarbamazine is ineffective or cannot be used, but repeated courses may be necessary (AD Klion et al, Clin Infect Dis 1999; 29:680; TE Tabi et al, Am J Trop Med Hyg 2004; 71:211). Ivermectin has also been used to reduce microfilaremia, but albendazole is preferred because of its slower onset of action and lower risk of precipitating encephalopathy (AD Klion et al, J Infect Dis 1993; 168:202; M Kombila et al, Am J Trop Med Hyg 1998; 58:458). Diethylcarbamazine, 300 mg PO once/wk, has been recommended for prevention of loiasis (TB Nutman et al, N Engl J Med 1988; 319:752).

Table 4.9. Drugs for Parasitic Infections, continued

Infection	Drug	Adult dosage	Pediatric dosage
FILARIASIS (continued)[30]			
Mansonella ozzardi			
Drug of choice:	See footnote 35		
Mansonella perstans			
Drug of choice:	Albendazole[7,12]	400 mg PO bid × 10d	400 mg PO bid × 10d
OR	Mebendazole[7]	100 mg PO bid × 30d	100 mg PO bid × 30d
Mansonella streptocerca			
Drug of choice:[36]	Diethylcarbamazine*	6 mg/kg/d PO × 12d[33]	6 mg/kg/d PO × 12d[33]
OR	Ivermectin[7,16]	150 mcg/kg PO once	150 mcg/kg PO once
Tropical Pulmonary Eosinophilia (TPE)[37]			
Drug of choice:	Diethylcarbamazine*	6 mg/kg/d in 3 doses × 12–21d[33]	6 mg/kg/d in 3 doses × 12–21d[33]
Onchocerca volvulus (River blindness)			
Drug of choice:	Ivermectin[16,38]	150 mcg/kg PO once, repeated every 6–12 mos until asymptomatic	150 mcg/kg PO once, repeated every 6–12 mos until asymptomatic
FLUKE, hermaphroditic, infection			
Clonorchis sinensis (Chinese liver fluke)			
Drug of choice:	Praziquantel[39]	75 mg/kg/d PO in 3 doses × 2d	75 mg/kg/d PO in 3 doses × 2d
OR	Albendazole[7,12]	10 mg/kg/d PO × 7d	10 mg/kg/d PO × 7d

* Availability problems. See footnote on page 814.

35. Diethylcarbamazine has no effect. A single dose of ivermectin 200 mcg/kg PO reduces microfilaria densities and provides both short- and long-term reductions in *M. ozzardi* microfilaremia (AA Gonzalez et al, W Indian Med J 1999; 48:231).

36. Diethylcarbamazine is potentially curative due to activity against both adult worms and microfilariae. Ivermectin is active only against microfilariae.

37. Diethylcarbamazine is potentially curative and can be treated with a repeated course of diethylcarbamazine. Relapses occur and can be treated with a repeated course of diethylcarbamazine.

37. AK Boggild et al, Clin Infect Dis 2004; 39:1123.

38. Diethylcarbamazine should not be used for treatment of this disease because rapid killing of the worms can lead to blindness. Periodic treatment with ivermectin (every 3–12 months), 150 mcg/kg PO, can prevent blindness due to ocular onchocerciasis (DN Udall, Clin Infect Dis 2007; 44:53). Skin reactions after ivermectin treatment are often reported in persons with high microfilarial skin densities. Ivermectin has been inadvertently given to pregnant women during mass treatment programs; the rates of congenital abnormalities were similar in treated and untreated women. Because of the high risk of blindness from onchocerciasis, the use of ivermectin after the first trimester is considered acceptable according to the WHO. Doxycycline (100 mg/day PO for 6 weeks), followed by a single 150 mcg/kg PO dose of ivermectin, resulted in up to 19 months of amicrofilaridermia and 100% elimination of *Wolbachia* species (A Hoerauf et al, Lancet 2001; 357:1415).

39. Praziquantel should be taken with liquids during a meal.

Table 4.9. Drugs for Parasitic Infections, continued

Infection	Drug	Adult dosage	Pediatric dosage
FLUKE, hermaphroditic, infection, continued			
Fasciola hepatica (sheep liver fluke)			
Drug of choice:[40]	Triclabendazole*	10 mg/kg PO once or twice[41]	10 mg/kg PO once or twice[41]
Alternative:	Bithionol*	30–50 mg/kg on alternate days × 10–15 doses	30–50 mg/kg on alternate days × 10–15 doses
OR	Nitazoxanide[5,7]	500 mg PO bid × 7d	1–3yrs: 100 mg PO q12h × 7d 4–11yrs: 200 mg PO q12h × 7d >12yrs: 500 mg PO q12h × 7d
Fasciolopsis buski, Heterophyes heterophyes, Metagonimus yokogawai (intestinal flukes)			
Drug of choice:	Praziquantel[7,39]	75 mg/kg/d PO in 3 doses × 1d	75 mg/kg/d PO in 3 doses × 1d
Metorchis conjunctus (North American liver fluke)			
Drug of choice:	Praziquantel[7,39]	75 mg/kg/d PO in 3 doses × 1d	75 mg/kg/d PO in 3 doses × 1d
Nanophyetus salmincola			
Drug of choice:	Praziquantel[7,39]	60 mg/kg/d PO in 3 doses × 1d	60 mg/kg/d PO in 3 doses × 1d
Opisthorchis viverrini (Southeast Asian liver fluke)			
Drug of choice:	Praziquantel[39]	75 mg/kg/d PO in 3 doses × 2d	75 mg/kg/d PO in 3 doses × 2d
Paragonimus westermani (lung fluke)			
Drug of choice:	Praziquantel[7,39]	75 mg/kg/d PO in 3 doses × 2d	75 mg/kg/d PO in 3 doses × 2d
Alternative:[42]	Bithionol*	30–50 mg/kg on alternate days × 10–15 doses	30–50 mg/kg on alternate days × 10–15 doses

*Availability problems. See table on page 814.

40. Unlike infections with other flukes, *Fasciola hepatica* infections may not respond to praziquantel. Triclabendazole (*Egaten*—Novartis) appears to be safe and effective, but data are limited (DY Aksoy et al, Clin Microbiol Infect 2005; 11:859). It is available from Victoria Pharmacy, Zurich, Switzerland (**www.pharmaworld.com**; 41–1-211-24-32) and should be given with food for better absorption. Nitazoxanide also appears to have efficacy in treating fascioliasis in adults and in children (L Favennec et al, Aliment Pharmacol Ther 2003; 17:265; JF Rossignol et al, Trans R Soc Trop Med Hyg 1998; 92:103; SM Kabil et al, Curr Ther Res 2000; 61:339).

41. J Keiser et al, Expert Opin Investig Drugs 2005; 14:1513.

42. Triclabendazole may be effective in a dosage of 5 mg/kg PO once/d × 3d or 10 mg/kg PO bid × 1d (M Calvopiña et al, Trans R Soc Trop Med Hyg 1998; 92:566). See footnote 40 for availability.

Table 4.9. Drugs for Parasitic Infections, continued

Infection	Drug	Adult dosage	Pediatric dosage
GIARDIASIS (*Giardia duodenalis*)			
Drug of choice:	Metronidazole[7]	250 mg PO tid × 5–7d	15 mg/kg/d PO in 3 doses × 5–7d
OR	Tinidazole[6]	2 g PO once	50 mg/kg PO once (max. 2 g)
OR	Nitazoxanide[5]	500 mg PO bid × 3d	1–3yrs: 100 mg PO q12h × 3d 4–11yrs: 200 mg PO q12h × 3d >12yrs: 500 mg PO q12h × 3d
Alternative:[43]	Paromomycin[3,7,44]	25–35 mg/kg/d PO in 3 doses × 5–10d	25–35 mg/kg/d PO in 3 doses × 5–10d
OR	Furazolidone*	100 mg PO qid × 7–10d	6 mg/kg/d PO in 4 doses × 7–10d
OR	Quinacrine[4,45]*	100 mg PO tid × 5d	2 mg/kg/d PO in 3 doses × 5d (max 300 mg/d)
GNATHOSTOMIASIS (*Gnathostoma spingerum*)[46]			
Treatment of choice:	Albendazole[7,12]	400 mg PO bid × 21d	400 mg PO bid × 21d
OR	Ivermectin[7,16]	200 mcg/kg/d PO × 2d	200 mcg/kg/d PO × 2d
Either	± Surgical removal		
GONGYLONEMIASIS (*Gongylonema sp.*)[47]			
Treatment of choice:	Surgical removal		
OR	Albendazole[7,12]	400 mg/d PO × 3d	400 mg/d PO × 3d

* Availability problems. See table on page 814.

43. Another alternative is albendazole 400 mg/d PO × 5d in adults and 10 mg/kg/d PO × 5d in children (K Yereli et al, Clin Microbiol Infect 2004; 10:527; O Karabay et al, World J Gastroenterol 2004; 10:1215). Combination treatment with standard doses of metronidazole and quinacrine × 3wks has been effective for a small number of refractory infections (TE Nash et al, Clin Infect Dis 2001; 33:22). In one study, nitazoxanide was used successfully in high doses to treat a case of *Giardia* resistant to metronidazole and albendazole (P Abboud et al, Clin Infect Dis 2001; 32:1792).

44. Poorly absorbed; may be useful for treatment of giardiasis in pregnancy.

45. Quinacrine should be taken with liquids after a meal.

46. P Nontasut et al, Southeast Asian J Trop Med Pub Health 2005; 36:650; M de Gorgolas et al, J Travel Med 2003; 10:358. All patients should be treated with medication whether surgery is attempted or not.

47. ME Wilson et al, Clin Infect Dis 2001; 32:1378; G Molavi et al, J Helminth 2006; 80:425.

Table 4.9. Drugs for Parasitic Infections, continued

Infection	Drug	Adult dosage	Pediatric dosage
HOOKWORM infection (*Ancylostoma duodenale, Necator americanus*)			
Drug of choice:	Albendazole[7,12]	400 mg PO once	400 mg PO once
OR	Mebendazole	100 mg PO bid × 3d or 500 mg once	100 mg PO bid × 3d or 500 mg once
OR	Pyrantel pamoate[7,13]*	11 mg/kg (max. 1g) PO × 3d	11 mg/kg (max. 1g) PO × 3d
Hydatid cyst, see TAPEWORM infection			
Hymenolepis nana, see TAPEWORM infection			
ISOSPORIASIS (*Isospora belli*)			
Drug of choice:[48]	Trimethoprim-sulfamethoxazole[7]	TMP 160 mg/SMX 800 mg (1 DS tab) PO bid × 10d	TMP 5 mg/kg/d/SMX 25 mg/kg/d PO in 2 doses × 10d
LEISHMANIA[49,50]			
Visceral[49,50]			
Drug of choice:	Liposomal amphotericin B[51]	3 mg/kg/d IV d 1–5, 14 and 21[52]	3 mg/kg/d IV d 1–5, 14 and 21[52]
OR	Sodium stibogluconate*	20 mg Sb/kg/d IV or IM × 28d	20 mg Sb/kg/d IV or IM × 28d
OR	Miltefosine[53]*	2.5 mg/kg/d PO (max 150 mg/d) × 28d	2.5 mg/kg/d PO (max 150 mg/d) × 28d

* Availability problems. See table on page 814.

48. Usually a self-limited illness in immunocompetent patients. Immunosuppressed patients may need higher doses, longer duration (TMP/SMX qid × 10d, followed by bid × 3wks) and long-term maintenance. In sulfonamide-sensitive patients, pyrimethamine 50–75 mg daily in divided doses (plus leucovorin 10–25 mg/d) has been effective.

49. To maximize effectiveness and minimize toxicity, the choice of drug, dosage, and duration of therapy should be individualized based on the region of disease acquisition, a likely infecting species, and host factors such as immune status (BL Herwaldt, Lancet 1999; 354:1191). Some of the listed drugs and regimens are effective only against certain *Leishmania* species/strains and only in certain areas of the world (J Arevalo et al, Clin Infect Dis 2007; 195:1846). Medical Letter consultants recommend consultation with physicians experienced in management of this disease.

50. Visceral infection is most commonly due to the Old World species *L. donovani* (kala-azar) and *L. infantum* and the New World species *L. chagasi.*

51. Liposomal amphotericin B (*AmBisome*) is the only lipid formulation of amphotericin B FDA-approved for treatment of visceral leishmania, largely based on clinical trials in patients infected with *L. infantum* (A Meyerhoff, Clin Infect Dis 1999; 28:42). Two other amphotericin B lipid formulations, amphotericin B lipid complex (*Abelcet*) and amphotericin B cholesteryl sulfate (*Amphotec*) have been used, but are considered investigational for this condition and may not be as effective (C Bern et al, Clin Infect Dis 2006; 43:917).

52. The FDA-approved dosage regimen for immunocompromised patients (e.g., HIV infected) is 4 mg/kg/d IV on days 1–5, 10, 17, 24, 31 and 38. The relapse rate is high; maintenance therapy (secondary prevention) may be indicated, but there is no consensus as to dosage or duration.

53. Effective for both antimony-sensitive and -resistant *L. donovani* (Indian); miltefosine (*Impavido*) is manufactured in 10- or 50-mg capsules by Zentaris (Frankfurt, Germany) at **info@zentaris.com**) and is available through consultation with the CDC. The drug is contraindicated in pregnancy; a negative pregnancy test before drug initiation and effective contraception during and for 2 months after treatment is recommended (H Murray et al, Lancet 2005; 366:1561). In a placebo-controlled trial in patients ≥12 years old, oral miltefosine 2.5 mg/kg/d × 28d was also effective for treatment of cutaneous leishmaniasis due to *L.(V) braziliensis* or *L. mexicana* in Guatemala (J Soto et al, Clin Infect Dis 2004; 38:1266). "Motion sickness," nausea, headache and increased creatinine are the most frequent adverse effects (J Soto and P Soto, Expert Rev Anti Infect Ther 2006; 4:177).

Table 4.9. Drugs for Parasitic Infections, continued

Infection	Drug	Adult dosage	Pediatric dosage
LEISHMANIA, continued			
Alternative:	Meglumine antimonate*	20 mg Sb/kg/d IV or IM × 28d	20 mg Sb/kg/d IV or IM × 28d
OR	Amphotericin B[7]	1 mg/kg IV daily x 15–20d or every second day for up to 8 wks	1 mg/kg IV daily × 15–20d or every second day for up to 8 wks
OR	Paromomycin[7,13,54]*	15 mg/kg IM × 21d	15 mg/kd IM × 21d
Cutaneous[49,55]			
Drugs of choice:	Sodium stibogluconate*	20 mg Sb/kg/d IV or IM × 20d	20 mg Sb/kg/d IV or IM × 20d
OR	Meglumine antimonate*	20 mg Sb/kg/d IV or IM × 20d	20 mg Sb/kg/d IV or IM × 20d
OR	Miltefosine[53]*	2.5 mg/kg/d PO (max 150 mg/d) × 28d	2.5 mg/kg/d PO (max 150 mg/d) × 28d
Alternative:[56]	Paromomycin[7,13,54]*	Topically 2x/d × 10–20d	Topically 2x/d × 10–20d
OR	Pentamidine[7]	2–3 mg/kg IV or IM daily or every second day × 4–7 doses[57]	2–3 mg/kg IV or IM daily or every second day × 4–7 doses[57]

* Availability problems. See table on page 814.

54. Paromomycin IM has been effective against leishmania in India; it has not yet been tested in South America or the Mediterranean and there is insufficient data to support its use in pregnancy (S Sundar et al, N Engl J Med 2007; 356:2371). Topical paromomycin should be used only in geographic regions where cutaneous leishmaniasis species have low potential for mucosal spread. A formulation of 15% paromomycin/12% methylbenzethonium chloride (*Leshcutan*) in soft white paraffin for topical use has been reported to be partially effective against cutaneous leishmaniasis due to *L. major* in Israel and *L. mexicana* and *L. (V.) braziliensis* in Guatemala, where mucosal spread is very rare (BA Arana et al, Am J Trop Med Hyg 2001; 65:466). The methylbenzethonium is irritating to the skin; lesions may worsen before they improve.

55. Cutaneous infection is most commonly due to the Old World species *L. major* and *L. tropica* and the New World species *L. mexicana, L. (Viannia) braziliensis,* and others.

56. Although azole drugs (fluconazole, ketoconazole, itraconazole) have been used to treat cutaneous disease, they are not reliably effective and have no efficacy against mucosal disease (AJ Magill, Infect Dis Clin North Am 2005; 19:241). For treatment of *L. major* cutaneous lesions, a study in Saudi Arabia found that oral fluconazole, 200 mg once/d × 6wks appeared to speed healing (AA Alrajhi et al, N Engl J Med 2002; 346:891). Thermotherapy may be an option for cutaneous *L. tropica* infection (R Reithinger et al, Clin Infect Dis 2005; 40:1148). A device that generates focused and controlled heating of the skin has been approved by the FDA for this indication (*ThermoMed*-ThermoSurgery Technologies Inc., Phoenix, AZ, 602-264-7300; **www.thermosurgery.com**).

57. At this dosage pentamidine has been effective in Colombia predominantly against *L. (V.) panamensis* (J Soto-Mancipe et al, Clin Infect Dis 1993; 16:417; J Soto et al, Am J Trop Med Hyg 1994; 50:107). Activity against other species is not well established.

Table 4.9. Drugs for Parasitic Infections, continued

Infection	Drug	Adult dosage	Pediatric dosage
LEISHMANIA, continued			
Mucosal[49,58]			
Drug of choice:	Sodium stibogluconate*	20 mg Sb/kg/d IV or IM × 28d	20 mg Sb/kg/d IV or IM × 28d
OR	Meglumine antimonate*	20 mg Sb/kg/d IV or IM × 28d	20 mg Sb/kg/d IV or IM × 28d
OR	Amphotericin B[7]	0.5–1 mg/kg IV daily or every second day for up to 8wks	0.5–1 mg/kg IV daily or every second day for up to 8wks
OR	Miltefosine[53]*	2.5 mg/kg/d PO (max 150 mg/d) × 28d	2.5 mg/kg/d PO (max 150 mg/d) × 28d
LICE infestation (_Pediculus humanus, P. capitis, Phthirus pubis_)[59]			
Drug of choice:	0.5% Malathion[60]	Topically	Topically
OR	1% Permethrin[61]	Topically	Topically
Alternative:	Pyrethrins with piperonyl butoxide[61]	Topically	Topically
OR	Ivermectin[7,16,62]	200 mcg/kg PO	>15kg: 200 mcg/kg PO
Loa loa, see FILARIASIS			

*Availability problems. See table on page 814.

58. Mucosal infection is most commonly due to the New World species _L. (V.) braziliensis, L. (V.) panamensis_, or _L. (V.) guyanensis_.

59. Pediculocides should not be used for infestations of the eyelashes. Such infestations are treated with petrolatum ointment applied 2–4x/d × 8–10d. Oral TMP/SMX has also been used (TL Meinking and D Taplin, Curr Probl Dermatol 1996; 24:157). For pubic lice, treat with 5% permethrin or ivermectin as for scabies (see page 9). TMP/SMX has also been effective when used together with permethrin for head lice (RB Hipolito et al, Pediatrics 2001; 107:E30).

60. Malathion is both ovicidal and pediculocidal; 2 applications at least 7 days apart are generally necessary to kill all lice and nits.

61. Permethrin and pyrethrin are pediculocidal; retreatment in 7–10d is needed to eradicate the infestation. Some lice are resistant to pyrethrins and permethrin (TL Meinking et al, Arch Dermatol 2002; 138:220).

62. Ivermectin is pediculocidal, but more than one dose is generally necessary to eradicate the infestation (KN Jones and JC English 3rd, Clin Infect Dis 2003; 36:1355). The number of doses and interval between doses has not been established, but in one study of body lice, 3 doses administered at 7-day intervals were effective (C Fouault et al, J Infect Dis 2006; 193:474).

Table 4.9. Drugs for Parasitic Infections, continued

Infection	Drug	Adult dosage	Pediatric dosage
MALARIA, Treatment of (*Plasmodium falciparum*,[63] *P. vivax*,[64] *P. ovale*, and *P. malariae*[65])			
ORAL[66]			
P. falciparum or unidentified species acquired in areas of chloroquine-resistant *P. falciparum*[63]			
Drug of choice:[67]	Atovaquone/proguanil[68]	2 adult tabs bid[69] or 4 adult tabs once/d × 3d	<5kg: not indicated 5–8kg: 2 peds tabs once/d × 3d 9–10kg: 3 peds tabs once/d × 3d 11–20kg: 1 adult tab once/d × 3d 21–30kg: 2 adult tabs once/d × 3d 31–40kg: 3 adult tabs once/d × 3d >40kg: 4 adult tabs once/d × 3d

* Availability problems. See table on page 814.

63. Chloroquine-resistant *P. falciparum* occurs in all malarious areas except Central America (including Panama north and west of the Canal Zone), Mexico, Haiti, the Dominican Republic, Paraguay, northern Argentina, North and South Korea, Georgia, Armenia, most of rural China and some countries in the Middle East (chloroquine resistance has been reported in Yemen, Oman, Saudi Arabia and Iran). For treatment of multiple-drug-resistant *P. falciparum* in Southeast Asia, especially Thailand, where mefloquine resistance is frequent, atovaquone/proguanil, quinine plus either doxycycline or clindamycin, or artemether/lumefantrine may be used.

64. *P. vivax* with decreased susceptibility to chloroquine is a significant problem in Papua-New Guinea and Indonesia. There are also a few reports of resistance from Myanmar, India, the Solomon Islands, Vanuatu, Guyana, Brazil, Colombia and Peru (JK Baird et al, Curr Infect Dis Rep 2007; 9:39).

65. Chloroquine-resistant *P. malariae* has been reported from Sumatra (JD Maguire et al, Lancet 2002; 360:58).

66. Uncomplicated or mild malaria may be treated with oral drugs. Severe malaria (e.g. impaired consciousness, parasitemia >5%, shock, etc.) should be treated with parenteral drugs (KS Griffin et al, JAMA 2007; 297:2264).

67. Primaquine is given for prevention of relapse after infection with *P. vivax* or *P. ovale*. Some experts also prescribe primaquine phosphate 30 mg base/d (0.6 mg base/kg/d for children) for 14d after departure from areas where these species are endemic (Presumptive Anti-Relapse Therapy [PART], "terminal prophylaxis"). Since this is not always effective as prophylaxis (E Schwartz et al, N Engl J Med 2003; 349:1510), others prefer to rely on surveillance to detect cases when they occur, particularly when exposure was limited or doubtful. See also footnote 79.

68. Atovaquone/proguanil is available as a fixed-dose combination tablet: adult tablets (*Malarone*; 250 mg atovaquone/100 mg proguanil) and pediatric tablets (*Malarone Pediatric*; 62.5 mg atovaquone/25 mg proguanil). To enhance absorption and reduce nausea and vomiting, it should be taken with food or a milky drink. Safety in pregnancy is unknown; outcomes were normal in 24 women treated with the combination in the 2nd and 3rd trimester (R McGready et al, Eur J Clin Pharmacol 2003; 59:545). The drug should not be given to patients with severe renal impairment (creatinine clearance <30mL/min). There have been isolated case reports of resistance in *P. falciparum* in Africa, but Medical Letter consultants do not believe there is a high risk for acquisition of *Malarone*-resistant disease (E Schwartz et al, Clin Infect Dis 2003; 37:450; A Farnert et al, BMJ 2003; 326:628; S Kuhn et al, Am J Trop Med Hyg 2005; 72:407; CT Happi et al, Malaria Journal 2006; 5:82).

69. Although approved for once-daily dosing, Medical Letter consultants usually divide the dose in two to decrease nausea and vomiting.

Table 4.9. Drugs for Parasitic Infections, continued

Infection	Drug	Adult dosage	Pediatric dosage
MALARIA, Treatment of, continued			
OR	Quinine sulfate	650 mg q8h × 3 or 7d[70]	30 mg/kg/d in 3 doses × 3 or 7d[70]
	plus		
	doxycycline[7,21,71]	100 mg bid × 7d	4 mg/kg/d in 2 doses × 7d
	or plus		
	tetracycline[7,21]	250 mg qid × 7d	6.25 mg/kg/d in 4 doses × 7d
	or plus		
	clindamycin[7,18,72]	20 mg/kg/d in 3 doses × 7d[73]	20 mg/kg/d in 3 doses × 7d
Alternative:[67]	Mefloquine[74,75]	750 mg followed 12 hrs later by 500 mg	15 mg/kg followed 12 hrs later by 10 mg/kg

*Availability problems. See table on page 814.

70. Available in the US in a 324-mg capsule; 2 capsules suffice for adult dosage. In Southeast Asia, relative resistance to quinine has increased and treatment should be continued for 7d. Quinine should be taken with or after meals to decrease gastrointestinal adverse effects.

71. Doxycycline should be taken with adequate water to avoid esophageal irritation. It can be taken with food to minimize gastrointestinal adverse effects.

72. For use in pregnancy and in children <8 yrs.

73. B Lell and PG Kremsner, Antimicrob Agents Chemother 2002; 46:2315; M Ramharter et al, Clin Infect Dis 2005; 40:1777.

74. At this dosage, adverse effects include nausea, vomiting, diarrhea and dizziness. Disturbed sense of balance, toxic psychosis and seizures can also occur. Mefloquine should not be used for treatment of malaria in pregnancy unless there is no other treatment option because of increased risk for stillbirth (F Nosten et al, Clin Infect Dis 1999; 28:808). It should be avoided for treatment of malaria in persons with active depression or with a history of psychosis or seizures and should be used with caution in persons with any psychiatric illness. Mefloquine can be given to patients taking β-blockers if they do not have an underlying arrhythmia; it should not be used in patients with conduction abnormalities. Mefloquine should not be given together with quinine or quinidine, and caution is required in using quinine or quinidine to treat patients with malaria who have taken mefloquine for prophylaxis. Mefloquine should not be taken on an empty stomach; it should be taken with at least 8 oz of water.

75. *P. falciparum* with resistance to mefloquine is a significant problem in the malarious areas of Thailand and in areas of Myanmar and Cambodia that border on Thailand. It has also been reported on the borders between Myanmar and China, Laos and Myanmar, and in Southern Vietnam. In the US, a 250-mg tablet of mefloquine contains 228 mg mefloquine base. Outside the US, each 275-mg tablet contains 250 mg base.

Table 4.9. Drugs for Parasitic Infections, continued

Infection	Drug	Adult dosage	Pediatric dosage
MALARIA, Treatment of, continued			
OR	Artemether/ lumefantrine[76,77]*	6 doses over 3d (4 tabs/dose at 0, 8, 24, 36, 48 and 60 hours)	6 doses over 3d at same intervals as adults; <15kg: 1 tab/dose 15–25kg: 2 tabs/dose 25–35kg: 3 tabs/dose >35kg: 4 tabs/dose
OR	Artesunate[76]* **plus** see footnote 78	4 mg/kg/d × 3d	4 mg/kg/d × 3d
P. vivax acquired in areas of chloroquine-resistant *P. vivax*[64] Drug of choice:[67]	Mefloquine[74]	750 mg PO followed 12 hrs later by 500 mg	15 mg/kg PO followed 12 hrs later by 10 mg/kg
OR	Atovaquone/proguanil[68]	2 adult tabs bid[69] or 4 adult tabs once/d × 3d	<5kg: not indicated 5–8kg: 2 peds tabs once/d × 3d 9–10kg: 3 peds tabs once/d × 3d 11–20kg: 1 adult tab once/d × 3d 21–30kg: 2 adult tabs once/d × 3d 31–40kg: 3 adult tabs once/d × 3d >40kg: 4 adult tabs once/d × 3d
	either followed by primaquine phosphate[79]	30 mg base/d PO × 14d	0.6 mg/kg/d PO × 14d

*Availability problems. See table on page 814.

76. The artemisinin-derivatives, artemether and artesunate, are both frequently used globally in combination regimens to treat malaria. Both are available in oral, parenteral and rectal formulations, but manufacturing standards are not consistent (HA Karunajeewa et al, JAMA 2007; 297:2381; EA Ashley and NJ White, Curr Opin Infect Dis 2005; 18:531). In the US, only the IV formulation of artesunate is available; it can be obtained through the CDC under an IND for patients with severe disease who do not have timely access, cannot tolerate, or fail to respond to IV quinidine (**www.cdc.gov/malaria/features/artesunate_now_available.htm**). To avoid development of resistance, monotherapy should be avoided (PE Duffy and CH Sibley, Lancet 2005; 366:1908). In animal studies, artemisinins have been embryotoxic and caused a low incidence of teratogenicity; no adverse pregnancy outcomes have been observed in limited studies in humans (S Dellicour et al, Malaria J 2007;6:15).

77. Artemether/lumefantrine is available as a fixed-dose combination tablet (Coartem in countries with endemic malaria, *Riamet* in Europe and countries without endemic malaria); each tablet contains 20 mg artemether and 120 mg lumefantrine (M van Vugt et al, Am J Trop Med Hyg 1999; 60:936). It is contraindicated during the first trimester of pregnancy; safety during the second and third trimester is not known. The tablets should be taken with food. Artemether/lumefantrine should not be used in patients with cardiac arrhythmias, bradycardia, severe cardiac disease or QT prolongation. Concomitant use of drugs that prolong the QT interval or are metabolized by CYP2D6 is contraindicated.

78. Adults treated with artesunate should also receive oral treatment doses of either atovaquone/proguanil, doxycycline, clindamycin or mefloquine; children should take either atovaquone/proguanil, clindamycin or mefloquine (F Nosten et al, Lancet 2000; 356:297; M van Vugt, Clin Infect Dis 2002; 35:1498; F Smithuis et al, Trans R Soc Trop Med Hyg 2004; 98:182). If artesunate is given IV, oral medication should be started when the patient is able to tolerate it (SEAQUAMAT group, Lancet 2005; 366:717).

79. Primaquine phosphate can cause hemolytic anemia, especially in patients whose red cells are deficient in G-6-PD. This deficiency is most common in African, Asian and Mediterranean peoples. Patients should be screened for G-6-PD deficiency before treatment. Primaquine should not be used during pregnancy. It should be taken with food to minimize nausea and abdominal pain. Primaquine-tolerant *P. vivax* can be found globally. Relapses of primaquine-resistant strains may be retreated with 30 mg (base) × 28d.

Table 4.9. Drugs for Parasitic Infections, continued

Infection	Drug	Adult dosage	Pediatric dosage
MALARIA, Treatment of, continued			
Alternative:[67]	Chloroquine phosphate[80]	25 mg base/kg PO in 3 doses over 48 hrs[81]	25 mg base/kg PO in 3 doses over 48 hrs[81]
OR	Quinine sulfate **plus**	650 mg PO q8h × 3–7d70	30 mg/kg/d PO in 3 doses × 3–7d70
	doxycycline[7,21,71] **either followed by**	100 mg PO bid × 7d	4 mg/kg/d PO in 2 doses × 7d
	primaquine	30 mg base/d PO × 14d	0.6 mg/kg/d PO × 14d phosphate[79]
All *Plasmodium* species except chloroquine-resistant *P. falciparum*[63] and chloroquine-resistant *P. vivax*[64]			
Drug of choice:[57]	Chloroquine phosphate[80]	1 g (600 mg base) PO, then 500 mg(300 mg base) 6 hrs later, then 500mg (300 mg base) at 24 and 48 hrs[81]	10 mg base/kg (max. 600 mg base) PO, then 5 mg base/kg 6 hrs later, then 5 mg base/kg at 24 and 48 hrs[81]
PARENTERAL [66]			
All *Plasmodium* species (Chloroquine-sensitive and resistant)			
Drug of choice:[67,82]	Quinidine gluconate[83]	10 mg/kg IV loading dose (max. 600 mg) in normal saline over 1–2 hrs, followed by continuous infusion of 0.02 mg/kg/min until PO therapy can be started	10 mg/kg IV loading dose (max. 600 mg) in normal saline over 1–2 hrs, followed by continuous infusion of 0.02 mg/kg/min until PO therapy can be started

*Availability problems. See table on page 814.

80. Chloroquine should be taken with food to decrease gastrointestinal adverse effects. If chloroquine phosphate is not available, hydroxychloroquine sulfate is as effective; 400 mg of hydroxychloroquine sulfate is equivalent to 500 mg of chloroquine phosphate.

81. Chloroquine combined with primaquine was effective in 85% of patients with *P. vivax* resistant to chloroquine and could be a reasonable choice in areas where other alternatives are not available (JK Baird et al, J Infect Dis 1995; 171:1678).

82. Exchange transfusion is controversial, but has been helpful for some patients with high-density (>10%) parasitemia, altered mental status, pulmonary edema or renal complications (VI Powell and K Grima, Transfus Med Rev 2002; 16:239; MS Riddle et al, Clin Infect Dis 2002; 34:1192).

83. Continuous EKG, blood pressure and glucose monitoring are recommended, especially in pregnant women and young children. For problems with quinidine availability, call the manufacturer (Eli Lilly, 800-821-0538) or the CDC Malaria Hotline (770-488-7788). Quinidine may have greater antimalarial activity than quinine. The loading dose should be decreased or omitted in patients who have received quinine or mefloquine. If more than 48 hours of parenteral treatment is required, the quinine or quinidine dose should be reduced by 30–50%.

Table 4.9. Drugs for Parasitic Infections, continued

Infection	Drug	Adult dosage	Pediatric dosage
PARENTERAL[66], continued			
OR	Quinine dihydrochloride[83]*	20 mg/kg IV loading dose in 5% dextrose over 4 hrs, followed by 10 mg/kg over 2–4 hrs q8h (max. 1800 mg/d) until PO therapy can be started	20 mg/kg IV loading dose in 5% dextrose over 4 hrs, followed by 10 mg/kg over 2–4 hrs q8h (max. 1800 mg/d) until PO therapy can be started
OR	Artesunate[76]*	2.4 mg/kg/dose IV × 3d at 0, 12, 24, and 48 hrs	2.4 mg/kg/dose IV × 3d at 0, 12, 24, and 48 hrs
	plus see footnote 78		
MALARIA, Prevention of[84]			
All *Plasmodium* species in chloroquine-sensitive areas[63,64,65] Drug of choice:[67,85]	Chloroquine phosphate[80,86]	500 mg (300 mg base) PO once/wk[87]	5 mg/kg base PO once/wk, up to adult dose of 300 mg base[87]
All *Plasmodium* species in chloroquine-resistant areas[63,64,65] Drug of choice:[67]	Atovaquone/proguanil[68]	1 adult tab/d[88]	5–8kg: 1/2 peds tab/d[68,88] 9–10kg: 3/4 peds tab/d[68,88] 11–20kg: 1 peds tab/d[68,88] 21–30kg: 2 peds tabs/d[68,88] 31–40kg: 3 peds tabs/d[68,88] >40kg: 1 adult tab/d[68,88]

*Availability problems. See table on page 814.

84. No drug guarantees protection against malaria. Travelers should be advised to seek medical attention if fever develops after they return. Insect repellents, insecticide-impregnated bed nets and proper clothing are important adjuncts for malaria prophylaxis (Med Lett Drugs Ther 2005; 47:100). Malaria in pregnancy is particularly serious for both mother and fetus; prophylaxis is indicated if exposure cannot be avoided.

85. Alternatives for patients who are unable to take chloroquine include atovaquone/proguanil, mefloquine, doxycycline or primaquine dosed as for chloroquine-resistant areas.

86. Has been used extensively and safely for prophylaxis in pregnancy.

87. Beginning 1–2wks before travel and continuing weekly for the duration of stay and for 4wks after leaving.

88. Beginning 1–2d before travel and continuing for the duration of stay and for 1wk after leaving. In one study of malaria prophylaxis, atovaquone/proguanil was better tolerated than mefloquine in nonimmune travelers (D Overbosch et al, Clin Infect Dis 2001; 33:1015). The protective efficacy of *Malarone* against *P. vivax* is variable ranging from 84% in Indonesian New Guinea (J Ling et al, Clin Infect Dis 2002; 35:825) to 100% in Colombia (J Soto et al, Am J Trop Med Hyg 2006; 75:430). Some Medical Letter consultants prefer alternate drugs if traveling to areas where *P. vivax* predominates.

Table 4.9. Drugs for Parasitic Infections, continued

Infection	Drug	Adult dosage	Pediatric dosage
MALARIA, Prevention of[64]**, continued**			
OR	Doxycycline[7,21,71]	100 mg PO daily[89]	2 mg/kg/d PO, up to 100 mg/d[89]
OR	Mefloquine[74,75,90]	250 mg PO once/wk[91]	5–10kg: 1/8 tab once/wk[91]
			11–20kg: 1/4 tab once/wk[91]
			21–30kg: 1/2 tab once/wk[91]
			31–45kg: 3/4 tab once/wk[91]
			>45kg: 1 tab once/wk[91]
Alternative:[92]	Primaquine[7,79] phosphate	30 mg base PO daily[93]	0.6 mg/kg base PO daily[93]
MALARIA, Prevention of relapses: P. vivax and P. ovale[67]			
Drug of choice:	Primaquine phosphate[79]	30 mg base/d PO × 14d	0.6 mg base/kg/d PO × 14d
MALARIA, Self-Presumptive Treatment[94]			
Drug of Choice:	Atovaquone/proguanil[7,68]	4 adult tabs once/d × 3d[69]	<5kg: not indicated
			5–8kg: 2 peds tabs once/d × 3d
			9–10kg: 3 peds tabs once/d × 3d
			11–20kg: 1 adult tab once/d × 3d
			21–30kg: 2 adult tabs once/d × 3d
			31–40kg: 3 adult tabs once/d × 3d
			>40kg: 4 adult tabs once/d × 3d[69]
OR	Quinine sulfate	650 mg PO q8h × 3 or 7d[70]	30 mg/kg/d PO in 3 doses × 3 or 7d[70]
	plus		
	doxycycline[7,21,71]	100 mg PO bid × 7d	4 mg/kg/d PO in 2 doses × 7d
OR	Artesunate[76]*	4 mg/kg/d PO × 3d	4 mg/kg/d PO × 3d
	plus see footnote 78		

*Availability problems. See table on page 814.

89. Beginning 1–2d before travel and continuing for the duration of stay and for 4wks after leaving. Use of tetracyclines is contraindicated in pregnancy and in children <8 years old. Doxycycline can cause gastrointestinal disturbances, vaginal moniliasis and photosensitivity reactions.

90. Mefloquine has not been approved for use during pregnancy. However, it has been reported to be safe for prophylactic use during the second and third trimester of pregnancy and possibly during early pregnancy as well (CDC Health Information for International Travel, 2008, page 228; BL Smoak et al, J Infect Dis 1997; 176:831). For pediatric doses <1/2 tablet, it is advisable to have a pharmacist crush the tablet, estimate doses by weighing, and package them in gelatin capsules. There is no data for use in children <5 kg, but based on dosages in other weight groups, a dose of 5 mg/kg can be used. Not recommended for use in travelers with active depression or with a history of psychosis or seizures and should be used with caution in persons with psychiatric illness. Mefloquine can be given to patients taking β-blockers if they do not have an underlying arrhythmia; it should not be used in patients with conduction abnormalities.

91. Beginning 1–2wks before travel and continuing weekly for the duration of stay and for 4wks after leaving. Most adverse events occur within 3 doses. Some Medical Letter consultants favor starting mefloquine 3 weeks prior to travel and monitoring the patient for adverse events, this allows time to change to an alternative regimen if mefloquine is not tolerated.

Table 4.9. Drugs for Parasitic Infections, continued

Infection	Drug	Adult dosage	Pediatric dosage
MICROSPORIDIOSIS			
Ocular (*Encephalitozoon hellem, E. cuniculi, Vittaforma corneae [Nosema corneum]*)			
Drug of choice:	Albendazole[7,12] **plus** fumagillin[95]*	400 mg PO bid	
Intestinal (*E. bieneusi, E. [Septata] intestinalis*)			
E. bieneusi			
Drug of choice:	Fumagillin[96]*	20 mg PO tid × 14d	
E. intestinalis			
Drug of choice:	Albendazole[7,12]	400 mg PO bid × 21d	
Disseminated (*E. hellem, E. cuniculi, E. intestinalis, Pleistophora sp., Trachipleistophora sp.* and *Brachiola vesicularum*)			
Drug of choice:[97]	Albendazole[7,12]*	400 mg PO bid	
Mites, see SCABIES			
MONILIFORMIS *moniliformis* infection			
Drug of choice:	Pyrantel pamoate[7,13]*	11 mg/kg PO once, repeat twice, 2wks apart	11 mg/kg PO once, repeat twice, 2wks apart

* Availability problems. See table on page 814.

92. The combination of weekly chloroquine (300 mg base) and daily proguanil (200 mg) is recommended by the World Health Organization (**www.WHO.int**) for use in selected areas; this combination is no longer recommended by the CDC. Proguanil (*Paludrine*—AstraZeneca, United Kingdom) is not available alone in the US but is widely available in Canada and Europe. Prophylaxis is recommended during exposure and for 4 weeks afterwards. Proguanil has been used in pregnancy without evidence of toxicity (PA Phillips-Howard and D Wood, Drug Saf 1996; 14:131).

93. Studies have shown that daily primaquine beginning 1d before departure and continued until 3–7d after leaving the malarious area provides effective prophylaxis against chloroquine-resistant *P. falciparum* (JK Baird et al, Clin Infect Dis 2003; 37:1659). Some studies have shown less efficacy against *P. vivax.* Nausea and abdominal pain can be diminished by taking with food.

94. A traveler can be given a course of medication for presumptive self-treatment of febrile illness. The drug given for self-treatment should be different from that used for prophylaxis. This approach should be used only in very rare circumstances when a traveler would not be able to get medical care promptly.

95. CM Chan et al, Ophthalmology 2003; 110:1420. Ocular lesions due to *E. hellem* in HIV-infected patients have responded to fumagillin eyedrops prepared from *Fumidil-B* (bicyclohexyl ammonium fumagillin) used to control a microsporidial disease of honey bees (MJ Garvey et al, Ann Pharmacother 1995; 29:872), available from Leiter's Park Avenue Pharmacy (see footnote 1). For lesions due to *V. corneae,* topical therapy is generally not effective and keratoplasty may be required (RM Davis et al, Ophthalmology 1990; 97:953).

96. Oral fumagillin (*Flisint*—Sanofi-Aventis, France) has been effective in treating *E. bieneusi* (J-M Molina et al, N Engl J Med 2002; 346:1963), but has been associated with thrombocytopenia and neutropenia. Highly active antiretroviral therapy (HAART) may lead to microbiologic and clinical response in HIV-infected patients with microsporidial diarrhea. Octreotide (*Sandostatin*) has provided symptomatic relief in some patients with large-volume diarrhea.

97. J-M Molina et al, J Infect Dis 1995; 171:245. There is no established treatment for *Pleistophora.* For disseminated disease due to *Trachipleistophora* or *Brachiola,* itraconazole 400 mg PO once/d plus albendazole may also be tried (CM Coyle et al, N Engl J Med 2004; 351:42).

Table 4.9. Drugs for Parasitic Infections, continued

Infection	Drug	Adult dosage	Pediatric dosage
Naegleria species, see AMEBIC MENINGOENCEPHALITIS, PRIMARY			
Necator americanus, see HOOKWORM infection			
OESOPHAGOSTOMUM bifurcum			
Drug of choice:	See footnote 98		
Onchocerca volvulus, see FILARIASIS			
Opisthorchis viverrini, see FLUKE infection			
Paragonimus westermani, see FLUKE infection			
Pediculus capitis, humanus, Phthirus pubis, see LICE			
Pinworm, see ENTEROBIUS			
PNEUMOCYSTIS JIROVECI (formerly *carinii*) pneumonia (PCP)[99]			
Drug of choice:	Trimethoprim/ sulfamethoxazole	TMP 15 mg/SMX 75 mg/kg/d, PO or IV in 3 or 4 doses × 21d	TMP 15 mg/SMX 75 mg/kg/d, PO or IV in 3 or 4 doses × 21d
Alternative:	Primaquine[7,79]	30 mg base PO daily × 21d	0.3 mg/kg base PO daily × 21d
	plus clindamycin[7,18]	600 mg IV q6h × 21d, or 300–450 mg PO q6h × 21d	15–25 mg/kg IV q6h × 21d, or 10 mg/kg PO q6h × 21d
OR	Trimethoprim[7]	5 mg/kg PO tid × 21d	5 mg/kg PO tid × 21d
	plus dapsone[7]	100 mg daily × 21d	2 mg/kg/d PO × 21d
OR	Pentamidine	3–4 mg/kg IV daily × 21d	3–4 mg/kg IV daily × 21d
OR	Atovaquone	750 mg PO bid × 21d	1–3mos: 30 mg/kg/d PO × 21d 4–24mos: 45 mg/kg/d PO × 21d >24mos: 30 mg/d PO × 21d

*Availability problems. See table on page 814.

98. Albendazole or pyrantel pamoate may be effective (JB Ziem et al, Ann Trop Med Parasitol 2004; 98:385).

99. Pneumocystis has been reclassified as a fungus. In severe disease with room air $PO_2 \leq 70$ mmHg or Aa gradient ≥ 35 mmHg, prednisone should also be used (S Gagnon et al, N Engl J Med 1990; 323:1444; E Caumes et al, Clin Infect Dis 1994; 18:319).

Table 4.9. Drugs for Parasitic Infections, continued

Infection	Drug	Adult dosage	Pediatric dosage
PNEUMOCYSTIS JIROVECI, continued			
Primary and secondary prophylaxis[100]			
Drug of Choice:	Trimethoprim/ sulfamethoxazole	1 tab (single or double strength) daily or 1 DS tab PO 3d/wk	TMP 150 mg/SMX 750 mg/m²/d PO in 2 doses 3d/wk
Alternative:	Dapsone[7]	50 mg PO bid or 100 mg PO daily	2 mg/kg/d (max. 100 mg) PO or 4 mg/kg (max. 200 mg) PO each wk
OR	Dapsone[7] **plus** pyrimethamine[101]	50 mg PO daily or 200 mg PO each wk 50 mg PO or 75 mg PO each wk	
OR	Pentamidine	300 mg aerosol inhaled monthly via *Respirgard II* nebulizer	≥5yrs: 300 mg inhaled monthly via *Respirgard II* nebulizer
OR	Atovaquone[7,20]	1500 mg PO daily	1–3mos: 30 mg/kg/d PO 4–24mos: 45 mg/kg/d PO >24mos: 30 mg/kg/d PO
River Blindness, see FILARIASIS			
Roundworm, see ASCARIASIS			
Sappinia diploidea, See AMEBIC MENINGOENCEPHALITIS, PRIMARY			
SCABIES (*Sarcoptes scabiei*)			
Drug of choice:	5% Permethrin	Topically once[102]	Topically once[102]
Alternative:[103]	Ivermectin[7,16,104]	200 mcg/kg PO once[102]	200 mcg/kg PO once[102]
	10% Crotamiton	Topically once/d × 2	Topically once/d PO × 2

* Availability problems. See table on page 814.
100. Primary/secondary prophylaxis in patients with HIV can be discontinued after CD4 count increases to >200 × 10⁶/L for >3mos.
101. Plus leucovorin 25 mg with each dose of pyrimethamine. Pyrimethamine should be taken with food to minimize gastrointestinal adverse effects.
102. Treatment may need to be repeated in 10–14 days. A second ivermectin dose taken 2 weeks later increases the cure rate to 95%, which is equivalent to that of 5% permethrin (V Usha et al, J Am Acad Dermatol 2000; 42:236; O Chosidow, N Engl J Med 2006; 354:1718; J Heukelbach and H Feldmeier, Lancet 2006; 367:1767).
103. Lindane (γ-benzene hexachloride) should be reserved for treatment of patients who fail to respond to other drugs. The FDA has recommended it not be used for immunocompromised patients, young children, the elderly, pregnant and breast-feeding women, and patients weighing <50 kg.
104. Ivermectin, either alone or in combination with a topical scabicide, is the drug of choice for crusted scabies in immunocompromised patients (P del Giudice, Curr Opin Infect Dis 2004; 15:123).

Table 4.9. Drugs for Parasitic Infections, continued

Infection	Drug	Adult dosage	Pediatric dosage
SCHISTOSOMIASIS (*Bilharziasis*)			
S. haematobium			
Drug of choice:	Praziquantel[139]	40 mg/kg/d PO in 2 doses × 1d	40 mg/kg/d PO in 2 doses × 1d
S. japonicum			
Drug of choice:	Praziquantel[139]	60 mg/kg/d PO in 3 doses × 1d	60 mg/kg/d PO in 3 doses × 1d
S. mansoni			
Drug of choice:	Praziquantel[139]	40 mg/kg/d PO in 2 doses × 1d	40 mg/kg/d PO in 2 doses × 1d
Alternative:	Oxamniquine[105]*	15 mg/kg PO once[106]	20 mg/kg/d PO in 2 doses × 1d[106]
S. mekongi			
Drug of choice:	Praziquantel[139]	60 mg/kg/d PO in 3 doses × 1d	60 mg/kg/d PO in 3 doses × 1d
Sleeping sickness, see TRYPANOSOMIASIS			
STRONGYLOIDIASIS (*Strongyloides stercoralis*)			
Drug of choice:[107]	Ivermectin[16]	200 mcg/kg/d PO × 2d	200 mcg/kg/d PO × 2d
Alternative:	Albendazole[7,12]	400 mg PO bid × 7d	400 mg PO bid × 7d
TAPEWORM infection			
–Adult (intestinal stage)			
Diphyllobothrium latum (fish), ***Taenia saginata*** (beef), ***Taenia solium*** (pork), ***Dipylidium caninum*** (dog)			
Drug of choice:	Praziquantel[7,39]	5–10 mg/kg PO once	5–10 mg/kg PO once
Alternative:	Niclosamide[108]*	2 g PO once	50 mg/kg PO once

*Availability problems. See table on page 814.

105. Oxamniquine, which is not available in the US, is generally not as effective as praziquantel. It has been useful, however, in some areas in which praziquantel is less effective (ML Ferrari et al, Bull World Health Organ 2003; 81:190; A Harder, Parasitol Res 2002; 88:395). Oxamniquine is contraindicated in pregnancy. It should be taken after food.

106. In East Africa, the dose should be increased to 30 mg/kg, and in Egypt and South Africa to 30 mg/kg/d × 2d. Some experts recommend 40–60 mg/kg over 2–3d in all of Africa (KC Shekhar, Drugs 1991; 42:379).

107. In immunocompromised patients or disseminated disease, it may be necessary to prolong or repeat therapy, or to use other agents. Veterinary parenteral and enema formulations of ivermectin have been used in severely ill patients with hyperinfection who were unable to take or reliably absorb oral medications (J Orem et al, Clin Infect Dis 2003; 37:152; PE Tarr;Am J Trop Med Hyg 2003; 68:453; FM Marty et al, Clin Infect Dis 2005; 41:e5). In disseminated strongyloidiasis, combination therapy with albendazole and ivermectin has been suggested (S Lim et al, CMAJ 2004; 171:479).

108. Niclosamide must be chewed thoroughly before swallowing and washed down with water.

Table 4.9. Drugs for Parasitic Infections, continued

Infection	Drug	Adult dosage	Pediatric dosage
TAPEWORM infection, continued			
***Hymenolepis nana* (dwarf tapeworm)**			
Drug of choice:	Praziquantel[7,39]	25 mg/kg PO once	25 mg/kg PO once
Alternative:	Nitazoxanide[5,7]	500 mg PO once/d or bid × 3d[109]	1–3yrs: 100 mg PO bid × 3d[109] 4–11yrs: 200 mg PO bid × 3d[109]
–Larval (tissue stage)			
Echinococcus granulosus (hydatid cyst)			
Drug of choice:[110]	Albendazole[12]	400 mg PO bid × 1–6mos	15 mg/kg/d (max. 800 mg) × 1–6mos
Echinococcus multilocularis			
Treatment of choice:	See footnote 111		
Taenia solium (Cysticercosis)			
Treatment of choice:	See footnote 112		
Alternative:	Albendazole[12]	400 mg PO bid × 8–30d; can be repeated as necessary	15 mg/kg/d (max. 800 mg) PO in 2 doses × 8–30d; can be repeated as necessary
OR	Praziquantel[7,39]	100 mg/kg/d PO in 3 doses × 1 day then 50 mg/kg/d in 3 doses × 29 days	100 mg/kg/d PO in 3 doses × 1 day then 50 mg/kg/d in 3 doses × 29 days

Toxocariasis, see VISCERAL LARVA MIGRANS

* Availability problems. See table on page 814.

109. JO Juan et al, Trans R Soc Trop Med Hyg 2002; 96:193; JC Chero et al, Trans R Soc Trop Med Hyg 2007; 101:203; E Diaz et al, Am J Trop Med Hyg 2003; 68:384.

110. Patients may benefit from surgical resection or percutaneous drainage of cysts. Praziquantel is useful preoperatively or in case of spillage of cyst contents during surgery. Percutaneous aspiration-injection-reaspiration (PAIR) with ultrasound guidance plus albendazole therapy has been effective for management of hepatic hydatid cyst disease (RA Smego, Jr. et al, Clin Infect Dis 2003; 37:1073; S Nepalia et al, J Assoc Physicians India 2006; 54:458; E Zerem and R Jusufovic Surg Endosc 2006; 20:1543).

111. Surgical excision is the only reliable means of cure. Reports have suggested that in nonresectable cases use of albendazole (400 mg bid) can stabilize and sometimes cure infection (P Craig, Curr Opin Infect Dis 2003; 16:437; O Lidove et al, Am J Med 2005; 118:195).

112. Initial therapy for patients with inflamed parenchymal cysticercosis should focus on symptomatic treatment with anti-seizure medication (LS Yancey et al, Curr Infect Dis Rep 2005; 7:39; AH del Brutto et al, Ann Intern Med 2006; 145:43). Patients with live parenchymal cysts who have seizures should be treated with albendazole together with steroids (dexamethasone 6 mg/d or prednisone 40–60 mg/d) and an anti-seizure medication (HH Garcia et al, N Engl J Med 2004; 350:249). Patients with subarachnoid cysts or giant cysts in the fissures should be treated for at least 30d (JV Proaño et al, N Engl J Med 2001; 345:879). Surgical intervention (especially neuroendoscopic removal) or CSF diversion followed by albendazole and steroids is indicated for obstructive hydrocephalus. Arachnoiditis, vasculitis or cerebral edema is treated with prednisone 60 mg/d or dexamethasone 4–6 mg/d together with albendazole or praziquantel (AC White, Jr., Annu Rev Med 2000; 51:187). Any cysticercocidal drug may cause irreparable damage when used to treat ocular or spinal cysts, even when corticosteroids are used. An ophthalmic exam should always precede treatment to rule out intraocular cysts.

Table 4.9. Drugs for Parasitic Infections, continued

Infection	Drug	Adult dosage	Pediatric dosage
TOXOPLASMOSIS (*Toxoplasma gondii*)			
Drug of choice:[113]	Pyrimethamine[114]	25–100 mg/d PO × 3–4wks	2 mg/kg/d PO × 2d, then 1 mg/kg/d (max. 25 mg/d) × 4wks[115]
	plus		
	sulfadiazine[116]	1–1.5 g PO qid × 3–4wks	100–200 mg/kg/d PO × 3–4wks
TRICHINELLOSIS (*Trichinella spiralis*)			
Drug of choice:	Steroids for severe symptoms		
	plus		
	Albendazole[7,12]	400 mg PO bid × 8–14d	400 mg PO bid × 8–14d
Alternative:	Mebendazole[7]	200–400 mg PO tid × 3d, then 400–500 mg tid × 10d	200–400 mg PO tid × 3d, then 400–500 mg tid × 10d
TRICHOMONIASIS (*Trichomonas vaginalis*)			
Drug of choice:[117]	Metronidazole	2 g PO once or 500 mg bid × 7d	15 mg/kg/d PO in 3 doses × 7d
OR	Tinidazole[6]	2 g PO once	50 mg/kg once (max. 2 g)

* Availability problems. See table on page 814.

113. To treat CNS toxoplasmosis in HIV-infected patients, some clinicians have used pyrimethamine 50–100 mg/d (after a loading dose of 200 mg) with sulfadiazine and, when sulfonamide sensitivity developed, have given clindamycin 1.8–2.4 g/d in divided doses instead of the sulfonamide. Treatment is usually given for at least 4–6 weeks. Atovaquone (1500 mg PO bid) plus pyrimethamine (200 mg loading dose, followed by 75 mg/d PO) for 6 weeks appears to be an effective alternative in sulfa-intolerant patients (K Chirgwin et al, Clin Infect Dis 2002; 34:1243). Atovaquone must be taken with a meal to enhance absorption. Treatment is followed by chronic suppression with lower dosage regimens of the same drugs. For primary prophylaxis in HIV patients with <100 × 10⁶/L CD4 cells, either trimethoprim-sulfamethoxazole, pyrimethamine with dapsone, or atovaquone with or without pyrimethamine can be used. Primary or secondary prophylaxis may be discontinued when the CD4 count increases to >200 × 10⁶/L for >3mos (MMWR Morb Mortal Wkly Rep 2004; 53 [RR15]:1). In ocular toxoplasmosis with macular involvement, corticosteroids are recommended in addition to antiparasitic therapy for an anti-inflammatory effect. In one randomized single-blind study, trimethoprim/sulfamethoxazole was reported to be as effective as pyrimethamine/sulfadiazine for treatment of ocular toxoplasmosis (M Soheilian et al, Ophthalmology 2005; 112:1876). Women who develop toxoplasmosis during the first trimester of pregnancy should be treated with spiramycin (3–4 g/d). After the first trimester, if there is no documented transmission to the fetus, spiramycin can be continued until term. If transmission has occurred in utero, therapy with pyrimethamine and sulfadiazine should be started (JG Montoya and O Liesenfeld, Lancet 2004; 363:1965). Pyrimethamine is a potential teratogen and should be used only after the first trimester.

114. Plus leucovorin 10–25 mg with each dose of pyrimethamine. Pyrimethamine should be taken with food to minimize gastrointestinal adverse effects.

115. Congenitally infected newborns should be treated with pyrimethamine every 2 or 3 days and a sulfonamide daily for about one year (JS Remington and JO Klein, eds, *Infectious Disease of the Fetus and Newborn Infant*, 6th ed, Philadelphia:Saunders, 2006, page 1038).

116. Sulfadiazine should be taken on an empty stomach with adequate water.

117. Sexual partners should be treated simultaneously with same dosage. Metronidazole-resistant strains have been reported and can be treated with higher doses of metronidazole (2–4 g/d × 7–14d) or with tinidazole (MMWR Morb Mortal Wkly Rep 2006; 55 [RR11]:1).

Table 4.9. Drugs for Parasitic Infections, continued

Infection	Drug	Adult dosage	Pediatric dosage
TRICHOSTRONGYLUS infection			
Drug of choice:	Pyrantel pamoate[7,13]*	11 mg/kg base PO once (max. 1 g)	11 mg/kg PO once (max. 1 g)
Alternative:	Mebendazole[7]	100 mg PO bid × 3d	100 mg PO bid × 3d
OR	Albendazole[7,12]	400 mg PO once	400 mg PO once
TRICHURIASIS (*Trichuris trichura*, whipworm)			
Drug of choice:	Mebendazole	100 mg PO bid × 3d or 500 mg once	100 mg PO bid × 3d or 500 mg once
	Albendazole[7,12]	400 mg PO × 3d	400 mg PO × 3d
OR	Ivermectin[7,16]	200 mcg/kg PO daily × 3d	200 mcg/kg/d PO × 3d
TRYPANOSOMIASIS[118]			
T. cruzi (American trypanosomiasis, Chagas' disease)			
Drug of choice:	Nifurtimox*	8–10 mg/kg/d PO in 3–4 doses × 90–120d	1–10yrs: 15–20 mg/kg/d PO in 4 doses × 90–120d
			11–16yrs: 12.5–15 mg/kg/d in 4 doses × 90–120d
OR	Benznidazole[119]*	5–7 mg/kg/d PO in 2 doses × 30–90d	<12yrs: 10 mg/kg/d PO in 2 doses × 30–90d
			>12 yrs: 5–7 mg/kg/d in 2 doses × 30–90d
T. brucei gambiense (West African trypanosomiasis, sleeping sickness) **hemolymphatic stage**			
Drug of choice:[120]	Pentamidine[7]	4 mg/kg/d IM × 7d	4 mg/kg/d IM × 7d
Alternative:	Suramin*	100–200 mg (test dose) IV, then 1g IV on days 1,3,7,14 and 21	20 mg/kg on d 1,3,7,14 and 21

* Availability problems. See table on page 814.

118. MP Barrett et al, Lancet 2003; 362:1469. Treatment of chronic or indeterminate Chagas' disease with benznidazole has been associated with reduced progression and increased negative seroconversion (R Viotti et al, Ann Intern Med 2006; 144:724).

119. Benznidazole should be taken with meals to minimize gastrointestinal adverse effects. It is contraindicated during pregnancy.

120. Pentamidine and suramin have equal efficacy, but pentamidine is better tolerated.

Table 4.9. Drugs for Parasitic Infections, continued

Infection	Drug	Adult dosage	Pediatric dosage
TRYPANOSOMIASIS[118] , continued			
Late disease with CNS involvement			
Drug of Choice:	Eflornithine[121]*	400 mg/kg/d IV in 4 doses × 14d	400 mg/kg/d IV in 4 doses × 14d
OR	Melarsoprol[122]	2.2 mg/kg/d IV × 10d	2.2 mg/kg/d IV × 10d
T. b. rhodesiense (East African trypanosomiasis, sleeping sickness)			
hemolymphatic stage			
Drug of choice:	Suramin*	100–200 mg (test dose) IV, then 1 g IV on days 1,3,7,14 and 21	20 mg/kg on d 1,3,7,14 and 21
Late disease with CNS involvement			
Drug of choice:	Melarsoprol[122]	2–3.6 mg/kg/d IV x 3d; after 7d 3.6 mg/kg/d × 3d; repeat again after 7d	2–3.6 mg/kg/d × 3d; after 7d 3.6 mg/kg/d × 3d; repeat again after 7d
VISCERAL LARVA MIGRANS[123] *(Toxocariasis)*			
Drug of choice:	Albendazole[7,12]	400 mg PO bid × 5d	400 mg PO bid × 5d
OR	Mebendazole[7]	100–200 mg PO bid × 5d	100–200 mg PO bid × 5d
Whipworm, see TRICHURIASIS			
Wuchereria bancrofti, see FILARIASIS			

* Availability problems. See table on page 814.

121. Eflornithine is highly effective in *T.b. gambiense*, but not in *T.b. rhodesiense* infections. In one study of treatment of CNS disease due to *T.b. gambiense*, there were fewer serious complications with eflornithine than with melarsoprol (F Chappuis et al, Clin Infect Dis 2005; 41:748). Eflornithine is available in limited supply only from the WHO. It is contraindicated during pregnancy.

122. E Schmid et al, J Infect Dis 2005; 191:1922. Corticosteroids have been used to prevent arsenical encephalopathy (J Pepin et al, Trans R Soc Trop Med Hyg 1995; 89:92). Up to 20% of patients with *T.b. gambiense* fail to respond to melarsoprol (MP Barrett, Lancet 1999; 353:1113). In one study, a combination of low-dose melarsoprol (1.2 mg/kg/d IV) and nifurtimox (7.5 mg/kg PO bid) × 10d was more effective than standard-dose melarsoprol alone (S Bisser et al, J Infect Dis 2007; 195:322).

123. Optimum duration of therapy is not known; some Medical Letter consultants would treat x 20d. For severe symptoms or eye involvement, corticosteroids can be used in addition (D Despommier, Clin Microbiol Rev 2003; 16:265).

Table 4.10. Safety of Antiparasitic Drugs in Pregnancy

Drug	Toxicity in Pregnancy	Recommendations
Albendazole (Albenza)	Teratogenic and embryotoxic in animals	Caution*
Amphotericin B (Fungizone, and others)	None known	Caution*
Amphotericin B liposomal (AmBisome)	None known	Caution*
Artemether/lumefantrine (Coartem, Riamet)[1]	Embryotoxic and teratogenic in animals	Caution*
Artesunate[1]	Embryotoxic and teratogenic in animals	Caution*
Atovaquone (Mepron)	Maternal and fetal toxicity in animals	Caution*
Atovaquone/proguanil (Malarone)[2]	Maternal and fetal toxicity in animals	Caution*
Azithromycin (Zithromax, and others)	None known	Probably safe
Benznidazole (Rochagan)	Unknown	Contraindicated
Chloroquine (Aralen, and others)	None known with doses recommended for malaria prophylaxis	Probably safe in low doses
Clarithromycin (Biaxin, and others)	Teratogenic in animals	Contraindicated
Clindamycin (Cleocin, and others)	None known	Caution*
Crotamiton (Eurax)	Unknown	Caution*
Dapsone	None known; carcinogenic in rats and mice; hemolytic reactions in neonates	Caution*, especially at term
Diethylcarbamazine (DEC; Hetrazan)	Not known; abortifacient in one study in rabbits	Contraindicated
Diloxanide (Furamide)	Safety not established	Caution*
Doxycycline (Vibramycin, and others)	Tooth discoloration and dysplasia, inhibition of bone growth in fetus; hepatic toxicity and azotemia with IV use in pregnant patients with decreased renal function or with overdosage	Contraindicated
Eflornithine (Ornidyl)	Embryocidal in animals	Contraindicated
Fluconazole (Diflucan, and others)	Teratogenic	Contraindicated for high dose; caution* for single dose
Flucytosine (Ancoban)	Teratogenic in rats	Contraindicated

Table 4.10. Safety of Antiparasitic Drugs in Pregnancy, continued

Drug	Toxicity in Pregnancy	Recommendations
Furazolidone (*Furoxone*)	None known; carcinogenic in rodents; hemolysis with G-6-PD deficiency in newborn	Caution*; contraindicated at term
Hydroxychloroquine (*Plaquenil*)	None known with doses recommended for malaria prophylaxis	Probably safe in low doses
Itraconazole (*Sporanox*, and others)	Teratogenic and embryotoxic in rats	Caution*
Iodoquinol (*Yodoxin*, and others)	Unknown	Caution*
Ivermectin (*Stromectol*)	Teratogenic in animals	Contraindicated
Ketoconazole (*Nizoral*, and others)	Teratogenic and embryotoxic in rats	Contraindicated; topical probably safe
Lindane	Absorbed from the skin; potential CNS toxicity in fetus	Contraindicated
Malathion, topical (*Ovide*)	None known	Probably safe
Mebendazole (*Vermox*)	Teratogenic and embryotoxic in rats	Caution*
Mefloquine (*Lariam*)[3]	Teratogenic in animals	Caution*
Meglumine (*Glucantine*)	Not known	Caution*
Metronidazole (*Flagyl*, and others)	None known – carcinogenic in rats and mice	Caution*
Miconazole (*Monistat i.v.*)	None known	Caution*
Miltefosine (*Impavido*)	Teratogenic in rats and induces abortions in animals	Contraindicated; effective contraception must be used for 2 months after the last dose
Niclosamide (*Niclocide*)	Not absorbed; no known toxicity in fetus	Probably safe
Nitazoxanide (*Alinia*)	None known	Caution*
Oxamniquine (*Vansil*)	Embryocidal in animals	Contraindicated
Paromomycin (*Humatin*)	Poorly absorbed; toxicity in fetus unknown	Oral capsules probably safe
Pentamidine (*Pentam 300, NebuPent*, and others)	Safety not established	Caution*
Permethrin (*Nix*, and others)	Poorly absorbed; no known toxicity in fetus	Probably safe
Praziquantel (*Biltricide*)	Not known	Probably safe
Primaquine	Hemolysis in G-6-PD deficiency	Contraindicated
Pyrantel pamoate (*Antiminth*, and others)	Absorbed in small amounts; no known toxicity in fetus	Probably safe

Table 4.10. Safety of Antiparasitic Drugs in Pregnancy, continued

Drug	Toxicity in Pregnancy	Recommendations
Pyrethrins and piperonyl butoxide (*RID*, and others)	Poorly absorbed; no known toxicity in fetus	Probably safe
Pyrimethamine (*Daraprim*)[4]	Teratogenic in animals	Caution*; contraindicated during 1st trimester
Quinacrine (*Atabrine*)	Safety not established	Caution*
Quinidine	Large doses can cause abortion	Probably safe
Quinine (*Qualaquin*)	Large doses can cause abortion; auditory nerve hypoplasia, deafness in fetus; visual changes, limb anomalies, visceral defects also reported	Caution*
Sodium stibogluconate (*Pentostam*)	Not known	Caution*
Sulfonamides	Teratogenic in some animal studies; hemolysis in newborn with G-6-PD deficiency; increased risk of kernicterus in newborn	Caution*; contraindicated at term
Suramin sodium (*Germanin*)	Teratogenic in mice	Caution*
Tetracycline (*Sumycin*, and others)	Tooth discoloration and dysplasia, inhibition of bone growth in fetus; hepatic toxicity and azotemia with IV use in pregnant patients with decreased renal function or with overdosage	Contraindicated
Tinidazole (*Tindamax*)	Increased fetal mortality in rats	Caution*
Trimethoprim (*Proloprim*, and others)	Folate antagonism; teratogenic in rats	Caution*
Trimethoprim-sulfamethoxazole (*Bactrim*, and others)	Same as sulfonamides and trimethoprim	Caution*; contraindicated at term

*Use only for strong clinical indication in absence of suitable alternative.
1. See also footnote 76 in Table 4.9. In animal studies, artemisinins have been embryotoxic and caused a low incidence of teratogenicity; no adverse pregnancy outcomes have been observed in limited studies in humans (S Dellicour et al, Malaria J, 2007;6:15).
2. See also footnote 68 in Table 4.9.
3. See also footnotes 74 and 90 in Table 4.9.
4. See also footnote 113 in Table 4.9.

Table 4.11. Manufacturers of Some Antiparasitic Drugs

albendazole – *Albenza* (GlaxoSmithKline)
§ *Albenza* (GlaxoSmithKline) – albendazole
Alinia (Romark) – nitazoxanide
AmBisome (Gilead) – amphotericin B, liposomal
• amphotericin B – *Fungizone* (Apothecon), others
amphotericin B, liposomal – *AmBisome* (Gilead)
Ancobon (Valeant) – flucytosine
§ *Antiminth* (Pfizer) – pyrantel pamoate
• *Aralen* (Sanofi) – chloroquine HCl and chloroquine phosphate
§ artemether – *Artenam* (Arenco, Belgium)
§ artemether/lumefantrine – *Coartem, Riamet* (Novartis)
§ *Artenam* (Arenco, Belgium) – artemether
§ artesunate – (Guilin No. 1 Factory, People's Republic of China)
atovaquone – *Mepron* (GlaxoSmithKline)
atovaquone/proguanil – *Malarone* (GlaxoSmithKline)
azithromycin – *Zithromax* (Pfizer), others
• *Bactrim* (Roche) – TMP/Sulfa
§ benznidazole – *Rochagan* (Brazil)
§ *Biaxin* (Abbott) – clarithromycin
§ *Biltricide* (Bayer) – praziquantel
† bithional – *Bitin* (Tanabe, Japan)
† *Bitin* (Tanabe, Japan) – bithional
§ *Brolene* (Aventis, Canada) – propamidine isethionate
chloroquine HCl and chloroquine phosphate – *Aralen* (Sanofi), others
clarithromycin – *Biaxin* (Abbott), others
• *Cleocin* (Pfizer) – clindamycin

clindamycin – *Cleocin* (Pfizer), others
Coartem (Novartis) – artemether/lumefantrine
crotamiton – *Eurax* (Westwood-Squibb)
dapsone – (Jacobus)
§ *Daraprim* (GlaxoSmithKline) – pyrimethamine USP
† diethylcarbamazine citrate (DEC) – *Hetrazan*
• *Diflucan* (Pfizer) – fluconazole
§ diloxanide furoate – *Furamide* (Boots, United Kingdom)
doxycycline – *Vibramycin* (Pfizer), others
eflornithine (Difluoromethylornithine, DFMO) – *Ornidyl* (Aventis)
§ *Egaten* (Novartis) – triclabendazole
Elimite (Allergan) – permethrin
Ergamisol (Janssen) – levamisole
Eurax (Westwood-Squibb) – crotamiton
• *Flagyl* (Pfizer) – metronidazole
§ *Flisint* (Sanofi-Aventis, France) – fumagillin
fluconazole – *Diflucan* (Pfizer), others
flucytosine – *Ancobon* (Valeant)
§ fumagillin – *Flisint* (Sanofi-Aventis, France)
• *Fungizone* (Apothecon) – amphotericin
§ *Furamide* (Boots, United Kingdom) – diloxanide furoate
§ furazolidone – *Furozone* (Roberts)
§ *Furozone* (Roberts) – furazolidone
† *Germanin* (Bayer, Germany) – suramin sodium
§ *Glucantime* (Aventis, France) – meglumine antimonate
† *Hetrazan* – diethylcarbamazine citrate (DEC)

---

* Available in the US only from the manufacturer.
§ Not available in the US; may be available through a compounding pharmacy.
† Available from the CDC Drug Service, Centers for Disease Control and Prevention, Atlanta, Georgia 30333; 404-639-3670 (evenings, weekends, or holidays: 770-488-7100).
• Also available generically.

Table 4.11. Manufacturers of Some Antiparasitic Drugs, continued

Humatin (Monarch) – paromomycin
§ *Impavido* (Zentaris, Germany) – miltefosine
iodoquinol – *Yodoxin* (Glenwood), others
itraconazole – *Sporanox* (Janssen-Ortho), others
ivermectin – *Stromectol* (Merck)
ketoconazole – *Nizoral* (Janssen), others
† *Lampit* (Bayer, Germany) – nifurtimox
Lariam (Roche) – mefloquine
§ *Leshcutan* (Teva, Israel) – topical paromomycin
levamisole – *Ergamisol* (Janssen)
lumefantrine/artemether – *Coartem, Riamet* (Novartis)
Malarone (GlaxoSmithKline) – atovaquone/proguanil
malathion – *Ovide* (Medicis)
mebendazole – *Vermox* (McNeil), others
mefloquine – *Lariam* (Roche)
§ meglumine antimonate – *Glucantime* (Aventis, France)
† melarsoprol – *Mel-B*
† *Mel-B* – melarsoprol
Mepron (GlaxoSmithKline) – atovaquone
metronidazole – *Flagyl* (Pfizer), others
§ miconazole – *Monistat i.v.*
§ miltefosine – *Impavido* (Zentaris, Germany)
§ *Monistat i.v.* – miconazole
NebuPent (Fujisawa) – pentamidine isethionate
Neutrexin (US Bioscience) – trimetrexate
§ niclosamide – *Yomesan* (Bayer, Germany)

† nifurtimox – *Lampit* (Bayer, Germany)
nitazoxanide – *Alinia* (Romark)
• *Nizoral* (Janssen) – ketoconazole
§ *Nix* (GlaxoSmithKline) – permethrin
§ ornidazole – *Tiberal* (Roche, France)
Ornidyl (Aventis) – eflornithine (Difluoromethylornithine, DFMO)
Ovide (Medicis) – malathion
§ oxamniquine – *Vansil* (Pfizer)
§ *Paludrine* (AstraZeneca, United Kingdom) – proguanil
§ paromomycin – *Humatin* (Monarch); *Leshcutan* (Teva, Israel; (topical formulation not available in US)
Pentam 300 (Fujisawa) – pentamidine isethionate
pentamidine isethionate – *Pentam 300* (Fujisawa), *NebuPent* (Fujisawa)
† *Pentostam* (GlaxoSmithKline, United Kingdom) – sodium stibogluconate
permethrin – *Nix* (GlaxoSmithKline), *Elimite* (Allergan)
§ praziquantel – *Biltricide* (Bayer)
primaquine phosphate USP
§ proguanil – *Paludrine* (AstraZeneca, United Kingdom)
proguanil/atovaquone – *Malarone* (GlaxoSmithKline)
§ propamidine isethionate – *Brolene* (Aventis, Canada)
§ pyrantel pamoate – *Antiminth* (Pfizer)
pyrethrins and piperonyl butoxide – *RID* (Pfizer), others
pyrimethamine USP – *Daraprim* (GlaxoSmithKline)
Qualaquin – quinine sulfate (Mutual Pharmaceutical Co/AR Scientific)
* quinidine gluconate (Eli Lilly)
§ quinine dihydrochloride

* Available in the US only from the manufacturer.
§ Not available in the US; may be available through a compounding pharmacy.
† Available from the CDC Drug Service, Centers for Disease Control and Prevention, Atlanta, Georgia 30333; 404-639-3670 (evenings, weekends, or holidays: 770-488-7100).
• Also available generically.

Table 4.11. Manufacturers of Some Antiparasitic Drugs, continued

quinine sulfate – *Qualaquin* (Mutual Pharmaceutical Co/AR Scientific)

Riamet (Novartis) – artemether/lumefantrine

- *RID* (Pfizer) – pyrethrins and piperonyl butoxide
- *Rifadin* (Aventis) – rifampin

rifampin – *Rifadin* (Aventis), others

§ *Rochagan* (Brazil) – benznidazole

* *Rovamycine* (Aventis) – spiramycin

† sodium stibogluconate – *Pentostam* (GlaxoSmithKline, United Kingdom)

* spiramycin – *Rovamycine* (Aventis)

- *Sporanox* (Janssen-Ortho) – itraconazole
- *Stromectol* (Merck) – ivermectin

sulfadiazine – (Eon)

† suramin sodium – *Germanin* (Bayer, Germany)

§ *Tiberal* (Roche, France) – ornidazole

Tindamax (Mission) – tinidazole

tinidazole – *Tindamax* (Mission)

TMP/Sulfa – *Bactrim* (Roche), others

§ triclabendazole – *Egaten* (Novartis)

trimetrexate – *Neutrexin* (US Bioscience)

§ *Vansil* (Pfizer) – oxamniquine

- *Vermox* (McNeil) – mebendazole
- *Vibramycin* (Pfizer) – doxycycline
- *Yodoxin* (Glenwood) – iodoquinol

§ *Yomesan* (Bayer, Germany) – niclosamide

- *Zithromax* (Pfizer) – azithromycin

*Available in the US only from the manufacturer.

§ Not available in the US; may be available through a compounding pharmacy.

†Available from the CDC Drug Service, Centers for Disease Control and Prevention, Atlanta, Georgia 30333; 404-639-3670 (evenings, weekends, or holidays: 770-488-7100).

• Also available generically.

MedWatch—The FDA Safety Information and Adverse Event Reporting Program

MedWatch, the Food and Drug Administration (FDA) Safety Information and Adverse Event Reporting Program, is an outreach program for the health care system, including physicians, nurses, pharmacists, and patients, to enhance the effectiveness of the FDA's risk management activities for all regulated clinical medical products. These products include prescription and over-the-counter drugs, biologicals, medical and radiation-emitting devices, and special nutritional products (eg, dietary supplements, infant formulas).

The MedWatch program has 2 goals: (1) to provide clinically useful and timely safety information about safety alerts, recalls and withdrawals to health care professionals and their patients; and (2) to encourage and facilitate reporting of serious adverse events. Reports are used by the FDA as a data source to identify and evaluate new safety concerns with drugs and devices after they are approved and more widely used in clinical practice. With this new information, the FDA can develop, with the manufacturer, a modified product, revised and strengthened professional labeling and patient instructions, and a modified use strategy that will lead to a safer product.

Health care professionals and consumers are encouraged to report problems and adverse events. The MedWatch voluntary form is a 1-page, postage-paid form (see Fig 4.1, p 818). An outline version that can be completed and submitted immediately to the FDA is available at the MedWatch Web site (**www.fda.gov/medwatch**). This form then can be returned by fax (800-FDA-0178) or mail. A toll-free number (800-FDA-1088) is available for health care professionals and consumers to report by phone or request blank forms with instructions.

Vaccine-related adverse events are not reported to MedWatch but should be reported to the Vaccine Adverse Event Reporting System (**http://vaers.hhs.gov/**) (see Reporting of Adverse Events, p 42).

FIG 4.1 MEDWATCH REPORTING FORM

MEDWATCH

The FDA Safety Information and
Adverse Event Reporting Program

For VOLUNTARY reporting of
adverse events, product problems and
product use errors

Page ____ of ____

A. PATIENT INFORMATION

1. Patient Identifier

In confidence

2. Age at Time of Event, or
   Date of Birth:

3. Sex
   ☐ Female
   ☐ Male

4. Weight
   _____ lb
   or _____ kg

B. ADVERSE EVENT, PRODUCT PROBLEM OR ERROR

Check all that apply:

1. ☐ Adverse Event   ☐ Product Problem (e.g., defects/malfunctions)
   ☐ Product Use Error   ☐ Problem with Different Manufacturer of Same Medicine

2. Outcomes Attributed to Adverse Event
   (Check all that apply)
   ☐ Death: _____ (mm/dd/yyyy)
   ☐ Life-threatening
   ☐ Hospitalization - initial or prolonged
   ☐ Required Intervention to Prevent Permanent Impairment/Damage (Devices)
   ☐ Disability or Permanent Damage
   ☐ Congenital Anomaly/Birth Defect
   ☐ Other Serious (Important Medical Events)

3. Date of Event (mm/dd/yyyy)

4. Date of this Report (mm/dd/yyyy)

5. Describe Event, Problem or Product Use Error

6. Relevant Tests/Laboratory Data, Including Dates

7. Other Relevant History, Including Preexisting Medical Conditions (e.g., allergies, race, pregnancy, smoking and alcohol use, liver/kidney problems, etc.)

C. PRODUCT AVAILABILITY

Product Available for Evaluation? (Do not send product to FDA)

☐ Yes   ☐ No   ☐ Returned to Manufacturer on: _____ (mm/dd/yyyy)

PLEASE TYPE OR USE BLACK INK

D. SUSPECT PRODUCT(S)

1. Name, Strength, Manufacturer (from product label)
   #1
   #2

2. Dose or Amount | Frequency | Route
   #1
   #2

3. Dates of Use (if unknown, give duration) from/to (or best estimate)
   #1
   #2

4. Diagnosis or Reason for Use (Indication)
   #1
   #2

5. Event Abated After Use Stopped or Dose Reduced?
   #1 ☐ Yes ☐ No ☐ Doesn't Apply
   #2 ☐ Yes ☐ No ☐ Doesn't Apply

8. Event Reappeared After Reintroduction?
   #1 ☐ Yes ☐ No ☐ Doesn't Apply
   #2 ☐ Yes ☐ No ☐ Doesn't Apply

6. Lot # | 7. Expiration Date
   #1 | #1
   #2 | #2

9. NDC # or Unique ID

E. SUSPECT MEDICAL DEVICE

1. Brand Name

2. Common Device Name

3. Manufacturer Name, City and State

4. Model #   Lot #
   Catalog #   Expiration Date (mm/dd/yyyy)
   Serial #   Other #

5. Operator of Device
   ☐ Health Professional
   ☐ Lay User/Patient
   ☐ Other:

6. If Implanted, Give Date (mm/dd/yyyy)

7. If Explanted, Give Date (mm/dd/yyyy)

8. Is this a Single-use Device that was Reprocessed and Reused on a Patient?
   ☐ Yes   ☐ No

9. If Yes to Item No. 8, Enter Name and Address of Reprocessor

F. OTHER (CONCOMITANT) MEDICAL PRODUCTS

Product names and therapy dates (exclude treatment of event)

G. REPORTER (See confidentiality section on back)

1. Name and Address

   Phone #   E-mail

2. Health Professional?   ☐ Yes ☐ No

3. Occupation

4. Also Reported to:
   ☐ Manufacturer
   ☐ User Facility
   ☐ Distributor/Importer

5. If you do NOT want your identity disclosed to the manufacturer, place an "X" in this box: ☐

FORM FDA 3500 (10/05)   Submission of a report does not constitute an admission that medical personnel or the product caused or contributed to the event.

Antimicrobial Prophylaxis

ANTIMICROBIAL PROPHYLAXIS

Antimicrobial agents commonly are prescribed to prevent infections in infants and children. The efficacy of prophylactic antimicrobial agents has been documented for some conditions but is unsubstantiated for many. *Prophylaxis* is defined as the use of antimicrobial drugs in the absence of suspected or documented infection to prevent development of an infection.

Effective chemoprophylaxis should be directed at specific pathogens, for infection-prone body sites, in vulnerable hosts. Examples are shown in Table 5.1 (p 820). In any situation in which prophylactic antimicrobial therapy is being considered, the risk of emergence of resistant organisms and the possibility of an adverse event must be weighed against potential benefits. Prophylactic agents should have as narrow a spectrum of antimicrobial activity as possible and should be used for as brief a period of time as possible. Uses of antimicrobial agents in doses or routes of administration other than oral, intramuscular, or intravenous, such as "antibiotic solutions" for irrigation or instillation, should not be considered prophylaxis and generally are unproven as efficacious for prevention of infection.

Infection-Prone Body Sites

Prevention of infection of vulnerable body sites is most likely to be successful if (1) the period of risk is defined and brief; (2) the expected pathogens have predictable antimicrobial susceptibility; and (3) the site is accessible to adequate antimicrobial concentrations.

Acute Otitis Media. Acute otitis media recurs less frequently in otitis-prone children treated prophylactically with antimicrobial agents. Studies have demonstrated that amoxicillin, sulfisoxazole, and trimethoprim-sulfamethoxazole are effective. However, antimicrobial prophylaxis may alter the nasopharyngeal flora and foster colonization with resistant organisms, compromising long-term efficacy of the prophylactic drug. Continuous orally administered antimicrobial prophylaxis should be reserved for control of recurrent acute otitis media, only when defined as 3 or more distinct and well-documented episodes during a period of 6 months or 4 or more episodes during a period of 12 months. Although prophylactic administration of an antimicrobial agent limited to a period of time when a person is at high risk of otitis media, such as during acute viral respiratory tract infection, has been suggested, this method has not been evaluated critically.

Urinary Tract Infection. The role of chemoprophylaxis for urinary tract infection has come under increasing scrutiny. The effectiveness of therapy depends on the rate of emergence of antimicrobial resistance in the gastrointestinal tract flora, which is the usual source of bacteria causing urinary tract infection.

Table 5.1. Antimicrobial Chemoprophylaxis[a]

Site-Related Infections	Exposed Host	Vulnerable Host (Pathogen)

Otitis media
Urinary tract
    infection
Endocarditis
	Bordetella pertussis exposure
	Neisseria meningitidis exposure
	Traveler's diarrhea
	   (*Escherichia coli, Shigella*
	   species, *Salmonella* species)
	Perinatal group B *Streptococcus*
	   (mother/infant) exposure
	Bite wound (human, animal,
	   reptile)
	Infants born to HIV-infected
	   mothers
		Oncology patients (*Pneumocystis jirovecii,*
		   fungi)
		HIV-infected children; (*Pneumocystis jirovecii;*
		   polysaccharide encapsulated bacteria)
		Preterm neonates (*Candida* species)
		Anatomic or functional asplenia
		   (polysaccharide-encapsulated bacteria)
		Chronic granulomatous disease (*Staphylo-
		   coccus aureus* and certain other catalase-
		   positive bacteria and fungi)
		Congenital immune deficiencies (various
		   pathogens)

HIV indicates human immunodeficiency virus.

[a]Prophylactic regimens are described in each pathogen- or disease-specific chapter in Section 3.

Exposure to Specific Pathogens

Prophylaxis may be appropriate or indicated if an increased risk of serious infection with a specific pathogen exists and a specific antimicrobial agent has been demonstrated to decrease the risk of infection by that pathogen. It is assumed that the benefit of prevention of infection is greater than the risk of adverse effects of the antimicrobial agent or the risk of subsequent infection by antimicrobial-resistant organisms. For some pathogens, such as *Neisseria meningitidis,* that colonize the upper respiratory tract, elimination of the carrier state that precedes infection can be difficult and may require use of a particular antimicrobial agent, such as rifampin, that achieves microbiologically effective concentrations in nasopharyngeal secretions, a property often lacking among antimicrobial agents ordinarily used to treat meningococcal infections.

Vulnerable Hosts

Attempts to prevent serious infections in vulnerable patients with antimicrobial prophylaxis have been successful in carefully defined populations that are known to be at risk of infection caused by defined pathogens. In some situations, such as prophylaxis of pneumococcal bacteremia in asplenic children, resistance to beta-lactam agents may lead to decreased effectiveness of continuous prophylaxis, while in other situations such as prophylaxis of *Pneumocystis* infections, anti-infective resistance has not appeared to develop despite years of continuous prophylaxis.

ANTIMICROBIAL PROPHYLAXIS IN PEDIATRIC SURGICAL PATIENTS

A major use of antimicrobial agents in hospitalized children is for prevention of post-operative wound infections through perioperative prophylaxis, generally for procedures with high infection rates, procedures involving implantation of prosthetic material, and procedures in which the consequences of infection are likely to be serious. Because of this common use, consensus recommendations for prevention of surgical site infections in adults and children have been developed. Although few data exist specifically for pediatric surgical prophylaxis, the principles of antimicrobial agent selection and exposure at the surgical site should apply reasonably to children. The consequences of inappropriate prophylactic use of antimicrobial agents include increased costs as a result of unnecessary drug use, potential emergence of resistant organisms, and unnecessary adverse events.

Guidelines for Appropriate Use

Guidelines for prevention of surgical site infections have been published.[1] General principles are presented with the understanding that future studies in children or application to settings unique to infants and children may justify modification of these recommendations.

Indications for Prophylaxis

Systemic prophylaxis is indicated when the probability or morbidity of postoperative infection is high and benefits of preventing wound infection outweigh potential risks from adverse drug reactions or emergence of resistant organisms. The latter poses a potential risk not only to the recipient but also to other hospitalized patients in whom a health care-associated infection caused by resistant organisms can develop. Procedures in which the benefits justify the risks incurred in antimicrobial prophylaxis are procedures associated with an increased incidence of postoperative infection and procedures in which the likelihood of infection may not be great but the adverse consequences of infection are extreme, such as with prosthetic materials.

Major determinants of postoperative surgical site infection include: number of micro-organisms in the wound during the procedure, virulence of microorganisms, presence of foreign material in the wound, and host risk factors. The classification of surgical procedures is based on an estimation of bacterial contamination and, thus, risk of subsequent infection. The 4 classes are: (1) clean wounds; (2) clean-contaminated wounds; (3) contaminated wounds; and (4) dirty and infected wounds. Additional independent factors include site of operation, duration of the procedure, and patient's preoperative health status. A patient risk index, which incorporates the American Society of Anesthesiologists preoperative physical status assessment score and the duration of the operation, in addition to the aforementioned wound classification, has been demonstrated to be a good predictor of postoperative surgical site infection.[2]

---

[1]Antimicrobial prophylaxis for surgery. *Treat Guidel Med Lett.* 2006;4(52):83–88

[2]Gaynes RP, Culver DH, Horan TC, Edwards JR, Richards C, Tolson JS. Surgical site infection (SSI) rates in the United States, 1992–1998: the National Nosocomial Surveillance System basic SSI risk index. *Clin Infect Dis.* 2001;33(suppl2):S69–S77

CLEAN WOUNDS

Clean wounds are uninfected operative wounds in which no inflammation is encountered and the respiratory, alimentary, and genitourinary tracts or oropharyngeal cavity are not entered. The operative procedures are elective, and wounds are closed primarily and, if necessary, drained with closed drainage. No break in aseptic technique occurs. Operative incisional wounds that follow nonpenetrating (blunt) abdominal trauma should be included in this category, provided that the surgical procedure does not entail entry into the gastrointestinal or genitourinary tracts. The benefits of systemic antimicrobial prophylaxis do not justify the potential risks associated with antimicrobial use in most clean wound procedures, because the risk of infection is low (1%–2%). Some exceptions exist in which either the risks or consequences of infection are high. Examples are implantation of intravascular prosthetic material (eg, insertion of a prosthetic heart valve) or a prosthetic joint, open-heart surgery for repair of structural defects, body cavity exploration in neonates, and most neurosurgical operations. Prophylaxis generally is given in these circumstances.

CLEAN-CONTAMINATED WOUNDS

In clean-contaminated operative wounds, the respiratory, alimentary, or genitourinary tracts are entered under controlled conditions with no significant contamination. Operations involving the gastrointestinal tract, the biliary tract, appendix, vagina, or oropharynx and urgent or emergency surgery in an otherwise clean procedure are included in this category, provided that no evidence of infection is encountered and no major break in aseptic technique occurs. Prophylaxis is limited to procedures in which a substantial amount of wound contamination is expected. The overall risk of infection for the surgical site is 3% to 15%. On the basis of data from adults, procedures for which prophylaxis is indicated for pediatric patients include the following: (1) all gastrointestinal tract procedures in which there is obstruction, when the patient is receiving H_2 receptor antagonists or proton pump blockers, or when the patient has a permanent foreign body; (2) selected biliary tract operations (eg, when there is obstruction from common bile duct stones); and (3) urinary tract surgery or instrumentation in the presence of bacteriuria or obstructive uropathy.

CONTAMINATED WOUNDS

Contaminated wounds are previously sterile tissue sites that are likely to be heavily contaminated with bacteria, and include open, fresh, accidental wounds; operative wounds in the setting of major breaks in aseptic technique or gross spillage from the gastrointestinal tract; exposed viscera at birth from congenital anomalies; penetrating trauma of fewer than 4 hours' duration; and incisions in which acute nonpurulent inflammation is encountered. The estimated rate of infection for the surgical site is 15%. In contaminated wound procedures, antimicrobial prophylaxis is appropriate for some patients with acute nonpurulent inflammation isolated to and contained within an inflamed viscus (such as acute appendicitis or cholecystitis). For wounds in which contaminating bacteria have had an opportunity to establish inflammation and ongoing infection, antimicrobial therapy should be considered treatment rather than prophylaxis.

DIRTY AND INFECTED WOUNDS

Dirty and infected wounds include penetrating trauma of more than 4 hours' duration, wounds with retained devitalized tissue, and wounds involving existing clinical infection or perforated viscera. This definition suggests that the organisms causing postoperative infection were present in the operative field before surgery. The estimated rate of infection for the surgical site is 40%. In dirty and infected wound procedures, such as procedures for a perforated abdominal viscus, a compound fracture, a laceration attributable to an animal or human bite, or major break in sterile technique, antimicrobial agents are given as treatment rather than prophylaxis.

Timing of Administration of Prophylactic Antimicrobial Agents

Effective prophylaxis occurs only when adequate drug concentrations in tissues are present when bacterial contamination occurs intraoperatively. Administration of an antimicrobial agent within 2 hours before surgery has been demonstrated to decrease the risk of wound infection. Accordingly, administration is recommended at least 30 minutes before surgical incision to ensure adequate tissue concentrations at the start of the procedure, although with antimicrobial agents requiring longer administration times, such as glycopeptides and aminoglycosides, the dose should be completed 30 minutes before the surgery begins.

Duration of Administration of Antimicrobial Agents

A single dose of an antimicrobial agent that provides adequate tissue concentrations throughout the surgical procedure is sufficient. When surgery is prolonged (more than 4 hours), major blood loss occurs, or an antimicrobial agent with a short half-life is used, redosing every 1 to 2 half-lives of the drug should provide adequate antimicrobial concentrations during the procedure. Postoperative doses after closure generally are not recommended.

Recommended Antimicrobial Agents

An antimicrobial agent is chosen on the basis of bacterial pathogens most likely to cause infectious complications after the specific procedure, the antimicrobial susceptibility pattern of these pathogens, and the safety and efficacy of the drug. New, more broad-spectrum and more costly antimicrobial agents generally are not recommended unless prophylactic efficacy has been proven to be superior to drugs of established benefit or there is a shift in organisms causing surgical site infections or in their antimicrobial resistance patterns. Antimicrobial agents administered prophylactically do not have to be active in vitro against every potential organism to be effective. Doses and routes of administration are determined on the basis of the need to achieve therapeutic blood and tissue concentrations throughout the procedure. Antimicrobial prophylaxis for most surgical procedures (including gastric, biliary, thoracic [noncardiac], vascular, neurosurgical, and orthopedic operations) can be achieved effectively using an agent such as a first-generation cephalosporin (eg, cefazolin). For colorectal surgery or appendectomy, effective prophylaxis requires antimicrobial agents that are active against aerobic and anaerobic intestinal flora. Table 5.2 (p 824) provides recommendations for drugs, including preoperative doses, to be used in children undergoing surgical manipulation or invasive procedures.

Table 5.2. Recommendations for Preoperative Antimicrobial Prophylaxis[a]

Operation	Likely Pathogens	Recommended Drugs	Preoperative Dose
Neonatal (≤72 h of age)— all major procedures	Group B streptococci, enteric gram-negative bacilli, enterococci	Ampicillin **PLUS** gentamicin	50 mg/kg 2.5–3 mg/kg
Neonatal (>72 h of age)— all major procedures	Prophylaxis targeted to colonizing organisms, nosocomial organisms, and operative site		
Cardiac (prosthetic valve or pacemaker)	*Staphylococcus epidermidis, Staphylococcus aureus, Corynebacterium* species, enteric gram-negative bacilli	Cefazolin **OR,** if MRSA[a] or MRSE is likely, vancomycin	25 mg/kg 10 mg/kg
Gastrointestinal			
Esophageal and gastroduodenal	Enteric gram-negative bacilli, gram-positive cocci	Cefazolin (high risk only[b])	25 mg/kg
Biliary tract	Enteric gram-negative bacilli, enterococci, clostridia	Cefazolin[c]	25 mg/kg
Colorectal or appendectomy (nonperforated)	Enteric gram-negative bacilli, enterococci, anaerobes	Cefoxitin; if high risk, gentamicin **PLUS** clindamycin or metronidazole ± ampicillin	40 mg/kg 2 mg/kg 10 mg/kg 10 mg/kg 50 mg/kg
Ruptured viscus	Enteric gram-negative bacilli, anaerobes, enterococci	Cefoxitin ± gentamicin **OR** gentamicin **PLUS** clindamycin **OR** meropenem	40 mg/kg 2 mg/kg 2 mg/kg 10 mg/kg 20 mg/kg
Genitourinary	Enteric gram-negative bacilli, enterococci	Ampicillin **PLUS** gentamicin	50 mg/kg 2 mg/kg

Table 5.2. Recommendations for Preoperative Antimicrobial Prophylaxis,[a] continued

Operation	Likely Pathogens	Recommended Drugs	Preoperative Dose
Head and neck surgery (incision through oral or pharyngeal mucosa)	Anaerobes, enteric gram-negative bacilli, *S aureus*	Gentamicin **PLUS** clindamycin **OR** cefazolin	2 mg/kg 10 mg/kg 25 mg/kg
Neurosurgery (craniotomy, ventricular shunt placement)	*S epidermidis, S aureus*	Cefazolin **OR**, if MRSA or MRSE is likely, vancomycin	25 mg/kg 10 mg/kg
Ophthalmic	*S epidermidis, S aureus, streptococci,* enteric gram-negative bacilli, *Pseudomonas* species	Gentamicin, ciprofloxacin, ofloxacin, moxifloxacin, tobramycin, **OR** neomycin–gramicidin–polymyxin B, **OR** cefazolin	Multiple drops topically for 2–24 h before procedure 100 mg, subconjunctivally
Orthopedic (internal fixation of fractures or prosthetic joints)	*S epidermidis, S aureus*	Cefazolin **OR**, if MRSA or MRSE is likely, vancomycin	25 mg/kg 10 mg/kg
Thoracic (noncardiac)	*S epidermidis, S aureus,* streptococci, gram-negative enteric bacilli	Cefazolin **OR**, if MRSA or MRSE is likely, vancomycin	25 mg/kg 10 mg/kg
Traumatic wound (nonbites)	*S aureus,* group A streptococci, *Clostridium* species	Cefazolin	25 mg/kg

[a]MRSA indicates methicillin-resistant *Staphylococcus aureus*; MRSE indicates methicillin-resistant *S epidermidis*.
[b]Esophageal obstruction, decreased gastric acidity or gastrointestinal motility; morbid obesity.
[c]Acute cholecystitis, nonfunctioning gallbladder, obstructive jaundice, common duct stones.

Physicians should be aware of potential interactions and adverse effects associated with prophylactic antimicrobial agents and other medications the patient may be receiving. Routine use of extended-spectrum cephalosporins for surgical prophylaxis generally is not recommended. Routine use of vancomycin for prophylaxis is not recommended, although for children known to be colonized or previously infected by methicillin-resistant *Staphylococcus aureus*, vancomycin may be considered.

PREVENTION OF BACTERIAL ENDOCARDITIS

The Committee on Rheumatic Fever, Endocarditis, and Kawasaki Disease of the American Heart Association issues detailed recommendations on the rationale, indications, and antimicrobial regimens for prevention of bacterial endocarditis for people at increased risk. The most recent recommendations were published in 2007.[1] The committee noted that recent data have cast doubt on the benefits of dental prophylaxis because bacteremia associated with most dental procedures represents only a fraction of the bacteremias that occur with daily living such as brushing teeth, chewing, and other oral hygiene measures. The committee has restricted recommendations for prophylaxis to a narrower group of individuals with cardiac abnormalities and for fewer procedures than in the past. While previous recommendations stressed prophylaxis for people undergoing procedures most likely to produce bacteremia, this revision stresses cardiac conditions in which an episode of infective endocarditis would have high risk of adverse outcome. Furthermore, prophylaxis is recommended only for certain dental procedures. Prophylaxis is no longer recommended solely to prevent endocarditis for procedures involving the respiratory, gastrointestinal and genitourinary tracts. The cardiac conditions and procedures for which endocarditis prophylaxis is recommended and specific prophylactic regimens, are shown below and in Table 5.3 (p 827). Health care professionals should consult the published recommendations for further details (**http://circ.ahajournals.org/cgi/content/full/116/15/1736**).

Cardiac conditions associated with the highest risk of adverse outcome from endocarditis for which prophylaxis with dental procedures is reasonable include the following[2]:
- Prosthetic cardiac valve or prosthetic material used for repair of valve.
- Previous infective endocarditis.
- Congenital heart disease (CHD)[2]:
  - Unrepaired cyanotic CHD, including palliative shunts and conduits.
  - Completely repaired congenital heart defect with prosthetic material or device, whether placed by surgery or by catheter intervention, during the first 6 months after the procedure.[3]

---

[1]Wilson W, Taubert KA, Gewitz M, et al. Prevention of Infective Endocarditis. Guidelines from the American Heart Association Rheumatic Fever, Endocarditis, and Kawasaki Diseases Committee, Council on Cardiovascular Disease in the Young, and the Council on Clinical Cardiology, Council on Cardiovascular Surgery and Anesthesia, and the Quality of Care and Outcomes Research Interdisciplinary Working Group. *Circulation.* 2007;116(15):1736–1754

[2]Except for the conditions listed, antimicrobial prophylaxis no longer is recommended for any other form of CHD.

[3]Prophylaxis is recommended, because endothelialization of prosthetic material occurs within 6 months after the procedure.

Table 5.3. Regimens for Antimicrobial Prophylaxis for a Dental Procedure

Situation	Agent	Regimen: Single Dose 30 to 60 min Before Procedure	
		Children	Adults
Oral	Amoxicillin	50 mg/kg	2 g
Unable to take oral medication	Ampicillin	50 mg/kg, IM or IV	2 g, IM or IV
	OR		
	Cefazolin or ceftriaxone	50 mg/kg, IM or IV	1 g, IM or IV
Allergic to penicillins or oral ampicillin	Cephalexin[a,b]	50 mg/kg	2 g
	OR		
	Clindamycin	20 mg/kg	600 mg
	OR		
	Azithromycin or clarithromycin	15 mg/kg	500 mg
Allergic to penicillins or ampicillin and unable to take oral medication	Cefazolin or ceftriaxone[b]	50 mg/kg, IM or IV	1 g, IM or IV
	OR		
	Clindamycin	20 mg/kg, IM or IV	600 mg, IM or IV

IM, indicates intramuscular; IV, intravenous.

[a]Or other first- or second-generation oral cephalosporin in equivalent pediatric or adult dosage.

[b]Cephalosporins should not be used in an individual with a history of anaphylaxis, angioedema, or urticaria with penicillins or ampicillin.

- Repaired CHD with residual defect(s) at the site or adjacent to the site of a prosthetic patch or prosthetic device (which inhibit endothelialization).
- Cardiac transplantation with subsequent cardiac valvulopathy.

Dental procedures for which endocarditis prophylaxis is reasonable for patients listed above include the following:

- All dental procedures that involve manipulation of gingival tissue or the periapical region of teeth or perforation of the oral mucosa. The following procedures and events do not require prophylaxis: routine anesthetic injections through noninfected tissue, taking dental radiographs, placement of removable prosthodontic or orthodontic appliances, adjustment of orthodontic appliances, placement of orthodontic brackets, shedding of deciduous teeth, and bleeding from trauma to the lips or oral mucosa.

PREVENTION OF NEONATAL OPHTHALMIA

Ophthalmia neonatorum is defined as conjunctivitis occurring within the first 4 weeks of life. The major causes of ophthalmia neonatorum are presented in Table 5.4 (p 829). The prevalence of infection with *Chlamydia trachomatis* and *Neisseria gonorrhoeae* in newborn infants is related directly to the prevalence of infection among pregnant women, whether pregnant women are screened and treated, and whether newborn infants are given ophthalmia prophylaxis. To prevent ophthalmia neonatorum, a prophylactic agent should be in instilled into the eyes of newborn infants. Ocular prophylaxis with these agents does not prevent perinatal transmission of *C trachomatis* from mother to infant. Screening of pregnant women for chlamydial and gonococcal infection followed by appropriate treatment and follow-up of all infected women and their partner(s) can minimize the risk of perinatal transmission (see Chlamydial Infections, p 252, and Gonococcal Infections, p 305). Not all women receive prenatal care, so ocular prophylaxis is warranted for all newborn infants.

Gonococcal Ophthalmia

For newborn infants, 0.5% erythromycin ointment or 1% tetracycline ophthalmic ointment are considered equally effective for prophylaxis of ocular gonorrheal infection. Each is available in single-dose forms, which are recommended, if possible. Use of povidone-iodine in a 2.5% solution also may be useful, but a product for this purpose is not available in the United States. Healthy infants born to women with untreated gonococcal infection should receive 1 dose of ceftriaxone (25–50 mg/kg, intravenously [IV] or intramuscularly [IM], not to exceed 125 mg) or 1 dose of cefotaxime (100 mg/kg, IV or IM). Topical antimicrobial therapy alone is inadequate. Topical therapy also is not necessary if systemic therapy is administered. Infants who have gonococcal ophthalmia should be hospitalized, evaluated for signs of disseminated infection, and treated (see Gonococcal Infections, p 305).

Chlamydial Ophthalmia

Neonatal ophthalmia attributable to *C trachomatis*, although not as severe as gonococcal conjunctivitis, is common in the United States, and suspected cases should be evaluated and treated (see Chlamydial Infections, p 252). Chlamydial conjunctivitis in the neonate, which differs from that in adults, is characterized by lack of follicular response, but the presence of mucopurulent discharge, eyelid swelling, and propensity to form membranes on the palpebral conjunctiva. Neonatal ocular prophylaxis with silver nitrate solution or erythromycin ointment for prevention of gonococcal ophthalmia does not prevent perinatal transmission of *C trachomatis* from mother to infant. Topical therapy does not treat pneumonia, which requires oral therapy, which should be given to newborn infants with laboratory-proven chlamydial conjunctivitis (see Chlamydial Infections, p 252).

Nongonococcal, Nonchlamydial Ophthalmia

Neonatal ophthalmia can be caused by many different bacterial respiratory tract pathogens (see Table 5.4, p 829). Silver nitrate, povidone-iodine, and probably erythromycin are effective for preventing nongonococcal, nonchlamydial conjunctivitis during the first 2 weeks of life.

Administration of Neonatal Ophthalmic Prophylaxis. Before administering local prophylaxis, each eyelid should be wiped gently with sterile cotton. Two drops of a 1% silver nitrate solution or a 1-cm ribbon of antimicrobial ointment (0.5% erythromycin or 1% tetracycline) is placed in each lower conjunctival sac. The eyelids then should be massaged gently to spread the ointment. After 1 minute, ointment may be wiped away with sterile cotton. None of the prophylactic agents should be flushed from the eyes after instillation, because flushing can decrease the efficacy of prophylaxis.

Table 5.4. Major and Minor Pathogens in Ophthalmia Neonatorum

Etiology of Ophthalmia Neonatorum	Proportion of Cases	Incubation Period (Days)	Severity of Conjunctivitis[a]	Associated Problems
Chlamydia trachomatis	2%–40%	5–14	+	Pneumonitis 3 wk–3 mo (see Chlamydial Infections, p 252)
Neisseria gonorrhoeae	Less than 1%	2–7	+++	Disseminated infection (see Gonococcal Infections, p 305)
Other bacterial microbes[b]	30%–50%	5–14	+	Variable
Herpes simplex virus[c]	Less than 1%	6–14	+	Disseminated infection (see Herpes Simplex, p 363); keratitis and ulceration also possible
Chemical	Varies with silver nitrate use	1	+	...

[a] + indicates mild; +++, severe.
[b] *Staphylococcus* species; *Streptococcus pneumoniae; Haemophilus influenzae,* nontypeable; *Streptococcus mitis;* group A and B streptococci; *Neisseria cinerea; Corynebacterium* species; *Moraxella catarrhalis; Escherichia coli; Klebsiella pneumoniae; Pseudomonas aeruginosa.*
[c] Herpetic conjunctivitis in the neonate is rare but can be associated with significant morbidity. See Herpes Simplex Virus Infections (p 363).

Infants born by cesarean delivery should receive prophylaxis against neonatal gonococcal ophthalmia. Although gonococcal and chlamydial infections usually are transmitted to the infant during passage through the birth canal, infection by the ascending route also occurs.

Prophylaxis should be given shortly after birth. Delaying prophylaxis for as long as 1 hour after birth to facilitate parent-infant bonding is unlikely to influence efficacy. Longer delays have not been studied for efficacy. Hospitals should establish a process to ensure that infants are given prophylaxis appropriately.

APPENDIX I

Directory of Resources[a]

Organization	Telephone/Fax Number	Website
AIDSinfo PO Box 6303 Rockville, MD 20849-6303 USA	1-800-HIV-0440 (1-800-448-0440, USA & Canada) 1-301-519-0459 (International) TTY: 1-888-480-3739 1-301-519-6616 (Fax)	www.aidsinfo.nih.gov
American Academy of Pediatrics (AAP) 141 Northwest Point Blvd Elk Grove Village, IL 60007-1098 USA	1-847-434-4000 or 1-800-433-9016 1-847-434-8000 (Fax) Publications/Customer Service: 1-866-THEAAP1 (1-866-843-2271)	www.aap.org
Canadian Paediatric Society (CPS) 2305 St Laurent Blvd Ottawa, Ontario K1G 4J8 Canada	1-613-526-9397 1-613-526-3332 (Fax)	www.cps.ca
Centers for Disease Control and Prevention (CDC)[b] 1600 Clifton Rd Atlanta, GA 30333	1-404-639-3311	www.cdc.gov
• **24-Hour Service**		
• Advisory Committee on Immunization Practices	1-404-639-2888 1-404-639-8836	www.cdc.gov/vaccines/recs/ACIP
• Botulism case consultation and antitoxin	1-770-488-7100	
• Division of Bacterial and Mycotic Diseases	1-404-639-1603	www.cdc.gov/ncidod/dbmd
• Division of Parasitic Diseases	1-770-488-7775 OR 1-770-488-7760	www.cdc.gov/ncidod/dpd/default.htm
• Division of Tuberculosis Elimination	1-404-639-8120	www.cdc.gov/nchstp/tb/default.htm
• Division of Vector-Borne Infectious Diseases	1-970-221-6400	www.cdc.gov/ncidod/dvbid/index.htm
• Division of Viral Hepatitis	1-888-4-HEP-CDC (1-888-443-7232)	www.cdc.gov/ncidod/diseases/hepatitis
• Division of Viral and Rickettsial Diseases	1-404-639-3574	www.cdc.gov/ncidod/dvrd/index.htm

Directory of Resources,[a] continued

Organization	Telephone/Fax Number	Website
Centers for Disease Control and Prevention (CDC),[b] continued		
• Contact Center	1-800-CDC-INFO (1-800-232-4636)	www.cdc.gov/netinfo.htm
• Drug Service (weekdays, 8 am to 4:30 pm ET)	1-404-639-3670	www.cdc.gov/ncidod/srp/drugs/drug-service.html
• Drug Service (weekends, nights, holidays)	1-404-639-2888	www.cdc.gov/ncidod/srp/drugs/drug-service.html
• Immunization, Infectious Diseases, and Other Health Information—	1-800-232-SHOT (1-800-232-7468)	
Voice Information System		www.cdc.gov/vaccines
Immunization Web Site		www.cdc.gov/flu
Influenza (seasonal) materials		www.cdc.gov/malaria
Malaria Hotline	1-770-488-7788	www.ashastd.org/learn/learn_hiv_aids_sup.cfm
National STD/AIDS Hotline	1-800-227-8922	www.cdc.gov/ncird/index.html
National Center for Immunization and Respiratory Diseases	1-404-639-8200	
	English Hotline: 1-800-232-4636	
	Spanish Hotline: 1-800-232-0233	
	1-888-CDC-FAXX (Fax) (1-888-232-3299)	
• National Prevention Information Network	1-800-458-5231	www.cdcnpin.org
• National Vaccine Injury Compensation Program (for information on filing claims)	1-800-338-2382	www.hrsa.gov/osp/vicp/
• Public Inquiries	1-404-639-3534	
• Publications	1-800-232-2522	www.cdc.gov/publications.htm#pubs
	1-404-639-8828 (Fax)	
• Traveler's Health Hotline and Fax	1-877-FYI-TRIP (877-394-8747)	www.cdc.gov/travel
	1-888-232-3299 (Fax toll free)	
• Vaccine Information Statements		www.cdc.gov/vaccines/pubs/default.htm
• VFC Operations Guide		www.cdc.gov/vaccines/programs/vfc/operations-guide.htm
• Voice/Fax Information Service (including international travel and immunization)	1-404-332-4555 (Voice)	www.cdc.gov/travel
	1-404-332-4565 (Fax)	

Directory of Resources,[a] continued

Organization	Telephone/Fax Number	Website
Food and Drug Administration (FDA) 5600 Fishers Ln Rockville, MD 20857-0001	1-888-463-6332	www.fda.gov
• Center for Biologics Evaluation and Research	1-301-827-2000 OR 1-800-835-4709	www.fda.gov/cber
• Center for Drug Evaluation and Research Division of Special Pathogen and Immunologic Drug Products	1-301-827-4570 1-301-796-1600 1-301-827-2475 (Fax)	www.fda.gov/cder
• HIV/AIDS Office of Special Health Issues • Kids' Vaccinations • MedWatch	1-301-827-4460 1-800-FDA-1088 (1-800-332-1088) 1-800-FDA-0178 (Fax) (1-800-332-0178)	www.fda.gov/oashi/aids/hiv.html www.fda.gov/fdac/reprints/vaccine.html www.fda.gov/medwatch
• Vaccine Adverse Event Reporting System (VAERS)	1-800-822-7967	www.fda.gov/cber/vaers/vaers.htm
Immunization Action Coalition (IAC) 1573 Selby Ave, Ste 234 St Paul, MN 55104	1-651-647-9009 1-651-647-9131 (Fax)	www.immunize.org
Infectious Diseases Society of America (IDSA) 66 Canal Center Plaza, Ste 600 Alexandria, VA 22314	1-703-299-0200 1-703-299-0204 (Fax)	www.idsociety.org
Institute of Medicine (IOM) The National Academies 500 Fifth St, NW Washington, DC 20001	1-202-334-2352	www.iom.edu

Directory of Resources,[a] continued

Organization	Telephone/Fax Number	Website
National Institutes of Health (NIH) 9000 Rockville Pike Bethesda, MD 20892	1-301-496-4000	www.nih.gov
• National Institute of Allergy and Infectious Diseases (NIAID)	1-301-496-2263	• www3.niaid.nih.gov
• NIAID Collaborative Antiviral Study Group • National Library of Medicine 8600 Rockville Pike Bethesda, MD 20894	• 1-205-934-5316 • 1-888-346-3656	• www.niaid.nih.gov/daids/pdatguide/casg.htm • www.nlm.nih.gov
National Network for Immunization Information (NNii) 301 University Blvd CH 2.218 Galveston, TX 77555-0351	1-409-772-0199 1-409-747-4995 (Fax)	www.immunizationinfo.org
National Vaccine Program Office (NVPO)	1-202-260-1253	www.hhs.gov/nvpo/
Pediatric AIDS Drug Trials—Information		
• Pediatric Branch, National Cancer Institute • Pediatric Clinical Trials Group (NIAID-sponsored)	1-301-496-4256 1-800-TRIALS-A (1-800-874-2572)	http://home.ccr.cancer.gov/oncology/pediatric/ http://www3.niaid.nih.gov/
Pediatric Infectious Diseases Society 66 Canal Center Plaza, Ste 600 Alexandria, VA 22314	1-703-299-6764 1-703-299-0473 (Fax)	www.pids.org
Women, Children, and HIV		www.womenchildrenhiv.org/wchiv?page_wx-00-00
World Health Organization (WHO) Avenue Appia 20 1211 Geneva 27 Switzerland	(+41 22) 791 21 11 (+41 22) 791 3111 (Fax)	www.who.int

[a] Internet addresses and telephone/fax numbers are current at the time of publication.

[b] See Appendix XII for services of the CDC or visit www.cdc.gov.

APPENDIX II

FDA Licensure Dates of Selected Vaccines in the United States[a]

Vaccine	Year Licensed
Diphtheria and tetanus toxoids and acellular pertussis (DTaP)	1991
Diphtheria and tetanus toxoids and whole-cell pertussis (DTP)	1970
Diphtheria and tetanus toxoids for children 7 y of age or older and adults (Td)	1953
Diphtheria and tetanus toxoids for children younger than 7 y of age (DT)	1970
DTaP-HepB-IPV (Pediarix)	2002
DTaP/Hib (TriHIBit)	1996
DTaP-IPV (Kinrix)	2008
DTaP-IPV/Hib (Pentacel)	2008
Haemophilus influenzae type b (Hib)	
Polysaccharide	1985
Conjugate (18 mo of age or older)	1987
Conjugate (6 wk of age or older)	1990
Hepatitis A (HepA)	1995
Hepatitis B (HepB)	
Plasma-derived	1981
Recombinant	1986
HepA-HepB (Twinrix)	2001
Hib/HepB (Comvax)	1996
Human papillomavirus (HPV)	2006
Influenza	
Inactivated (TIV)[b]	1945
Live, intranasal (LAIV)	2003
Meningococcal	
Polysaccharide (quadrivalent) (MPSV4)	1978
Conjugate (quadrivalent) (MCV4)	2005
Measles-mumps-rubella (MMR)	1963/1971
Measles-mumps-rubella-varicella (MMRV) (ProQuad)	2005
Pneumococcal	
Polysaccharide (14-valent)	1977
Polysaccharide (23-valent) (PPSV23)	1983
Conjugate (7-valent) (PCV7)	2000
Poliomyelitis	
Inactivated (IPV)	1987
Oral (trivalent) (OPV)	1963

FDA Licensure Dates of Selected Vaccines in the United States, continued

Vaccine	Year Licensed
Rabies	1980
Rotavirus (RV5) (RotaTeq)	2006
Rotavirus (RV1) (Rotarix)	2008
Tetanus toxoid, reduced diphtheria toxoid, and acellular pertussis (Tdap)	
Boostrix	2005
Adacel	2005
Tetanus (TT)	1943
Varicella (VAR)	1995
Zoster (ZOS)	2006

[a]The US Food and Drug Administration (FDA) maintains and updates a Web site listing vaccines licensed for immunization in the United States (**www.fda.gov/cber/vaccine/licvacc.htm**)
[b]Additional vaccines licensed subsequently.

APPENDIX III

CPT and ICD-9-CM Codes for Commonly Administered Pediatric Vaccines/Toxoids and Immune Globulins

CPT Code

Immune Globulin		Manufacturer	Brand	ICD-9-CM Code
90378	Respiratory syncytial virus immune globulin (RSV-IgIM), for intramuscular use, 50 mg, each	MedImmune	Synagis	V04.82
90379	Respiratory syncytial virus immune globulin (RSV-IgIV), human, for intravenous use	MedImmune	Respigam	V04.82

Vaccine	REMEMBER: Report with immunization administration code(s) (90465–90474)*	Manufacturer	Brand	ICD-9-CM Code
90633	Hepatitis A vaccine, pediatric/adolescent dosage, 2 dose, for intramuscular use	GlaxoSmithKline Merck	Havrix Vaqta	V05.3
90634	Hepatitis A vaccine, pediatric/adolescent dosage, 3 dose, for intramuscular use	GlaxoSmithKline	Havrix	V05.3
90645	Hemophilus influenza B vaccine (Hib), HbOC conjugate, 4 dose, for intramuscular use	Wyeth	HibTITER	V03.81
90647	Hemophilus influenza B vaccine (Hib), PRP-OMP conjugate, 3 dose, for intramuscular use	Merck	PedvaxHIB	V03.81
90648	Hemophilus influenza B vaccine (Hib), PRP-T conjugate, 4 dose, for intramuscular use	sanofi pasteur	ActHIB	V03.81
90649	Human Papilloma virus (HPV) vaccine, types 6, 11, 16, 18 (quadrivalent), 3 dose schedule, for intramuscular use	Merck	Gardasil	V04.89
90650	Human Papilloma virus (HPV) vaccine, types 16 and 18, bivalent, 3 dose schedule, for intramuscular use	✔	✔	V04.89
90655	Influenza virus vaccine, split virus, preservative free, for children 6–35 months of age, for intramuscular use	sanofi pasteur	Fluzone No Preservative Pediatric	V04.81

CPT and ICD-9-CM Codes for Commonly Administered Pediatric Vaccines/Toxoids and Immune Globulins, continued

CPT Code

Vaccine	REMEMBER: Report with immunization administration code(s) (90465–90474)*	Manufacturer	Brand	ICD-9-CM Code
90656	Influenza virus vaccine, split virus, preservative free, when administered to 3 years of age and above, for intramuscular use	sanofi pasteur Chiron GlaxoSmithKline	Fluzone No Preservative Fluvirin Fluarix	V04.81
90657	Influenza virus vaccine, split virus, 6–35 months dosage, for intramuscular use	sanofi pasteur	Fluzone	V04.81
90658	Influenza virus vaccine, split virus, 3 years and older dosage, for intramuscular use	sanofi pasteur Chiron	Fluzone Fluvirin	V04.81
90660	Influenza virus vaccine, live, intranasal use	MedImmune	FluMist	V04.81
90661	Influenza virus vaccine, derived from cell cultures, subunit, preservative and antibiotic free, for intramuscular use	⚡	⚡	V04.81
90662	Influenza virus vaccine, split virus, preservative free, enhanced immunogenicity via increased antigen content, for intramuscular use	⚡	⚡	V04.81
90663	Influenza virus vaccine, pandemic formulation	⚡	⚡	V04.81
90669	Pneumococcal conjugate vaccine, for children under 5 years, for intramuscular use	Wyeth	Prevnar	V03.82
90680	Rotavirus vaccine, pentavalent, 3 dose schedule, live, for oral use	Merck	Rotateq	V04.89
90681	Rotavirus vaccine, human, attenuated, 2 dose schedule, live, for oral use	GlaxoSmithKline	Rotarix	V04.89
90696	Diphtheria, tetanus toxoids, and acellular pertussis vaccine and poliovirus vaccine, inactivated (DTaP-IPV), when administered to children 4 years through 6 years of age, for intramuscular use	GlaxoSmithKline	Kinrix	V06.3
90698	Diphtheria, tetanus toxoids, acellular pertussis vaccine, haemophilus influenza Type B, and poliovirus vaccine, inactivated (DTaP-Hib-IPV), for intramuscular use	sanofi pasteur	Pentacel	V06.8

CPT and ICD-9-CM Codes for Commonly Administered Pediatric Vaccines/Toxoids and Immune Globulins, continued

CPT Code Vaccine	REMEMBER: Report with immunization administration code(s) (90465–90474)*	Manufacturer	Brand	ICD-9-CM Code
90700	Diphtheria, tetanus toxoids, and acellular pertussis vaccine (DTaP), when administered to younger than seven years, for intramuscular use	sanofi pasteur sanofi pasteur GlaxoSmithKline	Daptacel Tripedia Infanrix	V06.1
90702	Diphtheria and tetanus toxoids (DT), adsorbed when administered to younger than seven years, for intramuscular use	sanofi pasteur	Diphtheria and Tetanus Toxoids Adsorbed	V06.5
90707	Measles, mumps, and rubella virus vaccine (MMR), live, for subcutaneous use	Merck	M-M-R II	V06.4
90710	Measles, mumps, rubella, and varicella vaccine (MMRV), live, for subcutaneous use	Merck	ProQuad	V06.8
90713	Poliovirus vaccine (IPV), inactivated, for subcutaneous or intramuscular use	sanofi pasteur	Ipol	V04.0
90714	Tetanus and diphtheria toxoids (Td) adsorbed, preservative free, when administered to seven years or older, for intramuscular use	sanofi pasteur	Decavac	V06.5
90715	Tetanus, diphtheria toxoids and acellular pertussis vaccine (Tdap), when administered to 7 years or older, for intramuscular use	sanofi pasteur GlaxoSmithKline	Adacel Boostrix	V06.1
90716	Varicella virus vaccine, live, for subcutaneous use	Merck	Varivax	V05.4
90718	Tetanus and diphtheria toxoids (Td) adsorbed when administered to 7 years or older, for intramuscular use	sanofi pasteur	Tetanus and Diphtheria Toxoids Adsorbed for Adult Use	V06.5
90721	Diphtheria, tetanus toxoids, and acellular pertussis vaccine and Hemophilus influenza B vaccine (DTaP-Hib)	sanofi pasteur	TriHIBit	V06.8
90723	Diphtheria, tetanus toxoids, acellular pertussis vaccine, Hepatitis B, and poliovirus vaccine (DTaP-Hep B-IPV), for intramuscular use	GlaxoSmithKline	Pediarix	V06.8

CPT and ICD-9-CM Codes for Commonly Administered Pediatric Vaccines/ Toxoids and Immune Globulins, continued

CPT Code

Vaccine	REMEMBER: Report with immunization administration code(s) (90465–90474)*	Manufacturer	Brand	ICD-9-CM Code
90732	Pneumococcal polysaccharide vaccine, 23-valent, adult or immunosuppressed patient dosage, when administered to 2 years or older, for subcutaneous or intramuscular use	Merck	Pneumovax	V03.82
90733	Meningococcal polysaccharide vaccine, for subcutaneous use	sanofi pasteur	Menomune	V03.89

Vaccine		Manufacturer	Brand	ICD-9-CM Code
90734	Meningococcal conjugate vaccine, serogroups A, C, Y and W-135 (tetravalent), for intramuscular use	sanofi pasteur	Menactra	V03.89
90740	Hepatitis B vaccine, dialysis or immunosuppressed patient dosage, 3 dose, for intramuscular use	Merck	Recombivax HB	V05.3
90743	Hepatitis B vaccine, adolescent, 2 dose, for intramuscular use	Merck	Recombivax HB	V05.3
90744	Hepatitis B, pediatric/adolescent dosage, 3 dose, for intramuscular use	Merck GlaxoSmithKline	Recombivax HB Engerix-B	V05.3
90746	Hepatitis B vaccine, adult dosage, for intramuscular use	Merck GlaxoSmithKline	Recombivax HB Engerix-B	V05.3
90747	Hepatitis B vaccine, dialysis or immunosuppressed patient dosage, 4 dose, for intramuscular use	GlaxoSmithKline	Engerix-B	V05.3
90748	Hepatitis B and Hib (Hep B-Hib), for intramuscular use	Merck	Comvax	V06.8
90749	**Unlisted vaccine or toxoid**	**Please**	**See**	**ICD-9-CM**

CPT and ICD-9-CM Codes for Commonly Administered Pediatric Vaccines/Toxoids and Immune Globulins, continued

CPT Code

*Immunization Administration Codes

Immunization Administration Under Age 8 With Physician Counseling

CPT Code	
90465	Immunization administration, first injection
90466	Immunization admin, each additional injection
90467	Immunization admin by intranasal/oral route, first administration
90468	Immunization admin by intranasal/oral route, each additional administration

Immunization Administration

CPT Code	
90471	Immunization administration, one vaccine
90472	Immunization administration, each additional vaccine
90473	Immunization administration by intranasal/oral route; one vaccine
90474	Immunization administration by intranasal/oral route; each additional vaccine

✔ Vaccine pending FDA licensure; CPT code released 7/1/07 and implemented 1/1/08 [**http://www.ama-assn.org/ama/pub/category/10902.html**]

Developed and maintained by the American Academy of Pediatrics (AAP). For reporting purposes only.

For an updated table including changes and new codes, see **http://practice.aap.org/content.aspx?aid=2334.**

·······················

APPENDIX IV

National Childhood Vaccine Injury Act.
Reporting and Vaccine Injury Table.

This table includes adverse events that are reportable to the Vaccine Adverse Event Reporting System (VAERS) (see Vaccine Safety and Contraindications, p 40) as well as vaccines covered by the National Vaccine Injury Compensation Program (VICP), including all Food and Drug Administration (FDA)-licensed and Advisory Committee on Immunization Practices (ACIP)-approved vaccine(s) and combination products that have one or more vaccines listed in the Vaccine Injury Table.

Whenever a vaccine is added to the VICP, a person who believes he or she has been injured by a vaccine may file a claim for injuries that have occurred as long as 8 years before the effective date of the excise tax. Therefore, human papillomavirus (HPV) vaccine given in 2006 and thereafter will be covered by the VICP. The same is the case for meningococcal vaccines administered as long as 8 years before the February 1, 2007, effective date. A vaccine officially is added to the Vaccine Injury Table once an excise tax is applied. The intervals from immunization to the onset of an event for reporting to VAERS and for possible compensation by the Compensation Program are listed in the accompanying tables. Information for filing a claim can be obtained through the VICP Web site (**www.hrsa.gov/vaccinecompensation**).

Vaccine Injury Table[a]

Vaccine	Adverse Event	Time Interval
I. Tetanus toxoid-containing vaccines (eg, DTaP, Tdap, DTP-Hib; DT, Td, or TT)	A. Anaphylaxis or anaphylactic shock	0–7 days
	B. Brachial neuritis	0–28 days
	C. Any acute complication or sequela (including death) of above events	Not applicable
II. Pertussis antigen-containing vaccines (eg, DTaP, Tdap, DTP, P, DTP-Hib)	A. Anaphylaxis or anaphylactic shock	0–7 days
	B. Encephalopathy (or encephalitis)	0–7 days
	C. Any acute complication or sequela (including death) of above events	Not applicable
III. Measles, mumps, and rubella virus-containing vaccines in any combination (eg, MMR, MR, M, R)	A. Anaphylaxis or anaphylactic shock	0–7 days
	B. Encephalopathy (or encephalitis)	0–15 days
	C. Any acute complication or sequela (including death) of above events	Not applicable
IV. Rubella virus-containing vaccines (eg, MMR, MR, R)	A. Chronic arthritis	0–42 days
	B. Any acute complication or sequela (including death) of above event	Not applicable
V. Measles virus-containing vaccines (eg, MMR, MR, M)	A. Thrombocytopenic purpura	0–30 days
	B. Vaccine-Strain Measles Viral Infection in an immunodeficient recipient	0–6 mo
	C. Any acute complication or sequela (including death) of above events	Not applicable
VI. Polio live virus-containing vaccines (OPV)	A. Paralytic polio	
	• in a nonimmunodeficient recipient	0–30 days
	• in an immunodeficient recipient	0–6 mo
	• in a vaccine associated community case	Not applicable
	B. Vaccine-strain polio viral infection	
	• in a nonimmunodeficient recipient	0–30 days
	• in an immunodeficient recipient	0–6 mo
	• in a vaccine associated community case	Not applicable
	C. Any acute complication or sequela (including death) of above events	Not applicable
VII. Polio inactivated-virus-containing vaccines (eg, IPV)	A. Anaphylaxis or anaphylactic shock	0–4 hours
	B. Any acute complication or sequela (including death) of above event	Not applicable
VIII. Hepatitis B antigen-containing vaccines	A. Anaphylaxis or anaphylactic shock	0–4 hours
	B. Any acute complication or sequela (including death) of above event	Not applicable

Vaccine Injury Table,[a] continued

Vaccine	Adverse Event	Time Interval
IX. *Haemophilus influenzae* type b (polysaccharide conjugate vaccines)	A. No condition specified for compensation	Not applicable
X. Varicella vaccine	A. No condition specified for compensation	Not applicable
XI. Rotavirus vaccine	A. No condition specified for compensation	Not applicable
XII. Pneumococcal conjugate vaccines	A. No condition specified for compensation	Not applicable
XII. Any new vaccine recommended by the Centers for Disease Control and Prevention for routine administration to children, after publication by Secretary of Health and Human Services of a notice of coverage[b,c]	A. No condition specified for compensation	Not applicable

DTaP indicates diphtheria and tetanus toxoids and acellular pertussis; Tdap, tetanus toxoid, reduced diphtheria toxoid, and acellular pertussis; DTP, diphtheria and tetanus toxoids and pertussis; Hib, *Haemophilus influenzae* type b; DT, diphtheria and tetanus toxoids; Td, diphtheria and tetanus toxoids (for children 7 years of age or older and adults); TT, tetanus toxoid vaccine; P, pertussis; MMR, measles-mumps-rubella; MR, measles-rubella; M, measles; R, rubella; OPV, oral poliovirus; IPV, inactivated poliovirus.

[a]Effective date November 10, 2008.

[b]As of December 1, 2004, **hepatitis A vaccines (HAVs)** have been added to the Vaccine Injury Table under this category. As of July 1, 2005, **trivalent influenza vaccines (TIV, LAIV)** have been added to the Table under this category. Trivalent influenza vaccines are given annually during the influenza season either by needle and syringe or in a nasal spray. All influenza vaccines routinely administered in the United States are trivalent vaccines covered in this category.

[c]As of February 1, 2007, **meningococcal vaccines (MCV4, MPSV4)** and **human papillomavirus virus (HPV)** vaccines have been added to the Table under this category.

....

APPENDIX V

Nationally Notifiable Infectious Diseases in the United States

Public health officials at state health departments and the Centers for Disease Control and Prevention (CDC) collaborate in determining which diseases should be nationally notifiable (see Table, p 846). The Council of State and Territorial Epidemiologists, with advice from the CDC, makes recommendations annually for additions and deletions to the list of nationally notifiable diseases. A disease may be added to the list as a new pathogen emerges or may be deleted as its incidence decreases. However, reporting of nationally notifiable diseases to the CDC by the states is voluntary. Reporting is mandated (ie, by state legislation or regulation) by individual states. The list of diseases that are considered notifiable, therefore, varies slightly by state. Additional and specific requirements should be obtained from the appropriate state health department. All states generally report diseases that are quarantined internationally (ie, cholera, plague, and yellow fever) in compliance with the World Health Organization's International Health Regulations (**www.cdc.gov/mmwr/preview/mmwrhtml/mm5628a5.htm**).

When health care professionals suspect or diagnose a disease considered notifiable in the state, they should report the case by telephone or by mail to the local, county, or state health department. Clinical laboratories also report results consistent with reportable diseases. Staff members in the county or state health department implement disease-control measures as needed. The written case report is forwarded to the state health department.

The CDC acts as a common agent for states and territories for collecting information and reporting of nationally notifiable diseases. Reports of occurrences of nationally notifiable diseases are transmitted to the CDC each week from the 50 states, 2 cities (Washington, DC, and New York, NY), and 5 territories (American Samoa, Commonwealth of Northern Mariana Islands, Guam, Puerto Rico, and the Virgin Islands). Provisional data are published weekly in the *Morbidity and Mortality Weekly Report;* final data are published each year by the CDC in the annual "Summary of Notifiable Diseases, United States." The timelines of the provisional weekly reports provide information that the CDC and state or local epidemiologists use to detect disease occurrence and more effectively interrupt outbreaks. Reporting provides the timely information needed to measure and demonstrate the effect of changed immunization laws or a new therapeutic modality. The finalized annual data provide information on reported disease incidence that is necessary for study of epidemiologic trends and development of disease-prevention policies. The CDC is the sole repository for these national data, which are used widely by schools of medicine and public health, communications media, and pharmaceutical or other companies producing health-related products as well as by local, state, and federal health agencies and other agencies or people concerned with the trends of reportable conditions in the United States.

Table. Infectious Diseases Designated as Notifiable at the National Level—United States, 2009[a]

Acquired immunodeficiency Syndrome (AIDS)

Anthrax

Arboviral neuroinvasive and non-neuroinvasive diseases
- California serogroup virus disease
- Eastern equine encephalitis virus disease
- Powassan virus disease
- St Louis encephalitis virus disease
- West Nile virus disease
- Western equine encephalitis virus disease

Botulism
- Botulism, foodborne
- Botulism, infant
- Botulism, other (wound and unspecified)

Brucellosis

Chancroid

Chlamydia trachomatis, genital infections

Cholera

Coccidioidomycosis

Cryptosporidiosis

Cyclosporiasis

Diphtheria

Ehrlichiosis/anaplasmosis
- *Ehrlichia chaffeensis*
- *Ehrlichia ewingii*
- *Anaplasma phagocytophilum*
- Undetermined

Giardiasis

Gonorrhea

Haemophilus influenzae, invasive disease

Hansen disease (leprosy)

Hantavirus pulmonary syndrome

Hemolytic uremic syndrome, postdiarrheal

- Hepatitis, viral, acute
- Hepatitis A, acute
- Hepatitis B, acute
- Hepatitis B virus, perinatal infection
- Hepatitis C, acute

Hepatitis, viral, chronic
- Chronic hepatitis B
- Hepatitis C virus infection (past or present)

HIV infection
- HIV infection, adult/adolescent (13 y of age or older)
- HIV infection, child (age ≥18 mo and <13 y)

Influenza-associated pediatric mortality

Legionellosis

Listeriosis

Lyme disease

Malaria

Measles

Meningococcal disease

Mumps

Novel influenza A virus infections

Pertussis

Plague

Poliomyelitis, paralytic

Poliovirus infection, nonparalytic

Psittacosis

Q fever
- Acute
- Chronic

Rabies
- Rabies, animal
- Rabies, human

Rocky Mountain spotted fever

Rubella

Rubella, congenital syndrome

Salmonellosis

Severe acute respiratory syndrome-associated coronavirus (SARS-CoV) disease

Shiga toxin-producing *Escherichia coli* (STEC)

Shigellosis

Smallpox

Streptococcal disease, invasive, group A

Streptococcal toxic shock syndrome

Streptococcus pneumoniae, drug resistant, invasive disease

Streptococcus pneumoniae, invasive nondrug resistant, in children younger than 5 y of age

Syphilis
- Syphilis, primary
- Syphilis, secondary
- Syphilis, latent
- Syphilis, early latent
- Syphilis, late latent
- Syphilis, latent, unknown duration
- Neurosyphilis
- Syphilis, late, nonneurologic
- Syphilitic stillbirth

Syphilis, congenital

Tetanus

Toxic-shock syndrome (other than streptococcal)

Trichinellosis (trichinosis)

Tuberculosis

Tularemia

Typhoid fever

Vancomycin-intermediate *Staphylococcus aureus* (VISA)

Vancomycin-resistant *Staphylococcus aureus* (VRSA)

Varicella (morbidity)

Varicella (deaths only)

Vibriosis

Yellow fever

[a]www.cdc.gov/ncphi/disss/nndss/phs/infdis2009.htm

· ·

APPENDIX VI

Guide to Contraindications and Precautions to Immunizations, 2009

This information is based on recommendations of the Advisory Committee on Immunization Practices (ACIP) of the Centers for Disease Control and Prevention and the Committee on Infectious Diseases of the American Academy of Pediatrics (AAP). Sometimes, these recommendations vary from those in the manufacturers' package inserts. For more detailed information, health care professionals should consult published recommendations of the ACIP and AAP, manufacturers' package inserts, and **www.cdc. gov/nip/recs/contraindications_vacc.htm.** These guidelines, originally issued in 1993, have been updated to give current recommendations as of 2009 (based on information available as of January 2009).

Guide to Contraindications and Precautions to Immunizations, 2009

Vaccine	Contraindications	Precautions[a]	Not Contraindications (Vaccines May Be Given if Indicated)
General for all vaccines (DTaP, DT, Td, Tdap, IPV, MMR, MMRV, Hib, pneumococcal, meningococcal, hepatitis B, varicella, hepatitis A, influenza, zoster, rotavirus, HPV)	Anaphylactic reaction to a vaccine contraindicates further doses of that vaccine Anaphylactic reaction to a vaccine constituent contraindicates the use of vaccines containing that substance	Moderate or severe illnesses with or without fever Latex allergy[b]	Mild to moderate local reaction (soreness, redness, swelling) after a dose of an injectable antigen Low-grade or moderate fever after a previous vaccine dose Mild acute illness with or without low-grade fever Current antimicrobial therapy Convalescent phase of illnesses Preterm birth (same dosage and indications as for healthy, full-term infants) Recent exposure to an infectious disease History of penicillin or other nonspecific allergies or fact that relatives have such allergies Pregnancy of mother or household contact Unimmunized household contact Immunodeficient household contact Breastfeeding (nursing infant OR lactating mother)
DTaP	Encephalopathy within 7 days of administration of previous dose of DTaP/DTP	Temperature of 40.5°C (104.8°F) within 48 h after immunization with a previous dose of DTaP/DTP Collapse or shock-like state (hypotonic-hyporesponsive episode) within 48 h of receiving a previous dose of DTaP/DTP Seizures within 3 days of receiving a previous dose of DTaP/DTP[c] Persistent inconsolable crying lasting 3 h, within 48 h of receiving a previous dose of DTaP/DTP GBS within 6 wk after a dose[d]	Family history of seizures[c] Family history of sudden infant death syndrome Family history of an adverse event after DTaP/DTP administration

Guide to Contraindications and Precautions to Immunizations, 2009, continued

Vaccine	Contraindications	Precautions[a]	Not Contraindications (Vaccines May Be Given if Indicated)
DT, Td	Severe allergic reaction after a previous dose or to a vaccine component	GBS 6 wk or less after previous dose of tetanus toxoid-containing vaccine Moderate or severe acute illness with or without fever	
IPV	Anaphylactic reactions to neomycin, streptomycin, or polymyxin B	Pregnancy	…
MCV4 and MPSV4	Severe allergic reaction to any component of the vaccine, including diphtheria toxoid, or to dry natural rubber latex		
MMR[e,f]	Pregnancy Anaphylactic reaction to neomycin or gelatin Known altered immunodeficiency (hematologic and solid tumors, congenital immunodeficiency, severe HIV infection, and long-term immunosuppressive therapy)	Recent (within 3–11 mo, depending on product and dose) Immune Globulin administration[g] (see Table 3.35, p 450) Thrombocytopenia or history of thrombocytopenic purpura[g] Tuberculosis or positive PPD test result[h]	Simultaneous tuberculin skin testing[i] Breastfeeding Pregnancy of mother of recipient Immunodeficient family member or household contact Infection with HIV Nonanaphylactic reactions to gelatin or neomycin
Hib	None	…	…
Hepatitis B	Severe allergic reaction after a previous dose or to a vaccine component	Preterm birth[j]	Pregnancy
PCV7 and PPSV23	Severe allergic reaction to previous dose or vaccine component	Moderate or severe acute illness with or without fever	

Guide to Contraindications and Precautions to Immunizations, 2009, continued

Vaccine	Contraindications	Precautions[a]	Not Contraindications (Vaccines May Be Given if Indicated)
Tdap	Serious allergic reaction to any vaccine component History of encephalopathy (eg, coma, prolonged seizures) within 7 days of administration of a pertussis vaccine that is not attributable to another identifiable cause	GBS 6 wk or less after previous dose of a tetanus toxoid vaccine. Progressive neurologic disorder, uncontrolled epilepsy, or progressive encephalopathy until the condition has stabilized.	Temperature 105°F (40.5°C) or greater within 48 h after DTP/DTaP immunization not attributable to another cause Collapse or shock-like state (hypotonic hyporesponsive episode) within 48 h after DTP/DTaP immunization. Persistent crying lasting 3 h or longer, occurring within 48 h after DTP/DTaP immunization. Convulsions with or without fever, occurring within 3 days after DTP/DTaP immunization. History of ELS reaction after pediatric DTP/DTaP or Td immunization that was not an Arthus hypersensitivity reaction. Stable neurologic disorder, including well-controlled seizures, history of seizure disorder, and cerebral palsy. Brachial neuritis Latex allergy other than anaphylactic allergies (eg, a history of contact to latex gloves). The tip and rubber plunger of the Boostrix needleless syringe contain latex. This Boostrix product should not be administered to adolescents with a history of a severe (anaphylactic) allergy to latex but may be administered to people with less severe allergies (eg, contact allergy to latex gloves). The Boostrix single-dose vial and Adacel preparations do not contain latex. Pregnancy. Breastfeeding. Immunosuppression, including people with human immunodeficiency virus infection. Tdap poses no known safety concern for immunosuppressed people. The immunogenicity of Tdap in people with immunosuppression has not been studied and could be suboptimal. Intercurrent minor illness. Antimicrobial use.

Guide to Contraindications and Precautions to Immunizations, 2009, continued

Vaccine	Contraindications	Precautions[a]	Not Contraindications (Vaccines May Be Given if Indicated)
Varicella[e]	Pregnancy Severe allergic reaction after a previous dose or to a vaccine component (ie, neomycin or gelatin) Infection with HIV[k] Known altered immunodeficiency (hematologic and solid tumors, congenital immunodeficiency, and long-term immunosuppressive therapy)[l]	Recent Immune Globulin administration (see Table 3.34, p 448) Family history of immunodeficiency[m]	Pregnancy of mother of recipient Immunodeficiency in a household contact Household contact with HIV
Hepatitis A	Severe allergic reaction after a previous dose or to a vaccine component (ie, to 2-phenoxyethanol or alum)	Pregnancy	…
Influenza (inactivated)	Severe allergic reaction to a previous dose or vaccine component including eggs	GBS within 6 wk after a previous influenza immunization	Pregnancy
Influenza (live-attenuated)	Severe allergic reaction to a previous dose or vaccine component (including eggs); pregnancy; people with any underlying medical conditions that serve as an indication to give routine inactivated influenza immunization; children 2 through 4 years of age with health care professional or medical history documentation of wheezing within the past 12 mo; receiving aspirin; history of GBS after influenza vaccine	GBS within 6 wk after a previous influenza immunization	

Guide to Contraindications and Precautions to Immunizations, 2009, continued

Vaccine	Contraindications	Precautions[a]	Not Contraindications (Vaccines May Be Given if Indicated)
Rotavirus	Severe allergic reaction after a previous dose or to a vaccine component	Altered immunocompetence Moderate to severe acute gastroenteritis Moderate to severe febrile illness Chronic gastrointestinal disease Intussusception	Breastfeeding Immunodeficient family member or household contact
HPV	Severe allergic reaction after a previous dose or to a vaccine component	Administration to people with moderate or severe acute illness	Administration to people with minor acute illnesses
Zoster	Severe allergic reaction after any component of the vaccine; primary or acquired immunodeficiency disease; pregnancy	Severe acute illness	Mild acute illness

DTaP indicates diphtheria and tetanus toxoids and acellular pertussis; DT, pediatric diphtheria-tetanus toxoid; Td, adult tetanus-diphtheria toxoid; Tdap, tetanus toxoid, reduced diphtheria toxoid, and acellular pertussis; IPV, inactivated poliovirus; MMR, measles-mumps-rubella; Hib, *Haemophilus influenzae* type b; DTP, diphtheria and tetanus toxoids and pertussis; GBS, Guillain-Barré syndrome; MCV4, tetravalent (A, C, Y, W-135) meningococcal conjugate vaccine; MPSV4, tetravalent meningococcal polysaccharide vaccine; PPD, purified protein derivative (tuberculin); HIV, human immunodeficiency virus; PCV7, pneumococcal conjugate vaccine; PPSV23, pneumococcal polysaccharide vaccine; HPV, human papillomavirus.

[a]The events or conditions listed as precautions, although not contraindications, should be reviewed carefully. The benefits and risks of administering a specific vaccine to a person under the circumstances should be considered. If the risks are believed to outweigh the benefits, the immunization should be withheld; if the benefits are believed to outweigh the risks (eg, during an outbreak or foreign travel), the immunization should be given. Whether and when to administer DTaP to children with proven or suspected underlying neurologic disorders should be decided on an individual basis.

[b]If a person reports a severe (anaphylactic) allergy to latex, vaccines supplied in vials or syringes that contain natural rubber should not be administered unless the benefits of immunization outweigh the risks of an allergic reaction to the vaccine. For latex allergies other than anaphylactic allergies (eg, a history of contact allergy to latex gloves), vaccines supplied in vials or syringes that contain dry natural rubber or latex can be administered.

[c]Acetaminophen given before administering DTaP and thereafter every 4 hours for 24 hours should be considered for children with a personal or family (ie, siblings or parents) history of seizures.

[d]The decision to give additional doses of DTaP should be made on the basis of consideration of the benefit of further immunization versus the risk of recurrence of GBS. For example, completion of the primary series in children is justified.

[e]The administration of multiple live-virus vaccines within 30 days (4 weeks) of one another if not given on the same day may result in suboptimal immune response. Data substantiate this risk for MMR and varicella vaccine, which should therefore be given on the same day or more than 4 weeks apart.

[f]An anaphylactic reaction to egg ingestion previously was considered a contraindication unless skin testing and, if indicated, desensitization had been performed. However, skin testing no longer is recommended as of 1997.

Guide to Contraindications and Precautions to Immunizations, 2009, continued

Vaccine	Contraindications	Precautions[a]	Not Contraindications (Vaccines May Be Given if Indicated)

[a] The decision to immunize should be made on the basis of consideration of the benefits of immunity to measles, mumps, and rubella versus the risk of recurrence or exacerbation of thrombocytopenia after immunization or from natural infections of measles or rubella. In most instances, the benefits of immunization will be much greater than the potential risks and justify giving MMR, particularly in view of the even greater risk of thrombocytopenia after measles or rubella disease. However, if a previous episode of thrombocytopenia occurred in temporal proximity to immunization, not giving a subsequent dose may be prudent.

[b] A theoretical basis exists for concern that measles vaccine might exacerbate tuberculosis. Consequently, before administering MMR to people with untreated active tuberculosis, initiating antituberculosis therapy is advisable.

[c] Measles immunization may suppress tuberculin reactivity temporarily. MMR vaccine may be given after, or on the same day as, tuberculin skin testing. If MMR has been given recently, postpone the tuberculin skin test until 4 to 6 weeks after administration of MMR.

For preterm infants weighing less than 2 kg at birth and born to hepatitis B surface antigen (HBsAg)-negative mothers, initiation of immunization should be delayed until just before hospital discharge if the infant weighs 2 kg or more, or until approximately 2 months of age, when other routine immunizations are given, to improve response. All preterm infants born to HBsAg-positive mothers should receive immunoprophylaxis (Hepatitis B Immune Globulin and vaccine) beginning as soon as possible after birth, followed by appropriate postimmunization testing.

[k] Varicella vaccine should be considered for asymptomatic or mildly symptomatic HIV-infected children, specifically children in Centers for Disease Control and Prevention class N1 or A1, with age-specific T-lymphocyte percentages of 15% or higher.

[l] Varicella vaccine should not be administered to people who have cellular immunodeficiencies, but people with impaired humoral immunity may be immunized.

[m] Varicella vaccine should not be administered to a person who has a family history of congenital or hereditary immunodeficiency in parents or siblings unless that person's immune competence has been substantiated clinically or verified by a laboratory.

· ·

APPENDIX VII

Standards for Child and Adolescent Immunization Practices[1]

Recommended by the **National Vaccine Advisory Committee**
Approved by the **United States Public Health Service**
Endorsed by the **American Academy of Pediatrics**

The Standards represent consensus of the National Vaccine Advisory Committee (NVAC) and are endorsed by a variety of medical and public health organizations, including the American Academy of Pediatrics. The Standards constitute the most essential and desirable immunization practices and represent an important element in our national strategy to protect America's children against vaccine-preventable diseases. The Standards can be useful in helping health care professionals identify needed changes in their office practices and obtain resources to implement the desirable immunization practices.

Since the Standards were published initially in 1992, vaccine delivery in the United States has changed in several important ways. First, immunization coverage rates among preschool children have increased substantially and now are monitored by the National Immunization Survey. Second, immunization of children has shifted markedly from the public to the private sector, with an emphasis on immunization in the context of primary care and the medical home.[2] The Vaccines for Children Program has provided critical support to this shift by covering the cost of immunizations for the most economically disadvantaged children and adolescents. Third, development and introduction of performance measures, such as the National Committee for Quality Assurance's HEDIS (Health Employer Data and Information Set), have focused national attention on the quality of preventive care, including immunization. Finally, high-quality research in health services has helped to refine strategies for raising and sustaining immunization coverage levels among children, adolescents, and adults.

Health care professionals who immunize children and adolescents continue to face important challenges. These challenges include a diminishing level of experience with diseases that vaccines prevent among patients, parents, and physicians, the ready availability of vaccine-related information that may be inaccurate or misleading, the increasing complexity of the immunization schedule, the failure of many health plans to pay for the costs associated with immunization, and the focus on adolescent immunization.

The Standards are directed toward *health care professionals*, an inclusive term for the many people in clinical settings who share in the responsibility for immunization of children and adolescents: physicians, nurses, other practitioners (eg, nurse practitioners, physician assistants), medical assistants, and clerical staff. In addition to this primary audience, the Standards are intended to be useful to public health professionals, policy makers, health plan administrators, employers who purchase health care coverage, and others whose efforts shape and support the delivery of immunization services.

---

[1]The National Vaccine Advisory Committee. Standards for Pediatric and Adolescent Immunization Practices. *Pediatrics.* 2003;112(4):958–963

[2]American Academy of Pediatrics, Medical Home Initiatives for Children With Special Needs Project Advisory Committee. The medical home. *Pediatrics.* 2002;110(1):184–186 (Reaffirmed May 2008)

The use of the term *standards* should not be confused with a minimum standard of care. Rather, these Standards represent the most desirable immunization practices, which health care professionals should strive to achieve. Given current resource limitations, some health care professionals may find it difficult to implement all of the Standards, resulting from circumstances over which they have little control. The expectation is that, by summarizing the best immunization practices in a clear and concise format, the Standards will assist these health care professionals in securing resources necessary to implement this set of recommendations.

By adopting these Standards, health care professionals can enhance their own policies and practices, making achievement of immunization objectives for children and adolescents as outlined in *Healthy People 2010* both feasible and likely. Achieving these objectives will improve the health and welfare of all children and adolescents as well as the communities in which they live. Provided here are the Standards and resource information. Supporting information for each Standard can be found at **www.aap.org** and in *Pediatrics*.[1]

Standards For Child And Adolescent Immunization Practices

AVAILABILITY OF VACCINES

1. Vaccination services are readily available.
2. Vaccinations are coordinated with other health care services and provided within a medical home when possible.
3. Barriers to vaccination are identified and minimized.
4. Patient costs are minimized. (For information about the Vaccines for Children Program, see **www.cdc.gov/nip/vfc.**)

ASSESSMENT OF VACCINATION STATUS

5. Health care professionals review the vaccination and health status of patients at every encounter to determine which vaccines are indicated (see Fig 1.1–1.3, p 24–28).
6. Health care professionals assess for and follow only medically accepted contraindications (see Vaccine Contraindications and Precautions, p 46).

EFFECTIVE COMMUNICATION ABOUT VACCINE BENEFITS AND RISKS

7. Parents/guardians and patients are educated about the benefits and risks of vaccination in a culturally appropriate manner and in easy-to-understand language (see Table 1.2, p 6; Informing Patients and Parents, p 5; and Risks and Adverse Events, p 40).

PROPER STORAGE AND ADMINISTRATION OF VACCINES AND DOCUMENTATION OF VACCINATIONS

8. Health care professionals follow appropriate procedures for vaccine storage and handling (see Vaccine Handling and Storage, p 13).

---

[1]The National Vaccine Advisory Committee. Standards for Child and Adolescent Immunization Practices. *Pediatrics.* 2003;112(4):958–963

9. Up-to-date, written vaccination protocols are accessible at all locations where vaccines are administered.

10. People who administer vaccines and staff members who manage or support vaccine administration are knowledgeable and receive ongoing education. (Information about training programs is available at **www.cdc.gov/vaccines/ed/default.htm.**)

11. Health care professionals simultaneously administer as many indicated vaccine doses as possible.

12. Vaccination records for patients are accurate, complete, and easily accessible (see Record Keeping and Immunization Registries, p 38).

13. Health care professionals report adverse events following vaccination promptly and accurately to the Vaccine Adverse Event Reporting System (VAERS) and are aware of a separate program, the Vaccine Injury Compensation Program (VICP) (see Vaccine Safety and Contraindications, p 40).

14. All personnel who have contact with patients are appropriately vaccinated (see **www. cdc.gov/vaccines/recs/schedules/adult-schedule.htm**).

IMPLEMENTATION OF STRATEGIES TO IMPROVE VACCINATION COVERAGE

15. Systems are used to remind parents/guardians, patients, and health care professionals when vaccinations are due and to recall those who are overdue.

16. Office- or clinic-based patient record reviews and vaccination coverage assessments are performed annually.

17. Health care professionals practice community-based approaches.

....
Appendix VIII

Prevention of Disease From Potentially Contaminated Food Products[1]

Foodborne diseases are associated with significant morbidity and mortality in people of all ages. The Centers for Disease Control and Prevention (CDC) estimates that there are more than 76 million cases of foodborne diseases in the United States each year, resulting in approximately 325 000 hospitalizations and 5000 deaths. Young children, the elderly, and especially immunocompromised people particularly are susceptible to illness and complications caused by many of the organisms associated with foodborne illness. Four general rules to maintain safety of foods are:
- Wash hands and surfaces often.
- Separate—don't cross contaminate.
- Refrigerate foods promptly.
- Cook food to the proper temperature.

The following preventive measures can be implemented to decrease the risk of infection and disease from potentially contaminated food.

Unpasteurized milk and cheese. The American Academy of Pediatrics (AAP) strongly endorses the use of pasteurized milk and recommends that parents and public health officials be fully informed of the important risks associated with consumption of unpasteurized milk. Interstate sale of raw milk is banned by the US Food and Drug Administration (FDA). Children should not consume unpasteurized milk or products made from unpasteurized milk, such as cheese and butter, from species including cows, sheep, and goats. Serious systemic infections attributable to *Salmonella* species, *Campylobacter* species, *Mycobacterium bovis*, *Listeria monocytogenes*, *Brucella* species, *Escherichia coli* O157:H7, and *Yersinia enterocolitica* have been attributed to consumption of unpasteurized milk, including certified raw milk. In particular, an increasing number of outbreaks of campylobacteriosis among children are associated with school field trips to farms and consumption of raw milk. Raw milk consumption should be prohibited during educational trips. Cheese made from unpasteurized milk has been associated with illness attributable to *Brucella* species, *L monocytogenes*, *Salmonella* species, and *E coli* O157.

Eggs. Children should not eat raw or undercooked eggs, unpasteurized powdered eggs, or products containing raw eggs or undercooked eggs. Ingestion of raw or improperly cooked eggs can result in severe salmonellosis. Examples of foods that may contain raw or undercooked eggs include some homemade frostings and mayonnaise, ice cream from uncooked custard, tiramisu, eggs prepared "sunny-side up," fresh Caesar salad dressing, Hollandaise sauce, and cookie and cake batter.

Raw and undercooked meat. Children should not eat raw or undercooked meat or meat products, particularly hamburger. Various raw or undercooked meat products have been associated with disease, such as poultry with *Salmonella* or *Campylobacter* species; ground beef with *E coli* O157:H7 and other enterohemorrhagic *E coli* (also known as Shiga-toxin

---

[1]Centers for Disease Control and Prevention. Diagnosis and management of foodborne illnesses: a primer for physicians. *MMWR Recomm Rep.* 2001;50(RR-2):1–69. Additional information can be found at **www.cdc.gov/foodsafety, www.foodsafety.gov,** and **www.fsis.usda.gov/home/index.asp.**

producing *E coli*) or *Salmonella* species; hot dogs with *Listeria* species; pork with trichinosis; and wild game with brucellosis, tularemia, or trichinosis. Ground meats should be cooked to an internal temperature of 160°F. Using a food thermometer is the only sure way of knowing that food has reached a high enough temperature to destroy bacteria. Color is not a reliable indicator that ground beef patties have been cooked to a temperature high enough to kill harmful bacteria such as *E coli* O157:H7. Knives, cutting boards, plates, and other utensils used for raw meats should not be used for preparation of fresh fruits or vegetables until the utensils have been cleaned properly.

Unpasteurized juices. Children should drink only pasteurized juice products unless the fruit is washed and freshly squeezed (eg, orange juice) immediately before consumption. Consumption of packaged fruit and vegetable juices that have not undergone pasteurization or a comparable treatment have been associated with foodborne illness attributable to *E coli* O157:H7 and *Salmonella* species. To identify a packaged juice that has not undergone pasteurization or a comparable treatment, consumers should look for a warning statement that the product has not been pasteurized.

Seed sprouts. The FDA and the CDC have reaffirmed health advisories that people who are at high risk of severe foodborne disease, including children, people with compromised immune systems, and elderly people, should avoid eating raw seed sprouts until intervention methods are implemented to improve the safety of these products.[1] Raw seed sprouts have been associated with outbreaks of illness attributable to *Salmonella* species and *E coli* O157:H7.

Fresh fruits, vegetables, and nuts. Many fresh fruits and vegetables have been associated with disease attributable to *Cryptosporidium* species, *Cyclospora* species, noroviruses, hepatitis A virus, *Giardia* species, *E coli*, *Salmonella* species, and *Shigella* species. Washing can decrease but not eliminate contamination of fruits and vegetables. All fruits and vegetables should be washed with cool tap water immediately before consumption. Produce should be scrubbed with a clean produce brush. Knives, cutting boards, utensils, and plates used for raw meats should not be used for preparation of fresh fruits or vegetables until the utensils have been cleaned properly. Raw shelled nuts have been associated with outbreaks of salmonellosis.

Raw shellfish and fish. Children should not eat raw shellfish, especially raw oysters. Raw shellfish, including mussels, clams, oysters, scallops, and other mollusks, have been associated with many pathogens and toxins (see Appendix IX, p 860). *Vibrio* species contaminating raw shellfish may cause severe disease in people with liver disease or other conditions associated with decreased immune function. Some experts caution against children ingesting raw fish which has been associated with transmission of parasites.

Honey. Children younger than 1 year of age should not be given honey. Honey has been shown to contain spores of *Clostridium botulinum*. Light and dark corn syrups are manufactured under sanitary conditions, and although the manufacturer cannot ensure that any product will be free of *C botulinum* spores, no cases associated with light and dark corn syrups have been documented.

---

[1] For additional information, contact the FDA Food Information Line at 1-800-FDA-4010 or the US Department of Agriculture at 1-800-535-4555 or 1-202-720-2791 or visit the following Web sites: **www.usda.gov** and **www.foodsafety.gov.**

Food irradiation.[1] There is no process to eliminate all foodborne diseases; however, food safety experts believe that irradiation of food can be an effective tool in helping control foodborne pathogens. Irradiation involves exposing food briefly to radiant energy (such as gamma rays, x-rays, or high-voltage electrons) and often is referred to as "cold pasteurization." More than 40 countries worldwide have approved the use of irradiation for various types of foods. In addition, every governmental and professional organization that has reviewed the efficacy and safety of food irradiation has endorsed its use. Irradiated meat and some produce items are available to US consumers. The risk of foodborne illness in children can be decreased significantly with the routine consumption of irradiated meat, poultry, and produce.

---

[1]**www.fsis.usda.gov/Fact_Sheets/Irradiation_Resources/index.asp**

APPENDIX IX

Clinical Syndromes Associated With Foodborne Diseases[1]

Foodborne disease results from consumption of contaminated foods or beverages and causes morbidity and mortality in children and adults in developing and developed countries. The epidemiology of foodborne disease is complex and dynamic because of the large number of pathogens, the variety of disease manifestations, the increasing prevalence of immunocompromised children and adults, changes in dietary habits, and trends toward centralized food production and widespread distribution.

To aid in diagnosis, foodborne disease syndromes are categorized by incubation period, duration, causative agent, and foods commonly associated with specific etiologic agents (see Table, p 861). Diagnosis can be confirmed by laboratory testing of stool, vomitus, or blood, depending on the causative agent. An outbreak should be considered when 2 or more people who have ingested the same food develop an acute illness characterized by nausea, vomiting, diarrhea, or neurologic signs or symptoms. If an outbreak is suspected, local or state public health officials should be notified immediately so they can work with local health care professionals, coordinate laboratory testing not available locally, and conduct epidemiologic investigations to curtail the outbreak.

---

[1]Centers for Disease Control and Prevention. Surveillance for foodborne-disease outbreaks—United States, 1998–2002. *MMWR Surveill Summ.* 2006;55(SS-10):1–42. Additional information can be found at **www.cdc.gov/foodsafety** and **www.fsis.usda.gov/home/index.asp.**

Clinical Syndromes Associated With Foodborne Diseases

Clinical Syndrome	Causative Agents	Incubation Period	Commonly Associated Vehicles[a]
Nausea and vomiting	*Staphylococcus aureus* (preformed toxins, A, B, C, D, E)	<1–6 h	Ham, poultry, cream-filled pastries, potato and egg salads, mushrooms
	Bacillus cereus (emetic toxin)		Fried rice, meats
	Heavy metals (copper, tin, cadmium, iron, zinc)		Acidic beverages, metallic container
Flushing, dizziness, burning of mouth and throat, headache, gastrointestinal symptoms, urticaria	Histamine (scombroid)	<1 h	Fish (bluefish, bonita, mackerel, mahi-mahi, marlin, tuna)
Neurologic, including paresthesias Gastrointestinal tract symptoms	Ciguateratoxin	<1–6 h	Fish (amberjack, barracuda, grouper, snapper)
	Neurotoxic shellfish toxin (brevetoxin)		Shellfish
	Domoic acid		Mussels
	Monosodium glutamate		Chinese food
Neurologic, including confusion, salivation, hallucinations; gastrointestinal tract manifestations	Mushroom toxins (early onset)	0–2 h	Mushrooms
Neuromuscular weakness, gastrointestinal tract manifestations	*Clostridium botulinum* (descending paralysis)	12–48 h	Home-canned vegetables, fruits and fish, salted fish, meats, bottled garlic, potatoes baked in aluminum foil, cheese sauce, honey (infants)
	Tetrodotoxin (ascending paralysis)	<30 min	Puffer fish
	Paralytic shellfish toxins (saxitoxins, etc)	0.5–3 h	Shellfish (clams, muscles, oysters, scallops, other mollusks)
Abdominal cramps and watery diarrhea, vomiting	*B cereus* enterotoxin	6–24 h	Meats, stews, gravies, vanilla sauce
	Clostridium perfringens enterotoxin	6–24 h	Meat, poultry, gravy, dried or precooked foods
	Norovirus	16–72 h	Shellfish, salads, ice, cookies, water, sandwiches, fruit
	Rotavirus	1–3 days	Fecally contaminated foods (salads, fruits)
	Enterotoxigenic *Escherichia coli*	1–4 days	Fruits, vegetables, water
	Vibrio cholerae 01 and 039	1–5 days	Shellfish (including crabs and shrimp), fish, water
	V cholerae non-01		Shellfish
	Cyclospora species	1–14 days	Raspberries, vegetables, water

Clinical Syndromes Associated With Foodborne Diseases, continued

Clinical Syndrome	Incubation Period	Causative Agents	Commonly Associated Vehicles[a]
Diarrhea, fever, abdominal cramps, blood and mucus in stools	2–14 days 1–4 wk 16–≥72 h	*Cryptosporidium* species *Giardia intestinalis* *Salmonella* species	Vegetables, fruits, milk, water Water; food sources Poultry; pork; beef; eggs; dairy products, including ice cream; vegetables (alfalfa sprouts and fresh produce); fruit, including unpasteurized juices; peanut butter
Bloody diarrhea, abdominal cramps	1–3 days 2–4 wk 72–120 h	*Shigella* species Amebiasis Enterohemorrhagic *E coli*	Water, milk, other contaminated food Fecally contaminated food or water Beef (hamburger); raw milk; roast beef; salami; salad dressings; lettuce; unpasteurized juices, including apple cider; alfalfa and radish sprouts; water
Hepatorenal failure, watery diarrhea	6–24 h	Mushroom toxins (late onset)	Mushrooms (especially *Amanita* species)
Gastrointestinal tract manifestations, then symmetric descending paralysis including ophthalmoplegias and other bulbar symptoms (diplopia) blurred vision, dry mouth, dysarthria	12–48 h	*Clostridium botulinum*	Home-canned vegetables, fruits and fish, salted fish, meats, bottled garlic, potatoes baked in aluminum foil, cheese sauce, honey (infants)
Chronic, urgent diarrhea	Varied	Brainerd diarrhea	Unknown vehicle, but may include unpasteurized milk, and contaminated water
Other extraintestinal manifestations Fever, chills, headache, pharyngitis, arthralgia	Varied	*Brucella* species Group A streptococcus	Goat cheese, queso fresco, raw milk, meats Egg and potato salads
Fever, malaise, anorexia, jaundice		Hepatitis A virus	Shellfish, raw produce (ie, strawberries, lettuce, green onions)
Meningoencephalitis sepsis		*Listeria monocytogenes*	Cheese, raw milk, hot dogs, cole slaw, ready-to eat delicatessen meats
Muscle soreness and pain Bullous skin lesions, hypotension Fever, lymphadenopathy, neurologic (reactivation)		*Trichinella spiralis* *Vibrio vulnificus* *Toxoplasma gondii*	Pork, wild game, meat Shellfish (especially oysters) Beef, pork, lamb, venison

Clinical Syndromes Associated With Foodborne Diseases, continued

Clinical Syndrome	Incubation Period	Causative Agents	Commonly Associated Vehicles[a]
Sepsis, meningitis		*Enterobacter sakazakii*	Powdered infant formula
		Salmonella species	Powdered infant formula
Seizures, behavioral disturbances and other neurologic signs and symptoms		*Taenia* species (neurocysticercosis)	Food contaminated with feces from a human carrier of adult pork tapeworm
Epigastric discomfort, abdominal pain, cholangitis, obstructive jaundice, pancreatitis		*Clonorchis sinensis*	Fish
		Opisthorchis species	Fish
Guillain-Barré syndrome (ascending paralysis)	Varied	*Campylobacter jejuni*	Poultry, raw milk, water
		Shigella	Egg salad, vegetables, scallions
		Enteroinvasive *E coli*	Vegetables, hamburger, raw milk
		Yersinia enterocolitica	Pork chiterlings, tofu, raw milk
		Vibrio parahaemolyticus	Fish, shellfish
Hemolytic-uremic syndrome (acute renal failure, hemolytic anemia, thrombocytopenia)	Varied	Enterohemorrhagic *E coli* (especially serotype O157:H7)	Beef (hamburger); raw milk; roast beef; salami, salad dressings; lettuce; unpasteurized juices, including apple cider; alfalfa and radish sprouts; water
		Shigella dysenteriae 1	Water, milk, other contaminated food
Reactive arthritis	Varied	*Campylobacter* species	Water, milk, other contaminated food
		Salmonella species	Poultry; pork; beef; eggs; dairy products, including ice cream; vegetables (alfalfa sprouts and fresh produce); fruit, including unpasteurized juices; peanut butter
		Shigella species	Poultry, raw milk, water
		Yersinia enterocolitica	Pork chiterlings, tofu, raw milk

[a]List of vehicles in several categories is not exhaustive, because any number of foods can be fecally contaminated.

····················
APPENDIX X

Diseases Transmitted by Animals (Zoonoses)

Important zoonoses that may be encountered in North America are listed in this Appendix and reviewed in the *Red Book* (see disease-specific chapters in Section 3 for further information). Morbidity resulting from selected zoonotic diseases in the United States is reported annually by the Centers for Disease Control and Prevention (see "Summary of Notifiable Diseases" at **www.cdc.gov/epo/dphsi/annsum**). Information also can be obtained via the Web site of the National Center for Zoonotic, Vector-borne, and Enteric Diseases: **www.cdc.gov/nczved** or through the main Centers for Disease Control and Prevention Web site: **www.cdc.gov.**

Table. Diseases Transmitted by Animals

Disease and/or Organism	Common Animal Sources/Reservoirs	Vector or Modes of Transmission
Bacterial Diseases		
Aeromonas species	Aquatic animals, especially shellfish	Wound infection, ingestion of contaminated food or water
Anthrax (*Bacillus anthracis*)	Herbivores (cattle, goats, sheep)	Direct contact with infected animals or contact with animal products (eg, hides) contaminated with *B anthracis* spores
Bartonellosis (*Bartonella* species, *B vinsonii vinsonii, B vinsonii berkhoffi, B v arupensis, B koehleri, B rochalaime, B quintana*)	Dogs, cattle, cats, body lice	Bites of arthropods suspected, but evidence is lacking in many species
Brucellosis (*Brucella* species)	Cattle, goats, sheep, swine, rarely dogs, elk, bison, deer	Direct contact with birth products, ingestion of contaminated dairy products, inhalation of aerosols, through skin wounds
Campylobacteriosis (*Campylobacter jejuni*)	Poultry, dogs (especially puppies), kittens, ferrets, hamsters, birds	Ingestion of contaminated food, water, milk, direct contact (particularly with animals with diarrhea), person-to-person (fecal-oral)
Capnocytophaga caninorsus	Dogs, rarely cats	Bites, scratches, and contact
Cat-scratch disease (*Bartonella henselae*)	Cats, infrequently other animals (less than 10%)	Scratches, bites; fleas play a role in cat-to-cat transmission (evidence for transmission from cat fleas to humans is lacking)
Erysipelothrix rhusiopathiae	Pigs, sheep, cattle, horses, birds, fish, shellfish	Direct contact with animal or contaminated animal product
Hemolytic-uremic syndrome (eg, Shiga toxin-producing *Escherichia coli*) (STEC)	Cattle, sheep, goats, deer	Ingestion of undercooked contaminated ground beef, unpasteurized milk, or other contaminated foods or water, person-to-person contact (fecal-oral), petting zoo contact, county fairs (fecal-oral)
Leptospirosis (*Leptospira* species)	Dogs, rats, livestock, other wild animals	Contact with or ingestion of water, food, or soil contaminated with urine
Lyme disease (*Borrelia burgdorferi*)	Mice, squirrels, shrews, and other small vertebrates	Black legged or deer tick bites (*Ixodes scapularis* or *I pacificus*)

Table. Diseases Transmitted by Animals, continued

Disease and/or Organism	Common Animal Sources/Reservoirs	Vector or Modes of Transmission
Mycobacteriosis (*Mycobacterium marinum*, others)	Fish (and cleaning aquaria)	Skin injury or contamination of existing wound
Mycobacterium tuberculosis	Elephants, giraffes, rhinoceroses, bison, deer, elk	Airborne
Pasteurella multocida	Cats, dogs, other animals	Bites, scratches, licks
Plague (*Yersinia pestis*)	Rodents, cats, ground squirrels, prairie dogs	Bite of rodent fleas, (especially tropical rat fleas, *Xenopsylla cheopis*), direct contact with infected animals, person-to-person with pneumonic plague
Rat-bite fever (*Streptobacillus moniliformis*, *Spirillum minus*)	Rodents (especially rats, occasionally squirrels), cats, weasels, gerbils	Bites, secretions, and contaminated food, milk, and water
Relapsing fever (tickborne) (*Borrelia* species)	Wild rodents	Soft tick bites (*Ornithodoros* species)
Salmonellosis (*Salmonella* species)	Poultry, lizards, snakes, salamanders, iguanas, dogs, cats, rodents, ferrets, turtles, other wild and domestic animals, hamsters, hedgehogs, Komodo dragons	Ingestion of contaminated food, milk, and water; direct contact; contact with fecally contaminated surfaces; person-to-person (fecal-oral)
Streptococcus iniae	Fish grown by aquaculture	Skin injury during handling of fish
Tetanus (*Clostridium tetani*)	Any animal, usually indirect via soil containing animal feces	Wound infection, skin injury or soft tissue injury with inoculation of bacteria (as from soil or a contaminated object), contaminated bites
Tularemia (*Francisella tularensis*)	Wild rabbits, hares, voles, sheep, cattle, muskrats, moles, cats, hamsters	Wood tick bites (*Dermacentor andersoni*), dog tick bites (*D variabilis*), Lone-star tick bites (*Amblyomma americanum*), deerfly bites, direct contact with infected animal, ingestion of contaminated water, mechanical transmission from claws or teeth (cats), aerosolization of tissues or excreta
Vibrio species	Shellfish	Skin injury or contamination of existing wound, ingestion of contaminated food

Table. Diseases Transmitted by Animals, continued

Disease and/or Organism	Common Animal Sources/Reservoirs	Vector or Modes of Transmission
Yersiniosis (Yersinia enterocolitica, Yersinia pseudotuberculosis)	Swine, deer, elk, horses, goats, sheep, cattle, rodents, birds, rabbits	Ingestion of contaminated food, water, or milk; rarely direct contact, person-to-person (fecal-oral)
Fungal Diseases		
Cryptococcosis (Cryptococcus neoformans)	Excreta of birds, particularly pigeons	Inhalation of aerosols from accumulations of bird feces
Histoplasmosis (Histoplasma capsulatum)	Excreta of bats, birds, particularly starlings	Inhalation of aerosols from accumulations of bat and bird feces
Ringworm/tinea corporis (Microsporum and Trichophyton species)	Cats, dogs, fowl, pigs, moles, horses, rodents, cattle, monkeys, goats	Direct contact
Parasitic Diseases		
Anisakiasis (Anisakis species)	Saltwater and anadromous fish	Ingestion of undercooked or raw fish (eg, sushi)
Babesiosis (several Babesia species)	Mice, dogs, wildlife	Tick bite, (I pacificus suspected)
Balantidiasis (Balantidium coli)	Swine	Ingestion of contaminated food or water
Baylisascariasis (Baylisascaris procyonis)	Raccoon	Ingestion of eggs shed in raccoon feces
Dwarf tapeworm (Hymenolepis nana)	Rodents	Ingestion of eggs from feces (contaminated food, water), person-to-person (fecal-oral)
Cryptosporidiosis (Cryptosporidium species)	Domestic animals (particularly cattle, sheep, goats, birds, reptiles), young animals	Ingestion of contaminated water or foods, person-to-person (fecal-oral)
Cutaneous larva migrans (Ancylostoma species)	Dogs, cats	Penetration of skin by larvae, which develop in soil contaminated with animal feces
Cysticercosis/pork tapeworm (Taenia solium)	Swine (intermediate host)	Ingestion of eggs from fecal-oral contact or contaminated food, water; ingestion of cysts in raw or undercooked meat (adult tapeworm infection)
Dog tapeworm (Dipylidium caninum)	Dogs, cats	Ingestion of fleas infected with larvae

Table. Diseases Transmitted by Animals, continued

Disease and/or Organism	Common Animal Sources/Reservoirs	Vector or Modes of Transmission
Echinococcosis, hydatid disease (*Echinococcus* species)	Dogs, foxes, possibly other carnivores, coyotes, wolves, moose, caribou, rodents, sheep (the most common intermediate host worldwide), also swine, cattle, horses, camels	Ingestion of eggs shed in animal feces
Fish tapeworm (*Diphyllobothrium latum*)	Saltwater and freshwater fish	Ingestion of larvae in raw or undercooked fish
Giardiasis (*Giardia intestinalis*)	Wild and domestic animals, including dogs, cats, beavers, muskrats	Ingestion of cysts in contaminated food, water, person-to-person
Hookworm (*Ancylostoma caninum*, *A braziliense*)	Dogs	Penetration of skin by larvae, which develop in soil contaminated with animal feces
Taeniasis, beef (*Taenia saginata*)	Cattle	Ingestion of larvae in undercooked beef
Toxoplasmosis (*Toxoplasma gondii*)	Cats, livestock	Ingestion of oocysts from cat feces, consumption of cysts in undercooked meat, contact with birth products of cats
Trichinosis (*Trichinella spiralis*)	Swine, horses, bears, seals, walruses	Ingestion of larvae in raw or undercooked meat
Visceral larva migrans (*Toxocara canis* and *Toxocara cati*)	Dogs, cats	Ingestion of eggs, usually from soil contaminated by animal feces
Chlamydial and Rickettsial Diseases		
Human ehrlichiosis (*Ehrlichia chaffeensis* and *E ewingii*)	Deer, dogs, gray foxes, goats	Tick bites (lone-star ticks, *Amblyomma americanum*)
Human anaplasmosis (*Anaplasma phagocytophilum*)	Deer, dogs, elk, wild rodents, horses, ruminants	Black-legged tick bites (*Ixodes scapularis*) and western black-legged tick bites (*I pacificus*)
Psittacosis (*Chlamydophila psittaci*)	Pet birds (especially psittacine birds) and poultry	Inhalation of aerosols from feces of infected birds
Q fever (*Coxiella burnetii*)	Sheep, goats, cows, cats, dogs, wild rodents, birds	Direct contact and aerosols from birth products or animal tissues or products (Possible role of ticks not well defined)
Rickettsialpox (*Rickettsia akari*)	House mice	Mite bites (house mouse mite, *Liponyssoides sanguineus*)

Table. Diseases Transmitted by Animals, continued

Disease and/or Organism	Common Animal Sources/Reservoirs	Vector or Modes of Transmission
Rocky Mountain spotted fever (*Rickettsia rickettsii*)	Dogs, wild rodents, rabbits	Tick bites; rarely by direct contamination with infectious material from ticks (American dog tick, *Dermacentor variabilis*; Rocky Mountain wood tick, *D andersoni*; and brown dog tick, *Rhipicephalus sanguineus*)
Rickettsia parkeri infection (Maculatum disease, American boutonneuse fever)	Unknown, perhaps small wild rodents	Gulf coast ticks, *Amblyomma maculatum*
Typhus, fleaborne endemic typhus (*Rickettsia typhi*)	Rats, opossums, cats, dogs	Rat flea feces scratched into abrasions; less common, other fleas (Oriental rat flea, *Xenopsylla cheopis*)
Typhus, louseborne epidemic typhus (*Rickettsia prowazekii*)	Flying squirrels	Person-to-person via body louse, contact with flying squirrels, their nests, or ectoparasites (role and species of ectoparasites undefined)
Viral Diseases		
Colorado tick fever	Wild rodents, (squirrels, chipmunks)	Tick bites (Rocky Mountain wood tick, *Dermacentor andersoni*)
Encephalitis		
LaCrosse (the most common member of the California encephalitis group)	Wild rodents	Mosquito bites (*Aedes triseriatus*)
Eastern equine	Wild birds, poultry, horses	Mosquito bites (*Coquillettidia* species, *Aedes* species)
Western equine	Wild birds, poultry, horses	Mosquito bites (*Culex tarsalis*)
St Louis	Wild birds, poultry	Mosquito bites (*Culex pipiens, Culex* species)
Venezuelan equine	Rodents, horses	Mosquito bites (34 species in 8 genera)
Powassan	Rodents, rabbits	Tick bites (groundhog tick, *Ixodes cookei*)
West Nile	Wild birds, horses	Mosquito bites (*Culex* species)
Nipah virus	Undetermined, possibly bats and pigs	Close contact with infected pigs
Hendra virus	Flying foxes; horses become infected	Contact with body fluids of infected horses
Hantaviruses	Wild rodents	Inhalation of aerosols of infected secreta and excreta
B virus (formerly herpesvirus simiae)	Macaque monkeys	Bite or exposure to secretions

Table. Diseases Transmitted by Animals, continued

Disease and/or Organism	Common Animal Sources/Reservoirs	Vector or Modes of Transmission
Lymphocytic choriomeningitis	Rodents, particularly hamsters, mice	Direct contact, inhalation of aerosols, ingestion of food contaminated with rodent excreta
Rabies (Lyssavirus)	In the United States, primarily wildlife (bats, raccoons, skunks, foxes, ferrets) or, less frequently, domestic animals (dogs, cats, cattle, goats, bear, ponies)	Bites, rarely contact of open wounds with infected materials (eg, saliva, neural tissue)
Monkeypox	Prairie dogs, African rodents	Direct contact, bite, scratch
Influenza (H5N1)	Chickens, birds, swine	Contact with infected animals or aerosols (markets, slaughter house)
Orf (pox virus of sheep)	Sheep	Contact with sheep saliva
Severe acute respiratory virus (coronavirus)	Civet cats, potentially other animal species	Unclear; person-to-person (respiratory, contact)

APPENDIX XI

State Immunization Requirements for School Attendance

The United States relies on child care and elementary and secondary school entry immunization requirements to achieve and sustain high levels of immunization coverage. This strategy has proven successful not only in dramatically decreasing communicable disease in settings where children gather and transmit infection but also in decreasing the opportunity for transmission of vaccine-preventable diseases to the unimmunized, the underimmunized, and the immunologically frail. All states require immunization of children at the time of entry into school, and most states require immunization for entry into licensed child care facilities. In addition, many states require immunization of children throughout grade school, older children in upper grades, and young adults entering college. The most up-to-date information about which vaccines are required in a specific state, permissible exemptions, and minor's consent to immunization can be obtained from the immunization program manager of each state health department, from a number of local health departments, and from **www.immunize.org/laws** and the State and Territorial Health Organization (**www.astho.org**).

The Centers for Disease Control and Prevention (CDC) collects state-specific data on current school entry laws and regulations (child care and Head Start, kindergarten, first grade, and middle school), immunization coverage levels, and exemption rates through state-based surveys. The most recent surveillance results can be accessed online through the CDC at **www.cdc.gov/vaccines/stats-surv/schoolsurv/default.htm.**

....
APPENDIX XII

Services of the Centers for Disease Control and Prevention (CDC)

The Centers for Disease Control and Prevention (CDC), US Public Health Service, Department of Health and Human Services, is the federal agency charged with protecting the public health of the nation by preventing disease and other disabling conditions. The CDC administers national programs for prevention and control of the following: (1) infectious diseases; (2) vaccine-preventable diseases; (3) occupational diseases and injury; (4) chronic diseases; (5) environment-related injury and illness; and (6) birth defects and developmental disabilities. The CDC also provides consultation to other nations and participates with international agencies in the control of preventable diseases. In addition, the CDC directs and enforces foreign quarantine activities and regulations and provides consultation and assistance in upgrading the performance of clinical laboratories.

The CDC provides a number of services related to infectious disease management and control. Although the CDC principally is a resource for state and local health departments, it also offers direct and indirect services to hospitals and practicing health care professionals. The range of services includes reference laboratory diagnosis and epidemiologic consultation, both usually arranged through state health departments.

The CDC Drug Service supplies some specific prophylactic or therapeutic drugs and biological agents. Specific immunobiological products available include botulinal equine (trivalent, ABE) antitoxin, Vaccinia Immune Globulin (VIG), botulinus pentavalent toxoid, and vaccinia vaccine. In addition, several drugs for treatment of parasitic disease, which currently are not approved for use in the United States, are handled under an investigational new drug permit. These antiparasitic drugs include bithionol, dehydroemetine, diethylcarbamazine citrate, melarsoprol, nifurtimox, sodium stibogluconate, and suramin.

Requests for biological products, antiparasitic drugs, and related information should be directed to the CDC Drug Service (see Appendix I, Directory of Resources, p 831).

Index

Page numbers followed by "t" indicate a table. Page numbers followed by "f" indicate a figure. Page numbers followed by "n" indicate a footnote.

N

Naegleria fowleri infections, 208–210, 785t
Nafcillin
dosage of
beyond newborn period, 755t
for neonates, 745t
for staphylococcal infections, 608, 610t
Naftifine
adverse events from, 774t
for candidiasis, 247
for pityriasis versicolor, 521
for tinea corporis, 663
for tinea cruris, 664
topical, 774t
Nail infections, tinea pedis, 665–666
Nairovirus infections, hemorrhagic fevers from, 327–329
Nanophyetus salmincola infections, 792t
Nasal congestion, from influenza, 400
Nasal discharge, from rhinovirus infections, 569
Nasopharyngeal carcinoma, from Epstein-Barr virus infections, 289
Nasopharyngitis. *See also* Pharyngitis
from diphtheria, 280
Natamycin
for amebic meningoencephalitis, 210
for *Naegleria fowleri* infections, 210
National Alliance for Hispanic Health, Web site, www.hispanichealth.org, 54
National Center for Immunization and Respiratory Diseases (CDC), Web site, www. cdc.gov/ncird/index.html, 832t
National Childhood Vaccine Injury Act (NCVIA)
notification requirements of, 5, 6t
recordkeeping requirements of, 6, 6t
reporting adverse events, 42, 43f
reporting and compensation table, 842, 843t–844t
Web site, www.hrsa.gov/vaccinecompensation, 842, 843t–844t
National Committee for Quality Assurance, Health Employer Data and Information Set (HEDIS), 854
National Disaster Medical System, Web site, www.ndms.dhhs.gov, 107t
National Hansen's Disease Program, 425–426
National Healthy Mothers, Healthy Babies Coalition, information sources of, Web site, www.hmhb.org, 54
National Immunization Hotline, 4
National Immunization Program (NIP), 4
National Institute of Allergy and Infectious Diseases, 834t
Web sites
www3.niaid.nih.gov, 834t
www3.niaid.nih.gov/topics/vaccines/default.htm, 55

National Institutes of Health (NIH), Web site, www.nih.gov, 834t
National Library of Medicine, Web site, www.nih.gov, 834t
National Medical Association, Web site, www.nmanet.org, 54
National Network for Immunization Information, 53, 834t
Web site, www.immunizationinfo.org, 4, 54, 834t
National Prevention Information Network (CDC), Web site, www.cdcnpin.org, 832t
National Prion Disease Pathology Surveillance Center, 549
National STD/AIDS Hotline, Web site, www.ashastd.org/learn/learn_hiv_aids_sup.cfm, 832t
National Vaccine Advisory Committee (NVAC)
immunization standards of, 854–856
recordkeeping standard of, Web site, www.cdc.gov/vaccines/programs/iis/default.htm, 38–39
National Vaccine Injury Compensation Program (VICP), 5–6, 6t, 45–46, 832t, 842, 843t–844t
National Vaccine Program Office, 834t
Web site, www.hhs.gov/nvpo/, 55, 834t
Native American children, vaccines for, 88–90
Nausea and vomiting
from *Anaplasma* infections, 284
from animal sera, 65
from anthrax, 211
from arbovirus infections, 215
from astrovirus infections, 225
from babesiosis, 226
from *Bacillus cereus* infections, 227
from *Balantidium coli* infections, 231
from biological terrorism, 106
from *Blastocystis hominis* infections, 233–234
from calicivirus infections, 241
in child care facilities, 128t
from cholera, 727
from *Clostridium perfringens* infections, 265
from cryptosporidiosis, 272
from cyclosporiasis, 274
from *Ehrlichia* infections, 284
from enterovirus infections, 287
from *Escherichia coli* infections, 292
from foodborne diseases, 861t
from hantavirus pulmonary syndrome, 321
from *Helicobacter pylori* infections, 324
from hepatitis A, 329
from hepatitis B, 337
from hookworm infections, 375
from influenza, 400
from isosporiasis, 412
from Kawasaki disease, 413

S

More must-have infectious disease resources from the AAP

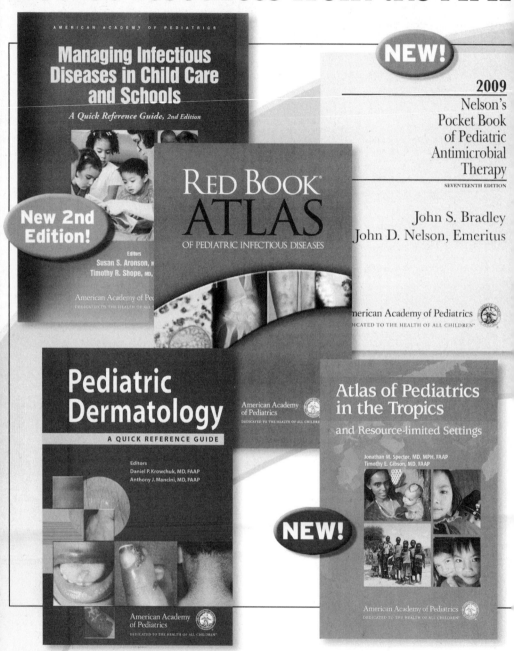
Order online at www.aap.org/bookstore
or call toll-free 888/227-1770.

American Academy of Pediatrics
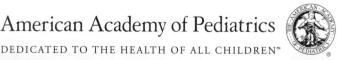
DEDICATED TO THE HEALTH OF ALL CHILDREN™